Transesophageal Echocardiography Multimedia Manual

Transesophageal Echocardiography Multimedia Manual
A Perioperative Transdisciplinary Approach

Second Edition

Edited by

André Y. Denault
Montreal Heart Institute
Centre Hospitalier de l'Université de Montréal
Montreal, Quebec, Canada

Pierre Couture
Montreal Heart Institute
Université de Montréal
Montreal, Quebec, Canada

Annette Vegas
Toronto General Hospital
University of Toronto
Toronto, Ontario, Canada

Jean Buithieu
McGill University Health Center
Montreal, Quebec, Canada

Jean-Claude Tardif
Montreal Heart Institute Research Center
Université de Montréal
Montreal, Quebec, Canada

informa
healthcare

New York London

First published in 2005 by Marcel Dekker, Inc. This edition published in 2011 by Informa Healthcare, Telephone House, 69-77 Paul Street, London EC2A 4LQ, UK.
Simultaneously published in the USA by Informa Healthcare, 52 Vanderbilt Avenue, 7th floor, New York, NY 10017, USA.

No claim to original U.S. Government works.

A CIP record for this book is available from the British Library.

ISBN-13: 978-1-420-08070-4

Orders may be sent to: Informa Healthcare, Sheepen Place, Colchester, Essex CO3 3LP, UK
Telephone: +44 (0)20 7017 5540
Email: CSDhealthcarebooks@informa.com
Website: http://informahealthcarebooks.com/

For corporate sales please contact: CorporateBooksIHC@informa.com
For foreign rights please contact: RightsIHC@informa.com
For reprint permissions please contact: PermissionsIHC@informa.com

Typeset by MPS Limited, a Macmillan Company
Printed and bound in India by Replika Press Pvt. Ltd.

This book is dedicated to

*my wife Denise and children Jean-Simon, Gabrielle, and Julien who have supported
me with love and patience (André Y. Denault);*

Frédéric and Noémi (Pierre Couture);

*my family Patrick, Lena, and Derek for their unconditional love
and encouragement (Annette Vegas);*

my wife Véronique and my parents Tuong and Thai (Jean Buithieu);

*Michèle, Jean-Daniel, and Pier-Luc, who have been so supportive and so
patient with me (Jean-Claude Tardif);*

our families and teachers who have prepared us for this work;

our students;

*and above all our patients for whom we hope and believe that transesophageal
echocardiography and perioperative echocardiography will improve their care.*

Foreword

When it was released in 2005, the first edition of *Transesophageal Echocardiography Multimedia Manual* was instantly praised as one of the most comprehensive pedagogical endeavor into the then-fairly-new field of perioperative echocardiography. So, when they decided, five years later, to undertake the challenge of creating a new and improved version of their work, André Denault and his team had to know that they would be held to the highest standard, the one that they themselves created. To be truly innovative and useful to beginners and experts alike, the new edition would have to include basic echographic notions while encompassing most major advances in the field of transesophageal echocardiography (TEE). Moreover, all this material would have to be showcased in an up-to-date and appealing format using the most advanced pedagogical tools available. Well, we can now state that the challenge has been met successfully and that this second edition of *Transesophageal Echocardiography Multimedia Manual* should become an instant classic for everybody who is seriously interested in TEE and perioperative echocardiography.

Dr. Denault and his fellow editors have been able to assemble a team of experts coming from several countries, giving their work a truly international flavor. Also, since contributors belong to various disciplines, namely anesthesiology, cardiology, surgery, and radiology, their work is uniquely positioned to provide the reader with a truly multidisciplinary approach to perioperative problems. The new edition contains more chapters, figures, and tables than the previous one. It includes new topics while expanding on issues that were already covered in the first edition. The DVD, with its numerous 3D animations and systematic approach to various physiological and pathological situations, will also allow the reader to complement and elaborate on the book's content.

The numerous editors and authors of this new edition of *Transesophageal Echocardiography Multimedia Manual* have to be commended for their contribution to the teaching of TEE and sustained commitment toward improving perioperative care.

Pierre Drolet, MD, FRCPC
Chairman, Department of Anesthesiology,
Université de Montréal, Quebec, Canada

Preface to the second edition

Since its introduction two decades ago, perioperative transesophageal echocardiography (TEE) has become a valuable adjunct in the management of cardiac surgery patients. Over the past five years there has been a rapid expansion in the use of TEE, to encompass newer cardiac surgical techniques, more diverse surgical procedures, and in the intensive care unit. This Second Edition of the *Transesophageal Echocardiography Multimedia Manual* is now geared to present these new developments and challenges for the anesthesiologist, cardiologist, cardiac surgeon and those interested in perioperative TEE.

Every chapter in this edition has been updated and six new chapters have been added which emphasize the role of TEE in (1) new cardiac surgical techniques (minimally invasive, transcatheter valves), (2) non cardiac surgery (transplant, endovascular, electrophysiology procedures) and (3) complementary imaging techniques (transthoracic, epicardial, three-dimensional echocardiography). This transdisciplinary book remains unique in that it contains the experience of individuals trained in anesthesiology, cardiology, critical care, internal medicine, cardiac and vascular surgery, lung and hepatic transplantation, radiology, pathology, physics, and computer technology.

As in the first edition, detailed figures present complementary information that provides the context to assist the clinician practicing perioperative TEE. But if "an image is worth a thousand words," what about a video? Transesophageal echocardiography is a dynamic process and most of our two-dimensional examples are presented in their original video format accompanied by sketches, three-dimensional orientation, Doppler information, hemodynamic, radiologic and anatomical correlation in a user-friendly companion DVD. The content of the DVD has expanded to include the key elements of several common surgical procedures and a multiple choice exam created by the cardiac anesthesiologists of St. Boniface General Hospital in Winnipeg under the supervision of G. Scott Mackenzie. This exam is inspired by the format of the National Board of Echocardiography. In addition, a web link to the Universities of Montreal, McGill and Toronto will offer continuing medical education (AMA certification) credits for those who use the TEE Multimedia Manual as an educational resource.

Such work would not have been possible without the collaboration of several individuals. First, we welcome Dr. Annette Vegas from the Toronto General Hospital who agreed to share her knowledge and passion for TEE and join the editorial team. Annette has significantly contributed to TEE education in Canada through the organization of an annual TEE Symposium in Toronto and by producing an outstanding pocket TEE manual. The editorial team includes Dr. Pierre Couture, who pioneered the development of perioperative TEE in Quebec and has been my most significant collaborator in TEE since 1993. I am also privileged to benefit from the expertise of Drs. Jean Buithieu and Jean-Claude Tardif, who contributed to the creation and revision of the second edition. My assistant, Denis Babin, supplied his enormous skill and talent in organizing, digitalizing, and his determination to make the dream a reality. I am grateful to my anesthesiologist colleagues and the surgical team of the Montreal Heart Institute who have always mutually shared their knowledge and informed me of interesting cases. Dr. Michel Pellerin, chief of cardiac surgery at the Montreal Heart Institute, remains a significant contributor by teaching us surgical anatomy and sharing his video material. Finally, Dr. Yoan Lamarche, a cardiac surgeon trained in TEE and in critical care medicine, provided us with a unique surgical perspective by stressing the key issues that the cardiac surgeon wants to resolve when a TEE exam is performed.

In addition to the authors of this TEE manual, there are several individuals in the operating room who have collaborated in the creation of this book. These individuals made suggestions for chapter content, figures, video clips, and DVD creation which greatly facilitated our work. Their names are listed on the following page. Financial support for the DVD, which accompanies this book, was provided with the support of Robert Busilacchi, Danielle Pagé and Dr. Annie Dore, through an educational grant from the Montreal Heart Institute, and by the Montreal Heart Institute Foundation. Sponsorship from Philips has allowed us to insert their brilliantly educational transesophageal echocardiography three-dimensional normal exam in the DVD. Finally, educational grants from General Electric, Sonosite, the Foundation of the Association des Anesthésiologistes du Québec (AAQ), and Organon through the Department of Anesthesiology at the University of Montreal, were pivotal in supporting image preparation for the manual.

I sincerely hope that this TEE manual will help to improve your care in providing echocardiographic diagnosis and monitoring, and that it will be useful in your teaching of perioperative echocardiography.

André Y. Denault, M.D., Ph.D., ABIM-CCM, FRCPC, FASE

Acknowledgments

Luce Begin
Sylvain Bélisle
Jean-Sébastien Bilodeau
Robert Blain
Denis Bouchard
Michèle Brault
Monique Brouillard
Diane Campeau
Jennifer Cogan
Philippe Demers
Nathalie De Mey
Sarah Dery
Sylvain Durocher
Amélie Gariepy
Alain Girard
Yves Hébert
Gisèle Hemmings
Stuart Herd
Normand Hey
Christophe Heyllbroeck
Christian Jodoin
Suzanne Kaprélian
Jean Leclerc
Tack Ki Leung
Patrick Limoges
Ariane Marelli
Avrum Morrow
Antoinette Paolitto
Pierre Pagé
Guy Pelletier
Louis Perrault
Nancy Poirier
Terry Potts
Baqir Qizilbash
Anan Raghunathan
Catherine Roy
Philippe Sahab
Sophie St-Onge
Jean Taillefer
France Thériault
Pierrette Thivierge
Karine Toledano
Ann Wright
Les inhalothérapeutes du bloc opératoire de l'ICM
Fonds de la Recherche en Santé du Québec

Educational grant from: Foundation of the Association des Anesthésiologistes du Québec, Bourse Organon du département d'anesthésiologie de l'Université de Montréal, Danielle Pagé from the Montreal Heart Institute Foundation, Robert Busilacchi and Annie Dore from the Montreal Heart Institute Educational Services.

Industrial support (unrestricted grant) from: Suzan Clair from General Electric, Joseph Bestavros and Suzie Grisolia from Sonosite, Sylvain Brunet from Philips, Réal Côté from Fresenius.

Contents

Contributors

Robert Amyot, MD, FRCPC Associate Professor, Department of Medicine, Division of Cardiology, Hôpital du Sacré-Coeur de Montréal, Université de Montréal, Montreal, Canada

Marie Arsenault, MD, FRCPC Director of Echocardiography Laboratory, Institut Universitaire de Cardiologie et de Pneumologie de Québec, Université Laval, Quebec City, Canada

Christian Ayoub, MD, B.Pharm, FRCPC Clinical Assistant Professor, Department of Cardiac Anesthesiology, Montreal Heart Institute, Department of Anesthesiology, Maisonneuve-Rosemont Hospital, Université de Montréal, Montreal, Canada

Daniel Bainbridge, MD, FRCPC Director of Cardiac Anesthesiology, London Health Sciences Centre, Associate Professor, Department of Anesthesiology and Perioperative Medicine, University of Western Ontario, London, Canada

Miguel A. Barrero Garcia, MD Cardiologist, Centre hospitalier régional de Trois Rivières, Quebec, Clinical Lecturer, Université de Montréal, Montreal, Canada

Arsène-J. Basmadjian, MD, MSc, FACC, FRCPC Director of Echocardiography and Non-Invasive Cardiology, Montreal Heart Institute, Associate Professor, Department of Medicine, Division of Cardiology, Université de Montréal, Montreal, Canada

Yanick Beaulieu, MD, FRCPC Cardiologist – Echocardiographer / Intensivist, Director of the Bedside Ultrasound Curriculum, Hôpital du Sacré-Coeur de Montréal, Assistant Professor, Department of Medicine, Université de Montréal, Montreal, Canada

François A. Béïque, MD, FRCPC Director of Cardiac Anesthesia, Sir Mortimer B. Davis Jewish General Hospital, Associate Professor, Department of Anesthesiology, McGill University, Montreal, Canada

Denis Bouchard, MD, CM, MSc, FRCSC Program Director of Cardiac Surgery, Montreal Heart Institute, Associate Professor, Department of Surgery, Université de Montréal, Montreal, Canada

John Bowering, MD, FRCP Associate Professor, Department of Anesthesiology, Providence Health Care, University of British Columbia, Vancouver, Canada

Richard Bowry, MBBS, FRCA Medical Director of Cardiovascular Intensive Care, Department of Anesthesiology, St. Michael's Hospital, Assistant Professor, Department of Anesthesiology, University of Toronto, Toronto, Canada

Jean Buithieu, MD, FRCPC Director of Echocardiography and Non-Invasive Cardiology, McGill University Health Center, Assistant Professor, Department of Medicine, Division of Cardiology, McGill University, Montreal, Canada

Jean S. Bussières, MD, FRCPC, DABA Anesthesiologist, Anesthesiology Research Team Director, Department of Anesthesiology, Institut Universitaire de Cardiologie et de Pneumologie de Québec, Associate Clinical Professor, Université Laval, Quebec City, Canada

Michel Carrier, MD, FRCSC Professor of Surgery, Department of Cardiac Surgery, Montreal Heart Institute, Université de Montréal, Montreal, Canada

Raymond Cartier, MD, FRCSC Professor of Cardiac Surgery, Department of Cardiac Surgery, Montreal Heart Institute, Université de Montréal, Montreal, Canada

Jean Champagne, MD, FRCPC Associate Professor, Department of Medicine, Division of Cardiology and Electrophysiology, Institut Universitaire de Cardiologie et de Pneumologie de Québec, Université Laval, Quebec City, Canada

Carl Chartrand-Lefebvre, MD FRCPC Associate Professor, Department of Radiology, Centre Hospitalier de l'Université de Montréal (CHUM) and Montreal Heart Institute, Université de Montréal, Montreal, Canada

Pierre-Guy Chassot, MD Former Chief of Cardiovascular Anesthesia, University Hospital Lausanne, Privat-Docent, Faculty of Biology and Medicine, University of Lausanne, Lausanne, Switzerland

Robert Chen, MD, FRCPC Cardiac Anesthesia Fellowship Program Director, St. Michael's Hospital, Assistant Professor, Department of Anaesthesiology, University of Toronto, Toronto, Canada

Anson Cheung, MD, FRCSC Surgical Director of Cardiac Transplant, Clinical Associate Professor of Surgery, Division of Cardiothoracic Surgery, St. Paul's Hospital, University of British Columbia, Vancouver, Canada

Chris Christodoulou, MBChB Cum Laude, DA (UK), FRCPC Assistant Professor, University of Manitoba, Winnipeg, Canada

Guy Cloutier, P.Eng, PhD Director of the Laboratory of Biorheology and Medical Ultrasonics, Research Center of Université de Montréal Hospital Center (CRCHUM); Professor of Radiology and Biomedical Engineering, Université de Montréal, Montreal, Canada.

José W. Coddens, MD Staff Anesthesiologist, Responsible for the Section Cardiovascular and Thoracic Anesthesia, Responsible for the Section Perioperative Echocardiography, Department of Anesthesia and Intensive Care Medicine, Onze Lieve Vrouw Clinic, Aalst, Belgium

Annie V. Côté, MD, FRCPC Assistant-Professor, Department of Cardiac Anesthesiology, McGill University Health Center, Montreal, Canada

Geneviève Côté, MD, MSc, FRCPC Pediatric Cardiac Anesthesiologist, Assistant Professor, Department of Pediatric Anesthesia, Centre Hospitalier Universitaire (CHU) Mère-Enfant Sainte-Justine, Université de Montréal, Montreal, Canada

Jean-Marc Côté, MD, FRCPC Pediatric Cardiologist, Associate Professor, Department of Pediatrics, Centre Hospitalier Universitaire de Québec (CHUQ), Université Laval, Quebec City, Canada

Stéphane Coutu, MD, FRCPC Associate Professor, Department of Anesthesiology, Centre Hospitalier Universitaire de Sherbrooke (CHUS), Université de Sherbrooke, Sherbrooke, Canada

Pierre Couture, MD, FRCPC Cardiac Anesthesiology Department, Montreal Heart Institute, Associate Clinical Professor, Department of Cardiac Anesthesiology, Université de Montréal, Montreal, Canada

Robert James Cusimano, MD, BSc, MSc, FACS, FRCSC Peter Munk Cardiac Centre, Associate Professor, Department of Surgery, Division of Cardiac Surgery, University of Toronto, Toronto, Canada

Roland DeBrouwere, MD, FRCPC Assistant Professor, University of Manitoba, Winnipeg, Canada

André Y. Denault, MD, PhD, ABIM-CCM, FRCPC, FASE Associate Professor, Department of Cardiac Anesthesiology, Montreal Heart Institute, Division of Critical Care of the Department of Medicine, Centre Hospitalier de l'Université de Montréal (CHUM), Université de Montréal, Montreal, Canada

Alain Deschamps, PhD, MD, FRCPC Director of Research of the Department of Anesthesiology, Montreal Heart Institute, Associate Professor, Department of Anesthesiology, Université de Montréal, Montreal Canada

Ariel Diaz, MD, MSc Cardiologist, Centre hospitalier régional de Trois Rivières, Quebec, Clinical Lecturer, Université de Montréal, Montreal, Canada

Maria Di Lorenzo, MD, FRCPC Cardiologist, Echocardiographist, Hôpital du Sacré-Coeur de Montréal, Assistant Professor, Department of Medicine, Division of Cardiology, Université de Montréal, Montreal, Canada

George Djaiani, MD, DEAA, FRCA, FRCPC Cardiac Anesthesia Fellowship Research Program Director, Associate Professor, Department of Anesthesia and Pain Management, Toronto General Hospital, University Health Network, University of Toronto, Toronto, Canada

Annie Dore, MD, FRCPC Director of Education, Montreal Heart Institute, Associate Professor, Department of Medicine, Université de Montréal, Montreal, Canada

Anique Ducharme, MD, MSc, FRCPC Director of the Heart Failure Clinic, Montreal Heart Institute, Associate Professor, Department of Medicine, Division of Cardiology, Université de Montréal, Montreal, Canada

Jean G. Dumesnil, CQ, MD, FRCPC, FACC Cardiologist, Institut Universitaire de Cardiologie et de Pneumologie de Québec /Québec Heart and Lung Institute, Professor of Medicine, Université Laval, Quebec City, Canada

Nicolas Dürrleman, MD Department of Cardiac, Thoracic and Vascular Surgery, Private Hospital Les Franciscaines, Nîmes, France

James P. Enns, BSc (Med), MD, FRCPC Assistant Professor, University of Manitoba, Winnipeg, Canada

Ashraf Fayad, MD, FRCPC, FASE, FACC Director of Echocardiography Fellowship for Non-Cardiac Surgery, Associate Professor, Department of Anesthesiology, University of Ottawa, Ottawa, Canada

Pasquale Ferraro, MD, FRCSC Associate Professor, Chief Division of Thoracic Surgery, Alfonso Minicozzi and Family Chair in Lung Transplantation, Surgical Director Lung Transplant Program, Centre Hospitalier de l'Université de Montréal (CHUM), Université de Montréal, Montreal, Canada

Alain Gauvin, MSc, MCCPM, DABR, DABMP Lecturer, Department of Radiology, Université de Montréal, Montreal, Canada

Michel Germain, MD, FRCPC, BA.Sc, B.Eng Staff Anesthesiologist, Royal Victoria Hospital, McGill University Health Center, Assistant Professor, Department of Anesthesiology, McGill University, Montreal, Canada

Martin Girard, MD, FRCPC Associate Clinical Professor, Department of Anesthesiology, Division of Critical Care of the Department of Medicine, Centre Hospitalier de l'Université de Montréal (CHUM), Université de Montréal, Montreal, Canada

Hilary P. Grocott, MD, FRCPC, FASE Professor of Anesthesia and Surgery, University of Manitoba, Winnipeg, Canada

Craig Guenther, MD, FRCPC Associate Clinical Professor, Anesthesiology and Pain Medicine, University of Alberta, Edmonton, Canada

François Haddad, MD, FRCPC Attending Cardiologist, Heart Failure and Transplant Program, Stanford University, Palo Alto, California, U.S.A.

Jane Heggie, MD, FRCP Assistant Professor of Anaesthesia, Director of Anaesthesia Fellowship Programs, Toronto General Hospital, University Health Network, University of Toronto, Toronto, Canada

George N. Honos, MD, FRCPC, FACC Head of Division of Cardiology, Medical Director of Cardiovascular Program, Centre Hospitalier de l'Université de Montréal (CHUM), Associate Professor of Medicine, Université de Montréal, Montreal, Canada

Mark Hynes, MD, FRCPC Department of Cardiac Anesthesiology, University of Ottawa Heart Institute, Assistant Professor, Department of Anesthesiology, University of Ottawa, Ottawa, Canada

Reda Ibrahim, MD, FRCPC Interventional Cardiology and Director of the Medical Care Unit, Montreal Heart Institute, Assistant Professor, Department of Medicine, Division of Cardiology, Université de Montréal, Montreal, Canada

Ivan Iglesias, MD, FRCPC, FASE Intraoperative Echocardiography Program Coordinator, Associate Professor, Department of Anaesthesia and Perioperative Medicine, London Health Sciences Centre, University of Western Ontario, London, Canada

Marjan Jariani, MD, FRCPC Assistant Professor, Department of Anesthesia, University of Toronto, Cardiovascular ICU and Transesophageal Echocardiography, Toronto General Hospital, University Health Network, Toronto, Canada

Philippe L.-L'Allier, MD, FRCPC Interventional Cardiologist and Director of the Coronary Care Unit, Department of Medicine, Division of Cardiology, Montreal Heart Institute, Associate Professor, Université de Montréal, Montreal, Canada

Yoan Lamarche, MD, MSc, FRCSC Cardiac surgeon and critical care physician, Department of Cardiac Surgery, Montreal Heart Institute and Hôpital du Sacré-Coeur de Montréal, Adjunct Clinical Professor, Université de Montréal, Montreal, Canada

Stéphane Lambert, MD, CM, FRCPC Assistant Professor, Division of Cardiac Anesthesiology, University of Ottawa Heart Institute, Ottawa, Canada

Réal Lebeau, MD Assistant Professor, Department of Medicine, Division of Cardiology, Hôpital du Sacré-Coeur de Montréal, Université de Montréal, Montreal, Canada

Jean-Sébastien Lebon, MD, FRCPC, B.Pharm Assistant Professor, Department of Cardiac Anesthesiology, Montreal Heart Institute, Université de Montréal, Montreal, Canada

Trevor W. R. Lee, MD, FRCPC, FASE, CPE Head, Department of Anesthesia and Perioperative Medicine, St. Boniface General Hospital, Assistant Professor, University of Manitoba, Winnipeg, Canada

G. Scott MacKenzie, MD, FRCPC Medical Director, Cardiac Anesthesia, WRHA/St. Boniface Cardiac Sciences Program, St. Boniface General Hospital, Winnipeg, Canada

Doug Maguire, MD, FRCPC Assistant Professor, University of Manitoba, Winnipeg, Canada

Warner M. Mampuya, MD, PhD, FRCPC Cardiology Fellow, Centre Hospitalier Universitaire de Sherbrooke, Université de Sherbrooke, Sherbrooke, Canada

François Marcotte, MD, FRCPC, FACC, FASE Cardiologist, Montreal Heart Institute, Associate Professor, Department of Medicine, Université de Montréal, Montreal, Canada

André Martineau, MD, FRCP Department of Anesthesiology, Institut Universitaire de Cardiologie et de Pneumologie de Québec, Laval Hospital, Université Laval, Quebec City, Canada

Luc Massicotte, MD Associate Professor, Department of Anesthesiology, Saint-Luc Hospital, Centre Hospitalier de l'Université de Montréal (CHUM), Université de Montréal, Montreal, Canada

Patrick Mathieu, MD, MSc, FRCSC Director of the Laboratoire d'Études Moléculaires des Valvulopathies (LEMV), Research Center Institut Universitaire de Cardiologie et de Pneumologie de Québec, Associate Professor, Department of Surgery, Université Laval, Quebec City, Canada

Massimiliano Meineri, MD Assistant Professor of Anesthesia, University of Toronto, Staff Anesthesiologist, Toronto General Hospital, Toronto, Canada

Bradley I. Munt, MD, FRCPC, FACC Cardiologist, St. Paul's Hospital, Vancouver, Canada

John M. Murkin, MD, FRCPC Professor of Anesthesiology, Director of Cardiac Anesthesia Research, Department of Anesthesiology and Perioperative Medicine, London Health Sciences Center, University of Western Ontario, London, Canada

Viviane T. Q. Nguyen, MD, FRCPC Heart Failure and Transplant Program Director, Assistant Professor of Medicine, Division of Cardiology, McGill University Health Center, McGill University, Montreal, Canada

Georghios Nicolaou, MBBCh, FRCPC Director and Fellowship Coordinator of Thoracic and Vascular Anesthesia, Associate Professor and Chief of Anesthesia, Victoria Hospital, Department of Anesthesia and Perioperative Medicine, London Health Sciences Center, University of Western Ontario, London, Canada

Michel Pellerin, MD, FRCSC Head of Department of Surgery, Montreal Heart Institute, Michal & Renata Hornstein Chair in Cardiac Surgery, Professor of Surgery, Université de Montréal, Montreal, Canada

Michel-Antoine Perrault, MD, FRCPC Clinical Assistant Professor, Department of Anesthesiology, Centre Hospitalier Universitaire de Sherbrooke (CHUS), Sherbrooke, Canada

Philippe Pibarot, DVM, PhD, FACC, FAHA Chair of the Canada Research Chair in Valvular Heart Disease, Full Professor, Institut Universitaire de Cardiologie et de Pneumologie de Québec (IUCPQ), Université Laval, Quebec City, Canada

François Plante, MD, FRCPC Associate Clinical Professor, Department of Anesthesiology, Centre Hospitalier de l'Université de Montréal (CHUM), Université de Montréal, Montreal, Canada

Mackenzie Quantz, MD Division of Cardiac Surgery, London Health Sciences Centre, Associate Professor, University of Western Ontario, London, Canada

Chinniampalayam Rajamohan, MBBS, DA, MD, DNB, FCPS, FRCA, FRCPC Assistant Professor, University of Manitoba, Winnipeg, Canada

Anthony Ralph-Edwards, MD Division of Cardiovascular Surgery, Toronto General Hospital, University of Toronto, Toronto, Canada

Antoine G. Rochon, MD, FRCPC Cardiac Anesthesiology Fellowship Program Director, Perioperative Transesophageal Echocardiography Training Program Director, Assistant Professor, Department of Anesthesiology, Montreal Heart Institute, Université de Montréal, Montreal, Canada

André Saint-Pierre, MD, FRCPC Medical Director, Operating Suite, Institut Universitaire de Cardiologie et de Pneumologie de Québec, Clinical Professor, Department of Anesthesiology, Université Laval, Quebec City, Canada

Claude Sauvé, MD, FRCPC Director of Echocardiography Laboratory, Hôpital du Sacré-Coeur de Montréal, Associate Professor, Department of Medicine, Division of Cardiology, Université de Montréal, Montreal, Canada

John Scatliff, MD, FRCPC Assistant Professor, University of Manitoba, Winnipeg, Canada

Yan-Fen Shi, MD Cardiologist, Research Centre, Montreal Heart Institute, Research Associate, Department of Medicine, Division of Cardiology, Université de Montréal, Montreal, Canada

Peter Slinger, MD, FRCPC Staff Anesthesiologist, Toronto General Hospital, Professor of Anesthesia, University of Toronto, Toronto, Canada

Oren K. Steinmetz, MDCM, FRCSC Chief of Division of Vascular Surgery, Associate Professor, Department of Surgery, McGill University Health Centre and McGill University, Montreal, Canada

Johann Strumpher, MD Assistant Professor, University of Manitoba, Winnipeg, Canada

Jean-Claude Tardif, MD, FACC, FRCPC, FCAHS Director of the Research Center, Montreal Heart Institute, Professor, Department of Medicine, Université de Montréal, Montreal, Canada

Eric Therasse, MD, FRCPC Associate Professor, Department of Radiology, Centre Hospitalier de l'Université de Montréal (CHUM) and Montreal Heart Institute, Université de Montréal, Montreal, Canada

Ian R. Thomson, MD Professor, University of Manitoba, Winnipeg, Canada

Claude Tousignant, MD, FRCPC Assistant Professor, Department of Anesthesia and Critical Care, Director, Perioperative Echocardiography, St. Michael's Hospital, University of Toronto, Toronto, Canada

Franck Vandenbroucke-Menu, MD Assistant Professor, Department of Surgery, Université de Montréal, Hepatobiliary and Pancreatic Surgery and Liver Transplantation Service, Centre Hospitalier de l'Université de Montréal (CHUM), Centre de Recherche du CHUM (CRCHUM), Montreal, Canada

Michel J. Van Dyck, MD Staff Anesthesiologist, Cliniques universitaires Saint-Luc, Department of Acute Medicine, Division of Cardiac Anesthesiology, Université Catholique de Louvain (UCL), Brussels, Belgium

Hugo Vanermen, MD Head of the Department of Cardiovascular and Thoracic Surgery Unit, OLV Hospital, KUL University, Aalst, Belgium

Adriaan van Rensburg, MD Department of Anaesthesia, Toronto General Hospital, University of Toronto, Toronto, Canada

Annette Vegas, MD, FRCPC Staff Anesthesiologist, Director of Perioperative Transesophageal Echocardiography, Department of Anesthesiology, Toronto General Hospital, Associate Professor, University of Toronto, Toronto, Canada

Professor Antoine Vieillard-Baron, MD, PhD Chief of Intensive Care Unit, Hôpital Ambroise Paré, Boulogne, France, Assistance Publique des Hôpitaux de Paris, Faculté de Médecine Paris-Ile-de-France-Ouest, Université Versailles Saint-Quentin-en-Yvelines, France

Christine Watremez, MD Department of Anesthesiology, Cliniques Universitaires Saint-Luc, Brussels, Belgium

Terrence M. Yau, MD, MSc, FRCSC Angelo and Lorenza DeGasperis Chair in Cardiovascular Surgery Research, Director of Research, Division of Cardiovascular Surgery, Toronto General Hospital, Professor, Department of Surgery, University of Toronto, Toronto, Canada

R. Shawn Young, MD, FRCPC Medical Director, Anesthesia, Victoria General Hospital, Assistant Professor of Anesthesia, University of Manitoba, Winnipeg, Canada

Abbreviations

2D	two-dimensional
3D	three-dimensional
ε	strain
ε_L	Lagrangian strain
ε_N	natural or Eulerian strain
ρ	density
λ	wavelength
A	anterior
A-mode	amplitude mode
AA	apical anterior
AAA	abdominal aortic aneurysm
AC	accessory chamber
AC	atrial contraction
ACC	American College of Cardiology
ACGME	Accreditation Council for Graduate of Medical Education
ACT	activated clotting time
AF	atrial fibrillation
AHA	American Heart Association
AI	apical inferior
AIDS	acquired immunodeficiency syndrome
AL	antero-lateral
AL	apical lateral
AMA	American Medical Association
AML	anterior mitral leaflet
AMP	adenosine monophosphate
AMVL	anterior mitral valve leaflet
Ao	aorta
AoPV	aortic bioprosthetic valve
AoV	aortic valve
AP	antero-posterior
APE	acute pulmonary embolism
AR	aortic regurgitation
AR	atrial reversal
ARDS	acute respiratory distress syndrome
ARDS	adult respiratory distress syndrome
AS	anteroseptal
AS	aortic stenosis
AS	apical septal
ASA	American Society of Anesthesiologists
ASA	atrial septal aneurysm
ASC	ascending
ASD	atrial septal defect
ASE	American Society of Echocardiography
ASYNC	asynchronous
AT	acceleration time
AV	aortic valve
AV	atrioventricular
AVA	aortic valve area
AVC	aortic valve closure
AVJ	aorto-ventricular junction
AVO	aortic valve opening
AVR	aortic valve replacement

B-mode	brightness mode
BA	basal anterior
BAL	basal anterolateral
BAS	basal anteroseptal
BCA	brachiocephalic artery
BD	bile duct
BIL	basal inferior
BIS	basal inferoseptal
BP	blood pressure
BSA	body surface area
BTTAI	blunt traumatic thoracic aortic injury
BVR	balloon valvuloplasty registry
c	propagation speed
CABG	coronary artery bypass graft
CAD	coronary artery disease
CAP	congenital absence of the pericardium
CAS	Canadian Anesthesia Society
CFI	color flow imaging
CHF	congestive heart failure
CI	cardiac index
CJA	color jet area
CME	continuous medical education
CO	cardiac output
COPD	chronic obstructive pulmonary disease
CI	cardiac index
CP	constrictive pericarditis
CPB	cardiopulmonary bypass
CPS	cardiopulmonary surgery
CRT	cardiac resynchronization therapy
CS	coronary sinus
CSA	cross-sectional area
CSE	Canadian Society of Echocardiography
CRT	cardiac resynchronization therapy
CT	computed tomography
CT	celiac trunk
CTEPH	chronic thromboembolic pulmonary hypertension
CTF	celiac trunk flow
CVCAS	Cardiovascular Section of the Canadian Anesthesia Society
CVP	central venous pressure
CW	continuous wave
CXR	chest X-ray
d	depth
D	diastolic
D	diastasis
DA	dopamine
dB	decibel
dBP	diastolic blood pressure
DCM	dilated cardiomyopathy
DD	diastolic dysfunction
DESC	descending
DFT	diastolic filling time
DHCA	deep hypothermic cardiac arrest
dIVC	distensibility index of IVC
DT	deceleration time
DVI	dimensionless velocity index
E	peak early diastolic velocity of the mitral valve inflow
EAU	epiaortic ultrasonographic
EAU	epiaortic ultrasound
EC	endocardial cushion(s)
ECMO	extracorporeal membrane oxygenation
ED	end-diastolic
ED	end-diastole
EDA	end-diastolic area

EDP	end-diastolic pressure
EDV	end-diastolic volume
EE	epicardial echocardiography
EF	ejection fraction
EF	early filling
EI	eccentricity index
EKG	electrocardiogram
Eln	elastance
E_{max}	maximum time varying elastance
EMD	pseudo-electromechanical dissociation
EOA	effective orifice area
EP	ejection period
EPSS	E point septal separation
ERO	effective regurgitant orifice
EROA	effective regurgitant orifice area
ES	end-systole
ESA	end-systolic area
ESC	European Society of Cardiology
E'es	end-systolic elastance
ET	ejection time
$ETCO_2$	end-tidal CO_2
ETT	endotracheal tube
EXT SYNC	external synchronization
f	frequency
FAA	functional aortic annulus
FAC	fractional area change
FDA	Food and Drug Administration
FL	false lumen
FO	foramen oval
FO	fossa ovalis
FOCCUS	FOcused Critical Care Ultrasound Study
FOCUS	FOcused Cardiac Ultrasound Study
FP	foramen primum
Fr	frame rate
FS	fractional shortening
FVR	flow velocity ratio
GE	gastroesophaeal
GI	gastrointestinal
gm	gram
H	hour
HA	hepatic artery
HCM	hypertrophic cardiomyopathy
HCUs	hand-carried ultrasound devices
HOCM	hypertrophic obstructive cardiomyopathy
HPS	hepatopulmonary syndrome
HR	heart rate
HV	hepatic vein
HVF	hepatic venous flow
Hz	Hertz
I	inferior
I	intensity
IA	innominate artery
IAB	intra-aortic balloon
IABP	intra-aortic balloon pump
IAS	interatrial septal
ICA	internal carotid artery
ICE	intracardiac echocardiography
ICU	intensive care unit
IE	inner edge
IF	intimal flap
IH	intramural hematoma
IMR	ischemic mitral regurgitation

IOE	intraoperative echocardiography
IPPV	intermittent positive pressure ventilation
IRI	ischemia reperfusion injury
IS	inferoseptal
ISHLT	International Society of Heart and Lung Transplant
IVA	isovolumic acceleration
IVC	inferior vena cava
IVC	isovolumic contraction
IVCT	isovolumic contraction time
IVMD	interventricular mechanical delay
IVR	isovolumic relaxation
IVRT	isovolumic relaxation time
IVS	interventricular septum
IVST	interventricular septal thickness
IVUS	intravascular ultrasound
J/sec	Joule per second
k	compressibility or elasticity
L	left
L	length
L_0	unstressed length
LA	left atrial
LA	left atrium
LAA	left atrial appendage
LAD	left anterior descending
LAFB	left atrio-femoral bypass
LAP	left atrial pressure
LAX	long axis
LBBB	left bundle branch block
LBVC	left brachiocephalic vein
LCA	left coronary artery
LCC	left coronary cusp
LCCA	left common carotid artery
LCPC	left coronary prosthetic cusp
LCX	left circumflex
LDR	late diastolic reversal
LE	low esophageal
LE	leading edge
LGC	lateral gain control
LHV	left hepatic vein
LIJV	left internal jugular vein
LIMA	left internal mammary artery
LLPV	left lower pulmonary vein
LMCA	left main coronary artery
LPA	left pulmonary artery
LPV	left portal vein
LRA	left renal artery
LRV	left renal vein
LSCA	left subclavian artery
LSCV	left subclavian vein
LSVC	left superior vena cava
LUPV	left upper pulmonary vein
LV	left ventricle
LV	left ventricular
LVAD	left ventricular assist device
LVD	left ventricular diameter
LVEDA	left ventricular end-diastolic area
LVEDD	left ventricular end-diastolic dimension
LVEDP	left ventricular end-diastolic pressure
LVEDV	left ventricular end-diastolic volume
LVEF	left ventricular ejection fraction
LVES	left ventricular end systolic
LVESA	left ventricular end-systolic area

LVESCO	left ventricular end-systolic cardiac output
LVESD	left ventricular end-systolic dimension
LVESP	left ventricular end-systolic pressure
LVESV	left ventricular end-systolic volume
LVET	left ventricular ejection time
LVgram	left ventricular ventriculogram
LVH	left ventricular hypertrophy
LViDd	left ventricular internal diameter in diastole
LVNC	left ventricular myocardial noncompaction
LVOT	left ventricular outflow tract
LVOTO	left ventricular outflow tract obstruction
LVPEP	left ventricular pre-ejection period
LVSV	left ventricular stroke volume
LVSW	left ventricular stroke work
LVWS	left ventricular wall stress
M	meter
M-mode	motion mode
MA	mid anterior
MAL	mid inferolateral
MAM	mitral annular motion
MAP	mean arterial pressure
MAR	mitral annuloplasty ring
MAS	mid anteroseptal
MAV	mitral annular velocities
Max	maximum
mDT	mitral deceleration time of the E velocity
ME	mid-esophageal
MI	mechanical index
MI	myocardial infarction
MI	mid inferior
MIDCAB	minimally invasive direct coronary artery bypass
MIS	mid inferoseptal
ML	medio-lateral
MLT	mitral leaflet tenting
Mn	mean
MOC	maintenance of competence
MPA	main pulmonary artery
MPAP	mean pulmonary artery pressure
MPI	myocardial performance index
MR	mitral regurgitation
MRI	magnetic resonance imaging
MS	mitral stenosis
MV	mitral valve
MVA	mitral valve area
MVP	mitral valve prolapse
MVR	mitral valve replacement
NA	noradrenaline
NBE	National Board of Echocardiography
NCC	non-coronary cusp
NCPC	non-coronary prosthetic cusp
NIRS	near-infrared spectroscopy monitoring
NYHA	New York Heart Association
OE	outer edge
OLV	one lung ventilation
OHT	orthotopic heart transplantation
OLT	orthotopic liver transplantation
OLV	one lung ventilation
OPCAB	off-pump coronary artery bypass surgery
OP-CABG	off-pump coronary artery bypass grafting
OR	operating room
P	pressure
Pa	Pascal

Pa	arterial pressure
PA	pulmonary artery
Pabd	abdominal pressure
PAC	pulmonary artery catheter
PADC	pulmonary artery decompression catheter
PAEDP	pulmonary artery end-diastolic pressure
Paf or Pfa	femoral arterial pressure
PAL	passive leg raising
PaO$_2$	oxygen partial pressure
Paop	pulmonary artery occlusion pressure
PAP or Pap	pulmonary artery pressure
PASP	pulmonary artery systolic pressure
PAVR	percutaneous aortic valve replacement
Paw	airway pressure
Pcs	coronary sinus pressure
PCWP	pulmonary capillary wedge pressure
PD	pulse duration
PDA	patent ductus arteriosus
PE	pericardial effusions
PE	pulmonary embolism
PEEP	positive end-expiratory pressure
PEP	pre-ejection period
PET	positron emission tomography
PFO	patent foramen ovale
PG	pressure gradient
PGD	primary graft dysfunction
PHT	pressure half-time
PISA	proximal isovelocity surface area
PLL	posterior leaflet length
PLR	passive leg raising
Plv	left ventricular pressure
PM	postero-medial
PML	posterior mitral valve leaflet
PML	posterior mitral leaflet
Pms	Mean systemic pressure
Ppa	pulmonary artery pressure
PPH	primary pulmonary hypertension
PPHTN	portopulmonary hypertension
PPL	paraprosthetic leak
PPM	patient-prosthesis mismatch
PPV	positive-pressure ventilation
PPVR	percutaneous pulmonic valve replacement
PR	pressure recovery
PR	pulmonic regurgitation
Pra	right atrial pressure
Pra	radial artery pressure
PRF	pulse repetition frequency
PROX	proximal
PRP	pulse repetition period
PRS	postreperfusion syndrome
Prv	right ventricular pressure
PS	pulmonic stenosis
PST	post-systolic thickening
PTE	pulmonary thromboendarterectomy
PV	portal vein
PV	pulmonic valve
PVAC	pulmonic valve anterior cusp
PVD	peripheral vascular disease
PVF	pulmonary venous flow
PVL	paravalvular leak
PVLC	pulmonic valve left cusp
PVR	pulmonary vascular resistance
PW	pulsed wave

PWT	posterior wall thickness
PWTd	posterior wall thickness in diastole
Q	volumetric flow rate
Q	quality factor
Qp	pulmonary blood flow
Qs	systemic blood flow
R	right
RA	right atrial
RA	right atrium
RAA	right atrial appendage
RAF	renal artery flow
RAP	right atrial pressure
RBBB	right bundle branch block
RCA	right coronary artery
RCC	right coronary cusp
RCC	retrograde cardioplegia catheter
RCM	restrictive cardiomyopathy
RCPC	right coronary prosthetic cusp
Reg Vol	regurgitant volume
REJV	right external jugular vein
RESP	respiration
RF	radio-frequency
RF	regurgitant fraction
RHT	regurgitant pressure half-time
RHV	right hepatic vein
RICA	right internal carotid artery
RIJV	right internal jugular vein
RLPV	right lower pulmonary vein
RPA	right pulmonary artery
RPV	right portal vein
RUPV	right upper pulmonary vein
RV	right ventricle
RV	right ventricular
RVAD	right ventricular assist device
RVEDA	right ventricular end-diastolic area
RVEDD	right ventricular end-diastolic diameter
RVEDD	right ventricular end-diastolic dimension
RVEDP	right ventricular end-diastolic pressure
RVEF	right ventricular ejection fraction
RVD	right ventricular diameter
RVG	radionuclide ventriculography
RVH	right ventricular hypertrophy
RVOT	right ventricular outflow tract
Rvr	resistance to venous return
RVSP	right ventricular systolic pressure
RWMA	regional wall motion abnormalities
RVH	right ventricular hypertrophy
RVWT	right ventricular wall thickness
S	systolic
S	systole
Sa	systolic annular
SA	stroke area
SAM	septal myectomy
SAM	systolic anterior motion
SaO_2	oxygen saturation
SAP	systolic arterial pressure
SAX	short axis
SBP or sBP	systolic aortic blood pressure
SCA	Society of Cardiovascular Anesthesiologists
ScO_2	regional brain saturation
SD	standard deviation(s)
S/D:	systolic to diastolic ratio

SEC	spontaneous echo contrast
SI	strain imaging
SL	septal to lateral
SLCL	septal to leaflet coaptation length
Sm	systolic mitral
SMA	superior mesenteric artery
SMAV	systolic mitral annular velocity
SP	septum primum
SPECT	single photon emission computer tomography
SPL	spatial pulse length
SPPA	spatial peak pulse average
SPTA	spatial peak/temporal average
SPWMD	septal-to-posterior wall motion delay
SR	strain rate
SS	septum secundum
STJ	sinotabular junction
SV	stroke volume
SVC	superior vena cava
SVR	systemic vascular resistance
SWT	septal wall thickness
SWTd	septal wall thickness in diastole
t	time-of-flight
T	temperature
T	transmitted intensity
TAAA	thoracoabdominal aortic aneurysm
TAPSE	tricuspid annular plane systolic excursion
TAV	tricuspid annular velocity
TAVI	transcatheter aortic valve implantation
TAVR	transcatheter aortic valve replacement
TD	thermal dilution
TDI	tissue Doppler imaging
TE	trailing edge
TECAB	total endoscopic coronary artery bypass
TEE	transesophageal echocardiography
TG	transgastric
TGA	transposition of great arteries
TGC	time gain control
THV	transcatheter heart valve
TI	thermal index
TIAs	transient ischemic attacks
TIS	soft tissue thermal index
TL	true lumen
TMF	transmitral flow
TOF	tetralogy of Fallot
TPF	transpulmonary flow
TR	tricuspid regurgitation
TRPA	transplanted right pulmonary artery
TS	tricuspid stenosis
TSI	tissue synchronization imaging
TT	tissue tracking
TTE	transthoracic echocardiography
TTF	transtricuspid flow
TV	tricuspid valve
TVA	tricuspid valve area
TVAL	tricuspid valve anterior leaflet
TVPL	tricuspid valve posterior leaflet
TVSL	tricuspid valve septal leaflet
UE	upper esophageal
V	mean velocity
VA	ventriculoatrial
VAD	ventricular assist device

VAE	venous air embolism
Var-ed	end-diastolic peak aortic regurgitant velocity
VC	valve compliance
VC	vena contracta
Vel	velocity
VF	venous flow
V_m	mean velocity
VM	minute ventilation
V_{max}	maximal velocity
V_{mr}	peak mitral regurgitant velocity
V_{ms}	peak mitral stenosis velocity
V_p	velocity of propagation
V_{pda}	peak velocity of the patent ductus arteriosus
V_{peak}	peak velocity
Vpr-e	early peak pulmonary regurgitant velocity
Vpr-ed	end-diastolic peak pulmonary regurgitant velocity
VR	venous return
VSD	ventricular septal defect
V_{vsd}	peak ventricular septal defect velocity
VT.1/2	velocity half time
VTI	velocity-time integral
V_{tr}	peak tricuspid regurgitant velocity
VV	ventricular-to-ventricular
W	Watt
WMSI	wall motion score index
WS	wall stress
Z	acoustic impedance (rayls)

How to Use the Transesophageal Echocardiography Multimedia Manual

The manual was designed to facilitate the learning of transesophageal echocardiography (TEE). To this end, TEE images are accompanied by explanatory two-dimensional (2D) diagrams and 3D icons for spatial orientation. Both diagram and icon borders share a unique thick black line meant to allow the reader to exactly realign the 2D diagram on the 3D icon. Superposition of both lines gives the spatial orientation of the TEE image.

The manual is accompanied by a DVD-ROM where all the figures and the related video clips are stored. Several figures are accompanied by echocardiographic, hemodynamic, radiological, anatomical/surgical data, and other video clips. Moreover, three-dimensional (3D) animations are provided to clarify the spatial orientation of the TEE images. As anatomical variations can occur between patients, the suggested 3D planes represent our best understanding of the images orientation. To maximize the learning experience with this multimedia manual, we strongly recommend that reading be performed with simultaneously running the DVD.

SKETCH (BLACK LINE) AND 3D ICON (TRIANGLE) CORRELATION AND SUPERPOSITION

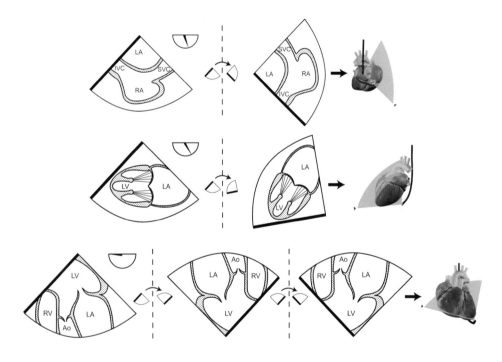

 This symbol used in the legend indicates the presence of additional video clips in relation to the figure available on the accompany DVD.

 The human body icon indicates how the patient was positioned relative to the camera when intraoperative images or videos were obtained.

Principles of Ultrasound

Alain Gauvin and Guy Cloutier
Université de Montréal, Montreal, Quebec, Canada

Michel Germain
McGill University, Montreal, Quebec, Canada

COMPRESSION AND RAREFACTION

Ultrasound consists of mechanical sound waves whose frequencies are above the audible range, that is, $\geq$20,000 Hz (Hz stands for the number of wave cycles per second). Sound is defined as a mechanical wave that propagates in a medium due to molecular interaction. The mode of propagation of ultrasound is related to successive molecular compressions and rarefactions occurring in that medium (Fig. 1.1). When individual molecular motion is in the same direction as the wave propagation, it forms a longitudinal wave. When molecular motion is perpendicular to wave direction, it is a transverse (or shear) wave. Solids, such as biological tissues, can experience both transverse (or shear) and longitudinal waves. Ultrasound in fluids and gases mostly experiences longitudinal propagation because of the lack of strong coupling between the molecules. Recent research suggests that shear waves may become clinically useful to characterize the viscoelastic properties of biological tissues and be used in sonoelasticity imaging and dynamic elastography.

To understand ultrasound production, one can imagine a small transducer driving an oscillating surface in contact with gas molecules, as illustrated in Figure 1.2. As the surface moves forward, it pushes gas molecules in front of it, creating a zone of compression (Fig. 1.2A). The oscillating surface then retracts, during which time the newly created zone of compression moves forward. However, this backward motion of the surface also causes a rarefaction of local gas molecules (Fig. 1.2B). In the time elapsed between Figure 1.2A and B, the zone of increased density initially created moves forward at propagation speed denoted as *c*. If the oscillation of this surface, which can be referred to as the source, is sustained, a continuous traveling wave, made by alternating compressions and rarefactions, is established.

At a given point in space, the rarefactions and compressions are accompanied by local oscillation of molecules in a direction parallel to the axis of propagation of the wave forming a mechanical longitudinal wave. During the transition from compression to rarefaction, molecules, initially located in a compressive region, on average, move backward (with respect to the direction of propagation of ultrasound) so that the local density of molecules is reduced. The process repeats itself as long as the surface is in oscillating motion. It is, therefore, the momentum (or the mechanical motion of molecules initially at rest) that propagates, not the molecules themselves which merely oscillate back and forth when insonified.

The velocity of the molecules reaches its maximum when the local density is half that of the maximum density for a sinusoidal wave, which occurs midway between a maximum and a minimum density. Molecules eventually come to a stop, at which point their local density is at its minimum, right in the middle of the rarefaction zone. Motion then resumes, and the velocity reaches its maximum midway in the transitory period, as noted previously. This corresponds to the intercept points of the wave with the distance axis (Fig. 1.1B), while the minimum average velocity is encountered at the peaks (negative and positive) of the same wave. Finally, molecules again come to rest when the density is at its highest. Therefore, at any given point in space, molecules experience all density states at different times (Fig. 1.2).

In conclusion, these compressions and rarefactions are made possible by the elastic nature of the material, arising from intermolecular interactions. It is this elasticity, together with the density of the material, which mainly governs the properties of the medium with respect to longitudinal wave propagation.

Frequency, Wavelength, and Propagation Speed in Biological Tissues

Ultrasound can be described by the following: period, frequency, amplitude, power, pressure, intensity, wavelength, and propagation speed. These variables can be determined by the sound source or the medium in which it travels (Table 1.1).

Frequency

Once a traveling wave has established a given spatial position (Fig. 1.1), it will find itself crossed by alternating

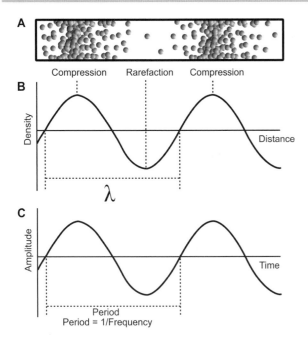

Figure 1.1 Ultrasound wave. (A) Representation of alternating molecular compressions and rarefactions in a longitudinal wave. **(B)** Corresponding 2D plot of molecular density as a function of distance along the propagation direction. The wavelength, λ, is the distance corresponding to one cycle of the longitudinal wave. **(C)** Plot of amplitude of the wave as a function of time. The period is the time corresponding to one cycle of the longitudinal wave.

compressions and rarefactions, at a pace determined by the frequency (f). Hertz (Hz) represents the number of cycles per second (unit of $1/\sec = \sec^{-1}$) (a cycle being a complete back-and-forth motion) of the oscillating surface that gives rise to the mechanical waves. One MegaHertz (MHz) corresponds to 1,000,000 (or 1 million) cycles per second. The frequency is determined by

the source, which, in this case, is the oscillating surface. Nevertheless, attenuation by the medium and nonlinear propagation effects can modify the shape and frequency of the transmitted waves.

The time interval, or the duration of a cycle, is the period, which is inversely related to the frequency (Fig. 1.1). The frequency of ultrasound used for medical imaging usually ranges from 2 to 15 MHz, although it can be higher for some special imaging techniques, such as endovascular ultrasound and ultrasound biomicroscopy, where frequencies typically vary from 20 to 60 MHz. Endovascular ultrasound [also known as intravascular ultrasound (IVUS)] produces images from inside a blood vessel with a catheter, whereas ultrasound biomicroscopy is mainly used, so far, for preclinical studies in small animals.

Wavelength

The wavelength (λ) corresponds to the distance separating two adjacent maximums or minimums of a wave (Fig. 1.1). Therefore, λ represents the spatial spacing of points of similar intensity along the wave at a given instant, while the period represents the temporal spacing of points, also with similar intensity, at a given location (Fig. 1.1).

Propagation Speed

A given location in space is crossed by a number of cycles per second given by f, these cycles being spaced by a distance given by λ. The product of both values yields the propagation speed, c, of the wave.

$$c = f\lambda \qquad (1.1)$$

An analogy would be evenly spaced cars driving on a highway at the same speed; the speed is the distance between each car multiplied by the number of cars per time unit passing an observer at rest along the road. The propagation speed, c, is generally a property of the medium and is independent of

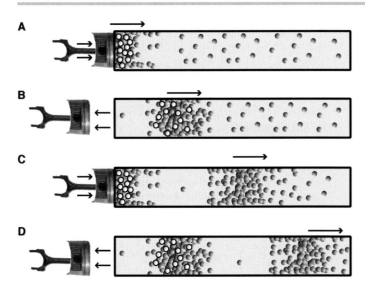

Figure 1.2 Generation of ultrasound wave. Representation of the density of gas molecules subjected to the oscillation of a column of gas from a small transducer at one end. **(A)** The surface has moved forward from a rest position creating a zone of increased molecule density (compression). **(B)** The surface has retracted and now leaves a zone of decreased density (rarefaction). **(C)** The initial compression and rarefaction in has traveled further. **(D)** Note the particles themselves oscillate locally and do not traverse the length of the column. *Source:* Courtesy of Dr. Dan Russell, Kettering University, www.kettering.edu/~drussell/Demos/waves/wavemotion.

Table 1.1 Various Parameters for Describing Waves

Parameters	Symbol	Basic units	Units	Mainly determined by
Period	τ	Time	sec, μsec	Sound source
Frequency	f	1/Time	Hz, MHz, sec^{-1}	Sound source
Amplitude	A	Pressure or density	Pa or g/cm^3	Sound source
Power	W	Work/time	J/sec, W	Sound source
Pressure	P	Force/area	N/m^2, Pa, MPa	Sound source
Intensity	I	Power/area	W/cm^2	Sound source
Wavelength	λ	Distance	m, cm, mm	Source and medium
Propagation speed	c	Distance/time	m/sec	Medium

Table 1.2 Ultrasound Properties of Some Common Materials

Material	Density (g/cm^3)	c (m/sec)	Z (rayls $\times$ 10^{-5})	Attenuation coefficient (dB/cm at 1 MHz)
Air	0.0000012	331	0.0004	12
Fat	0.95	1450	1.38	0.63
Muscle	1.1	1580	1.70	0.5–1.0
Skull bone	1.91	4080	7.80	20

Abbreviations: c, speed of sound; dB, decibel; Z, acoustic impedance, which is the product of density and speed of sound.

frequency, f. It is determined by the stiffness (K) and density (ρ) of the medium, through the equation

$$c = \sqrt{\frac{K}{\rho}} \qquad (1.2)$$

Stiffness, K, is the pressure increase required to cause a relative decrease in volume. It is the inverse of compressibility, which itself corresponds to the relative decrease of volume caused by external pressure. For example, air is compressible, bone is not. Density, ρ, is the concentration of mass or weight, and its unit is kg/cm^3. It is a property of the medium through which sound travels. As frequency, f, is mainly determined by the ultrasound source, specifying its value and the nature of the medium generally determines the wavelength, λ, through equation (1.1).

The speed of sound, c, varies with different material (Table 1.2), typically a few hundred m/sec for gases (330 m/sec in air), 1000 to 2000 m/sec for liquids (1480 m/sec in pure water at 20°C), and 1540 m/sec in soft biological tissues. The actual speed at a given point can vary a few percent above or below this accepted value depending on the local density and compressibility of the tissue. According to equation (1.2), the value of c is inversely proportional to the density of the material. It is of note that the speed of sound in air (low density) is much lower than that observed in solids (high density). This is because the relative difference in stiffness of air, compared with solids, is much more important than their relative density differences.

Other Properties of Ultrasound Waves

Amplitude

Longitudinal waves are characterized by molecular motion within a medium. The amplitude of this motion can be defined as the range of change of a certain property of the medium around its mean value, which is the density of molecules (Fig. 1.1). Acoustic amplitude in the context of ultrasound usually has units of pressure or voltage. An amplitude of zero generally corresponds to the average value of the property or to the normal value of the property when no motion exists. In other words, the amplitude is the deviation of the property around its mean value.

Power

As already discussed, a medium crossed by ultrasound will undergo localized compressions and rarefactions of the density of its molecules. In order for compressions to occur locally, supplementary energy must be provided, so a sound wave constitutes a form of energy transport, that energy being carried from the source into the medium. It is possible to characterize the power of the source, or the amount of energy it transfers to the medium per unit of time [in the International Unit System, the power of the source is given in joules per second (J/sec) or watt (W)]. In medical imaging, the power is influenced by many operating parameters and its value is generally difficult to measure but is proportional to the intensity defined in the following text.

Pressure

Compressions and rarefactions accompany the propagation of a sound wave and can be described as density differences along the direction of the wave propagation. However, varying densities also correspond to different pressures, which can be defined as force per unit area. Thus, one can also describe the manifestation of a longitudinal wave by the higher-than-average and lower-than-average pressure. The unit of pressure is Pascals.

The pressure (P) is related to the intensity of the beam (I) by the proportionality relationship

$$I \propto P^2 \qquad (1.3)$$

Intensity

The power was previously described as the energy per unit of time transferred from the source to the medium. The source (the transducer in an actual ultrasound imaging system) has a certain area. When the ultrasound energy is transmitted from the source, the amount of power crossing a certain area varies considerably with respect to the position of the transducer, due to the directional dependence of ultrasound emission and attenuation. Intensity is the parameter used to describe that spatial dependence, and it is defined as the energy per unit of time (or power) that crosses a small surface located at the point where intensity is sought.

For concerns related to the safety of diagnostic ultrasound, the intensity, or pressure, of the sound wave is an important parameter to consider. However, other parameters that pertain to patient safety can be displayed on the screen of medical ultrasound instruments, namely the thermal index (TI) and the mechanical index (MI). Different forms of TI are proposed in the ultrasound literature. In general terms, the TI can be defined as the ratio of the transmitted ultrasonic power to the power required to raise the temperature of the medium by 1°C under the same conditions. The TI is proportional to frequency, with higher frequencies more likely to produce local tissue heating. The MI is a parameter that reflects the potential for cavitation, or bubble formation in zones of rarefactions, which has been hypothesized as a potential mechanism for biologically harmful effects. The MI increases together with the transmitted power of the transducer and is inversely related to the square root of the frequency. More specifically, it is given by the rarefactional peak pressure at a point along the ultrasound beam axis where the pulse intensity is maximum, divided by the square root of the transmitted frequency, f. For safety reasons, it is more relevant to measure the MI than the power of the source. It is common for instruments to display the MI, as it allows the operator to understand the effect of common operating parameters, such as the transmitting power on the MI (Fig. 1.3). In a comparable fashion, the soft tissue thermal index (TIS), which corresponds to the thermal index evaluated in soft tissues, can often be visualized on some instruments, and it is influenced by similar operating factors (Fig. 1.3).

Depending on the type of clinical scan (obstetric, cardiac, peripheral, etc.), the maximum values of mechanical and thermal indices are usually limited by the instrument. Consequently, the potential for harmful effects is limited and possibly nonexistent. However, epidemiological demonstrations of noncausality are very difficult to obtain, and the existence of such risk should not be ruled out.

Specular Reflection

Acoustic Impedance

The acoustic impedance (Z) is the resistance to sound transmission in a medium. It is not measured but calculated as the product of tissue density (ρ) and tissue propagation speed, c.

$$Z = \rho \times c \qquad (1.4)$$

As both ρ and c are constants of a material, so is Z (equation 1.4). When ultrasound propagates from one medium to another, the impedance generally changes at the interface between media. When the boundary is perpendicular to the direction of propagation, part of the incoming ultrasound energy is reflected back, whereas the remainder penetrates the new medium and pursues its course. The relative amount of reflected energy depends on the impedance difference, as described later in this chapter. When the ultrasound wavelength, λ, is much smaller than the size of the interface, this phenomenon is termed specular reflection. Conversely, when λ is much larger than the size of the interface, it is termed nonspecular reflection or scattering. The term backscatter is also generally used to designate scatter emitted toward the ultrasound transducer.

Angle Dependence

With any angle of incidence θ with respect to the impedance boundary, the reflected beam is oriented with the same angle of incidence θ. Ultrasound imaging is based on the detection of the reflected ultrasound energy from internal boundaries and structures, as these generally have different impedance values. A smooth structure at 90° with respect to the incident beam yields specular reflection and is, therefore, seen on the image display (Fig. 1.4). If, however, the same structure has a different orientation, specular reflection will neither be returned to the transducer nor displayed.

Given the largely complex shapes of boundaries inside the human body, it might, therefore, seem like specular reflection alone would not yield much information, as surfaces are generally not perpendicular with respect to the incident beam. However, most surfaces also have a structural pattern that can be described on a scale smaller than the macroscopic boundary of the organ to which they belong. Consequently, this microstructural pattern gives rise to nonspecular reflections that cover a broad angular distribution, thus allowing imaging of the interfaces even if the angle of incidence differs from 90° (90° still being the optimal angle to obtain the maximal amount of energy reflected back to the transducer). This explains why nonspecular reflections, known as scattering, play the biggest role in the generation of ultrasound images (Fig. 1.5). It is also relevant to mention that, in practice, by using a range of incident angles, one can detect perfect flat specular reflectors due to the complex pattern of intensities and divergence of the ultrasound beam (see Chapter 3). Indeed, side lobes of the ultrasound beam may help to identify specular flat surfaces even if the transducer is not perfectly aligned perpendicular to the searched interface.

Nonspecular reflection allows the return of ultrasound to the transducer through multiple paths, each with a varying number of scatter interactions, and also allows for destructive and constructive interferences

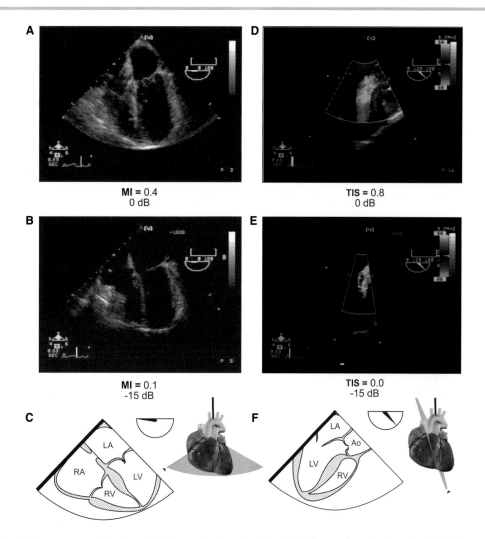

Figure 1.3 Transmitting power and indices. ME four-chamber (**A–C**) and ME long axis color Doppler (**D–F**) views are shown. (**A,D**) Transmitting power is expressed in decibels (dB), a value of 0 dB indicates the emitting source is at 100% of its power. (**B,E**) When transmitting power is reduced, it is expressed in negative dB, both the MI and TIS decrease. *Abbreviations*: Ao, aorta; LA, left atrium; LV, left ventricle; ME, mid-esophageal; MI, mechanical index; RA, right atrium; RV, right ventricle; TIS, soft tissue thermal index.

of ultrasound reaching the transducer. This produces the speckle appearance of ultrasound images, for which a relatively uniform tissue, such as the liver, gives a nonuniform pattern (Fig. 1.5). Speckle may be seen as artifactual and does not directly reflect the location of scatters from which echoes seem to arise.

Acoustic Impedance Mismatch

When ultrasound crosses a boundary, either side of which acoustic impedance differs, the intensity of the reflected ultrasound depends on the difference between acoustic impedance of the two media: this is termed the acoustic-impedance mismatch. With a 90° angle of incidence, the proportion of the transmitted intensity that is reflected back (R) at the interface is given by

$$R = \left(\frac{Z_2 - Z_1}{Z_2 + Z_1}\right)^2 \qquad (1.5)$$

where Z_1 and Z_2 represent the impedance of the medium before and after the boundary. Therefore, the transmitted intensity (T) is simply the remaining fraction of the initial intensity value, or

$$T = 1 - R = 1 - \left(\frac{Z_2 - Z_1}{Z_2 + Z_1}\right)^2 = \frac{4Z_1 Z_2}{(Z_2 + Z_1)^2}. \qquad (1.6)$$

According to the aforementioned definitions of the reflected and transmitted signal intensities, some examples can be given to understand better the mechanisms of ultrasound propagation in the human body. For instance, let us consider the impedance of air Z_1 (0.004×10^{-5} rayls) that is much smaller than that of fat Z_2 (1.38×10^{-5} rayls). The reflected intensity at this interface will be close to one, and such a boundary essentially reflects all incoming ultrasound energy (T is close to zero, see equation 1.6) (Fig. 1.6). Another interface involving a large reflected fraction of the incoming wave is that of bone/tissue because of the

A

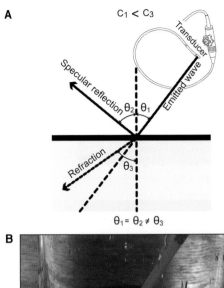

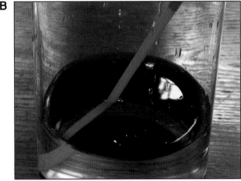

$$\theta_1 = \theta_2 \neq \theta_3$$

B

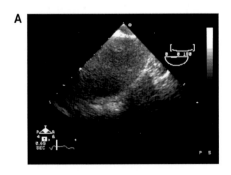

Figure 1.4 Refraction phenomenon. (A) A wave reflected at a boundary on either side of which are two different impedance values is reflected with an incidence angle (θ_2) identical to the one of the incoming beam (θ_1), but away from the transducer. However, part of the wave penetrates the second medium, but changes speed and propagation direction or angle (θ_3) according to Snell's law (C, propagation speed). **(B)** The visible light from the immersed part of the straw follows a different path than the light from the non-immersed part: air and water are two different media in this case. The refraction creates the illusion of a broken straw.

high impedance of bone (7.80×10^{-5} rayls) with respect to biological tissues. This particular situation poses a special problem for cardiac imaging, as the heart is "shielded" by the rib cage during transthoracic echocardiography (TTE).

Scattering, Refraction, and Attenuation

Scattering

As ultrasound interacts with a medium, most of the energy is absorbed and the rest is reflected or scattered. When ultrasound interacts with structures much smaller than the wavelength, nonspecular reflection or scattering occurs, as described previously. Such interaction involves the absorption of ultrasound, followed by its reemission in all directions. In ultrasound imaging, this situation is typical of parenchymal tissue, in which complex structures exist at a microscopic level.

Refraction

Refraction is a change in the direction of travel of an ultrasound wave as it moves into a different medium (Fig. 1.4). When applied to light, the same phenomenon causes the distorted appearance of objects that are partly immersed in water (Fig. 1.4B).

Refraction, therefore, implies a deviation of the beam from its original direction of propagation. Fundamental to the understanding of refraction is the fact that frequency, f, does not normally change when ultrasound passes from one medium to the next, as it is determined by the source. As seen previously, small velocity differences, however, do exist, and in order for equation (1.1) ($c = f\lambda$) to be true, wavelength, λ, must be modified by the medium change (Fig. 1.7). This, in turn, can only hold true if one considers a change in the orientation of the beam at an interface (Fig. 1.4).

$$\frac{\sin \theta_1}{\sin \theta_2} = \frac{c_1}{c_2}. \tag{1.7}$$

Equation (1.7) represents Snell's law, which quantifies the deviation of the penetrating beam in Figure 1.4. In ultrasound imaging, it is generally assumed that the beam is traveling in a straight line with respect to the source and refraction can cause structures to be spatially positioned at the wrong location, thereby causing image artifacts. However, as all biological tissues, with the exception of bone cause relatively small changes in speed of sound (that is assumed at 1540 m/sec by most ultrasound scanners), image distortions are limited.

A

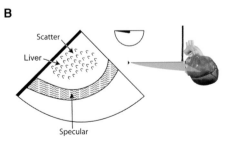

B

Figure 1.5 Specular reflection and scattering. (A,B) Transgastric ultrasound image of the liver shows its boundary as a specular reflection and its tissue as non specular reflections or scattering resulting in a speckled appearance.

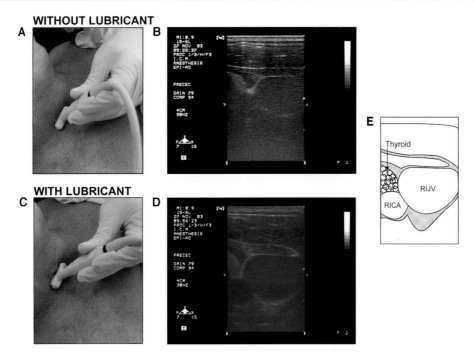

WITHOUT LUBRICANT

WITH LUBRICANT

Figure 1.6 Acoustic mismatch. An example of different acoustic mismatch obtained with a 10 MHz transducer used during insertion of a central venous catheter. Compare the image without lubricant (**A,B**) to the image using lubricant (**C–E**). The lubricant reduces the acoustic impedance mismatch because the impedance of the lubricant is much higher than air. Therefore, the amount of transmitted intensity is increased and the ultrasound image is clearer. *Abbreviations*: RICA, right internal carotid artery; RIJV, right internal jugular vein.

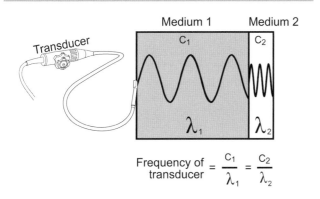

Figure 1.7 Ultrasound characteristics in different medium. The speed of sound is how fast the disturbance is passed from molecule to molecule and is determined only by the medium. Two different media are shown with their own velocity of propagation (c_1 and c_2). The frequency, f, does not change when ultrasound passes from one medium to the next, as it is determined by the source. Wavelength, λ, however, will be modified by the medium change according to the formula: $f = c/\lambda$.

Attenuation

Typical media are not perfectly elastic, which implies that some energy is converted to heat. The ultrasound beam is, therefore, attenuated through the loss of energy in the medium. Mechanisms of attenuation in biological tissues include reflection, absorption, and scattering. As a part of the energy is removed from the beam, the intensity decreases as ultrasound travels, so density difference between maximum and minimum amplitudes is correspondingly decreased (Fig. 1.8). At a given frequency, f, the amount of energy loss per distance traveled through the medium can vary depending on the human tissues concerned. For example, the attenuation in muscle is twice that of liver and soft biological tissues. The frequency, f, of the ultrasound beam is another important parameter to consider. As frequency, f, is increased, so is the attenuation. This explains why ultrasound images are more attenuated as a function of depth at higher frequencies. It is interesting to note that attenuation due to scattering actually decreases with increasing f. However, the decrease in attenuation scattering is not sufficient to compensate for the increase in absorption at higher frequencies. Therefore, the total attenuation increases with frequency f (Fig. 1.9).

To describe attenuation, it is necessary to look at the ratio of intensities at two points along the beam. Intensity changes can span a very large range. Therefore it is convenient to express it on a logarithm scale.

There is a convention to indicate that a given attenuation has been obtained from the log of a ratio rather than the ratio itself, and this consists of converting the ratio in units of ''bel.'' Generally, the prefix

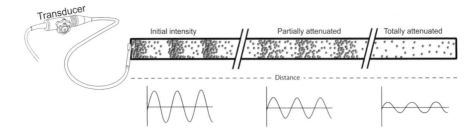

Figure 1.8 Attenuation. As the wave travels through the medium it undergoes attenuation, the relative difference of density between compressions and rarefactions, or intensity, decreases. There is a loss in sound signal strength due to reflection, scattering or absorption of the sound wave.

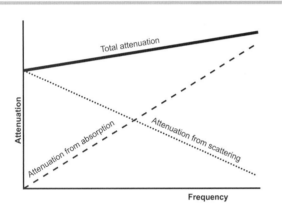

Figure 1.9 Components of attenuation. Total attenuation arises from both absorption and scattering, which are modified by a change in frequency. With increasing frequency, attenuation due to absorption increases (worsens) while that due to scattering decreases (improves). Overall, the effect of absorption predominates such that overall attenuation increases (worsens) with a higher imaging frequency.

Table 1.3 Relative Ultrasound Intensity Changes for Various Decibel (dB) Values, Both Negative and Positive

dB	Relative intensity
−40	0.0001
−30	0.001
−20	0.01
−10	0.1
−3	0.5
−2	0.63
−1	0.79
0	1.0
1	1.26
2	1.59
3	2.00
10	10
20	100
30	1,000
40	10,000

Note that a reduction of −10 dB and −3 dB means that the intensity is reduced by one-tenth and one-half. A 3 dB and a 10 dB change means that the intensity will double or increase ten times.

"deci" is applied on the bel, and the resulting unit, the decibel, is used with the abbreviation dB. From this discussion, the calculation of attenuation in dB is given by

$$\text{Attenuation(dB)} = 10 \log\left(\frac{I_2}{I_1}\right) \quad (1.8)$$

where I indicates the intensity (Table 1.3). The attenuation in decibel has a negative value and is expressed as a function of depth. If the pressure is considered instead of the intensity, the multiplicative factor of 20 should be used instead of 10, as described in equation (1.3): $I \propto P^2$.

The attenuation in human tissue is fairly constant per unit of depth, being about 0.5 dB/cm at 1 MHz (see Table 1.2 for attenuation values of different materials). Multiple attenuations in dB can be arithmetically added to yield the overall attenuation. Therefore, one can simply obtain the overall attenuation of a beam crossing a certain thickness (th) measured in centi-

meters (cm), using

$$\text{Attenuation(th)} = 0.5\frac{\text{dB}}{\text{cm}} \times \text{th(cm)}. \quad (1.9)$$

To account for frequency f, a first-order approximation can be used by considering a linear relationship between attenuation and f. Consequently, equation (1.9) can be rewritten, for all frequencies (measured in MHz), as

$$\text{Attenuation} = 0.5\frac{\text{dB}}{\text{MHz} \times \text{cm}} \times d(\text{cm}) \times f(\text{MHz}). \quad (1.10)$$

where d is the distance traveled in the medium. Note that this corresponds to twice the depth indicated on the screen of an ultrasound scanner: indeed, it has to be taken into account that ultrasound has to travel from the probe to the target point, and back to the probe, with the resulting attenuation as a function of depth. Consequently, attenuation can be approximated as being proportional to both depth and frequency f (Fig. 1.10).

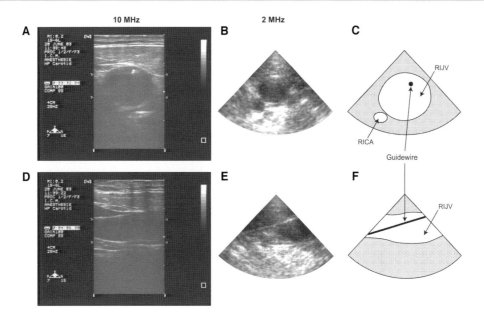

Figure 1.10 Imaging ultrasound frequency. Surface images of the RIJV and RICA in a transverse plane (**A–C**) and a longitudinal plane (**D–F**) are shown. The selection of probe frequency determines the relative importance of either better resolution or improved penetration for structural imaging. The images obtained with the 10 MHz transducer (**A,D**) provide more anatomical details but the deeper RICA is not clearly seen as with the 2 MHz probe (**B,E**) because of greater attenuation. Abbreviations: RIJV, right internal jugular vein; RICA, right internal carotid artery.

IMAGING

The imaging process can be presented in several modes of data acquisition and display. This includes the A-, B-, C-, and M-modes and three-dimensional (3D) imaging (Fig. 1.11). Transducers, which are described in greater detail in Chapter 3, are driven by an electrical signal (voltage) to produce ultrasound waves. An interesting feature of transducers is their bifunctionality, allowing them not only to emit but also to receive ultrasound and create an electrical signal from it, although the voltage involved in that process is much weaker than that used for emission.

A transducer releases a pulse, or a small sequence of successive compressions and rarefactions created by the oscillating surface of the transducer. The oscillating surface then comes to rest, putting itself in "listening" mode, while the rarefaction and compression waves travel away from the transducer. The wavefront eventually meets a reflector, or a zone of acoustic impedance difference, which returns a fraction of the incident ultrasound wave energy, thus creating an echo, while the nonreflected component pursues its course. As further reflectors are met, the same process is repeated, with more echoes being returned to the transducer, until those from the maximum depth (set as an operating parameter) are received. At this point, a new pulse is released and a new series of echoes is received. In the ultrasound scanning system (Fig. 1.12), the transducer spends relatively little time emitting ultrasound and is, most of the time, listening for returning echoes.

Such an echo train of returning periodic echoes is detected by the transducer, which converts it to an electrical signal. Successive electrical signals are then created and are separated by time intervals corresponding to the time taken by ultrasound pulses to travel between those reflectors, also termed time-of-flight. The relationship between the time-of-flight (t), propagation speed, c, and the distance (d) traveled by ultrasound is given by

$$d = ct \qquad (1.11)$$

The time of arrival of an echo at the transducer is related to the depth at which the reflecting structure is located. To determine the depth of a reflecting structure, it is important to take into account the fact that the ultrasound echo has to accomplish a round trip and, consequently, twice the time is required.

Equation (1.11) also expresses the need to know precisely the propagation speed of ultrasound in order for an accurate value of depth to be calculated. Fortunately, propagation speeds in most tissues are closely represented by an accepted average value of 1540 m/sec, and this is necessary to allow ultrasound images to be relatively free of geometrical distortion. In fact, most large geometrical distortions occur from other causes, such as refraction.

Advantages and Limitations of A-, B-, and M-Mode Ultrasonography

A-Mode

The bidirectional mode of operation of a transducer is fundamental to the process of ultrasound image formation, of which A-mode (for amplitude mode) is the

A

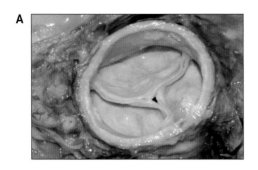

B

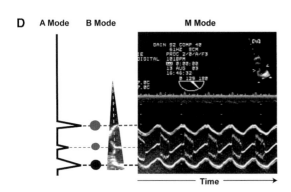

C

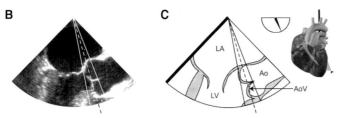

D

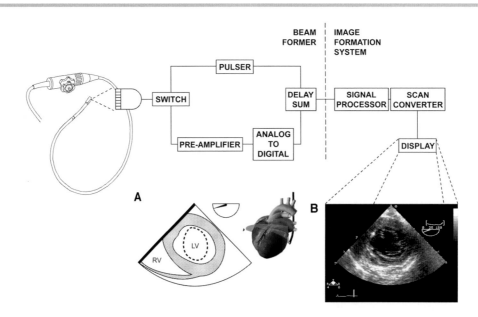

Figure 1.11 Ultrasound imaging modes. The B (brightness), M (motion) and A (amplitude) modes are illustrated. (**A**) The real object, an AoV, is displayed. (**B,C**) Brightness mode displays the intensity of the echo signals on a bidimensional map. (**D**) The A-mode displays each ultrasound boundary reflector as a peak corresponding to the strength of the reflected ultrasound. In M-mode, a small slice of the 2D object is displayed on a format where the abscissa represents the time dimension and the ordinate represents the spatial dimension. This displays accurate motion of the anatomical structures. *Abbreviations*: Ao, aorta; AoV, aortic valve; LA, left atrium; LV, left ventricle. *Source*: Photo A courtesy of Dr. Nicolas Dürrleman.

Figure 1.12 Ultrasound scanning system. Schematics of an ultrasound scanner, divided into two subgroups; the beam former and the image formation system. On the beam former side, the electronics illustrated exist for each element of the transducer array, and connect to the delay/sum module. The latter then connects to the image formation modules. (**A,B**) Transgastric LV short axis view is shown. *Abbreviations*: LV, left ventricle; RV, right ventricle.

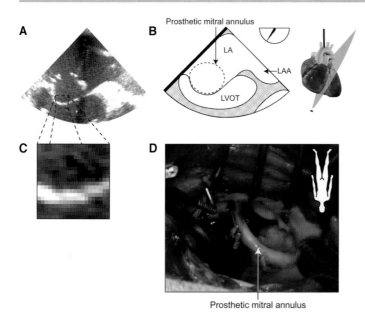

A **B**

Prosthetic mitral annulus

LA

LAA

LVOT

C **D**

Prosthetic mitral annulus

Figure 1.13 Matrix representation of an ultrasound image. (**A–C**) A matrix is a 2D arrangement of rows and columns of pixels easily evident at higher magnification (**C**) compared with the anatomical correlation (**D**). *Abbreviations*: LA, left atrium; LAA, left atrial appendage; LVOT, left ventricular outflow tract. *Source*: Photo D courtesy of Dr. Michel Pellerin.

most elementary form (Fig. 1.11D). The amplitude mode (or A-mode) owes its name to the fact that it displays each ultrasound boundary reflector as a peak corresponding to the amplitude of the reflected ultrasound echo envelope. The A-mode allows identification of changes in echogenicity (or the presence of ultrasound reflecting structures) of a patient's internal organ. However, the information is unidimensional as only the depth and relative strength (itself an indication of the impedance difference) of reflecting structures can be determined (Fig. 1.11). No precise determination of the shape of these structures can be achieved. With the exception of ophthalmology and research applications in tissue characterization, A-mode is rarely used in medical imaging.

B-Mode

The brightness mode (or B-mode) represents each ultrasound boundary reflector as a luminous dot whose brightness is proportional to the strength of the received echo. The B-mode can allow for two-dimensional (2D) echogenicity maps to be acquired. It can be obtained by juxtaposing multiple B-mode lines, where each one is plotted on an image matrix with intensity proportional to the echo strength (Fig. 1.11D). A matrix is a 2D arrangement of values positioned in rows and columns (Fig. 1.13). The ultrasound beam for B-mode imaging is kept narrow enough by focusing so that the interrogated tissue (the tissue that returns an echo) is confined laterally for a given scan line. By moving the scan line mechanically or electronically, 2D maps of echo strength can be obtained. During the receiving of a given scan line, all echoes are assumed to originate from points along that line, whose precise distance from the transducer can be determined using equation (1.11). The vast majority of contemporary B-mode systems now direct

the beam by using a nonmechanical technique in a manner that will be described in detail in Chapter 3.

M-Mode

In M-mode (motion mode), a B line is displayed on a 2D B-mode map (image matrix) with brightness indicating the echo strength or the amplitude (Fig. 1.11D). However, the other dimension direction corresponds to time rather than lateral distance, as in A- or B-mode. Consequently, this mode is used to show the motion of reflectors as a function of time by continuously retracing a line such as that acquired in B-mode, but maintaining the location to which this line corresponds with respect to the patient, thus insonifying the same column of tissue every time (in a true B-mode image acquisition, this line is swept in the patient). Each of these lines is traced vertically in the image, and shifted laterally on the screen from one line to the next. Once the full width of the image has been swept in this way, the process is repeated for a new image.

This mode is commonly used for dimensional measurements at specific times of the cardiac cycle and for the analysis of valve leaflets, wall and abnormal structure motions. Refreshing of B-mode images (i.e., its frame rate that is typically 30–90 images/s) limits visualizing rapidly moving structures, such as heart valves. Consequently, M-mode is often preferred because of the higher temporal resolution of this modality, which can be below 1 ms.

Other Modes

Other modes of imaging such as C-mode, duplex, continuous wave (CW) Doppler, pulsed wave (PW) Doppler, color Doppler, power Doppler, tissue Doppler, harmonic imaging, 3D imaging, and elastography are not described here and are beyond the scope of this chapter.

Instrumentation

Transducers

Whatever the type of transducer used, a 2D scanner image involves the gathering of multiple B-mode lines to construct the final image. Modern transducers are actually made of many crystal elements arranged as an array within a portable assembly. Each element is selectively fired using a scheme described in Chapter 3. It is common to refer to the assembly as the probe. Modern transducers can generate a beam of ultrasound, and send it in a selectable direction, in a manner compatible with the description of B-mode acquisition given earlier.

Transmitting/Receiving Electronics

The dual use of the transducer for both ultrasound transmitting and receiving implies that some switching must take place. In addition, the different signal strengths involved between transmission and reception imply that different electronics must be used for each role. The beam former is the first stage of the transmitting/receiving electronics, and handles output/input to/from the transducer elements. Switching allows for the selection of the proper module within the beam former, depending on whether the system is transmitting or receiving (Fig. 1.12).

When the system is in transmitting mode, the beam former generates the signal to be sent to the different transducer elements. Focusing of the transmitted beam can be achieved by correctly selecting the delays of the electrical impulses fired by each crystal element. The output for each element has to be amplified so that a large voltage (typically 100–200 V) can be applied to the transducer elements, a task performed by the "pulser," which connects to the switching module.

When the system is in receiving mode, the weak voltage detected must first be amplified using a pre-amplifier. That amplification process is weighted as a function of the time-of-flight, increasing the applied gain as a greater time-of-flight implies a greater attenuation for which this needs to be compensated. The signal is then converted into digital form, as most modern systems process that way.

Further processing is applied to combine the signal from the different transducer elements (or individual crystals) to form a single A-mode scan line, a step termed focusing in reception. It involves the summing of the signals from many transducer elements, each of those signals being applied at a variable time delay prior to recombination. Delays for each element are typically time variable, to allow dynamic focusing with time delays best suited for each depth at which an echo is detected.

Apodization is also performed by most beam formers. This refers to the process that consists of multiplying the echo of each element of the array by a "weight." This allows performance shaping of the ultrasound beam and modification of the size of the side lobes. The output of the beam former stage is a cyclical electrical signal containing information on both phase and amplitude of received echoes. It is termed radio-frequency (RF) signal, and is sometimes used in advanced applications, but the majority of systems simply extract the envelope of this signal, which looks at the intensity of the signal along that scan line.

The stage following the beam former is the signal processor, which first applies time gain control (TGC) to amplify the scan line increasingly as a function of depth. The TGC settings are normally user-adjustable (Fig. 1.14). The signal is then converted to its logarithm form, which effectively compresses the range of signal values encountered. This procedure allows the

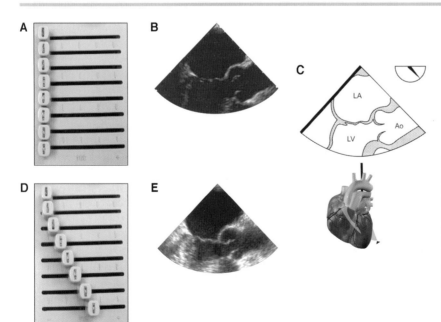

Figure 1.14 Time gain compensation. (**A–E**) The effects of TGC adjustments to a mid-esophageal aortic valve long-axis view are shown. Each TGC control slider is assigned to a selected depth. (**A–C**) The TGC control sliders are set to the left at 0. As the depth increases towards the bottom, the image brightness is less because of attenuation. (**D–E**) The TGC adjustments are made to change the brightness to that of the near field, creating a more homogenous image. *Abbreviations*: Ao, aorta; LA, left atrium; LV, left ventricle; TGC, time gain compensation.

display of both large amplitude echoes from reflectors and weak scattering from small cellular elements on a single 2D display. The signal is then rectified, and the envelope of the signal is obtained with a Hilbert transform mathematical operation. An overall description of a typical ultrasound scanner is provided in Chapter 3.

Scan Converters

The scan lines have to be stored and combined so that a 2D image can be obtained and displayed. This task is left to the scan converter, a device that represents the overall image as a matrix. Interpolation between the various A-lines of data has to be performed to obtain a matrix of typically 512 × 512 pixels. Modern scan converters also support a variety of postacquisition image processing, and are integrated with storage and transmission peripherals (e.g., network card).

Signal Processing, Image Resolution, and Display

Time Gain Control

There are two sets of gain control for the receiving amplifier: the overall gain control (Fig. 1.15), which affects all echoes equally, and the TGC (Fig. 1.14), which modifies the performance of the amplifier as a function of depth.

The TGCs are divided into two types. The first TGC amplification of the received signal is weighted according to the time-of-flight. The gain applied between the nearest and furthest echoes may be linear or follow a predetermined nonlinear function to emphasize, for example, the echo signals away from the transducer. This step is also used to adjust the dynamic range of the displayed images. For this purpose, the maximum and minimum gains in dB applied as a function of depth can be predetermined. This allows limiting the range of echo strengths to display the B-mode images, and consequently the echo contrasts, which may help to emphasize diagnostic features.

The second type of TGC consists of a series of cursors (also known as sliders or potentiometers) that are usually available beside the monitor to modulate the amplification as a function of depth (or time-of-flight). These cursors are easily accessible and their positions are changed by the clinician or technician according to the physiological structures being investigated (Fig. 1.14). From top to bottom, sliders of the TGC control apply a gain (proportional to the position of the slider from left to right) that corresponds to the axial position within the image (the top slider affects the portion of the image closer to the transducer and vice versa).

Image Resolution

Resolution is the ability to distinguish small objects located close to each other. The resolution of ultrasound imaging systems is not characterized as an overall resolution value but as separate directional components, which are the axial resolution (along the direction propagation of ultrasound), the lateral resolution (perpendicular to it), and the resolution in elevation (perpendicular to the long axis of the ultrasound probe). The axial resolution is a function of the crystal characteristics of each transducer element affecting its frequency bandwidth and a function of the shape of transmitted signals firing each element. The lateral resolution of the beam is determined by the firing sequence (focusing in either transmission, reception, or both) and by the line density of the image, whereas in the elevation direction, the

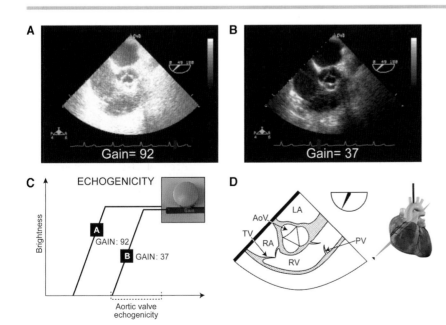

Figure 1.15 Overall gain control. (A,B,D) The effect of varying gain on echogenicity (visual quality of the image) is shown in these midesophageal AoV short-axis views. Compare the gain of 92 (**A**) with the lower gain of 37 (**B**). (**C**) Adjusting total gain modifies the relative position of the center of the slope with respect to the available range. Brightness is therefore enhanced within that range. However, echo signals below the chosen minimal threshold will appear as black pixels, while those exceeding the maximal range will be uniformly displayed as dense white pixels. *Abbreviations*: AoV, aortic valve; LA, left atrium; PV, pulmonic valve; RA, right atrium; RV, right ventricle; TV, tricuspid valve.

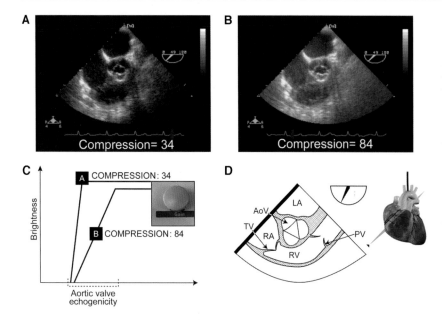

Figure 1.16 Dynamic range compression. (**A,B,D**) The effect of varying compression on echogenicity (visual quality of the image) is shown in these mid-esophageal AoV short-axis views. Compare the compression of 34 (**A**) with the higher compression at 84 (**B**). (**C**) Compression range modifies the slope of the relationship between brightness and echo strength. Further, it also alters the range of echo signal strength which can be displayed by the scale of brightness. Contrast is therefore enhanced within that range. For instance, the brightness difference between blood and the AoV is more pronounced with lower compression (slope A). Reducing compression range increases the slope such that larger differences in brightness will occur for the same difference in echo strength. Increasing compression range reduces the perceived difference in brightness because the slope is more flat. *Abbreviations*: AoV, aortic valve; LA, left atrium; PV, pulmonic valve; RA, right atrium; RV, right ventricle; TV, tricuspid valve.

Table 1.4   Various Parameters for Pulsed Ultrasound

Parameters	Basic units	Units	Determined by	Common values
Pulse repetition period	Time	sec, ms, μsec	Sound source	0.1–1.0 ms
Pulse repetition frequency	1/Time	sec⁻¹, Hz	Sound source	1–10 kHz
Pulse duration	Time	sec, ms, μsec	Sound source	0.5–3.0 μsec
Duty factor	None	None	Sound source	0.001–0.01
Spatial pulse length	Distance	mm, cm	Source and medium	0.1–1.0 mm

resolution or image thickness is determined by the size of the crystal elements and by the characteristics of acoustic lens positioned on the surface of the probe. For most scanners, the axial resolution, which is on the order of 1 mm, is better than the lateral and elevational resolutions. Image resolution is further discussed in Chapter 3.

Display

The ultrasound image is displayed on a computer monitor that allows the viewing of 2D echo images. Dynamic range compression determines the range of signal strength used to display received echo intensities and may affect overall image contrast (Fig. 1.16). For each new frame acquired by the system, the display is refreshed with the new image data. This is repeated many times per second, allowing for a real-time update of the image. Digital processing and storage capability are today available with most ultrasound systems.

Related Factors

Pulsing Characteristics

Pulsed wave (PW), as employed in B-mode can be characterized by the following parameters: the pulse duration (PD), pulse repetition period (PRP), pulse repetition frequency (PRF), duty factor, and spatial pulse length (SPL) (Table 1.4) (Fig. 1.17). The duty factor is the fraction of time that the ultrasound scanner is producing a pulse. It corresponds to the ratio of the PD to the PRP. The duty factor is important for safety issues as it affects the average echo intensity.

The PRF (1/PRP) can be defined as the number of pulses emitted by the transducer per unit of time; it depends on the maximum depth d_{max} and velocity of propagation (c) according to the following equation

$$\mathrm{PRF} = \frac{c}{2d_{max}}. \qquad (1.12)$$

Thus, it is clear that the number of pulses per time unit depends on the maximum depth for which echoes are to be measured (Fig. 1.18). This stems from the fact that the time elapsed between a pulse and the one following it (already defined as PRP) must be chosen so that it allows echoes from all depths of interest to reach the probe. The last echoes to be received are the furthest away from the probe and are emitted from locations at a depth of d_{max} with respect to the probe. If echoes are emitted from points located beyond d_{max}, they will reach the probe at the same time as echoes of the next pulse, which come from closer locations.

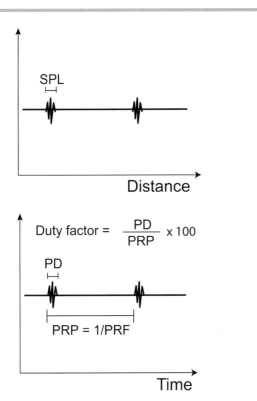

Figure 1.17 Pulsed Doppler characteristics. The pulse duration (PD) in time and spatial pulse length (SPL) in distance indicate when the pulse is on. The pulse repetition period (PRP) is the time from the start of one pulse to the next. The pulse repetition frequency (PRF) is the number of pulses in one second, irrespective of the number of cycles per pulse. The duty factor is the ratio of time that the transducer produces a pulse (or is on).

To illustrate this better, one can consider the case of a boat using, as is typical, a sound echo–based system to evaluate the depth. Such a system emits a pulse that propagates in water until it reflects at the bottom of the lake. It then comes back toward the surface and is eventually detected by the sound detector of the depth evaluation system. It will then translate the delay between the emission of the pulse and the reception of the echo into depth using equation (1.11), but dividing the distance by 2, as the back-and-forth course of the sound and its echo is in total twice the depth. Naturally, the system repeats its measurement to update the operator as the depth under the boat changes, so that the process is also described by equation (1.12), with PRF corresponding to the frequency of updates of the depth measurement system. For instance, if the PRF is chosen so that d_{max} equals 80 m. When a boat moves above depths greater than 80 m the returning echoes from these great depths will not come back in time and with the chosen PRF we will now proceed to emit a new echo without waiting further. If the depth is 100 m, the first echo will not return on time for the 80 m limit. A subsequent pulse will be issued while the first echo is still traveling toward the boat. That echo will reach the boat at the same time as an echo of the second pulse would if the

depth were 20 m, therefore leading the system to falsely indicate a depth of 20 m. This corresponds to the difference between the actual depth and the maximum depth allowed by the PRF. An alternate representation of this situation can demonstrate the same principle, using a diver rather than a pulse to evaluate the depth. If the diver swims at velocity c and a diver steps off the boat with a frequency (PRF) such that the maximum measurement depth is 80 m, one is not able to distinguish between the first diver coming back from a depth of 100 m and the second one who is now at 20 m.

In practice, echoes that originate from locations beyond d_{max} are detected by the probe, but are actually much weaker than the "new" proximal echoes from the next pulse, which arrive at the same time, so that their contribution is normally diluted by the new signal. However, very strong reflectors located at depths greater than d_{max} could cause an echo strong enough to be close in magnitude to low-depth echoes and, therefore, be represented at a depth much shallower than what should be seen. This is a potential cause of image artifact.

Frame Rate and Time to Generate One Frame

In B-mode, the exact number of lines from which the image (also called a frame) is made can vary, and this number is referred to as N_{line}. The number of frames per second (or the rate of image refresh on a B-mode ultrasound system) f_{frame} is given by

$$f_{frame} = \frac{PRF}{N_{line}}. \tag{1.13}$$

This explains why a small sector (lower N_{line}) will result in a higher frame rate, and why an increase in PRF will be associated with a shallower (less time is required to wait for distal echoes) image with an increased frame rate (Fig. 1.20). By combining equations (1.12) and (1.13), the latter can be rewritten as

$$f_{frame} = \frac{c}{2d_{max}N_{line}} = \frac{154,000 \, cm/s}{2d_{max}N_{line}}. \tag{1.14}$$

The average speed of ultrasound in tissues has been introduced in the second part of equation (1.14) to convert distance units to time units. The parameter d_{max} is the maximum depth of the image and is expressed in centimeters. The frame rate is typically displayed as a parameter on the monitor of ultrasound systems.

The time to generate one frame T_{frame} is simply

$$T_{frame} = \frac{1}{f_{frame}} = \frac{N_{line}}{PRF}. \tag{1.15}$$

and one can use equations (1.12) and (1.15) to rewrite equation (1.14):

$$T_{frame} = \frac{2d_{max}N_{line}}{c} = \frac{2d_{max}N_{line}}{154,000 \, cm/s}. \tag{1.16}$$

where d_{max} is again expressed in centimeters. As the depth decreases, less time is spent waiting for returning echoes, and T_{frame} decreases, while f_{frame} increases

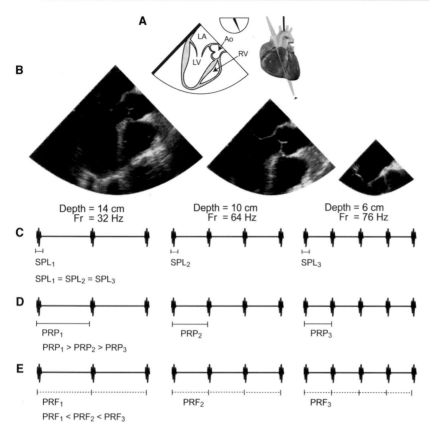

Figure 1.18 **Imaging depth.** (**A,B**) Mid-esophageal long axis and aortic valve long-axis views are obtained by changing depth. Maximal imaging depth is a function of the PRF. As depth is decreased the PRF increases with associated increase in Fr from 32 to 64 and 76 Hz. SPL is left identical between the three cases (**C**), the PRP decreases (**D**) and the PRF increases (**E**) as depth decreases. The duty factor (PD/PRP) would therefore increase as depth decreases. *Abbreviations*: Ao, aorta; Fr, frame rate; LA, left atrium; LV, left ventricle; PD, pulse duration; PRF, pulse repetition frequency; PRP, pulse repetition period; RV right ventricle; SPL, spatial pulse length.

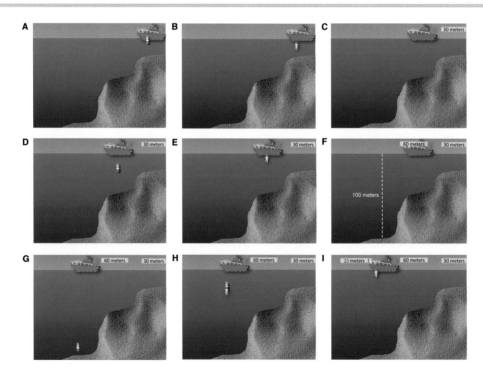

Figure 1.19 **PRF and aliasing.** (**A–G**) A diver swims at velocity c and another diver steps off the boat (**H**) with a frequency equivalent to a PRF of c/160 or a dmax of 80 m. At a depth of 100 m, it is not possible (**I**) to distinguish between the diver coming back from a depth of 100 m and the one at 20 m. *Abbreviations*: c, velocity of propagation; m, meters; PRF, pulse repetition frequency.

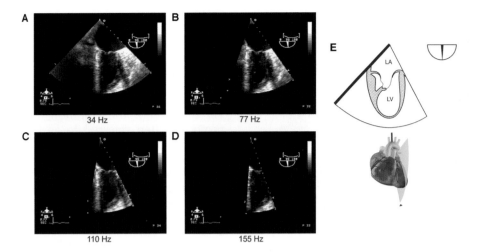

Figure 1.20 Sector width. (A–E) Mid-esophageal two-chamber views of the LV with different sectors are displayed. As the operator narrows the width of the sector scanned, the system takes less time to sweep the sector and thus refreshes the image more often. Therefore, a narrower sector yields a higher frame rate. *Abbreviations*: Hz, hertz; LA, left atrium; LV, left ventricle.

(Fig. 1.18). Decreasing the number of lines per image has the same effect (Fig. 1.20).

Number of Lines per Frame

The number of lines per frame can be rewritten from equations (1.15) and (1.16) as

$$N_{\text{line}} = \frac{154,000 \, \text{cm/s}}{2 f_{\text{frame}} d_{\text{max}}} = \frac{154,000 T_{\text{frame}}}{2 d_{\text{max}}}. \qquad (1.17)$$

If the depth increases, less lines can be acquired if a given frame rate is to be maintained. The number of lines covering a given area in an image influences the lateral resolution, which increases with the density of such lines. However, if the number of lines is modified with corresponding change of spatial coverage (scanning sector) to maintain the scan line density, lateral resolution is not affected, but the time to acquire a frame will be modified, as indicated by equation (1.16), with a corresponding change in frame rate (Fig. 1.20).

The scuba diver example can again be used to explain this concept. The various trajectories of descent of a scuba diver in a same diving session are compared with the number of lines acquired in a single frame in B-mode acquisition. If the scuba diver swims at a constant velocity (just as acoustic waves travel at a constant speed in a given medium), the number of diving trajectories taken increases as each dive ends at a shallower depth. If depth is increased, the number of diving trajectories will decrease if the duration of the diving session is unchanged.

Depth

As the ultrasound beam travels away from the transducer it becomes attenuated. Therefore, there is less and less power available downstream from the transducer for remote reflectors to return an echo, so echo

intensity decreases with the depth from which it originates. This can be compensated for by using the TGC control, so the distal echoes are more amplified than proximal ones. This, however, only works up to a point, when the echo signal is so weak that its electrical signal becomes similar in strength to electrical noise, the presence of which is unavoidable in any electronic system. This defines a maximum range for an ultrasound beam, which depends on the capability of the system to detect small echoes, and the frequency employed, through the influence of the latter on attenuation (Fig. 1.10). It is also possible to increase the time resolution by decreasing the image depth, as indicated on the screen by an increase in the frame rate (Fig. 1.18).

Temporal Resolution

The temporal resolution is given by equation (1.16) and is the time taken to generate one frame. As T_{frame} increases, the motion in the image field is not rendered as structures seem to move in a discontinuous fashion from one frame to the next. Improved temporal resolution occurs at the expense of lateral resolution (number of lines) and maximum depth from which echoes are measured. In cases where temporal resolution is called for, such as during TTE, this provides a strong incentive to bring the probe as close as possible to the anatomy of interest, thereby decreasing the maximum exploration depth (with respect to the probe). This is precisely what is done in transesophageal ultrasound. As indicated earlier, temporal resolution is maximal in M-mode as the number of lines is reduced to one.

Pixels

A pixel is the smallest element of a digital picture. Image data gathered from an ultrasound imaging

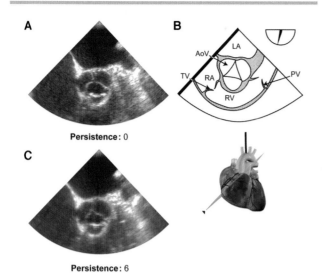

Figure 1.21   Persistence. (A–C) Digital post-processing can substantially impact the image appearance of these mid-esophageal AoV short-axis views. By averaging multiple images (persistence), the image appears smoother (**C**), at the cost of reduced time resolution. *Abbreviations*: AoV, aortic valve; LA, left atrium; PV, pulmonic valve; RA, right atrium; RV, right ventricle; TV, tricuspid valve.

system ultimately end up being represented as a matrix, typically of 512 × 512 pixels, which is then displayed on a computer screen in real time. As the acquired lines do not follow the columns or rows of the matrix, an interpolation process needs to be used to resample the image to the image pixels. The number of available pixels is normally such that no resolution loss is incurred from that process. Such digital images lend themselves well to postprocessing, which can sometimes enhance the appearance of images, and make important details more conspicuous (Fig. 1.21).

The image is normally displayed with the points located nearest the probe on top on the monitor image. Simple ultrasound images are generally displayed as gray scale, with a pixel value in the range of 0 to 255 (8 bits). However, a narrower range is generally selected for display, through windowing, which allows for that narrower range of pixel values to be represented by the full brightness range of the monitor, at the expense of contrast for pixel values outside of that range, which are either black or white. However, Doppler images need to be represented in color. To accomplish this, such images are rendered using 16 to 24 bits.

The DICOM standard allows for images to be sent in digital form to an external device over conventional, nonproprietary networks. This is accomplished via the use of the common TCP/IP transmission protocol (often referred to as the Internet protocol) over that network. This group of protocols enables devices from different manufacturers to exchange images, including all attached demographic data and other acquisition information that accompany images. Image management systems, such as picture archiving and communication systems (PACS), can then take over the distribution, display, and archival of images. Both static and dynamic images (which consist of successive static images acquired one after another over a short period of time) can be sent using DICOM, although dynamic data, such as that obtained in echocardiography, requires a considerable amount of disk storage space, and this constitutes an emerging challenge for PACS.

CONCLUSION

The operation of ultrasound imaging systems is based on principles directly derived from the physics and technology of medical ultrasound. A proficient use of such systems strongly depends on mastering these principles.

REFERENCE

1. McDicken WN. Diagnostic Ultrasonics. Principles and Use of Instruments. 3rd ed. Edinburgh: Churchill Livingstone, 1991.

FURTHER READING

Zagzebski JA. Essentials of Ultrasound Physics. St. Louis: Mosby-Year Book Inc., 1996.
Kremkau FW. Diagnostic Ultrasound: Principles and Instruments. 6th ed. Philadelphia: W.B. Saunders, 2002.
Bushberg JT, Seibert JA, Leidholt EM, et al. The Essential Physics of Medical Imaging. 2nd ed. Philadelphia: Lippincott Williams & Wilkins, 2002.

2

Basic Principles of Doppler Ultrasound

Pierre-Guy Chassot
University of Lausanne, Lausanne, Switzerland

Claude Tousignant
St. Michael's Hospital, University of Toronto, Toronto, Ontario, Canada

DOPPLER EFFECT

The Doppler effect is a well-known phenomenon: the sound of a train whistle has a higher pitch when the train is traveling toward the listener than when moving away, though the emitting frequency remains the same. In 1842, the Austrian physicist Johann-Christian Doppler, studying the direction of movement of stars, mathematically described this frequency shift of recorded waves when a luminous or acoustic source, in relative motion, is compared with the stationary observer.

The speed of traveling waves (c), such as light, sound, or ultrasound, is constant through a determined medium and depends on the characteristics of this medium. When the emitting source is in motion, regardless of its speed, the sound waves are "compressed" in front of the transmitter, which is "catching up" with the transmitted waves it has produced (Fig. 2.1A). When the source moves slightly toward the stationary receiver before emitting the next wave, the two wave peaks are closer together when they reach the receiver (observer), where the wavelength (λ) is shortened and the frequency (f) is increased (1). This happens because the product of λ and f is a constant wave propagation of speed c:

$$c = f \times \lambda \qquad (2.1)$$

If the source moves away, the opposite occurs: λ increases and f decreases. The Doppler shift is the difference between the frequency generated by the source (f_0) and the frequency observed by the listener (f_1):

$$\Delta f = f_1 - f_0 \qquad (2.2)$$

This shift is proportional to the ratio of the velocity of the object (v) to the speed of the sound, c, and to the generated frequency, f_0, but is independent of the amplitude of the wave:

$$\Delta f = \frac{v \times f_0}{c} \qquad (2.3)$$

The formula can be rearranged to determine the velocity of the object, v:

$$v = \frac{c \times \Delta f}{f_0} \qquad (2.4)$$

The same phenomenon occurs if the moving object is the target of an ultrasound wave emitted by a fixed source: the emitted ultrasound wave and the echo reflected wave returning to the transducer have different frequencies (Fig. 2.2). They are also linked by the previous Doppler equation, but the frequency shift (Δf) occurs twice, in the emitted and in the reflected waves:

$$\Delta f = f_1 - f_0$$
$$\Delta f = \frac{v}{c} \times 2f_0 \qquad (2.5)$$

The velocity of ultrasound in human soft tissues is constant; it lies between 1540 and 1580 m/sec (2). In blood, the acknowledged value is 1540 m/sec. The frequency shift can be positive or negative depending on whether the target is moving toward or away from the receiver. The Doppler equation is completed by an angle correction and can be rearranged to determine the velocity of the target:

$$v = \frac{c \times (\pm \Delta f)}{2f_0 \cos \theta} \qquad (2.6)$$

where θ is the angle between the motion of the target and the interrogating ultrasound beam, v is the velocity of the target (e.g., moving red blood cells), c is the speed of ultrasound (1540 m/sec), and f_0 is the emitting frequency of the ultrasound transducer.

The angle, θ, between the direction of the target and the interrogating beam has to be introduced in the formula to determine velocity accurately. The maximal frequency shift is observed when the transducer's orientation is parallel to the blood flow: if the angle is

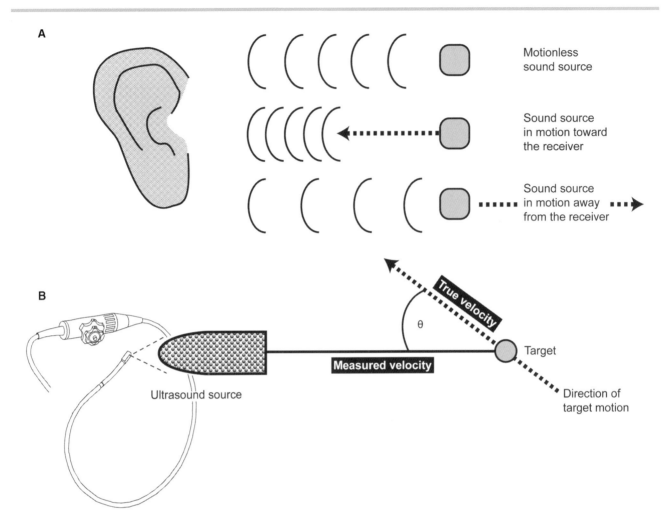

Figure 2.1 Doppler effect. (A) When a sound source is in motion toward the observer, its emitting frequency is increased compared with the same sound wave emitted from a stationary source. If the sound source is in motion away from the observer, its emitting frequency is decreased compared with the same sound wave emitted from a stationary source. **(B)** Illustration of the effect of angle (θ) between the direction of the interrogating Doppler beam and target motion on velocity.

zero, the cosine is 1 (Fig. 2.1B). On the other hand, perpendicular orientation of the interrogating beam to the axis of the flow gives no Doppler shift because the cosine of 90° equals zero. The underestimation of measured velocity induced by a 20° angle deviation (cosine 0.94) is <6% (~5 cm/s) and considered as negligible for clinical purposes (1). Increasing the angle to 30° (cosine 0.87) increases the error to 13%. Although ultrasound systems can perform a correction for the angle of incidence in the Doppler formula calculation, this correction is done only in the displayed two-dimensional (2D) plane. Therefore, this angle correction is not recommended because it creates a false sense of precision (3).

Given typical blood flow velocities (0.2–6.0 m/sec), the speed of the ultrasound in tissues (1540 m/sec), and emitting frequencies of the cardiac transducers (2–10 MHz), the Doppler shift falls within the human audible range (4–10 kHz) and can be heard through the ultrasound machine's loudspeaker. This sound is mathematically reproduced by the addition or multiplication of emitted and received waves. The product of this operation is a new wave with an f equal to the Doppler shift (4). Echocardiography is based on the time-delay measurement between the emission of a short pulse of ultrasound and the detected returning echo. 2D echo is essentially based on variations in amplitude (or intensity) of returning waves, whereas Doppler echo analysis is based principally on variations in frequency (Fig. 2.2). Doppler analysis and 2D display require different conditions for optimal results. The best 2D image is obtained with a high-frequency transducer (>5 MHz) and an interrogating beam perpendicular to the structure. The Doppler shift is maximal when the ultrasound beam is parallel to the flow and when the emitting f is low (1–2 MHz) (5). In clinical practice, the setup of the ultrasound machine has to be properly adjusted for each function.

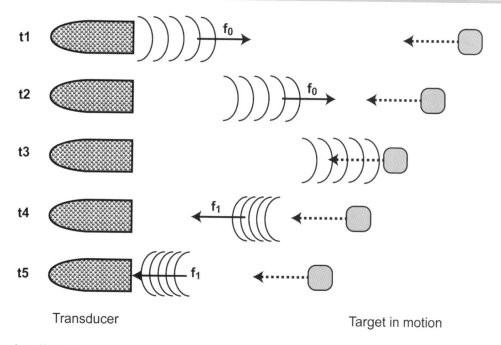

Figure 2.2 Doppler effect. The target in motion toward the transducer reflects the emitted sound wave of frequency (f_0) with an increased frequency (f_1). The delay of the time (t) sequence from (t_1–t_5) of the events determines the depth (distance) of the target.

All moving structures and elements can induce a Doppler shift when hit by an ultrasound wave. Blood cell velocities represent a high-frequency, low-amplitude signal compared with the velocity of surrounding tissue, which is characterized by dense high-amplitude (>80 dB) but slow-moving low-frequency (<200 Hz) echoes. Echoes from heart structures are considered as "noise" in conventional Doppler systems and are eliminated by a high-pass filter that removes frequencies below 200 Hz. Alternatively, a low-pass filter eliminates high frequencies (noise) to enhance tissue velocities (6). Tissue Doppler imaging is devoted to the analysis of the information contained in the low-frequency band of velocities as tissue velocities rarely exceed 10 cm/s (7).

INSTRUMENTATION

Blood flow can be evaluated by continuous wave (CW) or pulsed wave (PW) Doppler that is shown on the screen using spectral display and color Doppler using PW. The beam axis, sampling volume, and color image are overlaid on the regular 2D images (duplex scanning) to isolate the targeted blood flow anatomically. To spare computer working time being shared between the different modes, the 2D images are renewed at a much lower rate than the Doppler sampling rate.

Three technical concepts have to be explained before embarking further on the description of instruments: the pulse repetition frequency (PRF), the frame rate, and the Nyquist limit. The PRF is the number of times a PW Doppler instrument transmits and receives

pulses of ultrasound in one second. The rate of the emitting-receiving cycles is 1000 to 6000/sec. The PRF decreases with increasing depth of analysis as returning echoes take more time to reach the transducer from a remote target. It also decreases with increased transducer emitting frequency (f) as described in the Doppler formula, where Δf and f_0 vary reciprocally for the same target velocity. The frame rate is the frequency of image renewal on the screen; it varies from 6 to 120 images/sec. This depends on the number of scan lines used for investigating the field (the larger the field, the slower the frame rate) and on the additional data processing such as simultaneous color Doppler and 2D images (8). The Nyquist limit is linked to a phenomenon called "aliasing."

ALIASING

Any pulsating system observing an oscillating object will record anomalous images if its sampling rate is close to the vibration frequency of the observed structure. The Doppler effect, generated by moving blood cells ($\Delta f = 4000$–$10,000$ cycles/sec), has an oscillating frequency approaching the PRF of the observing instrument (PRF $= 1000$–6000 impulses/sec). This proximity induces an artifact due to the insufficient sampling, called aliasing. It is well illustrated by the apparent counter-rotation of a carriage wheel in a Western movie, when the number of rotations per second is superior to the number of images per second taken by the movie camera (9). When the wheel

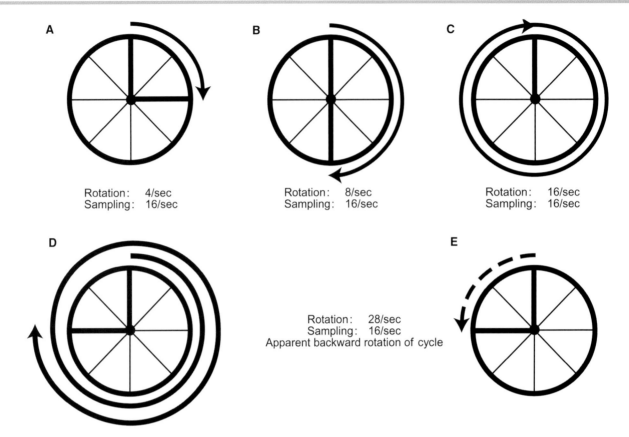

Figure 2.3 Aliasing in movie image. The rotating speed of the wheel is increasing from 4, 8 and 16 rotations per second, whereas the sampling rate of the camera is fixed at 16 images per second. (**A**) The wheel rotates at a rate equal to one-fourth of the camera sampling rate: the index spoke has turned one-fourth of a complete rotation with each camera image and moved from the 12 hour (h) to the 3 h position. (**B**) The wheel rotates at a rate equal to one-half of the camera sampling rate: the index spoke has turned one-half of a turn with each camera image and moved from the 12 h to the 6 h position. However, it is not possible to tell if that movement direction was clockwise or counterclockwise. (**C**) Both the wheel and the camera have the same rate and the wheel has done a complete turn with each camera image, but seems immobile because each camera frame always finds the wheel in the same position. (**D**) Aliasing occurs when the sampling rate of the camera (16/second) is lower than the rotating rate of the wheel (28/second). The wheel has performed one and three-quarters rotation during the time elapse between two camera images. (**E**) However the index spoke looks as though it has moved slowly backwards from the 12 h to the 9 h position.

revolution rate is much slower than the camera frame rate, the image is accurate. When the wheel rotates at a speed that is half the camera frame rate, the direction of rotation is no longer discernible because the wheel spokes are at 180° on each movie frame. If the rotation rate equals the sampling rate, the film will catch the spokes of the wheel at the same place in each cycle and the wheel will appear motionless. Finally, when the rotation rate exceeds the sampling rate, the wheel will appear to be reversing and will rotate at an inaccurate and slow speed (Fig. 2.3).

This sampling phenomenon introduces a limit above which the precision of movement reporting is lost. The maximum frequency shift measurement is equivalent to one-half of the sampling frequency. This limit is called the "Nyquist limit":

$$\text{Nyquist limit} = \frac{\text{PRF}}{2} \qquad (2.7)$$

To represent a corrected frequency signal (fs), it must be sampled at least twice for each cycle of the signal; the PRF of the computer must be superior to two oscillating periods of the observed wave, in this instance, the Doppler shift Δf (10):

$$\text{PRF} > 2\text{fs} \quad \text{or} \quad \text{PRF} > 2\Delta f \qquad (2.8)$$

If the Doppler frequency shift is superior to one-half of the PRF, aliasing occurs (Fig. 2.4). The instrument reports a spurious value equal to the true Doppler shift minus the PRF: on the spectral frame, the velocity curve appears as artificially reversed on the opposite side of the baseline (Fig. 2.5). In color flow, aliasing appears as an area of reversed color (Fig. 2.6). By increasing the PRF, the Nyquist limit can be raised and the ability to obtain high-velocity recordings is also increased. This is done by the technique called high-PRF PW Doppler that is however less precise than the CW instrument. The use of

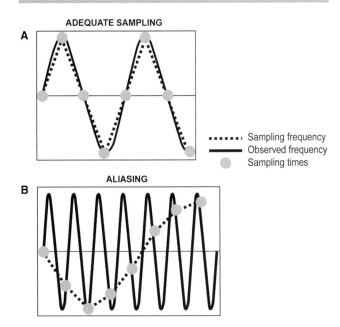

ADEQUATE SAMPLING

A

ALIASING

B

- ······ Sampling frequency
- —— Observed frequency
- ● Sampling times

Figure 2.4 Aliasing in computer sampling. (A) When the computer sampling rate (gray dots) is more then twice the observed wave frequency, it is sufficient enough to correctly reproduce the interrogated wave. **(B)** If the wave frequency is increased and the same sampling rate is unchanged from **(A)**, the calculated frequency by the computer (dotted lines) is completely different from the actual frequency of the wave (solid line). The latter frequency is markedly superior to the sampling rate; the recorded frequency is out of phase and much lower, creating aliasing.

CW Doppler is mandatory for analyzing high velocities accurately. The maximum velocity (V_{max}) that can be measured by PW without aliasing is given by the formula (4):

$$V_{max} = \frac{PRF \times c}{4f_0 \cos \theta} \qquad (2.9)$$

Aliasing can be limited by reducing the emitting frequency of the transducer, f_0, or increasing the PRF. For a specific Nyquist limit, the presence of aliasing flow does not always signify flow turbulence. It can also be seen in laminar flow with increased velocity beyond the Nyquist limit with flow acceleration (Fig. 2.6).

CONTINUOUS AND PULSED WAVE DOPPLER

The CW Doppler equipment transmits and receives the ultrasound signal continuously and simultaneously through two separate crystals: one for emitting and one for receiving (Fig. 2.7A). It records all velocities in the area of overlap between the emitted and the returning beams at any depth and at any frequency shift. No limitation for analysis of high velocities is present because its emission is continuous and has, therefore, an infinite PRF. However, it lacks the spatial resolution necessary to know the exact depth at

which the measurement is obtained. As emission and reception are continuous, the computer cannot define when or where the emitted waves are reflected by the moving target.

In PW Doppler, the transducer emits a short burst of ultrasound waves (three to six waves) and waits for the return of the reflected waves (Fig. 2.7B). As the transducer alternates between transmitting and receiving bursts of ultrasound energy, it is able to calculate the time delay for the echoes to return and interrogate the blood flow in a specific region (Fig. 2.5). It waits until the echo from a specific location reaches the transducer whereupon it opens an electronic gate to read the signal. The gate then shuts for a fixed duration after reading the signal (11). The duration of gate opening determines the length of the exploring window or sample volume (Fig. 2.7B). This volume appears as a box that can be moved along the Doppler cursor on the screen (depth of the sample) and its size can be modified (duration of echo listening). The sensitivity rises when the dimension of the window increases because a larger sample volume contains more blood cells and produces stronger signals, but the axial resolution is lessened because the location is less precise. The delay, Δt, is the time necessary for the ultrasound of known speed, c, to make a round-trip between the transmitter and its target. The delay determines the depth (D) of the target. Therefore, D is defined as

$$D = c \times \left(\frac{\Delta t}{2}\right) \qquad (2.10)$$

This precision in the location of the source of frequency shift has a drawback; it limits the velocity range that the instrument can read because of the following factors. First, the sampling rate will alter precision. This is because the frequency overlap between PRF and Doppler shift can give rise to aliasing, as explained earlier. Second, the emitting frequency of the probe will be important. For the same Doppler shift, the transducer must sample twice as fast for a 5-MHz as for a 2.5-MHz probe. Indeed at the same PRF, the maximum recordable velocity with a 5-MHz probe is half the velocity determined by a 2.5-MHz probe (7). Finally, the depth of the sampling gate will influence precision. The deeper the interrogated target, the longer will be the elapsed time between two pulse emissions. The maximum recordable velocity is lessened when the PRF decreases (2.3 m/sec at 8 cm with a 2.5-MHz probe and 0.65 cm/s at 16 cm with a 5.0-MHz probe) (5).

To enable the measurement of higher velocities, a modification called "high PRF" has been implemented on most echo machines. Using this system, the PRF is multiplied by 2, 3, or 4: a new burst of ultrasound waves is sent before the electronic receiving gate is opened to returning echoes. It, therefore, raises the number of sampling sites and introduces a "range ambiguity" as the computer is unable to identify the origin of the echo (1). Fortunately, the gates are pictured on the 2D images and the examiner can assume that the sampling volume lies where the

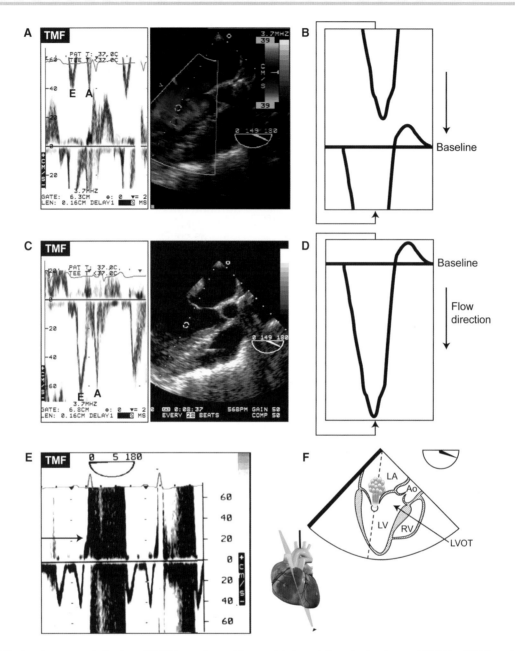

Figure 2.5 Aliasing in spectral display. (**A**) Mid-esophageal long-axis view of the mitral valve and TMF by PW Doppler sampling is shown. The scale on the left is lower than the maximum mitral velocity, resulting in aliasing. This is also shown on the schematic drawing of spectral display (**B**). (**C**) The aliasing is eliminated by elevating the baseline thus increasing the scale. The tip of the curve is readjusted into the forward direction and maximal velocity can be calculated, as shown on the schematic drawing (**D**). (**E**) PW Doppler image of MR with the site of TMFPW Doppler sampling (**F**) demonstrated. The velocity of the forward flow is correctly estimated (0.45 cm/s), but the high-velocity jet of MR (5–6 m/s) is buried in the aliasing signal (arrow).The maximal MR velocity is unrecordable. *Abbreviations*: A, peak late diastolic TMF velocity; Ao, aorta; E, peak early diastolic TMF velocity; LA, left atrium; LV, left ventricle; LVOT, left ventricular outflow tract; MR, mitral regurgitation; PW, pulsed wave; RV, right ventricle; TMF, transmitral flow.

recorded flow velocity is expected. The actual PRF is determined by the most proximal sample volume but the most distal PRF is used for sampling flow in the zone of interest (3).

An additional problem occurs with the PW technology. The bursts of ultrasound waves are produced at a certain rhythmic time period, introducing an additional frequency in the emission. The frequency of bursts of an ultrasound wave, f_0, is also Doppler-shifted by the moving blood. The resultant velocity profile is not as precise as CW Doppler and is affected by a significant spectral broadening (11).

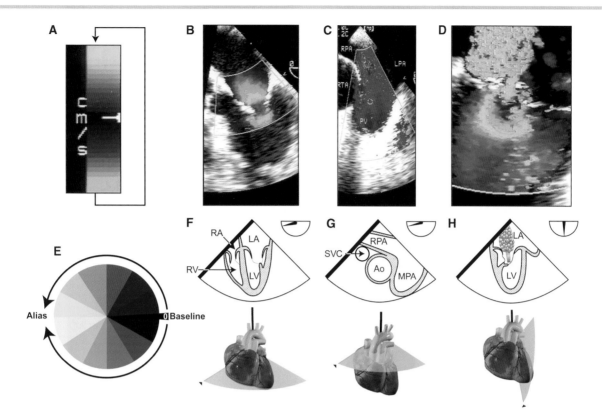

Figure 2.6 Color reversal with aliasing. In this color map (**A**), when the velocity is above the Nyquist limit, the color suddenly jumps from clear blue to bright yellow as shown by the color wheel below. (**B**) Zoom of ME four-chamber view with color Doppler showing accelerating flow through a restricted mitral valve orifice. (**C**) ME ascending Ao short-axis view with color Doppler shows a central acceleration zone (blue) in the MPA. (**D**) Proximal flow acceleration convergence zone on the ventricular side of a mitral regurgitation jet is shown in a zoom of a ME two-chamber color Doppler view. *Abbreviations*: Ao, aorta; LA, left atrium; LV, left ventricle; ME, mid-esophageal; MPA, main pulmonary artery; RA, right atrium; RPA, right pulmonary artery; RV, right ventricle; SVC, superior vena cava.

SPECTRAL DISPLAY

To display the Doppler information, the apparatus must reproduce the spectrum of the frequency shifts. This spectrum must be updated regularly during a cardiac cycle. The Doppler signal is a complex wave, containing information about the motion of all blood cells and tissue moving at different velocities. The received signal is a wave, out of phase with the original emitted signal. In the spectral mode, this shift is visually displayed as a power spectrum of frequencies against time. The ultrasound echoes go through a logarithmic amplifier that increases the amplitude of the weaker signals more than the stronger signals so that the amplitudes are comparable. The signal is processed in segments of 1–5 ms duration by the computer, and a mathematical calculation, called fast Fourier transform, is performed on each segment to resolve the Doppler signal into its individual component frequencies.

This spectrum represents the relative magnitude (or amplitude) of each frequency component. The calculation of velocity (Doppler equation) is done automatically by the computer from these frequency shifts. Each segment of time is assigned a stack of vertical bins whose intensity is proportional to the strength of the signal or to the number of blood cells moving within the range of velocities represented by each bin (9) (Fig. 2.8). A trade-off exists between temporal and frequency resolution: the time period represented by each time slice is correlated with the ability to distinguish between two Doppler shifts.

The spectral display of the Doppler trace has time on the horizontal axis and flow velocity on the vertical axis. The gray scale is proportional to the number of blood cells moving at a certain speed: the darker the trace, the greater the number of blood cells. Usually, 16 to 32 shades of gray are used because human eye resolution can discern no more than 32 shades of gray. The width of the trace is proportional to the spread of frequency. With little difference in velocity, the band is narrow and the flow laminar, whereas multiple velocities produce a wide spectral spread (termed spectral broadening) and a filled-in trace on the screen with a turbulent flow (Figs. 2.9 and 2.10). By convention, the flow toward the transducer is depicted above the baseline and the flow away from it is below. A filtering technique (high-pass filter) removes the echoes of high intensity but low frequency (<200 Hz) due to the movements of the cardiac walls and valves.

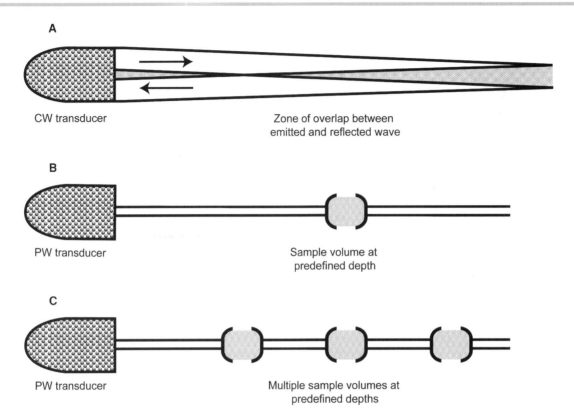

Figure 2.7 Transducer Doppler modes. (A) CW mode transducer with emitting and receiving beams; the area explored is the opacified area of overlap between the two beams. **(B)** PW mode transducer: the Doppler Effect is analyzed in a small zone of predefined depth and volume called the sample volume (opacified area). Depth is defined by the position of the cursor along the axial beam; the sample volume is chosen by widening or narrowing the window. **(C)** High pulsed repetition frequency sampling uses multiple sampling points in the PW mode. *Abbreviations*: CW, continuous wave; PW, pulsed wave.

On the spectral frame, the CW Doppler appears as a filled gray curve, showing all the velocities encountered on the ultrasound beam, whereas the PW velocity curve has a thin envelope representing the blood flow at a determined sampling site (Fig. 2.11). The maximal velocity measurement must be done at the outer edge of the trace. To display the entire flow curve, it is frequently necessary to displace the baseline in the direction opposite to the flow. In case of aliasing, the velocity curve appears artificially reversed on the opposite side of the baseline (Fig. 2.5). For blood flow toward the transducer, it will be plotted below the zero line as a negative shift. For high velocities, the wrapping around may occur many times so that the peak of the spectrum is buried in the superimposed traces and the maximal velocity is impossible to determine (Fig. 2.5E). By repositioning the baseline in the direction opposite to flow, some degree of aliasing may be unwrapped because higher velocities can be recorded in the direction of the flow.

COLOR DOPPLER

The PW Doppler analyzes the complete spectrum of blood flow velocities in a single sampling site. The technique can be expanded to the analysis of several samples along a line of information. This multigate Doppler technique allows flow mapping by measuring returning echoes sequentially at different successive times after transmission of a single burst of ultrasound. The scan line is interrogated many times, ranging from 3 to 16. The amount of time each line is sampled is called the packet size and is selected by the examiner or provided by the instrument. After having interrogated one scan line, the beam direction is changed to the next scan line and so on for the entire field. Every time a scan line is interrogated, an algorithm stores the Doppler data at each sample site along the line. Depending on the ultrasound system, the spacing between scan lines can be modified. This spacing is called line density. Spatial resolution increases with greater density of scan line, but the frame rate decreases simultaneously because processing times are longer. The number of sample sites per scan line varies among manufacturers, while the number of scan lines is determined by the color sector width and the line density.

Despite the power of recent microprocessors, this large amount of information significantly lowers the frame rate of the images displayed on the screen. Therefore, instead of determining the complete spectrum of frequencies, as in PW spectral display, an autocorrelator analyzes the resultant phase shift

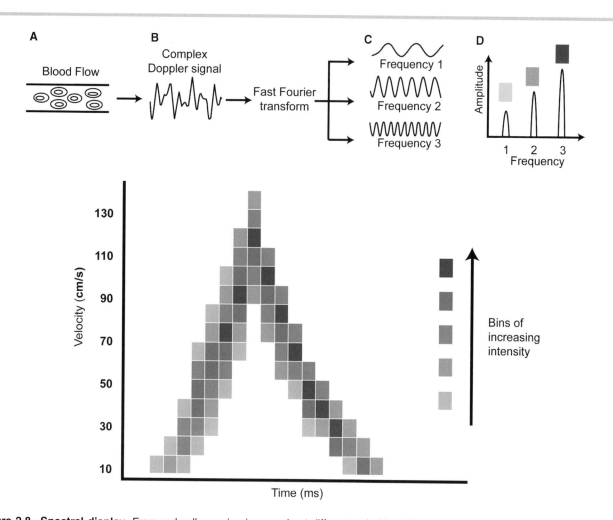

Figure 2.8 Spectral display. From red cells moving in vessels at different velocities (**A**), a complex Doppler signal is obtained (**B**). Using Fast-Fourier transformation, the sinusoidal components can be extracted (**C**) and the amplitude to frequency component can be displayed (**D**). From this information a spectral curve with vertical stacks of bins of varying intensity can be constructed. The shade of gray is proportional to the quantity of blood cells (amplitude) moving at a corresponding velocity (derived from the frequency shifts). The Doppler shift frequencies are calculated over 5-ms intervals. The width of the curve corresponds to the spectrum of different velocities of blood cells. *Source:* Adapted from Ref. 12.

between the emitted and received waveforms to generate a modal frequency representing the velocity of the majority of blood cells (13). If the packet size comprises eight pulses, for example, the first pulse travels the scan line and returns to the transducer. It is followed by the second pulse whose recorded frequency is slightly out of phase with the first pulse because the target is moving. The calculation is repeated for the eight pulses on the scan line (Fig. 2.12). If pulse two is ahead of pulse one, the target is moving toward the transducer and if pulse two lags behind pulse one, the target is flowing away. Echoes from subsequent pulses are correlated with echoes from previous pulses to determine the mean Doppler shift and its "variance," which is the difference between the highest and the lowest returning frequencies or the frequency spread of the spectrum. Averaging, by repetitive sampling, is performed to improve the statistics. The modal frequency can be

used in the Doppler equation to determine mean velocities and variance. For laminar flows, the value of the mean velocity is approximately the same as the peak velocity (14).

By converting the calculated values of mean velocity into colors, the blood flow velocity image can be overlaid onto a 2D gray-scale display. Blood flow moving toward the transducer is usually displayed in red and blood flow moving away from the transducer in blue (Fig. 2.13). Color maps identify the pattern of colors in use and are shown by a color bar appearing on the screen. It displays the color properties such as hue (amount of primary colors red, blue, or green), saturation (amount of white contained), and intensity (brightness). Lower velocities are displayed in dark colors located closer to the color bar's baseline. Higher velocities are displayed in brighter tones near the end of the scale. In "enhanced" color maps, the red gradually changes to yellow and the blue changes to

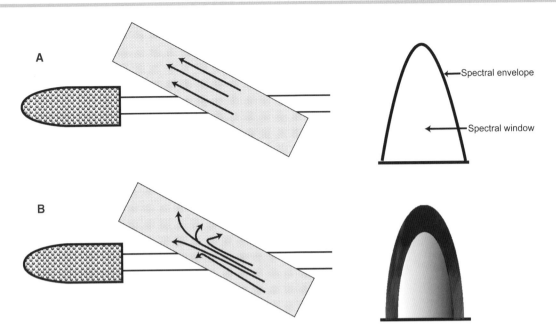

Figure 2.9 Spectral broadening. (A) Spectral Doppler in laminar flow shows a narrow envelope of measured velocities with a large spectral window (unfilled area of the curve) and no spectral broadening. **(B)** Patients with turbulent flow, or when using CW Doppler, have a less distinct spectral envelope and small spectral window (filled in area of curve). Any spectral Doppler display using either PW or CW Doppler with a filled in curve from a wide range of velocities has spectral broadening. *Abbreviations*: CW, continuous wave; PW, pulsed wave.

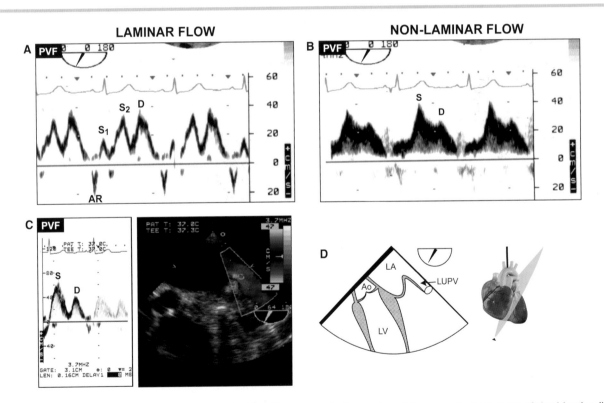

Figure 2.10 Laminar and non-laminar flow. (A) Laminar flow occurs in the center of the vessel where most of the blood cells are traveling at the same velocity. The PW Doppler spectral display shows a well-defined narrow envelope. **(B)** Non-laminar flow occurs near the wall of the vessel, resulting in many different velocities. The PW Doppler sampled here records a larger spectrum of velocities and the envelope is replaced by a large band of different velocities. **(C,D)** Mid-esophageal left atrial appendage view with interrogation of the LUPV is shown. As the sampling volume moves from the center to the side of the LUPV, flow profile changes from a narrow laminar tracing to a broader non-laminar pattern. *Abbreviations*: Ao, aorta; AR, peak atrial reversal PVF velocity; D, peak diastolic PVF velocity; LA, left atrium; LUPV, left upper pulmonary vein; LV, left ventricle; PVF, pulmonary venous flow; PW, pulsed wave; S, peak systolic PVF velocity.

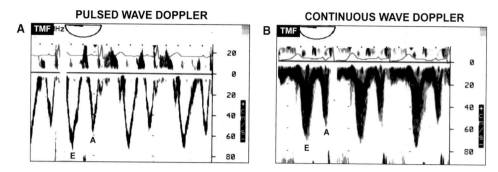

Figure 2.11 PW and CW Doppler flow. (A) PW Doppler examination of TMF is interrogated at a specific location by placing the sample volume between the tips of the MV leaflets. Because most blood cells are travelling at the same velocity the flow is laminar at this sampling site, and the envelope is narrow and well defined. **(B)** CW Doppler examination of TMF interrogates all velocities along the ultrasound beam, the envelope has significant spectral broadening, that is the curve is filled with different velocities. The maximal velocity is assumed to be at the narrowest area, that is, between the tips of the MV leaflets. *Abbreviations*: A, peak late diastolic TMF velocity; CW, continuous wave; E, peak early diastolic TMF velocity; MV, mitral valve; PW, pulsed wave; TMF, transmitral flow.

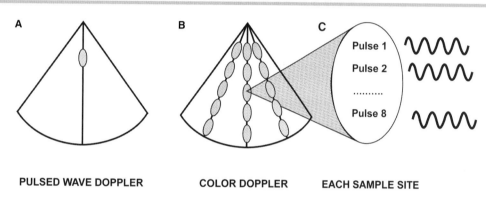

Figure 2.12 Color Doppler principle. (A) In pulsed wave Doppler one site is sampled on one scan line. **(B)** In Color Doppler imaging: several hundred sites are sampled on many scan lines. **(C)** Each area of the scanning lines is interrogated successively eight times according to the packet size. The packet size (dwell time or ensemble length) corresponds to the number of sound bursts transmitted per color sector line. Each successive wave is slightly out of phase compared with the preceding one. An algorithm processes the phase shift between the waves of the eight pulses and estimates the mean velocity by derivation at each sample site; it then assigns a color to each area. The larger the packet size, the more precise the results, but the lower the frame rate.

an intense luminous shade as the velocity increases (Fig. 2.13). This display is useful in operating rooms (ORs) because it increases the contrast with the surrounding light. The numbers seen at both ends of the color scale bar represent the limit of the recordable mean velocity, or Nyquist limit, rather than peak velocity estimates as in PW or CW Doppler (Fig. 2.13). Above this limit, aliasing appears as color reversal: the blood flowing toward the transducer, for example, changes abruptly from yellow to bright blue. By moving the color bar baseline toward the flow, the recordable velocity is increased in the flow direction but diminished in the opposite direction (Fig. 2.14).

Laminar flow appears as a homogeneous smooth pattern of red or blue; turbulent flow is displayed in a disorganized multicolored pattern called "mosaic," representing the many different velocities and directions of each sample site. The severity of turbulence is

illustrated with an orthogonal color, usually green, and can be laid across the standard red and blue velocity bars. An algorithm calculates the variance between individual velocities at each sampling site and adds the green if the irregularity is above a predetermined level. This particular display (Fig. 2.15) offers the advantage of "mapping" the turbulent areas inside the color flow. Under normal circumstances, intracardiac flows are laminar. Turbulent flow appears if there are pathological flows or abnormally high velocities.

The extent of calculations imposed by data processing is dependent on the dimensions of the field of investigation. With a wide sector, more lines are sampled. With a deeper sector, greater time is required for the echoes to return to the transducer. Decreasing the sector width and depth decreases the processing time and increases the frame rate that consequently varies from 6 to 90 images/sec. This is

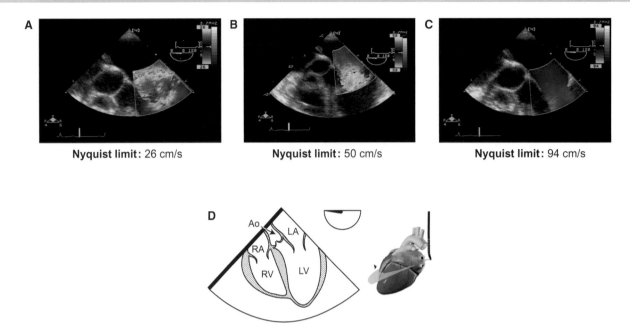

Nyquist limit: 26 cm/s   Nyquist limit: 50 cm/s   Nyquist limit: 94 cm/s

Figure 2.13 Color mapping. (A–D) Mid-esophageal five-chamber views with color Doppler interrogation of the mitral valve inflow are shown. The upper limit of the color coded scale is progressively increased from 26 cm/s (**A**), 50 cm/s (**B**), and 94 cm/s (**C**). Aliasing is reduced by increasing the Nyquist limit. *Abbreviations*: Ao, aorta; LA, left atrium; LV, left ventricle; RA, right atrium; RV, right ventricle.

critical for patients with rapid heart rates because important information can be missed if the frame rate is too low. Moreover, a minimum frame rate of 15 images/sec is required for the human eye to achieve the blending of images into smooth motion. Therefore, keeping the color sector as narrow as required often improves the temporal resolution of color imaging.

Another method of raising the frame rate is to decrease the packet size or to increase the PRF by adjusting the color scale to a higher mean velocity. Nevertheless, it decreases the system's sensitivity to low-velocity blood flow (Fig. 2.13). Using a transducer of lower frequency (<5 MHz) or reducing the emitting frequency of the probe will increase the PRF and the maximum velocity measurement capability at any depth. This decreases tissue attenuation because lower frequencies lose less energy than high-frequency waves while traveling through the organ. The depth at which transmission can interrogate the number of scan lines, the probe frequency, the PRF, and the frame rate are interdependent. It is up to the observer to find the optimal combination between these settings to obtain the most accurate flow information.

Sometimes, the interrogating beam can record frequency shift caused by wall motion, and colors can be assigned to moving structures. This phenomenon is called ghosting. It is minimized by a filtering process named clutter filter that attenuates the signals of low velocity and high intensity corresponding to tissues. However, it may eliminate the low-velocity blood flow images. This drop-out in low-velocity flow can also occur when using a high PRF because it increases the lowest readable flow velocity. These phenomena lead to a smaller-sized color flow jet and make it appear smaller than it actually is.

Color gain has to be properly adjusted. Setting the gain control too low prevents detection of low-amplitude signals, and blood flow patterns appear smaller than they are. A gain set too high causes a lot of color noise, which appear as random multicolored specks sprayed over cardiac chambers and tissues. Adequate gain is obtained by adjusting the control until noise becomes obvious and then reducing it to a point where the noise begins to disappear (Fig. 2.16). The gray-scale gain that displays the 2D tissue image over which the flow is superimposed must be kept low. If not, noise is generated restricting the dimensions of the color flow. Like all Doppler data, color flow accuracy is dependent on the angle between the flow direction and the beam axis. If this angle is too wide (>20°), the displayed color velocity will be mistakenly lower than the true flow velocity. If the beam and the flow are perpendicular, there is no Doppler effect and no color picture (Fig. 2.17). The adjustment of the transducer's focal zone is important in multigated Doppler systems because distal sensitivity and spatial resolution decrease as the focal zone is set in the near field. The distal area of flow can appear larger than it actually is because Doppler data are collected in the divergent part of the ultrasound beam. When using color flow, the focal zone must be kept at, or below, the interrogated area (1).

By displaying flow patterns, color provides an indicator of adequate positioning of the beam to perform quantitative spectral Doppler measurements.

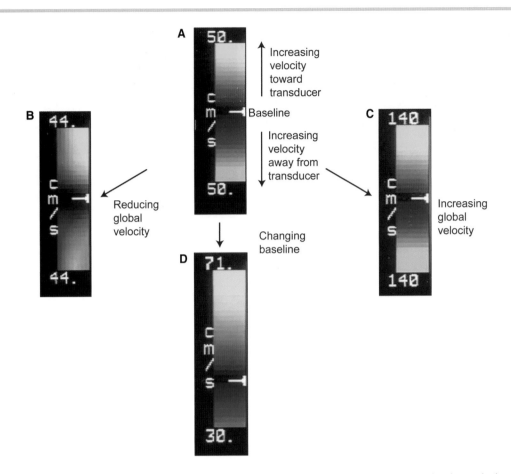

Figure 2.14 Color map scale. (A) An enhanced color map shows flow towards the transducer as red at low velocity, progressing to yellow at higher velocities, and blue when the flow is away from the transducer. The color becomes lighter with increasing velocity. The upper limit of mean velocity readable without aliasing is 50 cm/s under the present conditions (Nyquist limit). **(B)** Using a variance map, green is superimposed on the previous colors to illustrate the presence of turbulence, characterized by a large amount of variance in sampled velocities. **(C)** An increased Nyquist limit is obtained, by increasing the pulsed repetition frequency and/or decreasing the depth of the color field, the upper limit of velocity readable without aliasing can be significantly increased (140 cm/s). **(D)** To prevent or induce aliasing, the baseline of the color bar can be shifted in the direction of flow opposite to it. The maximal velocity recordable without aliasing is increased in one direction (71 cm/s) but decreased in the opposite (30 cm/s).

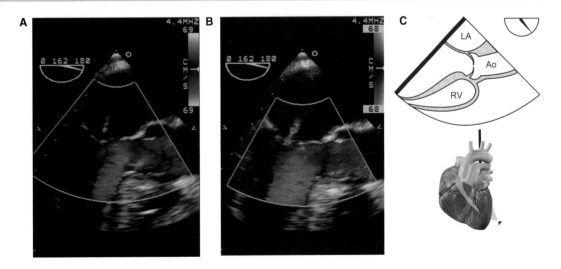

Figure 2.15 Variance. (A–C) Color Doppler mid-esophageal aortic valve long-axis views shown during systole with **(A)** velocity and **(B)** variance color maps. *Abbreviations*: Ao, aorta; LA, left atrium; LV, left ventricle; RV, right ventricle.

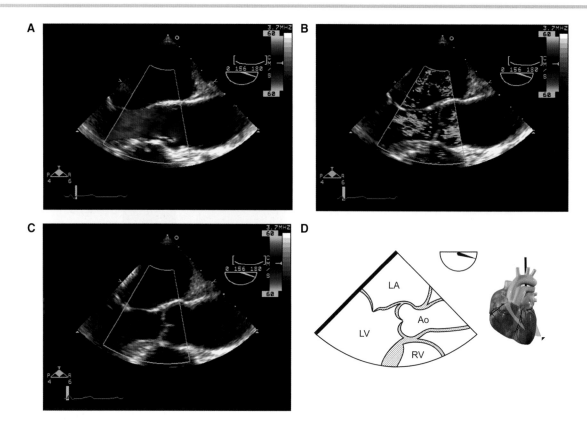

Figure 2.16   Color Doppler gain settings. (A–D) Mid-esophageal aortic valve long-axis views with color Doppler at optimal **(A)** and suboptimal; too high **(B)** or too low **(C)** gain settings. *Abbreviations*: Ao, aorta; LA, left atrium; LV, left ventricle; RV, right ventricle.

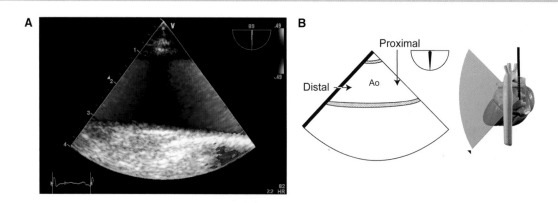

Figure 2.17   Color flow Doppler in the Ao. (A,B) Descending thoracic Ao long-axis view with color Doppler at 90° is shown. The flow is colored in red on the right-hand side of the screen where it comes toward the transducer but is blue on the left part of the screen, where it moves away from the transducer. Note also that when flow is at 90° to the direction of the ultrasound beam in the center of the screen, that there is no Doppler axial frequency shift and this no color flow displayed. *Abbreviation*: Ao, aorta.

As the images obtained are 2D, it is important to visualize the flows in different planes to reconstitute the 3D structure of a given flow jet. A flow in a vessel crossing the entire screen, although uniform, will appear under different colors as the angle of the flow with the different scan lines changes along its visible course. For instance, on a 90° image of the descending thoracic aorta, the flow will be colored in red on the right-hand side of the screen where it comes toward the transducer but in blue on the left part of the screen, where it moves away from the transducer (Fig. 2.17).

It is important to remember that color flow display is a velocity mapping and not an actual blood

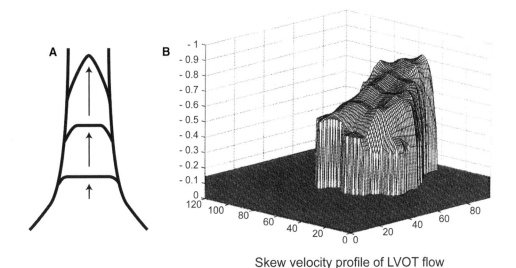

Skew velocity profile of LVOT flow

Figure 2.18   Flow profiles. (A) In a vessel, the flow front presents an aspect of increasing central acceleration with a parabolic profile. The flow front is convergent. **(B)** Three-dimensional (3D) aspect of the systolic flow in the LVOT, the flow front is complex and skewed with increasing speed near the septum. *Abbreviation*: LVOT, left ventricular outflow tract. *Source:* With permission from Ref. 16.

volume measurement. Area and brightness on the screen are determined only by the speed of blood, which is the result of an instantaneous pressure gradient between upstream and downstream cavities (15). A small mitral regurgitation (MR) orifice, in the context of a normal left ventricular (LV) function, will create a high-velocity jet (6 m/sec) into the left atrium (LA) appearing larger than the real regurgitant blood volume. This is due to the sweeping of left atrial blood by the regurgitant jet. Color image in severe MR with poor LV function will underestimate the amount of regurgitant blood because of smaller pressure gradient. Moreover, the velocity measured in a precise vessel does not take into account the real flow profile, which is not flat, except closer to the root of great vessels or when convergent. Most of the time, flow profile is parabolic or displays zones of acceleration near the curvatures (Fig. 2.18) (16). This limits the accuracy of velocity measurements, particularly when integrated into calculations such as cardiac output. Various positioning of the Doppler sample volume in the main pulmonary artery cross-sectional area, for example, introduces errors of ± 35% in cardiac output measurements (17). In turbulent flows, random swirls and eddies appear where there are wide fluctuations in direction and velocity of flow components. They are spread among a slow varying, forward motion of blood. Consequently, the measured velocity corresponds to the mean flow velocity.

DOPPLER TISSUE IMAGING

Doppler signals are generated not only by flowing red blood cells but also by cardiac walls and valvular motion. Tissues induce stronger backscatter echoes at lower frequency but these are usually filtered out to improve the blood flow image. These echoes appear only when color gain is too high or when filters are set too low. However, this drawback can be used to identify parietal movements and wall kinetics if the low-amplitude, high-frequency signals of blood cells are properly filtered (high-pass filtering system and low-clutter filter setting). Tissue Doppler mode records velocities as low as 0.1 cm/s. Depth resolution is inferior to that of conventional Doppler because velocity mapping requires longer pulses to be transmitted and longer gate times (7).

Tissue Doppler velocities can be measured along the myocardial wall (Fig. 2.19). Integration of the velocities yields tissue tracking (Fig. 2.20). Frame rate can be increased by sampling a single line in color M-mode. Using color M-mode, a myocardial velocity mapping can be obtained (Fig. 2.21A). It may be used to assess regional myocardial velocity gradients (18). Subepicardial layers usually have lower velocities than subendocardial layers (Fig. 2.21B). The instantaneous velocity gradients within the walls present different patterns for normal, ischemic, or dysfunctional myocardial muscle (see Chapter 9). Tissue Doppler imaging can also be used to analyze motion of specific structures such as the mitral or the tricuspid annulus displacement in the evaluation of diastolic function (Fig. 2.22). From tissue Doppler imaging, strain imaging can be obtained and displayed over 2D images as waveforms and as a color M-mode (Fig. 2.23). Normal tissue Doppler velocities are shown in Table 2.1.

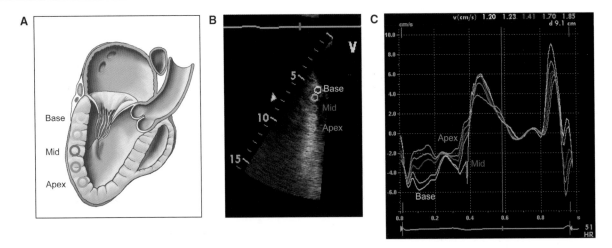

Figure 2.19   Tissue Doppler velocities. (A–C) TDI of the mid-esophageal long-axis view of the LV inferolateral wall in a 56-year-old man is shown. **(B)** Sample volumes are positioned in the basal (yellow), mid (red) and apical (orange) myocardial segments in this narrowed sector of the inferolateral LV wall. **(C)** A spectral display over one cardiac cycle shows the individual segment myocardial velocities (cm/s) after off-line postprocessing of TDI. Normally the basal segments have higher velocities than the apical segments. *Abbreviations*: LV, left ventricle; TDI, tissue Doppler imaging. *Source:* Part A courtesy of Gian-Marco Busato.

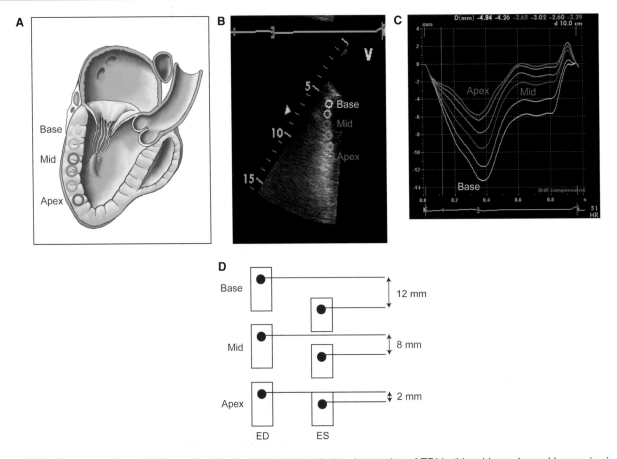

Figure 2.20   Tissue tracking. (A) Tissue tracking is obtained through time integration of TDI in this mid-esophageal long-axis view of the LV inferolateral wall in a 56-year-old man. **(B)** Sample volumes are positioned in the basal (yellow), mid (red) and apical (purple) myocardial segments in this narrowed sector of the inferolateral LV wall. **(C)** A spectral display over one cardiac cycle shows the individual segment myocardial displacement (mm) after off-line postprocessing of TDI. **(D)** Stylized myocardial segments (boxes) with markers (black circles) shown at end diastole (left) and at end systole (right). The boxes progress from base (top) to apex (bottom). Normally the basal segments have higher displacement than the apical segments. *Abbreviations*: ED, end-diastolic; ES, end-systolic; LV, left ventricle; TDI, tissue Doppler imaging. *Source:* Part A courtesy of Gian-Marco Busato.

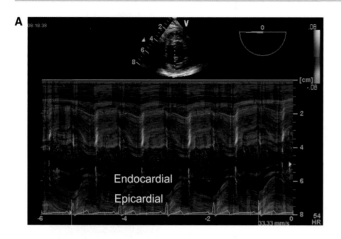
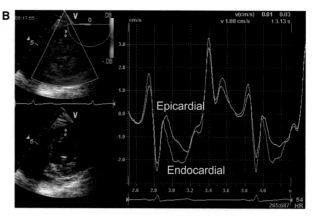

Figure 2.21 Tissue Doppler imaging. (A) Color M-mode of myocardial tissue velocities of the inferior and anterior walls of the LV. Velocities are encoded in color, with shades of red for positive velocities (toward the transducer) and shades of blue for negative velocities (away from the transducer). Because of radial displacement, note that the inferior wall has opposite color to the anterior wall. **(B)** Pulsed wave tissue Doppler tracing of the inferior wall, with negative velocities away from the transducer in systole. One sample volume is positioned in the epicardium (yellow) and one in the endocardium (green). The difference between the two velocity curves represents the myocardial velocity gradient, with the negative velocity lower in the epicardium compared to the endocardium. These instantaneous velocity gradients within the walls may demonstrate different patterns for normal, ischemic, or dysfunctional myocardial muscle. *Abbreviations*: LV, left ventricle; TDI, tissue Doppler imaging.

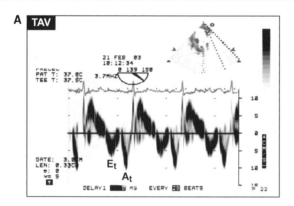
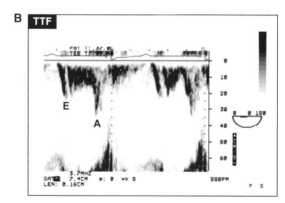
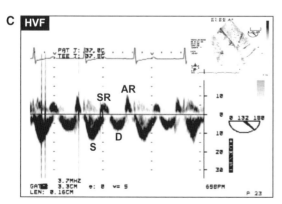
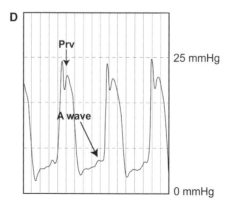

Figure 2.22 TDI and RV diastolic function. (A) Spectral TDI of TAV shows the atrial (At) is predominant over the early (Et) filling component. **(B)** Pulsed wave (PW) Doppler of TTF shows the atrial (A) is predominant over the early (E) filling component. **(C)** HVF demonstrates a systolic *S*, a systolic reversal *SR*, a diastolic *D*, and an atrial reversal *AR* waves. **(D)** Right ventricular pressure (Prv) waveform displays an A wave corresponding to atrial contraction. This combination is consistent with a mild filling abnormality of the RV. *Abbreviations*: HVF, hepatic venous flow; RV, right ventricle; TAV, tricuspid annular velocity; TDI, tissue Doppler imaging; TTF, transtricuspid flow.

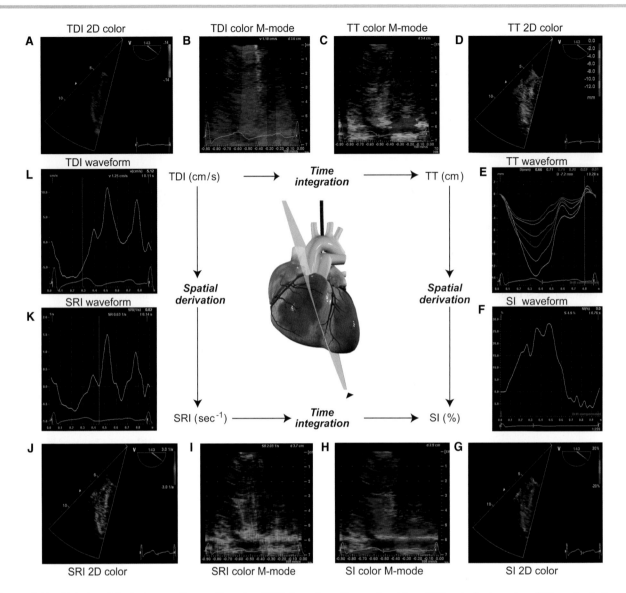

Figure 2.23 Relationship between tissue Doppler (TDI) imaging, tissue tracking (TT), strain imaging (SI) and strain rate imaging (SRI). (**A**) A color TDI sector is applied to the inferolateral wall. (**B**) To the right, the image represents the anatomical M mode traced from base to apex along the center of the myocardium. Below (**L**), a velocity trace is obtained by sampling in the color sector. (**C–E**) Velocity time integration yields displacement. The color has now been coded for displacement. The display to the left is the anatomical m mode of this color image from base to apex and below is the graphical display of displacement over time for various points along the myocardium from base to apex. (**F–H**) Integration of velocity differences over time yields strain. In the bottom right hand corner, the color has now been coded for strain. Sampling in the color sector yields the image above while the image on the left in the corresponding anatomical m mode display. (**I–K**) Spatial velocity differences yield strain rate. In the lower left hand corner, the color sector is now coded for strain rate. Sampling in the color sector yields a graphical display of strain rate over time. To the right is an anatomical m mode representation of strain rate. For all images, a mid-esophageal long-axis view at 143° with interrogation of the inferolateral wall was used.

STRAIN IMAGING

Strain imaging is among the new modalities that can be obtained using tissue Doppler and more recently 2D speckle tracking.

Strain

When stress is applied to a deformable physical body, it will change shape. Myocardial deformation can be described in much the same way. For example, if a muscle strip is excised and hung from a fixed point, its passive deformation can be observed by hanging various weights at the other end. Its active deformation, on the other hand, can be measured by stimulating the muscle (while loaded) and measuring the resulting change in length. We can loosely transpose these examples to physiological assessments of myocardial diastolic and systolic deformation, respectively.

Table 2.1 Velocity of Individual Segments

	Septum	Lateral	Inferior	Anterior
	Doppler tissue echocardiography			
	S wave			
Basal	5.97 ± 1.14	6.26 ± 2.44	6.52 ± 1.31	6.44 ± 2.32
Mid	6.29 ± 1.89	4.48 ± 0.92	5.21 ± 2.79	5.1 ± 1.16
Apical	4.42 ± 2.3	4.81 ± 1.97	2.97 ± 1.14	3.8 ± 2.66
	E wave			
Basal	7.91 ± 2.16	8.54 ± 2.77	9.01 ± 2.44	8.09 ± 2.48
Mid	8.39 ± 2.5	6.85 ± 1.86	6.82 ± 3.16	7.22 ± 2.04
Apical	6.03 ± 2.95	6.74 ± 2.58	4.76 ± 1.94	4.52 ± 2.95
	A wave			
Basal	5.99 ± 1.73	3.77 ± 1.95	5.84 ± 2.06	3.86 ± 1.75
Mid	4.87 ± 2.14	4.9 ± 1.72	2.62 ± 1.84	4.78 ± 1.7
Apical	2.69 ± 1.93	3.77 ± 2.1	3.08 ± 1.54	1.69 ± 1.45

Systolic (S), early (E), and late (A) velocities shown in cm/s.
Source: From Ref. 19 with permission.

Strain (ε) describes the extent of deformation. Lagrangian strain (ε_L) is defined as the difference in length from initial length (L_0) to stressed length (L) normalized over the original length (L_0). It is described by the following relationship:

$$\varepsilon_L = \frac{L - L_0}{L_0} \qquad (2.11)$$

For example, a 5-cm (L_0) muscle strip fixed at one end is loaded with a small weight. When stimulated to lift this weight, it shortens to 2.5 cm (L) (Fig. 2.24). The resulting strain, using equation (2.11), is −50%. The equation is arranged such that, by convention, shortening is a negative number and lengthening is a positive number (Fig. 2.24). Strain rate (SR) describes the rate at which strain occurs. Therefore, if the muscle contraction (negative strain) occurred over 0.25 seconds, the resulting strain rate would be −50%/0.25 sec or −0.5/0.25 sec, i.e., −2.0 sec^{-1} (20,21).

If the sampling rate of lengths is increased, we can calculate instantaneous strain normalized to a previously known initial length. If the time intervals (dt) are sufficiently short, precise outlines of strain can be determined. These can be summed up to obtain the total strain for the event (20). However, when the reference length is the previously measured length (previous time interval), this is known as natural (or Eulerian) strain (ε_N).

Natural strain does not depend on the measurement of L_0 (Lagrangian) and as a result may be more suitable for cardiac applications in a clinical setting (22). Instantaneous natural strain can be expressed as follows:

$$d\varepsilon_N(t) = \frac{L(t + dt) - L(t)}{L(t)} \qquad (2.12)$$

The total strain is the sum of these infinitesimal strains where

$$\varepsilon_N(t) = \int_{t_0}^{t} d\varepsilon_N(t) \qquad (2.13)$$

It is possible using magnetic resonance imaging (MRI) or myocardial ultrasonic crystals to measure lengths directly and, hence, Lagrangian strain (L_0 is taken at end diastole) (23,24). This is not practical in the OR. In a routine clinical setting, strain is subjectively assessed by observing wall thickening. For instance, in a transgastric view, we can use M-mode echocardiography to measure changes in thickness or radial function (25). For longitudinal function, the excursion of the mitral annulus can also be used. These methods, although useful, are crude and can be affected by translation or rotation. Furthermore, they do not discriminate between contracting segments and those that are passively pulled (Figs. 2.25–2.27). Therefore, length changes may not always be the result of the myocardial activity in the region in question. Poor edge definition is also a limiting factor. They are, at best, limited to peak changes and do not easily characterize the change in strain or its pattern of change throughout the heart cycle. To measure strain, velocity

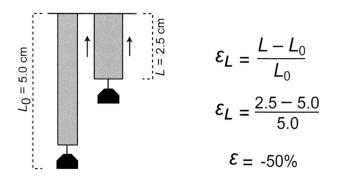

$$\varepsilon_L = \frac{L - L_0}{L_0}$$

$$\varepsilon_L = \frac{2.5 - 5.0}{5.0}$$

$$\varepsilon = -50\%$$

Figure 2.24 Lagrangian strain (ε_L) concept. Diagrammatic representation of a muscle strip fixed at the top end with weight attached to the bottom. The initial length (L_0) is 5 cm. The muscle shortens to 2.5 cm following stimulation (*right*). Inserting L_0 (5 cm) and L (2.5 cm) into the equation (*top right*), the calculated strain (ε_L) is −50%.

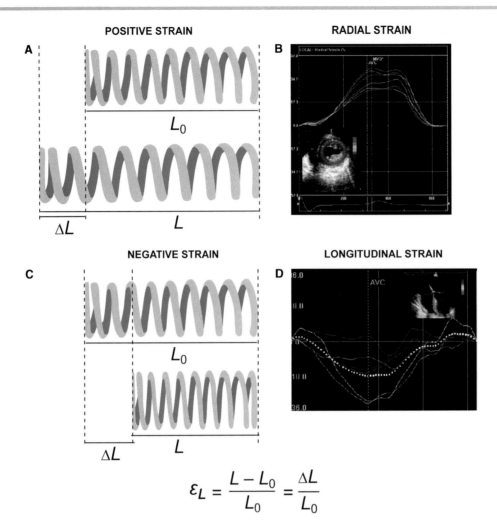

$$\varepsilon_L = \frac{L - L_0}{L_0} = \frac{\Delta L}{L_0}$$

Figure 2.25 Strain (ε), or deformation concept. (A,B) When the strain is positive, the initial length value (L_0) is smaller than the final one (L). For instance, in the transgastric mid short-axis view, the myocardial thickness increases during radial shortening. The radial strain obtained from this view will be positive (thickening). **(C,D)** The opposite applies for a negative strain. Typically, the longitudinal contraction of the left ventricle obtained from a mid-esophageal four-chamber view has a negative systolic strain.

differences employing echocardiography can be used as surrogates for length changes.

Strain Rate from Velocity Gradients

Tissue myocardial velocity gradients have been used to characterize deformation of the myocardium (26). Using tissue Doppler imaging, myocardial velocity can be determined for every point in the myocardium as long as the motion lies along the Doppler plane (Fig. 2.19). The velocity gradient can be used to describe deformation. SR defines a spatial velocity gradient that is determined from tissue Doppler using the following relationship:

$$SR = \frac{V_1 - V_2}{L} \tag{2.14}$$

SR is the velocity difference between two points; V_1 sampled at distance L_1 from the transducer and V_2 sampled at distance L_2 from the transducer normalized over the offset distance L, which is the result of $L_2 - L_1$. The offset distance L characterizes the distance between the two sampling points in the area of myocardium to be assessed (Fig. 2.28).

Natural strain, ε_N, is obtained by integrating instantaneous SR values from time t_0 to time t provided that the time interval (dt) is sufficiently short (20–22). It is described by the following relationship:

$$\varepsilon_N = \int_{t_0}^{t} SR dt \tag{2.15}$$

In the case for systolic myocardial strain, integration is begun at end diastole (t_0), the presumed unstressed

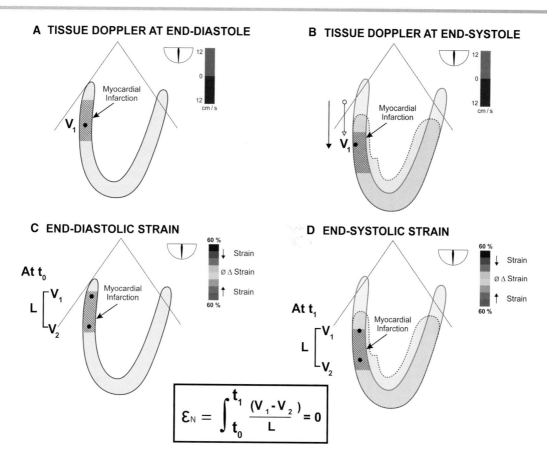

Figure 2.26 Tissue Doppler in myocardial infarction. Tissue Doppler velocity obtained during at end-diastole (**A**) and end-systole (**B**) in a patient with a localized myocardial infarction. In the area of myocardial infarction (shaded zone), there will be a measurable systolic velocity (V_1); a result of tethering as the abnormal segment is attached to normal myocardium. (**C,D**) Strain measurement at end-diastole (**C**) and end-systole (**D**). In diastole, a baseline velocity difference is obtained from two points (V_1 and V_2) separated by a set distance (L). t_0 is the time at end-diastole and the strain is zero. During systole, at another specific time (t_1 or end-systole), there has been no velocity difference and hence no strain. The tissue Doppler velocity-derived strain is zero because no deformation has occurred due to ischemia. Strain, unlike velocity, is not influenced by the tethering effect.

velocity difference. Natural strain, ε_N, has a nonlinear relationship to Lagrangian strain, ε_L, where (20)

$$\varepsilon_N(t) = \ln(1 + \varepsilon_L(t)) \qquad (2.16)$$

$$\varepsilon_L(t) = \exp(\varepsilon_N(t)) - 1 \qquad (2.17)$$

When deformations are small, the two are relatively similar; however, when larger, they may deviate significantly. It is, therefore, important to define the type of strain measured. To understand the difference between the two, we must understand the frames of reference. Lagrangian strain, ε_L, measures deformation from a single fixed point. Natural strain, ε_N, measures deformation from two predefined points or through velocity differences.

Let us examine the following analogy: suppose we float ping pong balls down a stream and describe their path as they follow the flow of water. We can look at it from two perspectives. First, Lagrangian strain, ε_L: as you sit on the shore, you can observe the ping pong balls' paths as they follow the water flow. You can sample the distance and time traveled as they move to and away from you. Therefore, it corresponds to an absolute measure with a predefined reference point. Second, natural strain, ε_N: suppose you and a friend were floating on fixed platforms separated by a specific distance. You could sample the ping pong balls' velocities at these two predetermined points as they pass you by. Therefore, you describe the flow via velocity differences at two predefined reference points.

Although water and myocardial tissue do not behave in the same way, for illustrative purposes, we can loosely transpose myocardial motion for the flowing water and myocardial landmarks for the ping pong balls. Using this analogy, one can describe the path, or deformation, of the heart much like that of the stream.

Strain and the Coordinate System in the Heart

Global and regional coordinate systems can be described for the heart. We are very familiar with global coordinate measurements in the determination of LV

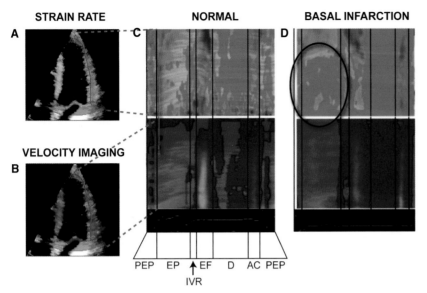

STRAIN RATE   NORMAL   BASAL INFARCTION

A

C

VELOCITY IMAGING

B

D

PEP   EP   EF   D   AC   PEP

IVR

Figure 2.27   Color M-mode TDI and strain rate imaging. Transthoracic apical four-chamber views with anterolateral wall analysis using SRI (**A**) and color TDI (**B**) are shown. Color M-mode of the SRI (**C,** upper) and TDI velocity imaging (**C,** lower) from the lateral wall are shown in a normal patient. In a patient with basal infarction (**D,** upper), SRI shows an abrupt change in color in the basal region (circled). However, the TDI velocity signal displays no abnormalities (**D,** lower) as it is influenced by tethering of the normal segments. *Abbreviations*: AC, atrial contraction; D, diastasis; EF, early filling; EP, ejection period; IVR, isovolumic relaxation; PEP, pre-ejection period; SRI, strain rate imaging; TDI, tissue Doppler imaging. *Source:* Courtesy of GE Healthcare.

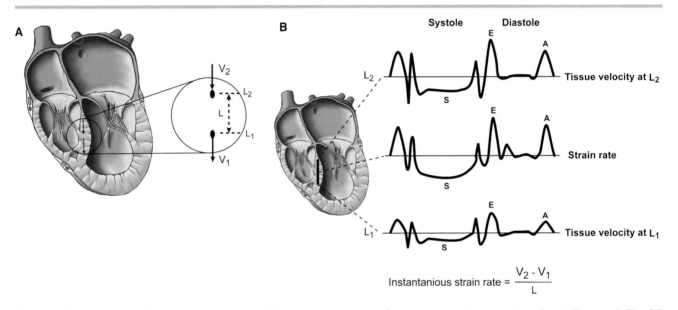

A

B

Systole   Diastole

E

A

L_2

S

Tissue velocity at L_2

E

A

S

Strain rate

E

A

L_1

S

Tissue velocity at L_1

$$\text{Instantanious strain rate} = \frac{V_2 - V_1}{L}$$

Figure 2.28   Strain rate. (A) Septal velocity-based SR measurement from a mid-esophageal four-chamber view is illustrated. The SR (1/sec) represents the difference in velocity (V_1 and V_2) at two points separated by a distance (L, the offset distance) corresponding to the difference from the transducer to points L_1 and L_2 ($L = L_1 - L_2$). **(B)** Velocity tracing at two specific points (L_1 and L_2) are shown. The SR tracing corresponds to the velocity difference at these two points divided by the length that separates them ($L_1 - L_2$). *Abbreviations*: A, atrial contraction; E, early filling; S, systolic; SR, strain rate. *Source:* Illustration courtesy of Gian-Marco Busato.

cavity size and ejection fraction. For example, we can determine the LV length (coordinate x) and its perpendicular measurements of LV diameters (coordinates z and y) (Fig. 2.29). For the purposes of SR echocardiography, we describe local myocardial coordinate systems. Using tissue Doppler, each coordinate must be measured separately (the Doppler axis). For example, if we measure strain at the level of the inferior wall in the transgastric short-axis view, we

are measuring radial strain or the amount of thickening of the ventricular wall in systole, a positive strain value (Fig. 2.30). If we then train our ultrasound beam laterally to the midseptal wall, we are measuring the amount of shortening in the circumferential axis, a negative value. Finally, in the two-chamber view, inferior wall sampling will measure shortening in the longitudinal axis (another negative value) (Fig. 2.30).

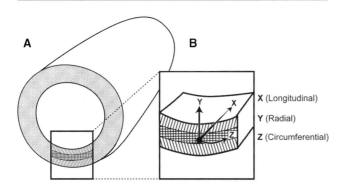

Figure 2.29 LV strain coordinates. (A,B) Schematic representation of the LV with coordinates *x, y* and *z* from a myocardial perspective. The local myocardial coordinates are demonstrated (inset) with corresponding axes. Strain and strain rate can be defined along the three coordinates. *Abbreviation*: LV, left ventricle.

Strain Rate from Velocity Differences Using Tissue Doppler

Color-coded analysis of myocardial motion was introduced in the early 1990s (18). This allowed for simultaneous myocardial velocity measurements at selected locations (26). When color tissue Doppler is applied to a specific area of myocardium, velocity and direction of motion are determined for each pixel displayed (Fig. 2.19). SR can be calculated by sampling velocities at two distinct points separated by a known distance as demonstrated in equation (2.14). Using specialized software, a sample volume of predetermined size can be placed on the area color coded for tissue Doppler. A specific offset distance can be selected. In Figure 2.30, the sample volume measures 6 × 6 mm with an offset of 12 mm for SR calculations. The SR is averaged over this sample volume and displayed graphically (Fig. 2.31). In Figure 2.30, the sample volume

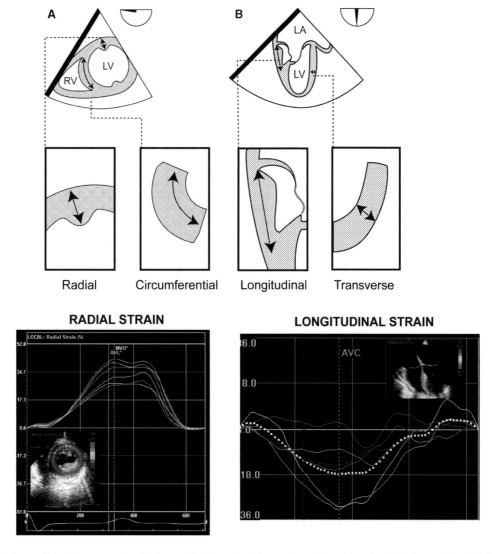

Figure 2.30 Strain motion. Transgastric mid short-axis (**A**) and mid-esophageal two-chamber (**B**) views of the LV demonstrating the myocardial motion in systole for radial, circumferential and longitudinal strain or strain rate. *Abbreviations*: LA, left atrium; LV, left ventricle; RV, right ventricle.

RADIAL STRAIN RATE   RADIAL STRAIN

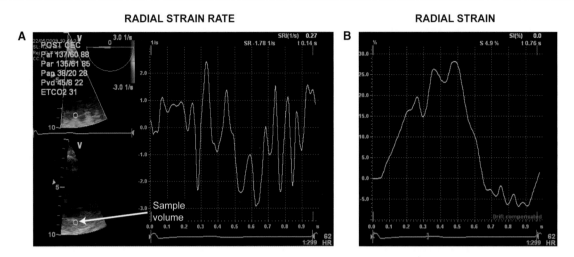

Figure 2.31   Strain rate and strain. (**A**) Transgastric mid short-axis views of the left ventricle with a 6 × 6 mm sample volume applied to the anterior wall (*lower panel*) in the region where color tissue Doppler has been applied (*upper panel*). The offset distance selected is 12 mm. Off-line processing of the SR is demonstrated graphically for this sample volume time (x axis) for one cardiac cycle on the right. (**B**) Integration of SR yields strain and is represented graphically over one cardiac cycle. *Abbreviation*: SR, strain rate.

RADIAL STRAIN RATE   RADIAL STRAIN   RADIAL STRAIN

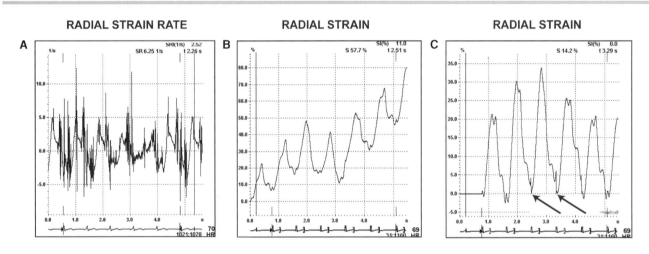

Figure 2.32   Strain rate and strain limitations. (**A**) Radial strain rate of the inferior wall of the left ventricle obtained with off-line processing is shown over five cardiac cycles. Strain rate calculations are inherently noisy therefore smoothing algorithms are frequently applied to minimize this problem. (**B**) Upward radial strain drift is demonstrated over five cardiac cycles. As there can be no net strain, correction must be applied. (**C**) The strain has been reset to zero at the beginning of each cardiac cycle (QRS) (arrows). *Abbreviation*: SR, strain rate.

can be moved anywhere where color tissue Doppler has been applied. SR integration then yields strain (equation 2.15), which is demonstrated for five consecutive cardiac cycles on the right side (Fig. 2.32).

Pitfalls of Strain and SR Measurements

Strain rate measurements are inherently prone to noise as they incorporate small random velocity changes that are magnified when velocity differences are calculated (20,21,27) (Fig. 2.32). Smaller offsets

(distance between V_1 and V_2, equation 2.14) also tend to increase noise (27). Increasing the sample size (larger averaging volume) will help reduce the noise. This, however, will come at the cost of decreasing spatial discrimination (larger myocardial segments assessed). Various smoothing algorithms can also be applied to the sample volume. Integration of SR to yield strain will yield a smoother trace as random noise tends to cancel out.

Doppler angle dependency is a limitation of strain and SR measurements when done using tissue

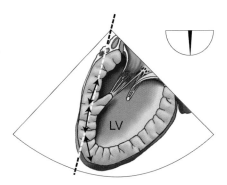

Figure 2.33 Longitudinal strain limitations. Diagrammatic representation of a mid-esophageal two-chamber view with three sets of arrows used to represent myocardial motion for the apex, mid and basal inferior walls of the LV. The dashed line corresponds to the tissue Doppler plane for which only the basal and mid portion of the inferior wall line up correctly. *Abbreviation:* LV, left ventricle. *Source:* Drawing courtesy of Gian-Marco Busato.

Doppler (Fig. 2.33). The measured velocities must line up with tissue motion to reflect true myocardial strain in the desired coordinate axis.

Solid structures are inherently incompressible. Conservation of mass dictates that there will be associated perpendicular changes in one direction (shortening, a negative value) when compared to another (thickening, a positive value). Deviations from proper alignment may result in erroneous strain measurements (27). For example, longitudinal strain with a negative value would be reduced if a component of radial strain were introduced (a positive value). Not all segments of the heart may be amenable to strain measurements. This is especially true when using transesophageal echocardiography (TEE). Limited probe movement when compared with transthoracic echocardiography (TTE) can significantly impair the ability to line up wall motion with the Doppler plane. Acoustic artifacts may interfere with or lead to erroneous velocity measurements and hence to erroneous strain measurements. Finally, strain and SR measurements must be performed offline, which is impractical and time consuming.

Optimizing SR and Strain Measurements

Ideally, myocardial motion should be correctly aligned with the Doppler angle. A 25° deviation can result in a 50% decline in strain (21,27). As the sample volume is fixed, it is important to ensure that it is of appropriate size for the area examined and that it remains within the myocardium throughout the cardiac cycle. Frame-by-frame manual tracking of the sample volume is possible; however, it remains extremely tedious and impractical. Maximizing frame rates for tissue Doppler measurements (>200/sec) will also ensure proper strain and SR measurements, increase temporal resolution as well as minimize strain drift. It will also ensure proper assessments of short-lived events such as isovolumic SR phases.

Myocardial Strain Distribution

During systole, the base of the heart descends toward the apex that remains fixed. Myocardial velocities progressively decrease from base to apex (28) (Fig. 2.19). Therefore, strain should be diminished near the apex. The literature varies on the distribution of strain and SR in the heart especially for the right ventricle (RV). Skulstad et al. found homogeneous strain throughout all segments of the LV anterior wall where only the most apical values were reduced (28). Kowalski et al. (29), on the other hand, found no strain gradient from base to apex in the septal, lateral, posterior, and anterior LV walls. Weideman et al. also found no gradient in the LV anterior and inferior walls of healthy children (30). The RV, on the other hand, demonstrates more variability. Weideman et al. found increasing strain in the mid-wall followed by a decrease at the apex (30–32). Conversely, Kowalski et al. found significantly higher strain and SR at the apex (28,29).

The disparities in measurements, however, may seem perplexing but they may be accounted for, in some cases, by technique. In TTE, the apical two- or four-chamber views will yield better alignment of the apex than for the base if the probe is not positioned properly. The opposite can be seen with TEE. Variable offset distances may yield different strains by varying or enhancing differences in the region examined. Additionally, longitudinal strain is smaller than radial strain by approximately 50% and of opposite value, further underscoring the importance of proper alignment (29–32).

Speckle Tracking

Other technologies have been developed, which circumvent the limitations in strain measurements using tissue Doppler. Speckle tracking is a technology based on tracking of features created by B-mode imaging (33–35). These features appear randomly, and therefore, each myocardial segment will have a unique pattern. Myocardial displacement based on this technology does not depend on the Doppler angle and allows for simultaneous 2D assessments (e.g., radial and longitudinal) over large areas. Unique myocardial features are tracked frame by frame using a search algorithm (Fig. 2.34), but this is computer intensive. The technology, however, is limited by frame rate and image quality. For example, a large 2D sector will result in a lower frame rate, which may, in turn, lead to an inability to track features. In other words, these features will have moved too far away during longer intervals and will be *lost* to tracking. Longer interval between frames will also result in a loss of discrimination of short-lived events such as isovolumic intervals. Artifacts may also lead to erroneous measurements.

For illustrative purposes, we will use the transgastric short-axis view of the LV. To acquire tissue displacement using speckle tracking, the endocardium is carefully traced (Fig. 2.35). Following this,

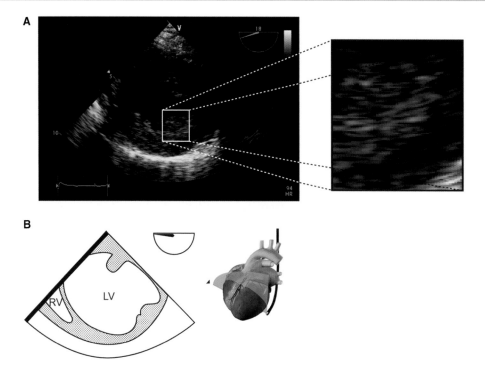

Figure 2.34   Speckle tracking. (A,B) In this transgastric mid short-axis view, an area of the anterior myocardium of the LV is magnified. Speckle tracking is based on pattern recognition, or cross-correlation, of the Kernel area. This is defined as the smallest difference in the total sum of pixel value. The program will then analyze global motion coherence, consistency of periodicity, three-point and Gaussian filtering and finally Fourier analysis. *Abbreviations*: LV, left ventricle; RV, right ventricle.

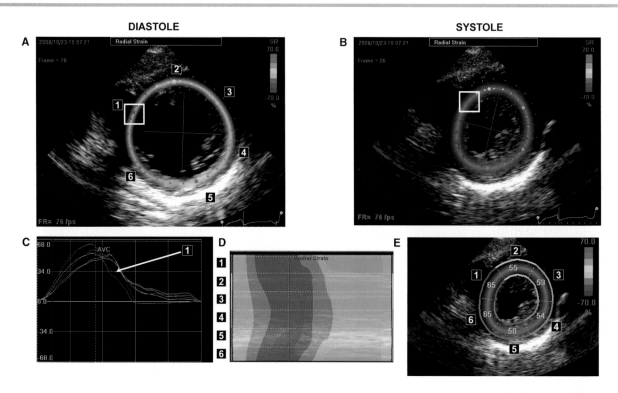

Figure 2.35   Speckle tracking strain displays. Transgastric mid short-axis views with displays of speckle tracking in diastole (**A**) and in systole (**B**) are shown. The myocardial segments are color-coded for strain (scale on right of image). In addition, a clockwise rotation can be appreciated (the crosshair has turned in systole (**A** to **B**)). (**C**) Individual strain curves over time averaged from six predefined areas of the myocardium (labeled 1 through 6). (**D**) Normal curved M-mode strain display from the infero-septal (1 red segment in (**E**) and at top in (**D**)) clockwise to the antero-septal wall (6 blue segment in (**E**) and bottom in (**D**)). (**E**) Peak systolic strain is displayed for the six regions.

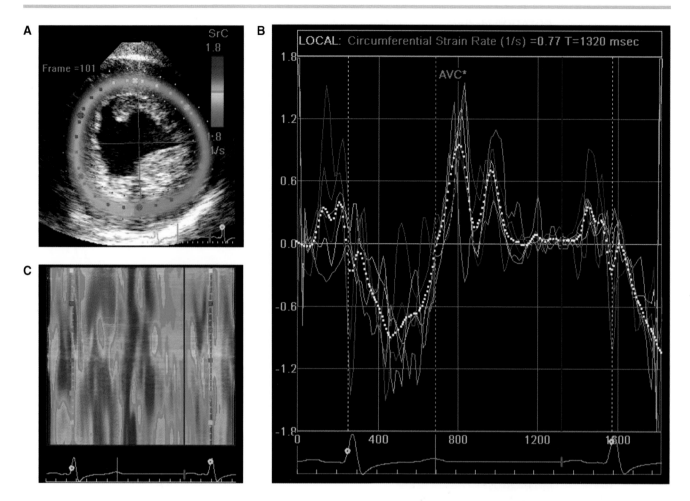

Figure 2.36 Speckle tracking strain rate displays. Transgastric mid short-axis view is used for the determination of circumferential strain rate (**A**) with graphical display, (**B**) matching curved M-mode and (**C**) spectral display.

an appropriate myocardial thickness is selected to define the area of interest within which calculations will be performed (Fig. 2.35). The heart is divided into standard segments that are usually color coded. The displacement of particular myocardial B-mode features is measured and a tracking score is provided by the computer, which indicates whether the myocardial features were reliably tracked during the process. A failure of proper tracking will result in erroneous measurements. The strain and SR will then be calculated from feature displacement and frame intervals and averaged over each myocardial segment. The resulting myocardial strain and SR can be displayed in one of several ways. Information can be displayed as color on 2D images (Fig. 2.35A and B), as individual lines per region (Fig. 2.35C), as curved M-mode (color carpet) where the change over time of the relevant myocardial segments are displayed (Fig. 2.35D), and as maximal strain per region of interest (Fig. 2.35E). Corresponding SR is displayed in Figure 2.36. These results are

inherently noisier than those of strain. Cardiac torsion and myocardial twisting can also be calculated using speckle tracking in the transgastric view (Fig. 2.37).

Mid-esophageal views can also be used to calculate myocardial deformation using speckle tracking. Myocardial shortening and thickening will be calculated as opposed to circumferential and radial, which were demonstrated in the transgastric views illustrated above.

Clinical Potential of Strain and SR Imaging

Myocardial (or annular) velocities are commonly used in the assessment of RV and LV systolic and diastolic function. They are, however, prone to errors due to translation and tethering. Myocardial velocities are insensitive to the severity of systolic dysfunction (Figs. 2.26 and 2.27) (28). Strain and SR echocardiography removes the limitations associated with velocity

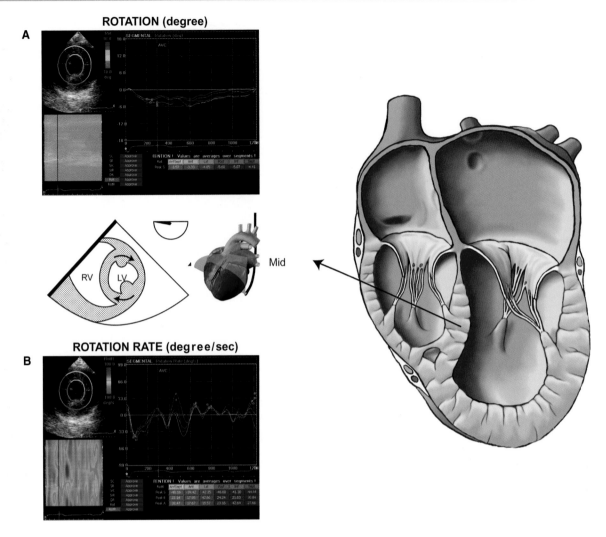

ROTATION (degree)

ROTATION RATE (degree/sec)

Figure 2.37   LV rotation. During systole, twisting of the heart can be observed through a central axis. When viewed from the apex (using transthoracic echocardiography), the LV rotates counter-clockwise at the apex and clockwise at the base in systole. The rotational (**A**) and rotation rate (**B**) can be calculated using speckle tracking in the transgastric views. *Source:* Drawing courtesy of Gian-Marco Busato.

measurements. Figure 2.38 summarizes the relationship between tissue velocities and SR.

What are we measuring with strain and SR? It is important to recognize that we are measuring local myocardial deformations that, on the whole, cannot be extrapolated to global ventricular function or easily compared with how the heart handles volume. Strain may represent a "regional ejection fraction." Myocardial deformation is dependent on preload and afterload as well as myocardial stiffness. SR represents the rate of deformation (or the rate of work) and *may* be less dependent on changes in preload and afterload (32). SR has correlated best with dP/dt, whereas strain was more closely associated with ejection fraction (36).

Multiple applications of strain and SR imaging can be brought to the perioperative period (see

Chapter 9). A full understanding of limitations, as well as the significance of the measurements, is required. The application of this technology in the OR may seem cumbersome and limited, however, it will open up more avenues of assessments, thereby greatly enhancing the role of the perioperative echocardiographer.

CONCLUSION

In the clinical setting, Doppler has two main applications: detection and quantification of normal and disturbed blood flow or myocardial motion. The Doppler technique has high detection sensitivity and specificity. Color Doppler allows fast localization of abnormal flows and provides a spatial display in 2D. Quantification is, however, better performed using PW and

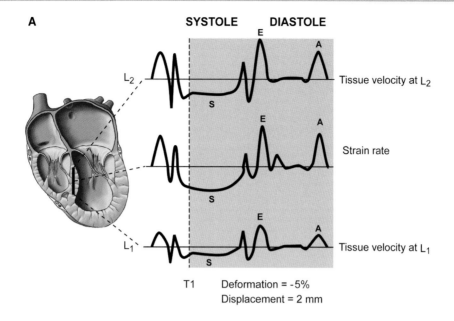

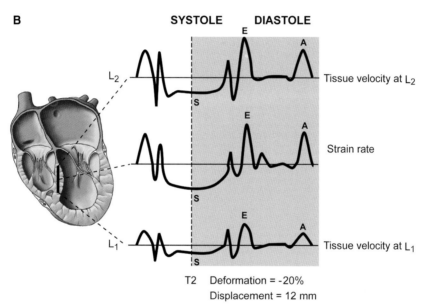

Figure 2.38 Relationship summary between tissue velocity, displacement, strain rate (SR) and strain. Mid-esophageal four-chamber view shows where tissue Doppler velocities and strain rate are obtained for the septal wall at two different time periods. (**A**) During early systole (S), at a specific time (t_t), the septum has moved 2 mm away from the transducer. This was obtained with tissue tracking through time integration of the velocity signal. (**B**) At the same time, a −5% deformation is noted. This was obtained with strain through time integration of the SR signal. (**C**) Later in systole, the septum has moved 12 mm away from the transducer. (**D**) At the same time, a −20% deformation was noted. These time-varying values can be also demonstrated with individual waveforms or using curved M-mode. *Abbreviation*: A, peak late diastolic tissue velocity or strain rate; E, peak early diastolic tissue velocity or strain rate. *Source: Drawing courtesy of Gian-Marco Busato.*

CW Doppler and spectral display. The PW Doppler is primarily used for flow sampling in specific areas such as cardiac valves or large arteries and veins. Most normal velocities are within the range of measurement free of aliasing. The CW Doppler must be utilized for measurement of high velocities across restrictive orifices such as stenotic or regurgitant valves. It is more reliable for use in hemodynamic calculations and should be used for all velocities >1.2 m/sec. Finally, tissue velocities, strain, and SR measurements are newer modalities that will increase our ability to quantify myocardial deformation and function. Normal regional displacement, strain, and SR are shown in Tables 2.2 and 2.3.

Table 2.2 Strain Rate of Individual Segments

	Septum	Lateral	Inferior	Anterior
Peak systolic wave (Ssr)				
Basal	0.99 ± 0.49	1.5 ± 0.74	0.88 ± 0.39	1.64 ± 0.9
Mid	1.25 ± 0.73	1.29 ± 0.58	0.95 ± 0.54	0.98 ± 0.68
Apical	1.15 ± 0.5	1.09 ± 0.59	1.38 ± 0.45	1.05 ± 0.63
Early diastolic wave (Esr)				
Basal	1.95 ± 0.89	1.92 ± 1.11	1.85 ± 0.89	2.03 ± 0.99
Mid	1.94 ± 0.97	1.71 ± 0.66	1.92 ± 1.2	1.7 ± 0.82
Apical	1.91 ± 0.66	1.81 ± 0.87	2.29 ± 0.88	1.76 ± 0.98
Late diastolic wave (Asr)				
Basal	1.54 ± 0.93	0.93 ± 0.59	1.18 ± 0.78	1.49 ± 0.96
Mid	1.29 ± 0.86	1.48 ± 0.77	0.78 ± 0.62	1.04 ± 0.57
Apical	0.95 ± 0.54	1.07 ± 0.68	1.68 ± 0.76	0.68 ± 0.65

Peak systolic (Ssr), early (Esr), and late (Asr) diastolic strain rates shown in 1/sec.
Source: From Ref. 19 with permission.

Table 2.3 Displacement and Systolic Strain of Individual Segments

	Septum	Lateral	Inferior	Anterior
Displacement (D)				
Basal	1.2 ± 0.19	0.93 ± 0.22	1.33 ± 0.22	1.05 ± 0.27
Mid	1.13 ± 0.27	0.91 ± 0.18	0.62 ± 0.22	1.04 ± 0.19
Apical	0.65 ± 0.24	0.82 ± 0.27	0.55 ± 0.18	0.41 ± 0.25
Systolic strain (E)				
Basal	17.5 ± 5.32	18.22 ± 6.79	14.97 ± 5.74	22.19 ± 7.75
Mid	18.27 ± 6.93	18.83 ± 5.29	14.2 ± 5.14	17.95 ± 5.53
Apical	19.31 ± 6.07	17.56 ± 5.85	23.6 ± 5.17	13.17 ± 5.83

Displacement shown in centimeters. Systolic strain shown in percent.
Source: From Ref. 19 with permission.

ACKNOWLEDGMENTS

The author is particularly grateful to Dr Dominique Bettex (University Hospital Zürich, Switzerland) and Mrs Cristine Dardel (CHUV, Lausanne, Switzerland) for their invaluable help in correcting the manuscript.

REFERENCES

1. Labovitz AJ, Williams GA. Doppler Echocardiography. The Quantitative Approach. 3rd ed. Philadelphia: Lea & Febiger, 1992.
2. Goldman DE, Jueter DF. Tabular data of the velocity and absorption of high-frequency sound in mammalian tissues. J Acoust Soc Am 1956; 28:35–37.
3. Quinones MA, Otto CM, Stoddard M, et al. Recommendations for quantification of Doppler echocardiography: a report from the Doppler Quantification Task Force of the Nomenclature and Standards Committee of the American Society of Echocardiography. J Am Soc Echocardiogr 2002; 15:167–184.
4. Sehgal CM. Principles of ultrasonic imaging and Doppler ultrasond. In: St John Sutton MG, Oldershaw PJ, Kotler MN, eds. Textbook of Echocardiography and Doppler in Adults and Children. 2nd ed. Cambridge, MA: Blackwell Science, 1996:3–30.
5. Chassot PG. Principes physiques de l'échocardiographie. In: Bettex D, Chassot PG, eds. Échocardiographie trans-oesophagienne en anesthésie-réanimation. Paris: Masson, 1997:13–39.
6. Hedrick WR, Hykes DL, Starchman DE. Ultrasound Physics and Instrumentation. 3rd ed. St. Louis: Mosby, 1995.
7. Garcia-Fernandez MA, Zamorano J, Azevedo J. Doppler tissue imaging in ischemic heart disease. In: Garcia-Fernandez MA, Zamorano J, Azevedo J, eds. Doppler Tissue Imaging Echocardiography. Madrid: McGraw-Hill, 1998:7–21.
8. Feigenbaum H. Instrumentation. In: Feigenbaum H, ed. Echocardiography. Philadelphia: Lea & Febiger, 1994:1–67.
9. DeMaria E. Cardiac Doppler: The Basics. Andover: Hewlett Packard Co, 1984:1–35.
10. Bom K, de Boo J, Rijsterborgh H. On the aliasing problem in pulsed Doppler cardiac studies. J Clin Ultrasound 1984; 12:559–567.
11. Baker DW, Rubenstein SA, Lorch GS. Pulsed Doppler echocardiography: principles and applications. Am J Med 1977; 63:69–80.
12. Pellett AA, Kerut EK. The Doppler velocity waveform. Echocardiography 2006; 23:528–530.
13. Wells PNT. Colour flow mapping: principles and limitations. In: Roelandt JRT, Sutherland GR, Iliceto S, eds. Cardiac Ultrasound. Edinburgh: Churchill Livingstone, 1993:43–51.
14. Nanda NC. Basics in Doppler echocardiography. In: Nanda NC, ed. Atlas of Color Doppler Echocardiography. Philadelphia: Lea & Febiger, 1989:1–5.
15. Feigenbaum H. Echocardiography. 5th ed. Baltimore: Williams & Williams, 1994.

16. Berg S, Torp H, Haugen BO, et al. Volumetric blood flow measurement with the use of dynamic 3-dimensional ultrasound color flow imaging. J Am Soc Echocardiogr 2000; 13:393–402.

17. Muhiudeen IA, Kuecherer HF, Lee E, et al. Intraoperative estimation of cardiac output by transesophageal pulsed Doppler echocardiography. Anesthesiology 1991; 74:9–14.

18. Sutherland GR, Stewart MJ, Groundstroem KW, et al. Color Doppler myocardial imaging: a new technique for the assessment of myocardial function. J Am Soc Echocardiogr 1994; 7:441–458.

19. Sun JP, Popovic ZB, Greenberg NL, et al. Noninvasive quantification of regional myocardial function using Doppler-derived velocity, displacement, strain rate, and strain in healthy volunteers: effects of aging. J Am Soc Echocardiogr 2004; 17:132–138.

20. D'hooge J, Heimdal A, Jamal F, et al. Regional strain and strain rate measurements by cardiac ultrasound: principles, implementation and limitations. Eur J Echocardiogr 2000; 1:154–170.

21. Pislaru C, Abraham TP, Belohlavek M. Strain and strain rate echocardiography. Curr Opin Cardiol 2002; 17: 443–454.

22. D'hooge J, Jamal F, Bijnens B, et al. Calculation of strain values from strain rate curves: how should this be done? IEEE 2, Conference Proceeding. IEEE Ultrasonics Symposium 2000:1269–1272.

23. Urheim S, Edvardsen T, Steine K, et al. Postsystolic shortening of ischemic myocardium: a mechanism of abnormal intraventricular filling. Am J Physiol Heart Circ Physiol 2003; 284:H2343–H2350.

24. Axel L, Goncalves RC, Bloomgarden D. Regional heart wall motion: two-dimensional analysis and functional imaging with MR imaging. Radiology 1992; 183:745–750.

25. Guth B, Savage R, White F, et al. Detection of ischemic wall dysfunction: comparison between M-mode echocardiography and sonomicrometry. Am Heart J 1984; 107:449–457.

26. Uematsu M, Miyatake K, Tanaka N, et al. Myocardial velocity gradient as a new indicator of regional left ventricular contraction: detection by a two-dimensional tissue Doppler imaging technique. J Am Coll Cardiol 1995; 26:217–223.

27. Urheim S, Edvardsen T, Torp H, et al. Myocardial strain by Doppler echocardiography. Validation of a new method to quantify regional myocardial function. Circulation 2000; 102:1158–1164.

28. Skulstad H, Urheim S, Edvardsen T, et al. Grading of myocardial dysfunction by tissue Doppler echocardiography: a comparison between velocity, displacement, and strain imaging in acute ischemia. J Am Coll Cardiol 2006; 47:1672–1682.

29. Kowalski M, Kukulski T, Jamal F, et al. Can natural strain and strain rate quantify regional myocardial deformation? A study in healthy subjects. Ultrasound Med Biol 2001; 27:1087–1097.

30. Weidemann F, Eyskens B, Jamal F, et al. Quantification of regional left and right ventricular radial and longitudinal function in healthy children using ultrasound-based strain rate and strain imaging. J Am Soc Echocardiogr 2002; 15:20–28.

31. Yip G, Abraham T, Belohlavek M, et al. Clinical applications of strain rate imaging. J Am Soc Echocardiogr 2003; 16:1334–1342.

32. Sutherland GR, Di Salvo G, Claus P, et al. Strain and strain rate imaging: a new clinical approach to quantifying regional myocardial function. J Am Soc Echocardiogr 2004; 17:788–802.

33. Leitman M, Lysyansky P, Sidenko S, et al. Two-dimensional strain-a novel software for real-time quantitative echocardiographic assessment of myocardial function. J Am Soc Echocardiogr 2004; 17:1021–1029.

34. Becker M, Hoffmann R, Kuhl HP, et al. Analysis of myocardial deformation based on ultrasonic pixel tracking to determine transmurality in chronic myocardial infarction. Eur Heart J 2006; 27:2560–2566.

35. Amundsen BH, Helle-Valle T, Edvardsen T, et al. Noninvasive myocardial strain measurement by speckle tracking echocardiography: validation against sonomicrometry and tagged magnetic resonance imaging. J Am Coll Cardiol 2006; 47:789–793.

36. Weidemann F, Jamal F, Sutherland GR, et al. Myocardial function defined by strain rate and strain during alterations in inotropic states and heart rate. Am J Physiol Heart Circ Physiol 2002; 283:H792–H799.

3

Transducers

François Haddad
Stanford University, Palo Alto, California, U.S.A.

Warner Mampuya
Université de Sherbrooke, Sherbrooke, Quebec, Canada

Craig Guenther
University of Alberta, Edmonton, Alberta, Canada

Bradley I. Munt and John Bowering
Providence Health Care, University of British Columbia, Vancouver, Canada

INTRODUCTION

A transducer is a device capable of converting one form of energy into another. Ultrasound transducers convert electrical energy into ultrasound energy or vice versa (Fig. 3.1). This chapter will review the structure and operation of transducers as they relate to clinical echocardiography.

PIEZOELECTRIC PRINCIPLE

Ultrasound transducers operate according to the piezoelectric principle. Piezoelectric is derived from the Greek words piezo meaning to press and electron meaning amber (a gemstone derived from hardened sap attracting small objects when rub with fur) (1). The piezoelectric effect is the phenomenon whereby some materials (quartz, ceramics, lithium sulfate, and others) are able to generate an electric current when deformed by mechanical pressure or stress (1, 2). The same materials, when submitted to an alternating electrical current, change shape and can be made to vibrate, deform, and generate sound wave pulses, that is, the opposite of the first principle (Fig. 3.2).

This is the basis of the transducer's construction and function. When we apply this principle to clinical echocardiography, we can understand how an ultrasound transducer can be used to generate ultrasound waves from electrical stimulation and how an electrical current can be generated from the mechanical stimulation caused by the returning ultrasound echoes.

STRUCTURE OF THE TRANSDUCER

Structure of a Single Element Transducer

The simplest transducer is composed of a single piezoelectric element or crystal. In practice, single crystals are used for A- and M-mode recordings. The transducer contains seven important components (3, 4) (Fig. 3.3):

1. The piezoelectric element generates acoustic pulses and electrical signals when submitted to electrical or mechanical stimulation.
2. The electrodes transmit the electric current to and from the piezoelectric element and record the voltage generated by the returning echoes.
3. The backing material shortens the time during which the crystal vibrates following excitation, thus shortening the spatial pulse length and improving axial resolution. It is usually composed of a mixture of tungsten and rubber.
4. The matching layer reduces the acoustic impedance mismatch between the patient and the transducer, thereby attenuating reflected ultrasound waves at the transducer-patient interface.
5. The acoustic insulation prevents the transmission of vibration to the transducer housing.
6. The face plate allows for improved contact of the probe with the patient.
7. A casing provides protection for all the probe components.

Assembly and Array

A transducer assembly is composed of an element, or a set of piezoelectric elements, with damping and matching material in a case (1). Almost all imaging transducers used in clinical echocardiography today are transducer arrays that contain many elements in a given configuration. If the elements are placed side by side, the transducer is referred to as a linear array as used in an epiaortic probe (Fig. 3.4). The elements can be arranged in a curve (convex or curved array) or a circle (annular array) (Fig. 3.4). The term phasing is applied to array transducers (phased array) and implies both focusing and steering of the ultrasound

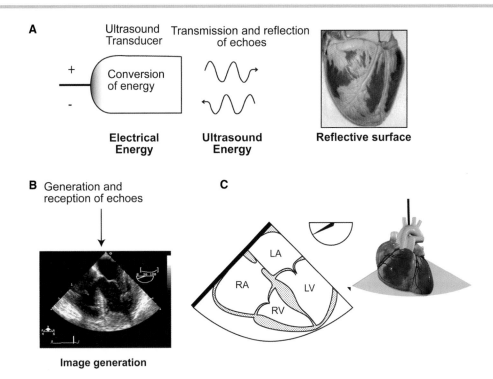

Figure 3.1 **Ultrasound transducer.** (**A**) An ultrasound transducer converts electrical energy into ultrasound energy and *vice versa*. The heart represents the reflective surface where transmission and reflection of echoes will occur. (**B,C**) The ultrasound image is generated from conversion of the incoming ultrasound energy into electrical energy. Shown here is a mid-esophageal four-chamber view. *Abbreviations:* LA, left atrium; LV, left ventricle; RA, right atrium; RV, right ventricle.

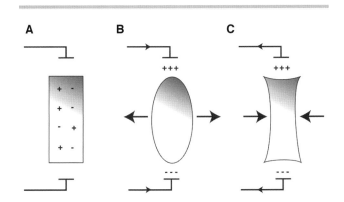

Figure 3.2 **Piezoelectric effect.** (**A**) The piezoelectric effect describes the relation between a mechanical stress and an electrical voltage in solids. (**B**) The reverse piezoelectric effect occurs as crystals in an ultrasound transducer deform or change shape when they have a voltage applied to generate sound wave pulses. (**C**) The piezoelectric effect occurs when ultrasound transducer crystals are struck by a returning sound wave to produce an electric impulse. The arrows represent pressure (sound wave), while (+) and (−) represent electrical charges.

beam (see the following section). Transesophageal echocardiography (TEE) transducers are phased array, comprising from 64 to 256 piezoelectric elements (Fig. 3.3).

MODE OF OPERATION OF TRANSDUCERS

This section answers three questions:

1. How does a transducer emit or capture (receive) an ultrasound wave (transducer operation)?
2. What are the main characteristics of an ultrasound beam (structure and focus)?
3. How can a good quality ultrasound image be generated by combining a set of focused beams (the principle of scanning and steering)?

Emission of Ultrasound Energy

To understand the fundamental principles of transducer function, one has to keep in mind the important characteristics of an ultrasound wave (see Chapter 1).

Mode of Generation of the Electrical Impulse

Transducers can operate in two different generation modes: burst excited or shock excited. In the burst-excited mode, transducers convert an alternating electrical voltage burst into an ultrasound pulse by inducing conformational changes in the piezoelectric elements. The transducer can also convert incoming ultrasound echoes into alternating electrical voltage bursts. Most modern transducers operate in burst-excited mode because this provides the possibility of selecting the operating frequency from the bandwidth. Typically,

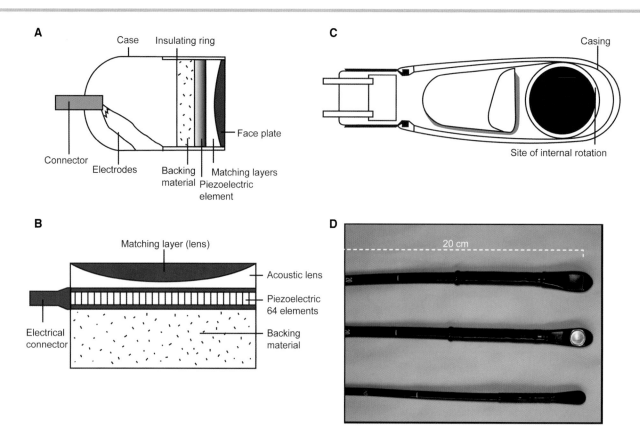

Figure 3.3 Transducer structure. (**A**) The structure of a single disk shaped ultrasound transducer. See text for details. (**B,C**) Transesophageal ultrasound transducer. (**D**) Transesophageal 3D matrix, multiplane and pediatric transducers. *Source*: Adapted from Ref. 4.

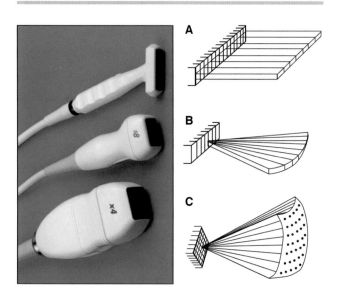

Figure 3.4 Ultrasound arrays. Epiaortic probe with linear sequential array of up to 512 elements (**A**), transthoracic probe with linear phased array of up to 128 elements (**B**) and 3D transthoracic probe with matrix array of up to 2500 elements (**C**) are shown.

transducers are driven by one to three cycles of alternating current to generate an image. In the shock-excited mode, a transducer converts a uniphasic voltage impulse into ultrasound pulses, while returning echoes are converted into alternating electrical voltage bursts.

Operating Frequency

The operating, or resonant, frequency of the system is the preferred vibrating frequency of the transducer that provides the maximum efficiency of operation. This frequency depends on the following two factors:

1. Piezoelectric element thickness, which corresponds to one-half of the pulse wavelength
2. Propagation speed in the crystal

Wavelength and frequency are reciprocally related; the thinner the element, the higher the transducer frequency. The typical thickness for a piezoelectric element is between 0.2 and 1 mm (1).

As propagation speed = wavelength × frequency and the element thickness = 1/2 × wavelength; therefore,

$$\text{Frequency} = \frac{\text{propagation speed}}{2 \times \text{element thickness}} \qquad (3.1)$$

Frequency Bandwidth

Under ideal circumstances, when a transducer produces a pulse, its frequency will equal the operating frequency. However, in reality, a pulse contains different frequencies. The bandwidth refers to the range of frequencies in which amplitude exceeds a given value, contained in the ultrasound pulse. The bandwidth is inversely related to spatial pulse length. Therefore, sound pulses with a short duration (shorter spatial pulse length) are composed of more frequencies. Pulses with greater spatial length will have fewer frequencies. The range of frequencies can also be described by the quality factor, Q, as

$$Q = \frac{\text{operating frequency}}{\text{bandwidth}} \qquad (3.2)$$

A lower Q factor generates images with better detail resolution. A transducer with a high (wide) bandwidth can, under certain circumstances, operate at different frequencies. This property provides the advantage of choosing the appropriate operating frequency depending on the desired axial resolution and penetration (a compromise). The bandwidth concept is also important for new imaging modalities such as harmonic imaging, which will be discussed briefly at the end of the chapter.

Transducer Damping

Transducer damping is the process in which the number of cycles in each pulse is reduced (Fig. 3.5). This is achieved by placement of specific backing material behind the piezoelectric crystal. The advantage of damping is to improve detail resolution by reducing the spatial pulse length. However, damping has the disadvantage of decreasing the ultrasound amplitude, which reduces the ability of the system to detect weak returning echoes and decreases its sensitivity. A system that has poorly damped crystals will have a higher sensitivity but lower detail resolution and a smaller bandwidth.

Impedance Matching

The transducer element has acoustic impedance ~25 times greater than that of the human body (5). This acoustic impedance mismatch can generate a large reflective loss at the transducer-skin interface. To reduce this loss, a matching layer is placed between the skin and the transducer, which has an impedance intermediate between those of the crystal and tissue. Its thickness is equal to one-quarter of the wavelength of the transducer's center frequency (3). This specific thickness provides constructive interference in the layers, thereby improving sound transmission. Multiple matching layers have the advantage of increasing sensitivity as well as bandwidth.

When the ultrasound wave is emitted from the transducer and strikes air, which has low impedance, the difference in impedance between the two interfaces reflects most of the ultrasound wave away from the patient. This is minimized by the use of a coupling medium such as aqueous gel (see Fig. 1.6).

Electrical Matching

Electrical matching represents the electrical compatibility between the transducer and the diagnostic instrument. Suboptimal electrical matching could lower the transducer sensitivity and explain why a particular transducer performs better in a certain electrical environment on a different pulser machine. Electrical matching is accomplished by tuning the transducer's impedance to that of the pulse/receiver of the diagnostic machine. This tuning is not a user-variable function and has to be designed into the transducer on the basis of a good understanding of the pulse/receiver characteristics of the echographic instrument (3).

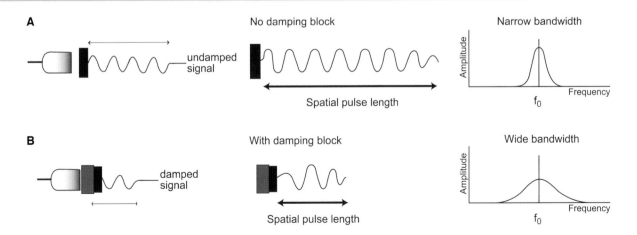

Figure 3.5 Damping material. The SPL is altered by the absence (**A**) or the presence (**B**) of a dampening block. The presence of a dampening block reduces the SPL which improves detail resolution. It also increases the frequency bandwidth but decreases the ability of the system to detect weak distal echoes through a reduction of the amplitude. *Abbreviations:* f_0, resonant frequency of the transducer; SPL, spatial pulse length.

Ultrasound Beam, Focusing, and Scanning

Ultrasound waves propagate in the acoustic medium as part of a beam. The ultrasound beam determines the area of the heart from which returning echoes will be recorded.

Structure

The ultrasound beam is composed of a main beam, or central beam, as well as side lobes, or grating lobes. The main beam generates the desired image, whereas the side lobes can be responsible for artifact imaging (Fig. 3.6). The main beam represents the part in which the intensity of the acoustic wave is greater than a determined percentage of a spatial peak value. The side lobes represent a weaker beam of sounds that propagate in a different direction than that of the main beam.

Main Beam

In a simple disk transducer, the convergent portion of the beam is referred to as the near or Fresnel zone. The point where the beam begins to diverge is the transition zone. Beyond the transition zone lies the far or Fraunhöfer zone (Fig. 3.6). The shape of the ultrasound beam is important because it determines the area from which echoes can be recorded as well as the intensity and lateral resolution of the system.

As the pulse travels through the near zone, its diameter decreases; as it travels through the far zone, its diameter increases. The length of the near zone is determined by the operating frequency and the diameter (or aperture) of the transducer element(s). Both an increase in the operating frequency and diameter of the transducer will increase the near zone length or focal depth (Fig. 3.7). This relation is expressed as follows (6):

$$\text{Focal depth} = \frac{\text{diameter}^2 \times \text{frequency}}{61.6} \qquad (3.3)$$

or by using wavelength instead of frequency:

$$\text{Focal depth} = \frac{\text{diameter}^2}{4 \times \text{wavelength}} \qquad (3.4)$$

At a sufficient distance from the near zone, increasing the operating frequency or the aperture can decrease the beam diameter. Therefore, the width of the ultrasound beam depends on (*i*) the distance from the element, (*ii*) the diameter of the piezoelectric element, and (*iii*) the wavelength and the operating frequency. The concept of beam width is important because objects that are imaged at the end of the near zone where the beam width is narrow will generate images with a better lateral resolution. Beam width can be further reduced through focusing.

Although the ultrasound beam is often displayed in two dimensions (2D), it has a three-dimensional (3D)

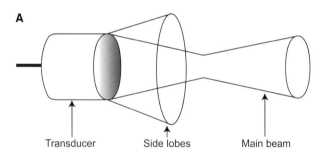

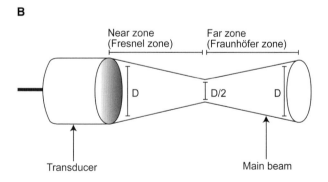

Figure 3.6 Ultrasound beam. (**A**) The single disc transducer creates an ultrasound beam comprised of a main beam and side lobes. (**B**) The near (Fresnel) and far (Fraunhöfer) zones of the main beam are shown. The diameter (D) of the near zone decreases until it reaches a value of one-half its initial D (= D/2) in the transition zone. It then increases in the far zone until it reaches its original diameter at twice the near zone length.

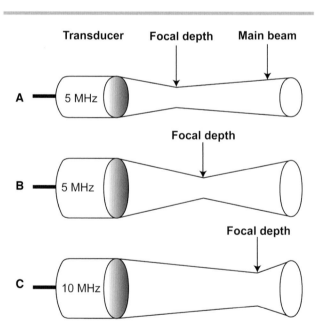

Figure 3.7 Beam shape. In an unfocused beam the length of the near zone and convergence angle in the far field depends on the transducer diameter and frequency. Compared with transducer (**A**), an increased diameter (**B**) increases the distance from the focal depth. As the frequency increases from a 5-MHz transducer (**B**) to a 10-MHz transducer (**C**) the near field is also lengthened. The near field distance is proportional to the diameter² and the frequency.

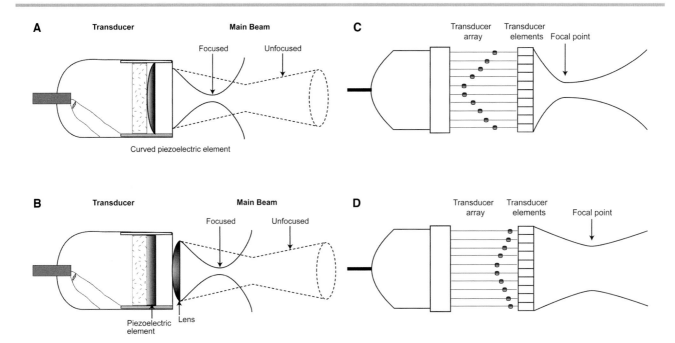

Figure 3.8 Beam focusing. Mechanical methods of ultrasound beam focusing using a curved piezoelectric crystal (**A**) or a flat crystal with a concave lens (**B**). The time-delay pattern using electronic methods of ultrasound beam activation determines the specific focus point and focal length. (**C**) A long delay in activation of the elements results in a greater curvature moving the focus region closer to the transducer. (**D**) The delay between element activation is decreased, producing a narrower curvature moving the focus region further away.

volume. The thickness of the ultrasound beam, also called the z-axis or elevation axis, is important because it determines the extent of section thickness artifact. This artifact occurs when the third dimension of the beam is collapsed to zero (1). The off-axis echoes often disappear when changing the position of the scan plane. These thickness artifacts can sometimes be seen when imaging the aortic arch and should not be confused with abnormal thickness of the aortic wall.

Focusing

Focusing consists of concentrating the beam to a smaller cross-sectional area—the focal region—to improve resolution. This process brings the end of the near zone closer to the transducer. The focal length, defined as the distance from the transducer to the focal region, is equal to, or shorter than, the near-zone length of the unfocused beam. The beam width decreases from the transducer to the focal region but increases beyond in the far zone. Beam focusing can be achieved by either mechanical or electronic means (Fig. 3.8).

With simple disk transducers, two methods of focusing have been described. Internal focusing that is achieved by applying a radius of curvature to the piezoelectric crystal and external focusing when the piezoelectric element is kept flat while a concave acoustic lens is placed in front of the crystal (Fig. 3.8).

Using multiple piezoelectric elements organized in a transducer array, focusing is achieved by electronic phasing. This consists of the successive activation of the different elements of the transducer array following a specific time-delay pattern. Varying activation time pattern creates different specific focus regions and allows the generation of multiple foci regions without modifying the curvature of a mechanical element (Fig. 3.8).

It is important to note that beam width changes as the focal length is increased. To maintain the same focal width, the number of elements activated has to change according to the focal length. For short focal lengths, a small number of the elements are activated, while for a focus placed further from the transducer, a larger percentage of the elements must be activated (Fig. 3.9). The ability to change the number of activated elements is referred to as variable or dynamic aperture. Likewise, the concept of dynamic reception focus refers to the ability to adjust the focus of the "listening" capability of the transducer to a given depth. This is analogous to the automatic focusing device in movie cameras, which changes the focus while tracking a moving object.

Side Lobes

As mentioned previously, side lobes represent weaker beams of sound that propagate in a direction different from that of the main beam originating from a single element. Grating lobes also represent weaker beams of sound that propagate in a direction different from that of the main beam. Grating lobes in contrast to side lobes are a result of the multi-element structure of the transducer array (1). If the side lobes or grating lobe beam encounter a strong reflector, their echoes may be imaged, particularly if they propagate in a

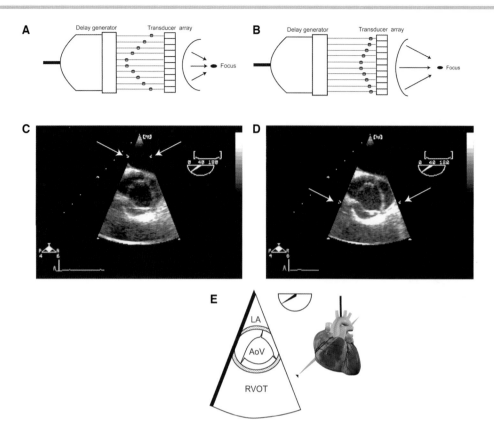

Figure 3.9 Beam focusing. (A–B) Dynamic aperture describes the activation of a different number of piezoelectric elements to maintain the focal width. **(C–D)** Examples of two mid-esophageal AoV short-axis views with different focus location obtained with electronic focusing. Notice the difference when the focus zone is not centered on the structure of interest, the AoV **(C)**, compared with an improved detail resolution when it is positioned over the AoV **(D)**. *Abbreviations:* AoV, aortic valve; LA, left atrium; RVOT, right ventricular outflow tract.

poorly echogenic region. Because the system assumes that the echoes originate from the main beam, the image is displayed in a position that differs from its true location and will usually cross anatomical boundaries. These artifacts are called side lobes or grating lobes artifacts (see Chapter 7).

In a transducer array, grating lobe artifacts can be minimized by dividing the elements into smaller pieces, a process known as subdicing (7). Further reduction of this artifact is achieved by applying different voltages to these elements. They usually disappear with readjustment of depth, angle, emitting frequency of the transducer, or by adjusting the mode of harmonic imaging.

Image Scanning

Scanning (or steering) is the process by which pulses are sent through many paths required to generate the cross-sectional image. The cross-sectional image is then assembled from the reconstruction of the focused ultrasound beams. Ultrasound beam scanning can be achieved by mechanical steering, electronic scanning, and electronic phasing. Mechanical steering is accomplished by oscillating or rotating a transducer element. This method is used with the intravascular ultrasound probe, where the ultrasound beam is made to turn

360° by rotating either the crystal or an ultrasound reflector or mirror. In electronic scanning (Fig. 3.10), the ultrasound beam is created by successively activating different subsets of transducer elements within an array, where each subset acts as a larger transducer element. Phasic scanning (Fig. 3.10) uses small time differences (phases) in stimulating piezoelectric element activity to generate beams with various orientations. Modern ultrasound transducers operate using mostly electronic scanning and phasing.

Generation of the Image

The initial step of ultrasound image generation involves the application of a short pulse of voltage to the electrodes of the piezoelectric crystal, resulting in vibration and a pulse wave of very short duration. The ultrasound pulse waves are then propagated into the surrounding medium where they will be both reflected and transmitted by the tissue interfaces encountered. The portion of sound energy returned to the transducer (the echo) causes conformational changes in the piezoelectric crystal, generating in turn an electrical charge on its surface. Because of its weak strength, this signal is then amplified. The receiver circuit can then determine the amplitude of

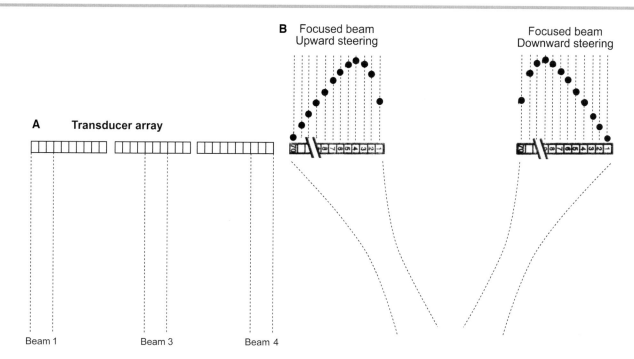

Figure 3.10 Beam steering. The difference between electronic scanning and phasing. (**A**) With electronic scanning, only a subset of piezoelectric crystals are successively activated. (**B**) During electronic phasing, sequential activation of all the piezoelectric crystals allows steering of the ultrasound beam.

the echo, its total travel time away from the transducer as well as the depth of the reflecting tissue. The amplitude of the echo determines the shade of gray it is assigned in the image. Each pulse produced by the ultrasound machine creates a single line of information. Only one pulse is required for each scan line, but with multifocus beam systems and color Doppler, numerous pulses can be used to generate each scan line. To produce an adequate image, 128 lines of information are normally used (Fig. 3.11).

To reduce the flicker of the image, 20 to 30 frames of information are required per second of viewing. The term pulse repetition frequency (PRF) is applied to the number of pulses generated in one second. Most modern transducers emit several thousand pulses per second. All echoes from one pulse must be received by the transducer before subsequent pulses can be emitted.

STRUCTURAL AND FUNCTIONAL CLASSIFICATION OF TRANSDUCERS

Table 3.1 classifies the transducer arrays according to their configuration, scanning, focusing, and image properties. One of the most common transducer arrays used in echocardiography is the vector array, in which phasing is applied to a linear sequenced array to generate focused pulses in different directions.

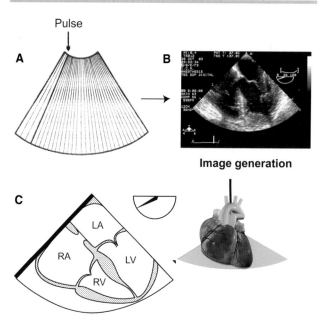

Figure 3.11 Image generation. (**A**) Each line in the image is created by a pulse. (**B,C**) Summation of all the lines creates the final 2D image of the mid-esophageal four-chamber view. *Abbreviations:* LA, left atrium; LV, left ventricle; RA, right atrium; RV, right ventricle.

Table 3.1 Transducer Arrays

Transducer array	Scanning or steering	Focusing	Image display
Mechanical sector	Motor drive	Curved lens or element	Sector
Linear array	Electronic sequencing	Electronic phasing	Rectangular
Phased linear array	Electronic sequencing	Electronic phasing	Parallelogram
Convex array	Electronic sequencing	Intrinsic property due to its configuration	Sector
Phased convex array	Electronic sequencing	Electronic phasing	Sector
Annular array	Motor drive	Electronic phasing	Sector
Vector array	Electronic sequencing and electronic phasing	Electronic phasing	Sector

IMAGE QUALITY

Resolution is a characteristic that describes the quality of the image. It allows echoes to be distinguished in terms of space, intensity, and time and displayed in their correct anatomic position. These are known as spatial, contrast, and temporal resolution, respectively.

Resolution

Detail Resolution

Detail, linear, or spatial resolution refers to the ability of the imaging system to represent two closely related but spatially distinct objects (ultrasound reflectors) as separate (or resolved) nonoverlapping echoes. As spatial resolution is the minimum reflector separation required to discriminate between two objects, the smaller the value of resolution, the better the imaging system. There are three components to spatial resolution: axial, lateral, and elevational (Fig. 3.12).

Axial. Axial (longitudinal, depth) resolution is the ability to separate two objects spatially along the direction of the ultrasound beam (scan line). It is affected by the spatial pulse length (SPL, the length that a pulse takes up), equal to the product of wavelength (λ) by the number of cycles in the pulse (n).

$$\text{Axial resolution} = \frac{\text{SPL}}{2} = \frac{\lambda n}{2} \qquad (3.5)$$

Therefore, axial resolution is improved by decreasing both the wavelength and the number of cycles per pulse. The latter is determined by the damping material in the transducer and, currently, cannot be modified by the user. On the other hand, wavelength can be reduced by increasing the transducer imaging frequency, an operation that is easily accessible to the imaging system operator (Fig. 3.13). However, the drawback in increasing frequency for better resolution is higher attenuation with imaging depth and consequently a reduction in penetration capability.

Lateral. Lateral resolution represents the ability to discriminate between two objects lying perpendicular to the ultrasound beam direction (scan line). It is determined by the beam width: if the spatial separation between two objects is greater than the beam width, two different echoes can be generated and resolved as the beam is scanned across them. Because beam width

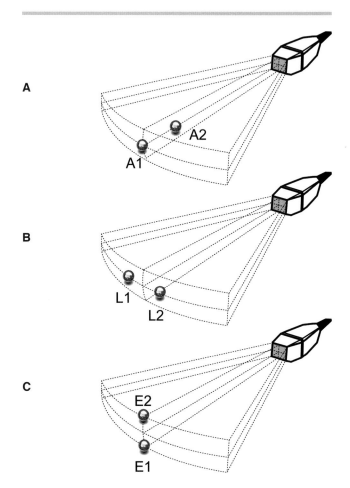

Figure 3.12 Types of spatial resolution. Spatial resolution is the ability to create images of small structures accurately in their correct anatomic position and involves three components: (**A**) axial (A1 and A2), (**B**) lateral (L1 and L2) and (**C**) elevational (E1 and E2).

changes with the distance from the transducer, so does lateral resolution. In an unfocused beam, the best lateral resolution is seen at the transition or focal zone (Fig. 3.7). At the focal zone, the lateral resolution will be determined by the probe frequency or wavelength (λ), the focal length (L) and the diameter (aperture) of the element.

$$\text{Lateral resolution} = \text{beam width} = \frac{2.4\lambda L}{d} \qquad (3.6)$$

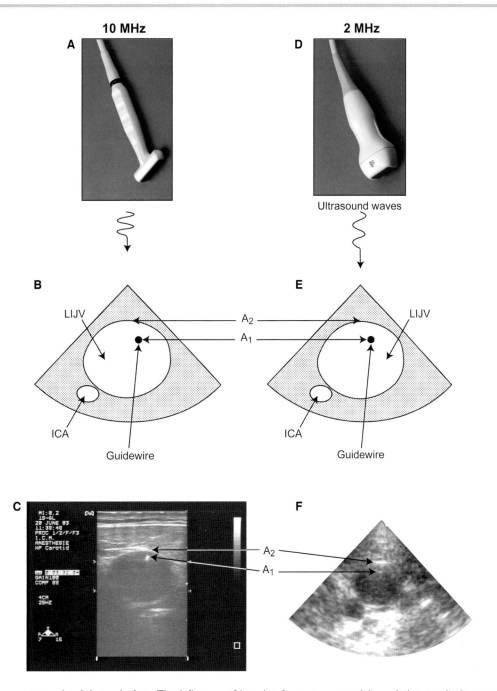

Figure 3.13 **Frequency and axial resolution.** The influence of imaging frequency on axial resolution results in separate echoes of closely spaced reflectors (A1 and A2). In this example, the 10-MHz probe (**A–C**) allows better discrimination of the LIJV and the guidewire compared with the 2-MHz transducer (**D–F**). However, with higher frequency of imaging, beam attenuation is higher, resulting in less penetration: the deeper ICA is less well visualized in (**C**) compared to (**F**). *Abbreviations:* ICA, internal carotid artery; LIJV, left internal jugular vein.

Lateral resolution can be improved by reducing the beam diameter through focusing (Fig. 3.8). In the focused beam, the best lateral resolution will be found at the focal point.

Relationship between axial and lateral resolution. Axial and lateral resolutions are not independent of each other. Indeed, beam width, and therefore, lateral resolution, is influenced by the pulse bandwidth. The pulse bandwidth is related to spatial pulse length, which is a determinant of axial resolution.

Elevational. Elevational resolution is the ability to separate reflectors that are in different 2D planes (Fig. 3.12). The sound beam has a thickness of 3 to 10 mm depending on depth and the specific transducer. Structures may be present in the thickness of the beam or side lobes and may be represented as artifacts on the display. Echoes arising from near the edge of the beam are displayed as if they are located in the main beam.

Contrast Resolution

Contrast resolution refers to the ability to discriminate subtle echo-strength (or intensity) differences between two adjacent reflectors. Depending on the respective difference in amplitude signal of separate echoes, the echographic system assigns a different shade of gray, that is, a different number of bits per pixel. Weak echoes are assigned darker shades of gray, while strong reflectors are placed at the white end of the scale. Contrast resolution will be improved by increasing the number of bits per pixel or by having a greater number of gray shades available.

Compression is an operator-adjustable function that can adjust the dynamic range of signal amplitude, that is, it can change the value assigned to the highest and lowest value of the returning signal amplitude. By adjusting the level of compression, the operator can choose the best dynamic range to optimize the contrast resolution of the image (see Fig. 1.16). As the dynamic range is decreased, a smaller difference in intensity is required to be assigned a different shade of gray. Contrast resolution has a direct influence on detail resolution because it influences the recognition of overlapping pulses. With better contrast, a system can recognize important wave overlap. The better the contrast resolution, the greater is the spatial resolution.

Temporal Resolution

Temporal resolution refers to the ability of the echographic system to discriminate between two closely related events in time. Without temporal resolution, imaging of valve motion or heart contraction would be impossible. Temporal resolution is directly related to frame rate, which represents the number of ultrasound images (or frames) stored by seconds (see Chapter 1, section "Imaging—Related Factors"). As frame rate increases, the temporal resolution improves. Because each frame is made of scan lines, the PRF required will depend on the number of focus zones, lines per frame, and the frame rate. To improve temporal resolution, the operator can reduce the width of the sector image (see Fig. 1.20) or the number of focus areas.

Attenuation and Penetration

As ultrasound propagates in tissue, it loses energy progressively and attenuation occurs. The mechanisms involved in attenuation include the conversion of ultrasound energy to heat (a process called absorption) as well as reflection and scattering (see Chapter 1). Attenuation is frequency dependent, with the lower frequencies having a greater depth of penetration than higher frequencies.

$$\text{Penetration} = \frac{1}{\text{Operating frequency}} \quad (3.7)$$

In clinical echocardiography, the transducer frequency is chosen to provide the best axial resolution

Table 3.2 Axial Resolution, Penetration, and Frequency

Frequency (MHz)	Depth (cm)	Axial resolution (mm)
2.0	30	0.77
3.5	17	0.44
5.0	12	0.31
7.5	8	0.20
10.0	6	0.15
15.0	4	0.10

Table 3.3 Typical Operating Frequencies Used with Different Transducers

Transducer type	Usual probe frequency (MHz)
Transthoracic probe	
• Newborn	7.5–12.0
• Child	5.0–7.5
• Adult	2.5–3.5
Transesophageal probe	5.0–10.0
Intravascular ultrasound	10.0–40.0

while maintaining ultrasound penetration to a desirable depth. Table 3.2 lists the typical imaging depth and axial resolution of two-cycle pulses in tissue. Table 3.3 lists the typical operating frequencies used with different transducers.

HARMONIC IMAGING

Improved transducer technology has made tissue harmonic imaging possible. Harmonics are generated in the body by interaction of the ultrasound beam with tissue. When sound passes through tissue it compresses, increasing the speed of sound, and expands the tissue, lowering the speed of sound. The tissue distortion causes a resonance of twice or more of the fundamental frequency. These multiples of the fundamental frequency are called harmonics. Tissue harmonic imaging is a signal processing technique in which the transducer transmits at its fundamental frequency and receives at twice this frequency (second harmonic). The returning signal contains both the fundamental and harmonic frequencies. A receiving filter is set specifically to receive harmonic frequencies while filtering out the fundamental frequencies.

This method significantly improves the image quality in several ways. First, the source of harmonic frequencies is the target object and not the transducer. The travel distance to the receiver is, therefore, halved, reducing the potential for signal degradation. Most of the artifacts generated in the near field, before the ultrasound beam from the transducer reaches the object, are also eliminated. Moreover, grating lobe artifacts (additional side beams emitted from multiple-element array transducers) caused by strong reflectors are eliminated as those side beams are not sufficiently powerful to generate harmonic frequencies. Finally, because the minimum power required to generate harmonics will be reduced to the higher-intensity portion of the ultrasound beam, the resulting

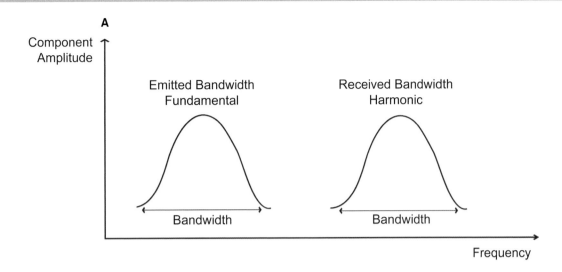

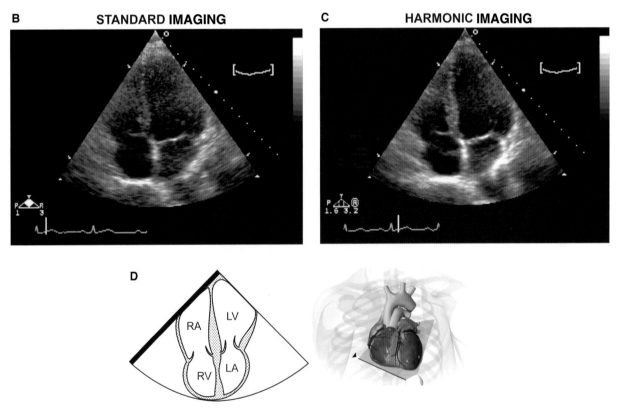

Figure 3.14 Harmonic imaging principle. (A) An ultrasound beam is emitted at a fundamental frequency but reflected echoes are selectively received at harmonics (multiples) of the fundamental frequency. This results in improved detail resolution because of the higher frequency. **(B–D)** Transthoracic apical four-chamber view shows the difference between fundamental **(B)** and harmonic **(C)** imaging. *Abbreviations:* LA, left atrium; LV, left ventricle; RA, right atrium; RV, right ventricle.

"harmonic-generating" beam will have a smaller beam width, improving resolution (Fig. 3.14).

3D IMAGING

Recent progress in matrix phased-array transducer (8) technology has opened a new era in real-time volumetric 3D echocardiography. The development of 3D fully sampled matrix array transducers has allowed real-time acquisition and online display of 3D images (Fig. 3.15). These transducers contain about 3000 piezoelectric elements and 150 computer boards. They combine novel electronic circuitry with miniaturized beam-forming technology in the tip of otherwise conventional probes. Parallel processing

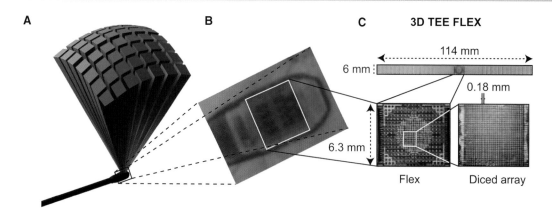

Figure 3.15   3D transducer and imaging. (**A**) The 3D TEE transducer contains a matrix array of individually functioning crystals. (**B**) Fluoroscopic image of a 3D TEE probe. (**C**) Close up view of the flex and the diced array. The thickness is shown on top. *Abbreviation:* TEE, transesophageal echocardiography. *Source:* Courtesy of Philips Healthcare.

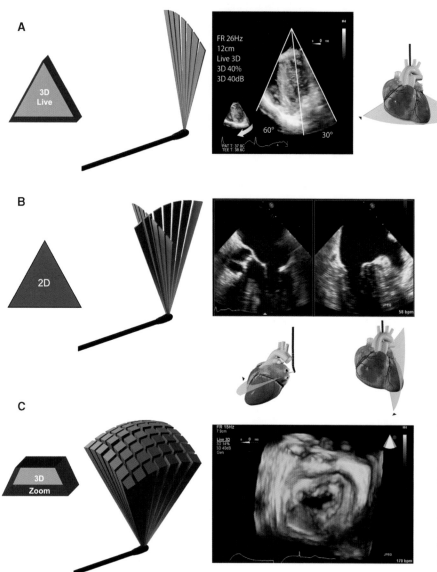

Figure 3.16   3D imaging modes. The 3D transesophageal transducer contains a matrix array of 2500 elements. (**A**) The 3D live imaging mode uses a plane with defined thickness shown in the ME four-chamber view. (**B**) The biplane mode displays two simultaneous 2D images shown in the ME five-chamber and two-chamber views. (**C**) The 3D zoom acquisition uses data from the selected part of the pyramidal volume as shown here for the mitral valve as viewed from the left atrium. Abbreviation: ME, mid-esophageal.

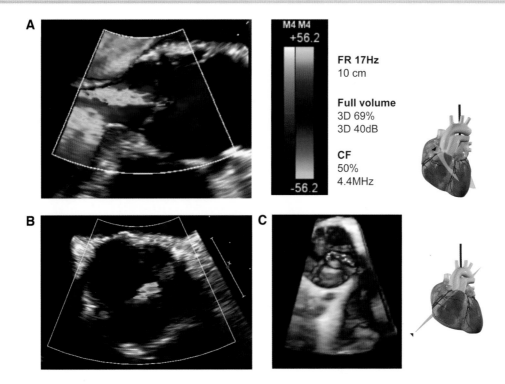

Figure 3.17   3D color Doppler. The use of 3D color Doppler requires acquisition of a gated full volume. (**A**) Mid-esophageal long-axis and (**B**) short-axis 2D color Doppler zoomed views of a jet of AR are shown originating from the commissure between the right and left coronary cusps. (**C**) 3D color Doppler view of the aortic valve as viewed from the aortic root side. *Abbreviations*: AR, aortic regurgitation; CF, color flow; FR, frequency.

technology is used to meet the challenge of processing the huge volume of information generated by matrix-array transducers. These transducers can scan a 3D volume by electronically steering the acoustic beam, allowing a scanning of a pyramidal volume in real time with acceptable resolution.

All major imaging companies are developing real-time 3D TEE systems, but currently the only commercially available technology is the X7-2t transducer (IE-33, Philips Healthcare, Bothell, Washington, U.S.). In addition to routine 2D scanning, the matrix probe allows scanning and display of two different 2D ultrasound planes simultaneously (Live xPlane mode) without moving the probe (Fig. 3.16A). There are four 3D acquisition modes:

1. Live 3D mode displays a real-time narrow angle 3D pyramidal volume with fixed dimensions of 30° by 60° (Fig. 3.16B). It can assess the heart using the standard TEE views.
2. Full-volume acquisition mode is an ECG-gated acquisition of a large 3D pyramidal volume with fixed dimensions of 90° by 90° (Fig. 3.16C).
3. 3D zoom mode displays a magnified subsection of 3D pyramidal volume that can vary in dimensions from 20° by 20° to 90° by 90° (Fig. 3.16D).
4. 3D full-volume color Doppler mode is a gated acquisition of a small 3D pyramidal volume with superimposed 3D representation of color Doppler

flow (Fig. 3.17). Current technology is limited and only allows creation of a small 3D volume at a low frame rate (<20 fps).

Appraisal of real-time 3D TEE is becoming more frequent in the medical literature as the technique is gaining in interest. There are more and more studies and case reports comparing 3D TEE and 2D TEE in the perioperative setting. There seems to be an agreement that 3D TEE allows better visualization of complex cardiac pathologies such as mitral valve disease and congenital heart disease. Some of the presumed advantages of 3D TEE over conventional TEE are extrapolated from studies comparing the latest to 3D transthoracic echocardiography generally done without the need of sedation. The role of 3D TEE in cardiac surgery has been recently reviewed (9) and will be discussed in the upcoming chapters.

REFERENCES

1. Kremkau FW. Diagnostic Ultrasound: Principles and Instruments. 6th ed. Philadelphia: W.B. Saunders, 2002.
2. Ballato A. Piezoelectricity: old effect, new thrusts. IEEE Trans Ultrason Ferroelectr Freq Control 1995; 42:916–926.
3. Weyman AE. Principles and Practice of Echocardiography. 2nd ed. Philadelphia: Lea & Febiger, 1994.
4. Rengasamy S, Subramaniam B. Basic physics of transesophageal echocardiography. Int Anesthesiol Clin 2008; 46:11–29.

5. Duck FA. Physical Properties of Tissue. New York: Academic Press, 1990.

6. Edelman K. Understanding Ultrasound Physics. Woodlands, TX: ESP, 2007.

7. Otto CM. Textbook of Clinical Echocardiography. 2nd ed. Philadelphia: W.B. Saunders, 2000.

8. Sugeng L, Coon P, Weinert L, et al. Use of real-time 3-dimensional transthoracic echocardiography in the evaluation of mitral valve disease. J Am Soc Echocardiogr 2006; 19:413–421.

9. Vegas A, Meineri M. Core review: three-dimensional transesophageal echocardiography is a major advance for intraoperative clinical management of patients undergoing cardiac surgery: a core review. Anesth Analg 2010; 110:1548–1573.

4

Normal Anatomy and Flow

George N. Honos, Nicolas Dürrleman, and André Y. Denault
Université de Montréal, Montreal, Quebec, Canada

Jean Buithieu
McGill University, Montreal, Quebec, Canada

NORMAL ANATOMY AND FLOW DURING THE COMPLETE EXAMINATION

Systematic Transesophageal Echocardiography Examination and Imaging Planes

Transesophageal Echocardiography Probe Manipulation

Following successful insertion into the patient's esophagus, the operator manipulates the transesophageal echocardiography (TEE) probe to obtain the desired cross-sectional images of the heart (1). Because of variation in the anatomic relationship between the esophagus and the heart, manipulation must be individualized and based on the images that unfold on the echo system's display. Moreover, unlike comprehensive transthoracic imaging, where a systematic approach is generally preferred, a TEE study should be tailored to address the clinical question first, followed by the acquisition of other standard views and Doppler information. This initial targeted approach is prudent to ensure that the TEE study is diagnostic in the event that the examination must be terminated quickly or postponed due to patient discomfort or clinical instability (2).

The TEE probe can be manipulated as follows to acquire images (Fig. 4.1):

- Advancement/withdrawal (to view inferior or superior structures, respectively)
- Rotation (clockwise to view rightward structures and counterclockwise to view leftward structures)
- Anteflexion and retroflexion of the probe shaft (to view structures toward the heart base or toward the apex)
- Leftward and rightward flexion of the probe shaft (used infrequently, with the advent of multiplane probes)
- Electronic image plane rotation (0–180°, where 0° represents a transverse plane, perpendicular to the length of the probe).

Manipulation of the TEE probe begins with advancement or withdrawal to specific levels within the upper gastrointestinal tract adjacent to the heart and vascular structures. Standard imaging plane levels (with their average distance from the incisors) include upper or high esophageal (25–28 cm), mid-esophageal (29–33 cm), gastroesophageal junction (34–37 cm), transgastric (38–42 cm), and deep transgastric (>42 cm).

At each imaging level, a multiplane TEE probe provides a continuous range of transverse and longitudinal images of the heart by electronic rotation of the transducer sector scan. Images can be acquired continuously through a 180° arc, producing an unlimited number of possible two-dimensional (2D) views of the heart. The electronic orientation of the ultrasound beam relative to the probe is usually indicated in degrees and with an icon on the ultrasound display. Finally, additional rotation (clockwise = rightward and counterclockwise = leftward) and flexion (anteflexion, retroflexion, leftward, and rightward flexion) of the probe shaft are used to optimize visualization of selected anatomic structures.

While there is considerable variation between patients, certain electronic imaging angles are useful as a starting point in most studies as they relate to specific transverse or longitudinal sections through the heart as listed in Table 4.1.

Conventions of Image Display

Modern ultrasound systems allow the acquired 2D images to be rotated electronically (up-down, left-right) before displaying them on screen. By convention, the American Society of Echocardiography (ASE) and the Society of Cardiovascular Anesthesiologists (SCA) recommend positioning the apex of the 2D sector at the top for transthoracic echocardiography (TTE) and for TEE, with left cardiac structures on the right of the display (Fig. 4.2). However, there are exceptions in certain circumstances, such as in pediatric echocardiograms where the apex of the 2D sector is displayed at the bottom of the screen for certain views.

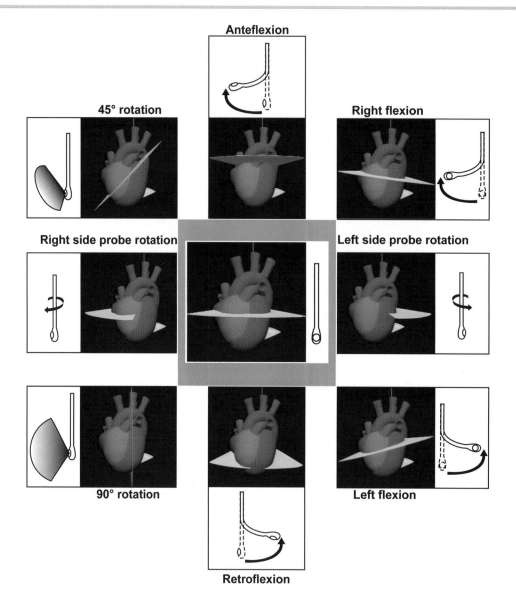

Figure 4.1   TEE probe manipulation. Graphical display of TEE probe manipulation and plane orientation is shown. *Abbreviation*: TEE, transesophageal echocardiography.

Table 4.1   TEE Probe Orientation

Orientation	Description and features of view
0°	Transverse plane to the probe LAX Horizontal to the plane of the body Oblique to cardiac SAX
45°	SAX view of cardiac basal structures (e.g., aortic valve)
90°	Longitudinal plane (parallel to the probe LAX) Sagittal (vertical) to the plane of the body Oblique to the cardiac LAX Parallel to the ascending aorta
135°	LAX view of cardiac structures (LV and LVOT)
180°	Mirror image of the 0° transverse plane

Abbreviations: LAX, long axis; LV, left ventricle; LVOT, left ventricular outflow tract; SAX, short axis.

Some centers (such as the Mayo Clinic) prefer flipping the TEE images sector with the apex down to reproduce the 2D cardiac views that are anatomically comparable with those obtained from transthoracic surface imaging. In this chapter, the more widespread SCA and ASE display orientation will be utilized for clarity and consistency.

Views and Structures

A comprehensive multiplane TEE examination, as recommended by the SCA and ASE, consists of acquiring 2D images and Doppler data by skillful manipulation of the multiplane TEE probe through a series of positions in the patient's esophagus and stomach (Fig. 4.3) (3). The operator systematically

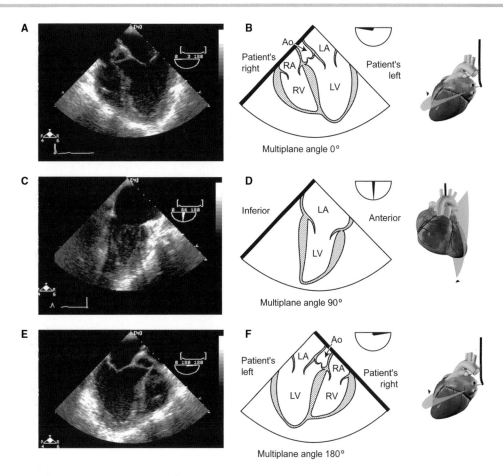

Figure 4.2 TEE display convention. Display convention of TEE images showing the mid-esophageal 0° (**A,B**), 90° (**C,D**) and 180° (**E,F**) views. The broader line on the 2D diagram display corresponds to the arrowhead on the 3D icon. By convention, the dark line corresponds to the right side of the ultrasound beam and the display. *Abbreviations*: Ao, aorta; LA, left atrium; LV, left ventricle; RA, right atrium; RV, right ventricle; TEE, transesophageal echocardiography.

progresses from views obtained with the transducer tip in the mid to gradually more distal esophagus, stomach fundus after gentle advancement across the cardia, and finally slow withdrawal of the probe while a complete scan of the thoracic aorta (Ao) is obtained from high esophageal views. An organized approach avoids excessive to and fro movement of the probe and reduces patient discomfort while ensuring that all cardiovascular structures are appropriately and consistently evaluated. A complete TEE examination usually takes 15–20 minutes in a nonteaching environment. An abbreviated, or problem-focused, TEE study may occasionally be appropriate in unstable or uncooperative patients, where the operator feels that there might not be sufficient time to obtain all possible views.

The TEE examination usually begins with the insertion of the probe tip to the mid-esophageal position and oriented anteriorly. From this position, at 0°, multiple basal cardiac structures are visualized.

Tip: The operator makes fine adjustments in probe tip insertion, rotation, and anteflexion to position the probe in the middle of the left atrium (LA), where optimal esophageal mucosal apposition with minimal interfering tissues will usually provide the best image quality. This is easier when the LA is large and is inversely more difficult to do in young normal patients because of a small LA window. This is a good time for the operator to adjust the image depth as well as gain settings on the echo system. These are likely to remain the same until imaging of the descending Ao is performed at a shallower depth just prior to study completion.

Mid-esophageal Views

The mid-esophageal four-chamber view depicts the left and right ventricles (LV, RV), LA and right atrium (RA), atrial septum, and mitral and tricuspid valves (MV, TV) (Figs. 4.3A1 and 4.4). However, the apex of the LV is usually foreshortened, precluding optimal

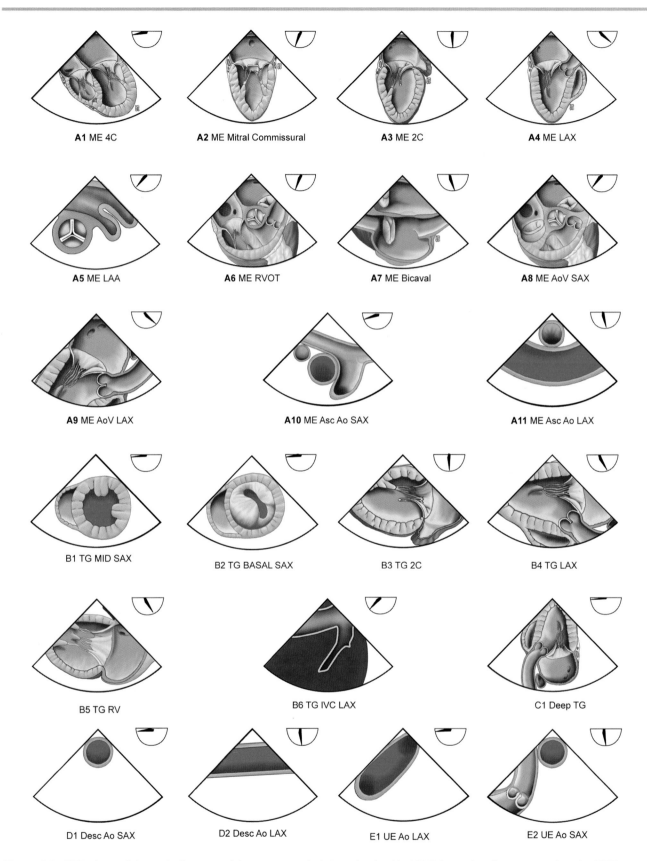

Figure 4.3   TEE views. Schematic diagrams of the recommended views (revised in 2008) for performing a comprehensive TEE exam. *Abbreviations*: Ao, aorta; Asc, ascending; AoV, aortic valve; C, chamber; Desc, descending; IVC, inferior vena cava; LAA, left atrial appendage; LAX, long axis; ME, mid-esophageal; RV, right ventricle; RVOT, right ventricular outflow; SAX, short axis; TEE, transesophageal echocardiography; TG, transgastric; UE, upper esophageal. *Source*: Adapted from Ref. 3 and www.asecho.org. Drawings courtesy of Gian-Marco Busato.

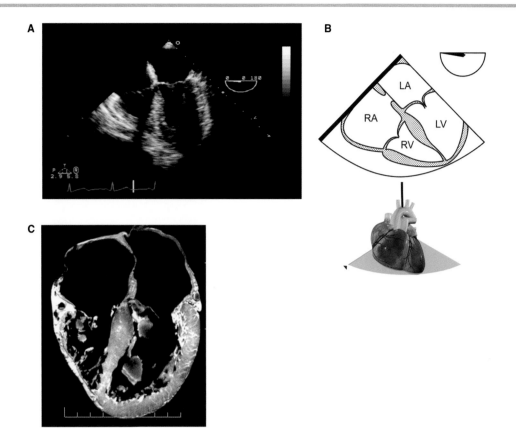

Figure 4.4 Mid-esophageal four-chamber view. This view at 0° (**A,B**) shows all four cardiac chambers compared with a magnetic resonance image (**C**). *Abbreviations*: LA, left atrium; LV, left ventricle; RA, right atrium; RV, right ventricle.

visualization of the true anatomical apex. This can sometimes be corrected by further probe retroflexion, but loss of esophageal mucosal contact and image degradation are common limiting factors. The study proceeds with the examination of the MV apparatus, a 0° to 135° sweep in 2D, to assess structure and mobility of leaflets, then 135° back sweep to 0° with color Doppler flow to detect and characterize mitral regurgitation (MR).

Transgastric Views

The probe is advanced from the mid-esophageal position through the lower esophageal sphincter into the stomach. At 0° with anteflexion of the probe tip and gentle advancement or withdrawal, a short-axis (SAX) view of the LV at the papillary muscle level is obtained (Figs. 4.3B1 and 4.5). From this position, withdrawal or anteflexion of the probe tip often allows a SAX view of the MV (Figs. 4.3B2 and 4.6), while further insertion or retroflexion of the probe tip will allow evaluation of the LV apex.

From the 0° SAX view of the LV, rotation of the plane to 90° provides a longitudinal two-chamber view of the LV (Figs. 4.3B3 and 4.7). Rightward (clockwise) rotation from this position results in a two-chamber view of the right heart chambers with the RA and RV together with the TV (Figs. 4.3B5 and 4.8).

From the two-chamber view of the LA and LV at 90°, further transducer rotation to 100° to 135° may yield a long-axis (LAX) view of the LV and left ventricular outflow tract (LVOT) (Figs. 4.3B4 and 4.9). From this position, parallel cursor alignment with the LVOT allows for continuous wave (CW) Doppler measurement of maximal flow velocity across the aortic valve (AoV) and pulsed wave (PW) Doppler measurement of LVOT velocity-time integral (VTI) for the assessment of cardiac output (CO) by volumetric Doppler method.

Thoracic Aorta Views

Gradual withdrawal of the TEE probe from the transgastric position allows for visualization of the descending thoracic Ao and aortic arch. With the transducer at 0°, the operator begins by probe withdrawal to the level of the cardia and rotation of the probe tip counterclockwise about 180° to visualize the descending thoracic Ao in a transverse view as a circular dark (blood filled) structure in the near field. The entire length of the descending thoracic

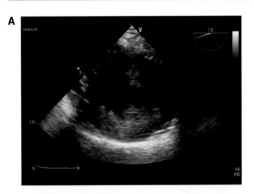

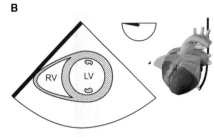

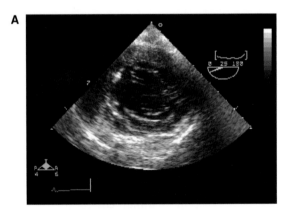

1 Tricuspid valve
2 Ventricular septum
3 Aortic valve
4 Mitral valve
5 Papillary muscles
6 Mitral aortic continuity
7 Left ventricular wall
8 Right ventricular wall

Figure 4.5 Transgastric mid short-axis view. This view at 18° (**A,B**) of the LV at the mid-papillary level with anatomical correlation (**C**) is seen. *Abbreviations*: LV, left ventricle; RV, right ventricle.

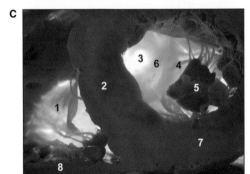

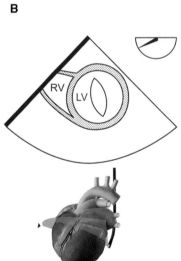

POSTERIOR

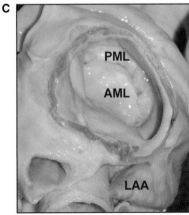

ANTERIOR

Figure 4.6 Transgastric basal short-axis view. This view at 0° (**A,B**) of the mitral valve with anatomical correlation (**C**) is shown. *Abbreviations*: AML, anterior mitral valve leaflet; LAA, left atrial appendage; LV, left ventricle; PML, posterior mitral valve leaflet; RV, right ventricle.

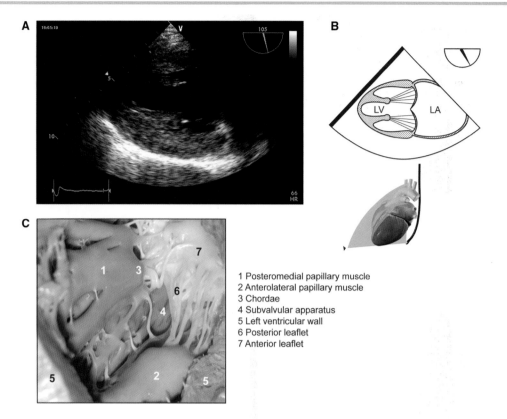

Figure 4.7 Transgastric two-chamber view. This view at 105° **(A,B)** of the LV with anatomical correlation **(C)** is shown. *Abbreviations*: LA, left atrium, LV, left ventricle.

1 Posteromedial papillary muscle
2 Anterolateral papillary muscle
3 Chordae
4 Subvalvular apparatus
5 Left ventricular wall
6 Posterior leaflet
7 Anterior leaflet

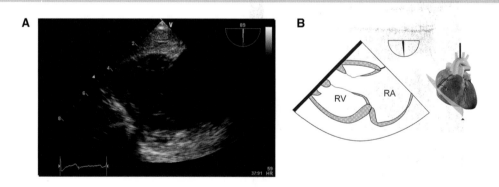

Figure 4.8 Transgastric right ventricular inflow view. (A,B) This view at 89° in a 20-year-old woman is shown. *Abbreviations*: RA, right atrium; RV, right ventricle.

Ao is then imaged with gradual pullback and slight clockwise rotation, keeping the Ao centered on the screen. The operator may switch between transverse at 0° (Figs. 4.3D1 and 4.10) and longitudinal at 90° (Figs. 4.3D2 and 4.10) views at different depths to better visualize any pathology.

The position of identified abnormalities is recorded in centimeters from the patient's incisors by reading the distance from the scale on the probe. During pullback, color Doppler flow imaging can assist in differentiating artifactual from true anatomical echo densities in the aortic lumen as well as depicting the site of reentry and true and false lumens of a dissected Ao.

When the probe tip withdrawal reaches the level of the aortic arch, pullback is stopped while clockwise

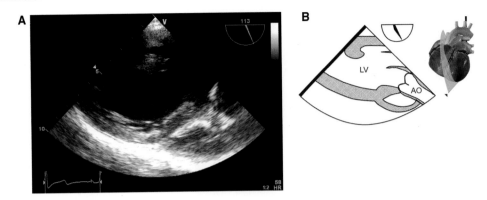

Figure 4.9 Transgastric long-axis view. (A,B) This view at 113° of the LV and aortic valve in a 20-year-old woman is shown. *Abbreviations*: Ao, aorta; LV, left ventricle.

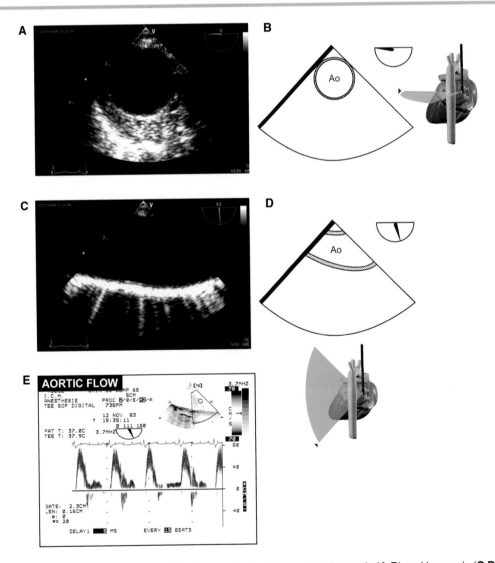

Figure 4.10 Descending thoracic aorta views. The descending Ao is imaged in short-axis (**A,B**) and long-axis (**C,D**) views. A pulsed wave Doppler signal of aortic flow is obtained by placing the sample volume in the proximal portion of the descending Ao (**E**). *Abbreviations*: Ao, aorta.

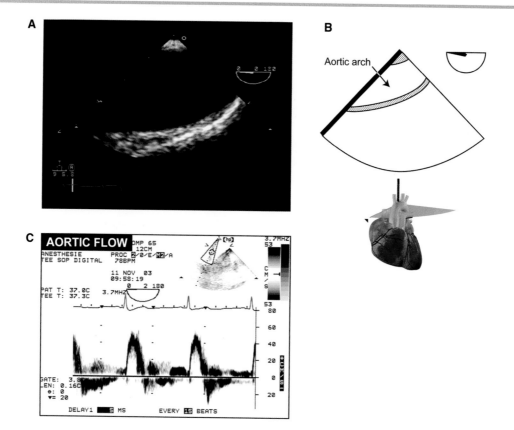

Figure 4.11 Upper esophageal aortic arch long-axis view. This view (**A,B**) with pulsed wave Doppler signal of aortic flow sampled from the mid portion of the aortic arch (**C**) is shown. ⌐

rotation provides a longitudinal view of the arch and (Figs. 4.3E1 and 4.11) further rotation reveals the distal ascending Ao.

Tip: During imaging of the Ao, the operator should optimize depth and gain settings to allow the Ao to fill about two-thirds of the imaging sector. Sometimes, all the walls of the Ao may not be viewed at the same time on the sector scan and, therefore, some left and right rotations may be necessary during the pullback to assess all the walls of the Ao completely.

Anatomy and Physiology

Cardiac Chambers

Left ventricle. It is important to describe size, wall thickness, and global and segmental systolic function of the LV. Analysis by TEE of the contractility of all 16 LV segments requires five views: three mid-esophageal views (four-chamber, two-chamber, and LAX views) and two transgastric views (mid and basal SAX views) (see Chapter 9). The apical segments are often difficult to evaluate because of the foreshortening of the LV. A visual assessment of global systolic function and ejection fraction should

be possible from the different views of the LV used for segmental wall motion assessment. Diastolic LV function can be assessed from spectral Doppler and color M-mode MV inflow, mitral annulus tissue Doppler, and pulmonary venous flow patterns (see Chapter 10).

Left ventricular outflow tract. The LVOT is imaged from the mid-esophageal position at 0° (Fig. 4.12) and at 135° (Figs. 4.3A4 and 4.13), as well as from the transgastric view at 110° (Figs. 4.3B4 and 4.9) and the deep transgastric view (Figs. 4.3C1 and 4.14). The latter two views allow the optimal ultrasound beam alignment for Doppler flow velocity measurement.

Right ventricle (inflow chamber, outflow tract). The RV has an inflow chamber and a right ventricular outflow tract (RVOT). The RV inflow chamber is imaged from the mid-esophageal position at 0° with slight retroflexion (four-chamber view) (Figs. 4.3A1 and 4.15) as well as from the transgastric position at 90° with rightward rotation (Fig. 4.8). Both inflow chamber and RVOT are seen simultaneously from the mid-esophageal position at 60° to 90° with slight rightward rotation (Figs. 4.3A6 and 4.16), or from a transgastric position at 60° to 90° (Fig. 4.17). The RVOT, pulmonic valve (PV), pulmonary artery trunk, and proximal right and left pulmonary arteries

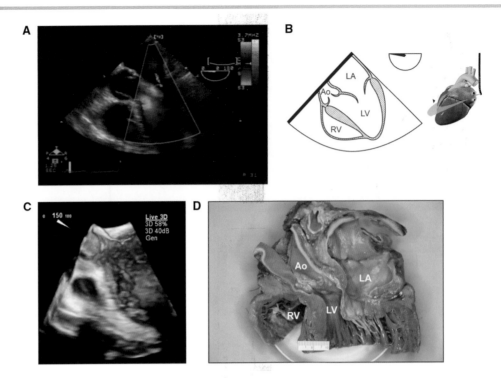

Figure 4.12   Modified ME four-chamber view. The ME long-axis view of the left ventricular outflow tract at 0° with color Doppler (**A,B**), 3D echocardiogram (**C**) and anatomical correlation (**D**) are shown. *Abbreviations*: Ao, aorta; LA, left atrium; LV, left ventricle; ME, mid-esophageal; RV, right ventricle.

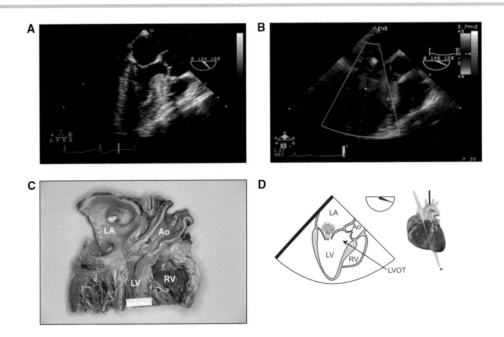

Figure 4.13   Mid-esophageal long-axis view. This view at 146° (**A**) of the LV with color Doppler (**B,D**) in the LVOT and anatomical correlation (**C**) are shown. *Abbreviations*: Ao, aorta; LA, left atrium; LV, left ventricle; LVOT, left ventricular outflow tract; RV, right ventricle.

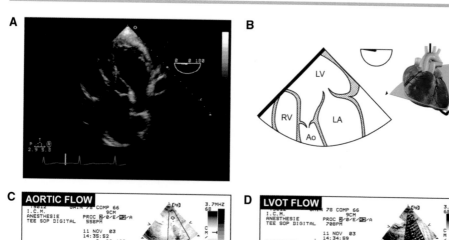

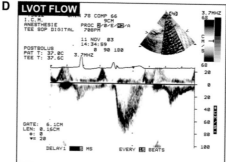

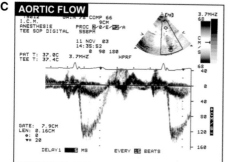

Figure 4.14 Deep transgastric long-axis view. This view at 0° (**A,B**) with pulsed wave Doppler interrogation of the ascending Ao flow (**C**) and LVOT flow (**D**) are shown. *Abbreviations*: Ao, aorta; LA, left atrium; LV, left ventricle; LVOT, left ventricular outflow tract RV, right ventricle.

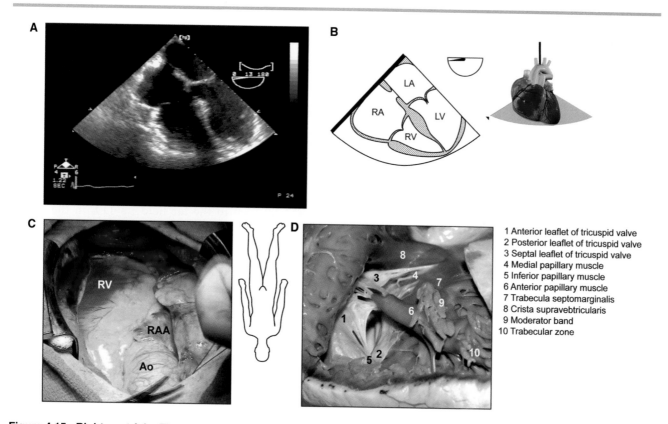

1 Anterior leaflet of tricuspid valve
2 Posterior leaflet of tricuspid valve
3 Septal leaflet of tricuspid valve
4 Medial papillary muscle
5 Inferior papillary muscle
6 Anterior papillary muscle
7 Trabecula septomarginalis
8 Crista supravebtricularis
9 Moderator band
10 Trabecular zone

Figure 4.15 Right ventricle. The mid-esophageal four-chamber view (**A,B**) of the RV compared with an intraoperative view (**C**) and anatomical correlation (**D**). *Abbreviations*: Ao, aorta; LA, left atrium; LV, left ventricle; RA, right atrium; RAA, right atrial appendage; RV, right ventricle. *Source*: Photo C courtesy of Dr. Michel Pellerin.

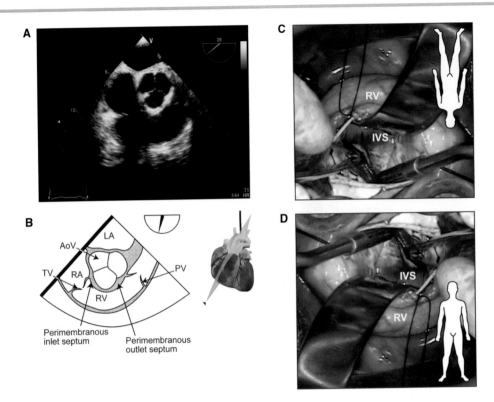

Figure 4.16 Mid-esophageal right ventricular inflow/outflow view. (A,B) This view at 72° is shown. The surgical view (**C**) is repositioned to correlate better with the echocardiographic window (**D**). *Abbreviations*: AoV, aortic valve; IVS, interventricular septum; LA, left atrium; PV, pulmonic valve; RA, right atrium; RV, right ventricle, TV, tricuspid valve. *Source*: Photo C courtesy of Dr. Nancy Poirier.

(RPA and LPA) are viewed from the mid-esophageal position with anteflexion (Figs. 4.3A6 and 4.18).

Left atrium. The LA, located anterior to the esophagus, can be easily imaged from all mid-esophageal views, including five-chamber, four-chamber, two-chamber, the LAX as well as the 90° bicaval positions (Figs. 4.3A7 and 4.19).

Right atrium. The RA is best visualized by TEE in the mid-esophageal four-chamber view at 0° with slight retroflexion (Figs. 4.3A1 and 4.15) and also in the 90° bicaval view (Figs. 4.3A7 and 4.19), and the RV inflow-outflow view at 60° to 90° (Figs. 4.3A6 and 4.16).

Cardiac Appendages

Left atrial appendage. The left atrial appendage (LAA) is imaged with an initial orientation of 0° to 45° (Fig. 4.3A5) and slight leftward (counter clockwise) rotation (Fig. 4.20). The best orientation is the one that is aligned with the LAA LAX with clear visualization of the LAA inlet.

Tip: Bilobed and multilobed cauliflower-like LAA are common, together with prominent pectinate muscle trabeculae. These findings may reduce the accuracy of TEE for detecting or excluding a thrombus unless the operator takes additional orthogonal views of the LAA at 90° up to 135° (Fig. 4.21) (4).

Spontaneous echo contrast within the LAA may be associated with an increased risk of embolic phenomena. This can be more or less prominent, depending on gain settings and the imaging frequency used. Considerable operator experience is, therefore, required to ensure a reliable assessment of the LAA.

Right atrial appendage. The right atrial appendage (RAA) is a broad-based outpouching of the RA (Fig. 4.22) seen in the far field by TEE in the 90° to 100° bicaval view of the atrial septum and RA.

Cardiac Septae

Ventricular septum. The ventricular septum is composed of a large muscular and a smaller membranous portion (Figs. 4.23 and 4.24). The trabecular muscular portion is easily assessed in the mid-esophageal four-chamber at 0° (Fig. 4.23) or LAX 135° views (Figs. 4.3A4 and 4.24) and the transgastric LAX view at 110° (Figs. 4.3B4 and 4.9). The posteroapical muscular septum, where most post-infarction ventricular septal rupture occurs with a serpiginous course, can also be assessed through the deep transgastric view at 0°.

The membranous septum is divided into an interventricular and an atrioventricular portion by the insertion of the tricuspid septal leaflet. The inlet

A

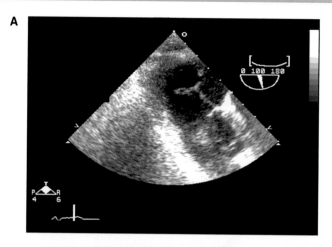

B

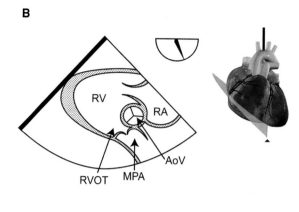

C

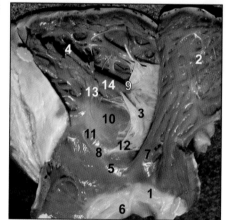

1 Pulmonary annulus
2 Right ventricular anterior wall
3 Tricuspid valve
4 Trabecular zone
5 Anterior limb of trabecula septomarginalis (TSM)
6 Pulmonic valve
7 Crista supraventricularis
8 Outflow component or infundibulum
9 Inlet component
10 Posterior limb of TSM
11 Body of TSM
12 Medial papillary muscle
13 Moderator band
14 Anterior papillary muscle

Figure 4.17   Modified transgastric right ventricular inflow/outflow view. This view (**A,B**) at 110° of the RV with corresponding anatomical correlation (**C**) is shown. *Abbreviations*: AoV, aortic valve; MPA, main pulmonary artery; RA, right atrium; RV, right ventricle; RVOT, right ventricular outflow tract.

portion beneath the TV is visualized in the mid-esophageal four-chamber view (Fig. 4.23), as well as the transgastric SAX view of the basal septum, both at 0°. The perimembranous atrioventricular portion is evaluated through the mid-esophageal five-chamber view at 0° near the LV outflow. It can also be assessed in the AoV SAX view at 45° near the base of the tricuspid septal leaflet (Fig. 4.16). The perimembranous outlet beneath the AoV is best evaluated through the mid-esophageal LAX view at 135° or sometimes through the transgastric LAX view at 110°.

Atrial septum. The atrial septum consists of a thin central fossa ovalis with thicker limbus regions anteriorly and posteriorly, and is viewed from the mid-esophageal probe position (Fig. 4.15).

The septum primum and the fossa ovalis are best seen in the four-chamber view at 0° (Fig. 4.15) with slight retroflexion and the bicaval view at 90° to 100° with rightward (clockwise) rotation (Fig. 4.19). The latter view is also best for visualizing the superior portion of the atrial septum and excluding a sinus venosus atrial septal defect with the occasionally associated right anomalous pulmonary venous return.

Another useful view for visualizing the interatrial septum is a clockwise rotation from the LVOT view with the probe in the midesophageal position at 135°. This view provides an axial assessment of the interatrial septum and is best for measuring the diameter of a secundum atrial septal defect and for ascertaining the adequacy of septal rims prior to percutaneous device closure. This view is also useful for verifying the stretch diameter of the defect and position of the (Amplatzer) device at insertion and in follow up as well as excluding residual interatrial shunting (see Chapter 29).

Veins

Pulmonary veins. The determination of normal pulmonary venous drainage is important in the assessment of congenital heart disease. Two methods can be consistently used to establish their normal connections to the LA. The first method starts in the mid-esophageal AoV SAX view at 45°, a central point in the heart. To image the left pulmonary veins, the probe will be rotated counterclockwise toward the

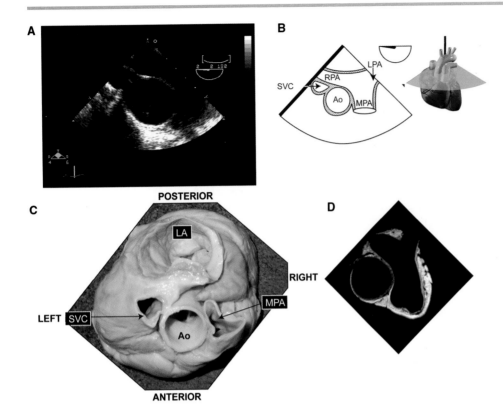

Figure 4.18   ME ascending aorta short-axis view. The ME view at 0° (**A,B**) of the great vessels compared with anatomical correlation (**C**) and magnetic resonance imaging (**D**). *Abbreviations*: Ao, aorta; LA, left atrium; LPA, left pulmonary artery; ME, mid-esophageal; MPA, main pulmonary artery; RPA, right pulmonary artery; SVC, superior vena cava.

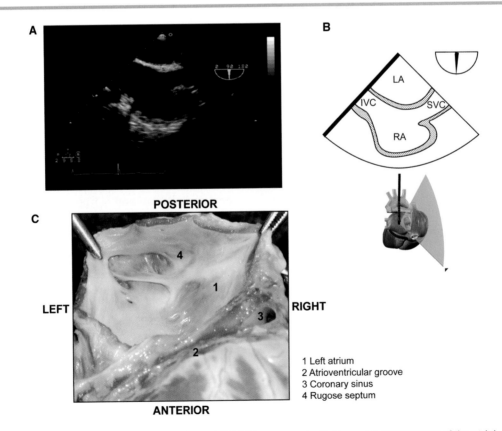

1 Left atrium
2 Atrioventricular groove
3 Coronary sinus
4 Rugose septum

Figure 4.19   Mid-esophageal bicaval view. This view at 90° (**A,B**) compared with the anatomical aspect of the atrial septum is viewed from the LA (**C**). *Abbreviations*: IVC, inferior vena cava; LA, left atrium; RA, right atrium; SVC, superior vena cava.

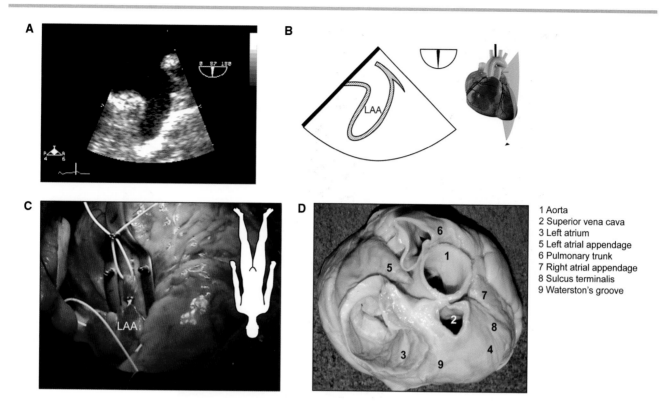

Figure 4.20 ME LAA view. (A,B) ME view of the LAA is viewed at 90°. (**C**) Intraoperative view of the LAA during off pump bypass surgery. (**D**) Anatomically the LAA is anterolateral to the left atrium and close to the left upper pulmonary vein. *Abbreviations*: ME, mid-esophageal; LAA, left atrial appendage. *Source*: Photo C courtesy of Dr. Raymond Cartier.

1 Aorta
2 Superior vena cava
3 Left atrium
5 Left atrial appendage
6 Pulmonary trunk
7 Right atrial appendage
8 Sulcus terminalis
9 Waterston's groove

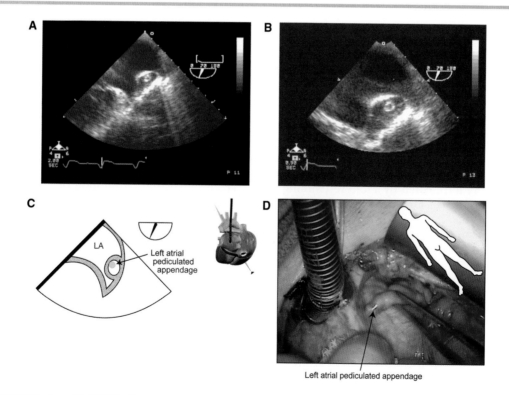

Left atrial pediculated appendage

Figure 4.21 ME LAA view. (A–C) ME view at 78° of the LAA in a 71-year-old woman scheduled for coronary revascularization, aortic and mitral valve replacement. A mobile mass is seen close to the LAA (**A–C**) which represents the tip of a multilobe LAA (**D**). *Abbreviations*: ME, mid-esophageal; LAA, left atrial appendage. *Source*: Photo D courtesy of Dr. Michel Pellerin.

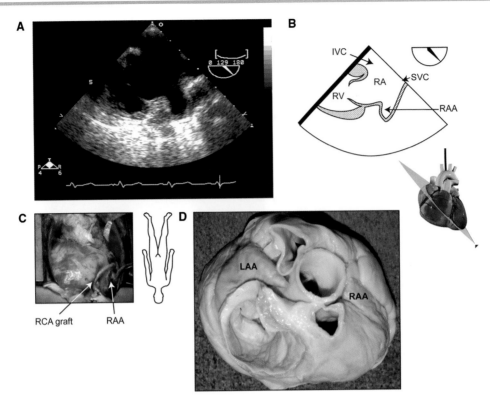

Figure 4.22 **RAA view.** Mid-esophageal view at 129° (**A,B**) of the RA and RAA is shown with an (**C**) intraoperative view in a patient undergoing coronary revascularization. (**D**) Anatomical location of both the RAA and LAA. *Abbreviations*: IVC, inferior vena cava; LAA, left atrial appendage; RA, right atrium; RAA, right atrial appendage; RCA, right coronary artery; RV, right ventricle; SVC, superior vena cava. *Source*: Photo C courtesy of Dr. Philippe Demers.

left. Alternatively, to assess the right pulmonary veins, the probe will be rotated clockwise toward the right. To facilitate the visualization of both upper and lower pulmonary veins, the rotation plane usually needs to be increased to 60° to 80°.

With a slight rotation toward the left, the left upper pulmonary vein (LUPV) in its LAX can be found next to the LAA from which it is separated by a linear echodensity terminated by a fold resembling a cotton tip, the limbus of the LUPV or "coumadin ridge" (Fig. 4.25).

Near the opening of the LUPV into the LA, the orifice of the left lower pulmonary vein (LLPV) will most often be viewed in its SAX and, therefore, is not as easy to visualize as the LUPV. The LLPV is usually viewed by advancing the TEE probe tip 1 to 2 cm from the plane in which the LUPV is best seen (Figs. 4.25 and 4.26). Occasionally, the LUPV and LLPV join each other prior to entering the LA as a single vessel in a "Y"-shaped configuration on TEE (Fig. 4.26).

With probe rotation toward the right from the AoV view, the right upper pulmonary vein (RUPV), like the LUPV, can be seen entering the LA in its LAX (Fig. 4.27). The right lower pulmonary vein (RLPV), like the LLPV, enters the LA in a horizontal plane inferiorly to the RUPV and is often viewed in its SAX.

It is best seen following optimal imaging of the RUPV by advancing the probe 1 to 2 cm and further right-ward rotation (Fig. 4.28). Occasionally, a right middle lobe pulmonary vein can be viewed entering the LA between the orifices of the RUPV and the RLPV.

The second method images the pulmonary veins at 0° in the transverse plane. All pulmonary veins should then be viewed in their longitudinal axis, which makes the recognition of the lower pulmonary veins easier than with the first method. Again, to image the left pulmonary veins, the probe will be rotated counterclockwise toward the left. Alternatively, to assess the right pulmonary veins, the probe will be rotated clockwise toward the right.

From a higher mid-esophageal position at 0°, the SAX view showing the superior vena cava (SVC), the Ao, and the longitudinal view of the RPA (Figs. 4.3A10 and 4.18), the probe is rotated toward the right and slowly advanced. Near the junction of the SVC with the RA, the RUPV will be seen entering the LA. In the advent of an anomalous right upper venous connection, the RUPV would be seen entering the SVC instead, causing turbulent flow in the usually laminar SVC flow. The RLPV can then be similarly visualized below the RUPV by advancing the probe at approximately the same angle. In this view, it may be easier to

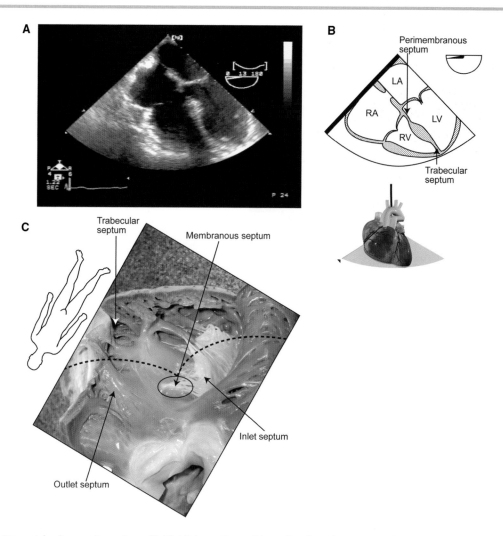

Figure 4.23 Interventricular septum view. (A,B) Mid-esophageal four-chamber view at 13° of the ventricular septum is shown. **(C)** Anatomical classification of the ventricular septum is divided into membranous, trabecular, inlet and outlet portions. *Abbreviations*: LA, left atrium; LV, left ventricle; RA, right atrium; RV, right ventricle.

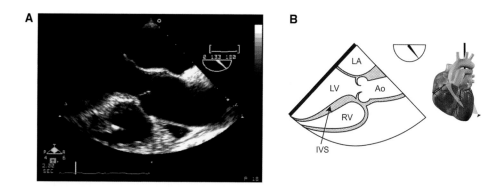

Figure 4.24 Mid-esophageal aortic valve long-axis view. (A,B) This view at 117° of the aortic root, proximal ascending Ao and IVS is shown. *Abbreviations*: Ao, aorta; IVS, interventricular septum; LA, left atrium; LV, left ventricle; RV, right ventricle.

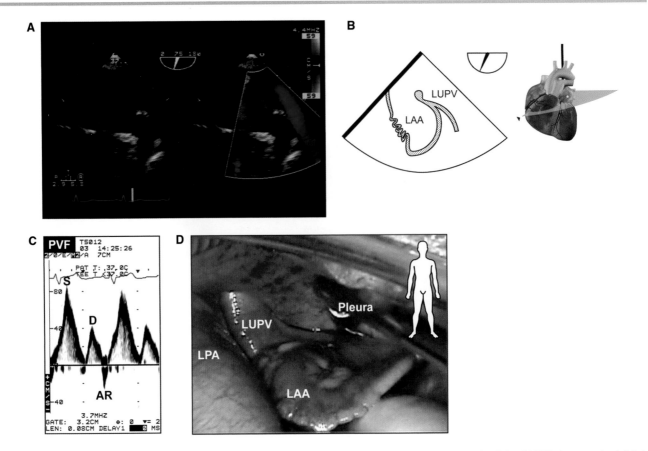

Figure 4.25 Pulmonary vein Doppler. Mid-esophageal color Doppler compare view at 75° (**A,B**) of the LUPV close to the LAA is shown with an intraoperative anatomical correlation (**D**). (**C**) Pulsed wave Doppler interrogation of PVF reveals normal S, D, and AR waves. *Abbreviations*: AR, atrial reversal; D, diastolic; LAA, left atrial appendage; LPA, left pulmonary artery; LUPV, left upper pulmonary vein; PVF, pulmonary venous flow; S, systolic. *Source*: Photo D courtesy of Dr. Michel Pellerin.

visualize than at 60° to 80° where it is seen in its short axis, and therefore, it is harder to track its course.

The LUPV is obtained starting from a high esophageal position at the level of the SAX view of the SVC, the Ao, and the longitudinal view of the RPA, but with the probe now rotated toward the left and slowly advanced. Again, the proximity of the LAA will help localize it (Fig. 4.25). The LLPV is then visualized in its LAX by advancing the probe at the same angle.

Superior and inferior vena cavae. As mentioned, the SVC is visualized in its transverse view from the high esophageal position posterior and to the right of the Ao (Fig. 4.18). This view is particularly helpful to see an intraluminal catheter or thrombus. The SVC, particularly its distal portion with its junction to the RA, can then be seen in its longitudinal axis in the mid-esophageal bicaval view at 90° (Fig. 4.19). A deep transgastric view can also be used to perform Doppler interrogation of the SVC (Fig. 4.29).

The proximal inferior vena cava (IVC) is seen from the mid-esophageal bicaval view at 90° (Figs. 4.3A7 and 4.19). The rest of the IVC can be assessed by advancing the probe to transgastric views, where its diameter can

be measured in response to respiratory variations. This view also provides an excellent Doppler interrogation angle of the hepatic veins as they merge with the IVC (Figs. 4.3B6 and 4.30).

Coronary sinus. The coronary sinus runs in the posterior atrioventricular groove and empties into the RA at the inferoposterior aspect of the interatrial septum near the attachment of the tricuspid septal leaflet (Fig. 4.31). The longitudinal image of the coronary sinus, running lateral to medial behind the inferior aspect of the LA, is obtained from the mid-esophageal four-chamber view with slight retroflexion of the probe tip (Fig. 4.32). A cross-sectional view of the coronary sinus appears in the lateral atrioventricular groove in the mid-esophageal two-chamber view at 90° (Fig. 4.32).

Arteries

Coronary arteries. The coronary ostia and proximal coronary arteries can be seen from the mid-esophageal SAX 45° view of the aortic annulus and aortic root. The left main coronary artery originates from the aortic root above the left coronary cusp and

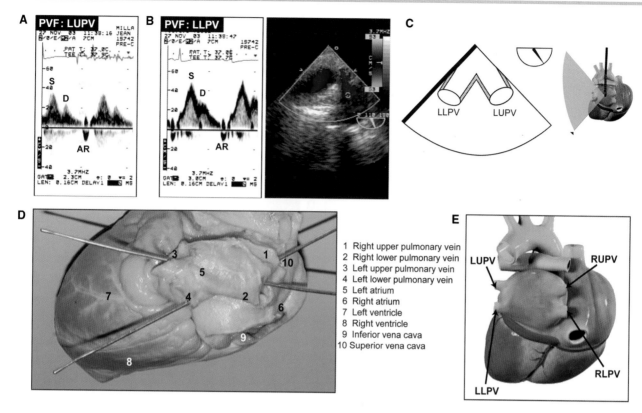

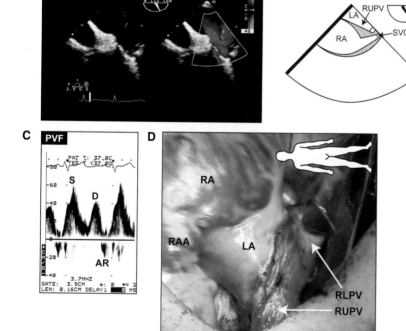

Figure 4.26 Pulmonary vein Doppler. (A–C) Pulsed wave Doppler interrogation of **(A)** the LUPV and **(B)** the LLPV from a mid-esophageal 110° view is shown. The normal S, diastolic D, and AR waves of PVF are shown. Compare the anatomical specimen **(D)** with the schematic representation of all pulmonary veins **(E)**. *Abbreviations*: AR, atrial reversal; D, diastolic; LAA, left atrial appendage; LLPV, left lower pulmonary vein; LUPV, left upper pulmonary vein; PVF, pulmonary venous flow; RLPV, right lower pulmonary vein; RUPV, right upper pulmonary vein; S, systolic. ⌐

Figure 4.27 Pulmonary vein Doppler. (A,B) Mid-esophageal color Doppler compare view at 118° of the RUPV positioned behind the RA and close to the SVC as seen on the intraoperative view **(D)**. **(C)** Pulsed wave Doppler interrogation of PVF shows a normal pattern of S, D, and AR waves. *Abbreviations*: AR, atrial reversal; D, diastolic; LA, left atrium; LUPV, left upper pulmonary vein; PVF, pulmonary venous flow; RA, right atrium; RAA, right atrial appendage; RLPV, right lower pulmonary vein; RUPV, right upper pulmonary vein; S, systolic; SVC, superior vena cava. *Source*: Photo D courtesy of Dr. Nancy Poirier. ⌐

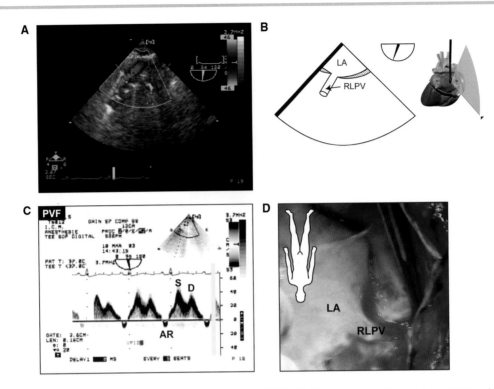

Figure 4.28 Pulmonary vein Doppler. Mid-esophageal view of the RLPV (**A,B**) compared with an intraoperative view (**D**). (**C**) Pulsed wave Doppler interrogation of PVF shows a normal pattern of S, D, and AR waves. *Abbreviations*: AR, atrial reversal; D, diastolic; LA, left atrium; PVF, pulmonary venous flow; RLPV, right lower pulmonary vein; S, systolic. *Source*: Photo D courtesy of Dr. Nancy Poirier.

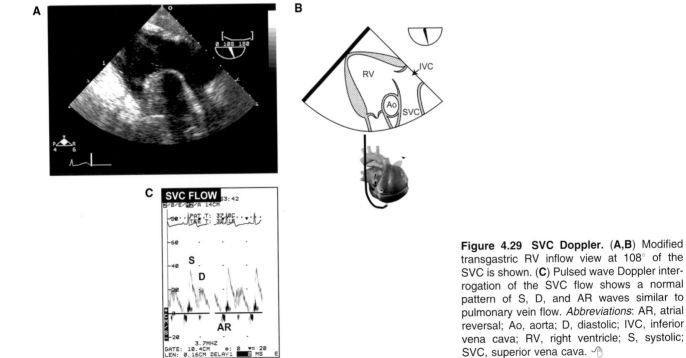

Figure 4.29 SVC Doppler. (**A,B**) Modified transgastric RV inflow view at 108° of the SVC is shown. (**C**) Pulsed wave Doppler interrogation of the SVC flow shows a normal pattern of S, D, and AR waves similar to pulmonary vein flow. *Abbreviations*: AR, atrial reversal; Ao, aorta; D, diastolic; IVC, inferior vena cava; RV, right ventricle; S, systolic; SVC, superior vena cava.

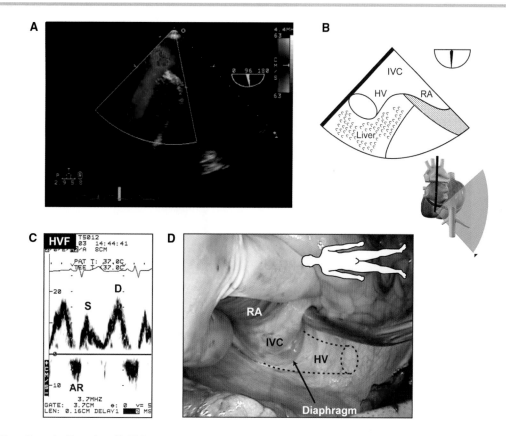

Figure 4.30 Hepatic vein Doppler. (A,B) Lower esophageal view of the IVC and HV compared with surgical correlation **(D)**. **(C)** Pulsed wave Doppler interrogation of HVF shows the S, D, and AR waves with an abnormal S/D ratio (<1). *Abbreviations*: AR, atrial reversal; D, diastolic; HV, hepatic vein; HVF, hepatic vein flow; IVC, inferior vena cava; RA, left atrium; S, systolic. *Source*: Photo D courtesy of Dr. Michel Pellerin.

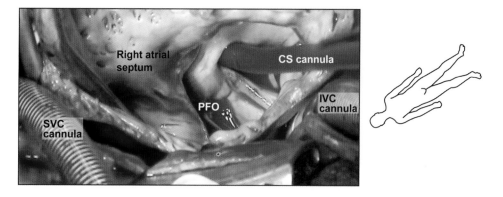

Figure 4.31 Right atrial surgical view. Intraoperative photo of a sinus venosus atrial septal defect and a PFO in a 48-year-old man are viewed from the right atrium. The IVC and SVC cannulae are seen. Note the proximity of the PFO and the CS with its retrograde cannula. *Abbreviations*: CS, coronary sinus; IVC, inferior vena cava; PFO, patent foramen ovale; SVC, superior vena cava. *Source*: Photo courtesy of Dr. Nancy Poirier.

runs laterally toward the right side of the image sector (Fig. 4.33). Slight adjustment of probe tip depth and flexion together with color Doppler flow imaging is often needed to optimize its visualization. The left main bifurcation and proximal portions of the circumflex and left anterior descending (LAD) coronary artery can be seen in many patients. The left circumflex artery can sometimes be followed in the left atrioventricular groove with the coronary sinus.

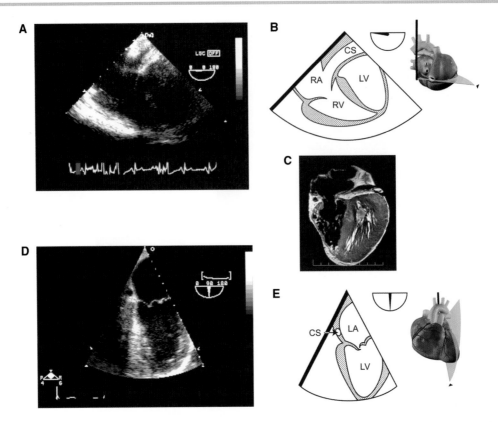

Figure 4.32   Coronary sinus views. Lower esophageal view at 0° (**A,B**) of the CS in long axis draining into the RA with magnetic resonance imaging correlation (**C**). Compare with the mid-esophageal two-chamber view at 90° (**D,E**) showing the CS in short axis. *Abbreviations*: CS, coronary sinus; LA, left atrium; LV, left ventricle; RA, right atrium; RV, right ventricle.

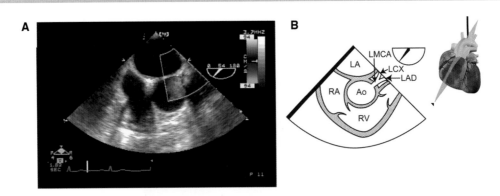

Figure 4.33   Left coronary artery view. (**A,B**) The LMCA is seen in this mid-esophageal aortic valve short-axis color Doppler view at 54°. *Abbreviations*: Ao, aorta; LA, left atrium; LAD, left anterior descending; LCX, left circumflex; LMCA, left main coronary artery; RA, right atrium; RV, right ventricle.

The right coronary artery (RCA) is more difficult to image with TEE. The RCA originates from the right sinus of Valsalva and runs anteriorly in the far field toward the bottom of the ultrasound sector away from the probe tip. It is, therefore, rare to be able to see more than the first centimeter or two of the RCA by TEE in the AoV SAX or LAX views (Fig. 4.34).

Tip: The noncoronary AoV cusp is always adjacent to the atrial septum and the right coronary cusp is always anterior in any ultrasound imaging view. The RCA always runs anteriorly in any echo imaging view.

Aorta. Multiplane TEE allows a near complete visualization of the Ao from the aortic root to

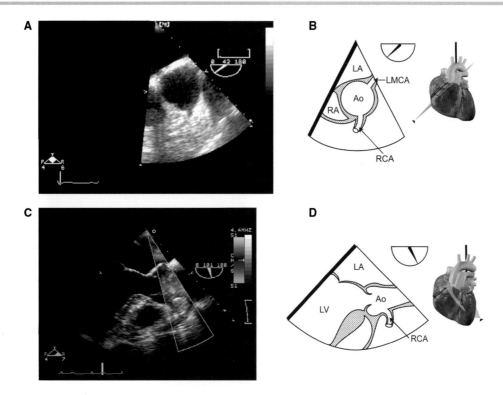

Figure 4.34 **Right coronary artery views.** The RCA is seen in the mid-esophageal short-axis (**A,B**) and long-axis color Doppler (**C,D**) views of the ascending aorta. *Abbreviations*: Ao, aorta; LA, left atrium; LMCA, left main coronary artery; LV, left ventricle; RA, right atrium; RCA, right coronary artery; RV, right ventricle. 🖱

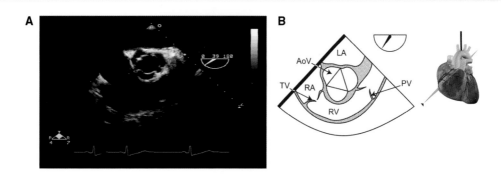

Figure 4.35 **Mid-esophageal AoV short-axis view. (A,B)** This view at 39° is shown during systole. *Abbreviations*: AoV, aortic valve; LA, left atrium; PV, pulmonic valve; RA, right atrium; RV, right ventricle; TV, tricuspid valve. 🖱

the upper abdominal descending Ao. Occasionally, the distal ascending Ao and proximal aortic arch may be masked by the interposition of the air-filled trachea and left mainstem bronchus between the esophagus and the Ao.

A SAX view of the aortic root is seen from the mid-esophageal 45° (0°–60°) position at about 30 cm from the incisors (Fig. 4.35). The rotation angle should be adjusted to optimize a circular view of the aortic

ring and three AoV cusps. Gentle probe withdrawal from this position and at 0° allows a SAX view of the proximal ascending Ao (Fig. 4.18).

The LAX view of the aortic root, sinuses of Valsalva, sinotubular junction (STJ), and proximal ascending Ao (Fig. 4.24) are imaged by rotating the angle to 135° (100°–150°). The mid-ascending Ao (Fig. 4.36) is imaged, often at a lower angle (100°), while withdrawing the probe. In this view, the

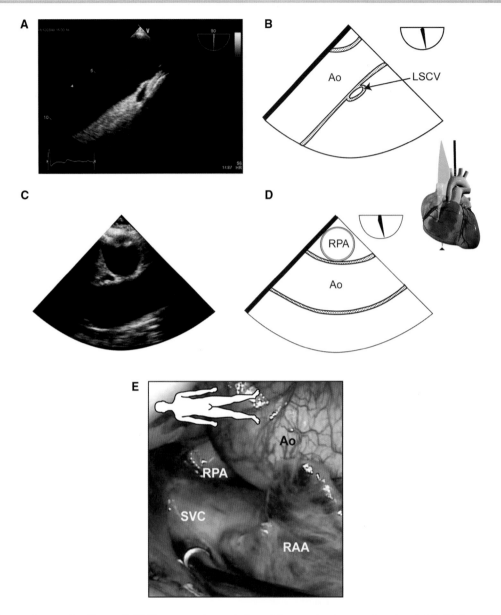

Figure 4.36   Ascending aorta views. (A,B) Upper esophageal view of the proximal ascending Ao at 90°. Mid-esophageal ascending Ao long-axis view at 90° (**C,D**) compared with an intraoperative view of the Ao (**E**). *Abbreviations*: Ao, aorta; LSVC, left subclavian vein; RAA, right atrial appendage; RPA, right pulmonary artery; SVC, superior vena cava. *Source*: Photo E courtesy of Dr. Michel Pellerin.

anterior and posterior walls of the Ao are parallel to each other and perpendicular to the ultrasound beam, allowing precise measurement of aortic dimensions.

The aortic arch initially lies anterior to the esophagus and continues to the left to become the descending thoracic Ao. The latter then winds around from the left side to the posterior aspect of the esophagus at the level of the diaphragm (see Fig. 23.3). It is customary to image the descending and abdominal Ao from distal to proximal. From the lower- to mid-esophageal four-chamber view at 0°, a slight quarter-turn toward the left will bring the lower descending thoracic Ao in view on its SAX (Fig. 4.10). While keeping the Ao in view, the probe tip is advanced gradually through the

lower esophageal sphincter into the stomach until the abdominal Ao moves away from the stomach and is no longer clearly visible. The upper abdominal and descending thoracic Ao is imaged by slowly withdrawing the TEE probe from this most distal point to the level of the distal aortic arch (about 10–15 cm). The ultrasound sector is centered on the Ao SAX view by gentle rightward (clockwise) rotation of the probe as it is withdrawn. A longitudinal view of the Ao can be obtained at any point, if desired, by changing the angle from 0° to 90° (Fig. 4.10).

Tip: The descending thoracic Ao lies immediately adjacent to the probe tip in the distal esophagus and appears in the near field of the ultrasound sector requiring several ultrasound system image adjustments for optimal visualization. Sector depth should be reduced to 6–8 cm, gain reduced, and focus adjusted to the near field. Finally, air within the esophagus can reduce image quality if the ultrasound probe tip is not apposed to the wall of the esophagus. Proper probe tip apposition can be ensured through the maintenance of slight probe tip flexion. However, because the descending Ao can be tortuous, alternation between slight anteflexion and retroflexion may occasionally be needed to ensure optimal image quality.

As the Ao and esophagus intertwine, it is difficult to localize abnormalities anatomically within the descending thoracic Ao. The level of any abnormality is typically described in centimeters from the incisors or sometimes from the left subclavian artery origin. The location is further described relative to the probe tip in the esophagus (e.g., near-field, far-field, left side, or right side of the Ao at 30 cm).

The aortic arch is viewed longitudinally at 0° with probe withdrawal from the descending Ao (Fig. 4.11). Its anterior course requires the combination of gentle withdrawal and simultaneous rightward rotation for optimal visualization. An aortic arch SAX view can then be obtained by plane rotation to 90° (Fig. 4.36). This is particularly useful to assess the whole anterior wall and the floor of the Ao. While rotating the probe toward the right, the origin of the left subclavian, left common carotid, and right brachiocephalic arteries may be seen at 90° (Fig. 4.37).

Tip: This view is obtained from a high esophageal position where the probe tip, applied against the posterior surface of the trachea, may cause discomfort and induce paroxysmal cough in lightly sedated patients. It is, therefore, best left until the end of examination and obtained just prior to probe withdrawal unless the patient is under deep sedation or anesthesia.

Valves

Mitral valve. Multiplane TEE can be used to image individual structures of the MV apparatus including the annulus, the anterior and posterior leaflets, the chordae tendinae, and the papillary muscles (Fig. 4.5) (see Chapter 16).

The anterior mitral leaflet (AML) has the larger surface area of the two leaflets but has a smaller

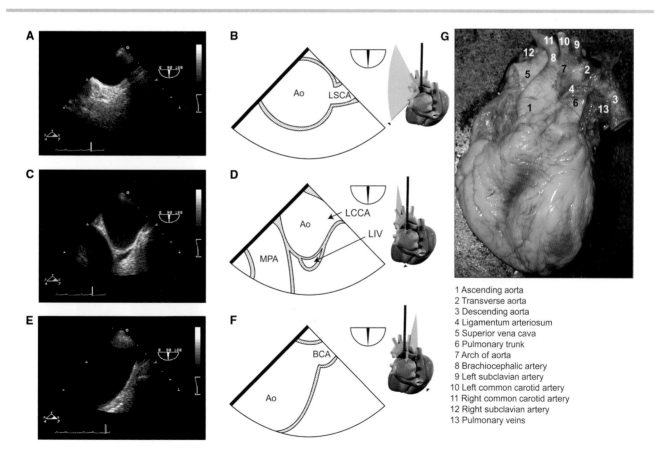

1 Ascending aorta
2 Transverse aorta
3 Descending aorta
4 Ligamentum arteriosum
5 Superior vena cava
6 Pulmonary trunk
7 Arch of aorta
8 Brachiocephalic artery
9 Left subclavian artery
10 Left common carotid artery
11 Right common carotid artery
12 Right subclavian artery
13 Pulmonary veins

Figure 4.37 Aortic arch and vessels. Upper esophageal view of the transverse Ao and proximal arch vessels (**A–F**) compared with anatomical correlation (**G**). The views of the proximal vessels are obtained with a left to right rotation of the transesophageal echocardiographic probe from an aortic arch short-axis view at 90°. *Abbreviations*: Ao, aorta; BCA, brachiocephalic artery; LCCA, left common carotid artery; LIV, left innominate vein; LSCA, left subclavian artery; MPA, main pulmonary artery.

perimeter of attachment to the MV annulus. For descriptive purposes, the AML surface is divided into three segments: the anterolateral (A1), the middle (A2), and the posteromedial segment (A3). The posterior mitral leaflet (PML) consists of three distinct scallops labeled anterolateral (P1), middle (P2), and posteromedial (P3). All aspects of the MV leaflets and annulus can be viewed during a TEE examination from the mid-esophageal probe position. Beginning at 0° (A2–P2) (see Fig. 16.2), the morphology of the leaflets by 2D echo is assessed as the angle is progressively changed through 30° (A3–A2–P1), 60° (P3–A2–P1), then 90° (P3–A2–A1), and finally 135° (P2–A2) (Fig. 4.38). The degree of MR is assessed by color Doppler flow as the angle is returned from 135° back to 0° keeping any MR jet into the LA centered in the display. The comprehensive back and forth sweep of the MV leaflets from the mid-esophageal level should be an integral part of all TEE examinations.

In addition to the mid-esophageal views, the MV leaflets can also be visualized from the transgastric probe position with anteflexion of the probe tip toward the base and slight withdrawal from the papillary muscle SAX plane (Figs. 4.3B2 and 4.6). In this view, the posteromedial MV commissure is the closest to the transducer while the anterolateral commissure is the furthest, opposite to the septum. This transgastric basal SAX view of the MV is excellent for localizing precisely MV leaflet abnormalities or the extent of MV annular calcifications. Rotating the angle to 90° from this position yields a two-chamber view with the posterior leaflet closest to the transducer at the top of the display and the anterior leaflet toward the bottom of the display (Figs. 4.3B3 and 4.7).

The chordae tendinae are best seen in the transgastric two-chamber view at 90°, where they are perpendicular to the ultrasound beam. In this view, the anterior chordae can be tracked from the anterolateral papillary muscle at the bottom of the screen while the posterior chordae originate from the posteromedial papillary muscle closer to the transducer (Fig. 4.7). The papillary muscles are best seen in the transgastric SAX view at 0° while evaluating the contractility of the LV mid-segments (Figs. 4.3B1 and 4.5).

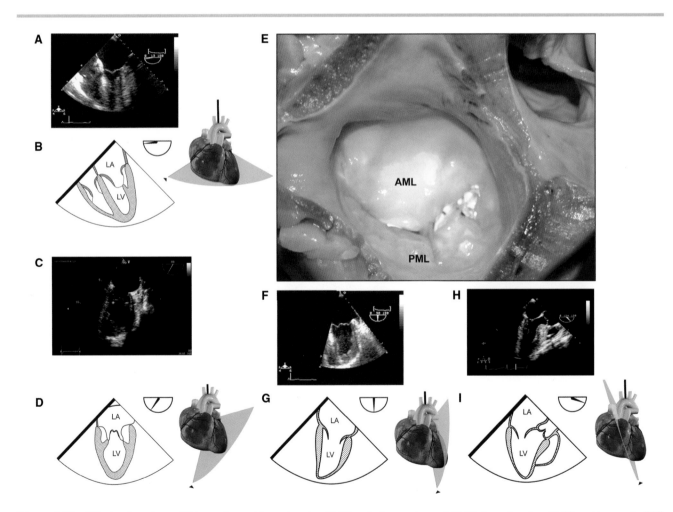

Figure 4.38 Mitral valve views. Mid-esophageal four-chamber (**A,B**), mitral commissural (**C,D**), two-chamber (**F,G**) and long-axis (**H,I**) views of the mitral valve compared with the surgical view (**E**). *Abbreviations*: AML, anterior mitral valve leaflet; LA, left atrium; LV, left ventricle; PML, posterior mitral valve leaflet.

AoV and aortic root. The aortic root comprises the AoV annulus, AoV cusps, the sinuses of Valsalva and coronary ostia, the STJ, and the proximal ascending Ao. Complete visualization of all these structures can be achieved from the mid-esophageal position. The presence and degree of aortic regurgitation (AR) with color Doppler flow can also be assessed from the mid-esophageal probe position. Spectral Doppler assessment of transaortic flow requires visualization of the LVOT, the AoV, and the proximal ascending Ao from a transgastric probe position where transaortic flow is parallel to the ultrasound beam (Fig. 4.14).

The aortic root is imaged in SAX from the mid-esophageal position with an angle rotation of about 45° to 90° slight anteflexion and sector depth of 10 to 12 cm (Figs. 4.3A8 and 4.34). In this view, the ultrasound beam is perfectly parallel to the AoV annulus and the three aortic cups are visualized symmetrically, with the noncoronary cusp adjacent to the atrial septum and the right coronary cusp seen anteriorly at the bottom of the display (Fig. 4.35). Planimetry of the aortic orifice area is frequently possible in this view and has been found to correlate well with that obtained using the continuity equation. Slight withdrawal and/or slight clockwise (rightward) rotation of the shaft brings the probe above the AoV to obtain the SAX view of the sinuses of Valsalva, the left and right coronary ostia, and proximal ascending Ao, respectively. Alternatively, further insertion and/or slight counterclockwise (leftward) rotation of the shaft below the AoV yields the LVOT in cross section.

Tip: The aortic cusp facing the interatrial septum is always the noncoronary cusp, and the one that is anterior is always the right coronary cusp in the absence of major congenital heart disease. This principle assists with aortic cusp identification independent of the imaging modality (TTE or TEE) being used.

A mid-esophageal longitudinal view of the AoV may be obtained at 0° with some probe withdrawal (Fig. 4.12) but is better imaged at 135° where the LVOT, the AoV, and the proximal Ao are viewed in the same plane (Fig. 4.13). Both positions allow for diagnosis and semi-quantification of AR with color Doppler flow.

The mid-esophageal 135° view is, however, best for making precise measurements of the aortic annulus, sinus of Valsalva, STJ, and proximal ascending Ao diameters as the ultrasound beam intersects these structures perpendicularly (see Fig. 23.1). This view corresponds to the transthoracic left parasternal LAX view (see Fig. 6.10), and it is important to get the most precise measurements of the LVOT diameter (Figs. 4.3A9 and 4.24).

Another is at 90° when, with slight leftward rotation, the imaging plane is parallel to the ascending Ao. It is this view that is most useful in excluding ascending aortic aneurysm as well as type A dissection (Figs. 4.3A11 and 4.36).

Longitudinal views of the aortic root in the far field of the display may sometimes be obtained from the transgastric probe position. Two options include further angle rotation to 90° to 120° from the transgastric two-chamber view, as previously described, or

a deep transgastric view obtained with further probe tip advancement and maximal anteflexion at an angle of 0° (Fig. 4.14). Color Doppler flow imaging is frequently useful to optimize PW and CW Doppler alignment with aortic outflow in these positions where the distal aortic root location does not generally allow optimal 2D structure visualization.

Tricuspid valve and pulmonic valve. The TV and PV are anterior structures that are more difficult to visualize with TEE (Fig. 4.39). Both valves are seen in the far field in the mid-esophageal 60° view (Fig. 4.16). In this position, the TV, RV, PV, and pulmonary artery trunk appear to wrap around the aortic root from left to right across the bottom of the display.

A similar view from a different imaging point can be obtained from a transgastric probe position at 90° with rightward rotation from the two-chamber view (Fig. 4.17). Sometimes, slight readjustment of the angle from 60° to 90° may be required to display the RA, TV, RV, and PV together.

The PV, main pulmonary artery, and bifurcation of the proximal RPA and LPA are best visualized at 0° in the proximal esophageal probe position with more anteflexion (Fig. 4.18). While rightward rotation of the probe often enables visualization of the RPA up to its first bifurcation in the near field of the display, only the first 1–2 cm of the LPA can be visualized most of the time.

DOPPLER FLOW PROFILES FOR NORMAL AND ABNORMAL PHYSIOLOGY

Phases of the Cardiac Cycle (Systole Vs. Diastole/Four Phases)

The cardiac cycle consists of two phases: systole and diastole. Systole is defined as the period between MV and AoV closures. It consists of an isovolumic contraction period (both atrioventricular and semilunar valves closed) followed by the ejection time (ET) during which blood is expelled from the ventricles into the great arteries. The amount of blood ejected per cardiac cycle, or stroke volume (SV), multiplied by the number of cardiac cycles per minute, or heart rate (HR), yields the CO.

Diastole is more complex and is divided into four phases: isovolumic relaxation, rapid filling, diastasis, and atrial contraction. It begins with AoV closure and ends with MV closure. The period between AoV closure and MV opening is defined as the isovolumic relaxation time (IVRT) and is a period of active (energy-requiring) and rapid ventricular relaxation. On MV opening, rapid initial filling of the ventricle from the atria occurs, driven by the pressure gradient between the two chambers. Normally 70% to 80% of ventricular filling occurs during this rapid filling phase. A period of near-pressure equalization between the atrium and ventricle follows (diastasis) when little forward flow occurs. Finally, atrial contraction follows with an additional 10% to 20% in ventricular filling (see Chapter 10).

While the systolic ET changes little with increasing HR, the diastolic phase of the cardiac cycle shortens

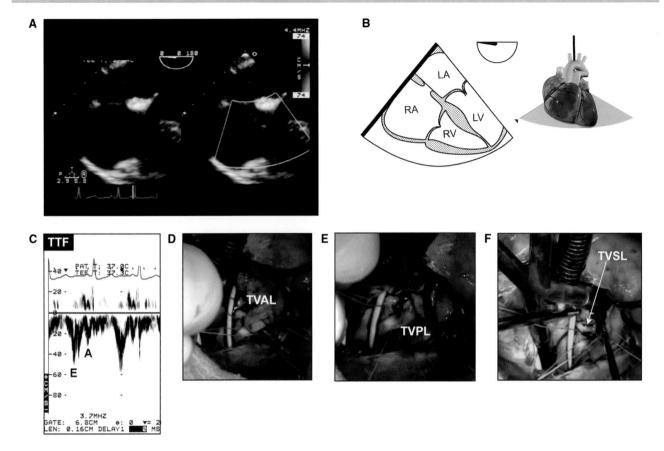

Figure 4.39 Tricuspid valve Doppler. (A,B) Mid-esophageal color Doppler compare view of the TV at 0° is shown. Pulsed wave Doppler interrogation (**C**) of TTF shows the E or early filling and A or atrial contraction waves. (**D–F**) Intraoperative views of the TV shown through the RA. *Abbreviations*: LA, left atrium; LV, left ventricle; RA, right atrium; RV, right ventricle; TTF, transtricuspid flow; TV, tricuspid valve; TVAL, tricuspid valve anterior leaflet; TVSL, tricuspid valve septal leaflet; TVPL, tricuspid valve posterior leaflet. ⌂

substantially with exercise. Therefore, any degree of diastolic dysfunction is more likely to become symptomatic with exercise as the ventricle is unable to fill adequately at normal pressures.

Normal Pressures in Cardiac Chambers and Great Vessels

It is important to be aware of the normal pressures in the cardiac chambers and great arteries during the systolic and diastolic phases of the cardiac cycle (all in mmHg) (Table 4.2).

Mitral Valve (See Chap. 17)

Mitral Regurgitation

From a mid-esophageal TEE probe position, regurgitant flow across the MV is directed toward the probe, unless it is extremely eccentric. Transesophageal examination constitutes an excellent modality to assess MR, especially with prosthetic valves. Color Doppler imaging is used to detect and semi-quantify MR on a scale of 1+ (trivial MR) to 4+ (severe MR). The width of the narrowest regurgitant color jet as it crosses the regurgitant orifice, or vena contracta, as

Table 4.2 Normal Pressure in Cardiac Chambers and Great Vessels

Pressure (mmHg)	Systolic	Diastolic	Mean
RA			1–8
RV	15–30	1–8	
PA	15–30	4–12	9–18
LA			2–12
LV	100–140	3–12	
Aorta	100–140	60–90	70–105

Abbreviations: LA, left atrial; LV, left ventricular; PA, pulmonary artery; RA, right atrial; RV, right ventricular.

well as the velocity of forward flow in early diastole are also useful in the primary assessment of MR severity, while more quantitative methods can be implemented (see Chapter 16 and Table 16.3).

Care must be taken to differentiate MR signals from obstructive outflow tract jets. As jets can be identified by the company they keep, systolic MR jets will be associated with mitral inflow (with E and A velocities) in diastole, while systolic obstructive outflow tract signals may be accompanied by aortic regurgitant signals. Also the aortic regurgitant signal will be separated from the mitral diastolic signals by the isovolumic contraction time (IVCT) and IVRT intervals (see Chapter 14). Because of the usual LV-LA pressure gradient in systole, most mitral regurgitant jet velocities are >4 m/sec, unless there is severe LV systolic dysfunction.

Mitral Stenosis

Optimal ultrasound beam alignment with the MV forward flow during TEE is also ideal for spectral Doppler (PW or CW) assessment of mitral stenosis (MS). Peak and mean transvalvular gradients, as well as mitral valve area (MVA), can be measured from the MV diastolic inflow velocity spectral trace using the modified Bernoulli equation and pressure half-time methods, respectively (see Chapter 16).

Left Ventricular Inflow

Abnormal Relaxation

Abnormal LV relaxation can be evaluated by PW Doppler interrogation of the MV inflow pattern. The PW Doppler sample volume must be carefully positioned between the MV leaflet tips while maintaining strict alignment with the direction of the mitral flow, often laterally directed because of the large anterior leaflet (see Chapter 10). From the spectral display obtained, a number of parameters can be evaluated, including the IVRT, the mitral deceleration time (mDT) of the E velocity, and the E/A velocity ratio. With delayed LV relaxation, the IVRT and deceleration time (DT) are prolonged, while the E/A velocity ratio is typically <1.0 as relatively more filling occurs in late diastole. However, these values may be affected by a number of additional factors, including left atrial and ventricular filling pressures, left ventricular passive compliance, HR, and age. Reliable Doppler assessment of diastolic function, therefore, requires an integrated approach together with a thorough understanding of diastolic physiology (see Chaper 10).

Restrictive Filling

At this stage, the reduced passive operating compliance properties of the chamber lead to rapidly equalizing pressures: filling occurs mostly in early diastole and ends abruptly prior to diastasis and atrial contraction where little additional flow into the LV occurs. Therefore, in restriction, the PW Doppler spectral display of mitral inflow usually shows prominent E and decreased A velocities (resulting in elevated E/A ratio), with shortened IVRT and DT.

Tricuspid Valve (See Chap. 18)

Assessment of TV gradients is more challenging with TEE as parallel alignment of the ultrasound beam with TV inflow is generally not ideal from any of the conventional views. Visualization of the TV inflow by color Doppler imaging is a key to minimizing errors in spectral Doppler measurement. The best opportunity for acceptable alignment might be with the mid-esophageal four-chamber view where fine adjustments of angle and probe tip flexion may reduce the ultrasound beam to TV flow angle to <20° (Fig. 4.39). Sometimes, the mid-esophageal position in the RV inflow-outflow view at 60° to 90° can be tried with slightly further probe tip insertion.

Tricuspid regurgitation (TR) can generally be assessed by TEE with color Doppler imaging from the TV views described above. The extent of the color regurgitant jet in the RA and the width of the TR vena contracta are used for semi-quantification in a manner similar to the evaluation of MR (see Chapter 18).

Tricuspid stenosis is rare in adults but may be seen with associated left-sided valve rheumatic involvement and with carcinoid syndrome and fenfluramine-phentermine (fen-phen) toxicity. Abnormal pressure gradients can also be found after valve repair and annuloplasty or replacement.

Aortic Valve (See Chap. 15)

Aortic Regurgitation

Aortic regurgitant jets can be visualized in mid-esophageal SAX and LAX views of the AoV at 45° and 135°, respectively. However, for quantitative assessment, the best alignment of the ultrasound beam with aortic regurgitant jets is usually obtained from LAX transgastric views at 100° to 110° or deep transgastric view at 0° for measurement of regurgitant flow pressure half-time, as well as for measurements of regurgitant volume by the continuity equation.

Aortic Stenosis

Assessment of aortic stenosis (AS) severity requires measurement of valvular peak and mean pressure gradients as well as additional measurement of LVOT diameter, velocity, and VTI for the estimation of AoV area by the continuity equation. Again, transgastric views at either LAX 100° to 110° or deep 0° are traditionally used to acquire these values, and to ensure that the aortic maximal gradient is obtained. CW Doppler interrogation from a high esophageal position looking down the distal ascending Ao should also be tried when windows are available (Fig. 4.14).

Pulmonic Valve (See Chap. 18)

Pulmonic Regurgitation

Pulmonic regurgitant jets can be visualized in a mid-esophageal SAX view of the AoV at 45° and at 110°. However, for quantitative assessment of pulmonary artery diastolic pressures, the best alignment of the ultrasound beam with pulmonic regurgitant jets is usually obtained from an upper esophageal view at 0° of the main pulmonary artery trunk (Fig. 4.18) or 60° to 90° of the pulmonary artery, and alternatively, from the transgastric view at 60° to 90° rotated to the right looking up toward the RVOT (Fig. 4.40).

Pulmonic Stenosis

Assessment of pulmonic stenosis (PS) severity requires measurement of valvular peak and mean pressure gradients as well as additional measurement of RVOT diameter, velocity, and VTI for the estimation of valve area by the continuity equation. Again, transgastric views at 60°–90° can be used to obtain these values (Fig. 4.40). The PV maximal gradient can also be measured from above the valve by CW Doppler interrogation through the upper esophageal position looking down the main pulmonary artery trunk at 0° (Fig. 4.18) or 90° (Figs. 4.40 and 18.7).

Left Ventricular Outflow Tract

See section "Cardiac Chambers" (Figs. 4.12 and 4.13).

Pulmonary Vein

The RUPV and LUPV usually present the best alignment for PW Doppler interrogation, with the sample volume positioned approximately 1 cm inside the vein from the ostium (Figs. 4.25–4.28). Normal pulmonary venous flow is multiphasic, with two peaks in systole (S_1 and S_2), one peak in diastole (D), and one retrograde peak during atrial contraction, called atrial reversal. The S_1 peak is related to atrial relaxation and may be proportional to the magnitude of atrial systole and, therefore, the atrial reversal wave. The S_2 velocity is influenced by the suction of blood from the pulmonary veins with LA expansion secondary to the MV annulus descent during ventricular systole and to RV contraction. The diastolic velocity (D) depends on the LA pressure drop after the MV opening and also on the LA to LV pressure gradient.

With normal LV filling pressures, there is more pulmonary venous flow in systole than in diastole, with the *S/D* ratio >1. In the case of a young adult with excellent ventricular relaxation, an *S/D* ratio <1 may be observed. The atrial reversal wave duration may also exceed the duration of the mitral A wave but never by >30 ms with normal left-sided filling

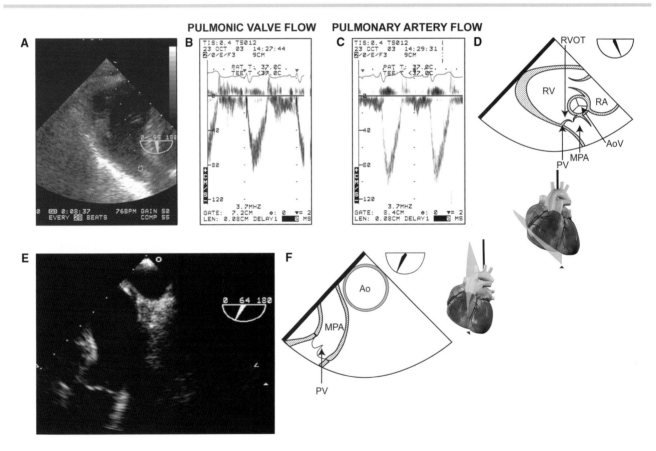

Figure 4.40 Pulmonic valve Doppler. (A–D) Pulsed wave Doppler interrogation of the PV and the MPA from the transgastric right ventricular inflow/outflow view at 94° are shown. **(E,F)** Upper esophageal aortic arch short-axis view shows the PV with good Doppler alignment. *Abbreviations*: Ao, aorta; AoV, aortic valve; MPA, main pulmonary artery; PV, pulmonic valve; RA, right atrium; RV, right ventricle; RVOT, right ventricular outflow tract.

pressures. In the case of abnormally decreased LV compliance or elevated LA or LV filling pressures, such as in moderate-to-severe MR or significant LV systolic or diastolic dysfunction, there will be diastolic flow prominence ($S/D < 1$). Severe MR can even cause systolic flow reversal.

Elevated LV end-diastolic pressures during atrial contraction cause preferential blood backflow in the pulmonary veins rather than downstream through the MV. This leads not only to increased atrial reversal velocity but also atrial reversal duration exceeding that of the mitral A wave by >30 ms (see Chapter 10).

Hepatic Vein

The hepatic veins are the equivalent of the pulmonary veins for the right heart (Fig. 4.30). Similarly, the hepatic venous spectral Doppler flow is multiphasic, with systolic, diastolic, and atrial reversal waves. However, with operating pressures on the right heart lower than on the left, there is often some mild systolic flow reversal before diastolic flow. The S/D ratio is usually >1 with normal right-sided filling pressures (see Chapter 10).

When the right-sided filling pressures are elevated, normal systolic flow prominence may be lost with, occasionally, even an absence of forward flow during systole. In such cases, the S/D ratio will be inverted (<1) (see Chapter 10). Tamponade physiology can also be accompanied by abnormal expiratory diastolic flow reversal (see Chapter 12).

Ascending Aorta

As stated earlier in the evaluation of AS, maximal aortic velocity and pressure gradient should be sought from a high esophageal window looking down the distal ascending Ao even if this is not always achievable because of interference from the air-filled trachea (Fig. 4.11).

Descending Ao-Flow Reversal and Aortic Regurgitation

Although the descending thoracic Ao easily lends itself to 2D examination because of its very close proximity to the esophagus, the direction of aortic flow is, however, often perpendicular to the direction of the ultrasound beam of the TEE probe. Therefore, precise measurements of the descending thoracic Ao pressure gradient (for coarctation evaluation, for instance) are usually precluded. Likewise, assessment of AR severity with measurement of the duration, velocity, and VTI of the diastolic flow reversal may be harder to achieve than by TTE (see Chapter 23).

Coronary Sinus

Coronary sinus Doppler examination is best conducted from the lower esophageal sphincter position while withdrawing the probe from the transgastric to the esophageal position in the longitudinal plane at 90°. The coronary sinus will appear in its SAX near the left atrioventricular groove (Fig. 4.32D and E). When the coronary sinus is positioned over the top center of the display, clockwise rotation of the probe shaft toward the right will follow the course of the coronary sinus towards its ostium in the RA. Most often, the coronary sinus will then be imaged in its LAX at 0°, with the coronary sinus flow going away from the probe. Coronary sinus spectral Doppler flow is similar to the multiphasic right-sided venous flow.

Pulmonary Artery

As stated previously in the evaluation of PS, maximal pulmonic velocity, and pressure gradient can be assessed from upper esophageal transverse plane at 0° looking down the PV. Alternatively, this can be achieved from below the valve through a modified transgastric view at 60° to 90° with the probe shaft rotated rightward.

CONCLUSION

Multiplane TEE enables a complete assessment of cardiac structure and function in most patients. Optimal use of TEE requires a thorough understanding of cardiac anatomy and pathophysiology together with considerable experience in TEE probe and ultrasound system manipulation (5). While a TEE study targeted at a specific clinical question is justified in certain circumstances, a comprehensive evaluation is encouraged in most patients. Finally, as with any imaging study in medicine, TEE should, preferably, only be performed if the results of the examination will have an impact on subsequent patient management.

REFERENCES

1. Frazin L, Talano JV, Stephanides L, et al. Esophageal echocardiography. Circulation 1976; 54:102–108.
2. Khandheria BK, Tajik AJ, Seward JB. Multiplane transesophageal echocardiography: examination technique, anatomic correlations, and image orientation. Crit Care Clin 1996; 12:203–233.
3. Shanewise JS, Cheung AT, Aronson S, et al. ASE/SCA guidelines for performing a comprehensive intraoperative multiplane transesophageal echocardiography examination: recommendations of the American Society of Echocardiography Council for Intraoperative Echocardiography and the Society of Cardiovascular Anesthesiologists Task Force for Certification in Perioperative Transesophageal Echocardiography. Anesth Analg 1999; 89:870–884.
4. Khandheria BK, Seward JB, Tajik AJ. Critical appraisal of transesophageal echocardiography: limitations and pitfalls. Crit Care Clin 1996; 12:235–251.
5. Toronto General Hospital Department of Anesthesia. Virtual TEE. Available at: http://pie.med.utoronto.ca/tee/TEE_ content/TEE_standardViews_intro.html.

5

Quantitative Echocardiography

Jean Buithieu
McGill University, Montreal, Quebec, Canada

Annette Vegas
University of Toronto, Toronto, Ontario, Canada

André Y. Denault
Université de Montréal, Montreal, Quebec, Canada

M-MODE AND TWO-DIMENSIONAL IMAGING

Edge Recognition

The edge between the left ventricular (LV) cavity and the myocardium is represented by the endocardial border that reflects echoes with a certain thickness. The leading edge of a structure is defined as the portion of the border closest to the transducer, while the trailing edge is the portion furthest from the transducer. In two-dimensional (2D) echocardiography, the inner edge is defined as the portion of the border closest to the center of the structure while the outer edge is the furthest from it (Fig. 5.1). Several conventions have been proposed to measure the size of cardiac structures, which differ on the basis of imaging mode, and whether to include the thickness of edge echoes in the measurements.

The *Standard Convention*, published in 1968, for M-mode echocardiography included the edge thickness in the measurement of wall thickness (1). The interventricular septum (IVS) was defined as the area from leading to trailing edge; the posterior wall as the area from the leading edge of the endocardium to the leading edge of the posterior pericardium. Good correlation of the posterior wall thickness (PWT) measurement was found by this method when compared with pathological specimens. Measuring the LV internal dimension by this method also correlated with measurements obtained by contrast ventriculography.

The *Penn Convention* was developed in 1977 to provide a better correlation between LV mass derived from M-mode echocardiographic calculations and gold standard pathology measurements (2). This convention excluded the edge thickness in the measurement of wall thickness. The septum and posterior wall were defined as the areas from trailing edge to leading edge (Fig. 5.1). The LV internal dimension, therefore, included the thickness of the endocardial borders.

Over the years the American Society of Echocardiography (ASE) has published guidelines to improve the consistency of echocardiographic measurements. In 1978, the initial ASE convention for M-mode echocardiography recommended using a leading edge to leading edge method for measuring cardiac structures (3). This ASE convention was based on a consensus of questionnaire surveys returned from various echocardiographic laboratories rather than on validated correlative data. The ASE guidelines from 1989 for left ventricle (LV) quantitation by 2D echocardiography suggested using the endocardial cavity (black-white) interface for measurements (4). This is the same recommendation that was in the 2005 consensus guidelines by the ASE and European Association for Echocardiography for the 2D measurements of cardiac structure for both transthoracic (TTE) and transesophageal echocardiography (TEE) (5).

Timing

The ASE recommends the timing of end-diastole and end-systole be preferably referenced to the mitral valve (MV) (4) or alternatively to chamber size rather than the electrocardiogram (EKG) (5). The end of diastole is timed at the frame where the MV leaflets initially coapt, marking MV closure. As EKG tracing quality may vary and, consequently, result in a variable R wave of the QRS complex, the ASE advises the end of diastole be best timed at the onset of the QRS complex.

The end of systole can be timed at the frame preceding the opening of the MV leaflets or at minimum LV cavity dimensions. When timing end-systole with aortic valve (AoV) closure, the ASE suggests making end-systolic measurements using the peak motion of the IVS. This is best seen using a transthoracic parasternal long-axis (LAX) M-mode echocardiogram where the peak downward motion of the IVS often slightly precedes the peak upward motion of the LV posterior wall. The apparent asynchrony of the inward motion of the two opposite walls may be

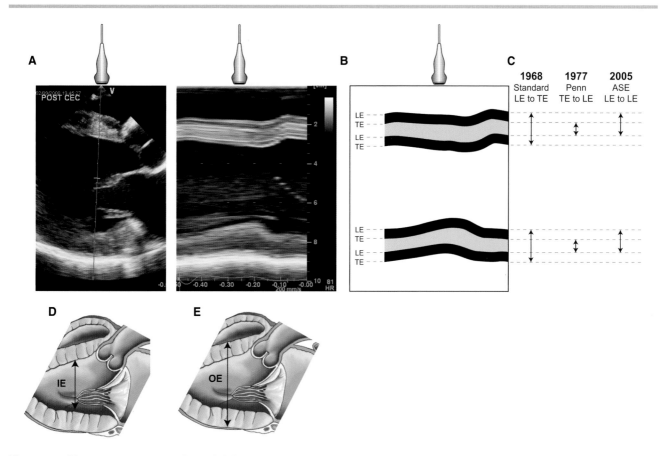

Figure 5.1 Measurement conventions. (A) Transthoracic parasternal long-axis view of the left ventricle with corresponding M-mode is shown. **(B)** The LE and TE are referenced to the transducer in M-mode schematic. **(C)** The various conventions for measuring cardiac structures in M-mode are shown. **(D,E)** The American Society of Echocardiography (ASE) current guidelines suggest measuring at the tissue blood interface in 2D image. *Abbreviations*: IE, inner edge; LE, leading edge; OE; outer edge; TE, trailing edge.

accentuated with abnormal septal wall motion associated with decreased regional wall contractility, bundle branch conduction delays, pacing, or cardiac surgery. In the presence of abnormal septal motion, with a delay of inward septal motion, the peak motion of the posterior wall should be used to time end-systole.

Referencing Centroids

The heart contracts in systole using at least five identified movements: (*i*) myocardial wall thickening in a radial fashion, toward the center of the ventricle, (*ii*) base-to-apex LAX shortening toward the apex, (*iii*) rotational motion around the long axis, (*iv*) some degree of tilting, that is, rotational motion around the minor axis, and (*v*) translation of the entire heart in space and torsion (Fig. 5.2). Evaluating the regional contractility of a three-dimensional (3D) spatial object, such as the heart, against time by a tomographic technique, such as 2D echocardiography, is bound by certain limitations. A valid system for assessment of regional wall motion abnormalities must first

compensate for global heart motion then evaluate both endocardial motion and myocardial thickening. In the quantitative assessment of regional wall function, reference centroids address the reference used to define the parameters of normal and abnormal function.

The pixel coordinate system of the video image frame appears easy to use for the comparison of the endocardial and epicardial contour traced at end-diastole and end-systole. This static reference system does not allow any correction of 3D translational and rotational heart motions. Potential error is introduced, as true assessment of wall thickening is not made perpendicular to the defined contours. A polar coordinate system is preferable using, as a reference, a center of mass point (centroid) within the LV internal cavity. If defined from internal cardiac landmarks, this centroid reference system would have the advantage of moving with the heart and allowing corrections for translational and rotational motions.

Different methods have been proposed to define the central reference point (centroid) for a given video-frame in time. The bisector of a line traced between an accepted landmark in the ventricular

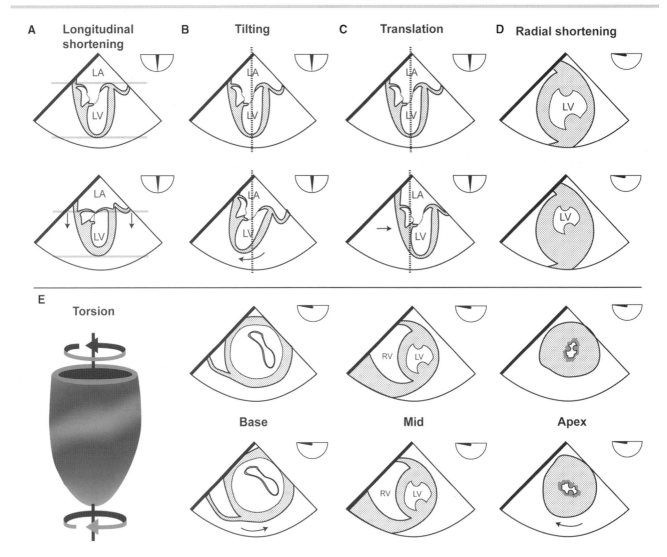

Figure 5.2 Schematic representations of heart movements. Heart movements include (**A**) base to apex longitudinal shortening, (**B**) tilting around the minor axis, (**C**) translation of the entire heart, (**D**) radial shortening rotation around the long axis, and (**E**) torsion. Normally when viewed from the apex, the base turns clockwise and the apex counterclockwise. (**E**) From a transgastric view, the opposite will be observed. *Abbreviations*: LA, left atrium; LV, left ventricle; RV, right ventricle.

wall and the furthest point on the opposing wall may divide the cavity in half, but it may also be easily skewed by the presence of asymmetrical distortion of the LV shape, such as with an LV aneurysm or a dyskinetic ventricle. Other methods consist of computing the centroid from either the whole endocardial or epicardial contour, using various algorithms (6).

As the heart moves during the cardiac cycle, the centroid determined for each video-frame during the contraction sequence will not be in the same position throughout this period. Therefore, it is also necessary to define the spatial centroid in time. In the fixed axis reference method, all wall motion is referenced to a fixed centroid in time, which may be the centroid of a chosen particular frame (e.g., the end-diastolic point) or the average (or integration) of all the centroids

found throughout the cardiac sequence. In the floating axis reference method, each video-frame keeps its own-derived centroid, and the centroid position is allowed to change (float) during the contraction sequence (Fig. 5.3).

As the type of centroid chosen influences the length of all the radii traced from the reference centroid to the myocardial border, each method has its own advantages and disadvantages. A floating centroid will better correct for the heart translation but will, for the same reason, underestimate the amount and location of a dyskinetic wall. Conversely, a fixed axis reference system will portray normal heart translation as abnormal wall motion, but may adequately detect nontranslating hypokinetic walls (Fig. 5.3). While none of the centroid methods are ideal for all

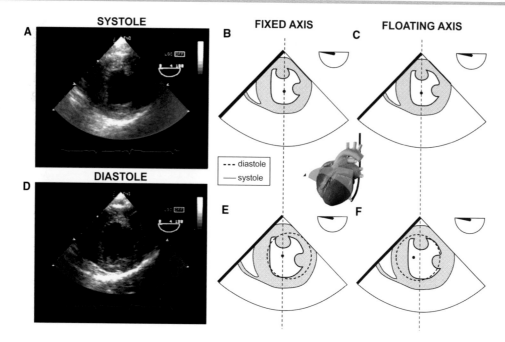

Figure 5.3   Abnormal septal motion. Transgastric mid short-axis view of a patient with a left bundle branch block results in abnormal septal motion shown during systole (**A–C**) and diastole (**D–F**). Using a fixed axis (**B,E**), the abnormal septal motion is identified without the rotational artifact. With a floating axis (**C,F**), the center of the image is displaced to the left but the normal segment appears hypokinetic. 🖱

situations, the comparison of results between data obtained with each method may shed some light on understanding the type and degree of heart motion contaminating the analysis of wall thickening. For instance, if there is no difference in short-axis (SAX) endocardial symmetrical motion between the fixed and the floating axis method, we can infer that no significant translation is present.

Parallel Chord and Centerline Methods

Once the most appropriate centroid reference system has been chosen, different approaches are proposed to measure the extent and severity of regional contractility. In SAX views of the LV, radial chords can be traced between the centroid and the endocardial contour and followed throughout the cardiac cycle to endocardial excursion. Alternatively, the difference in the radial chord length between the centroid and the endocardial and epicardial contours can be tracked to measure myocardial wall thickening. For two- and four-chamber views, the major LV long axis can be used to trace a series of parallel chords perpendicularly between the myocardial contour and the major axis. A variation combining parallel chords for the base and the mid-ventricle and radial chords for the apical region may help, imperfectly, to reduce the shortcomings of apical thickening assessment with the parallel chord method.

The centerline method traces the diastolic and systolic endocardial borders and the computer constructs a line, the centerline, midway between the traced endocardial LV contours (Fig. 5.4). The computer draws perpendicular chords connecting all the midpoints between the endocardial contour in diastole and systole. Endocardial excursion, starting from the end-diastolic contour, is measured along 100 perpendicular chords to the centerline, resulting in systematic assessment of regional wall motion. If a similar analysis is carried out conjointly with the epicardial contour in diastole and in systole, systematic assessment of regional wall thickening is also performed.

Cardiac Dimensions

Simple on-screen linear and area measurements can be performed using both M-mode and 2D echocardiography to assess the size of cardiac structures.

M-Mode

Because of its superior temporal and axial resolution, M-mode echocardiography has generally been the method of choice for measuring cardiac chamber size dimensions. The validity of M-mode measurements is based on a perpendicular alignment of the structures of interest with the line of the M-mode

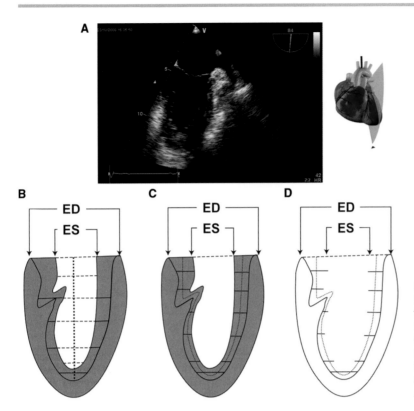

Figure 5.4 Centroid reference systems. (A–B) Parallel chords drawn from the centroid (long axis) trace the endocardial border during ES and ED in this mid-esophageal two-chamber view. **(C–D)** Centerline method traces ED and ES endocardial borders and the computer draws a centerline midway between these endocardial borders. Note there is slightly greater systolic thickening in the anterior wall. *Abbreviations*: ED, end-diastole; ES, end-systole.

cursor. The width of the M-mode echoes may be influenced by instrumentation and gain settings. The ASE recommends that all M-mode measurements of cardiac structures be made from leading edge to leading edge of the lines representing the structures' interface (7).

Transthoracic M-mode measurements. From a TTE parasternal SAX 2D view of the AoV and the left atrium (LA), the M-mode cursor is positioned through the center of the AoV (Fig. 5.5). The aortic root is measured at end-diastole (onset of QRS complex) from the leading edge of the anterior aortic wall to the leading edge of the posterior aortic wall. The normal value is 1.0 to 1.8 cm/m² in normal young adults (8). The LA is measured at end-systole at the peak of the anterior motion of the posterior wall of the aorta (Ao). The convention for M-mode measurement used to measure from the leading edge of the posterior aortic wall to the leading edge of the posterior LA wall, but the most recent guidelines recommend to measure from the trailing edge of the posterior wall of the Ao to the leading edge of the posterior wall of the LA, to avoid the variable extent of space between the LA and aortic root (5). The normal value is 3.8 ± 0.98 cm for the LA (9).

From a TTE parasternal LAX 2D view of the LV just beneath the MV leaflets, the M-mode cursor is positioned through the center of the LV cavity (Fig. 5.5). Measurements at end-diastole are performed at the onset of QRS complex and at end-systole at the peak posterior displacement of the ventricular septum. The interventricular septal wall thickness (SWT) is measured from the leading edge of the IVS to the leading edge of the endocardial border of the interventricular septal wall. The left ventricular dimension at end-diastole (LVEDD) or end-systole (LVESD) is measured from the leading edge of the endocardial border of the interventricular septal wall to the leading edge of the endocardial border of the posterior wall. The PWT is measured from the leading edge of the endocardial border of the posterior wall to the leading edge of the epicardial surface of the posterior wall. The right ventricular end-diastolic dimension (RVEDD) is measured from the leading edge of the endocardial border of the right ventricular anterior wall to the leading edge of the right endocardial border of the IVS.

Two-Dimensional Measurements

When the cardiac structures of interest cannot be positioned perpendicular to the line of M-mode interrogation, 2D echocardiographic measurements are preferred. The ASE recommends measuring cardiac structures by 2D echocardiography from inner edge to inner edge (black-white interface), as opposed to the leading edge to leading edge method in M-mode echocardiography (4,5,10). Normal values have been reported for TEE, which differ slightly from those of TTE (8,9,11) (Fig. 5.6). The ASE quantification guidelines published in 2005 suggest using the same values for equivalent TTE and TEE views (5).

LV measurements. The ASE recommends measuring the LV dimensions from the mid-esophageal

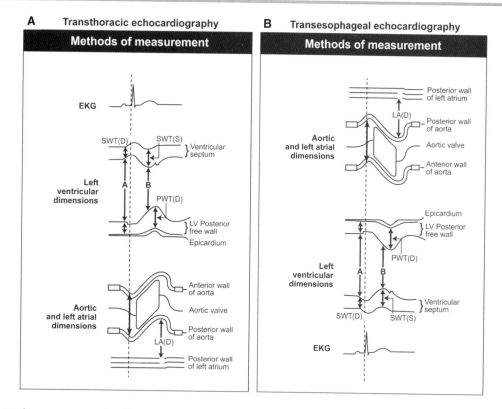

Figure 5.5 M-mode measurements. Recommended M-mode measurements of ventricular, aortic and atrial dimensions from (**A**) transthoracic and (**B**) transesophageal echocardiography are shown. *Abbreviations*: A, left ventricular end-diastolic dimension; B, left ventricular end-diastolic dimension; EKG, electrocardiogram; D, diastole; LA, left atrium; LV, left ventricle; PWT, posterior wall thickness; S, systole; SWT, septal wall thickness.

and transgastric two-chamber views, as the apex of the LV is frequently foreshortened in the mid-esophageal four-chamber view (5) (Fig. 5.7). The major, or long, axis is measured from inner edge of the true apical endocardium to the middle of the MV annulus. The minor, or short, axis of the LV is measured at the mitral chordal level, perpendicular to the long axis, from the endocardium of the anterior to inferior walls (Fig. 5.7). The minor axis can also be measured in the anterior-posterior and medial-lateral planes from an LV transgastric SAX view at 0° at the level of the papillary muscles. The ASE describes partition values for LV size with severe dilatation in short axis at end-diastole (LVEDD) in females of ≥6.2 cm and males ≥6.9 cm (Fig. 5.8).

Right ventricle measurements. The right ventricle (RV) is a complex structure that is difficult to image, adequately, in a single TEE plane. The ASE recommends measuring the RV dimensions from a mid-esophageal four-chamber view at 0° (5). The major, or long, axis of the RV is measured from inner edge of the true apical endocardium to the middle of the tricuspid valve (TV) annulus as determined from the base of the TV leaflets (Fig. 5.9). The minor, or short, axis of the RV is measured in the lateral to septal plane perpendicular to the hypothetical long axis at two levels, at a point located at the junction between the basal and the middle third of the RV and at the base of

the TV. The ASE describes partition values for RV size with severe dilatation at end-diastole at the base of ≥3.9 cm, in mid short axis of ≥4.2 cm, and base to apex length of ≥9.2 cm.

Left and right atrial measurements. Because of the proximity of the LA to the TEE probe it is difficult to image the entire LA. The major, or long, axis of the LA and RA can be measured in the superior-inferior plane from a mid-esophageal four-chamber view at 0°, from inner edge of the dome of the atria to the middle of the atrioventricular valve annulus. This measurement is however not part of the current guidelines (5). The minor, or short, axis of the LA and RA is measured in the lateral to septal plane perpendicular to the hypothetical long axis at a point located halfway (Fig. 5.10). Alterations in size of the atria may be asymmetric so linear measurements may be less accurate than estimating LA volume. The ASE defines severely abnormal dimensions of the LA as left atrial diameter ≥4.7 cm (women), ≥5.2 cm (men), an LA area of >40 cm², and indexed LA volume more than 40 mL/m² in both genders (5).

Left ventricular outflow tract and aorta diameter measurements. The diameter of the Ao is measured at various locations corresponding to the different portions of the Ao. The ASE recommends measuring the aortic root from the 2D image of the mid-esophageal AoV LAX view at ~100° to 135° (Fig. 5.11).

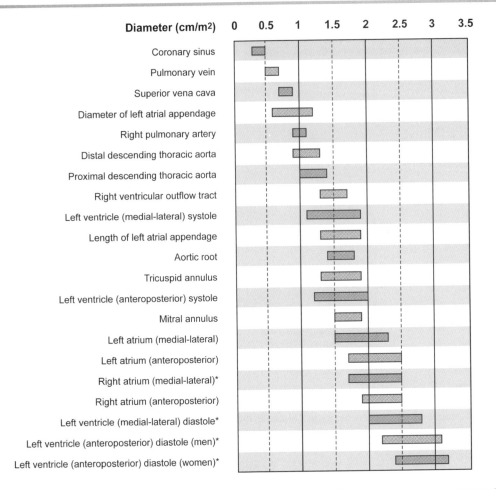

Figure 5.6 TEE reference values. The dimensions of cardiac structures indexed to body surface area as measured using TEE are shown. *Abbreviation*: TEE, transesophageal echocardiography. *Source*: Adapted from Refs. 5 and 11.

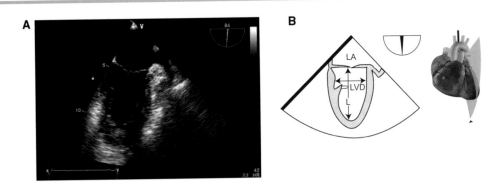

Figure 5.7 LV dimensions. (A,B) Transesophageal echocardiographic measurements, at end-diastole, of LV length (L) and minor diameter (LVD) are acquired from an optimized mid-esophageal two-chamber view at 60–90°. *Abbreviations*: LA, left atrium, LV, left ventricle (see Fig. 5.8 for LVD reference values). *Source*: Adapted from Ref. 5.

Measurements made during end-systole and end-diastole are relatively similar. Measurements are taken using an inner edge to inner edge technique at the left ventricular outflow tract (LVOT), base of the aortic cusps, sinus of Valsalva, sinotubular junction, and the proximal ascending Ao. The TEE probe is withdrawn to obtain a better image of the ascending Ao in long axis and measure the middle and distal

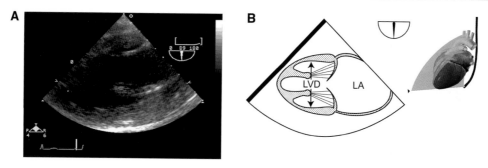

		Reference range	Mildly abnormal	Moderatly abnormal	Severely abnormal
LV dimension					
LV diastolic diameter, cm	W	3.9-5.3	5.4-5.7	5.8-6.1	≥ 6.2
	M	4.2-5.9	6.0-6.3	6.4-6.8	≥ 6.9
LV diastolic diameter/BSA, cm/m²	W	2.4-3.2	3.3-3.4	3.5-3.7	≥ 3.8
	M	2.2-3.1	3.2-3.4	3.5-3.6	≥ 3.7
LV diastolic diameter/height, cm/m	W	2.5-3.2	3.3-3.4	3.5-3.6	≥ 3.7
	M	2.4-3.3	3.4-3.5	3.6-3.7	≥ 3.8
LV volume					
LV diastolic volume, mL	W	56-104	105-117	118-130	>131
	M	67-155	156-178	179-201	>201
LV diastolic volume/BSA, mL/m²	W	35-75	76-86	87-96	≥ 97
	M	35-75	76-86	87-96	≥ 97
LV systolic volume, mL	W	19-49	50-59	60-69	≥ 70
	M	22-58	59-70	71-82	≥ 83
LV systolic volume/BSA, mL/m²	W	12-30	31-36	37-42	≥ 43
	M	12-30	31-36	37-42	≥ 43

Figure 5.8 LV dimensions. (A,B) Transesophageal echocardiographic measurements, at end-diastole, of LV minor-axis diameter (LVD) are obtained from a transgastric two-chamber view of the LV at 90–110°. **(C)** The table shows values of LVD and LV volume, by sex, as absolute values (mL) and indexed to BSA (mL/m²) and height (cm/m). *Abbreviations*: BSA, body surface area; LA, left atrium; LV, left ventricle; M, man; W, woman. *Source*: Adapted with permission from Ref. 5.

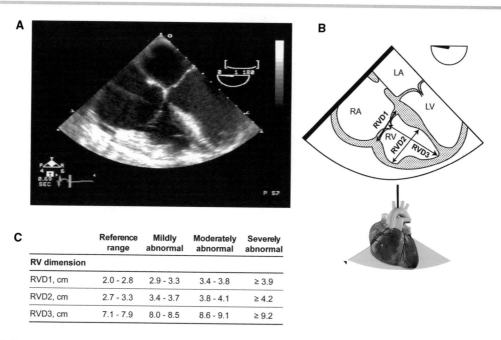

	Reference range	Mildly abnormal	Moderately abnormal	Severely abnormal
RV dimension				
RVD1, cm	2.0 - 2.8	2.9 - 3.3	3.4 - 3.8	≥ 3.9
RVD2, cm	2.7 - 3.3	3.4 - 3.7	3.8 - 4.1	≥ 4.2
RVD3, cm	7.1 - 7.9	8.0 - 8.5	8.6 - 9.1	≥ 9.2

Figure 5.9 RV dimensions. (A,B) Transesophageal echocardiographic measurements, at end-diastole, of various RV diameters (RVD) obtained from a mid-esophageal four-chamber view optimized to the maximum RV size by varying angles 0°–20°. **(C)** The table shows normal and abnormal values for RVD1, RVD2, and RVD3. *Abbreviations*: LA, left atrium; LV, left ventricle, RA, right atrium; RV, right ventricle. *Source*: Adapted with permission from Refs. 5 and 12.

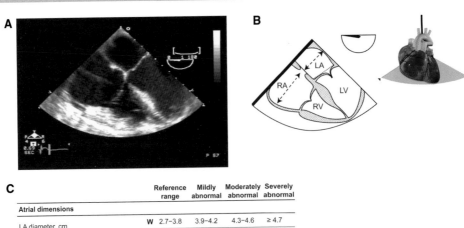

		Reference range	Mildly abnormal	Moderately abnormal	Severely abnormal
Atrial dimensions					
LA diameter, cm	W	2.7–3.8	3.9–4.2	4.3–4.6	≥ 4.7
	M	3.0–4.0	4.1–4.6	4.7–5.2	≥ 5.2
LA diameter/BSA, cm/m²	W	1.5–2.3	2.4–2.6	2.7–2.9	≥ 3.0
	M	1.5–2.3	2.4–2.6	2.7–2.9	≥ 3.0
LA area, cm²	W	≤ 20	20-30	30-40	> 40
	M	≤ 20	≤ 20-30	30-40	> 40
LA volume, mL	W	22-52	53-62	63-72	≥ 73
	M	18-58	59-68	69-78	≥ 79
LA volume/BSA, mL/m²	W	16-28	29-33	34-39	≥ 40
	M	16-28	29-33	34-39	≥ 40
RA minor-axis dimension, cm	W	2.9–4.5	4.6–4.9	5.0–5.4	≥ 5.5
	M	2.9–4.5	4.6–4.9	5.0–5.4	≥ 5.5
RA minor-axis dimension/BSA, cm/m²	W	1.7–2.5	2.6–2.8	2.9–3.1	≥ 3.2
	M	1.7–2.5	2.6–2.8	2.9–3.1	≥ 3.2

Figure 5.10   Atrial dimensions. (A,B) Transesophageal echocardiographic measurements, at ventricular end-systole, of the RA and LA from the mid-esophageal four-chamber view optimally positioned to visualize both chambers. **(C)** Table of normal and abnormal values for atrial dimensions and volumes as absolute values and indexed to BSA. *Abbreviations*: BSA, body surface area; LA, left atrium; LV, left ventricle; RA, right atrium; RV, right ventricle. *Source*: Adapted with permission from Ref. 5.

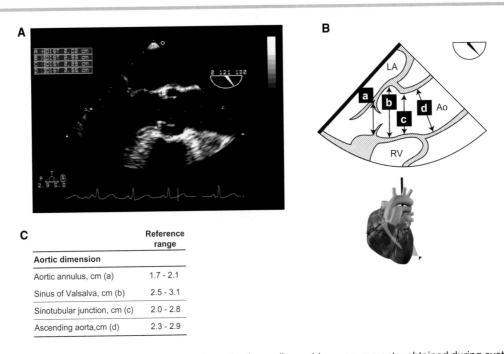

	Reference range
Aortic dimension	
Aortic annulus, cm (a)	1.7 - 2.1
Sinus of Valsalva, cm (b)	2.5 - 3.1
Sinotubular junction, cm (c)	2.0 - 2.8
Ascending aorta,cm (d)	2.3 - 2.9

Figure 5.11   Aortic root dimensions. (A,B) Transesophageal echocardiographic measurements, obtained during systole, from a mid-esophageal long- axis view at 110°–115 °. Measurements using the inner to inner edge technique are taken at the (a) aortic annulus, (b) sinus of Valsalva, (c) sinotubular junction and (d) ascending Ao. **(C)** Table of normal absolute values is shown. *Abbreviations*: Ao, aorta; LA, left atrium; RV, right ventricle. *Source*: from Ref. 13.

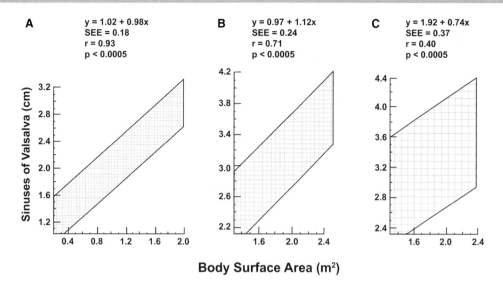

Body Surface Area (m²)

Figure 5.12 Aortic root dimensions. The 95% confidence intervals for aortic root diameter at the sinuses of Valsalva indexed to body surface area in children and adolescents (**A**), adults aged 20 to 39 years (**B**), and adults aged 40 years or older (**C**) are shown. *Source*: Adapted with permission from Ref. 5.

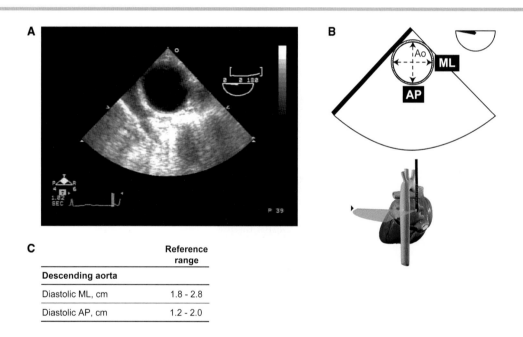

Descending aorta	Reference range
Diastolic ML, cm	1.8 - 2.8
Diastolic AP, cm	1.2 - 2.0

Figure 5.13 Descending aorta dimensions. (**A,B**) Transesophageal echocardiographic measurements, obtained during diastole, of the descending aorta AP and ML dimensions from a mid-esophageal short-axis view at 0°. (**C**) The normal absolute values (in cm) for a 25-year-old man with a body surface area of 1.8 cm² are shown. *Abbreviations*: Ao, aorta; AP, anteroposterior; ML, medial-lateral. *Source*: from Ref. 8.

ascending Ao. These measurements are made using the largest aortic diameter perpendicular to the long axis of the Ao. Abnormalities in Ao size are best indexed to age and body surface area (BSA) (14) (Fig. 5.12).

From the upper esophageal (UE) position at 90°, the transverse arch in short axis can be measured before the origin of the brachiocephalic trunk, and between the brachiocephalic trunk and the left common

carotid artery (see Fig. 4.37). Advancing the TEE probe at 0° from the high esophageal position to the transgastric position, the diameter of the descending thoracic and upper abdominal Ao is measured (Fig. 5.13).

RV outflow tract and pulmonary artery diameter measurements.   The right ventricular outflow tract (RVOT), which includes the pulmonic valve (PV), is best imaged using TEE in the RV inflow-outflow view at

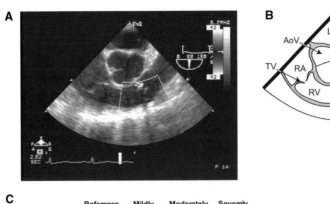
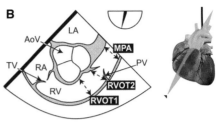

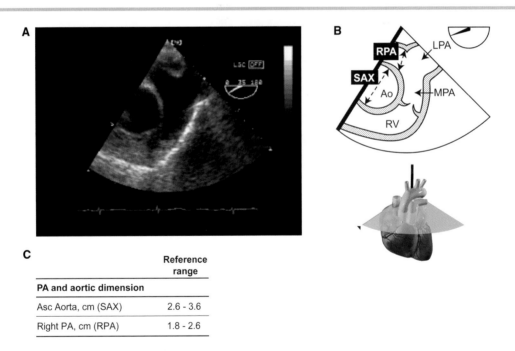

	Reference range	Mildly abnormal	Moderately abnormal	Severely abnormal
RV dimension				
RVOT1, cm	2.5 - 2.9	3.0 - 3.2	3.3 - 3.5	≥ 3.6
RVOT2, cm	1.7 - 2.3	2.4 - 2.7	2.8 - 3.1	≥ 3.2
MPA, cm	1.5 - 2.1	2.2 - 2.5	2.6 - 2.9	≥ 3.0

Figure 5.14 RVOT dimensions. (A,B) Transesophageal echocardiographic measurements, during end-diastole, of the RVOT at two levels (RVOT1, RVOT2) and the MPA from the mid-esophageal right ventricular inflow/outflow view at 88°. **(C)** The normal and abnormal absolute values (in cm) are presented. *Abbreviations*: AoV, aortic valve; LA, left atrium; LV, left ventricle; MPA, main pulmonary artery; PV, pulmonic valve; RA, right atrium; RV, right ventricle; RVOT, right ventricular outflow tract; TV, tricuspid valve. *Source*: Adapted with permission from Refs. 5 and 12.

	Reference range
PA and aortic dimension	
Asc Aorta, cm (SAX)	2.6 - 3.6
Right PA, cm (RPA)	1.8 - 2.6

Figure 5.15 PA and ascending aorta dimensions. (A,B) Transesophageal echocardiographic measurement obtained during systole of the RPA and ascending Ao from a mid-esophageal ascending Ao SAX view at 0°. **(C)** The normal absolute values (in cm) for a 25-year-old man with a body surface area of 1.8 cm² are shown. *Abbreviations*: Ao, aorta; LPA, left pulmonary artery; MPA, main pulmonary artery; PA, pulmonary artery; RPA, right pulmonary artery; RV, right ventricle; SAX, short axis. *Source*: from Ref. 8.

60° to 75° (Fig. 5.14). The ASE recommends measuring the diameter of the RVOT during end-diastole at two levels, at the subpulmonary (RVOT1, severely dilated ≥3.6 cm) and at the pulmonic annulus (RVOT2, severely dilated ≥ 3.2 cm) (5). Measurement of the main pulmonary artery trunk diameter (severely dilated ≥3.0 cm) can also be obtained in this view. The diameter of the origin of the right and left pulmonary arteries is more easily obtained in a slightly more superior esophageal position at 0° (Fig. 5.15).

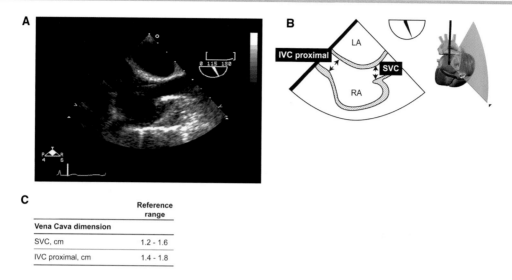

Figure 5.16   Vena cavae dimensions. (A,B) Transesophageal echocardiographic measurements, during systole, of the proximal vena cavae at the junction of the RA from a mid-esophageal bicaval view at 90°. **(C)** Normal absolute values (in cm) are shown. *Abbreviations*: IVC, inferior vena cava; LA, left atrium; RA, right atrium; SVC, superior vena cava. *Source*: from Refs. 11 and 13.

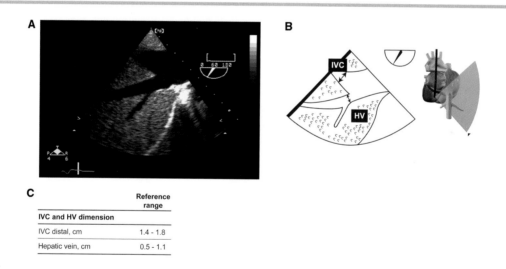

Figure 5.17   IVC and hepatic vein HV dimensions. (A,B) TEE measurements, during systole, of the distal IVC and HV from a modified transgastric view at 60° with the TEE probe turned towards the liver. **(C)** Normal absolute values (in cm) are shown. *Abbreviations*: HV, hepatic vein, IVC, inferior vena cava; TEE, transesophageal echocardiography. *Source*: from Ref. 13.

Inferior vena cava, superior vena cava, and hepatic vein measurements. Both the proximal superior vena cava (SVC) and inferior vena cava (IVC) can easily be imaged and measured in the mid-esophageal bicaval view at 90° (Fig. 5.16). The IVC and the hepatic veins can also be measured from a modified TG view (0–60°) with the TEE probe directed toward the liver (Fig. 5.17). Caval diameter is affected by alterations in right atrial pressure (RAP). The normal IVC diameter is <1.7 cm, though values up to 2.3 cm may occur in athletes (5).

Atrioventricular valve annular diameters measurements. The TV annulus diameter is obtained from the mid-esophageal four-chamber view at 0°. Annular measurements vary slightly between systole and diastole. The measurements frequently recorded in TTE are 28 ± 5 mm measured during systole that correlates with the early diastolic measurement in the TEE mid-esophageal four-chamber view in normal adults (11). The best TEE correlation of TV annular measurements with surgical comparison is in the transgastric right ventricular LAX view (15). The two diameters of the saddle-shaped MV annulus may be obtained from the mid-esophageal four-chamber view at 0° and from the two-chamber view at 90°.

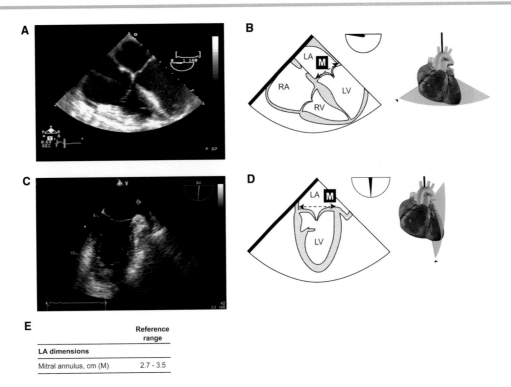

Figure 5.18   Mitral annular dimensions. (A–D) Transesophageal echocardiographic measurements, during systole, of the mitral valve annulus (M) from the mid-esophageal four-chamber view **(A,B)** at 0° and two-chamber view **(C,D)** at 90°. **(E)** Normal absolute value (in cm) is shown. *Abbreviations*: LA, left atrium; LV, left ventricle; RA, right atrium; RV, right ventricle. *Source*: from Ref. 11.

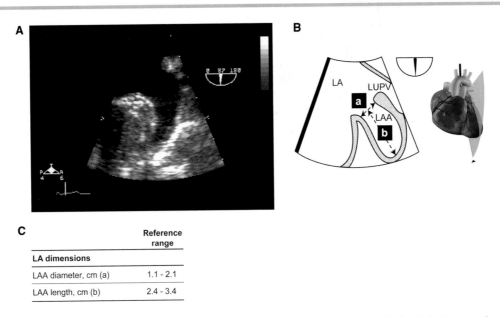

Figure 5.19   LAA dimensions. (A,B) Transesophageal echocardiographic measurements, obtained during systole, of the LAA and LUPV from a zoomed mid-esophageal two-chamber view at 90°. The LAA diameter (a) is taken at the ostium bounded by the "coumadin ridge," the tissue separating the LUPV and the lower transverse pericardial sinus. The length of the LAA (b) extends from the LAA tip to the ostial line. **(C)** Normal absolute values (in cm) are shown. *Abbreviations*: LA, left atrium; LAA, Left atrial appendage; LUPV, left upper pulmonary vein. *Source*: from Ref. 11.

Measurements should be taken from the base of the leaflets (Fig. 5.18).

Pulmonary vein, left atrial appendage, and coronary sinus measurements.   The left atrial appendage (LAA)

is best imaged in the mid-esophageal two-chamber at 90° or mitral commissural view at 60° to 75° as a triangle-shaped structure just above the MV annulus (Fig. 5.19). With the LAA on display the cephalad

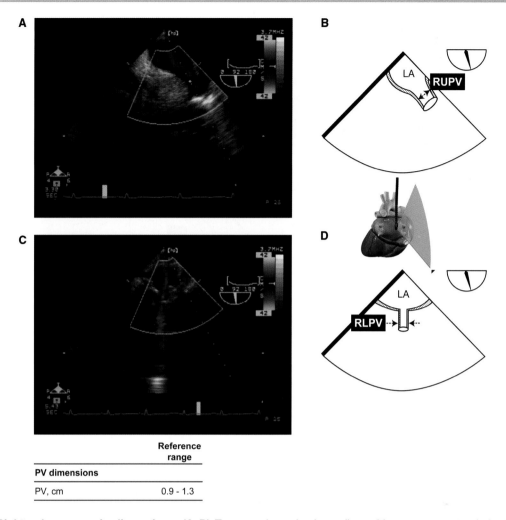

Figure 5.20 Right pulmonary vein dimensions. (A–D) Transesophageal echocardiographic measurements, during systole, of the RUPV from a modified bicaval view (**A,B**) at 98° and RLPV from a mid-esophageal view (**C,D**). The measurement is made at 1 cm from where the pulmonary veins enter the LA. *Abbreviations*: LA, left atrium; RLPV, right lower pulmonary vein; RUPV, right upper pulmonary vein. *Source*: from Ref. 11.

positioned left upper pulmonary vein (LUPV) is viewed by slightly withdrawing the TEE probe. In this view, the dimensions of the LAA and diameter of the LUPV can easily be measured. The right-sided pulmonary veins are easier to identify using a bicaval view with right-sided rotation (Fig. 5.20). Finally, the coronary sinus diameter is measured from a LAX view of the coronary sinus obtained by advancing the probe from the mid-esophageal four-chamber view to the gastroesophageal junction (Fig. 5.21).

Chamber Volume Calculations

Various methods have been used to estimate LV volumes from linear and area cardiac chamber dimensions measured in M-mode and 2D echocardiography. These methods are based on the assumption that the LV has a symmetrical geometric form (Fig. 5.22). This assumption is correct if the heart is normal but may not hold true if the heart is deformed by an aneurysm, or becomes asymmetrical in systole because of regional wall motion abnormalities.

Cubic Method

Earlier correlation with LV volumes assessed by angiographic data (16) seemed to suggest a reasonable relationship with estimations derived from cubing the cavity dimensions. The cubic method assumes that the LV shape is approximated by a prolate symmetrical ellipse with a major axis (L) and two minor axes (d_1 and d_2) (Fig. 5. 22A). Mathematically, the volume of a prolate ellipse is given by the equation:

$$\text{Volume} = \pi \frac{4}{3} \times \frac{d_1}{2} \times \frac{d_2}{2} \times \frac{L}{2} \qquad (5.1)$$

Assuming that the LV has two identical minor axes ($d_1 = d_2$) and a major axis twice the size of the minor axis ($L = 2d$), the volume can be estimated by the following simplified equation:

$$\text{Volume} = d^3 \qquad (5.2)$$

where d represents the LV minor axis dimension in diastole (LVEDD) or in systole (LVESD). This LV

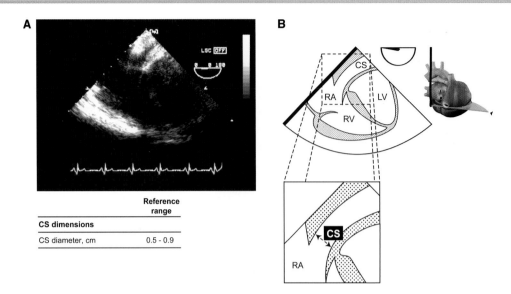

Figure 5.21   Coronary sinus dimensions. (A,B) TEE measurement of the CS can be obtained by advancing the TEE probe from the mid-esophageal four-chamber view. The CS is seen in long axis and is measured 1 cm proximal to where it enters the RA. *Abbreviations*: CS, coronary sinus; LV, left ventricle; RA, right atrium; RV, right ventricle; TEE, transesophageal echocardiography. *Source*: from Ref. 11.

Geometric Model	Algorithm	Formula
A	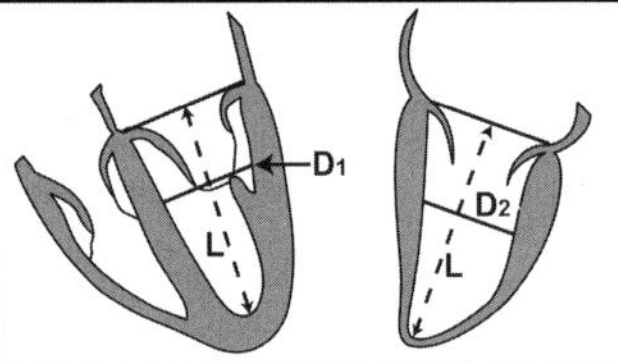 **Ellipsoid**	**Cubic** $$\text{Volume} = \pi \frac{4}{3} \times \frac{D_1}{2} \times \frac{D_2}{2} \times \frac{L}{2}$$
B	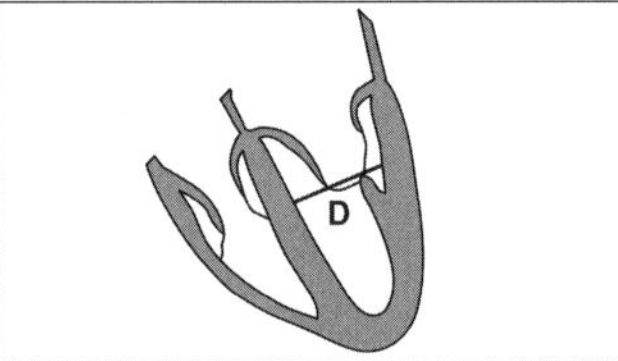 **Modified Ellipsoid**	**Teichholz** $$\text{Volume} = D^3 \times \frac{7.0}{2.4 + D}$$
C	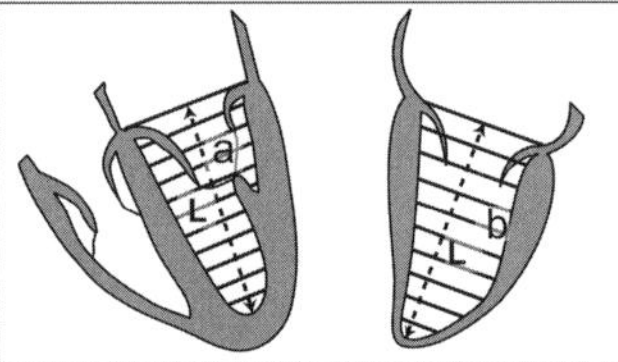 **Method of Discs**	**Simpson's** $$\text{Volume} = \frac{\pi}{4} \sum_{i=1}^{20} a_i\, b_i\, \frac{L}{20}$$
D	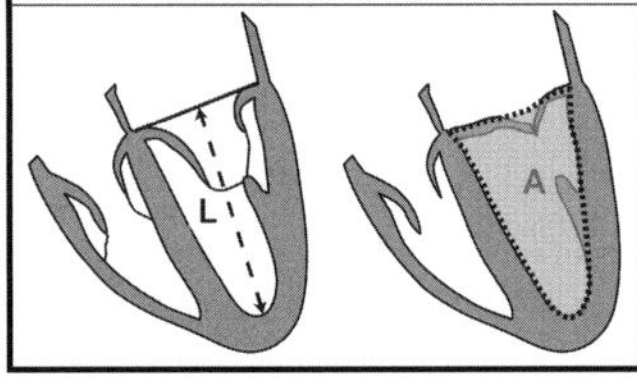 **Ellipsoid Single Plane**	**Area-Length** $$\text{Volume} = 0.85 \frac{A^2}{L}$$

Figure 5.22   Geometric models of LV volume. These geometric models and formulae are used to estimate LV volume. *Abbreviations*: A, area; D, diameter; L, length; LV, left ventricle.

volume estimate is relatively close in diastole but less so in systole or with LV dilatation.

Other investigators have introduced correction factors for change in ventricular assumed shape. The Teichholz method (17) seems to have the least imprecision (18) and has been incorporated in most commercialized echocardiography system on-line analysis software (Fig. 5.22B) as given by the equation:

$$\text{Volume} = d^3 \times \frac{7.0}{2.4 + d} \quad (5.3)$$

To minimize the error caused by too many geometric assumptions, investigators have developed different methods to estimate chamber volume that utilize multiple 2D measurements. The ASE currently recommends two methods to estimate left ventricular end-systolic (LVESV) or end-diastolic volume (LVEDV): the modified Simpson's biplane method and the single plane area-length method (4,5).

The Modified Simpson's Biplane Method

Simpson's rule states that the volume of a cavity is equal to the sum of the volumes of a series of smaller slices (disc summation method). The volume of each slice (disc) is obtained by knowing its surface area and thickness. The modified Simpson's biplane method applies this algorithm in the determination of LV volume from two orthogonal views; the four- and two-chamber views (see Fig. 10.12). The thickness of each disc is calculated by dividing the length (L) of the LV major axis into 20 equal segments ($L/20$). The surface area of each disc is obtained from measuring, on each of these 20 discs, the two orthogonal minor axes (a and b). Once the LV endocardial border has been manually traced in the four- and two-chamber views, most cardiac ultrasound systems will derive those two orthogonal diameters (a and b) by taking the distance between the opposite endocardial intercepts of lines drawn perpendicular to the long axis at each disc (Fig. 5.22C). Thus, the LV volume is automatically calculated with the formula:

$$\text{Volume} = \frac{\pi}{4} \sum_{i=1}^{20} a_i b_i \frac{L}{20} \quad (5.4)$$

where a is the diameter (cm) of the disc in the four-chamber view; b is the diameter (cm) of the disc in the two-chamber view; and L is the length (cm) of the LV long axis.

However, as this method assumes that the length of the LV is similar in the two orthogonal views, its accuracy decreases if the measurements of the major axis of the LV in the four- and two-chamber views differs by >20% (7).

The Single Plane Area-Length Method

As its name implies, this method uses the LV area from a single four- or two-chamber view and assumes that the two orthogonal views of the LV are symmetrical (Fig. 5.22D). The formula for calculating the LV volumes by this method is expressed by the equation:

$$\text{Volume} = 0.85 \frac{A^2}{L} \quad (5.5)$$

where A is the area (cm^2) of the LV in either the four- or two-chamber view and L is the length (cm) of the LV long axis.

Global LV Function

Several indices of LV global systolic function can be derived from simple linear and LV area measurements and calculation of LV volume. Single measurements of dimensions used to assess LV function are less accurate in the presence of regional wall motion abnormalities involving the other ventricular segments. It is important to note that some indices assess LV systolic performance and should not be confused with measurements of ejection fraction.

Stroke Volume, Cardiac Output, and Cardiac Index

The stroke volume (SV) is the blood volume ejected from the LV during each systole and can be calculated from the difference between the LVEDV and LVESV obtained by the previously described M-mode or 2D echocardiographic methods. Note that the SV can alternatively be calculated by Doppler volumetric method (see also equation 5.30 below).

The cardiac output (CO) is the amount of blood pumped by the heart per minute and most commonly reported in liters per minute:

$$\text{SV} = \text{LVEDV} - \text{LVESV} \quad (5.6)$$

$$\text{CO} = \text{SV} \times \text{HR} \times 0.001 \quad (5.7)$$

where CO is the cardiac output (L/min), SV is the stroke volume (mL), and HR is the heart rate (bpm).

The CO is often indexed to the patient's body size to facilitate comparison with reference values. The cardiac index (CI) is obtained by the equation:

$$\text{CI} = \frac{\text{CO}}{\text{BSA}} \quad (5.8)$$

where CI is the cardiac index (in L/min/m^2) and BSA is the body surface area (m^2).

Ejection Fraction

The left ventricular ejection fraction (LVEF) is defined as the percentage or fraction of the LVEDV that is ejected with each systole, that is, the ratio of the stroke volume to the end-diastolic volume. The LVEF (in %) can be expressed by the equation:

$$\begin{aligned} \text{LVEF} &= \frac{\text{SV}}{\text{LVEDV}} \times 100 \\ &= \frac{\text{LVEDV} - \text{LVESV}}{\text{LVEDV}} \times 100 \end{aligned} \quad (5.9)$$

where LVEF is the left ventricular ejection fraction (%); SV is the stroke volume (mL); LVEDV is the left ventricular end-diastolic volume (mL); and LVESV is the left ventricular end-systolic volume (mL). The normal LVEF is 55% to 75%.

Ejection fraction is a measure of myocardial performance and represents the efficiency of the global cardiac pump to eject part of its end-diastolic volume. Estimation of LVEF is affected by cardiac preload, afterload, and myocardial contractility (see Chapter 10). Ejection fraction does not necessarily mirror cardiac output. A patient may have a high ejection fraction but a small SV (and CO) as occurs in hypovolemia.

Linear Measurements

Simple linear measurements can be used in different formulae to assess global LV systolic performance. The ASE no longer recommends the use of linear measurements to assess ejection fraction. Fractional shortening (FS) and ejection fraction by Quinones method are discussed in Chapter 10 (see Fig. 10.14) (5).

Area Measurements

Fractional area change. The fractional area change (FAC) can be used for the estimation of left ventricular systolic performance and is further described in Chapter 10 (see Fig. 10.15).

Systolic Time Intervals

Left ventricular systolic performance can be also evaluated by measuring several systolic time intervals, particularly the pre-ejection period and left ventricular ejection time (LVET) as described in Chapter 10 (see Fig. 10.16).

The right and left ventricular myocardial performance index (MPI) incorporates both systolic and diastolic time intervals, and as these are more easily obtained on Doppler tracings, they will be covered further in Chapter 10 (see Fig. 10.18).

Wall Thickness and Mass

Wall Thickness

In 1935, Tennant and Wiggers (19) first described the immediate cessation of myocardial wall thickening after the ligation of a coronary artery in a canine model. Analysis has subsequently shown wall thickening to be an early sensitive marker of myocardial ischemia. This was initially reported by M-mode echocardiography, which could detect thickening of the myocardium directly, but only on a one-dimensional (1D) ice-pick view of the anteroseptal and inferolateral walls. With the advent of 2D echocardiography, this limitation was overcome by the ability to examine the entire myocardium utilizing multiple tomographic planes (20), and also by ensuring more accurate wall thickness measurements in a direction truly perpendicular to the wall. The percentage of LV wall thickening is helpful to compare the contractility of different myocardial segments. It is calculated according to the equation:

$$WT = \frac{EST - EDT}{EST} \times 100 \qquad (5.10)$$

where WT is the wall thickening (%), EST is the end-systolic thickness (cm), and EDT is the end-diastolic thickness (cm). Wall motion hypokinesia and akinesia are defined as <30% and <10% thickening respectively.

Wall Mass

Although an increase in LV wall thickness could reflect an increase in LV mass, redistribution of a normal LV mass over a smaller cavity may cause an apparent increase in wall thickness without constituting left ventricular hypertrophy (LVH). Left ventricular mass as determined by pathologists is better assessed by determining the LV muscle volume and converting the volume to a mass using the specific gravity of myocardium (1.040 g/mL). This is done by subtracting the LV endocardial, or chamber, volume from the epicardial or total volume.

Left ventricular mass can be determined from the M-mode end-diastolic measurement of the IVS wall thickness (IVST), the LVEDD, and the PWT using the ASE cube formula.

The ASE-Devereux method. The ASE cube method (equation 5.11A) uses a leading edge to leading edge technique for the M-mode measurements but results in a 25% overestimation of the true LV mass. Devereux and colleagues (21) proposed the following corrected formula (equation 5.11B) to derive the LV mass:

$$LV\ Mass_{ASE} = 1.04\left[(IVST + LVEDD + PWT)^3 \right.$$
$$\left. - (LVEDD)^3\right]$$
$$(5.11A)$$

$$LV\ Mass_{ASE-Devereux} = 1.04\left[(IVST + LVEDD + PWT)^3 \right.$$
$$\left. - (LVEDD)^3\right] \times 0.8 + 0.6$$
$$(5.11B)$$

Left ventricular mass, estimated by TEE wall thickness measurements (Fig. 5.23), is higher by an average of 6 g/m^2 (5). The classification of the type of LV hypertrophy is illustrated in Fig. 5.24.

Ventricular volume methods. Left ventricular mass can also be measured by 2D methods estimating total ventricular volume contained within the epicardial borders less the LV cavity volume delineated by the endocardial borders. Commonly used 2D techniques for estimating LV mass are based on the area-length formula and truncated ellipsoid method (Fig. 5.22) (4,5).

DOPPLER

The principles of Doppler are discussed in Chapter 2. Velocities, obtained through the spectral analysis of the Doppler echo signals, can be plotted on the y-axis against time on the x-axis to give a spectral (Doppler) display (Fig. 5.25). The direction of flow is indicated by positive (above the zero baseline) values for flow directed toward the probe. The timing and the duration of the flow are measured on the x-axis. The intensity of the signal indicates how many red blood cells were found to move at that velocity at that particular time. Blood flow is pulsatile and flow velocity varies during ejection. Laminar flow results in all similar velocities and the Doppler signal is a relatively thin wave form. Turbulent flow produces various velocities and

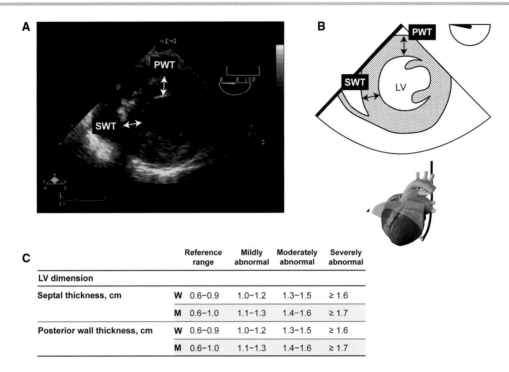

		Reference range	Mildly abnormal	Moderately abnormal	Severely abnormal
LV dimension					
Septal thickness, cm	W	0.6–0.9	1.0–1.2	1.3–1.5	≥ 1.6
	M	0.6–1.0	1.1–1.3	1.4–1.6	≥ 1.7
Posterior wall thickness, cm	W	0.6–0.9	1.0–1.2	1.3–1.5	≥ 1.6
	M	0.6–1.0	1.1–1.3	1.4–1.6	≥ 1.7

Figure 5.23 Wall thickness. (A,B) Transesophageal echocardiographic measurements of wall thickness of the LV septal wall and posterior wall obtained from a transgastric mid short-axis view at 0°. **(C)** Table of normal and abnormal values (in cm) for wall thickness is shown. *Abbreviations*: LV, left ventricle; PWT, posterior wall thickness; SWT, septal wall thickness. *Source*: Adapted from Ref. 5.

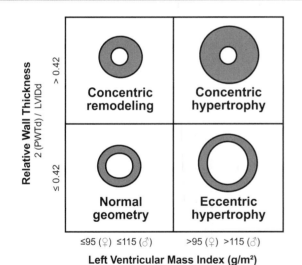

Left Ventricular Mass Index (g/m²)
0.8 X {1.04 [(LVIDd + PWTd + SWTd)³ – (LVIDd)³]} + 0.6 g

Figure 5.24 LV hypertrophy. Classification of LV hypertrophy is based on RWT and LV mass. Patients with normal LV mass can have either concentric remodeling (increased RWT > 0.42) or normal geometry (RWT ≤ 0.42). Patients with increased LV mass can have either concentric (RWT > 0.42) or eccentric (RWT ≤ 0.42) hypertrophy. These LV mass measurements are based on linear measurements. *Abbreviations*: gm, gram; LV, left ventricle; LVIDd, left ventricular internal diameter in diastole; m, meter; PWTd, posterior wall thickness in diastole; RWT, relative wall thickness; SWTd, septal wall thickness in diastole. *Source*: Adapted from Ref. 5.

different directions that result in a Doppler signal with multiple frequencies and marked spectral broadening.

The measured components of a spectral Doppler trace include the mean, peak, and modal velocities and the velocity-time integral (VTI). The peak velocity is the maximum velocity (either positive or negative) recorded during a flow period. All the measured velocities may be averaged over a flow period to give the mean velocity. By tracing the outline of the whole flow velocity signal most ultrasound systems can easily display these two values. The modal velocity is the dominant velocity that occurs most often and is identified by the brightest part of the PW spectral trace.

The VTI is the integrated area under the velocity time spectral Doppler trace and represents distance (distance/time × time). The VTI is sometimes referred to as *stroke distance* or the distance traveled by the sample volume with each heartbeat.

The acceleration time is the time from baseline to peak velocity and the deceleration time is the time from peak velocity to baseline (Figs. 5.25 and 5.26).

Doppler echocardiography measures velocity from which pressure, volume, and flow can be derived to form the basis of quantitative hemodynamics. In general, peak velocities are used to calculate pressure gradients and modal velocities to calculate flows.

Blood Flow

The blood flow through a vessel is not only determined by the pressure difference between two points

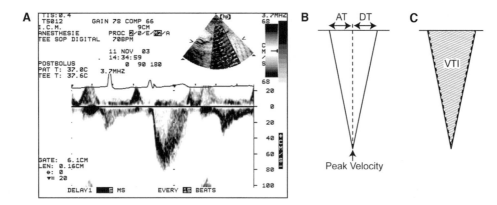

Figure 5.25 Spectral Doppler display. (A) Example of normal Doppler velocities and times recorded from pulsed wave Doppler in left ventricular outflow tract. **(B,C)** Schematic spectral Doppler display showing the peak velocity. *Abbreviations*: AT, acceleration time; DT, deceleration time; VTI, velocity-time integral.

(the driving pressure), but also by the resistance to flow that is influenced by the radius and the length of the vessel, and the viscosity of the blood. This can be described by the following equation (Poiseuille's law):

$$Q = \frac{\Delta P}{R} = \frac{\Delta P \pi r^4}{8Lv} \qquad (5.12)$$

where Q is the blood flow rate (mL/sec), ΔP is the pressure gradient (dynes/cm^2), R is the resistance to flow (g/cm^4/sec), r is the radius of the blood vessel (cm), L is the length of the blood vessel (cm) over which the pressure drop occurs, and v is the dynamic viscosity of blood (poise).

Conservation of Energy Principle and Pressure Difference (Gradient)

The driving pressure responsible for the movement of blood through the cardiovascular system can be derived from the application of the conservation of energy principle. This principle states that the total energy within a system is constant unless superimposed external forces are applied. This can be expressed by the Bernoulli equation:

Pressure difference = convective acceleration + flow acceleration + viscous friction

$$\Delta P = \frac{1}{2}\rho(V_2^2 - V_1^2) + \int_1^2 \frac{dv}{dt} ds + R(v) \qquad (5.13)$$

where ΔP is the pressure gradient (dynes/cm^2), ρ is the density of the fluid (g/cm^3), V_2 is the blood velocity at distal site (m/sec), V_1 is the blood velocity at proximal site (m/sec), dv is the change in velocity (cm/s) over the time period dt (sec); ds is the distance over which the pressure decreases (cm); and R is the viscous resistance in the vessel (g/cm^4/sec).

For most clinical settings, if one assumes that

1. The convective acceleration is only significant wherever there is a decrease in the cross-sectional area (CSA) of the vessel;

2. The flow acceleration is related to the pressure decrease necessary to overcome inertial forces and is negligible because acceleration is near zero at peak flow velocities;

3. The viscous friction is the loss of blood flow velocity because of friction between blood cellular elements and the vessel endoluminal surface, which is negligible for flat flow profile within the center of the vessel lumen.

After substituting known values for the mass density of normal blood ($\rho = 1.06 \times 10^3$ kg/m^3) and conversion factors where velocity in m/sec yields pressure drop in mmHg, the Bernoulli equation can be modified as follows:

$$\Delta P = 4(V_2^2 - V_1^2) \qquad (5.14)$$

When flow velocity V_1 proximal to a reduced orifice is low, and particularly small relative to the peak velocity V_2 across the reduced orifice, V_1 can be ignored and the modified Bernoulli equation is simplified to equation 5.15:

$$\Delta P = 4V_2^2 \qquad (5.15)$$

Several clinical situations do not meet the assumptions involved in the use of the simplified Bernoulli equation. In the hyperdynamic heart, or in the presence of subaortic dynamic obstruction, a $V_1 > 1.2$ m/sec is no longer negligible. Calculation of the pressure gradient, ignoring a high V_1, overestimates the true gradient. When there is significant anemia (decreased viscosity) or polycythemia (increased viscosity), ($\frac{1}{2}$)ρ can no longer be estimated by four. In the presence of long tubular obstructions (long coarctation), tunnel subaortic, or supra-valvular aortic stenosis (AS), the viscous friction is no longer negligible and cannot be ignored. Also, inertial forces may no longer be negligible in dysfunctional prosthetic valves.

In the case of AS, there is a pressure gradient across the AoV between the LV and Ao. As the peak blood flow velocity measured by CW Doppler

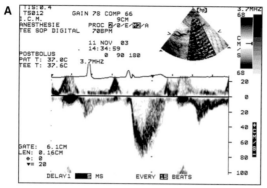

LVOT VELOCITY

Maximal velocity:	89 ± 14 cm/s
Acceleration time:	98 ± 20 ms
Ejection time:	311 ± 24 ms
Mean acceleration:	8.45 ± 2.43 m/s²
Velocity-time integral:	17 ± 3 cm

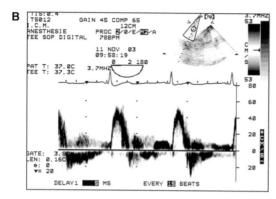

ASCENDING AORTIC VELOCITY

Maximal velocity:	66 ± 11 cm/s
Acceleration time:	61 ± 3 ms
Ejection time:	239 ± 43 ms
Mean acceleration:	7.23 ± 2.12 m/s²
Velocity-time integral:	10.5 ± 2.7 cm

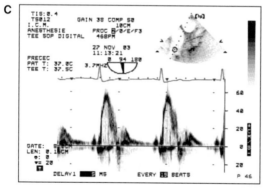

RVOT VELOCITY

Maximal velocity:	58 ± 1 cm/s
Acceleration time:	93 ± 6 ms
Ejection time:	277 ± 23 ms
Mean acceleration:	3.82 ± 0.76 m/s²
Velocity-time integral:	11.1 ± 1.7 cm

Figure 5.26   Doppler velocities. Normal values of Doppler velocities in a healthy young adult as recorded from the (**A**) LVOT, (**B**) the ascending aorta and (**C**) the RVOT (1 cm below the pulmonic valve). *Abbreviations*: LVOT, left ventricular outflow tract; RVOT, right ventricular outflow tract. *Source*: Part A from Ref. 22, Part B from Ref. 23, Part C from Ref. 24.

echocardiography is an instantaneous event, the pressure gradient derived from this measure is the peak instantaneous pressure gradient. Integrating all the instantaneous pressure gradients throughout a flow period results in the mean pressure gradient. These two gradients must be differentiated from the peak-to-peak gradient; a measurement in the catheterization laboratory consisting of measuring the difference between the peak LV pressure value and the peak aortic pressure value (see Fig. 14.17). This constitutes a nonphysiological measurement as these two events are not synchronous. Several studies have documented the excellent correlation between echo-Doppler-derived

and catheter-measured mean pressure gradients across AS (25), mitral stenosis (MS) (26), prosthetic valves (27), and TV (28).

Estimation of Intracardiac Pressures

No echocardiographic technique measures intracardiac pressures directly. Instead estimates of specific intracardiac pressures can be obtained using the Doppler velocity measurements of regurgitant jets and applying the pressure difference from the modified Bernoulli equation (equation 5.14). These estimates are valid only in the presence of an optimal spectral

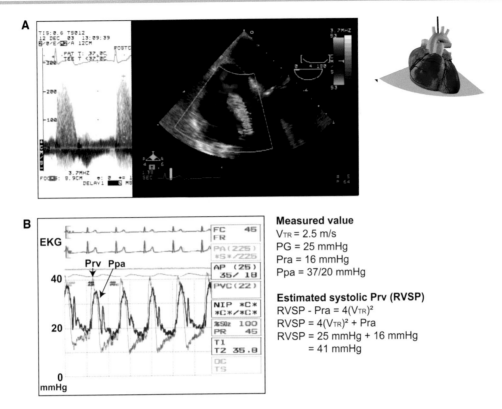

Figure 5.27   Right ventricular systolic pressure. (A) Estimation of RVSP using the PG obtained from TR and RAP. **(B)** Note that the RVSP is higher than the systolic pulmonary artery pressure (P_{PA}) due to a small gradient across the pulmonic valve. *Abbreviations*: EKG, electrocardiogram; LA, left atrium; LV, left ventricle; PG, pressure gradient; RA, right atrium; RAP or P_{RA}, right atrial pressure; RV, right ventricle; RVSP or P_{RV}, right ventricular systolic pressure; TR, tricuspid regurgitation; V, velocity; V_{TR}, peak tricuspid regurgitant velocity.

Doppler trace and absence of valvular or subvalvular stenosis.

Right Ventricular Systolic Pressure

The peak tricuspid regurgitant velocity reflects the peak pressure gradient between the RV and the RA (Fig. 5.27) during systole. The right ventricular systolic pressure (RVSP) is estimated using CW Doppler by the following equations:

$$RVSP - RAP = 4(V_{TR})^2$$
$$RVSP = 4(V_{TR})^2 + RAP \qquad (5.16)$$

where RVSP is the right ventricular systolic pressure (mmHg), V_{TR} is the peak tricuspid regurgitant velocity (m/sec), and RAP is the measured or estimated right atrial pressure (mmHg). This RVSP estimate is invalid in the presence of severe RV dysfunction, ventricular septal defect (VSD), or significant pulmonic valve regurgitation.

In the presence of a VSD, the peak systolic velocity obtained across a VSD reflects the peak pressure gradient between the LV and RV (Fig. 5.28). In the absence of left ventricular outflow (LVOT) obstruction (i.e., subvalvular, valvular, or supra-valvular AS), the peak LV systolic pressure can be approximated by the systolic aortic pressure, and secondarily by the arm systolic blood pressure (29), in the following equation:

$$sBP - RVSP = 4(V_{VSD})^2$$
$$RVSP = sBP - 4(V_{VSD})^2 \qquad (5.17)$$

where RVSP is the right ventricular systolic pressure (mmHg), V_{VSD} is the peak VSD velocity (m/sec), and sBP is the systolic arm blood pressure (mmHg).

Pulmonary Artery Systolic Pressure

In the absence of RVOT obstruction, such as pulmonic stenosis (PS), the PASP should be equal to the RSVP. In this setting, the two preceding equations can be rewritten as (30):

$$PASP = 4(V_{TR})^2 + RAP$$
$$PASP = sBP - 4(V_{VSD})^2 \qquad (5.18)$$

where PASP is the pulmonary artery systolic pressure (mmHg), V_{TR} is the peak tricuspid regurgitant velocity (m/sec), and RAP is the measured or estimated RAP (subsect. "Right Atrial Pressure") (mmHg). V_{VSD} is the peak VSD velocity (m/sec) and sBP is the systolic arm blood pressure (mmHg).

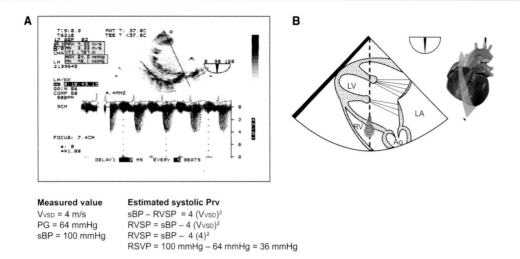

Measured value	Estimated systolic Prv
V_{VSD} = 4 m/s	sBP – RVSP = 4 $(V_{VSD})^2$
PG = 64 mmHg	RVSP = sBP – 4 $(V_{VSD})^2$
sBP = 100 mmHg	RVSP = sBP – 4 $(4)^2$
	RSVP = 100 mmHg – 64 mmHg = 36 mmHg

Figure 5.28 Right ventricular systolic pressure. This example shows the estimation of RVSP in the presence of a VSD. (**A,B**) Continuous wave Doppler spectral trace of flow between the RV and LV with a peak velocity (V_{VSD}) of 4m/s is from a transgastric two-chamber view. The measured peak PG is the pressure difference between the LV systolic pressure (estimated by sBP) and RVSP. Inserting the sBP value allows estimation of the RVSP. *Abbreviations*: Ao, aorta; LA, left atrium; LV, left ventricle; PG, pressure gradient; RV, right ventricle; RVSP, right ventricular systolic pressure; sBP, systolic blood pressure; VSD, ventricular septal defect.

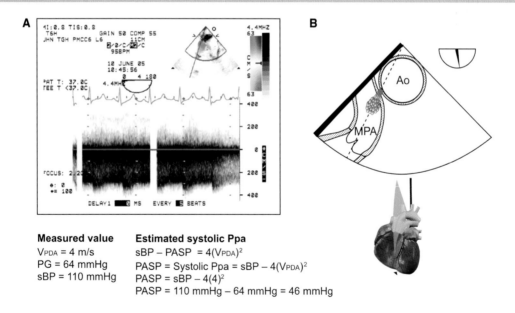

Measured value	Estimated systolic Ppa
V_{PDA} = 4 m/s	sBP – PASP = 4$(V_{PDA})^2$
PG = 64 mmHg	PASP = Systolic Ppa = sBP – 4$(V_{PDA})^2$
sBP = 110 mmHg	PASP = sBP – 4$(4)^2$
	PASP = 110 mmHg – 64 mmHg = 46 mmHg

Figure 5.29 Pulmonary artery systolic pressure. This example shows the estimation of PASP in the presence of a PDA. (**A**) Continuous wave Doppler spectral trace of flow between the Ao and MPA shows a peak velocity (V_{PDA}) of 4m/s. (**B**) As shown in this diagram the measured PG is the pressure difference between the aortic systolic pressure or systolic blood pressure (sBP) and the PASP. Inserting the sBP value allows estimation of the PASP. *Abbreviations*: Ao, aorta; MPA, mean pulmonary artery; PDA, patent ductus arteriosus; PASP, pulmonary artery systolic pressure; PG, pressure gradient.

In the presence of a patent ductus arteriosus (PDA) (between the thoracic Ao and the pulmonary artery), the peak velocity reflects the peak pressure gradient between the aortic and pulmonary artery pressures (Fig. 5.29) (31) as given in the following equation:

$$sBP - PASP = 4(V_{PDA})^2$$
$$PASP = sBP - 4(V_{PDA})^2 \quad (5.19)$$

where PASP is the pulmonary artery systolic pressure (mmHg), V_{PDA} is the peak PDA velocity (m/sec), and sBP is the systolic arm blood pressure (mmHg).

Mean Pulmonary Artery Pressure

The pulmonic valve regurgitant velocity represents the instantaneous pressure gradient between the main pulmonary artery and the RV during diastole

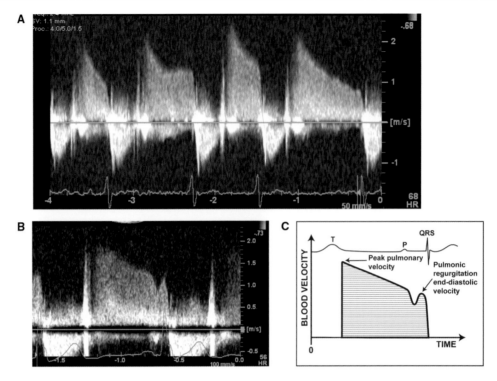

Figure 5.30   Pulmonary artery mean and end-diastolic pressures. Continuous wave Doppler of the PV for estimation of peak and end-diastolic PA pressures using the PR Doppler signal in a patient in atrial fibrillation (**A**) and in sinus rhythm (**B**). (**C**) Schematic of the ideal PR velocity signal with the sites of measurement for mean and end-diastolic velocity. The mean PA pressure is equal to 4 × the (peak pulmonary velocity)^2. *Abbreviations*: PA, pulmonary artery; PR, pulmonic regurgitation; PV, pulmonic valve.

(Fig. 5.30). The mean pulmonary artery pressure (MPAP) correlates to the peak PV regurgitant velocity in protodiastole (32):

$$\text{MPAP} = 4(V_{\text{PR-E}})^2 \qquad (5.20)$$

where MPAP is the mean pulmonary artery pressure (mmHg) and $V_{\text{PR-E}}$ is the early peak pulmonary regurgitant velocity (m/sec).

The MPAP has also been estimated using the right ventricular acceleration time (RV$_{\text{accel}}$ Time), from the onset of ejection to the peak RVOT velocity in a PW spectral Doppler of the RVOT (33,34). The Mahan (34) and Kitabatake (33) regression equations are:

$$\begin{aligned}
\text{Mahan MPAP} &= 79 - (0.45 \times A_{\text{c}}T_{\text{RV}}) \\
\text{Kitabatake MPAP} &= 90 - (0.62 \times A_{\text{c}}T_{\text{RV}})
\end{aligned} \qquad (5.21)$$

where MPAP is the mean pulmonary artery pressure (mmHg) and $A_{\text{c}}T_{\text{RV}}$ is the right ventricular acceleration time (ms), normal ≥ 120 ms. As suggested by these equations the $A_{\text{c}}T_{\text{RV}}$ is typically shortened in the presence of pulmonary hypertension. The $A_{\text{c}}T_{\text{RV}}$ is dependent on CO and heart rate. The MPAP estimated by the Mahan equation was studied in patients with a heart rate of 60 to 100 bpm, correction factors for heart rates beyond this range are required. When the right ventricular CO is increased by a left-to-right

shunt, the $A_{\text{c}}T_{\text{RV}}$ may not be shortened as much, despite a high pulmonary artery pressure.

Pulmonary Artery and Right Ventricular End-Diastolic Pressure

At the end of diastole, the RAP and the RV pressure are equalized, assuming there is no evidence of tricuspid valve stenosis. Therefore, the following equation can be rewritten as (32):

$$\begin{aligned}
\text{PAEDP} &= 4(V_{\text{PR-ED}})^2 + \text{RVEDP} \\
\text{PAEDP} &= 4(V_{\text{PR-ED}})^2 + \text{RAP}
\end{aligned} \qquad (5.22)$$

where PAEDP is the pulmonary artery end-diastolic pressure (mmHg), $V_{\text{PR-ED}}$ is the end-diastolic pulmonary regurgitant velocity (m/sec), RVEDP is the right ventricular end-diastolic pressure (mmHg), and RAP is the measured or estimated right atrial pressure (see below) (mmHg).

Right Atrial Pressure

Several methods have been proposed to approximate the RAP used in the preceding equations to estimate right-sided intracardiac pressures. The jugular venous pressure, estimated by physical examination or an empirical value of 10, was evaluated and compared with other regression equations (28).

A normal-sized IVC collapses with a rapid negative intrathoracic pressure during a sudden inspiration (*sniffing* maneuver). When the RAP increases, there is decreased venous return and compensatory increase in the IVC diameter that serves as a capacitance reservoir for the RA. Moreover, during sniffing, the decrease in IVC diameter is either blunted or absent with high RAP (35). Table 5.1 has been proposed to estimate mean RAP.

Correlation studies with catheterization have also shown that combined information from the IVC diameter and the hepatic venous Doppler profile can be used to assess RAP (36) (Table 5.2). The preceding estimate of RAP was however not prospectively validated in patients on positive pressure mechanical ventilation.

Left Ventricular End-Diastolic Pressure

The aortic regurgitant velocity reflects the instantaneous pressure gradient between the Ao and the LV

Table 5.1 Echocardiographic Estimation of RAP

Size of IVC (cm)	Collapse with *sniffing*	Suggested mRAP (mmHg)
<1.5	≥50%	0–5
1.5–2.5	≥50%	5–10
1.5–2.5	<50%	10–15
>2.5	<50%	15–20
>2.5	Fixed diameter	>20

Abbreviation: mRAP, mean right atrial pressure.

Table 5.2 Echocardiographic Estimation of RAP

Size of IVC (cm)	Collapse with *sniffing* (%)	Hepatic vein Doppler profile	Suggested mRAP (mmHg)
<1.5	≥50	S + AR > 0	5
<1.5	<50	S + AR > 0	10–14
>2.0	≥50	S + AR < 0	15–20
>2.0	<50	S + AR < 0	>20

Abbreviations: AR, atrial reversal; mRAP, mean right atrial pressure; S, systolic.

during diastole (Fig. 5.31). As the arm diastolic blood pressure approximates the left ventricular end-diastolic pressure (LVEDP) in the Ao we can, therefore, obtain this by the equation:

$$dBP - LVEDP = 4(V_{AR\text{-}ED})^2 \text{ or}$$
$$LVEDP = dBP - 4(V_{AR\text{-}ED})^2 \quad (5.23)$$

where LVEDP is the left ventricular end-diastolic pressure (mmHg), dBP is the diastolic blood pressure (mmHg), and $V_{AR\text{-}ED}$ is the end-diastolic aortic regurgitant velocity (m/sec).

Left Atrial Pressure

The mitral regurgitant velocity reflects the instantaneous pressure gradient between the LV and the LA during systole. If there is no LVOT obstruction (such as subvalvular, valvular, or supravalvular AS), the peak LV systolic pressure can be approximated by the

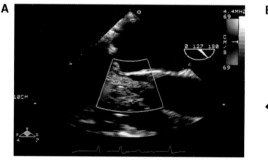
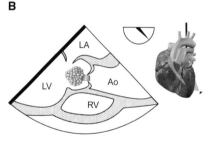

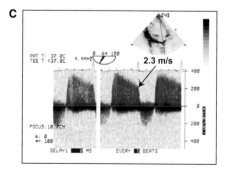

Measured value
V_{AR_ED} = 2.3 m/s
PG = 21 mmHg
dBP = 50 mmHg

Estimated LVEDP
dBP − LVEDP = 4 $(V_{AR\_ED})^2$
LVEDP = dBP − 4 $(V_{AR\_ED})^2$
LVEDP = 50 mmHg − 4 (2.3)²
LVEDP = 50 mmHg − 21 mmHg = 29 mmHg

Figure 5.31 Left ventricular end-diastolic pressure. Estimation of LVEDP using the PG obtained from the AR end-diastolic velocity ($V_{AR\ ED}$) and systemic aortic blood pressure. **(A,B)** Mid-esophageal aortic valve long-axis color Doppler view of a patient with AR. **(C)** The peak end-diastolic AR velocity is measured on the continuous wave Doppler signal in a transgastric view. The LVEDP is equal to the dBP minus the diastolic PG of the AR Doppler signal. *Abbreviations*: Ao, aorta; AR, aortic regurgitation; dBP, diastolic blood pressure; LA, left atrium; LV, left ventricle; LVEDP, left ventricular end-diastolic pressure; PG, pressure gradient; RV, right ventricle.

aortic systolic blood pressure. Therefore, left atrial pressure (LAP) can be estimated by the equation:

$$sBP - LAP = 4(V_{MR})^2$$
$$LAP = sBP - 4(V_{MR})^2$$

(5.24)

where LAP is the left atrial pressure (mmHg), sBP is the systolic aortic blood pressure (mmHg), and V_{MR} is the peak mitral regurgitant velocity (m/sec) (Fig. 5.32).

Several methods using other parameters obtained by PW Doppler, color M-mode, and tissue-Doppler echocardiography have also been proposed to estimate LAP. Using the velocity of the propagation of the E wave velocity by color M-mode, the LAP can be estimated by (37) using the equation:

$$LAP = 5.27(E/V_P) + 4.6\,mmHg$$

(5.25)

where LAP is the left atrial pressure (mmHg), E is the peak early diastolic velocity of the MV inflow (cm/s), and V_p is the velocity of propagation of the E wave (cm/s).

Volumetric Flow Calculations

Volumetric flow rate is the volume of fluid that passes through a given surface per unit time and can be

A

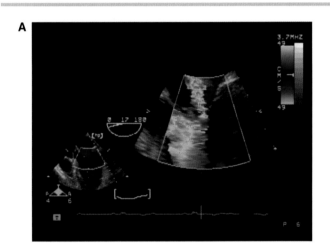

B

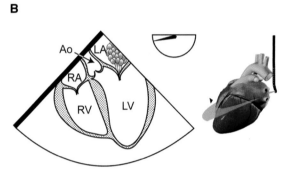

C

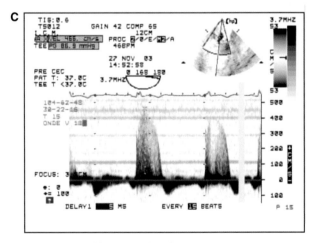

Measured values:
V_{MR} = 4.66 m/s
PG = 86.9 mmHg
Pa = 104/48 mmHg (not shown)
Paop V wave = 20 mmHg

D

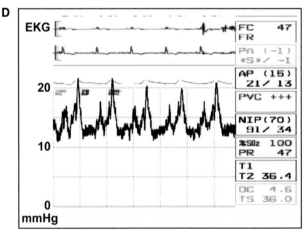

Doppler estimated LAP:
LAP = sBP - 4V_{MR}^2
    = 104 - 86.9 mmHg
    = 17.1 mmHg

Figure 5.32 Left atrial pressure. Estimation of LAP using the MR Doppler signal in a 70-year-old man scheduled for off-pump bypass surgery with a sBP of 104 mmHg. (**A,B**) Mid-esophageal four-chamber color Doppler view shows MR. (**C**) Continuous wave Doppler gives a peak PG of 86.9 mmHg between the LA and LV. This would yield a Doppler estimated LAP of 17.1 mmHg. (**D**) Hemodynamic pressure tracing of the pulmonary artery occlusion pressure (Paop) waveform is shown with a "v" wave of 20 mmHg. *Abbreviations*: Ao, aorta; EKG, electrocardiogram; LA, left atrium; LAP, left atrial pressure; LV, left ventricle; MR, mitral regurgitation; Pa, arterial pressure; PG, pressure gradient; RA, right atrium; RV, right ventricle; sBP, arterial systolic blood pressure; V, velocity.

calculated on the basis of the hydraulic principle. The measurement and comparison of volumetric flow rates at different locations within the cardiac pump form the basis of hemodynamic calculations essential to the assessment of SV and CO, valvular orifice areas, regurgitant volumes, and fractions as well as shunt fractions.

Hydraulic Principle

Assuming a constant mean flow velocity through a rigid circular tube of constant diameter and, therefore, fixed CSA, volumetric flow rate can be expressed by the hydraulic equation:

$$Q = V \times \text{CSA} \qquad (5.26)$$

where Q is the volumetric flow rate (L/sec), V is the mean velocity (cm/s), and CSA is the cross-sectional area of the orifice (cm^2).

During pulsatile flow periods, volumetric flow is calculated by the VTI, the stroke distance reached by the column of blood during the flow period, and calculation of volumetric flows is equivalent to determining the volume of a cylinder, where

$$\text{Volume} = \text{CSA} \times \text{Length} = \text{CSA} \times \text{VTI} \qquad (5.27)$$

If we assume a symmetrical circular orifice, the CSA can be obtained from the equation:

$$\text{CSA} = \pi r^2 = 0.785 d^2 \qquad (5.28)$$

where CSA is the cross-sectional area (cm^2), r is the radius of the circular orifice (cm), and d is the diameter of the circular orifice (cm).

Therefore, volumetric flow can be calculated from the simplified equation:

$$\text{Vol} = 0.785 d^2 \times \text{VTI} \qquad (5.29)$$

where Vol is the volume (mL), d is the diameter of orifice (cm), and VTI is the velocity-time integral (cm).

Clinically, the hydraulic equation is used to assess flow through an elastic blood vessel or a mobile, deformable, and not always circular valvular annulus. In practice the CSA does not remain constant and the sample volume may move during the flow period. Volumetric flow rates are particularly sensitive to inaccuracies in the orifice diameter measurement, as the error is magnified to the second power.

Stroke Volume and Cardiac Output

Volumetric flow across valves, either during systole or diastole, can be calculated using Doppler by measuring the annular diameter and VTI. When using the atrioventricular (mitral and tricuspid) valves, the flow is evaluated during diastole and the VTI is measured by tracing the PW spectral Doppler trace modal velocity, the most dense part of the flow velocity signal. When using the semilunar (aortic and pulmonary) valves, the VTI is obtained during systole by tracing the outer edge of the CW spectral Doppler trace. Annular measurements are made when the valves are open. The stroke volume, defined as the

Stroke volume = CSA x VTI

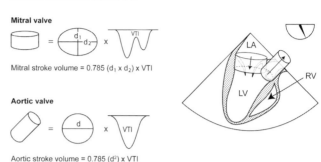

Mitral stroke volume = 0.785 (d$_1$ x d$_2$) x VTI

Aortic stroke volume = 0.785 (d^2) x VTI

Figure 5.33 Stroke volume. The measurements required to calculate the SV across the mitral and aortic valves are shown here. Note that two mitral annulus diameters (d1 and d2) are measured from the mid-esophageal four-chamber and two-chamber views to obtain the mitral SV. *Abbreviations*: CSA, cross sectional area; d, diameter; LA, left atrium; LV, left ventricle; SV, stroke volume; RV, right ventricle; VTI, velocity-time integral.

volume of blood ejected during one cardiac cycle, is calculated as:

$$\text{SV} = 0.785 d^2 \times \text{VTI} \qquad (5.30)$$

where SV is the stroke volume (mL), d is the diameter of orifice (cm), and VTI is the velocity-time integral (cm) (Fig. 5.33).

Stroke volume estimates obtained by Doppler do not make any geometric assumptions about the LV cavity. In assessing an asymmetric LV, where geometric assumptions introduce errors, SV measured by Doppler may present a theoretical advantage when compared with 2D echocardiography. The calculation of LVEF using the method of Dumesnil et al. (38) combines the measurement of SV by Doppler volumetric method and the end-diastolic volume by Teichholz's formula. To increase accuracy, it is suggested that you trace and average the VTI of at least 3 to 5 beats in normal sinus rhythm and up to 8 to 10 beats in atrial fibrillation.

By measuring the time interval between two consecutive beats, either on the EKG or on the Doppler tracing, one can deduce the heart rate by the following:

$$\text{HR} = 60,000/\text{time} \qquad (5.31)$$

where HR is the heart rate (bpm) and time is the time between two consecutive beats (ms).

Therefore, CO and CI can be deduced by the equations:

$$\text{CO} = 0.785 d^2 \times \text{VTI} \times \text{HR} \qquad (5.32)$$

$$\text{CI} = \text{CO}/\text{BSA} \qquad (5.33)$$

where CO is the cardiac output (mL/min), d is the diameter of orifice (cm), VTI is the velocity-time integral (cm), HR is the heart rate (bpm), CI is the cardiac index (mL/min/m^2), and BSA is the body surface area (m^2).

This equation assumes that the R—R interval is constant over a minute, and, consequently, the CO obtained by this method is sensitive to irregular rhythms such as atrial fibrillation and multifocal atrial tachycardias.

The Principle of Conservation of Mass and the Continuity Equation

The principle of conservation of mass states that provided there is no loss of fluid from the system between two points of interest, any mass or volume entering the system must flow out of it. The continuity equation is the mathematical expression of this principle:

$$Q_{in} = Q_{out}$$

where Q is the volumetric flow rate.

This equation can be clinically applied to the calculation of (*i*) native or prosthetic valvular areas and (*ii*) regurgitant orifices, volumes, and fractions.

Valvular Areas

Valvular Areas by the Continuity Equation Method

As the CSA of an orifice decreases, the mean velocity of the blood column must increase to maintain a constant flow rate to obey the principle of conservation of mass (volume). The CSA of a stenotic orifice can, therefore, be calculated from the maximal peak velocity across the orifice and the calculated volumetric flow proximal to the stenosis.

If

$$Q_{in} = CSA_{proximal} \times V_{proximal}$$

and

$$Q_{out} = CSA_{stenosis} \times V_{stenosis}$$

and

$$CSA_{stenosis} \times V_{stenosis} = CSA_{proximal} \times V_{proximal}$$

then

$$CSA_{stenosis} = CSA_{proximal} \frac{V_{proximal}}{V_{stenosis}}$$

Alternatively, the VTI can be substituted for the velocity:

$$CSA_{stenosis} = CSA_{proximal}$$

The aortic valve area (AVA) calculated by the continuity equation is obtained by the following equation:

$$AVA = 0.785 \, (d_{LVOT})^2 \frac{V_{LVOT}}{V_{maximal}}$$

or   (5.34)

$$AVA = 0.785 \, (d_{LVOT})^2 \frac{VTI_{LVOT}}{VTI_{maximal}}$$

where AVA is the aortic valve area (cm^2), d_{LVOT} is the diameter of the LVOT (cm), V_{LVOT} is the peak velocity

(m/sec) measured at the LVOT by PW Doppler, $V_{maximal}$ is the peak velocity (m/sec) across the valve, reflecting the smallest orifice, obtained by CW Doppler, VTI$_{LVOT}$ is the velocity-time integral (cm) obtained by tracing the LVOT PW spectral Doppler trace, and VTI$_{maximal}$ is the velocity-time integral (cm), obtained by tracing the CW spectral Doppler trace through the AoV.

The mitral valve area (MVA) can similarly be obtained by applying the continuity equation $Q_{mitral} = Q_{aortic}$, provided there is no significant MV or AoV regurgitation as given in the following equation:

$$MVA = 0.785 \, (d_{LVOT})^2 \frac{VTI_{LVOT}}{VTI_{mitral}} \qquad (5.35)$$

where VTI$_{mitral}$ (cm) is measured by CW Doppler across the mitral native or prosthetic valve during diastole.

Estimating valvular stenotic disease severity by the continuity equation is subject to limitations that include the accuracy of the LVOT diameter measurement, the absence of angulation between the maximal jet, and the Doppler ultrasound beam, optimal positioning of the sample volume before jet acceleration in the LVOT, as well as the consequence of low CO on the significance of the areas calculated. These limitations are reviewed in detail in Chapters 14 and 16.

Valvular Areas by the Pressure Half-Time Method

The presence of MS prevents the usual rapid equalization of intracardiac pressure between the LA and the LV. There is a resulting persisting increased pressure gradient during diastole across the MV and its rate of decline is prolonged proportionally to the severity of the stenosis. This can be assessed by the pressure half-time (PHT), defined as the time during which the pressure gradient decreases to one-half the initial value. The PHT is not equal to the velocity half-time, or the time it takes for the velocity to decrease by half. Recall pressure and velocity are related by the simplified Bernoulli equation, so the time it takes the pressure to decrease by half ($\frac{1}{2}P_{peak}$) is equal to the time for the diastolic velocity ($V_{\frac{1}{2}}$) to decrease to 0.707 of its initial value (V_{peak}).

$$
\begin{aligned}
PHT &= \tfrac{1}{2}P_{peak} \\
4(V_{\frac{1}{2}})^2 &= \tfrac{1}{2}(4 \times V_{peak}^2) \\
(V_{\frac{1}{2}})^2 &= \tfrac{1}{2}(V_{peak}^2) \\
V_{\frac{1}{2}} &= \sqrt{[\tfrac{1}{2}(V_{peak}^2)]} \\
V_{\frac{1}{2}} &= V_{peak}/\sqrt{2} \\
V_{\frac{1}{2}} &= V_{peak}/1.41 = 0.707 \times V_{peak}
\end{aligned}
\qquad (5.36)
$$

The PHT is related to the mitral deceleration time (Mdt), which is the time required for the peak early diastolic mitral velocity to fall to zero, extrapolated from its deceleration slope. The PHT is equal to $0.29 \times$ Mdt (Fig. 5.34).

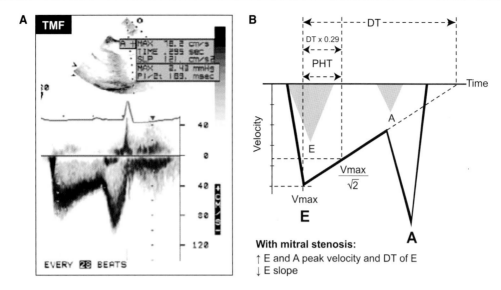

Figure 5.34 Pressure half-time concept. (A) Pulsed wave Doppler tracing of TMF is obtained during diastole in a patient with mitral stenosis. **(B)** An increase in the early (E) maximum and late (A) velocity (V) is observed. In addition a marked decrease or flattening of the slope of the deceleration portion of the E velocity or the DT is present. The velocity can be translated into pressure through the Bernoulli equation. The time it takes for the maximum pressure to decrease in half is known as the PHT. It is equal to the Vmax divided by $\sqrt{2}$ or 0.29 multiplied by the DT. *Abbreviations*: DT, deceleration time; PHT, pressure half-time; TMF, transmitral flow; Vmax, maximal velocity.

Hatle et al. (39) reported that PHT correlates with the MVA and is less influenced by flow across the valve. They reported a value of <60 ms in normal MV, increasing to 100 ms with mild stenosis and becoming progressively longer with increasing severity. A PHT >220 ms was usually associated with an MVA <1.00 cm^2, and equation 5.36 was derived from these studies (39):

$$\text{MVA} = \frac{220}{\text{PHT}} = \frac{759}{\text{Mdt}} \qquad (5.36)$$

where MVA is the mitral valve area (cm^2), PHT is the pressure half-time (ms), and Mdt is the mitral deceleration time (ms).

The MVA obtained by the PHT method is independent of the volumetric flow across the valve and, thus, less affected by the CO or coexistent significant MR. The PHT method is affected by conditions modifying the differential pressure between the LA and the LV, particularly those resulting in an elevation of LV diastolic pressure and reduced LV compliance. The applicability of the PHT method is, therefore, less valid following percutaneous balloon mitral valvuloplasty or cardiac surgery, and in the presence of severe aortic regurgitation or delayed LV relaxation. These limitations are reviewed in detail in Chapter 16.

Proximal Flow Convergence (Proximal Isovelocity Surface Area)

The proximal flow convergence method is another application of the principle of conservation of mass (volume) using a different hydraulic equation than that used with a circular orifice and the VTI. In the proximal isovelocity surface area (PISA) flow model, as the red blood cells

approach and converge toward a narrowed orifice, their velocity increases in a linear fashion, forming before the orifice, a series of concentric hemispheric shells of similar velocity (called isovelocity hemispheres). The closer the hemispheres are to the orifice and, therefore, the smaller the radius of the isovelocity hemisphere, the higher the corresponding velocity.

The flow rate at a given hemispheric shell velocity is shown by the following equation:

$$Q = \text{CSA} \times \text{Velocity} = 2\pi r^2 \times v_r \qquad (5.37)$$

where Q is the flow rate (mL/sec), $2\pi r^2$ is the area of the hemispheric shell from its radius r (cm); and v_r is the velocity (cm/s) at the radius r.

The flow at the narrowest orifice is given by the following equation:

$$Q = \text{CSA} \times V_{\text{max}} \qquad (5.38)$$

where Q is the flow rate (mL/sec), CSA is the cross-sectional area of the narrowest orifice (cm^2), and V_{max} is the maximal velocity across the orifice, obtained by CWD (cm/s).

Using the continuity equation, we can obtain the CSA by computing the equation:

$$\text{CSA} = 2\pi r^2 \frac{v_r}{V_{\text{MR max}}} \qquad (5.39)$$

In MR, where the surface surrounding the regurgitant orifice is relatively planar (Fig. 5.35A), the effective regurgitant orifice area (EROA) can be calculated by the PISA method:

$$\text{EROA} = 2\pi r^2 \frac{v_r}{V_{\text{MR max}}} \qquad (5.40)$$

A

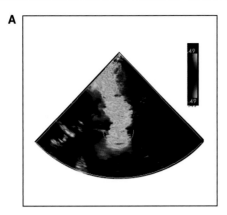

B

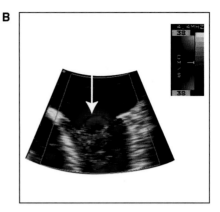

Mitral regurgitation
Flow proximal to MV = flow through MV
Area shell x Velocity shell = ERO x V$_{\text{MR max}}$
ERO = $\dfrac{2\pi r^2 \times \text{Aliasing Velocity}}{V_{\text{MR max}}}$

Mitral stenosis
Flow proximal to MV = flow through MV
Area shell x Velocity shell = MVA x V$_{\text{MS max}}$
MVA = $\dfrac{2\pi r^2 \times \text{Aliasing Velocity} \times \alpha/180}{V_{\text{MS max}}}$

Figure 5.35 PISA. (A,B) The PISA concept in two patients with MV disease from zoomed mid-esophageal four-chamber views are shown. Flow accelerates and converges before a narrow orifice to form a series of hemispheres (arrow). Each hemisphere surface has the same velocity (V) as indicated by the velocity scale. Flow at each hemisphere is estimated from the area of the sphere multiplied by the velocity. Calculation of the ERO area in MR (**A**) and the MVA in MS (**B**) is shown. Note that for the MVA in mitral stenosis (**B**), VMS max corresponds to the maximal early TMF diastolic velocity E. *Abbreviations*: α, angle; A, peak late diastolic TMF velocity; ERO, effective regurgitant orifice; MR, mitral regurgitation; MS, mitral stenosis; MV, mitral valve; MVA, mitral valve area; PISA, proximal isovelocity surface area; r, measured radius (cm) of the hemispheric shell of the aliased velocity; TMF, transmitral flow; V MS max, peak MS inflow velocity; V MR max, peak MR velocity.

where EROA is the effective regurgitant orifice area (cm^2), r is the measured radius (cm) of the hemispheric shell of the aliased velocity, v_r is the aliased velocity identified as the Nyquist limit (cm/s) at the radius r, and $V_{\text{MR max}}$ is the maximal systolic velocity across the regurgitant orifice, obtained by continuous wave (CW) Doppler (cm/s).

In the case of MS or TR, rather than being planar, the surface surrounding the narrowed orifice is funnel-shaped and distorts the PISA so that correction factors must be applied.

In the case of MS (Fig. 5.35B) (40):

$$\text{MVA} = 2\pi r^2 \frac{v_r}{V_{\text{MS max}}} \times \frac{\alpha}{180} \qquad (5.41)$$

where MVA is the mitral valve area (cm^2), r is the measured radius (cm) of the hemispheric shell of the aliased velocity, v_r is the aliased velocity identified as the Nyquist limit (cm/s) at the radius r, $V_{\text{MS max}}$ is the maximal diastolic E velocity across the mitral orifice, obtained by CW Doppler (cm/s), and a is the angle measured, in degrees, between the two mitral leaflets.

In the case of TR, two correction factors are required (41) as mentioned in the equation:

$$\text{ERO} = 2\pi r^2 \frac{v_r}{V_{\text{TR max}}} \times \frac{v_r}{V_{\text{TR max}} - v_r} \times \frac{\alpha}{180} \qquad (5.42)$$

where ERO is the effective regurgitant orifice area (cm^2), r is the measured radius (cm) of the hemispheric shell of the aliased velocity, v_r is the aliased

velocity identified as the Nyquist limit (cm/s) at the radius r, $V_{\text{TR max}}$ is the maximal systolic velocity across the regurgitant orifice, obtained by CW Doppler (cm/s), and α is the angle measured, in degrees, between the two tricuspid leaflets.

Regurgitant Volumes and Fractions

According to the principle of conservation of mass (volume), the volumetric flow across all the cardiac valves is equal as long as there is no regurgitation or intracardiac shunt. When valvular regurgitation occurs, a regurgitant volume is added to the forward SV present through the valve. Therefore, the SV measured across a regurgitant valve is higher compared with the other competent valves by a value equal to the regurgitant volume (Reg Vol). The Reg Vol can be calculated by the equation:

$$\text{Reg Vol} = \text{SV}_{\text{regurgitant valve}} - \text{SV}_{\text{competent valve}} \qquad (5.43)$$

The regurgitant fraction is the percentage of Reg Vol compared with total flow across the incompetent valve. This is mathematically expressed as follows:

$$\text{RF} = \frac{\text{Reg Vol}}{\text{SV}_{\text{Total}}} \times 100 \qquad (5.44)$$

where RF is the regurgitant fraction (%) and SV$_{\text{Total}}$ is the total stroke volume (mL), given by the Doppler-stroke volume across the incompetent valve or the SV obtained by 2D methods.

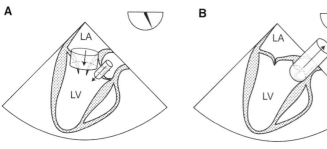

A

MV inflow stroke volume (SV$_{MV}$) = CSA x VTI

B

LVOT outflow stroke volume (SV$_{LVOT}$) = CSA x VTI

Regurgitant volume (Reg.Vol.) = SV$_{LVOT}$ − SV$_{MV}$
Regurgitant fraction = Reg.Vol./SV$_{LVOT}$

Figure 5.36 Volumetric measurements. (A,B) In the presence of aortic regurgitation the LVOT diameter can be measured from the mid-esophageal long-axis view and used to calculate the increased SV of the LVOT (SV$_{LVOT}$). The regurgitant volume corresponds to the difference between the SV$_{LVOT}$ and SV through the mitral valve (SV$_{MV}$). The regurgitant fraction is the ratio of the Reg. Vol. over SV$_{LVOT}$. *Abbreviations*: CSA, cross sectional area; LA, left atrium; LV, left ventricle; LVOT, left ventricular outflow tract; Reg. Vol., regurgitant volume; SV, stroke volume; VTI, velocity-time integral.

The amount of regurgitant volume or fraction indicates the severity of valvular regurgitation. Regurgitant volume can be estimated using either the volumetric method (Fig. 5.36) or flow convergence (PISA) method. Accuracy of the volumetric technique relies on correct Doppler sample volume positioning, diameter measurements, and stable cardiac rhythm.

The stroke volume across the aortic valve (SV$_{ao}$) is the same through the LVOT (SV$_{LVOT}$). It is obtained using the volumetric method and is given by the equation:

$$SV_{LVOT} = 0.785 \, (d_{LVOT})^2 \times VTI_{LVOT} \qquad (5.45)$$

The d_{LVOT} is the LVOT diameter (cm) measured at the base of the aortic cusps in the mid-esophageal AoV LAX view at 130° from inner edge to inner edge. The VTI$_{LVOT}$ is the velocity-time integral (cm) measured by PW Doppler in the deep transgastric view with the sample volume in the center of the LVOT, tracing the outer edge of the velocity Doppler signal envelope.

The stroke volume across the mitral valve (SV$_{MV}$) using the volumetric method is given by the equation:

$$SV_{MV} = 0.785 \, d_1 \times d_2 \times VTI_{MV} \qquad (5.46)$$

The diameters of the MV annulus are measured during diastole at the base of the leaflets from inner edge to inner edge in the mid-esophageal four-chamber view (d_1) and the mid-esophageal two-chamber view (d_2). The VTI$_{MV}$ is the velocity-time integral (cm) measured using PW Doppler with the sample volume in the center of the MV annulus, tracing the modal (densest) velocity on the diastolic Doppler signal envelope.

In the case of isolated aortic regurgitation (AR), the aortic regurgitant volume is given by the equation:

$$Aortic\ regurgitant\ volume = SV_{LVOT} - SV_{MV} \qquad (5.47)$$

In isolated mitral regurgitation (MR), the mitral regurgitant volume is given by the equation:

$$Mitral\ regurgitant\ volume = SV_{MV} - SV_{LVOT} \qquad (5.48)$$

Note that in both situations, the SV obtained by the difference between LVEDV and LVESV measured by 2D echocardiography corresponds to the sum of the forward SV and the regurgitant volume, and can be

substituted to the first SV of the equation. In this case, the calculated SV is not the effective forward flow.

With combined significant AR and MR, respective aortic and mitral regurgitant volumes cannot be determined by the preceding continuity equation applied to the mitral and aortic flow alone. In the absence of intracardiac shunt and pulmonic regurgitation, the forward SV can be obtained from the RVOT, considered as the competent valve and used to determine the regurgitant volume through the regurgitant valve.

Mitral regurgitant volume can alternatively be obtained using the convergence (PISA) method, as it invokes the continuity equation at the MV only and is not affected by the presence of AR. Once the mitral effective regurgitant orifice is calculated (see in the preceding text), the regurgitant volume is obtained by the equation:

$$Mitral\ regurgitant\ volume = ERO_{MV} \times VTI_{MR} \qquad (5.49)$$

where ERO is the effective regurgitant orifice (cm^2) and VTI$_{MR}$ is the velocity-time integral (cm) of the mitral regurgitant signal obtained by CW Doppler, tracing the peak (outer edge) of the Doppler signal envelope.

Shunt Fractions

According to the principle of conservation of mass (volume), the volumetric flow through the right heart should be equal to that through the left heart. However, in the presence of an intracardiac shunt, the SV will be greater on the side receiving the additional shunt volume. Because the left-sided intracardiac pressures are usually greater than on the right, intracardiac shunts are most often from left to right, and the pulmonary blood flow will be greater than the systemic blood flow. The magnitude of systemic-to-pulmonary intracardiac shunt can be quantified by determining the ratio of pulmonary blood flow (Q_p) to systemic blood flow (Q_s):

$$\frac{Q_P}{Q_s} = \frac{SV_{pulmonary}}{SV_{systemic}} \qquad (5.50)$$

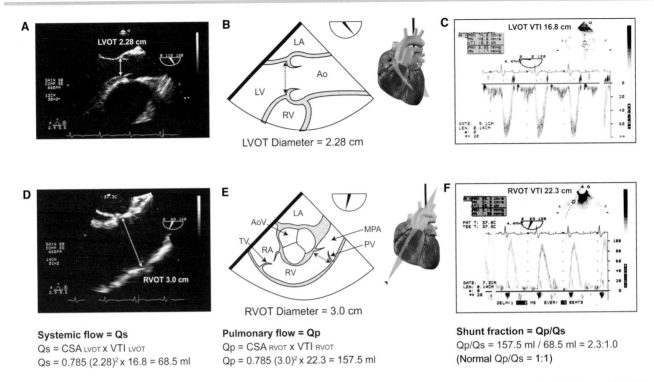

Systemic flow = Qs
Qs = CSA LVOT x VTI LVOT
Qs = 0.785 (2.28)² x 16.8 = 68.5 ml

Pulmonary flow = Qp
Qp = CSA RVOT x VTI RVOT
Qp = 0.785 (3.0)² x 22.3 = 157.5 ml

Shunt fraction = Qp/Qs
Qp/Qs = 157.5 ml / 68.5 ml = 2.3:1.0
(Normal Qp/Qs = 1:1)

Figure 5.37 Shunt fraction. Calculation of the shunt fraction in a patient before closure of an atrial septal defect is shown. **(A,B)** The LVOT diameter (D) is measured in the ME long-axis view. **(C)** The LVOT VTI is 16.8 cm. **(D,E)** From a ME right ventricular inflow/outflow view, the RVOT diameter is 3.0 cm. **(F)** The corresponding VTI is 22.3 cm. From these values, the pulmonary flow (Qp), the systemic flow (Qs) and the shunt fraction (Qp/Qs) can be calculated. *Abbreviations*: Ao, aorta; AoV, aortic valve; CSA, cross sectional area; LA, left atrium; LV, left ventricle; LVOT, left ventricular outflow tract; ME, mid-esophageal; MPA, main pulmonary artery; PV, pulmonic valve; RA, right atrium; RV, right ventricle; RVOT, right ventricular outflow tract; TV, tricuspid valve; VTI, velocity-time integral. 🖰

where Q_p is the pulmonary blood flow, including the added left-to-right shunt flow, Q_s is the systemic blood flow, and SV is the stroke volume by the hydraulic formula ($= 0.785\ d^2 \times$ VTI).

To reflect the magnitude of the shunt adequately, the pulmonary blood flow must be measured at a site distal to the shunt inflow, while the systemic blood flow should be measured at a site distal to the shunt outflow. The location of the shunt will determine where respective Q_p and Q_s measurements are made. For technical reasons, the preferred site of SV measurements appears to be at the LVOT or RVOT where the CSA diameter is best seen at the base of the semilunar cusps and the VTI outer edge is easily traced, as opposed to modal velocity in atrioventricular valves.

An example of calculating the shunt fraction pre- and post-ASD repair is presented in Fig. 5.37.

CONCLUSION

Transesophageal echocardiography is a powerful tool in the evaluation of cardiac structure and function through Doppler interrogation. Appreciation of the normal values is, however, important to interpret pathological conditions correctly.

REFERENCES

1. Feigenbaum H, Popp RL, Chip JN, et al. Left ventricular wall thickness measured by ultrasound. Arch Intern Med 1968; 121:391–395.
2. Devereux RB, Reichek N. Echocardiographic determination of left ventricular mass in man. Anatomic validation of the method. Circulation 1977; 55:613–618.
3. Wyatt HL, Heng MK, Meerbaum S, et al. Cross-sectional echocardiography. I. Analysis of mathematic models for quantifying mass of the left ventricle in dogs. Circulation 1979; 60:1104–1113.
4. Schiller NB, Shah PM, Crawford M, et al. Recommendations for quantitation of the left ventricle by two-dimensional echocardiography. American Society of Echocardiography Committee on Standards, Subcommittee on Quantitation of Two-Dimensional Echocardiograms. J Am Soc Echocardiogr 1989; 2:358–367.
5. Lang RM, Bierig M, Devereux RB, et al. Recommendations for chamber quantification: a report from the American Society of Echocardiography's Guidelines and Standards Committee and the Chamber Quantification Writing Group, developed in conjunction with the European Association of Echocardiography, a branch of the European Society of Cardiology. J Am Soc Echocardiogr 2005; 18: 1440–1463.
6. Wiske PS, Pearlman JD, Hogan RD, et al. Echocardiographic definition of the left ventricular centroid. II.

Determination of the optimal centroid during systole in normal and infarcted hearts. J Am Coll Cardiol 1990; 16:993–999.

7. Sahn DJ, DeMaria A, Kisslo J, et al. Recommendations regarding quantitation in M-mode echocardiography: results of a survey of echocardiographic measurements. Circulation 1978; 58:1072–1083.

8. Drexler M, Erbel R, Muller U, et al. Measurement of intracardiac dimensions and structures in normal young adult subjects by transesophageal echocardiography. Am J Cardiol 1990; 65:1491–1496.

9. Block M, Hourigan L, Bellows WH, et al. Comparison of left atrial dimensions by transesophageal and transthoracic echocardiography. J Am Soc Echocardiogr 2002; 15:143–149.

10. Schnittger I, Gordon EP, Fitzgerald PJ, et al. Standardized intracardiac measurements of two-dimensional echocardiography. J Am Coll Cardiol 1983; 2:934–938.

11. Cohen GI, White M, Sochowski RA, et al. Reference values for normal adult transesophageal echocardiographic measurements. J Am Soc Echocardiogr 1995; 8:221–230.

12. Haddad F, Hunt SA, Rosenthal DN, et al. Right ventricular function in cardiovascular disease. part I: Anatomy, physiology, aging, and functional assessment of the right ventricle. Circulation 2008; 117:1436–1448.

13. Weyman AE. Principles and practice of echocardiography. 2nd ed. Philadelphia: Lea & Febiger, 1994.

14. Roman MJ, Devereux RB, Kramer-Fox R, et al. Two-dimensional echocardiographic aortic root dimensions in normal children and adults. Am J Cardiol 1989; 64:507–512.

15. Maslow AD, Schwartz C, Singh AK. Assessment of the tricuspid valve: a comparison of four transesophageal echocardiographic windows. J Cardiothorac Vasc Anesth 2004; 18:719–724.

16. Feigenbaum H, Popp RL, Wolfe SB, et al. Ultrasound measurements of the left ventricle. A correlative study with angiocardiography. Arch Intern Med 1972; 129:461–467.

17. Teichholz LE, Kreulen T, Herman MV, et al. Problems in echocardiographic volume determinations: echocardiographic-angiographic correlations in the presence of absence of asynergy. Am J Cardiol 1976; 37:7–11.

18. Kronik G, Slany J, Mosslacher H. Comparative value of eight M-mode echocardiographic formulas for determining left ventricular stroke volume. A correlative study with thermodilution and left ventricular single-plane cineangiography. Circulation 1979; 60:1308–1316.

19. Tennant R, Wiggers CJ. The effect of coronary occlusion on myocardial contraction. Am J Physiol 1935; 112:351–361.

20. Pandian NG, Kerber RE. Two-dimensional echocardiography in experimental coronary stenosis. I. Sensitivity and specificity in detecting transient myocardial dyskinesis: comparison with sonomicrometers. Circulation 1982; 66:597–602.

21. Devereux RB, Alonso DR, Lutas EM, et al. Echocardiographic assessment of left ventricular hypertrophy: comparison to necropsy findings. Am J Cardiol 1986; 57:450–458.

22. Kupari M, Koskinen P. Systolic flow velocity profile in the left ventricular outflow tract in persons free of heart disease. Am J Cardiol 1993; 72:1172–1178.

23. Levy B, Targett RC, Bardou A, et al. Quantitative ascending aortic Doppler blood velocity in normal human subjects. Cardiovasc Res 1985; 19:383–393.

24. Targett RC, Heldt GP, McIlroy MB. Doppler blood velocity in the pulmonary artery of infants, children, and adults. Cardiovasc Res 1986; 20:816–821.

25. Currie PJ, Seward JB, Reeder GS, et al. Continuous-wave Doppler echocardiographic assessment of severity of calcific aortic stenosis: a simultaneous Doppler-catheter correlative study in 100 adult patients. Circulation 1985; 71:1162–1169.

26. Hatle L, Brubakk A, Tromsdal A, et al. Noninvasive assessment of pressure drop in mitral stenosis by Doppler ultrasound. Br Heart J 1978; 40:131–140.

27. Burstow DJ, Nishimura RA, Bailey KR, et al. Continuous wave Doppler echocardiographic measurement of prosthetic valve gradients. A simultaneous Doppler-catheter correlative study. Circulation 1989; 80:504–514.

28. Currie PJ, Seward JB, Chan KL, et al. Continuous wave Doppler determination of right ventricular pressure: a simultaneous Doppler-catheterization study in 127 patients. J Am Coll Cardiol 1985; 6:750–756.

29. Murphy DJ Jr, Ludomirsky A, Huhta JC. Continuous-wave Doppler in children with ventricular septal defect: noninvasive estimation of interventricular pressure gradient. Am J Cardiol 1986; 57:428–432.

30. Ge Z, Zhang Y, Kang W, et al. Noninvasive evaluation of right ventricular and pulmonary artery systolic pressures in patients with ventricular septal defects: simultaneous study of Doppler and catheterization data. Am Heart J 1993; 125:1073–1081.

31. Ge Z, Zhang Y, Fan D, et al. Simultaneous measurement of pulmonary artery diastolic pressure by Doppler echocardiography and catheterization in patients with patent ductus arteriosus. Am Heart J 1993; 125:263–266.

32. Masuyama T, Kodama K, Kitabatake A, et al. Continuous-wave Doppler echocardiographic detection of pulmonary regurgitation and its application to noninvasive estimation of pulmonary artery pressure. Circulation 1986; 74:484–492.

33. Kitabatake A, Inoue M, Asao M, et al. Noninvasive evaluation of pulmonary hypertension by a pulsed Doppler technique. Circulation 1983; 68:302–309.

34. Dabestani A, Mahan G, Gardin JM, et al. Evaluation of pulmonary artery pressure and resistance by pulsed Doppler echocardiography. Am J Cardiol 1987; 59:662–668.

35. Otto CM, Pearlman AS. Textbook of clinical echocardiography. Philadelphia: W.B. Saunders, 1995.

36. Ommen SR, Nishimura RA, Hurrell DG, et al. Assessment of RAP with 2-dimensional and Doppler echocardiography: a simultaneous catheterization and echocardiographic study. Mayo Clin Proc 2000; 75:24–29.

37. Garcia MJ, Ares MA, Asher C, et al. An index of early left ventricular filling that combined with pulsed Doppler peak E velocity may estimate capillary wedge pressure. J Am Coll Cardiol 1997; 29:448–454.

38. Dumesnil JG, Dion D, Yvorchuk K, et al. A new, simple and accurate method for determining ejection fraction by Doppler echocardiography. Can J Cardiol 1995; 11:1007–1014.

39. Hatle L, Angelsen B, Tromsdal A. Noninvasive assessment of atrioventricular pressure half-time by Doppler ultrasound. Circulation 1979; 60:1096–1104.

40. Rodriguez L, Thomas JD, Monterroso V, et al. Validation of the proximal flow convergence method. Calculation of orifice area in patients with mitral stenosis. Circulation 1993; 88:1157–1165.

41. Rivera JM, Vandervoort PM, Mele D, et al. Quantification of tricuspid regurgitation by means of the proximal flow convergence method: a clinical study. Am Heart J 1994; 127:1354–1362.

6

Goal-Oriented Transthoracic and Epicardial Echocardiography

Yanick Beaulieu

Hôpital du Sacré-Coeur de Montréal, Université de Montréal, Montreal, Quebec, Canada

Richard Bowry and Robert Chen

St. Michael's Hospital, University of Toronto, Toronto, Ontario, Canada

INTRODUCTION

Ultrasonography has become an invaluable tool in the management of critically ill patients. Its safety and portability allow for use at the bedside to provide rapid, detailed information regarding the function and anatomy of certain internal organs. Echocardiography can, noninvasively, elucidate cardiac function and structure. This information is vital in the management of hemodynamically unstable patients. Hand-carried ultrasound devices (HCUs) can provide immediate diagnostic information not assessable by physical examination alone.

In the anesthesia environment, bedside ultrasound has already gained important prominence for assessment of peripheral and/or central vessels to aid insertion of catheters and for performance of regional block anesthesia. With bedside ultrasound, the anesthesiologist can directly visualize nerves and their main surrounding structures (artery, veins, muscles, soft tissues), allowing precise insertion of the needle and direct visualization of local anesthetic spread around the nerves. The use of ultrasound has greatly improved the overall success and safety of these procedures.

This chapter will review the principles of the focused assessment of cardiac function by transthoracic and epicardial ultrasound.

BEDSIDE ECHOCARDIOGRAPHY

Performance and interpretation of a complete echocardiographic examination involves the assimilation of multiple and disparate types of data: chamber measurements, images, and hemodynamic assessment (derived using Doppler-based techniques) obtained in a continuous integrated fashion (1). Physician responsibilities in the echocardiographic examination include interpretation of all acquired images and measurements, generation of a report of those findings, and transmission of crucial findings to the attending physicians (1). To accomplish these roles, physicians engaged in echocardiography require specific training. Excellent guidelines exist, detailing the necessary skills to perform complete studies using transthoracic echocardiography (TTE) (2) and transesophageal echocardiography (TEE) (3). Any specialist, who aspires to become an "expert" echocardiographer, should follow these already well-established and recognized guidelines.

An approach that combines both physical examination and bedside echocardiography has improved clinical diagnosis and management in acutely ill patients. Such point-of-care echocardiographic examination is usually "directed" or "focused" toward a specific clinical question and is of significantly shorter duration (less than six minutes in some studies) than traditional echocardiography (4–6). The goal of such an exam is not to perform a complete, comprehensive study but instead to enhance or extend the physical examination.

Transthoracic echocardiography is noninvasive and more readily available than TEE and should, therefore, be the initial modality of choice to perform a goal-directed echocardiographic examination (7). It has not been widely applied in the intensive care unit (ICU) and operating room (OR) because only a few intensivists and anesthesiologists are trained in TTE (8). Bedside echocardiography has been performed increasingly over the last few years by the non-cardiologist, intensivist, and anesthesiologists to provide unobtainable diagnostic information by the physical examination alone (9–11).

FOCUS EXAMINATION

Indications

Focused, goal-directed TTE, termed *FOCUS* for FOcused Cardiac Ultrasound Study, or *FOCCUS* for FOcused Critical Care Ultrasound Study, is defined as a TTE done with specific, limited objectives (8). The

FOCUS objectives include assessment of left ventricular (LV) function, right ventricular (RV) function, assessment of the pericardial space for effusion and tamponade, and assessment of volume status. Additional FOCCUS objectives are beyond the scope of this chapter but would include assessment of lung pathology, abdominal fluid, vessels assessment, and so on. Also, in specific patients, a goal-directed color Doppler assessment of valves for massive regurgitation may be warranted. Detailed assessment of valvular function and the great vessels [aorta (Ao) and pulmonary artery] necessitates advanced skills and should not be a part of basic, limited echo training. It is crucial that if the physician performing the examination is unsure of all, or part, of the FOCUS exam findings, these should not be relied on for clinical decision making.

Training

In different studies, various curricula have been used to teach goal-directed echocardiography to non-cardiologists. Most of them comprise a combination of didactic and practical training. Echocardiography remains an imaging modality that is highly operator dependent for both acquisition and interpretation of the images. As there is no formal goal-directed echocardiography training program specifically for the clinical needs of intensivists, there is a risk of having inadequately trained medical personnel using the technology with potential adverse consequences.

Non-cardiologists wishing to use bedside echo in their ICU practice will need to undergo substantial training in acquiring the important echocardiographic views, interpreting the results, and, importantly, in understanding their limitations with the technique according to their level of training. Competency will have to be established according to predetermined levels of training (e.g., level 1 to 4). Some guidelines have already been proposed (12–14) including a consensus between the American College of Chest Physician and the Société de Réanimation de Langue Française (15).

It should not be the aim to train all acute care physicians to become expert echocardiographers. The initial step, entry level training, should be a part of critical care, emergency medicine, and anesthesiology fellowships. The objective of this basic training is to enhance the physical examination (often suboptimal in ICU patients) and not to replace a comprehensive echo examination.

A more advanced level of training would include a more complete TTE and/or TEE examination with requirements close to those proposed as level II by the American College Cardiology (ACC), American Heart Association (AHA), and American Society of Echocardiography (ASE) guidelines (16). Emphasis is placed on evaluation of hemodynamic parameters (for assessment of volume, cardiac output, pulmonary artery pressure) and for other types of cardiopulmonary abnormalities that are unique to the critical care patient (Table 6.1). Training is

Table 6.1 Indications for Echocardiography in the ICU

- Septic shock
- Acute circulatory failure
- Pulmonary embolism
- Cardiopulmonary interactions in mechanically ventilated patients
- Hemodynamic instability after cardiac surgery
- Hemodynamic instability after trauma
- Unexplained hypoxemia
- Atypical causes of cardiac dysfunction specific to ICU patients:
  Subarachnoid hemorrhage, cerebral death, metabolic problems, intoxication, myocarditis
- Noncardiogenic pulmonary edema (acute lung injury, ARDS)

Abbreviations: ARDS, acute respiratory distress syndrome; ICU, intensive care unit.

acquired by undertaking rotations with echo-trained intensivists in the ICU, cardiologists in the echocardiography laboratory, and anesthesiologists in the OR.

Technique

A focused echocardiographic examination can be performed with a high-end system or, most commonly, with a smaller portable ultrasound system. Whatever the type of ultrasound system used, it is important to ensure that the quality of the echocardiographic examination is adequate before concluding to a specific diagnosis. If the examination quality is inadequate and nondiagnostic, the clinician should ask for help from a more experienced echocardiographer or request another type of imaging modality to answer the clinical questions.

Despite being of a *limited* nature, the FOCUS examination is performed in a systematic three-step approach (Table 6.2):

1. Patient positioning: ensure the patient is optimally positioned for the area being studied
2. Image acquisition: adjust the basic image settings to display the image adequately
3. Image reading: possess sufficient knowledge to analyze the displayed image

The FOCUS examination includes the most important echocardiographic views, and scanning is performed from three main areas: the parasternal, apical, and subcostal areas (Figs. 6.1 and 6.2).

Specific Assessment

LV Systolic Function

In the ICU, clinical examination and invasive hemodynamic monitoring often fail to provide an adequate assessment of global ventricular function. Assessment of biventricular function is a primary indication for

Table 6.2 FOCUS Examination: The Systematic Three-Step Approach

Step 1: Position the patient

Step 2: Image acquisition
   a. Find the best ultrasonographic window available
   b. Optimize gain, depth, other controls
   c. Keep the area of interest in the center of the screen

Step 3: Image interpretation
   a. Identification of structures
   b. Systematic assessment of:
      LV size and function
      RV size and function
      Pericardial space for fluid and tamponade
      Color Doppler assessment of aortic, mitral, and tricuspid valves in specific cases
   c. Integration of findings in clinical decision making:
      Findings from the focused cardiac examination have to be correctly integrated in clinical decision making

Abbreviations: FOCUS, focused cardiac ultrasound study; LV, left ventricular; RV, right ventricular.
Source: With permission from the *FOCUS Pocket Guide*, courtesy of ICCU imaging inc.

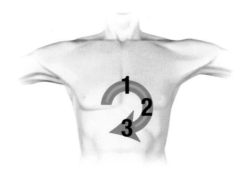

1 Parasternal long-axis and short-axis views
2 Apical four-chamber view
3 Subcostal four-chamber view

Figure 6.1 FOCUS. The FOCUS exam includes the most important echocardiographic views and scanning should be performed in a systematic, clockwise fashion, from three main areas: the parasternal (1), apical (2), and subcostal (3) areas. *Abbreviation*: FOCUS, focused cardiac ultrasound study. *Source*: Adapted from the *FOCUS pocket guide*, with permission from ICCU Imaging Inc.

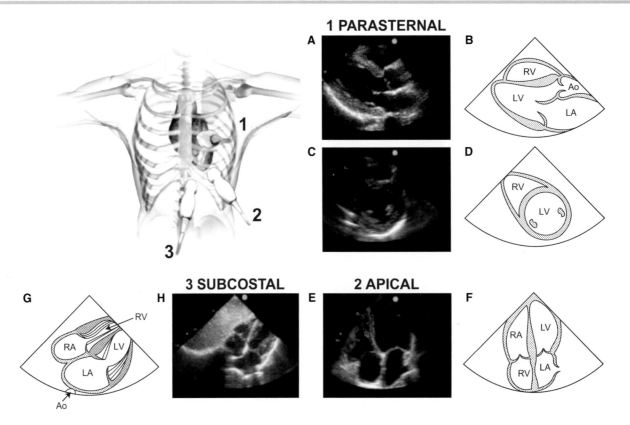

Figure 6.2 Basic FOCUS echocardiographic views. 1. Parasternal long-axis (**A,B**) and parasternal short-axis (**C,D**) views are shown. 2. Apical four-chamber view (**E,F**) and (3) Subcostal view (**G,H**) are shown. *Abbreviations*: Ao, aorta; LA, left atrium; FOCUS, focused cardiac ultrasound study; LV, left ventricle; RA, right atrium; RV, right ventricle. *Source*: Adapted from the *FOCUS pocket guide*, with permission from ICCU Imaging Inc.

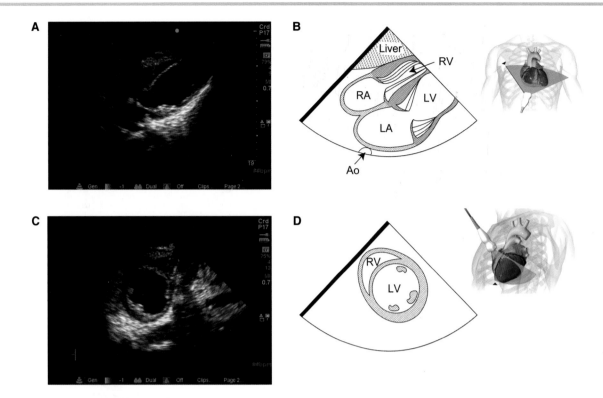

Figure 6.3 Takotsubo syndrome. Acute hemodynamic instability in a 73-year-old woman after duodenal perforation required investigation. (**A,B**) A FOCUS examination using a subcostal view revealed the presence of severe LV dysfunction with basal sparing typical of Takotsubo syndrome. (**C,D**) A parasternal short-axis view confirms the abnormal LV function. The patient recovered completely the following week. *Abbreviations*: FOCUS, focused cardiac ultrasound study; LA, left atrium; LV, left ventricle; RA, right atrium; RV, right ventricle.

echocardiographic studies in most ICU patients, particularly those with unexplained hemodynamic instability. Significant LV dysfunction is frequently seen in critically ill patients, and an accurate assessment helps guide resuscitation and ongoing medical management (Fig. 6.3).

Cardiac Arrest

In patients presenting with cardiac arrest, pulse assessment is used to detect the presence of underlying cardiac activity and the associated cardiac output. In a pulseless patient, bedside TTE is particularly useful in diagnosing pseudo-electromechanical dissociation (EMD), that is, the presence of some residual cardiac activity, as these patients have a better prognosis. Patients with pseudo-EMD may have extremes of severe LV dysfunction or hyperdynamic cardiac function from severe hypovolemia. Echocardiography can also be used for confirmation of asystole and ventricular fibrillation in patients where cardiac rhythm is difficult to assess.

Altered RV Size and Function

Altered RV size and function in the critical care setting can result from (*i*) increased RV afterload (increased pulmonary vascular resistance, mechanical ventilation) and/or (*ii*) depressed cardiac function (RV

infarct, sepsis). In unstable critically ill patients, the diagnosis of concomitant significant RV dysfunction may alter therapy (e.g., fluid loading, use of vasopressors, use of thrombolytics) and provide prognostic information (Fig. 6.4).

Pulmonary Embolism

Hemodynamic instability from acute cor pulmonale as a consequence of massive pulmonary embolism (PE) is a common occurrence. The diagnosis of acute cor pulmonale with bedside TTE has good positive predictive value for the indirect diagnosis of massive PE. Just the presence of acute RV dilatation and dysfunction, without actually imaging the embolus, is highly suggestive of the diagnosis (Fig. 6.4). Normal RV function does not rule out the presence of small emboli in patients with moderate-to-high clinical suspicion for PE. In a study by McConnell et al. (17), the presence of a distinct pattern of regional RV dysfunction, akinesia of the mid free wall but normal motion of the apex, was 77% sensitive and 94% specific for the diagnosis of acute PE using TTE.

Tamponade

Echocardiographic signs of tamponade show collapse of one or more cardiac chambers. Collapse of the RV free wall is seen in early diastole and the right atrium

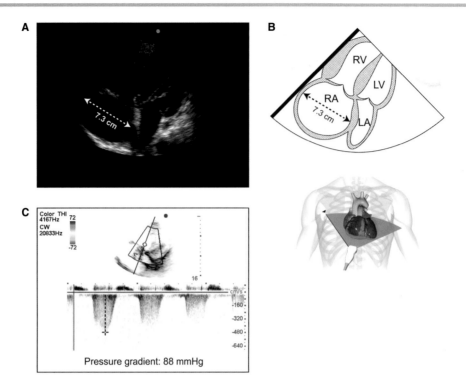

Figure 6.4 RV dysfunction and pulmonary hypertension. A 67-year-old man, in the emergency room, presented with hemodynamic instability. (**A,B**) FOCUS examination using a subcostal view revealed acute dilatation of the right atrium (RA) and the right ventricle (RV). The left ventricle (LV) was compressed. (**C**) Using continuous wave Doppler, a transtricuspid pressure gradient of 88 mmHg was present. Ancillary testing revealed the presence of pulmonary artery emboli. *Abbreviations*: FOCUS, focused cardiac ultrasound study; LA, left atrium; LV, left ventricle; RA, right atrium, RV, right ventricle. ⌐⊢

(RA) in late diastole. Hemodynamically significant effusion is diagnosed if the RA collapse lasts more than one-third of the R-R interval. The presence of a large effusion may cause the heart to swing in the pericardial cavity (see Chapter 12). A small amount of fluid may cause tamponade from rapid accumulation or a noncompliant pericardium. In poststernotomy patients, tamponade may be missed by TTE as the loculated clots may be located posterior to the heart in the far field. Doppler findings of tamponade, which rely on respiratory variation, may be difficult to interpret in mechanically ventilated patients with significant bronchospasm and pleural effusions (see Chapter 12).

Fluid Status and Fluid Responsiveness

Adequate determination of preload and volume status is important for proper management of critically ill patients. Invasive pressures measured at the bedside have a weak correlation to LV volume, potentially from differences in diastolic compliance. Key findings in favor of hypovolemia on two-dimensional (2D) imaging include (*i*) small hyperkinetic RV and LV, (*ii*) increased ejection fraction, (*iii*) dynamic LV obstruction, and (*iv*) small inferior vena cava (IVC) (<20 mm) with wide respiratory variation (Fig. 6.5) (see Chapter 10).

EPICARDIAL ECHOCARDIOGRAPHY

For the perioperative physician, an important advantage of achieving proficiency in FOCUS-style TTE is the immediate translation to epicardial and epiaortic scanning. Epicardial ultrasound guidelines for imaging are essentially those of a transthoracic exam. The TEE trained physician has the advantage of familiarity with the intra-operative environment and high frequency ultrasound imaging. The transesophageal sonographer must however rotate their "mental model" of the heart (Figs. 6.6–6.17). Time spent by both TEE and TTE sonographers learning anatomy and Doppler-based physiology is still valuable as it makes the epicardial and epiaortic examinations easier to learn.

Role

The use of perioperative epiaortic and epicardial echocardiography to assess mitral valve (MV) commissurotomy has been described since the early 1970s (18). Since the widespread adoption of TEE, these techniques are rarely used. In addition to the advantage of improved picture quality, TEE does not interfere with the surgery so it can be used as a continuous monitor. However, there are many patients in whom TEE is contraindicated, technically impossible (19), or

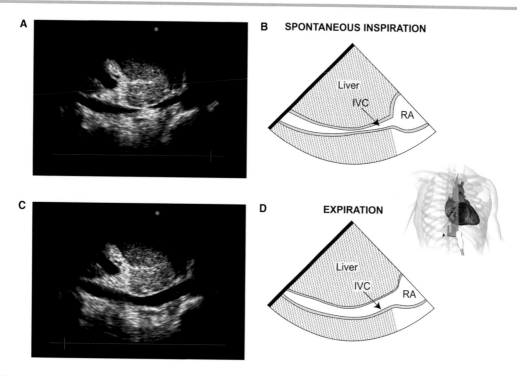

Figure 6.5 Echocardiographic sign of hypovolemia. Subcostal FOCUS view of the IVC shows typical fluid-responsiveness in a spontaneously breathing patient: IVC collapse during inspiration (**A,B**) and return to a normal size in expiration (**C,D**). *Abbreviations*: FOCUS, focused cardiac ultrasound study; IVC, inferior vena cava; RA, right atrium.

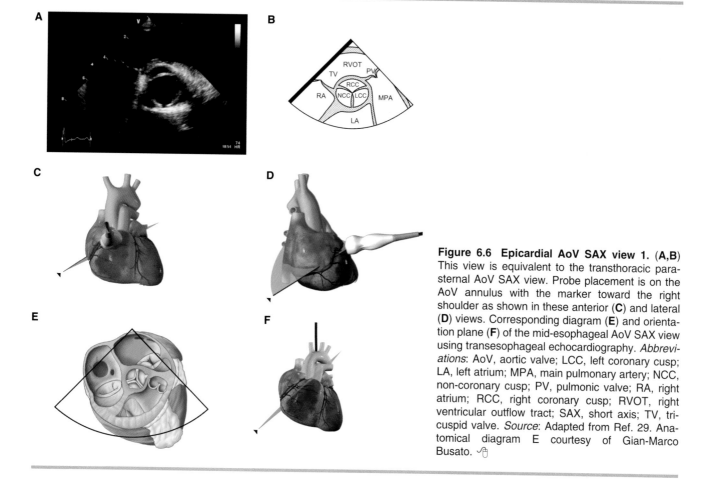

Figure 6.6 Epicardial AoV SAX view 1. (**A,B**) This view is equivalent to the transthoracic parasternal AoV SAX view. Probe placement is on the AoV annulus with the marker toward the right shoulder as shown in these anterior (**C**) and lateral (**D**) views. Corresponding diagram (**E**) and orientation plane (**F**) of the mid-esophageal AoV SAX view using transesophageal echocardiography. *Abbreviations*: AoV, aortic valve; LCC, left coronary cusp; LA, left atrium; MPA, main pulmonary artery; NCC, non-coronary cusp; PV, pulmonic valve; RA, right atrium; RCC, right coronary cusp; RVOT, right ventricular outflow tract; SAX, short axis; TV, tricuspid valve. *Source*: Adapted from Ref. 29. Anatomical diagram E courtesy of Gian-Marco Busato.

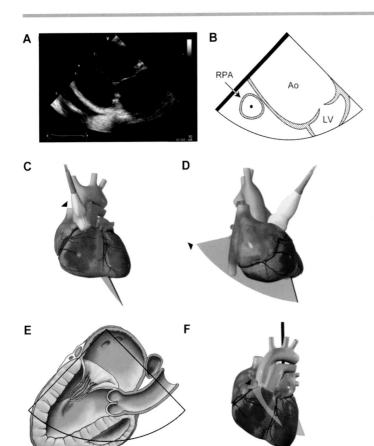

Figure 6.7   Epicardial AoV LAX view 2. (A,B) This view is equivalent to the transthoracic parasternal AoV LAX view. Probe placement is on the AoV annulus with the marker toward the left shoulder as shown in these anterior (**C**) and lateral (**D**) views. Corresponding diagram (**E**) and orientation plane (**F**) of the mid-esophageal AoV LAX view using transesophageal echocardiography. *Abbreviations*: Ao, aorta; AoV, aortic valve; LAX, long axis; LV, left ventricle; RPA, right pulmonary artery. *Source*: Adapted from Ref. 29. Anatomical diagram E courtesy of Gian-Marco Busato.

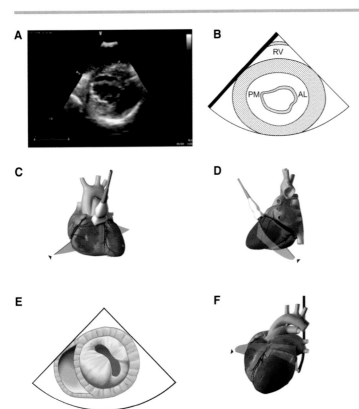

Figure 6.8   Epicardial LV basal SAX view 3. (A,B) This view is equivalent to the transthoracic parasternal LV basal SAX view. Probe placement is on the anterior RV with the marker toward the left as shown in these anterior (**C**) and posterior (**D**) views. Corresponding diagram (**E**) and orientation plane (**F**) of the transgastric basal SAX view using transesophageal echocardiography. *Abbreviations*: AL, anterolateral commissure; LV, left ventricle; PM, posteromedial commissure; RV, right ventricle; SAX, short axis. *Source*: Adapted from Ref. 29. Anatomical diagram E courtesy of Gian-Marco Busato.

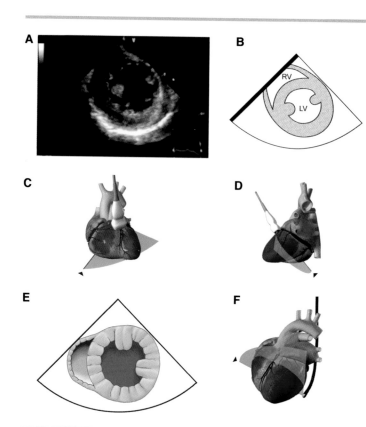

Figure 6.9 Epicardial LV mid-papillary SAX view 4. (A,B) This view is equivalent to the transthoracic parasternal LV mid-papillary SAX view. Probe placement is on the anterior RV with marker towards the left as shown in these anterior (**C**) and posterior (**D**) views. This differs from Figure 6.8 as the probe is directed more toward the apex of the LV. Corresponding diagram (**E**) and orientation plane (**F**) of the transgastric mid SAX view using transesophageal echocardiography. *Abbreviations*: LV, left ventricle; RV, right ventricle; SAX, short axis. *Source*: Adapted from Ref 29. Anatomical diagram E courtesy of Gian-Marco Busato.

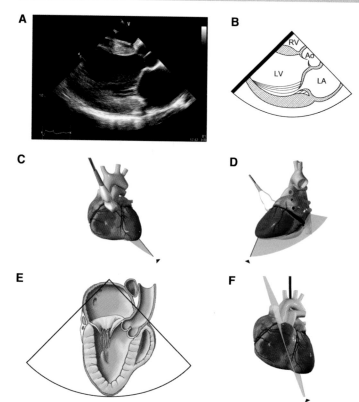

Figure 6.10 Epicardial LV LAX view 5. (A,B) This view is equivalent to the transthoracic parasternal LV LAX view. Probe placement is on the anterior RV with marker towards the right shoulder as shown in these anterior (**C**) and posterior (**D**) views. Corresponding diagram (**E**) and orientation plane (**F**) of the mid-esophageal LAX view using transesophageal echocardiography. *Abbreviations*: Ao, aorta; LA, left atrium; LAX; long axis; LV, left ventricle; RV, right ventricle. *Source*: Adapted from Ref 29. Anatomical diagram E courtesy of Gian-Marco Busato.

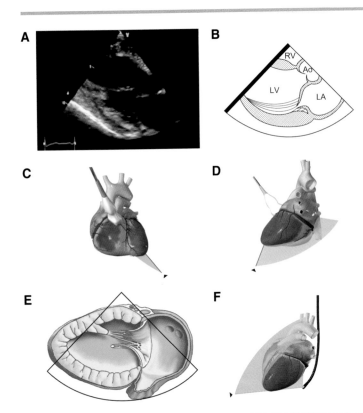

Figure 6.11 Epicardial LV mid-papillary LAX view 6. (A,B)
This view is equivalent to the transthoracic apical two-chamber view. Probe placement is on the anterior LV with marker midline cephalad as shown in these anterior (**C**) and posterior (**D**) views. Corresponding diagram (**E**) and orientation plane (**F**) of the transgastric two-chamber view using transesophageal echocardiography. *Abbreviations*: Ao, aorta; LA, left atrium; LAX, long axis; LV, left ventricle; RV, right ventricle. *Source*: Adapted from Ref 29. Anatomical diagram E courtesy of Gian-Marco Busato.

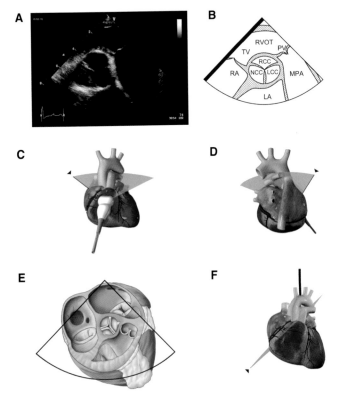

Figure 6.12 Epicardial RVOT view 7. (A,B) This view is equivalent to the transthoracic parasternal AoV SAX view. Probe placement is on the AoV annulus with the marker toward the left shoulder as shown in these anterior (**C**) and posterior (**D**) views. Corresponding diagram (**E**) and orientation plane (**F**) of the mid-esophageal right ventricular inflow/outflow view using TEE. Note that the orientation plane is more oblique in the TEE view than the epicardial view. *Abbreviations*: AoV, aortic valve; LA, left atrium; LCC, left coronary cusp; MPA, main pulmonary artery; NCC, non-coronary cusp; PV, pulmonic valve; RA, right atrium; RCC, right coronary cusp; RVOT, right ventricular outflow tract; SAX, short axis; TEE, transesophageal echocardiography; TV tricuspid valve. *Source*: Adapted from Ref 29. Anatomical diagram E courtesy of Gian-Marco Busato.

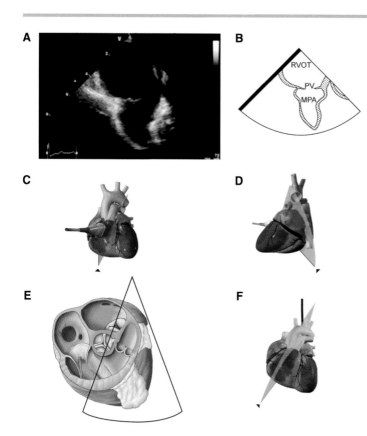

Figure 6.13 Alternative epicardial view RVOT. (A,B) This view is equivalent to the transthoracic parasternal SAX pulmonary artery view. Probe placement is on the RVOT with the marker toward the left shoulder as shown in these anterior (**C**) and posterior (**D**) views. The closest corresponding diagram (**E**) and orientation plane (**F**) is the mid-esophageal right ventricular inflow/outflow view with right-sided rotation using transesophageal echocardiography. *Abbreviations*: MPA, main pulmonary artery; PV, pulmonic valve; RVOT, right ventricular outflow tract; SAX, short axis. *Source*: Anatomical diagram E courtesy of Gian-Marco Busato.

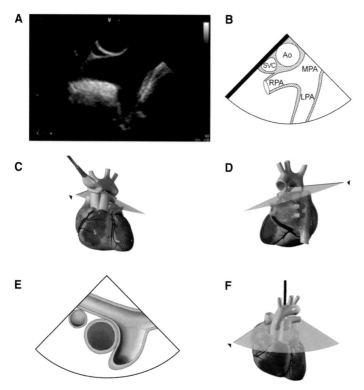

Figure 6.14 Alternative epicardial ascending Ao SAX view. (A,B) This view is equivalent to the transthoracic suprasternal Ao SAX view. Probe placement is on the ascending Ao with marker toward the left as shown in these anterior (**C**) and posterior (**D**) views. Corresponding diagram (**E**) and orientation plane (**F**) of the mid-esophageal ascending Ao SAX view using transesophageal echocardiography. *Abbreviations*: Ao, aorta; LPA, left pulmonary artery; MPA, main pulmonary artery; RPA, right pulmonary artery; SAX, short axis; SVC, superior vena cava. *Source*: Anatomical diagram E courtesy of Gian-Marco Busato.

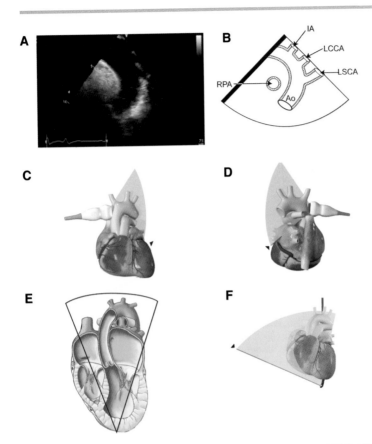

Figure 6.15 Alternative epicardial aortic arch LAX view. (**A,B**) This view is equivalent to the transthoracic suprasternal aortic LAX. Probe placement is on the ascending Ao with marker cephalad as shown in these anterior (**C**) and posterior (**D**) views. The closest corresponding diagram (**E**) and orientation plane (**F**) is the modified deep transgastric view at 80° of the aortic arch view using transesophageal echocardiography. *Abbreviations*: Ao, aorta; IA, innominate artery; LAX, long axis; LCCA, left common carotid artery; LSCA, left subclavian artery; RPA, right pulmonary artery. *Source*: Anatomical diagram E courtesy of Gian-Marco Busato.

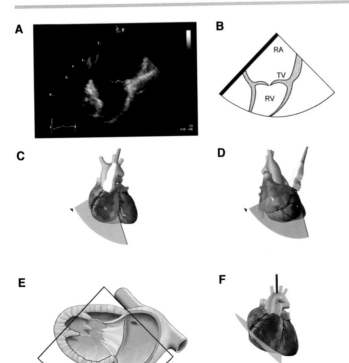

Figure 6.16 Epicardial alternative RV inflow view. (**A,B**) This view is equivalent to the transthoracic parasternal LAX view of the RV inflow. Probe placement is on the RV free wall with the marker toward the right shoulder as shown in these anterior (**C**) and lateral (**D**) views. Corresponding diagram (**E**) and orientation plane (**F**) is the transgastric RV inflow view using transesophageal echocardiography. *Abbreviations*: RA, right atrium; RV, right ventricle; TV, tricuspid valve. *Source*: Anatomical diagram E courtesy of Gian-Marco Busato.

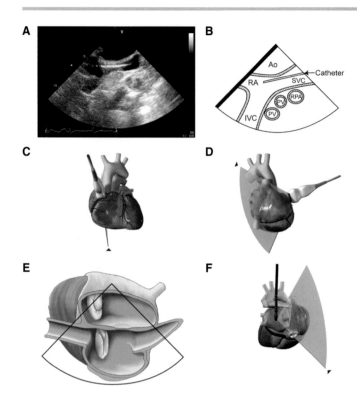

Figure 6.17 Epicardial alternative RA and bicaval view. (A, B) This view is equivalent to the transthoracic right parasternal right atrial and caval view. Probe placement is on the RV free wall with the marker toward the right shoulder with upwards tilt as shown in these anterior (**C**) and lateral (**D**) views. The closest corresponding diagram (**E**) and orientation plane (**F**) is the mid-esophageal bicaval view using transesophageal echocardiography. *Abbreviations*: IVC, inferior vena cava; PV; pulmonary vein; RA, right atrium; RPA, right pulmonary artery; RV, right ventricle; SVC, superior vena cava. *Source*: Anatomical diagram E courtesy of Gian-Marco Busato.

the equipment is unavailable. The ability to perform epiaortic and epicardial ultrasound will ensure that patients unsuitable for TEE are provided with the same high standard of intraoperative care.

Indications

There are also occasions where epiaortic and epicardial scanning can provide images and information unavailable with a complete TEE examination. Thus, for many patients, the surface techniques can be considered an adjunct to provide a more thorough assessment.

Assessment of Ascending Aortic Disease

The ascending Ao is assessed prior to arterial cannulation by either manual palpation or ultrasound. Although TEE is used for this role, the trachea and bronchi obscure the distal ascending Ao and it is possible to miss significant atheromatous disease. Epiaortic scanning has been shown to be superior to both TEE (multiplane and biplane) and manual palpation in identifying aortic atheroma (20–22) and is discussed more fully in Chapter 23 (23).

Pulmonary Artery Visualization

The pulmonic valve (PV) and artery can be clearly visualized with epicardial scanning. This allows detailed examination of the PV for endocarditis and function as well as identification of distal thrombus in

patients undergoing surgical management for pulmonary embolus (24) (Figs. 6.14 and 6.18).

Transvalvular Pressure Gradients and Paravalvular Leaks

It can often be difficult obtaining pressure gradients across the aortic valve (AoV) with TEE. This can result in significant underestimation of the transvalvular pressure gradient. Where this information will influence the surgery, epicardial scanning can be used to ensure an accurate assessment of the gradient (Figs. 6.7 and 6.19) (25–27). In certain patients, paravalvular leaks can be ruled out easily by using epicardial echocardiography (Fig. 6.20).

Technical Considerations

Maintaining Surgical Sterile Field

There are two alternatives to ensure that the surgical sterile field is maintained during the examination. They are the use of a sterile sheath with sterile ultrasound gel (Fig. 6.21) or the use of an ultrasound probe that can be sterilized. In view of the high cost of such probes, it is necessary to have proper facilities available to clean and sterilize them without causing damage. Despite the availability of remote pedals to operate the ultrasound machine, it is much easier to have two operators. This has the advantage of allowing one person to obtain the images without jeopardizing sterility while the second controls the

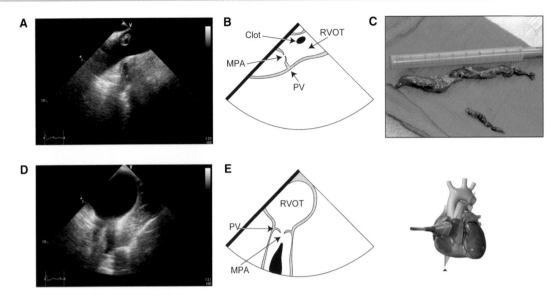

Figure 6.18 Epicardial RVOT view of pulmonary emboli. Epicardial echocardiography was used to localize the thrombus present in the RVOT (**A,B**) and the MPA (**D,E**) in a 49-year-old man with acute pulmonary emboli. (**C**) Anatomical specimen is shown. *Abbreviations*: MPA, main pulmonary artery; PV, pulmonic valve; RVOT, right ventricular outflow tract. *Source*: Courtesy of Drs. Gisèle Hemmings and Michel Pellerin.

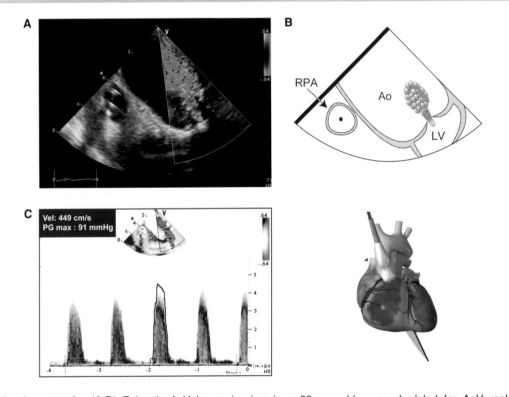

Figure 6.19 Aortic stenosis. (**A,B**) Epiaortic AoV long-axis view in a 58-year-old man scheduled for AoV replacement. The transesophageal echocardiographic views were not satisfactory. (**C**) The AoV PG is easily measured from this view. *Abbreviations*: Ao, aorta; AoV, aortic valve; LAX, long axis; LV, left ventricle; PG, pressure gradient; RPA, right pulmonary artery; Vel, velocity.

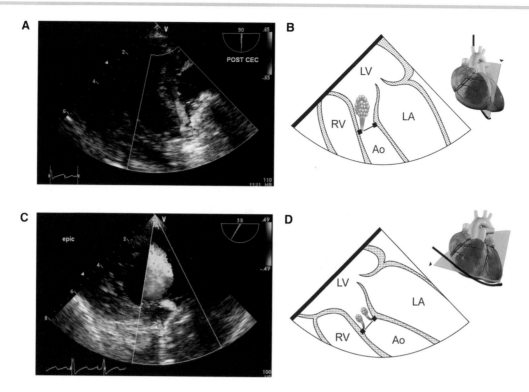

Figure 6.20 Aortic valve (AoV) replacement evaluation. (A,B) Transesophageal deep transgastric view at 0° in a 20-year-old woman after AoV replacement is shown. **(C,D)** Suspicion of paravalvular aortic regurgitation led to epicardial echocardiography using a transesophageal echocardiography probe. The abnormal jet was secondary to the normal closing volume and is well shown using this apical view. *Abbreviations*: Ao, aorta; AoV, aortic valve; LA, left atrium; LV, left ventricle; RV, right ventricle.

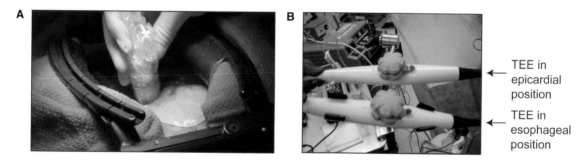

Figure 6.21 Methods used for epicardial echocardiography. (A) A high-frequency transthoracic probe in a sterile sheath is used and the cardiac surgeon is trained to identify the key structures. **(B)** In certain cases, an epicardial echocardiography is performed using a TEE probe. The exam is facilitated because the images are obtained by an experienced echocardiographer and requires minimal manipulation from the surgeon. *Abbreviation*: TEE, transesophageal echocardiography. *Source*: Courtesy of Dr. Michel Pellerin.

ultrasound machine. This will include image optimization, control of the Doppler cursor, and image storage.

Transducer Selection

When performing epiaortic and epicardial ultrasound, the structures of interest are typically near the transducer. This permits the use of high-frequency (6–10 MHz) transducers (Fig. 6.21A) to improve image quality as signal attenuation is less of a problem. Phased-array transducers are characterized with a small probe footprint. This is advantageous with epicardial scanning where the probe needs to be directed into cardiac grooves to obtain detailed images. The quality of the images will also differ. An epicardial finding of Lambl's excrescences or valvular vegetations could be invisible to the surface probe by the nature of their ultrasound resolution. This can be understood when you compare the

Table 6.3 Ultrasound Probe Comparison

	TTE	TEE	Epicardial
Probe frequency (MHz)	2.5–5.0	5.0–8.0	10.0
Theoretical resolution (2λ) (mm)	1.0	0.5	0.3
Limitations	Lung, pleural air, distal PA	Apex, distal PA	Surgical interruption
Contraindications	None	Anatomic	None

Abbreviations: TTE, transthoracic echocardiography; TEE, transesophageal echocardiography; PA, pulmonary artery.

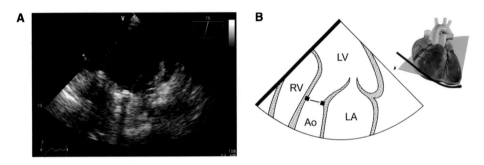

Figure 6.22   Apical LVOT view. (A,B) This view at 75° is obtained using a transesophageal echocardiography probe in a sterile sheath. With a smaller and more flexible probe, positioning at the LV apex is easier and therefore it is used in situations where there is a suspicion of prosthetic aortic valve malfunction. This approach can represent an alternative if the cardiac surgeon is not facile with epicardial echocardiography. *Abbreviations*: Ao, aorta; LA, left atrium; LV, left ventricle; LVOT, left ventricular outflow tract; RV, right ventricle.

typical transmission frequency of transthoracic, transesophageal and epicardial ultrasound probes (Table 6.3).

Image Acquisition

Unfortunately, the influence of near-field clutter can reduce image quality. Several approaches can be used to resolve this issue. These include filling the pericardium with warm saline so that the probe can be held a small distance away from the structure of interest. To that effect, using unagitated fluid will be important to prevent the occurrence of interfering microbubbles. It is also possible to create a "standoff" for the probe. This can be done using commercially available devices or placing extra ultrasound gel in the sterile sheath.

Linear array probes are less influenced by near-field clutter but typically have a large flat footprint. As a result, the probe is often too large to fit in the small spaces, or contact with the epicardial surface is poor. Filling the pericardium with warmed saline or using a TEE probe on the surface of the heart can circumvent these difficulties (Figs. 6.21B and 6.22).

Space Limitation

Image acquisition can be limited by the available space needed to manipulate the probe within the

pericardium. It is possible to obtain linear probes with malleable handles and smaller footprints that can be sterilized.

Technique

Performing an epicardial and epiaortic scan most often interrupts the usual flow of the surgical procedure. As a result, it is important that the examination be performed quickly, accurately, and without causing hemodynamic instability. In 2003, an examination protocol was created that examined the great vessels, valves, and ventricular function. This examination was performed in less than eight minutes and without causing hemodynamic instability (28). In 2007, the ASE and the Society of Cardiovascular Anesthesiologist (SCA) published their guidelines on the use of epicardial echocardiography and proposed a total of seven imaging planes (Figs. 6.6–6.12) consistent with the ASE recommendations for TTE (29). Additional views can also be used for specific purpose (Fig. 6.23) and are described in Figures 6.13 to 6.17. The ASE recommends that epicardial echocardiographic training should include the study of 25 epicardial examinations, of which five are personally directed under the supervision of an advanced echocardiographer.

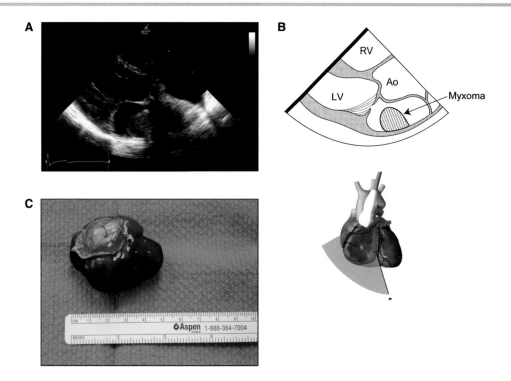

Figure 6.23 Left atrial myxoma. (A,B) Epicardial LV long-axis view before myxoma removal localizes fixation of the tumor on the interatrial septum. **(C)** Pathological specimen is shown. *Abbreviations*: Ao, aorta; LV, left ventricle; RV, right ventricle. *Source*: Courtesy of Dr Michel Pellerin.

CONCLUSION

The potential contribution of acute care physician-performed goal-directed echocardiography to enhance diagnostic ability, clinical management, and understanding of the critically ill patient is enormous, mostly when viewed as an addition to the physical examination. The challenge is to provide practical training programs that will ensure competency in performing focused, goal-directed echocardiography.

REFERENCES

1. Sanfilippo AJ, Bewick D, Chan KL, et al. Guidelines for the provision of echocardiography in Canada: recommendations of a joint Canadian Cardiovascular Society/Canadian Society of Echocardiography Consensus Panel. Can J Cardiol 2005; 21:763–780.
2. Cheitlin MD, Armstrong WF, Aurigemma GP, et al. ACC/AHA/ASE 2003 guideline update for the clinical application of echocardiography: summary article: a report of the American College of Cardiology/American Heart Association Task Force on Practice Guidelines (ACC/AHA/ASE Committee to Update the 1997 Guidelines for the Clinical Application of Echocardiography). Circulation 2003; 108:1146–1162.
3. Shanewise JS, Cheung AT, Aronson S, et al. ASE/SCA guidelines for performing a comprehensive intraoperative multiplane transesophageal echocardiography examination: recommendations of the American Society of Echocardiography Council for Intraoperative Echocardiography and the Society of Cardiovascular Anesthesiologists Task Force for Certification in Perioperative Transesophageal Echocardiography. Anesth Analg 1999; 89:870–884.
4. Spencer KT, Anderson AS, Bhargava A, et al. Physician-performed point-of-care echocardiography using a laptop platform compared with physical examination in the cardiovascular patient. J Am Coll Cardiol 2001; 37:2013–2018.
5. Rugolotto M, Chang CP, Hu B, et al. Clinical use of cardiac ultrasound performed with a hand-carried device in patients admitted for acute cardiac care. Am J Cardiol 2002; 90:1040–1042.
6. Gorcsan J III, Pandey P, Sade LE. Influence of hand-carried ultrasound on bedside patient treatment decisions for consultative cardiology. J Am Soc Echocardiogr 2004; 17:50–55.
7. Joseph MX, Disney PJ, Da Costa R, et al. Transthoracic echocardiography to identify or exclude cardiac cause of shock. Chest 2004; 126:1592–1597.
8. Manasia AR, Nagaraj HM, Kodali RB, et al. Feasibility and potential clinical utility of goal-directed transthoracic echocardiography performed by noncardiologist intensivists using a small hand-carried device (SonoHeart) in critically ill patients. J Cardiothorac Vasc Anesth 2005; 19:155–159.
9. Beaulieu Y, Marik PE. Bedside ultrasonography in the ICU: part 1. Chest 2005; 128:881–895.
10. Beaulieu Y, Marik PE. Bedside ultrasonography in the ICU: part 2. Chest 2005; 128:1766–1781.
11. Beaulieu Y. Bedside echocardiography in the assessment of the critically ill. Crit Care Med 2007; 35:S235–S249.
12. Langlois SP. Focused ultrasound training for clinicians. Crit Care Med 2007; 35:S138–S143.
13. Mazraeshahi RM, Farmer JC, Porembka DT. A suggested curriculum in echocardiography for critical care physicians. Crit Care Med 2007; 35:S431–S433.

14. Price S, Via G, Sloth E, et al. Echocardiography practice, training and accreditation in the intensive care: document for the World Interactive Network Focused on Critical Ultrasound (WINFOCUS). Cardiovasc Ultrasound 2008; 6:49.

15. Mayo PH, Beaulieu Y, Doelken P, et al. American College of Chest Physicians/La Société de Réanimation de Langue Française statement on competence in critical care ultrasonography. Chest 2009; 135:1050–1060.

16. Quinones MA, Douglas PS, Foster E, et al. American College of Cardiology/American Heart Association clinical competence statement on echocardiography: a report of the American College of Cardiology/American Heart Association/American College of Physicians—American Society of Internal Medicine Task Force on Clinical Competence. Circulation 2003; 107:1068–1089.

17. McConnell MV, Solomon SD, Rayan ME, et al. Regional right ventricular dysfunction detected by echocardiography in acute pulmonary embolism. Am J Cardiol 1996; 78:469–473.

18. Johnson ML, Holmes JH, Spangler RD, et al. Usefulness of echocardiography in patients undergoing mitral valve surgery. J Thorac Cardiovasc Surg 1972; 64:922–934.

19. Daniel WG, Erbel R, Kasper W, et al. Safety of transesophageal echocardiography. A multicenter survey of 10,419 examinations. Circulation 1991; 83:817–821.

20. Davila-Roman VG, Phillips KJ, Daily BB, et al. Intraoperative transesophageal echocardiography and epiaortic ultrasound for assessment of atherosclerosis of the thoracic aorta. J Am Coll Cardiol 1996; 28:942–947.

21. Sylivris S, Calafiore P, Matalanis G, et al. The intraoperative assessment of ascending aortic atheroma: epiaortic imaging is superior to both transesophageal echocardiography and direct palpation. J Cardiothorac Vasc Anesth 1997; 11:704–707.

22. Wilson MJ, Boyd SY, Lisagor PG, et al. Ascending aortic atheroma assessed intraoperatively by epiaortic and transesophageal echocardiography. Ann Thorac Surg 2000; 70:25–30.

23. Glas KE, Swaminathan M, Reeves ST, et al. Guidelines for the performance of a comprehensive intraoperative epiaortic ultrasonographic examination: recommendations of the American Society of Echocardiography and the Society of Cardiovascular Anesthesiologists; endorsed by the Society of Thoracic Surgeons. Anesth Analg 2008; 106:1376–1384.

24. Zlotnick AY, Lennon PF, Goldhaber SZ, et al. Intraoperative detection of pulmonary thromboemboli with epicardial echocardiography. Chest 1999; 115:1749–1751.

25. Edrich T, Shernan SK, Smith B, et al. Usefulness of intraoperative epiaortic echocardiography to resolve discrepancy between transthoracic and transesophageal measurements of aortic valve gradient—a case report. Can J Anaesth 2003; 50:293–296.

26. Frenk VE, Shernan SK, Eltzschig HK. Epicardial echocardiography: diagnostic utility for evaluating aortic valve disease during coronary surgery. J Clin Anesth 2003; 15: 271–274.

27. Hilberath JN, Shernan SK, Segal S, et al. The feasibility of epicardial echocardiography for measuring aortic valve area by the continuity equation. Anesth Analg 2009; 108:17–22.

28. Eltzschig HK, Kallmeyer IJ, Mihaljevic T, et al. A practical approach to a comprehensive epicardial and epiaortic echocardiographic examination. J Cardiothorac Vasc Anesth 2003; 17:422–429.

29. Reeves ST, Glas KE, Eltzschig H, et al. Guidelines for performing a comprehensive epicardial echocardiography examination: recommendations of the American Society of Echocardiography and the Society of Cardiovascular Anesthesiologists. J Am Soc Echocardiogr 2007; 20:427–437.

7

Imaging Artifacts and Pitfalls

Robert Amyot and Réal Lebeau
Université de Montréal, Montreal, Quebec, Canada

Stéphane Lambert
University of Ottawa Heart Institute, Ottawa, Ontario, Canada

INTRODUCTION

Kremkau and Taylor (1) define imaging artifacts as display phenomena that do not represent, properly, the structures to be imaged. Imaging pitfalls include artifacts, but also relate to the misinterpretation of a properly represented structure, whether normal or pathologic. These obstacles to accurate image analysis are commonly encountered during transesophageal echocardiography (TEE). They must be recognized to avoid diagnostic errors. Imaging artifacts generally fall into four categories:

1. Structures that appear to be there when in fact they are not
2. Structures that do not appear to be there when in fact they are
3. Structures that look different from reality
4. Structures that appear to be in the wrong location

A thorough understanding of the types and mechanisms of echocardiographic artifacts allows one to distinguish them from real structures. This chapter focuses on the most prevalent artifacts and pitfalls encountered during TEE.

IMAGE FEATURES AND ARTIFACTS

Reverberation

Strictly speaking, a reverberation is an acoustic phenomenon whereby sound waves bounce back and forth between structures. A simple example is shouting your name in the Grand Canyon and hearing it repeated over and over again. In echocardiography, reverberation artifacts result from multiple reflections of the ultrasound beam before returning to the transducer. As the imaging system assumes that the backscattered echo signal bounces off an object located within the ultrasound path and completes the round trip directly and unswervingly, the delay before the echo comes back to the transducer is interpreted as proportional to a straight-line distance between the object and the probe (1). Reverberation artifacts, therefore, are displayed at a greater depth than the actual object location. They may appear on the screen as nonspecific lines, bright areas, or a duplication of a whole structure located elsewhere on the screen. Moreover, the surface of the ultrasound transducer itself may act as a reflector and throw back part of the incoming signal that resumes its initial course and is backscattered a second time by the same target, and returns again to the transducer (2) (Fig. 7.1). Such reverberations are displayed at twice (or multiples of) the depth of the real object. Moreover, if a structure is moving, the velocity and movement amplitude of the artifact will be double (or multiples of) that of the object. In addition, color Doppler flow display in the vicinity of the actual target may be reflected in conjunction with the two-dimensional (2D) artifact. Finally, reverberations can also arise from other reflectors in the ultrasound field that may act in combination and create multiple reflection paths (Fig. 7.2).

Strongly reflective tissue-air and tissue-fluid interfaces with large impedance discontinuity, such as the aorta-lung interface (Fig. 7.3) and the anterior wall of the left atrium (LA) are often involved in these artifacts (3). The pericardium is another highly reflective surface with strong echogenicity that may reverberate the ultrasound beam. A typical example of reverberation is a linear artifact in the ascending aorta (Ao) lumen that must be differentiated from an aortic dissection flap (see Fig. 23.28).

Confirmation of the artifactual nature of an image requires a high index of suspicion and relies on several criteria that may, or may not, coexist: (a) indistinct boundaries, (b) nonplausible anatomy, (c) extension across normal surrounding structures, (d) disappearance with changes in sector depth setting, imaging planes, and transducer position (Fig. 7.4), (e) absence of independent motion, but rather movement paralleling that of the source of the reverberation (when identifiable), and (f) absence of influence on blood flow as assessed by color Doppler, showing flow crossing the artifact without turbulence or changes in direction or velocity (4). Foreign materials, most often catheters and prosthetic valves, typically contain metal, plastic, and/or pyrolytic carbon that strongly reverberate the ultrasound beam (5).

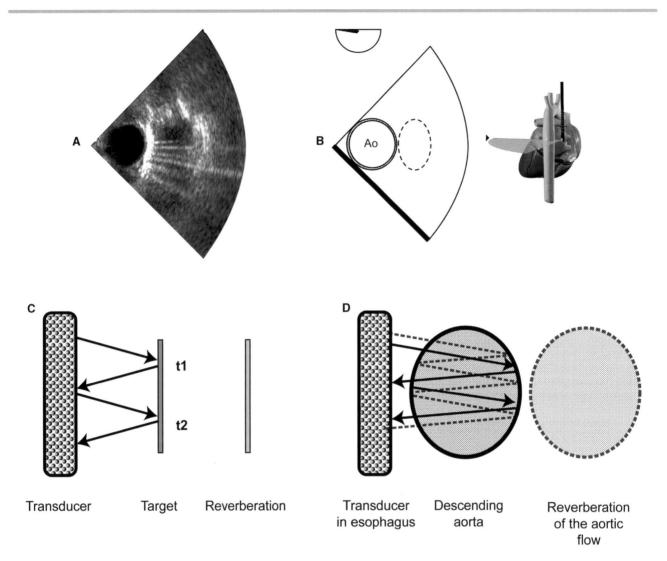

Figure 7.1   Reverberation. (A,B) A rotated mid-esophageal short-axis view of the aorta at 0° with a reverberation artifact is shown. **(C,D)** When a strong reflector is close to the transducer, the high-energy echo beam giving the image at the initial time (t1) is reflected on the front part of the transducer and then rerouted toward the reflector for a second time (t2). It gives a second image interpreted by the computer as being at a double distance of the first target, since t2 is twice t1. This will also be apparent for color Doppler. *Abbreviation*: Ao, aorta.

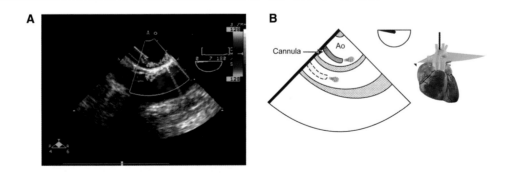

Figure 7.2   Reverberation. (A,B) Reverberation in both 2D and color Doppler signal of the Ao and the aortic cannula is displayed in this upper-esophageal aortic arch long-axis view at 7°. *Abbreviation*: Ao, aorta.

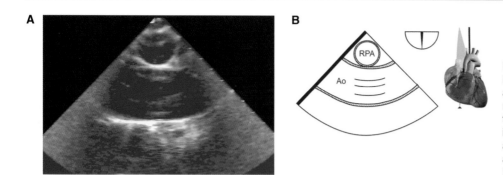

Figure 7.3 Reverberation. (A,B) Linear artifacts in the RPA and ascending Ao are generated by reverberation of the ultrasound on the strongly reflective aortic-lung interface as seen in this mid-esophageal ascending Ao long-axis view at 90°. *Abbreviations*: Ao, aorta; RPA, right pulmonary artery.

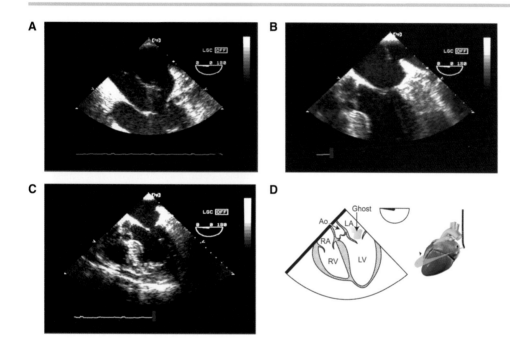

Figure 7.4 Ghosting phenomenon. (A–D) This mid-esophageal five-chamber view shows an ill defined ghost artifact located in the LA of a 57-year-old man undergoing coronary revascularization. As the sector depth is increased from (**A**) 8 cm to (**B**) 10 cm to (**C**) 16 cm there is a progressive disappearance of the artifact. *Abbreviations*: Ao, aorta; LA, left atrium; LGC, lateral gain control; LV, left ventricle; RA, right atrium; RV, right ventricle.

Multiple reflections of the ultrasound signal between different prosthetic components result in a dense succession of separate linear echoes extending from the prosthesis to the distal field (1,5) (Fig. 7.5).

Aliasing

Aliasing occurs in Doppler devices that operate in a pulsed mode: pulsed wave (PW) and color Doppler. These modalities have the ability to interrogate specific regions of interest within the ultrasound field. This sampling ability is achieved by transmitting ultrasound in intermittent short bursts rather than continuously, as in continuous wave (CW) Doppler. The transducer alternately acts as a transmitter and a receiver. Assuming the speed of sound remains constant in the thorax, the delay between pulse transmission and reception of the backscattered signal is proportional to the depth of the target. Therefore,

the sampling depth determines the rate of ultrasound burst transmission, or pulse repetition frequency (PRF) (see Chapter 1). Accordingly, Doppler shift can be measured only intermittently—when the system functions as an echo signal receiver—over a limited range of frequencies. Aliasing occurs when the frequency of the Doppler shift of the incoming echo exceeds the maximal frequency that the ultrasound system can properly assess. This frequency limit is known as the Nyquist limit and is equal to one-half of the PRF. The direction of the aliasing signal is displayed as opposite to the actual flow direction either on spectral display or on color-coded flow imaging display (3,6,7).

In PW Doppler mode, high velocities exceeding the Nyquist limit are depicted as a signal displayed on both sides of the baseline of the spectral display. A truncated part, where peak velocity exceeds the upper limit of the velocity scale, is displayed on the appropriate side of the baseline and, therefore, correctly reflects the direction of the actual flow; and a second

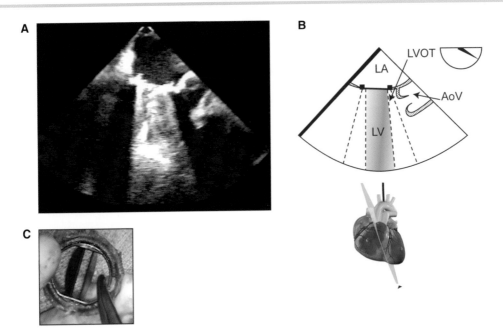

Figure 7.5 Reverberation and acoustic shadowing. (A,B) A dense succession of linear echoes extending from a mechanical bileaflet valve in the mitral position to the far field is seen in this mid-esophageal long-axis view. The prosthetic ring acts as an acoustic obstacle and the reverberation artifact is bordered by blind regions (shadowing) preventing visualization of the ventricular cavity and part of the basal ventricular septum. **(C)** Mechanical bileaflet prosthesis is examined after surgical removal. *Abbreviations*: AoV, aortic valve; LA, left atrium; LV, left ventricle; LVOT, left ventricular outflow tract. *Source*: Photo C courtesy of Dr. Michel Pellerin.

part, the aliasing signal, appearing and wrapping around on the opposite side of the baseline (Fig. 7.6). Therefore, aliasing prevents assessment of the peak velocity of the interrogated flow and may introduce confusion concerning its direction.

Shifting the baseline, to obtain a complete PW Doppler signal, and decreasing sampling depth may eliminate signal aliasing. Another approach to overcome aliasing is the utilization of high PRF Doppler mode where multiple sampling gates are aligned on an axis. Although this modality allows the increase of the Nyquist limit, it introduces range ambiguity, as it may become impossible to know which sampling gate recorded the highest displayed velocity.

In color Doppler mode, flow velocity, exceeding the maximal value of the color scale, is displayed by an abrupt change in color to the opposite end of the color-coded scale (wrap around phenomenon), wrongly suggesting a change in flow direction (Fig. 7.7). The color-flow signal may, therefore, display a mosaic of colors from both sides of the color-coded scale.

Ghosting

The terms "ghost artifact" and "ghosting" can lead to confusion, as they are used by different authors to identify distinct phenomena. For example, ghost artifact has been attributed to image duplication caused by refraction of the ultrasound beam (8). Reverberation artifacts have also been referred to as "ghosts" (Fig. 7.4) (6,9). Finally, ghosting has been used to describe at

least two types of artifacts in color Doppler imaging. One phenomenon is produced by the rapid motion of a target, such as cardiac valve leaflets, in conjunction with the reduced frame rate of color Doppler imaging causing color flashes (2). A second phenomenon refers to artifactual low-amplitude color echoes within the cardiac chambers in the presence of tachycardia (7). In the view of the authors, these terms should be avoided in favor of more specific terminology.

Mirror Images

The mirror image artifact is a form of reverberation artifact, which consists of the secondary representation of a target on the opposite side of a strongly reflective interface. It is caused by a significant difference in acoustic impedance between two adjacent structures and has been described, most commonly, around the diaphragm and pleura as the air-filled lungs act as total reflectors of the acoustic beam (1,9). Accordingly, the straight and regular interface between the thoracic Ao and the left lung behaves as a powerful ultrasound mirror (Fig. 7.2). Proximity of the reflector to the transducer allows for a high-energy echo reflection appearing in the usual depth range of the imaging sector (3). It is important to note that PW, CW, and color Doppler information of the actual target is also reflected and will be displayed in the artifactual image. In the presence of a curved, or irregular, reflective surface, the mirror image may be distorted, rendering its recognition more challenging.

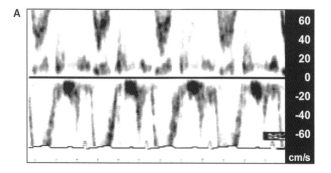

SCALE ADJUSTMENT

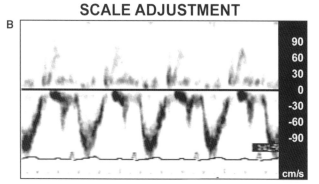

BASELINE SHIFT

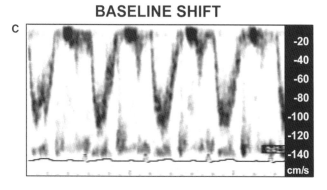

Figure 7.6 Spectral Doppler aliasing. (A–C) Pulsed wave Doppler signals of flow in the left ventricular outflow tract are shown. **(A)** The peak negative velocity (<0 cm/s or baseline) exceeds the upper limit of the velocity scale and a simultaneous aliasing signal appears on the opposite side of the baseline at the top of the display. **(B)** Altering the scale peak velocity from −60 to −90 cm/s or **(C)** shifting the baseline up to a maximum velocity of −140 cm/s eliminates the aliasing artifact.

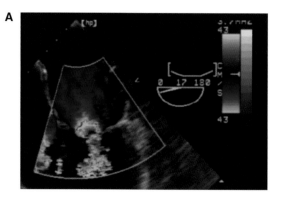

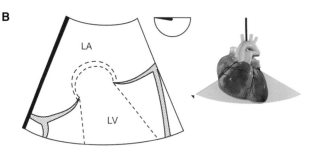

Figure 7.7 Color Doppler aliasing. (A,B) In color Doppler mode, acceleration of the blood flow through a stenotic mitral valve reaches velocities beyond the upper limit of the velocity scale. Aliasing appears as an abrupt change in color from light blue to yellow, which would suggest flow is going in the opposite direction. *Abbreviations*: LA, left atrium; LV, left ventricle.

Near-Field Clutter

Echocardiographic transducers are designed to generate an ultrasound beam providing optimal imaging in the center of the display sector. Near-field clutter arises from the complex and non uniform energy distribution in the portion of the sector adjacent to the transducer. Reverberation between near-field structures has also been involved in producing such interference and wave cancellation during transthoracic echocardiography (TTE) (10). Also contributing to limited visualization in the vicinity of the ultra-

sound probe are high-intensity echoes from reflectors in the proximal zone of the ultrasound beam where the intensity of the signal is maximal (6,11). Adjusting gain controls, use of the focal point, and introduction of multifrequency probes, with the highest frequencies dedicated to the near field, improve visualization close to the transducer and decrease near-field noise (Fig. 7.8).

Range Ambiguity

This phenomenon is an expected limitation of high PRF Doppler and may occur during conventional PW Doppler recording. The PW transducer acts as an echo receiver for a limited time between each transmission of ultrasound burst. The system assumes that the incoming echoes represent the backscattered signal of the most recently transmitted ultrasound pulse. This may not be the case, but rather represent the sum of returning echoes, that include backscattering of pulses sent in previous cycles, which have traveled to and from a target in the far field. These distal signals may display higher energy and represent higher velocities than the signal from the chosen sample volume. This situation is misleading as the displayed PW Doppler signal mostly represents echoes from blood flow further in the acoustic field while

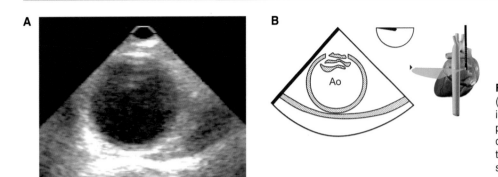

Figure 7.8 Near-field clutter.
(A,B) Linear echoes and poor image definition in the near field prevent optimal visualization of the descending aortic wall close to the transducer in this descending Ao short-axis view. *Abbreviation*: Ao, aorta.

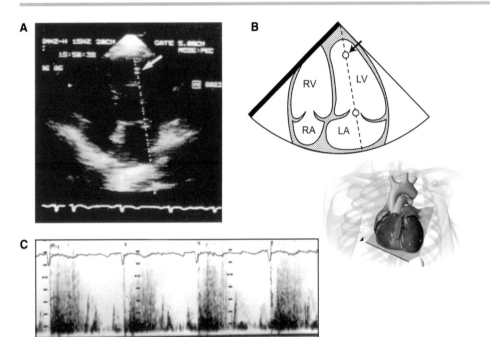

MR signal
0.2 m/sec

Figure 7.9 Range ambiguity. (A, B) The PW sample volume is located at the LV apex (arrow) in this transthoracic four-chamber view. **(C)** However, the PW Doppler signal also displays the MR flow from the far field. *Abbreviations*: LA, left atrium; LV, left ventricle; MR, mitral regurgitation; PW, pulsed wave; RA, right atrium; RV, right ventricle. *Source*: Adapted with permission from Ref. 6.

the sampling gate is in a more proximal location (Fig. 7.9) (6). When range ambiguity is suspected, the dominant source of the recorded signal may seem obvious; however, it may sometimes require a thorough examination for its identification.

Refraction

An ultrasound beam is transmitted in a straight line through a homogeneous medium. However, at the interface between two media of different acoustic impedance, both reflection and refraction of the ultrasound beam can occur (Fig. 7.10). On one hand, a proportion of the ultrasonic energy does not enter the second medium and bounce off the interface (reflection) and on the other hand, part of the ultrasonic energy propagates through the second medium deviated with respect to the axis of the incident beam in the first medium (refraction). The amplitude of this deviation of the refracted signal is a function of the difference between the speed of sound in both media. When part of the ultrasound beam is refracted,

A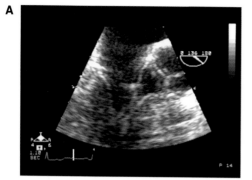

B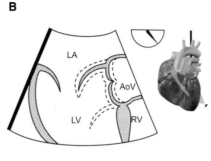

Figure 7.10 Refraction. (A,B) Mid-esophageal AoV long-axis view shows distortion and duplication through refraction of part of the ultra-sound beam. *Abbreviations*: AoV, aortic valve; LA, left atrium; LV, left ventricle; RV, right ventricle.

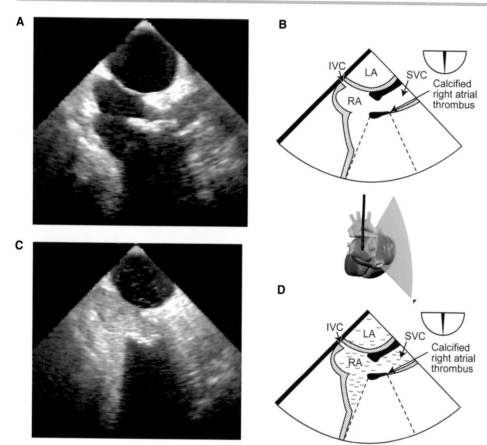

Figure 7.11 Acoustic shadowing. (A,B) In a mid-esophageal bicaval view calcified thrombus is located high in the RA at the junction with the SVC and obscures the far field. (C,D) Acoustic shadowing is clearly delineated after opacification of the RA by intravenous injection of agitated saline. Note the passage of a few microbubbles to the LA via a patent foramen ovale. *Abbreviations*: IVC, inferior vena cava; LA, left atrium; RA, right atrium; SVC, superior vena cava.

duplication, enlargement, or even contraction of imaged structures may occur (12).

This phenomenon is encountered most often during TTE where the ultrasound signal travels through media with various acoustic impedances, for example, costal cartilages, the chest wall, and the rectus abdominus muscle (subcostal window). Although less frequent, refraction may also cause significant image distortion during TEE by laterally displacing structures on the display (Fig. 7.10).

Shadowing

Acoustic shadowing describes a partial or total loss of echoes distal to a structure with high attenuation, typically containing metal or calcium. These structures usually produce strong ultrasound scattering and, most commonly, display high echogenicity. While shadowing often confirms the high density of a target, it prevents proper imaging behind this interposed acoustic obstacle (Figs. 7.5 and 7.11). The blind

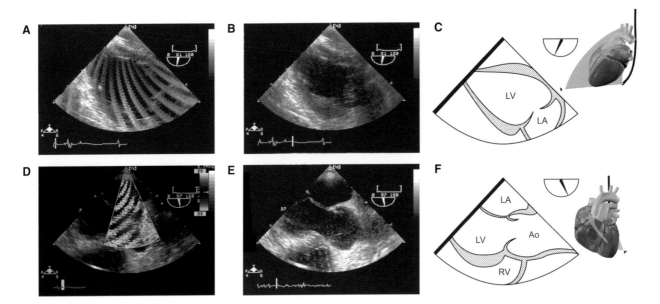

Figure 7.12 Electrocautery artifact. Characteristic, fan shaped electrocautery artifact is seen in a transgastric two-chamber view (**A–C**) and mid-esophageal long-axis view with color Doppler (**D–F**). *Abbreviations*: Ao, aorta; LA, left atrium; LV, left ventricle; RV, right ventricle.

region can usually be visualized from a different angle by positioning the transducer to avoid intervention of the shadowing object in the central axis of the ultrasound beam.

Electrocautery

Electrocautery produces a characteristic, fan-shaped interference pattern artifact precluding proper 2D and color Doppler imaging (Fig. 7.12). It is easily identified as this artifact appears only during electrocautery use. The screen is then covered by a geometric, regular display bearing no relation or resemblance to any anatomic structure. The artifact vanishes instantly when the electrocautery ceases to function. In some cases, the ultrasound probe can pick up electromagnetic interference from other electrical devices in the operating room. Once again, the pattern is usually easily recognizable.

Side Lobes

The geometry of the ultrasound field is determined by characteristics of the transducer and of the emitted signal. In the near field, there is minimal divergence of ultrasound energy from the main central beam. Conversely, at a distance from the transducer, the ultrasonic field progressively widens, as part of the ultrasound energy deviates from the main ultrasonic beam (Fig. 7.13). These regions of ultrasonic energy, lateral to the main beam in the far field, are termed "side lobes." Ultrasound systems are designed to suppress side lobes as they contribute to artifact generation. As a result, side lobes display less energy

than the primary beam and usually do not yield significant echoes. However, a strong reflector located in a side lobe may produce a backscattered signal with enough intensity to be detectable. As all incoming echoes are assumed to be generated in the main beam, a signal produced in a side lobe will be interpreted and imaged as if it were coming from a target located in the primary central ultrasonic beam. Such artifactual side lobe echoes are not detected when they are superimposed on properly imaged structures with high echogenicity (13). However, side lobe artifacts become obvious when they project over a relatively echo-free region of the heart (Fig. 7.13). Typically, they appear as "arc-shaped" images originating from a strong reflector and fading as they move away from that strong reflector. Decreasing the gain and use of second harmonic tissue imaging contributes to the reduction of side lobe artifacts (see Chapter 3).

Comet Tail

Comet tail artifacts are bright "tails" behind a strong reflector, characterized by multiple parallel bands (Fig. 7.14). These bands are produced by short-path reverberations at a point of extreme impedance mismatch. They were described in the noncardiac literature but they are usually seen on TEE, especially arising from prosthetic valves (14).

Ring Down

Ring down artifacts are another type of bright tail associated with gas bubbles. These were described in

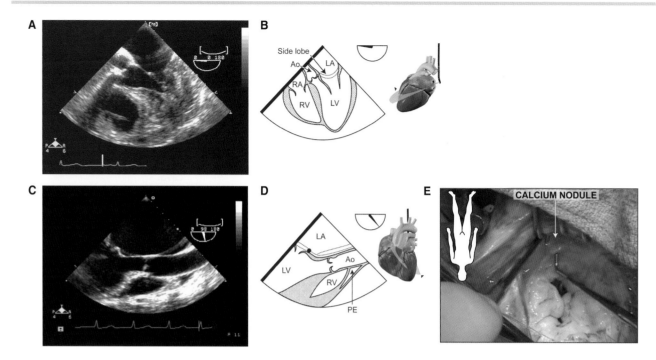

Figure 7.13 Side lobe artifact. (**A,B**) ME five-chamber view of a 77-year-old woman before AoV replacement shows a side lobe artifact beside the AoV that extends to the LA lateral wall. (**C,D**) ME long-axis view of a 53-year-old woman before mitral valve repair shows a side lobe artifact extending along the posterior aspect of the Ao. (**E**) Intraoperative view of calcium nodule responsible for the side lobe artifact. *Abbreviations*: Ao, aorta; AoV, aortic valve; LA, left atrium; LV, left ventricle; ME, mid-esophageal; PE, pericardial effusion; RA, right atrium; RV, right ventricle. *Source*: Photo C courtesy of Dr. Michel Pellerin.

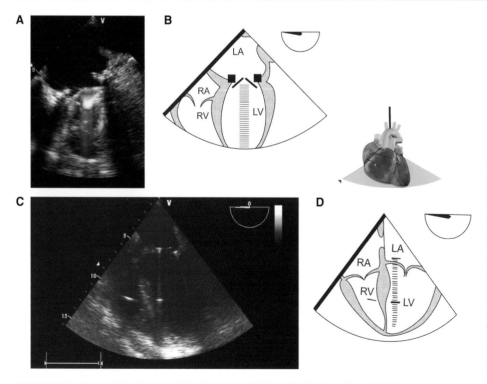

Figure 7.14 Comet tail artifacts. (**A,B**) These artifacts are bright tails behind a strong reflector, characterized by multiple parallel bands. In this case the strong reflector is a mechanical mitral prosthesis. (**C,D**) Mid-esophageal four-chamber view in a 40-year-old man during cardiac arrest shows a comet tail artifact originating from a calcified native MV. A strong reflector appears at an equal distance as from the transducer to the MV. *Abbreviations*: LA, left atrium; LV, left ventricle; MV, mitral valve; RA, right atrium; RV, right ventricle.

A

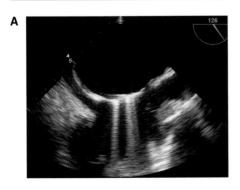

B

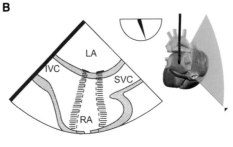

Figure 7.15 Ring down artifact.
(A,B) Mid-esophageal bicaval view shows residual air in the LA. Ring down artifact is specific to gas bubbles and can be seen when there is residual air in the heart following cardiotomy. *Abbreviations*: IVC, inferior vena cava; LA, left atrium; RA, right atrium; SVC, superior vena cava.

abdominal ultrasound but are also seen in the operating room post cardiotomy when there is residual air in the heart (Fig. 7.15) (15).

Beam Width

While not an artifact *per se*, divergence of the ultrasound beam can distort the appearance of cardiac structures in the far field, a phenomenon often referred to as "beam width" effect.

Quadrature-Channel Cross Talk

This phenomenon is easy to recognize and appears as two identical spectral Doppler signals on opposite sides of the baseline (Fig. 7.16). It arises from fundamental limitations in phase separation circuits, the mechanism by which echocardiography systems determine the direction of flow. This artifact occurs most frequently with high or very low velocity flow.

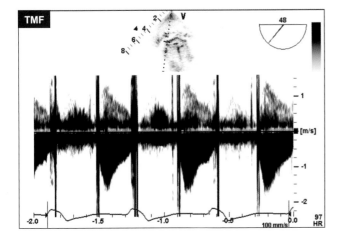

Figure 7.16 Quadrature channel cross-talk. This continuous wave Doppler spectral artifact looks like a mirror image of the initial signal and it is caused by phase separation circuits commonly used in echo machines. *Abbreviation*: TMF, transmitral flow.

Clinically, it is usually not a problem, as the direction of blood flow is known. However, in rare cases where bidirectional flow is questioned, such as atrial or ventricular septal defects, it can lead to confusion. The real signal is distinguished from the artifactual one as it is almost always the strongest (16).

MISINTERPRETATION OF NORMAL STRUCTURES

Trabeculations

Trabeculations are muscle bundles lining the inner surface of the heart. They are coarser in the right-sided chambers, conferring a more irregular texture to the endocardium of the right atrium (RA) and right ventricle (RV). Nevertheless, prominent left ventricular (LV) trabeculations are a common finding, occurring in 68% of normal hearts at autopsy (17). These prominent muscle bundles are multiple in 53% of the cases, although more than four prominent trabeculations are rarely observed in a single left ventricle (LV) (Fig. 7.17). The majority is located, at least in part, in the apical region and may be misinterpreted as apical thrombi. Normal contractility of the adjacent myocardium and similar echo density and texture to the surrounding ventricular wall militate in favor of a prominent trabeculation rather than a thrombus.

False Tendons

False tendons, also termed false chordae tendineae or aberrant ventricular bands, have been defined as "stringlike" structures with free intracavitary courses, unrelated to the atrioventricular valves, and connected to papillary muscles, ventricular walls, or both. False tendons may be multiple and are a common finding with a prevalence of 28% in the RV and 37% in the LV at pathologic examination (18). These linear, echodense fibromuscular structures are not associated with anatomic or physiologic cardiac anomalies, although they have been associated with innocent murmurs. Identification of false tendons is critical as they may simulate a subaortic membrane, the edge of a thrombus or mass, a flail aortic leaflet, or

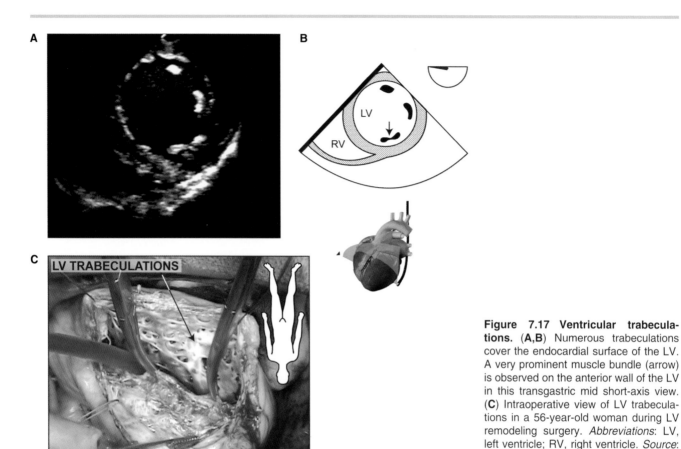

Figure 7.17 Ventricular trabeculations. (**A,B**) Numerous trabeculations cover the endocardial surface of the LV. A very prominent muscle bundle (arrow) is observed on the anterior wall of the LV in this transgastric mid short-axis view. (**C**) Intraoperative view of LV trabeculations in a 56-year-old woman during LV remodeling surgery. *Abbreviations*: LV, left ventricle; RV, right ventricle. *Source*: Photo C courtesy of Dr. Pierre Page.

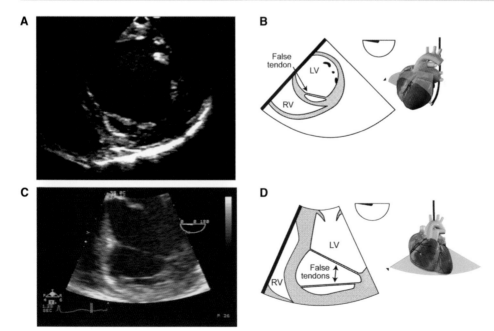

Figure 7.18 False tendon. (**A,B**) Transgastric mid short-axis view of the LV demonstrates a false tendon extending from the ventricular septum to the anterior wall. (**C,D**) Mid-esophageal four-chamber view shows two false tendons at the LV apex. *Abbreviations*: LV, left ventricle; RV, right ventricle.

asymmetric hypertrophic cardiomyopathy when parallel and close to the interventricular septum.

The presence of an echo-free space on both sides of the false tendon, and demonstration of blood flow around the band using color Doppler, may prove helpful in its distinction from pathologic structures. Their free intracavitary course differentiates them from ventricular trabeculations (Figs. 7.18 and 7.19).

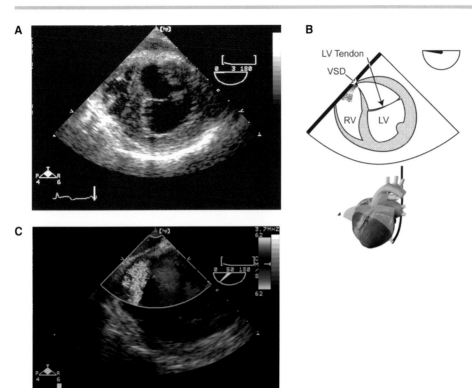

Figure 7.19 False tendon. Transgastric mid short-axis view (**A,B**) in a 67-year-old woman shows a LV tendon close to a VSD with a left-to-right shunt (**C**). *Abbreviations*: LV, left ventricle; RV, right ventricle; VSD, ventricular septal defect.

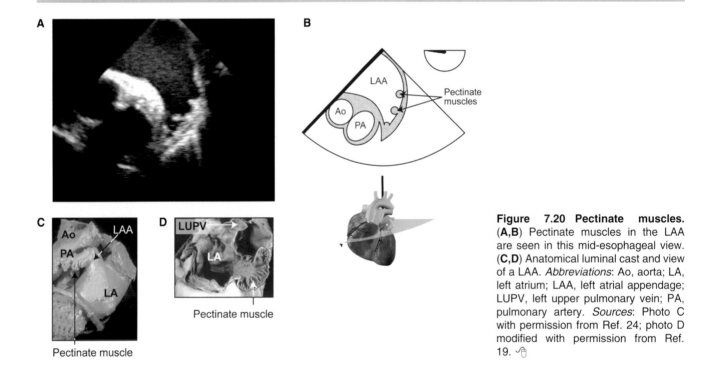

Figure 7.20 Pectinate muscles. (**A,B**) Pectinate muscles in the LAA are seen in this mid-esophageal view. (**C,D**) Anatomical luminal cast and view of a LAA. *Abbreviations*: Ao, aorta; LA, left atrium; LAA, left atrial appendage; LUPV, left upper pulmonary vein; PA, pulmonary artery. *Sources*: Photo C with permission from Ref. 24; photo D modified with permission from Ref. 19.

Pectinate Muscles

Pectinate muscles are parallel muscular ridges typically observed on the inner surface of both atrial appendages (Figs. 7.20 and 7.21). These trabeculations confer a characteristic crenelated appearance to the walls of both atrial appendages: they must be distinguished from thrombus or other pathologic cardiac masses. This is especially important when imaging the left atrial appendage (LAA), a recognized site of

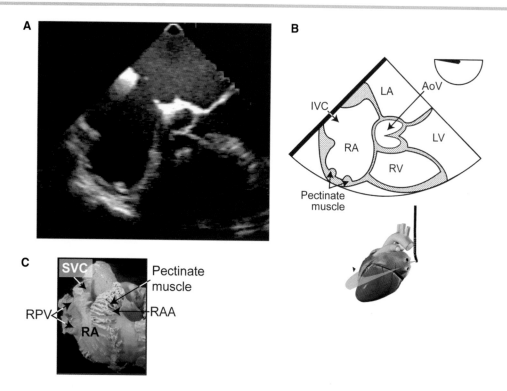

Figure 7.21 **Pectinate muscles.** (**A,B**) Pectinate muscles in the RA are seen in this mid-esophageal five-chamber view of the heart. (**C**) Anatomical luminal cast and view of a RAA. *Abbreviations*: AoV, aortic valve; IVC, inferior vena cava; LA, left atrium; LV, left ventricle; RA, right atrium; RAA, right atrial appendage; RPV, right pulmonary veins; RV, right ventricle; SVC, superior vena cava. *Source*: Photo C with permission from Ref. 24.

thrombus formation with potential for systemic embolization. The vast majority of normal adult subjects have multiple pectinate muscles of 1 mm in width in the LAA (20). Pectinate muscles and the underlying atrial wall share the same texture and echogenicity and display the same motion. Conversely, thrombi exhibit a different acoustic density from the atrial walls and may be pedunculated. Moreover, thrombi are usually found in conjunction with reduced Doppler velocities in the LAA and blood stasis in the LA in the context of arrhythmia, valvular disease, or reduced cardiac output (Fig. 7.22) (2,9,20).

Moderator Band

Usually classified as "anatomical or normal variant," the moderator band is a muscular structure located in the apical third of the RV. In the mid-esophageal four-chamber view, it presents as a prominent band stretching from the inferior interventricular septum to the lateral free wall of the RV (Fig. 7.23). Other muscular bands and large trabeculations are commonly visualized in the apical portion of the RV and must be distinguished from pathologic entities (2).

Lipomatous Hypertrophy of the Atrial Septum

Fatty deposits in the atrial septum may lead to high echogenicity and severe thickening of its muscular

region. Characteristic sparing of the central fossa ovalis membrane results in the typical bilobed, dumb-bell appearance of the atrial septum (Fig. 7.24). Severe adipose infiltration is rarely limited to the atrial septum and may involve the atrial wall, the atrioventricular groove, and the entire subepicardium (21). In some cases, it may even interfere with proper visualization of the RA and tricuspid valve (TV). Criteria for the diagnosis of this entity have been suggested: (*i*) characteristic bilobed appearance of the atrial septum, (*ii*) atrial septum thickness reaching ≥15 mm and (*iii*), absence of any other process more likely to cause septal infiltration (metastatic malignancy, amyloidosis) (6). Lipomatous hypertrophy of the atrial septum must be distinguished from metastases, mural thrombi, primary tumors of the heart, and other infiltrative processes.

Eustachian Valve

The Eustachian valve is an embryologic remnant commonly encountered in adult subjects. This rudimentary incomplete valve is located at the junction between the inferior vena cava (IVC) and the RA. It consists of a crescent-shaped ridge on the anterior aspect of the orifice of the IVC. It may be redundant and appear as a thin mobile membrane undulating in the RA. Unusually large Eustachian valves causing obstruction to blood flow from the

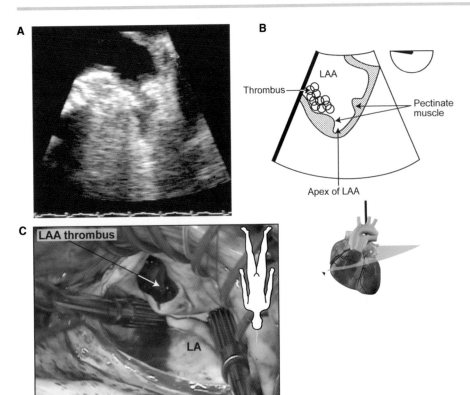

Figure 7.22 LAA thrombus. (A,B) A thrombus fills the LAA at the level of two prominent pectinate muscles in this zoomed view of the LAA. **(C)** Intraoperative view of a LAA thrombus is shown. *Abbreviations*: LA, left atrium; LAA, left atrial appendage. *Source*: Photo C courtesy of Dr. Michel Pellerin.

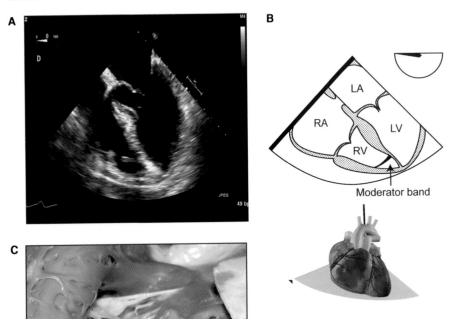

Figure 7.23 Moderator band. (A,B) Dilatation of the RV facilitates visualization of the moderator band and the densely trabeculated RV apex in this mid-esophageal four-chamber view. **(C)** Anatomical aspect of the moderator band. *Abbreviations*: LA, left atrium; LV, left ventricle; RA, right atrium; RV, right ventricle; TV, tricuspid valve. *Source*: Photo C courtesy of Dr. Nicolas Dürrleman.

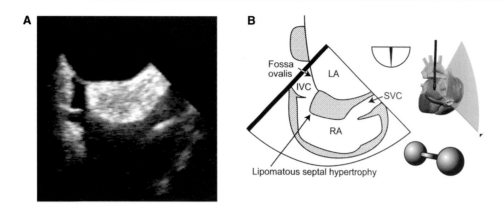

Figure 7.24 Lipomatous hypertrophy. (A,B) Mid-esophageal bicaval view shows lipomatous hypertrophy of the IAS in a 74-year-old woman. The IAS reaches 25 mm in thickness. The sparing of the fossa ovalis results in a typical dumbbell appearance of the IAS. *Abbreviations*: IAS, interatrial septum; IVC, inferior vena cava; LA, left atrium; RA, right atrium; SVC, superior vena cava.

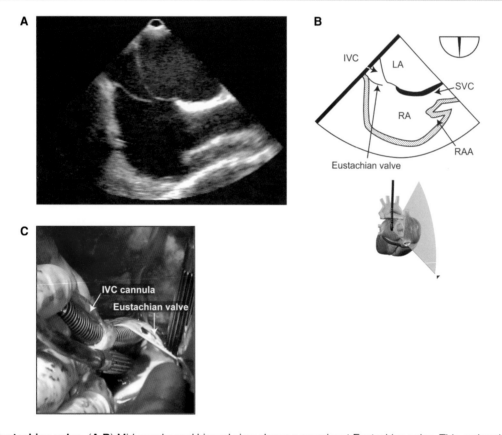

Figure 7.25 Eustachian valve. (A,B) Mid-esophageal bicaval view shows a prominent Eustachian valve. This embryologic remnant is inserted on the anterior aspect of the orifice of the IVC and was used in fetal life to direct flow from the IVC towards the foramen ovale. **(C)** Intraoperative view of the Eustachian valve. *Abbreviations*: IVC, inferior vena cava; LA, left atrium; RA, right atrium; RAA, right atrial appendage; SVC, superior vena cava.

IVC have been described (2). The Eustachian valve is best visualized when imaging both the superior and inferior venae cavae in longitudinal section. This imaging plane allows identification of its attachment, anteriorly at the orifice of the IVC (Fig. 7.25). It must not be confused with thrombi, central catheters, vegetations, tumors, or other pathologic processes.

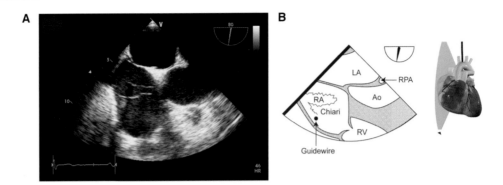

Figure 7.26   Chiari network. (A,B) Mid-esophageal view at 80° shows a Chiari network undulating in the RA. *Abbreviations*: Ao, aorta; HR, heart rate; IVC, inferior vena cava; LA, left atrium; RA, right atrium; RPA, right pulmonary artery; RV, right ventricle. ⌐🖱

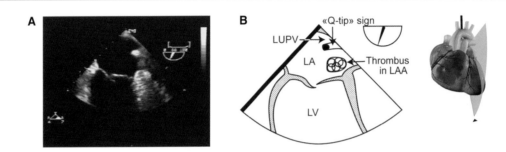

Figure 7.27   Coumadin ridge. (A,B) Mid-esophageal LAA view at 66° shows the "Q-tip" sign or appearance of the junction (or limbus) of the LAA and LUPV. Note also the thrombus in the LAA. *Abbreviations*: LA, left atrium; LAA, left atrial appendage; LUPV, left upper pulmonary vein; LV, left ventricle. ⌐🖱

Chiari Network

The Chiari network is an embryologic remnant found in 2% to 3% of normal hearts (6). This filamentous, fenestrated membrane is attached along the orifice of the coronary sinus (Fig. 7.26). It appears as a highly mobile structure within the RA, typically displaying random motion between two insertion points on the anterior aspect of the orifice of the IVC (like the Eustachian valve) and the superior aspect of the atrial septum. As mentioned for the Eustachian valve, the Chiari network must not be mistaken for a pathologic finding such as fibrinous thrombus or vegetations.

Coumadin Ridge

This is a ridge of tissue located between the LAA and the opening of the left upper pulmonary vein (LUPV), commonly called the Q-tip sign (Fig. 7.27). It can be more, or less, prominent in different patients. Its name comes from the fact that in early days of ultrasound, it was often mistaken for a thrombus, leading to initiation of anticoagulation therapy (22).

Thebesian Valve

The Thebesian valve is another remnant of embryonic tissue, guarding the entry to the coronary sinus. Its only clinical significance is that it may obstruct coronary sinus cannulation during retrograde cardioplegia (Fig. 7.28).

ECHO-FREE SPACES

Persistent Left Superior Vena Cava

Persistent left superior vena cava (SVC) occurs in 0.5% of otherwise normal subjects as an isolated finding. It is more frequent in patients with congenital heart disease, with a prevalence of 3% to 10% (6). It most commonly drains into the coronary sinus, which appears markedly dilated. Persistent left SVC presents as an echo-free space between the LAA and the LUPV. When imaged, in longitudinal section, it appears as a vascular structure anterior to the LA and connecting to the coronary sinus (Fig. 7.29) (9). Color Doppler confirms the presence of blood flow in its lumen, differentiating it from an abscess, a cystic cavity or a

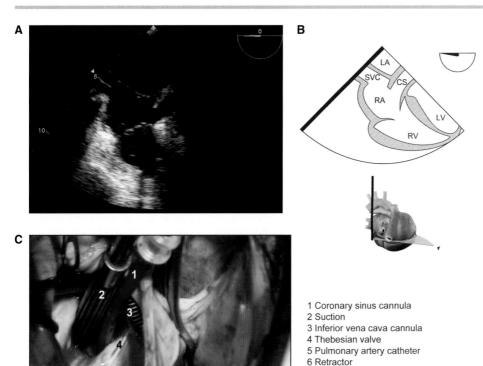

1 Coronary sinus cannula
2 Suction
3 Inferior vena cava cannula
4 Thebesian valve
5 Pulmonary artery catheter
6 Retractor

Figure 7.28 Thebesian valve. (A, B) This lower esophageal view at 0° near the gastro-esophageal junction shows the CS. The Thebesian valve is an embryonic tissue remnant at the entrance to the CS and it may interfere with CS cannulation during retrograde cardioplegia. (**C**) Intraoperative view of the Thebesian valve. *Abbreviations*: CS, coronary sinus; LA, left atrium; LV, left ventricle; RA, right atrium; RV, right ventricle; SVC, superior vena cava.

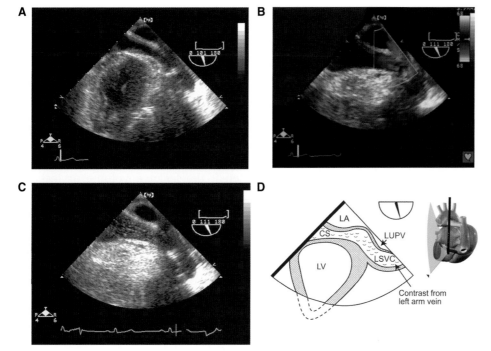

Figure 7.29 Left superior vena cava. (A,B) Lower esophageal and color Doppler views in a 48-year-old man show a persistent LSVC draining into a dilated CS. (**C,D**) Abnormal flow is also demonstrated using agitated saline injected into the left arm from the left subclavian vein with contrast material rapidly appearing in the CS. *Abbreviations*: CS, coronary sinus; LA, left atrium; LSVC, left superior vena cava; LUPV, left upper pulmonary vein; LV, left ventricle.

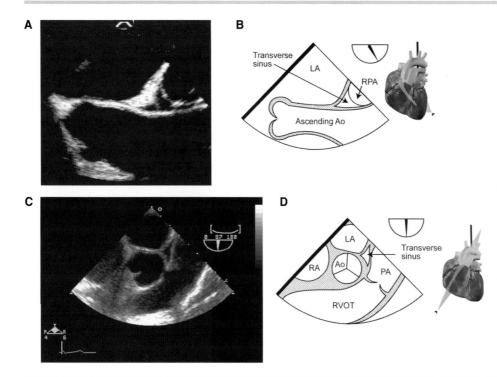

Figure 7.30 Transverse pericardial sinus. (**A,B**) The transverse pericardial sinus in this ME ascending Ao long-axis view at 120° is seen as a small triangular echo-free space between the ascending Ao and RPA. (**C,D**) ME right ventricular inflow/outflow view demonstrates the transverse sinus just beside the Ao. *Abbreviations*: Ao, aorta; ME, mid-esophageal; LA, left atrium; PA, pulmonary artery; RA, right atrium; RPA, right pulmonary artery; RVOT, right ventricular outflow tract.

fluid accumulation in a pericardial sinus. Another way to confirm the diagnosis is by injecting ultrasound contrast (such as agitated saline) in a left upper extremity vein, resulting in opacification of the persistent left SVC followed by the coronary sinus and the RA (Fig. 7.29). Identifying this abnormality in cardiac surgery is important, as cardioplegia administered through the coronary sinus in this situation could be inadequate.

Transverse Sinus of Pericardium

The transverse sinus consists of a pericardial reflection at the base of the heart. This blind segment, roughly triangular in cross section, is located superiorly to the oblique pericardial sinus. Echocardiographically, it appears as a small, echo-free space between the pulmonary artery, the ascending aorta, and the LA (Fig. 7.30). It must be distinguished from a cyst, an abscess, or an aortic dissection. In the presence of a pericardial effusion, the transverse sinus widens and epicardial fat lining the LAA, or the LAA itself, may manifest as irregular, high echogenicity indentations within the transverse sinus (Fig. 7.31). This pseudo-mass must be recognized to avoid misinterpreting it as a pathologic mass (6,9).

COLOR FLOW DOPPLER

Physiologic Regurgitation of Native and Prosthetic Valves

The heightened image quality of TEE confers a high sensitivity for even physiologic and trivial valvular regurgitation of native and prosthetic valves. Moreover, color Doppler imaging often detects an extremely short-lived, low-velocity backward movement of blood near the leaflets at valve closure. This phenomenon must be distinguished from valvular regurgitation. A small amount of regurgitation from morphologically normal native valves, especially from atrioventricular valves, is commonly detected on color Doppler imaging. Such physiologic regurgitation is characterized by a brief, short, and thin color jet. It is clinically inaudible and should be considered a normal variant (6,9).

Mere closure of mechanical prosthetic valves, and of some bioprosthetic valves, forces a small amount of blood backward: the closing volume or closing backflow. In addition, to avoid thrombus formation, bileaflet and tilting disk mechanical prosthesis are designed to generate a small degree of transprosthetic regurgitation after closure of the valve is completed: the leakage volume or leakage backflow (5,6,9). The pattern of this physiologic regurgitation varies according to the prosthesis model and manufacturer. Typically, tilting disk mechanical prosthetic valves display small peripheral regurgitation jets around the periphery of the disk and a more prominent central jet through the central disk orifice on color Doppler recording. However, bileaflet mechanical prosthetic valves produce more prominent peripheral regurgitation jets. These originate at the periphery of the central closure line and some are centrally oriented, yielding a typical regurgitation pattern on color Doppler imaging (Fig. 7.32) (6). The closing and leakage volumes of mechanical prosthetic valves are considered physiologic regurgitation jets without clinical significance.

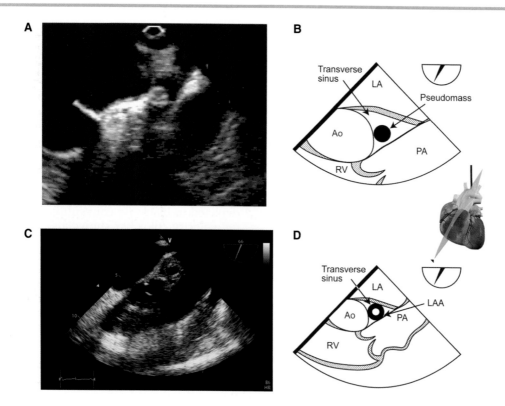

Figure 7.31 Transverse pericardial sinus. (A,B) Mid-esophageal right ventricular inflow/outflow view shows a pseudomass in a dilated transverse sinus. **(C,D)** This is a similar view from a 75-year-old woman with a pericardial effusion in which the pseudomass in the transverse sinus is the tip of the LAA. *Abbreviations*: Ao, aorta; LA, left atrium; LAA, left atrial appendage; PA, pulmonary artery; RV, right ventricle.

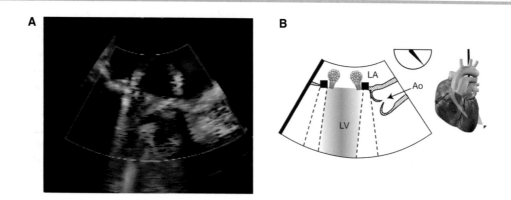

Figure 7.32 Normal prosthetic color Doppler flow. (A,B) This color Doppler mid-esophageal long-axis view demonstrates two small transvalvular regurgitation jets in a normally functioning mechanical bileaflet St. Jude prosthetic valve in the mitral position. Note also the shadowing and reverberation extending from the prosthetic valve to the far field. *Abbreviations*: Ao, aorta; LA, left atrium; LV, left ventricle.

Gain

Color flow Doppler is widely used for blood flow detection and characterization. Moreover, various quantitative and semiquantitative approaches for estimating the severity of valvular regurgitation and shunt lesions involve color Doppler mapping. Numerous factors may interfere with the proper assessment of such cardiac conditions by color Doppler, including the hemodynamic status at the time of the evaluation and instrument settings. Gain setting represents one of the most influential of these factors. Augmenting the color Doppler gain from low to high level has been shown to increase the color jet area by more than 100% (23).

To achieve sensitive, specific, and reproducible color Doppler evaluations, the gain setting must be optimized. Although no definitive standard criteria exist to ensure uniform color Doppler gain settings, a general principle is suggested. Starting from a low level, the color Doppler gain is progressively increased until background color noise artifacts appear. The gain is then slightly decreased to the highest level devoid of such color artifacts (see Fig. 2.16) (24). Perfect standardization, however, remains elusive because of individual differences in acoustic characteristics of the chest and the lack of uniform ultrasound system specifications from one manufacturer to another (24).

Frequency

Color jet area is determined by various technical factors in addition to color Doppler gain. These parameters may be overlooked because of a common tendency to focus exclusively on gain setting during an echocardiographic study. PRF and, to a lesser extent, transducer frequency are among these variables that need to be optimized. The size of the color jet area varies inversely with PRF and directly with transducer frequency.

At lower transducer frequency, lateral resolution is decreased. This reduced capability of precisely distinguishing velocities in two separate points explains the larger pixels on the color Doppler display. It also contributes, especially in conjunction with low color Doppler gain, to underestimate the turbulent flow component at the periphery of color jet areas. Therefore, the size of color flow areas appears smaller on the display with a lower frequency transducer (6,23). However, with more recent technology this factor is minimized as transesophageal probes transmit and receive ultrasounds over a broad range of frequencies simultaneously.

As previously explained in the section on aliasing, PRF represents a parameter inherent to color and PW Doppler. It describes the capability of these modalities of alternately transmitting ultrasound bursts and functioning as echo receiver. The most decisive factor limiting PRF is the depth of the region of interest. When interrogating structures in the far field, the interval before the backscattered signal reaches the transducer is obviously longer than for closer targets. The system must then act as an ultrasound receiver for a longer period before it sends another ultrasound burst. The depth of field limits the number of transmitted pulses per time unit and, therefore, the maximal PRF is lower.

The PRF has been demonstrated to be inversely related to color flow area for both laminar and turbulent flows. In an animal model, increasing the PRF from 4 to 8 kHz caused a 36% decrease in color jet size (23). However, predicting absolute and relative changes in color flow area with PRF adjustments is much more complex, as other system factors (gain, velocity scale, sector angle, instrument manufacturer, color algorithm, filter settings, etc.) may modulate the response to PRF changes. Moreover, the highest velocity that can be displayed without color aliasing varies inversely with transducer frequency and directly with PRF. A PRF corresponding to an aliasing velocity of 40 to 70 cm/s on the color Doppler scale is recommended (24).

Velocity Scale and Baseline Shift

The common default setting of the color Doppler places the baseline in the center of the velocity scale display. This baseline represents zero velocity and is depicted in black. By convention, the superior-half of the velocity color bar shows a scale in shades of red used by the system for mapping blood flowing toward the transducer. The velocity scale is surmounted by a positive number corresponding to the maximal velocity the system can display without signal aliasing. The lower half of the color bar is a scale in shades of blue utilized to depict blood moving away from the transducer. The number at the lower end of the velocity scale is equal to the number topping the scale, yet it is preceded by a negative sign implying opposite direction. This number corresponds to the maximal velocity of blood moving away from the probe that can be detected without signal aliasing. As stated in the previous section, the recommended aliasing velocity for color Doppler is between 40 and 70 cm/s (24).

Lowering the velocity scale (and therefore both positive and negative aliasing velocities) below this range may result in color flow mapping that proves difficult to interpret because of excessive signal aliasing and mosaic flow. Moreover, by lowering the maximal velocity of the scale, every tint of red and blue represents a lower velocity interval. Consequently, lower velocity blood flows are allocated brighter colors and become more obvious on the display. Conversely, increasing the aliasing velocity above the recommended range may result in color jet areas appearing smaller: as the color scale is stretched over a wider velocity range, the darker shades of red or blue are assigned higher velocities that consequently become more difficult to see on the display.

Shifting the baseline will result in an asymmetrical velocity scale display changing the maximal velocities at each end of the scale. Aliasing will occur at different velocities according to blood flow direction. For example, shifting the baseline upward results in a lower positive velocity at the top of the color Doppler scale and a more negative velocity at the bottom of the scale display. Accordingly, color Doppler aliasing occurs at a lower velocity for blood flow directed toward the transducer and, to the contrary, at a higher velocity in the case of blood flow moving away from the transducer. Therefore, shifting the baseline may prove helpful to eliminate signal aliasing in color flow and PW spectral Dopplers. It is also helpful in the quantification of color flow jet (most often regurgitant jets) where the baseline of the color scale will be moved in the direction of the flow to enable flow rate measurement by the proximal isovelocity surface area (PISA) method (see Chapter 5).

Sector Depth

Color jet size widens with increasing depth. Various factors contribute to this phenomenon. As previously discussed, the main determinant of the PRF is depth of field. Increasing the distance between the transducer and the region of interest reduces the PRF and, consequently, generates a larger color flow area. Another postulated mechanism is the widening of the ultrasound beam in the far field involving color Doppler mapping. These factors contribute to produce a color jet that may artifactually be larger than the actual, anatomical far field structure confining the flow.

SUMMARY

Sophisticated and accurate TEE appears to grant the operator a direct vision of a beating heart. One must remember, however, that this is not the case. The images are merely a complex graphic reconstruction of the heart through mathematical formulas and assumptions. Artifacts must be distinguished from properly displayed structures, and normal variants must not be confused with pathology. To avoid misinterpretations, appropriate instrument settings are of paramount importance. Comprehension of the mechanisms involved in artifact formation and familiarity with the technique are prerequisites before performing and interpreting transesophageal echoes. Finally, the operator must stay alert and take the time to explore unusual findings using all the necessary imaging planes and modalities. Only then will TEE achieve its full potential.

REFERENCES

1. Kremkau FW, Taylor KJ. Artifacts in ultrasound imaging. J Ultrasound Med 1986; 5:227–237.
2. Feigenbaum H. Echocardiography. 5th ed. Baltimore: Williams & Williams, 1994.
3. Appelbe AF, Walker PG, Yeoh JK, et al. Clinical significance and origin of artifacts in transesophageal echocardiography of the thoracic aorta. J Am Coll Cardiol 1993; 21:754–760.
4. Vignon P, Spencer KT, Rambaud G, et al. Differential transesophageal echocardiographic diagnosis between linear artifacts and intraluminal flap of aortic dissection or disruption. Chest 2001; 119:1778–1790.
5. Bach DS. Transesophageal echocardiographic (TEE) evaluation of prosthetic valves. Cardiol Clin 2000; 18:751–771.
6. Weyman AE. Principles and Practice of Echocardiography. 2nd ed. Philadelphia: Lea & Febiger, 1994.
7. Rao SR, Richardson SG, Simonetti J, et al. Problems and pitfalls in the performance and interpretation of color Doppler flow imaging: observations based on the influences of technical and physiological factors on the color Doppler examination of mitral regurgitation. Echocardiography 1990; 7:747–762.
8. Buttery B, Davison G. The ghost artifact. J Ultrasound Med 1984; 3:49–52.
9. Freeman WK, Seward JB, Khandheria BK, et al. Transesophageal Echocardiography. Boston: Little Brown, 1994.
10. Schmailzl KJG, Ormerod O. Ultrasound in Cardiology. Oxford: Blackwell Science, 1994.
11. Hozumi T, Yoshida K, Abe Y, et al. Visualization of clear echocardiographic images with near field noise reduction technique: experimental study and clinical experience. J Am Soc Echocardiogr 1998; 11:660–667.
12. Sauerbrei EE. Duplication of the aortic ring. An artifact in echocardiography. J Ultrasound Med 1989; 8:477–480.
13. Kremkau FW. Diagnostic Ultrasound: Principles and Instruments. 4th ed. Philadelphia: W.B. Saunders, 1993.
14. Thickman DI, Ziskin MC, Goldenberg NJ, et al. Clinical manifestations of the comet tail artifact. J Ultrasound Med 1983; 2:225–230.
15. Avruch L, Cooperberg PL. The ring-down artifact. J Ultrasound Med 1985; 4:21–28.
16. Nanda NC. Atlas of color Doppler echocardiography. Philadelphia: Lea & Febiger, 1989.
17. Boyd MT, Seward JB, Tajik AJ, et al. Frequency and location of prominent left ventricular trabeculations at autopsy in 474 normal human hearts: implications for evaluation of mural thrombi by two-dimensional echocardiography. J Am Coll Cardiol 1987; 9:323–326.
18. Keren A, Billingham ME, Popp RL. Echocardiographic recognition and implications of ventricular hypertrophic trabeculations and aberrant bands. Circulation 1984; 70:836–842.
19. Anderson RH, Levy J. Electrical Anatomy of the Atrial Chambers. Medtronic, 2000.
20. Veinot JP, Harrity PJ, Gentile F, et al. Anatomy of the normal left atrial appendage: a quantitative study of age-related changes in 500 autopsy hearts: implications for echocardiographic examination. Circulation 1997; 96: 3112–3115.
21. Shirani J, Roberts WC. Clinical, electrocardiographic and morphologic features of massive fatty deposits ("lipomatous hypertrophy") in the atrial septum. J Am Coll Cardiol 1993; 22:226–238.
22. Goldman JH, Foster E. Transesophageal echocardiographic (TEE) evaluation of intracardiac and pericardial masses. Cardiol Clin 2000; 18:849–860.
23. Stewart WJ, Cohen GI, Salcedo EE. Doppler color flow image size: dependence on instrument settings. Echocardiography 1991; 8:319–327.
24. Hoit BD, Jones M, Eidbo EE, et al. Sources of variability for Doppler color flow mapping of regurgitant jets in an animal model of mitral regurgitation. J Am Coll Cardiol 1989; 13:1631–1636.

8

Equipment, Complications, Infection Control, and Safety

Geneviève Côté and André Y. Denault

Université de Montréal, Montreal, Quebec, Canada

INTRODUCTION

Transesophageal echocardiography (TEE) is now widely used as a diagnostic and monitoring tool. The proximity of the probe location in the esophagus, immediately posterior to the heart, facilitates higher-quality image acquisition in comparison with the transthoracic technique where bones and lungs interfere. This chapter will discuss the biological effects of diagnostic ultrasound. The method, anatomy, preparation, and safety of the TEE examination will also be reviewed together with various complications.

BIOLOGICAL EFFECTS

Ultrasound is a valuable diagnostic modality. To date, there is no contraindication when medical benefit is expected. No confirmed biological effects, resulting from exposure to the present diagnostic ultrasound instruments in humans, including its use in diagnostic cardiac imagery, have been reported. Ultrasound operators have to understand potential bioeffects, assess the benefits versus the risks of a procedure for a patient, possess and maintain high levels of technical skill, and apply the "as low as reasonable achievable" (ALARA) principle. The bioeffects of ultrasound include thermal cavitation and other minor and experimentally observed bioeffects such as microstreaming and torque force. These are observed at a higher exposition level than the ultrasound level used for diagnostic echocardiography. Our discussion will focus on thermal and cavitation effects.

Thermal Bioeffect

The thermal effect is the most important bioeffect attributed to diagnostic ultrasound. This phenomenon is related to ultrasonic energy absorption and its conversion to heat. Increase in temperature, during tissue exposure to diagnostic ultrasound fields, depends on characteristics of the acoustic source, tissue properties, and exposure time (Table 8.1). Temperature elevation is offset by heat loss due to the blood flow through tissue and heat diffusion. Until now, epidemiological studies have shown no health-related problems associated with diagnostic ultrasound in humans.

The critical duration represents the duration of exposure for a given thermal elevation. The allowed time-temperature combination can be calculated for a given temperature T, between 39°C and 43°C (Table 8.2). According to the following equation, the duration varies from 1 to $\sim$250 minutes:

$$t_c = 4^{(43-T)} \tag{8.1}$$

where t_c is the duration of exposure (minutes) and T is the thermal elevation.

No thermal effects are expected at temperatures less than 38°C, regardless of exposure length. In animal studies where exposure was sustained for more than 50 hours, no significant biological effects were observed due to temperature elevation of less or equal to 2°C above normal. For example, the critical time for $T = 41°C$, an elevation of 4°C above normal, is 16 minutes. Exposure time becomes rapidly shorter with a further increase to 43°C, which brings the critical time to one minute. The probe and the patient's temperature are indicated on the display screen of the TEE ultrasound equipment (Fig. 8.1).

Calculation of the maximum temperature increase, resulting from ultrasound exposure in vivo, should not be assumed to be exact because of the uncertainties and approximations associated with thermal, acoustic, and structural characteristics of the tissue involved. Different tissues are generally heated by ultrasound in a similar manner, except for bone, which is so highly absorptive that it essentially stops the beam. Heating rate can be up to 50 times faster in bone than in typical soft tissue. Calculations can be used as a safety guide for clinical exposure where temperature measurements are not feasible. The rate of increase in temperature can be found by using the following equation:

$$\frac{dT}{dt} = \frac{2\alpha I}{C_v} \tag{8.2}$$

where dT/dt is the rate of increase in temperature, α is the absorption coefficient of the tissue for a given frequency, I is the intensity of ultrasound exposure, and C_v is the specific heat capacity of the tissue.

Of all ultrasound operating modes, Doppler presents the highest risk for inducing biological effects that are thermally mediated. With Doppler utilization, significant temperature increases occur at bone–soft tissue interfaces. Effects of elevated temperature may

Table 8.1 Acoustic Source and Tissue Properties Implicated in Temperature Increase

Acoustic source properties	Tissue properties
Frequency	Attenuation
Source dimensions	Absorption
Scan rate	Speed of sound
Power	Acoustic impedance
Pulse repetition frequency	Perfusion
Pulse duration	Thermal conductivity
Transducer self-heating	Anatomical structure
Wave shape	Nonlinearity parameters
	Cellular proliferation
	Potential for regeneration

Table 8.2 Maximum Exposure Time Allowed for Various Temperature Elevations Before Tissue Injury According to Equation (8.1)

Temperature (°C)	Exposure time (min)
39	256
40	64
41	16
42	4
43	1

be minimized by keeping dwell time as short as possible. The intensity released by an ultrasound transducer varies between 0.001 and 200 mW/cm², and it depends on the transmission level, compression, captor surface, and emission time. With pulsed wave (PW) Doppler, this energy can get as high as 1900 mW/cm². No biologic effect is observed with power between 100 and 200 mW/cm². As for current diagnostic systems, output ranges from 10 mW/cm² spatial peak/temporal average (SPTA) intensity for two-dimensional (2D) imaging to as high as 430 mW/cm² for PW Doppler. It is advisable to use the lowest level of energy for a short duration and to turn off the Doppler mode between examinations.

Risks of injury from heating depend on the temperature elevation and the dwell time. Thermal gradient has been proposed, theoretically, to increase the risk of potential injury. Therefore, it is advisable to shut down the ultrasound transducer when not in use during the bypass period in heart surgery. Concerns were raised about prolonged exposure in the hypothermic, hypoperfused, and hypoxemic patient. In general, adult tissues are more tolerant to temperature increase than fetal and neonatal tissues. Therefore, higher temperature and/or longer exposure would be required for thermal damage. Until now, reported lesions of the esophageal mucosa have been associated with local mechanical trauma attributed to difficult and extreme manipulation of the TEE probe, poor tolerance, and anatomical peculiarities of the patient, such as diverticula, esophageal stenosis, or vertebral osteophytes.

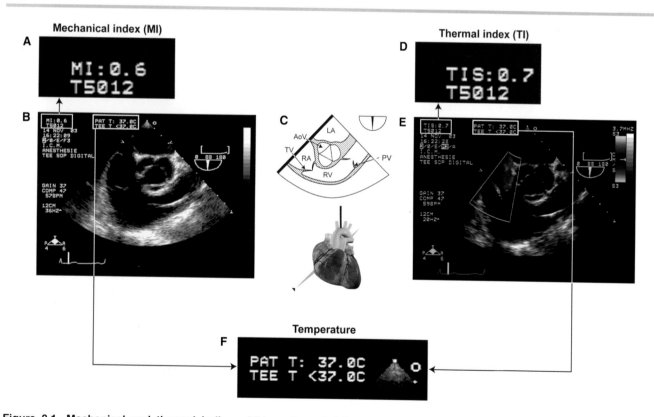

Figure 8.1 Mechanical and thermal indices. Mid-esophageal right ventricular inflow/outflow tract views in a 64-year-old man scheduled for revascularization. The (**A–C**) mechanical index (MI), (**D,E**) soft tissue thermal index (TIS) and (**F**) temperature (T) are indicated at the top of the display screen. *Abbreviations*: AoV, aortic valve; LA, left atrium; PV, pulmonic valve; RA, right atrium; RV, right ventricle; TEE, transesophageal echocardiography; TV, tricuspid valve.

Thermal Safety

The TEE probe contains a safety device that will shut down automatically in the event of overheating. It is recommended that the temperature of the transducer be checked before insertion in febrile critically ill patients or when TEE monitoring is expected to last for prolonged periods, and to modify the superior temperature limit otherwise the probe could turn itself off during the examination.

Cavitation

Gas-body activation and cavitation nuclei are sub-types of the general phenomenon of ultrasound cavitation. Cavitation corresponds to the oscillation, or vibration, of gas-filled bodies when exposed to ultrasound beam, making them potentially biologically active. Depending on their relationship with the ultrasound field, microbubbles resonate. This phenomenon induces expansion and reduction in microbubble size. Under certain conditions, bubbles contained in ultrasound contrast agents might be activated. The cavitation level appears to be relatively high in mammals. The resonance frequency is defined by the radius of the microbubble in the following equation:

$$F_0 = \frac{3260}{R_0} \qquad (8.3)$$

where F_0 is the resonance frequency (in Hz) and R_0 is the radius of the microbubble (in μm).

Until now, with the actual diagnostic system, cavitation has not been shown to occur in the human adult. Acoustic cavitation can alter mammalian tissues. Lung lesions are produced when animals are exposed to diagnostic pulsed ultrasound (1 MPa at 2 MHz). There have been no reports of lung hemorrhage with TEE use in humans. Direct mechanical action of cavitation yields pinpoint regions of destruction such as petechial hemorrhage. Concerns about the cavitation phenomenon arise especially with the fetus. The World Federation of Ultrasound Medicine and Biology 1998 recommendations state that the operator should minimize ultrasound exposure of human postnatal lungs.

Intensity Measurement and Quantification

The intensity (I) of ultrasound exposure can be expressed in several ways, with its unit in W/cm^2. The SPTA corresponds to the highest exposure within the beam averaged over the period of exposure. Another common measure is spatial peak pulse average (SPPA), defined as the average pulse intensity at the spatial location where the pulse intensity is maximum.

The thermal index (TI) and mechanical index (MI) define exposure level with diagnostic ultrasound (see Chapter 1) (1). The TI assesses the potential for ultrasonic heating and is related to the average intensity, and its value is indicated during Doppler examination (Fig. 8.1). The MI corresponds to cavitation effect that is related to peak pressure. This value is indicated during 2D examination (Fig. 8.1). These indices have incorporated factors such as tissue exposure to transmission period and the time the ultrasound beam dwells at a specific point (both being considerably shorter than the total examination time).

ELECTRICAL SAFETY

The risk of electrical harm with current ultrasound systems is very low. Erosion or perforation of its protective sheath can cause the loss of the system grounding. Loss of system electrical integrity increases the risk of thermal injury. Nowadays, operating room (OR) electrical systems are built in such a way that it takes two faults to induce an electrical shock. Also, when defibrillation is necessary, the echocardiography system does not have to be unplugged (<50 J). There have been reports of esophageal burns, perforation (1), and atrioesophageal fistula with intraoperative radiofrequency ablation (2,3). It is, therefore, recommended that TEE be avoided in patients undergoing radio frequency ablation. At the Montreal Heart Institute, we pull back the TEE probe above the left atrium (LA) during the procedure (Fig. 8.2). In addition, isolating devices in the oblique

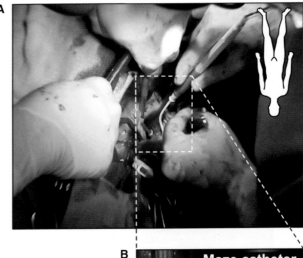

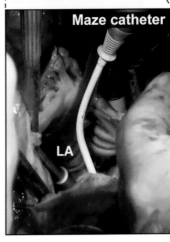

Figure 8.2 Maze procedure. (A,B) During closure of an atrial septal defect in a 48-year-old man, a Maze procedure is also performed for chronic atrial fibrillation. At that time the transesophageal echocardiography probe is pulled back above the LA to avoid esophageal damage. *Abbreviation*: LA, left atrium.

sinus behind the left atrial wall could be used to prevent passage of electrical and thermal energy through the left atrial wall toward the esophagus (2).

PERSONNEL AND EQUIPMENT

Various professional associations have published requirements for training, performance, and maintenance of TEE examination skills (4,5). The TEE examination is performed in various settings, in clinics with outpatients, in ORs, and in intensive care units (ICUs). Quality personnel, training, and monitoring

Table 8.3 Equipment and Set-up Required for TEE Examination

Crash cart
Instrument and accessories for intubation
Suction
Oxygen
Pulse oximetry
Capnography
Blood pressure monitor
EKG monitor
Bite block
Gloves, mask, protective glasses, gown
Medication
    Resuscitation drug
    Local anesthetic: lidocaine spray
    Sedation and analgesia: midazolam, propofol, fentanyl
    Sedation, analgesia and anesthesia antagonists: naloxone, narcan, intralipid
    Prophylaxis for aspiration
Cardiopulmonary resuscitation equipment and trained personnel

Abbreviations: TEE, transesophageal echocardiography; EKG, electrocardiogram.

can greatly reduce complications. Vigilance should be prime. Standard equipment should include all the proper material required for monitoring and patient resuscitation (Table 8.3).

PATIENT EVALUATION BEFORE THE PROCEDURE

Indications

The indications for TEE have increased over the years. Valuable information can be rapidly obtained in certain situations such as in the case of aortic dissection, native and prosthetic valvular dysfunctions, endocarditis, and source of emboli (4,6). It can also be used as a monitoring device in perioperative and emergency care. TEE is indicated whenever transthoracic echocardiography (TTE) is inconclusive and when further information could significantly alter the therapeutic management. The general approach to TEE is summarized in Figure 8.3, and the indications for use are reviewed in Chapter 31 and Table 8.4.

Evaluation

Before proceeding to the TEE examination, it is important that the patient be informed of the aims, technique, and risks of the procedure. The patient's informed consent should be documented in his/her medical record. The pre-procedure evaluation should include a review of the indications, present and past medical history, allergies, current medication, and pertinent physical examination findings. Potential contraindications to the examination should be

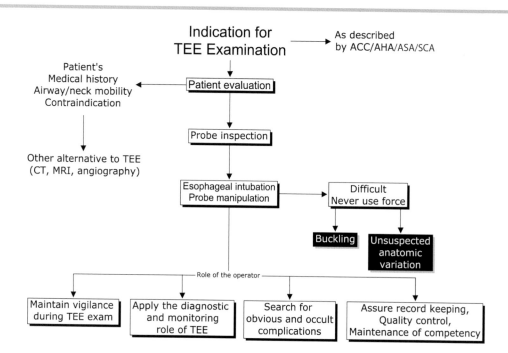

Figure 8.3 Use of TEE. A general approach to the use of TEE is presented. *Abbreviations*: ACC, American College of Cardiology; AHA, American Heart Association; ASA, American Society of Anesthesiologists; SCA, Society of Cardiovascular Anesthesiologists; TEE, transesophageal echocardiography.

Table 8.4 Patient Evaluation and Preparation for TEE Examination

Informed consent from patient
Careful medical history
- Absolute and relative contraindications (see Table 8.5)
- Medication use
- Drug allergy

Examination
- Teeth, oral/dental hygiene, throat neck deviation, and mobility
- Airway evaluation as for endotracheal intubation

Fasting status
- Absence of recent food ingestion within 6 hr and no fluid ingestion within 4 hr

Availability of adequate patient's safety monitoring
- Blood pressure, EKG, and saturometry monitoring devices
- Emergency resuscitation and suctioning equipment

Trained personnel

Abbreviations: EKG, electrocardiogram; TEE, transesophageal echocardiography.

anticipated (Table 8.5). Significant dysphagia is regarded as the indirect evidence of narrowing of the upper gastrointestinal (GI) tract and constitutes a relative contraindication to immediate insertion of the TEE probe. The diagnosis should be clarified by a barium swallow or a gastroenterology consultation. Adequate airway, mouth opening (sometimes reduced in diabetic patients with stiff joint syndrome), neck mobility, and stability are confirmed, particularly when cervical lesions are suspected such as with trauma or severe rheumatoid arthritis. Older patients are prone to occult esophageal lesion, arthritis, and

Table 8.5 Contraindications to TEE

Absolute contraindications
- Lack of informed consent
- Unwilling and uncooperative patient
- Lack of expertise in intubation of TEE
- Esophageal obstruction (cancer, stricture)
- Gastric volvulus
- Active upper gastrointestinal bleeding
- Perforated viscus (known or suspected)
- Full stomach
- Suspected neck injury
- Respiratory distress in the nonintubated patient (7)

Relative contraindications
Known esophageal pathology
- Esophageal varices without bleeding
- Esophageal diverticulum
- Esophageal fistula
- Esophagitis/inflammatory process
- Gastric herniation
- Scleroderma
- Carcinoma
- Penetrating or blunt thoracic esophageal trauma
- History of previous esophageal surgery
- Esophagectomy
- Fundoplication gastric surgery

Cervical abnormalities
- Severe cervical osteoarthritis/osteophytes/spondylosis
- Neck surgery
- Radiation therapy to the cervical area
- Severe oropharyngeal distortion

Previous radiation therapy to the mediastinum
Bleeding diathesis

Abbreviation: TEE, transesophageal echocardiography.

diabetic gastroparesis. Adult congenital heart patients may present with specific problems for sedation and airway management (8): for example, patients with Down's syndrome may have atlantoaxial instability, large tongue, subglottic stenosis, and pulmonary hypertension. Finally, full anticoagulation at therapeutic level warrants caution during TEE. In the OR, it is preferable to insert the TEE probe in patients requiring cardiopulmonary bypass before systemic anticoagulation (9).

Contraindications

Absolute contraindications include esophageal obstruction or interruption, gastric volvulus, active upper GI bleeding, and perforated viscus (Table 8.5). A nonfasting patient with a full stomach presents a major risk even in the case of an acute emergency such as aortic dissection. Prophylactic endotracheal intubation for airway protection against aspiration should be considered. In the presence of a history of significant trauma, cervical injury must be excluded before TEE examination. If cervical instability is present and TEE must be performed because information cannot be obtained otherwise, esophageal intubation under direct visualization with continuous cervical stabilization during the entire examination must be performed.

Relative contraindications are numerous (Table 8.5). They include various esophageal pathologies, previous gastroesophageal surgeries, bleeding diathesis, cervical abnormalities or anatomical distortion from arthritis, or radiation therapy. Relative contraindications may not preclude TEE examination but warrant careful evaluation of the risk-benefit ratio of the procedure and the possibility of using alternative diagnostic tests to obtain the relevant information. For instance, despite the fact that patients with liver failure present several relative contraindications such as esophageal varices, esophagitis, and acquired coagulopathy, TEE has, nevertheless, been cautiously used during liver transplantation (see Chapter 28).

PROPHYLAXIS PLANIFICATION

In preparation for TEE examination, the patient is fasting for at least six hours. In patients with gastroesophageal reflux and gastroparesis (common in the obese and diabetics), prophylaxis for aspiration should be considered, with H_2 blocker, substances neutralizing gastric pH (sodium citrate), and drugs that enhance gastric motility and emptying (metoclopramide). Endotracheal intubation should be further considered to protect the airways against potential aspiration in patients with severe symptoms or who still have a full stomach despite adequate preparation.

As with other diagnostic techniques, TEE is not exempt from possible bacteremia. Prophylaxis for endocarditis has been previously reviewed by the American Heart Association (AHA) (10) and updated in 2008 (11). While prophylaxis had been suggested in 2006 for patients with prosthetic valves, prior endocarditis, complex cyanotic congenital heart disease, surgically constructed systemic pulmonary shunts or conduits, congenital cardiac valve malformations and acquired valvular dysfunction, prior valve repair, hypertrophic cardiomyopathy with latent or resting obstruction, mitral valve prolapse with regurgitation, or thickened leaflets on echocardiography, the newest 2008 ACC/AHA Valvular Heart Disease Focused Update Recommendations no longer recommend antibioprophylaxis for nondental procedures such as TEE, esophagogastroduodenoscopy and colonoscopy in the absence of active infection (11).

Indeed, the risk of antibiotic-related adverse effects exceeds the benefit (if any) from prophylactic antibiotherapy. As this constituted quite a change from prior clinical practice and may not be easily adhered to without causing some discomfort amongst both patients and physicians, the writing committee specifically mentioned that the clinician should determine that the risks associated with antibiotherapy should be low before continuing a prophylaxis regimen. Clinical judgment should still be exerted in regards to the risk-benefit ratio of antibioprophylaxis.

For instance, antibiotics could be considered when TEE is performed in a patient with very poor oral hygiene and valvular disease.

MONITORING AND PATIENT POSITION DURING TEE EXAMINATION

When performing a TEE examination, basic monitoring of the patient is essential. In the OR at our institution, a satellite TEE display is positioned close to the hemodynamic monitor so that both are in the same visual field (Fig. 8.4). At a minimum, pulse oximetry, blood pressure, and electrocardiogram (EKG) must be monitored. Baseline vital signs are recorded before the beginning of the procedure. A reliable IV access must be secured for administration of sedation, anesthesia, or resuscitation drugs. Suctioning devices, supplementary oxygen, and resuscitation equipment should be readily available, as well as trained personnel to assist the procedure and help to monitor the patient.

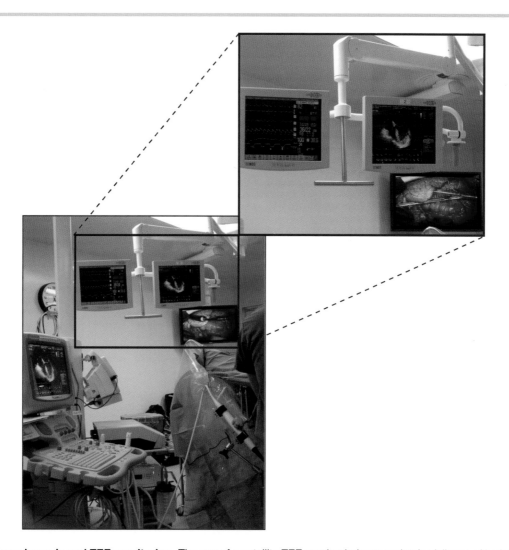

Figure 8.4   Hemodynamic and TEE monitoring. The use of a satellite TEE monitor helps to maintain vigilance of both hemodynamic and echocardiographic monitoring during an intraoperative TEE examination. *Abbreviation*: TEE, transesophageal echocardiography.

The performance of TEE under conscious sedation requires adequate knowledge of the pharmacodynamic and pharmacokinetic properties of sedative and narcotic agents. Guidelines on their utilization should be reviewed, particularly if given by nonanesthesiologists unfamiliar with them. Their dosage, utilization, and combination are beyond the scope of this chapter, but there have been several reviews on this subject (12–14). It has to be kept in mind that dosage has to be adjusted in the elderly or debilitated patient with reduced renal or liver function, and anticipate adverse reactions. Dosage is a delicate balance, and both reduced and excessive sedation can be associated with undesirable side effects (Fig. 8.5). Reversal agents for benzodiazepine and narcotic overdose, such as flumazenil and naloxone, respectively, should be readily available.

Oropharyngeal anesthesia with local anesthetic alone may not always succeed in adequately suppressing the gag reflex, particularly in patients aged 50 or less, and benefit from adding intravenous narcotic analgesia to improve patient tolerance to the procedure. If blood pressure remains stable, additional sedation with benzodiazepines may help alleviate the anxiety associated with the procedure and reduce the hemodynamic effects associated with esophageal intubation and probe manipulation. Additional superior laryngeal block can be performed if adequate local anesthesia and suppression of the gag reflex cannot be obtained. However, local anesthetic agents also have specific toxic dosages, and careful management is important. There have been many intoxication cases reported in the literature with TEE and upper GI endoscopy due to inappropriate administration of local anesthesia (15).

CHOICE OF TEE PROBE

The TEE probe consists of an ultrasound transducer installed at the distal extremity of a flexible endoscope. The maximal adult probe diameter is 0.9 to 1.6 cm and for the pediatric patient 0.5 to 0.6 cm. The probe total length varies between 70 and 120 cm. Two proximal control knobs permit anteroposterior and lateral motion of the head of the probe, of about 90° and 70°, respectively. The ultrasound probe uses an imaging frequency of 3 to 8 MHz (up to 10 MHz in pediatric probes). In our institution, we typically use a pediatric probe when the patient's weight is less than 45 kg.

ESOPHAGEAL INTUBATION

Insertion of the probe is attempted with control knobs in the neutral and unlocked position (Fig. 8.6). The distal end of the probe is lubricated with ultrasound gel and inserted through a mouth piece to protect the susceptible TEE shaft from teeth biting or jaw crushing (Fig. 8.7). The TEE examination can be performed under general anesthesia or conscious sedation in a cooperative patient. Under general anesthesia, blind intubation is commonly done using the second and third fingers as a guide or to pull up the mandible to assist TEE insertion while the probe is kept central to the tongue (Fig. 8.7). Unexpected difficult esophageal intubation may occur (Fig. 8.8), and some authors suggested that TEE placement under direct laryngoscopy reduces the incidence of oropharyngeal mucosal injury, odynophagia, and the number of insertion attempts (17) (Fig. 8.9). Occasionally, the endotracheal tube cuff may have to be deflated to facilitate insertion particularly when double-lumen

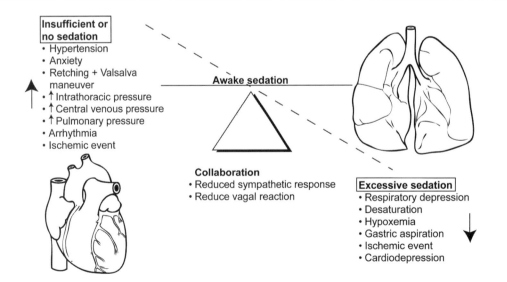

Figure 8.5   Sedation. The sedative agents have to be titrated for adequate performance of transesophageal echocardiography and this titration is a delicate balance between no sedation and excessive sedation. Insufficient, or absent sedation will lead, primarily, to cardiac symptoms such as tachycardia and hypertension. On the other hand, excessive sedation can lead to pulmonary symptoms such as respiratory depression and hypoxia.

A
NEUTRAL UNLOCKED

B
NEUTRAL LOCKED

C
NOT NEUTRAL UNLOCKED

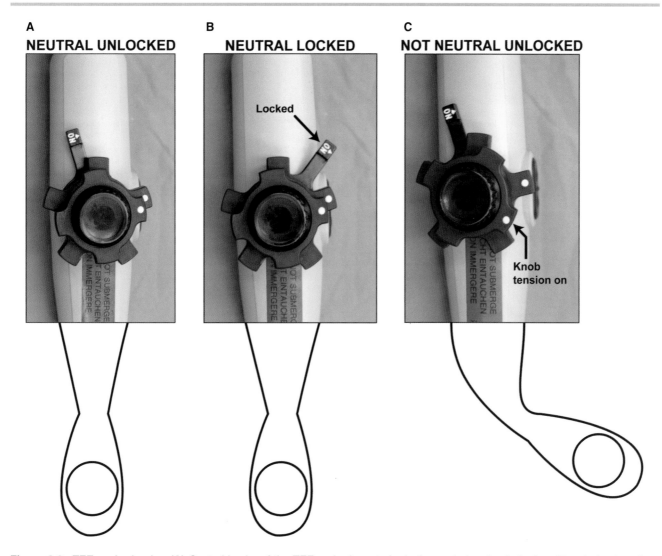

Figure 8.6 TEE probe knobs. (A) Control knobs of the TEE probe have to be in the neutral and unlocked position during insertion. **(B,C)** Inserting and manipulating the TEE probe in the neutral locked and not neutral unlocked position may result in esophageal damage. *Abbreviation*: TEE, transesophageal echocardiography.

tubes are used as in minimally invasive cardiac surgery (see Chapter 20).

Under conscious sedation, adequate local anesthesia combined with light sedation and reassurance can be sufficient for the patient to tolerate probe insertion and TEE examination. Placed in the left lateral decubitus, or sitting position, the patient is asked to try to swallow the probe. The deglutition maneuver closes the vocal cords, and the larynx moves forward to the posterior aspect of the tongue while the cricoid muscle relaxes. Local, or systemic, analgesia greatly contributes to patient tolerance by reducing retching and suppressing the gag reflex.

The probe insertion should be smooth and should not meet undue resistance. Forced insertion can cause vocal cord trauma or esophageal wall laceration. Mobilization of the probe is never performed with the probe in a locked and flexed position (Fig. 8.6). During insertion, the ultrasound system

display can be monitored to confirm the correct insertion of the TEE probe and to detect, rapidly, inadvertent tracheal intubation with associated image loss or appearance of tracheal rings (Fig. 8.10) (18,19). Under general anesthesia, this could be missed unless ventilation pressure modification is recognized. In the awake and sedated patient, tracheal intubation may be suspected in the event of stridor, coughing, and wheezing. In heavily sedated patients, tracheal placement may only be suspected by the presence of desaturation. The insertion and removal of the TEE probe can also be associated with displacement of the endotracheal tube.

COMPLICATIONS OF TEE

According to numerous studies, total complications, including minor and major events, vary between 0.6% and 3.5% (20–23). These results compare favorably

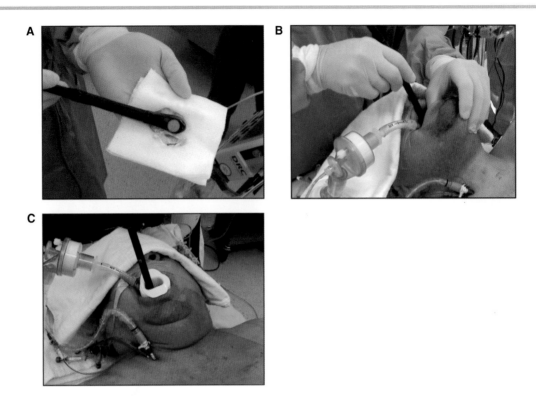

Figure 8.7   Demonstration of TEE probe insertion. (A,B) Lubricant is used prior to insertion of the TEE probe. **(C)** In anesthetized dentulous patients, a bite block is then fixed at the front of the mouth to prevent damage of the probe by teeth and to avoid endotracheal tube displacement. *Abbreviation*: TEE, transesophageal echocardiography. 🖱

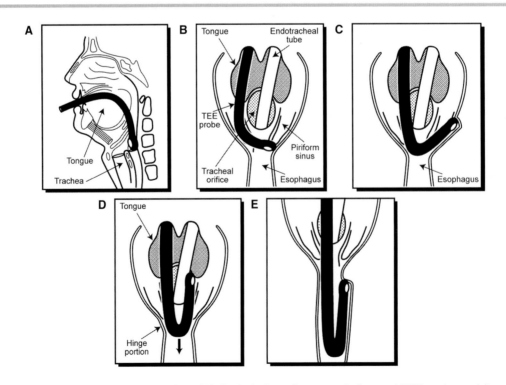

Figure 8.8   Buckling during TEE probe insertion. (A) Sagittal view of a correctly inserted TEE probe and its relationship with anatomical landmarks. **(B–E)** Coronal view of the oropharyngeal and upper esophageal area. **(B,C)** Difficult insertion of the TEE probe often results from a lateral insertion as opposed to the midline. If excessive force is used **(D)**, the probe could be inserted in a flexed position resulting in TEE probe buckling **(E)**. *Abbreviation*: TEE, transesophageal echocardiography. *Source*: Adapted from Ref. 16.

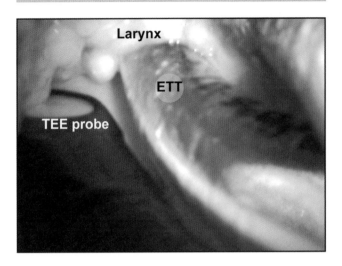

Figure 8.9 Anatomic view during TEE probe insertion. The insertion of a TEE probe under direct visualization using the fiberoptic laryngoscope (Glidescope) is shown. Resistance will be encountered when the probe is not directed in the midline position. *Abbreviations*: ETT, endotracheal tube; TEE, transesophageal echocardiography.

with those encountered for GI endoscopy. The TEE examination carried out in emergency settings has a higher complication rate of up to 12.6%. Several factors contribute to this situation, including the emergent need of the TEE, the hemodynamic status of the patient, the alteration of consciousness, and the risk of aspiration from a full stomach. The TEE-related complications are illustrated in Figure 8.11 and were recently reviewed (24). The use of direct laryngoscopy to insert the TEE probe has decreased the incidence of minor oropharyngeal trauma from 55% to 5% when compared to blind insertion (17).

Failure to introduce the probe correctly into the esophagus occurs in an estimated 1% to 2% of attempted procedures. Most of the time, it is attributed to the lack of patient collaboration or tolerance and to the operator's inexperience. In the setting of multiple unsuccessful attempts, it is sometimes

beneficial to reschedule the examination and plan it under general anesthesia and direct laryngoscopic visualization.

Excessive blind probe manipulation may result in buckling of the probe on itself when inserted into the esophagus (Fig. 8.8) (16,25). Forced withdrawal of a buckled probe may result in esophageal injury. The TEE probe must be delicately pushed into the stomach where it can unfold in a neutral straight position (Fig. 8.12). Further assistance with fluoroscopy and the presence of an anesthesiologist and a gastroenterologist endoscopist may, at times, be necessary. At no time should forceful manipulation or mobilization in a locked control knob position be attempted because of the risk of mucosal tear.

Secondary oropharyngeal or upper GI significant bleeding is rarely reported. However, unrecognized esophageal laceration and perforation (0.02–0.03%), leading to mediastinitis and sepsis, can be disastrous and sometimes only discovered at autopsy (Figs. 8.13 and 8.14) (24).

Transient hypoxemia can occur during TEE examination, with or without sedation and analgesia, and can be problematic for patients suffering from significant cardiac and/or pulmonary diseases. Hypoxemia correlates with the additive effects of narcotics and benzodiazepines, the presence of chronic obstructive pulmonary disease, and the size of the TEE probe. Alteration of the mental status after administration of sedation and analgesia also increases the risk of aspiration as the airway's protective reflexes are blunted. Methemoglobinemia can be induced by excessive administration of local anesthetic agent or in patients presenting with a certain enzymatic defect (cytochrome b5 reductase deficiency). The treatment is supportive and includes administration of methylene blue. An algorithm of hypoxia management during TEE insertion is presented in Figure 8.15.

Hemodynamic effects associated with TEE probe insertion and mobilization can be dramatic in awake and sedated patients. Tachycardia and hypertension can result in an ischemic event in susceptible subjects. Prominent gag reflexes and retching have been known to cause embolization of intracardiac mass and sudden death. Tachyarrhythmias have

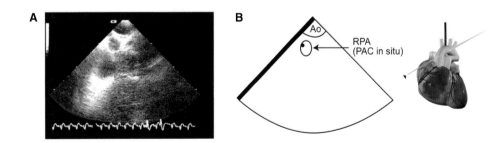

Figure 8.10 TEE probe malposition. (A,B) Transverse plane transtracheal image and diagram of the aortic arch and RPA with poorly visualized distal structures due to intratracheal malposition of the TEE probe. *Abbreviations*: RPA, right pulmonary artery; TEE, transesophageal echocardiography. *Source*: Adapted with permission from Ref. 19.

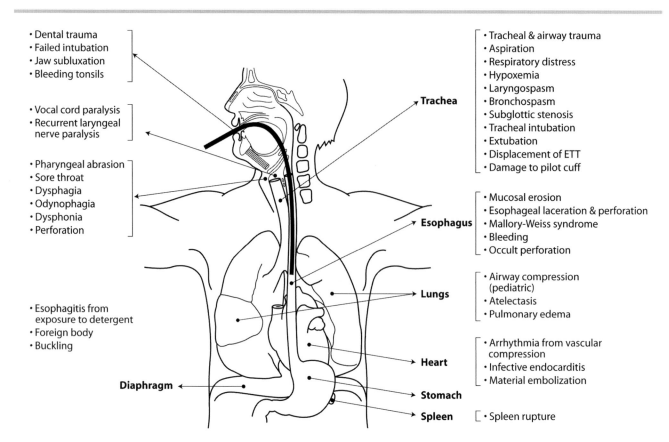

- Dental trauma
- Failed intubation
- Jaw subluxation
- Bleeding tonsils

- Vocal cord paralysis
- Recurrent laryngeal nerve paralysis

- Pharyngeal abrasion
- Sore throat
- Dysphagia
- Odynophagia
- Dysphonia
- Perforation

- Esophagitis from exposure to detergent
- Foreign body
- Buckling

Trachea
- Tracheal & airway trauma
- Aspiration
- Respiratory distress
- Hypoxemia
- Laryngospasm
- Bronchospasm
- Subglottic stenosis
- Tracheal intubation
- Extubation
- Displacement of ETT
- Damage to pilot cuff

Esophagus
- Mucosal erosion
- Esophageal laceration & perforation
- Mallory-Weiss syndrome
- Bleeding
- Occult perforation

Lungs
- Airway compression (pediatric)
- Atelectasis
- Pulmonary edema

Heart
- Arrhythmia from vascular compression
- Infective endocarditis
- Material embolization

Diaphragm

Stomach

Spleen
- Spleen rupture

Figure 8.11 TEE complications. Summary of TEE-related complications is shown. *Abbreviations*: ETT, endotracheal tube; TEE, transesophageal echocardiography.

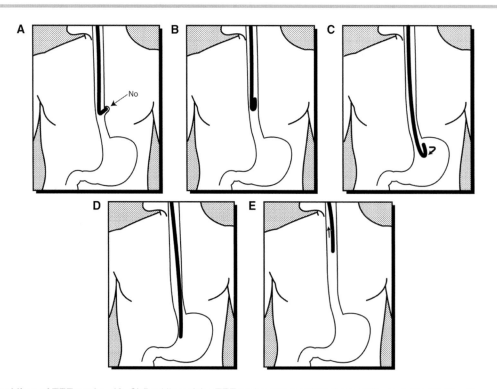

Figure 8.12 Buckling of TEE probe. (A–C) Buckling of the TEE probe can result in the inability to extract it from the esophagus. **(D,E)** If this condition is suspected, advancing the probe with retroflexion back to a straight position will lead to successful removal. *Abbreviation*: TEE, transesophageal echocardiography. *Source*: Adapted from Ref. 16.

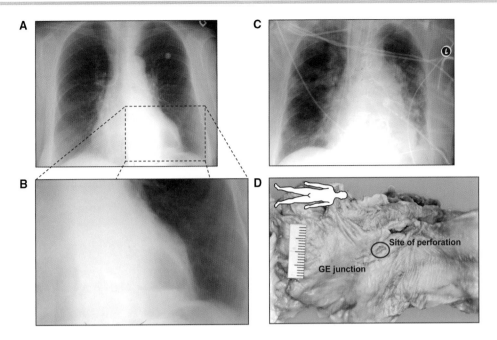

Figure 8.13 TEE probe complication: distal esophageal perforation. A 71-year-old woman is scheduled for aortic and mitral valve replacement with TEE monitoring. (**A,B**) On the preoperative chest X-ray a hiatal hernia was seen. (**C**) In the postoperative period she developed a left-sided pneumothorax and pleural effusion requiring a chest tube. She then went into multi-organ failure and died. (**D**) The autopsy showed distal esophageal perforation and a posterior mediastinal abscess. *Abbreviations*: GE, gastroesophageal; L, left; TEE, transesophageal echocardiography. *Source*: Photo D courtesy of Dr. Tack Ki Leung.

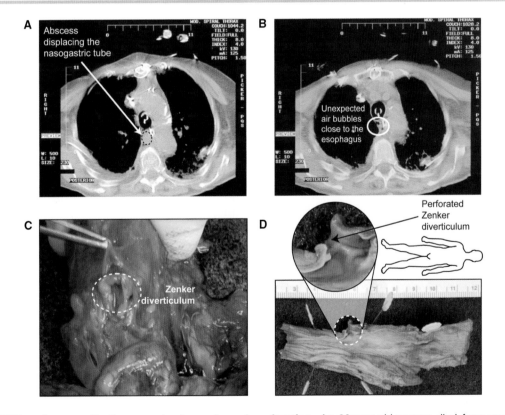

Figure 8.14 TEE probe complication: proximal esophageal perforation. An 82-year-old woman died from septic shock after cardiac surgery. Computed tomography scans show (**A**) an abscess displacing the nasogastric tube and (**B**) air bubbles close to the esophagus. (**C**) The autopsy demonstrated the presence of an unexpected perforated Zenker diverticulum. (**D**) A longitudinal view of the internal esophagus shows the perforated Zenker diverticulum. It was perforated presumably by the TEE probe either intraoperatively or post-operatively. *Abbreviation*: TEE, transesophageal echocardiography. *Source*: Adapted with permission from Ref. 24.

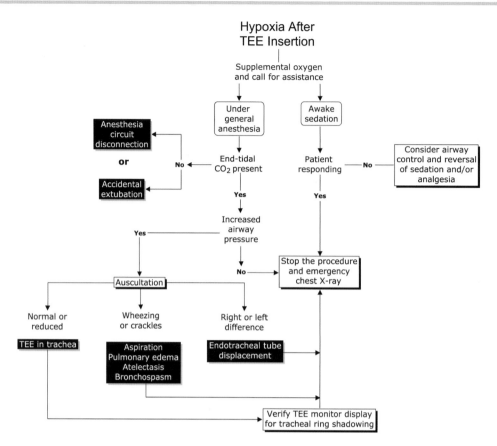

Figure 8.15 Hypoxia. Proposed management algorithm for hypoxia during TEE probe insertion is presented. *Abbreviations*: CO_2, carbon dioxide; TEE, transesophageal echocardiography.

also been reported during probe insertion and manipulation even under general anesthesia. Patients can also experience pain and vomiting. The TEE examination can exacerbate medical conditions such as cardiac and respiratory insufficiency, severe and uncontrolled high blood pressure, aortic dissection, pulmonary hypertension, and critical aortic stenosis.

PROBE MAINTENANCE AND INFECTION CONTROL

The TEE probe cleaning is necessary to prevent transmission of pathogens from one patient to the next. The emergence of multidrug-resistant bacteria, tuberculosis, prions, and various viruses emphasizes a methodical work flow pattern and the importance of adequate disinfection. The cleaning process must clearly define the clean and soiled areas and eliminate the possibility of recontamination (Fig. 8.16).

Immediately after use, and removal from the patient, the TEE probe shaft is separated from the ultrasound system and brought to the sink where it is washed with soap and running water. Gentle, but thorough, mechanical cleaning removes organic and inorganic debris and reduces the microbial

contamination by 99%. Care must be taken not to immerse the probe control knobs and electrical proximal connector. The probe is then soaked in a bath of 2% glutaraldehyde solution for 20 to 30 minutes. This solution is effective against infection propagation and serves as a second-line antibacterial and antiviral disinfectant (Tables 8.6 and 8.7). Finally, because of its potential for toxicity, the glutaraldehyde is rinsed off under running water and the probe is left to hang until dry. The distal end of the probe should be covered with a plastic cap, to protect the ultrasound transducer during storage, and installed in a protective supporting system (Fig. 8.17). Alternatively, a commercially available automated TEE probe-cleaning machine can be used in a centralized cleaning area (Fig. 8.18).

As an integral part of the reprocessing of the probe, the outer sheath, control knobs, and range of motion must routinely be inspected. With repeated abrasion from use, cleaning, and damage from teeth bites or jaw crushing, the outer sheath can develop fissures and false lumen. This may result in sequestration of soiled liquid or glutaraldehyde disinfectant that can later be remobilized during use in a different patient, causing either contamination or chemical burn. A break in the sheath integrity, caused by the steel wire of the inner probe control, is rarely

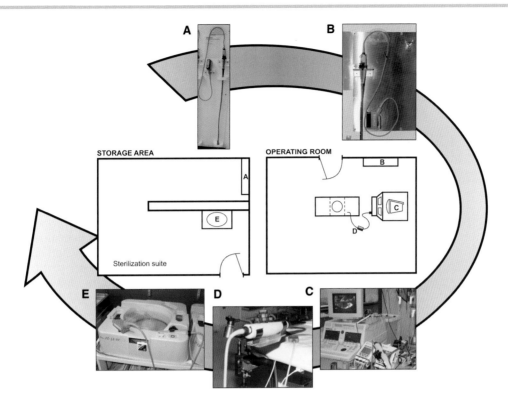

Figure 8.16   TEE probe turnover. Operating room maintenance and cleaning system for the TEE probe at the Montreal Heart Institute. (**A**) The TEE probes are stored in a rack system in a clean area outside the cardiac operating rooms. (**B**) Before surgery, a TEE probe is brought to the operating room where it is temporarily left on a supporting rack. (**C**) For use, the TEE probe is connected to the ultrasound system. (**D**) During monitoring, the TEE handle is supported by a custom-made stabilizer. (**E**) Once the exam is completed, the TEE probe is transferred back to the cleaning and sterilization suite. *Abbreviation*: TEE, transesophageal echocardiography.

Table 8.6   Cleaning and Disinfection of the TEE Probe

1. Always follow universal precautions.
2. All TEE and endoscopic equipments must be cleaned between each patient.
3. Cleaning should be done by properly trained staff.
4. Thorough, but gentle, mechanical cleaning under running water with soap or detergent to remove all gross organic material (secretions, saliva, and so on) from the probe.
5. Probe soaking in a bath of 2% glutaraldehyde for 20–30 min, and up to 45 min in case of HIV patients. Excessive soaking times may result in premature wear off of the TEE probe protective coating.
6. Probe rinsing to wash off all trace of glutaraldehyde.
7. Inspection of the TEE probe for potential tear/break and break in electrical integrity.

Abbreviations: HIV, human immunodeficiency virus; TEE, transesophageal echocardiography.

Table 8.7   Duration of Glutaraldehyde Exposition and Pathogen Destruction

Glutaraldehyde exposition (min)	Pathogens
1	Bacteria
2	100% sterile solution
2	Inactivates HIV and enteroviruses
2.5–5	Inactivates HBV
5–10	Low titer of mycobacterium tuberculosis

Abbreviations: HBV, hepatitis B virus; HIV, human immunodeficiency virus.

electrical safety checked regularly. Electrical and mechanical dysfunction, such as excessive or restricted probe motion upon manipulation of the control knobs, must be corrected before further use. Excessive motion range could result in buckling on TEE probe introduction. It is useful to have a maintenance log book for each TEE probe to keep a track of usage, cleaning, and periodic inspection.

Finally, with repeated plugging and unplugging of the TEE probe main electrical connector with the ultrasound platform electrical receptacle, defective probe function most commonly occurs secondary to worn-out and broken metal contacts, cracked shell, and accumulation of interfering dirt (Fig. 8.19).

encountered (26). Exaggerated flexion of the probe tip should be repaired as it can contribute to buckling.

After each use, inspection of the outer sheath integrity for breaks, fissure, or extruding wire should be systematically performed (Fig. 8.19). The plastic and rubber casing of the probe must be intact, and the

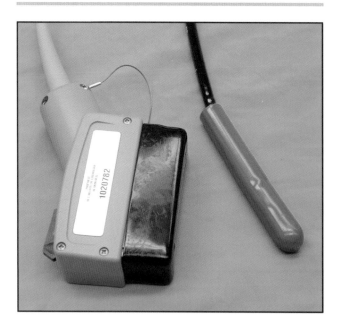

Figure 8.17 Protective covers for the transesophageal echocardiography probe.

CONCERNS OF HEALTH PERSONNEL

At all times, medical and paramedical staff should follow the rules for universal protection against transmittable diseases. Gloves, gowns, protective eyewear, and masks are worn to protect against splashing, spray, droplets, and other infectious materials that may be generated during coughing, retching, and vomiting by a patient during the procedure. Hepatitis vaccination is strongly recommended, as the infectious status of a patient is often unknown. Herpetic infection of a finger contaminated by oral secretions and herpetic conjunctivitis acquired during endoscopy by salivary spray occur frequently enough to deserve the sobriquet "endoscopist's eye." The utilization of a bite block protects the operator and the probe from being bitten by teeth or crushed by an edentulous jaw.

The glutaraldehyde solution has a toxic potential that should be made known to the personnel dedicated to probe manipulation and disinfection. Indeed, this product causes lung and mucosal toxicity, with dermatitis, conjunctivitis, nasal irritation, and asthma. Thus, the disinfection area should be well ventilated, and a lid should cover the glutaraldehyde container at all times to prevent propagation of toxic fumes to the whole room (Fig. 8.16).

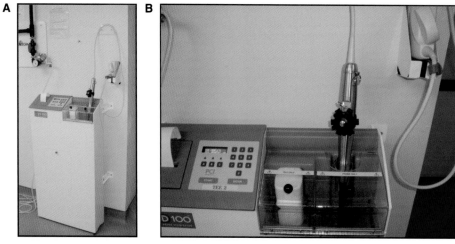

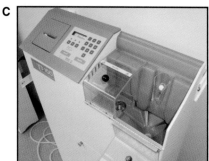

Figure 8.18 Automated TEE probe cleaner. (A–C) Automated TEE probe cleaning machine in a centralized cleaning area can process two TEE probes at the same time. *Abbreviation*: TEE, transesophageal echocardiography. *Source*: Courtesy of Dr Massimiliano Meineri, Toronto General Hospital.

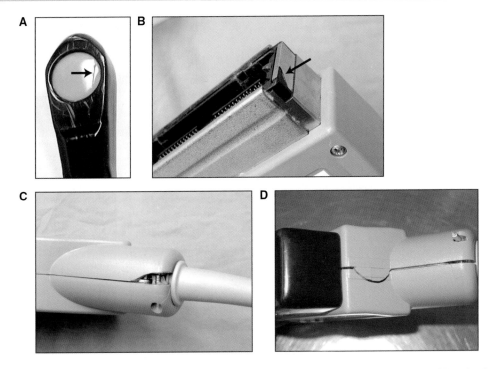

Figure 8.19 TEE probe damage. Damaged TEE probes include (**A**) linear fissure in the distal tip of the TEE probe (arrow), (**B**) broken connector plate (arrow) and (**C,D**) broken casing. *Abbreviation*: TEE, transesophageal echocardiography.

CONCLUSION

Since its inception as a diagnostic test, TEE examination has been clearly shown to yield important diagnostic information capable of altering cardiovascular disease management while being relatively easy to perform, with an excellent safety record, even in critically ill patients. However, this examination is, nevertheless, semi-invasive and has a definite potential for significant complications, particularly in ill-prepared procedures. It is, therefore, important for the clinician, who wishes to maximize the risk-benefit ratio of this test, to understand its indications, its limitations, to master the details of proper equipment usage, and to be alert to its potential complications by following a methodical and rigorous procedural technique meant to maximize patient safety.

REFERENCES

1. Doll N, Borger MA, Fabricius A, et al. Esophageal perforation during left atrial radiofrequency ablation: is the risk too high? J Thorac Cardiovasc Surg 2003; 125: 836–842.
2. Mohr FW, Fabricius AM, Falk V, et al. Curative treatment of atrial fibrillation with intraoperative radiofrequency ablation: short-term and midterm results. J Thorac Cardiovasc Surg 2002; 123:919–927.
3. Sonmez B, Demirsoy E, Yagan N, et al. A fatal complication due to radiofrequency ablation for atrial fibrillation: atrio-esophageal fistula. Ann Thorac Surg 2003; 76:281–283.
4. Flachskampf FA, Decoodt P, Fraser AG, et al. Guidelines from the working group. Recommendations for performing transesophageal echocardiography. Eur J Echocardiogr 2001; 2:8–21.
5. Quinones MA, Douglas PS, Foster E, et al. American College of Cardiology/American Heart Association clinical competence statement on echocardiography: a report of the American College of Cardiology/American Heart Association/American College of Physicians—American Society of Internal Medicine Task Force on Clinical Competence. Circulation 2003; 107:1068–1089.
6. Douglas PS, Khandheria B, Stainback RF, et al. ACCF/ASE/ACEP/ASNC/SCAI/SCCT/SCMR 2007 appropriateness criteria for transthoracic and transesophageal echocardiography: a report of the American College of Cardiology Foundation Quality Strategic Directions Committee Appropriateness Criteria Working Group, American Society of Echocardiography, American College of Emergency Physicians, American Society of Nuclear Cardiology, Society for Cardiovascular Angiography and Interventions, Society of Cardiovascular Computed Tomography, and the Society for Cardiovascular Magnetic Resonance endorsed by the American College of Chest Physicians and the Society of Critical Care Medicine. J Am Coll Cardiol 2007; 50:187–204.
7. Beique F, Ali M, Hynes M, et al. Canadian guidelines for training in adult perioperative transesophageal echocardiography. Recommendations of the Cardiovascular Section of the Canadian Anesthesiologists' Society and the Canadian Society of Echocardiography. Can J Cardiol 2006; 22:1015–1027.
8. Muhiudeen RI, Miller-Hance WC, Silverman NH. Intraoperative transesophageal echocardiography for pediatric patients with congenital heart disease. Anesth Analg 1998; 87:1058–1076.

9. St-Pierre J, Fortier LP, Couture P, et al. Massive gastrointestinal hemorrhage after transoesophageal echocardiography probe insertion. Can J Anaesth 1998; 45:1196–1199.

10. Wilson W, Taubert KA, Gewitz M, et al. Prevention of infective endocarditis: guidelines from the American Heart Association: a guideline from the American Heart Association Rheumatic Fever, Endocarditis, and Kawasaki Disease Committee, Council on Cardiovascular Disease in the Young, and the Council on Clinical Cardiology, Council on Cardiovascular Surgery and Anesthesia, and the Quality of Care and Outcomes Research Interdisciplinary Working Group. Circulation 2007; 116:1736–1754.

11. Nishimura RA, Carabello BA, Faxon DP, et al. ACC/AHA 2008 Guideline update on valvular heart disease: focused update on infective endocarditis: a report of the American College of Cardiology/American Heart Association Task Force on Practice Guidelines endorsed by the Society of Cardiovascular Anesthesiologists, Society for Cardiovascular Angiography and Interventions, and Society of Thoracic Surgeons. J Am Coll Cardiol 2008; 52:676–685.

12. Chang YY, Chang CI, Wang MJ, et al. Recommended practices for managing the patient receiving moderate sedation/analgesia. AORN J 2002; 75:642–652.

13. Gross JB, Bailey PL, Connis RT, et al. Practice guidelines for sedation and analgesia by non-anesthesiologists. Anesthesiology 2002; 96:1004–1017.

14. Waring JP, Baron TH, Hirota WK, et al. Guidelines for conscious sedation and monitoring during gastrointestinal endoscopy. Gastrointest Endosc 2003; 58:317–322.

15. Sharma SC, Rama PR, Miller GL, et al. Systemic absorption and toxicity from topically administered lidocaine during transesophageal echocardiography. J Am Soc Echocardiogr 1996; 9:710–711.

16. Orihashi K, Sueda T, Matsuura Y, et al. Buckling of transesophageal echocardiography probe: a pitfall at insertion in an anesthetized patient. Hiroshima J Med Sci 1993; 42:155–157.

17. Na S, Kim CS, Kim JY, et al. Rigid laryngoscope-assisted insertion of transesophageal echocardiography probe reduces oropharyngeal mucosal injury in anesthetized patients. Anesthesiology 2009; 110:38–40.

18. Fagan LF Jr, Weiss R, Castello R, et al. Transtracheal placement and imaging with a transesophageal echocardiographic probe. Am J Cardiol 1991; 67:909–910.

19. Sutton DC. Accidental transtracheal imaging with a transesophageal echocardiography probe. Anesth Analg 1997; 85:760–762.

20. Daniel WG, Erbel R, Kasper W, et al. Safety of transesophageal echocardiography. A multicenter survey of 10,419 examinations. Circulation 1991; 83:817–821.

21. Stevenson JG. Incidence of complications in pediatric transesophageal echocardiography: experience in 1650 cases. J Am Soc Echocardiogr 1999; 12:527–532.

22. Kallmeyer IJ, Collard CD, Fox JA, et al. The safety of intraoperative transesophageal echocardiography: a case series of 7200 cardiac surgical patients. Anesth Analg 2001; 92:1126–1130.

23. Piercy M, McNicol L, Dinh DT, et al. Major complications related to the use of transesophageal echocardiography in cardiac surgery. J Cardiothorac Vasc Anesth 2009; 23: 62–65.

24. Côté G, Denault A. Transesophageal echocardiography-related complications. Can J Anaesth 2008; 55:622–647.

25. Kronzon I, Cziner DG, Katz ES, et al. Buckling of the tip of the transesophageal echocardiography probe: a potentially dangerous technical malfunction. J Am Soc Echocardiogr 1992; 5:176–177.

26. Chan KL, Burwash I. Unusual structural abnormality in a biplane transesophageal transducer with normal imaging function. J Am Soc Echocardiogr 1998; 11:310–312.

Segmental Ventricular Function and Ischemia

Anique Ducharme, Ariel Diaz, and Jean-Claude Tardif
Université de Montréal, Montreal, Quebec, Canada

Adriaan Van Rensburg and Terrence Yau
University of Toronto, Toronto, Ontario, Canada

INTRODUCTION

Transesophageal echocardiography (TEE) is an invaluable tool, in the perioperative setting, in patients with inadequate transthoracic echocardiographic (TTE) images and in ventilated critically ill patients (1). Among its multiple intraoperative applications, TEE can be used to monitor global and regional ventricular function as well as the patient's volume status. The development of new ultrasound technology has permitted better identification and quantitative assessment of ventricular regional wall motion. This chapter focuses on the perioperative TEE evaluation of segmental ventricular function and detection of complications after myocardial infarction.

ANATOMY AND FUNCTION

Coronary Artery Distribution and Flow

Coronary anatomy varies but there is an overall pattern of coronary artery distribution. The left main coronary artery rises from the superior aspect of the left sinus of Valsalva and divides into the left anterior descending (LAD) and circumflex coronary arteries (Fig. 9.1). The LAD artery descends in the anterior interventricular groove down to the left ventricular (LV) apex contributing diagonal and septal branches. The circumflex artery continues, laterally, down the left atrioventricular groove giving rise to obtuse marginal branches (Fig. 9.2). The right coronary artery (RCA) rises from the superior aspect of the right sinus of Valsalva and extends inferomedially along the right atrioventricular groove (Fig. 9.3).

System dominance is defined by the artery providing the posterior descending artery that supplies the inferior aspect of the ventricular septum and the inferior free wall. The posterior descending artery arises from the RCA in 80% of patients and from the circumflex artery in 20%.

On the basis of studies correlating coronary angiography with echocardiography, a scheme was developed describing the specific coronary artery perfusing each LV segment (2) (Fig. 9.4). The LAD coronary artery supplies the anterior portion of the interventricular septum (IVS) through septal branches (Fig. 9.5), the anterior LV free wall through diagonal branches, and the septal and anterior portion of the apex. Because the basal portion of the anterior IVS is perfused by the first septal perforator, a wall motion abnormality in this region is consistent with stenosis of the proximal LAD artery. The circumflex artery perfuses the inferolateral (posterior) and anterolateral LV walls and the lateral apex. The RCA supplies the right ventricle (RV) through proximal and mid-ventricular branches, the LV inferior free wall, the inferior-half of the septum, and the inferior apex from the posterior descending artery. In the presence of coronary artery stenosis, wall motion abnormalities are more likely to occur at a fast, rather than slow, heart rate because of the shorter diastolic duration.

Myocardial Segmental Identification

Various methods for reporting the location of wall motion abnormalities during the echocardiographic examination are available. They differ mainly by the number of segments in which the left ventricle (LV) is divided (between 15 and 20) but are similar with regard to the general nomenclature of the segment. From base to apex, the LV is divided into basal, mid, and apical thirds corresponding to the proximal, middle, and apical segments of the coronary arteries. The most current scheme, approved by the American Society of Echocardiography (ASE) (2), divides the ventricle into 17 segments, 6 segments in both the basal and mid-portions (anteroseptal, inferoseptal, anterior, anterolateral, inferolateral, and inferior walls) and 5 at the apex (septal, anterior, lateral, inferior, and apical). As these segments can be recorded from three short-axis (SAX) and several longitudinal views, it is possible (and useful) to evaluate a segment from more than one view (Figs. 9.6 and 9.7).

The mid-esophageal four-chamber view allows simultaneous visualization of the LV and RV

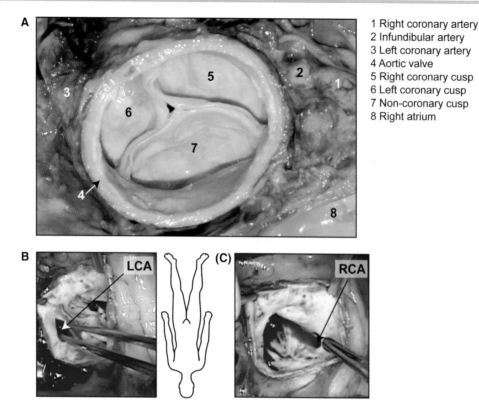

Figure 9.1 AoV and coronary ostia. Surgical anatomy view (**A**) of the AoV and the origins of the coronary arteries compared with intraoperative views (**B**) of the LCA and (**C**) RCA. *Abbreviations*: AoV, aortic valve; LCA, left coronary artery; RCA, right coronary artery.

(Fig. 9.6A). Because foreshortening of the LV and RV cavities occurs in this view, it is useful to use probe retroflexion to attenuate the problem, although this may result in degradation of image quality. This view permits assessment of segmental function of the mid-inferior septum and septal apex as perfused by the LAD coronary artery, the basal inferior septum supplied by the RCA artery, and the basal and mid-anterolateral walls supplied by the circumflex artery (Fig. 9.6). Rotation of the transducer to ~45° depicts the inferior septum to the left of the screen and the anterolateral wall to the right. With the transducer at 90°, the mid-esophageal two-chamber view allows visualization of the inferior wall supplied by the RCA, anterior wall perfused by the LAD artery, and adjacent portions of the apex that often has a dual coronary artery support. Further transducer rotation to 120° to 150° will result in a long-axis (LAX) view, with the anterior septum and inferolateral wall on the right and left, respectively.

Using the transgastric approach (Fig. 9.7), a series of SAX views can be obtained at 0° to 20° by modifying probe depth and anteflexion. For example, maximal anteflexion generally images the basal ventricular segments and the mitral valve (MV). A lesser degree of anteflexion or slight probe advancement will result in SAX views at the high and low papillary muscle levels.

In these SAX views, the inferior wall (#4, #10 and #15 supplied by the RCA) is seen at the top of the display, the anterior wall (#1, #7, and #13 supplied by the LAD artery) at the bottom, the inferolateral (#5 and #11) and anterolateral walls (# 6 and #12 supplied by the circumflex artery) to the right, and the anterior (#2 and #8 supplied by the LAD artery) and inferior (#3 and #9 supplied by the RCA) septums to the display lower left and upper left (Fig. 9.4). Further probe advancement will often result in a SAX view of the LV apical segments (#13–17). Because ventricular segments perfused by each of the three major coronary arteries are represented in the SAX view at the mid-papillary muscle level, it is commonly used in the intraoperative setting to evaluate global and segmental function (3).

Transducer rotation to 90° yields a transgastric two-chamber view, with the inferior (#4, #10, and #15 supplied by the RCA) and anterior (#1, #7, #13, and #17 supplied by the LAD artery) walls at the display top and bottom, respectively. It is usually possible to visualize the nontruncated, true LV apex (#17) on the display left in this view and to identify a wall motion abnormality, aneurysm, or thrombus. Further rotation to 120° to 150° will result in a LAX view, with the inferolateral wall on top and the anterior septum at the bottom of the display.

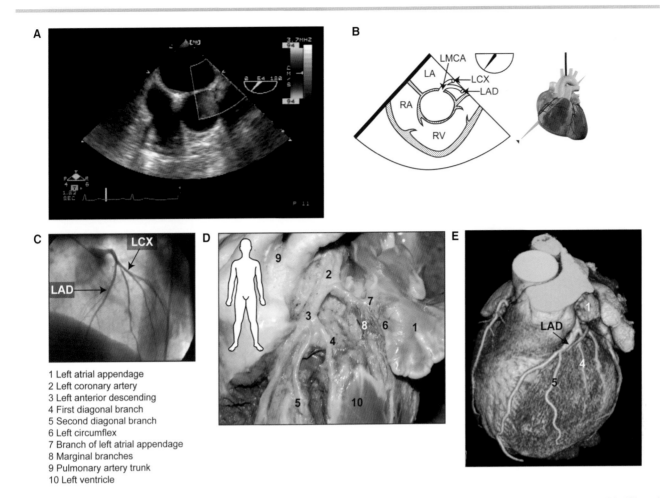

1 Left atrial appendage
2 Left coronary artery
3 Left anterior descending
4 First diagonal branch
5 Second diagonal branch
6 Left circumflex
7 Branch of left atrial appendage
8 Marginal branches
9 Pulmonary artery trunk
10 Left ventricle

Figure 9.2 Left coronary artery. Echocardiographic color Doppler mid-esophageal aortic valve short-axis (**A,B**), angiographic (**C**) and anatomical (**D**) and 256-slice ECG-gated computed tomography (**E**) views of the left coronary artery are shown. *Abbreviations*: D1, first diagonal; D2, second diagonal; LA, left atrium; LAA, left atrial appendage; LAD, left anterior descending; LCX, left circumflex; LMCA, left main coronary artery; RA, right atrium; RV, right ventricle. *Sources*: Photos C–E courtesy of Drs. Philippe L. L'Allier, Nicolas Dürrleman and Carl Chartrand-Lefebvre.

Normal Segmental Function

With ventricular contraction, a target point, chosen along the endocardial border interface, will move inward toward the center of the ventricle (endocardial excursion or radial shortening), resulting in reduced cavity area and increased distance between the endocardial and epicardial interfaces (wall thickening). During systole, a normally contracting myocardium is characterized by a radial shortening of more than 30% and myocardial thickening of 30% to 50% (3) (Table 9.1). It is important to take into account the heterogeneity of normal segmental function when assessing myocardial contractility. For example, the normally contracting basal inferior wall and basal IVS often appear to have reduced wall motion thickening compared with the other ventricular segments.

In addition, the presence of a left bundle branch block, right volume overload, constrictive pericarditis, artificial pacing, or the postoperative state after cardiac surgery often complicates the assessment of interventricular septal wall motion (Fig. 9.8).

Table 9.1 Wall Motion Scoring System

Movement	Radial displacement	Thickening
Normal or hyperkinesis = 1	>30%	Normal
Hypokinesis = 2	0–30%	+
Akinesis = 3	0%	Negligible
Dyskinesis = 4	Systolic lengthening	Paradoxical systolic motion
Aneurysmal = 5	Paradoxical displacement	Diastolic deformation

Adapted from Ref. 12.

Using an abnormality in wall motion as the sole criterion for the presence of ischemia has its limitations. The movement of a given ventricular segment is affected by the rotation and translation of the heart, and can be also be influenced by the adjacent muscle to which it is attached (tethering), resulting in overestimation of the extent of ischemia. Decreased myocardial thickening is more specific for ischemia (4) and, in extreme cases, systolic thinning can occur.

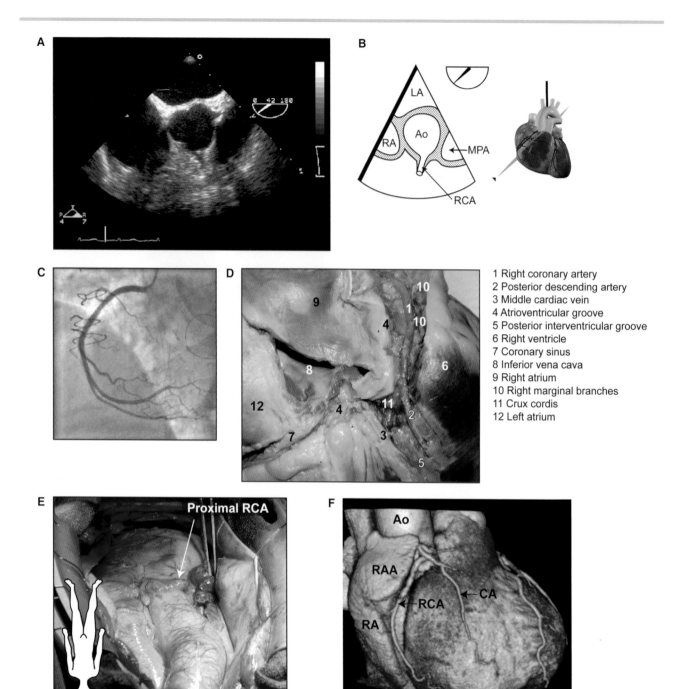

Figure 9.3   Right coronary artery. Echocardiographic mid-esophageal aortic valve short-axis (**A,B**), angiographic (**C**), anatomical (**D**), and intraoperative (**E**) and 256-slice ECG-gated computed tomography (**F**) views of the RCA are shown. *Abbreviations*: Ao, aorta; CA, conus artery; LA, left atrium; MPA, main pulmonary artery; RA, right atrium; RAA, right atrial appendage; RCA, right coronary artery. *Sources*: Photos C–F courtesy of Drs. Philippe L. L'Allier, Nicolas Dürrleman and Carl Chartrand-Lefebvre.

Indeed, the assessment of myocardial thickening is not affected by cardiac rotation and translation. Although the transgastric mid-papillary SAX view is the plane most commonly used to detect ischemia, one-third of regional wall motion abnormalities may not be detected in this view (5,6). A complete analysis of all 17 ventricular segments, as described earlier, should be carried out.

Both animal and clinical studies have documented that wall motion is rapidly altered after coronary artery occlusion. The first detectable abnormalities are cellular biochemical changes and a perfusion defect (detected by radionuclide techniques), followed by delayed myocardial relaxation and/or decreased compliance, and within minutes, reduced systolic wall thickening and endocardial motion. The electrocardiographic ST-T

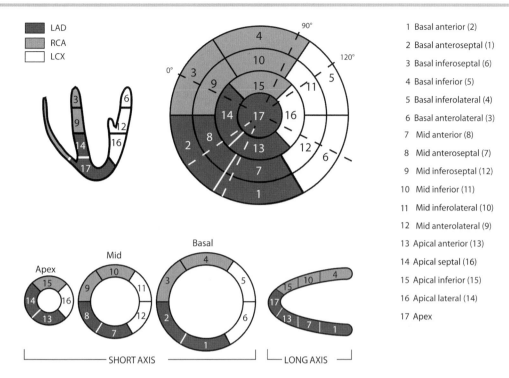

1 Basal anterior (2)

2 Basal anteroseptal (1)

3 Basal inferoseptal (6)

4 Basal inferior (5)

5 Basal inferolateral (4)

6 Basal anterolateral (3)

7 Mid anterior (8)

8 Mid anteroseptal (7)

9 Mid inferoseptal (12)

10 Mid inferior (11)

11 Mid inferolateral (10)

12 Mid anterolateral (9)

13 Apical anterior (13)

14 Apical septal (16)

15 Apical inferior (15)

16 Apical lateral (14)

17 Apex

Figure 9.4 Segmental model of the left ventricle. Transesophageal echocardiographic correlation of coronary artery distribution and the American Heart Association 17-segment model is shown. The corresponding segment numbers from the American Society of Echocardiography are in parentheses. *Abbreviations*: LAD, left anterior descending; LCX, left circumflex artery; RCA, right coronary artery. *Source*: Adapted from Ref. 2.

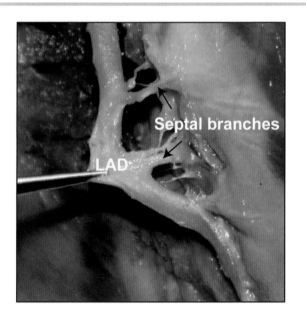

Figure 9.5 Septal branches. The septal branches of the LAD are displayed. *Abbreviation*: LAD, left anterior descending artery. *Source*: Courtesy of Nicolas Dürrleman.

changes and clinical symptoms of angina, if they appear, are late manifestations of ischemia. Although acute ischemia is usually manifested, echocardiographically as a regional wall motion abnormality, global ventricular dysfunction may result from high-grade obstruction of one or more arteries perfusing a large area, or the acute obstruction of one artery in the setting of previous infarction in other areas.

GLOBAL SYSTOLIC FUNCTION CHANGES

Global LV systolic function can be evaluated, either qualitatively or quantitatively, as described in Chapter 10. Global systolic function can be qualitatively classified as normal, mildly, moderately, or severely reduced, but this information is considered incomplete by most clinicians. In contrast, determination of the left ventricular ejection fraction (LVEF) has major prognostic significance in patients with coronary artery disease (CAD). In the clinical setting, visual estimation of the LVEF has become common practice. The correlation between the visual echocardiographic estimation (eye balling) and the radionuclide determination is surprisingly good, especially in patients with impaired LVEF. This method, however, requires experience, and clinicians should validate their own performance with quantitative methods.

All echocardiographic approaches for the assessment of regional and global ventricular function need to take into account the quality of endocardial border definition, the asynchronous contraction patterns observed with ventricular pacing or in the presence of conduction defects, the heterogeneity of normal ventricular function, and the observed abnormality in septal wall motion frequent in the postoperative period.

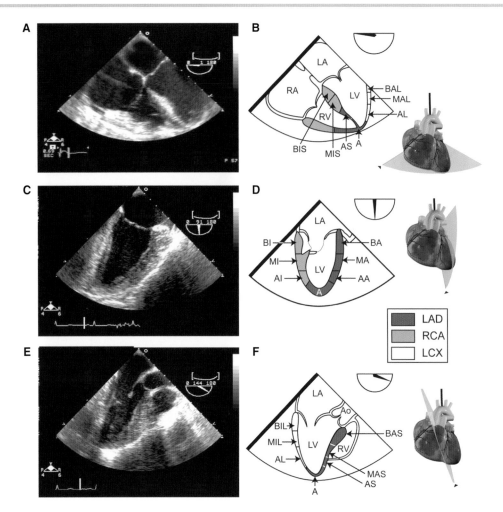

Figure 9.6 LV function. Mid-esophageal views to evaluate RV and LV function: (**A,B**) four-chamber, (**C,D**) two-chamber and (**E,F**) long-axis views. *Abbreviations*: A, apex; AA, apical anterior; AI, apical inferior; AL, apical lateral; Ao, aorta; AS, apical septal; BA, basal anterior; BAL, basal anterolateral; BAS, basal anteroseptal; BI, basal inferior; BIL, basal inferolateral; BIS, basal inferoseptal; LA, left atrium; LAD, left anterior descending; LCX, left circumflex artery; LV, left ventricle; MA, mid-anterior; MAL, mid-anterolateral; MAS, mid-anteroseptal; MI, mid-inferior; MIL, mid-inferolateral; MIS, mid-inferoseptal; RA, right atrium; RCA, right coronary artery; RV, right ventricle.

SEGMENTAL SYSTOLIC FUNCTION CHANGES

Studies and clinical experience have shown that segmental wall motion abnormalities occur in the area supplied by the obstructed artery within seconds after the interruption of myocardial blood flow, minutes before the development of any ischemic electrocardiographic changes and chest pain. Most quantitative methods are based on the evaluation of wall motion. A segmental wall motion abnormality is defined as hypokinesis when contraction is normally directed, but reduced in magnitude, akinesis when it is absent, or dyskinesis when there is systolic bulging (Table 9.1).

Compared with multilead electrocardiogram (EKG) monitoring and invasive hemodynamic monitoring, TEE has proved to be superior at detecting acute ischemia as reflected by new regional wall motion abnormalities (3,7). In a group of patients at high risk for intraoperative ischemia undergoing coronary artery bypass or major vascular surgery, Smith et al. (3) found that 24 (48%) of the 50 patients demonstrated new segmental wall motion abnormalities while only 6 (12%) patients presented new ischemic ST changes. Furthermore, Leung et al. (8) demonstrated that wall motion abnormalities occurred in the absence of hemodynamic changes and were predictive of adverse outcomes after cardiac surgery. Consistent with these observations, van Daele et al. (7) have shown the lack of sensitivity of hemodynamic measurements in predicting ischemia or postoperative cardiac complications.

Quantitative evaluation of regional LV systolic function requires high-quality images with good endocardial resolution. The centerline method is a quantitative approach for assessing regional ventricular function, which first involves the construction of a line halfway between the end-diastolic and end-systolic endocardial perimeters (9). The endocardial

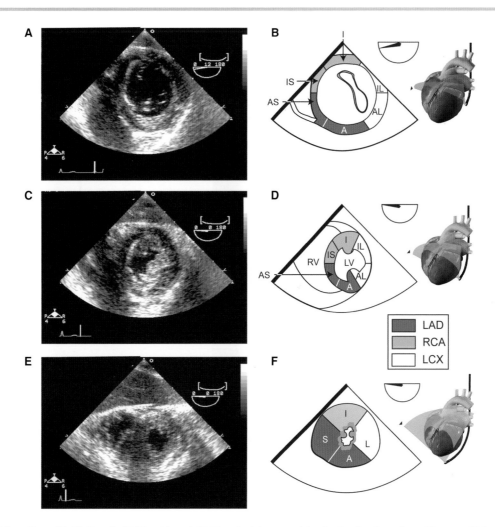

Figure 9.7 LV function. (A,B) Basal, **(C,D)** mid and **(E,F)** apical transgastric short-axis views in a 49-year-old female are shown. *Abbreviations*: A, anterior; AL, anterolateral; AS, anteroseptal; I, inferior; IL, inferolateral; IS, inferoseptal; L, lateral; LAD, left anterior descending; LCX, left circumflex artery; LV, left ventricle; RCA, right coronary artery; RV, right ventricle; S, septal.

excursion is determined along 100 equally spaced chords perpendicular to the centerline. Motion is then normalized for heart size by dividing by the length of the end-diastolic perimeter. The normalized length of each line is then converted into units of standard deviation (SD) from the mean excursion along a given chord, which allows the regional heterogeneity of ventricular contraction to be taken into account (see Fig. 5.4). By convention, negative and positive values indicate hypokinetic and hyperkinetic chords, respectively. The extent of abnormal wall motion is calculated as the number of chords with hypokinesis equal to or more severe than two SDs. The severity of wall motion abnormalities is calculated as the area under the curve below the zero SD line.

A few limitations and pitfalls of using TEE for the assessment of regional systolic function should be mentioned. The segmental wall motion analysis system must first compensate for global motion of the heart, usually by a floating frame (see Fig. 5.3). When

viable and nonischemic, the IVS thickens during systole but its asynchronous motion can begin slightly before or after the inward motion of the other walls (see Fig. 5.5). Experimental and clinical studies have also defined important regional differences in normal myocardial contraction (10). As mentioned previously, it is important to realize that contraction of the inferobasal wall is often slightly more limited than that of the other ventricular segments. Not all systolic wall motion abnormalities are indicative of ischemia as these may occur in patients with myocarditis, septic shock, ventricular pacing, and bundle branch block (Fig. 9.8). Tethering of nonischemic myocardium adjacent to an ischemic or infarcted myocardium is a frequent cause of overestimation of the infarct size with echocardiography compared with postmortem examination. Force et al. (11) found that although tethering does lead to an unavoidable overestimation of the infarct size, within 1 cm of the ischemic area, the amount of myocardium involved is small and

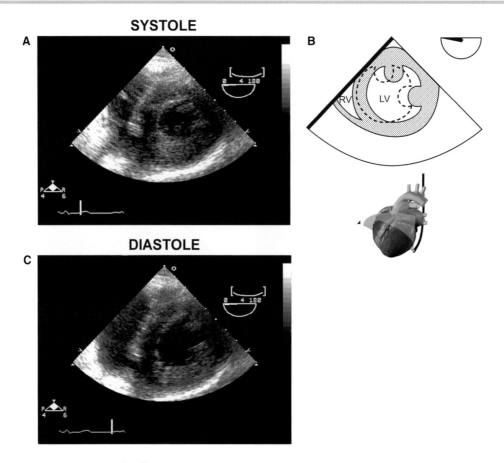

Figure 9.8 **Abnormal septal motion.** **(A–C)** A 57-year-old woman scheduled for coronary revascularization with a left bundle-branch block has abnormal septal motion (*dotted line*) as shown in these transgastric mid short-axis views. *Abbreviations*: LV, left ventricle; RV, right ventricle.

relatively predictable. Altered loading conditions may also result in segmental wall motion abnormalities or may unmask areas of scarring. For example, an acute elevation of the blood pressure may retard the contraction of an already damaged myocardial segment more than that of a normal one.

Identification of a persistent or new wall motion abnormality does not distinguish a stunned or hibernating region from infarcted or ischemic myocardium. Stunning, defined as prolonged postischemic contractile dysfunction of the myocardium, has been observed in several clinical situations including stress-induced angina, unstable angina, thrombolysis, percutaneous transluminal angioplasty, and coronary artery bypass surgery. Complete recovery of myocardial function may require from three days to several weeks in the presence of stunning. Hibernation is a state of persistently impaired myocardial and LV functions at rest due to reduced coronary blood flow that can be partially, or completely, restored to normal if the myocardial oxygen supply/demand relationship is favorably altered, either by improving blood flow (surgery, percutaneous coronary angioplasty) and/or by reducing demand.

Wall Motion Score Index

A semi-quantitative assessment of regional LV contraction is provided by the wall motion score index (WMSI). A score is assigned to the contractility of each segment of the 17 segment LV model (2) recommended by the ASE (12). A score of 1 is given to a normally contracting or hyperkinetic segment, 2 for an hypokinetic segment, 3 for akinesis, 4 in the presence of a dyskinetic segment, and 5 for an aneurysmal (diastolic deformation) segment (12) (Table 9.1). Of note, there is no specific score for compensatory hyperkinesis. The WMSI is equal to the sum of the regional scores divided by the number of evaluable segments and can vary between 1.0 (for normal ventricular contraction) and 3.9 (for severe systolic dysfunction). Because CAD causes segmental dysfunction, which can be accompanied by compensatory hyperkinesis of nonischemic segments, regional assessment of systolic function is more sensitive for the detection of ischemia than global approaches.

Furthermore, the prognostic value of the motion score has been shown in clinical studies. Among a group of patients admitted with acute myocardial infarction, those with favorable indices (best quintile) had an 8% incidence of cardiovascular death at one year. In contrast, patients with motion indexes in the worst quintile had a mortality of 51% at one year (13). Kan et al. (14) also examined the value of WMSI in patients with acute myocardial infarction and found a significantly higher mortality rate in the group with the most abnormal score indexes compared with those with more favorable ones (61% vs 3%, respectively).

Tissue Doppler Imaging

Tissue Doppler imaging (TDI) filters out high velocity blood signals in favor of low velocity, high amplitude signals from the myocardium to analyze direction and velocity of myocardial motion and quantify regional wall motion (see Chapter 2) (15). Combining this technology with pulsed wave (PW) Doppler allows for interrogation of a single point/segment within the ventricular wall. Simultaneous evaluation of multiple segments is not possible in real time PW spectral TDI, but can be performed off-line out of stored 2D TDI loops (Figs. 9.9 and 9.10). Typical velocities are affected by gender and age. Mean values of 7.5 cm/s and values below 5.5 cm/s are indicative of myocardial failure. Several studies evaluating TDI have reported a decrease in regional myocardial velocity during ischemic events (16–18).

A major limitation of this technology is that it is based on the Doppler equation, and the velocities measured are inaccurate if the Doppler beam is not parallel to the movement of the segment evaluated. Another limitation is that it cannot distinguish akinetic segments tethered by the contracting adjacent

myocardium. Furthermore, the high temporal but poor spatial resolution makes it difficult to differentiate between subendocardium and subepicardium.

Color Tissue Doppler Imaging

Color TDI superimposes color-coded tissue velocity onto a real time live 2D image. Color TDI evaluates mean velocities from each pixel so the velocity is lower than that of PW spectral TDI, which measures peak velocities at the sample volume. Color TDI compared with pulsed TDI has superior spatial resolution making it possible to evaluate multiple segments at the same time (Fig. 9.10). It can be displayed in different formats, as velocity against time for each segment or as a curved M-mode (Fig. 9.11).

Strain and Strain Rate

During the cardiac cycle, myocardial tissue changes length; shortening during systole and elongating in diastole. This change is called deformation, and strain is used to measure myocardial deformation (see Chapter 2). Strain is defined as a change of myocardial length in relation to its original length divided by the original length (see equation 2.11). Strain rate (SR) is defined as the rate of myocardial deformation (see equation 2.14).

Myocardial ischemia causes reductions in systolic strain and SR. It has been quoted, by some investigators, to be superior to TDI in detecting myocardial ischemia (15). Changes, indicative of myocardial ischemia, occurred earlier with strain and SR measurements than with TDI measurement.

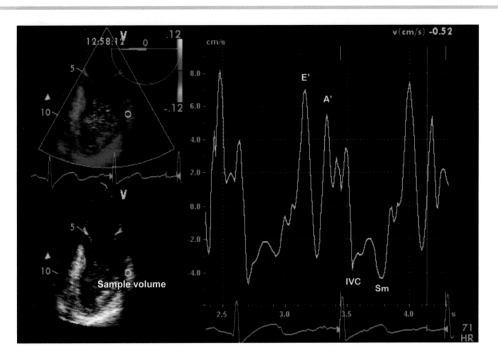

Figure 9.9 **TDI.** Normal velocities (cm/s) are displayed over time with evaluation of a left ventricular mid anterolateral wall segment using TDI obtained from a mid-esophageal four-chamber view. *Abbreviations*: A', late diastolic velocity; E', early diastolic peak velocity; HR, heart rate; IVC, isovolumic contraction; S_m, systolic mitral annular velocity, TDI, tissue Doppler imaging.

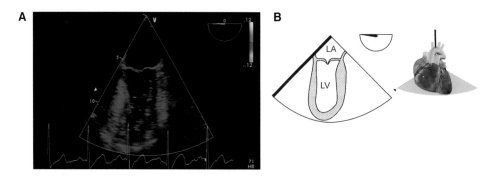

Figure 9.10 Color TDI. (A,B) Evaluation of segmental velocities of the LV using color TDI from an end-systolic frame of a mid-esophageal four-chamber view allows for instantaneous assessment of segmental velocities. The presence of uniform colors during any moment of the cardiac cycle suggests homogenous contraction and relaxation. *Abbreviations*: HR, heart rate; LA, left atrium; LV, left ventricle; TDI, tissue Doppler imaging.

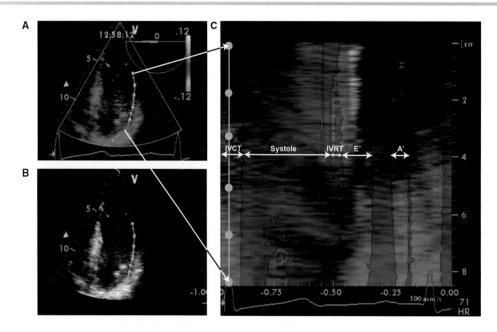

Figure 9.11 Color TDI curved M-mode. (A) Stored color TDI of a mid-esophageal four-chamber view. **(B)** Same image with the color overlay turned off: the precise location of the sample points are more easily visualized on the anterolateral wall of the LV. **(C)** Corresponding curved M-mode of the anterolateral wall is displayed for a single cardiac cycle. The duration of each period of the cardiac cycle can be precisely measured in this normal tracing. *Abbreviations*: *A'*, late diastolic velocity; *E'*, early diastolic velocity; HR, heart rate; ICVT, isovolumic contraction time; IVRT, isovolumic relaxation time; LV, left ventricle; TDI, tissue Doppler imaging.

By convention myocardial shortening has a negative SR and myocardial lengthening positive strain. This implies that radial strain (obtained in a transgastric mid SAX view) (Fig. 9.12) will be positive during systole and longitudinal strain (obtained in mid-esophageal views) will be positive during diastole (Fig. 9.13). Strain is calculated off-line from TDI or using 2D speckle tracking technology (see Chapter 2). Strain corresponds to the integration of SR over time. Strain and SR can be displayed against time or as a curved anatomic M-mode (Figs. 9.12 and 9.13). Values for strain and SR vary according to the type of strain

(radial or longitudinal) and the segment evaluated (see Table 2.2).

Myocardial deformation can provide information on local myocardial function in diseases such as cardiomyopathy (19,20). It has also demonstrated usefulness in the assessment of ischemic heart disease (21–24). Strain is reduced in ischemic myocardium or absent when infarcted (see Fig. 2.27) and, in some cases, will demonstrate dyskinesis (abnormal stretching or thinning in systole). The timing of events is also helpful. Post-systolic strain (following aortic valve closure for the LV) is a marker of ischemia (Fig. 9.14).

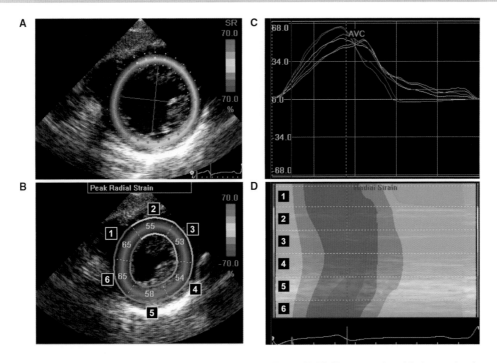

Figure 9.12 Radial strain by 2D speckle tracking in a normal patient. (A,B) Transgastric mid short-axis view with radial strain overlay. The peak radial strain has a positive value for all left ventricular (LV) segments because of myocardial thickening during systole. **(C,D)** The change in peak radial strain of each LV segment can be displayed as individual tracings over time **(C)** or as a curved M-mode map over time **(D)**.

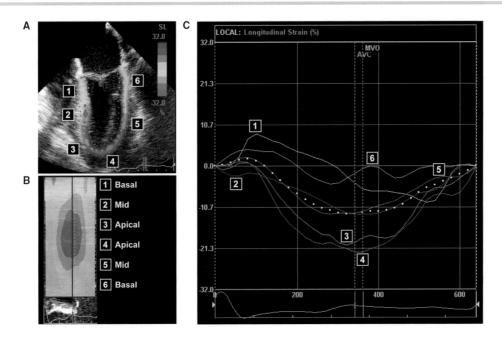

Figure 9.13 Longitudinal strain by 2D speckle tracking. (A–C) Mid-esophageal four-chamber view with peak longitudinal strain overlay. Both the curved M-mode mapping **(B)** and individual sampling curves **(C)** show that the basal regions (1,6) have lower strain value compared to the apical regions (3,4). *Abbreviations*: AVC, aortic valve closure; MVO, mitral valve opening; SL, strain longitudinal.

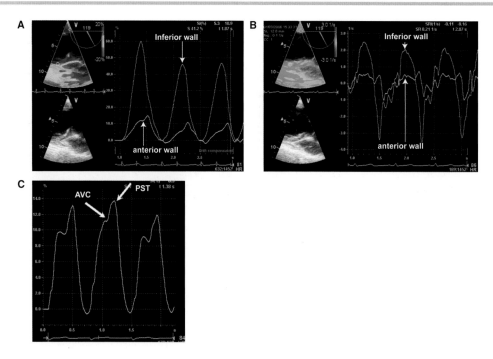

Figure 9.14 Ischemia and radial strain and strain rate by tissue Doppler. (A) Radial strain and **(B)** strain rate (SR) from a transgastric view at 119° in a patient with basal anterior wall ischemia. Compared with the inferior wall, note the reduced radial strain and SR of the anterior wall. **(C)** Radial strain in the inferior wall from a transgastric short axis view over three consecutive heart beats in a different patient with ischemia following air embolization. Approximate timing for the aortic valve closure (AVC) is demonstrated as well as post systolic thickening (PST) secondary to ischemia.

Stunned myocardium will demonstrate a strain pattern similar to ischemia, however, when inotropic administration is started the pattern normalizes. In contrast, ischemic myocardium will respond to inotropic stimulation by increasing post-systolic strain. The ratio of systolic strain to the sum of post-systolic strain and systolic strain has been shown to relate to the level of ischemia (24). SR imaging can also provide information on diastolic function.

The major limitation of strain and SR is that they are very sensitive to noise. Second, as with all Doppler applications, the accuracy depends on proper alignment of the ultrasound beam and the direction of tissue motion. However, this limitation is reduced with the use of 2D speckle tracking technology. Most ultrasound platforms do not allow online evaluation of these measurements. Very little data is currently available on the use and application of strain and SR during routine perioperative TEE.

Speckle Tracking

Speckle tracking is a technology based on tracking of features created by B-mode imaging (25–27) (see Chapter 2). These features appear randomly, and, therefore, each myocardial segment will have unique patterns. Myocardial velocity differences, based on this technology, do not depend on the Doppler angle and allow for simultaneous 2D assessments (e.g., radial and longitudinal) over large areas. Figures 9.12 and 28.20 are two examples of a normal and abnormal mid-papillary

transgastric view and Figure 9.13 from a four-chamber view using speckle tracking.

Three-Dimensional Echocardiography

The recent availability of three-dimensional (3D) technology for TEE has opened up a new approach to LV assessment. It has been shown to provide accurate analysis of LV morphology and function, compared with cardiac computed tomography (CT) and magnetic resonance imaging (MRI) (28). A 3D dataset has to be acquired then exported to the analytical software (Fig. 9.15). A mathematical model and a cast are created (Fig. 9.16). The cast is divided into the standard 17 segments. A change in volume for each segment can be calculated and plotted for each cardiac cycle. This application has mainly been used, so far, to assess the effectiveness of cardiac resynchronization therapy in patients with congestive heart failure. The development of a technology that allows live 3D LV reconstruction and on line analysis would be of great value.

Dobutamine Stress Echocardiography

Perioperatively, it is extremely difficult to determine whether a new segmental wall motion abnormality represents inadequate revascularization, ongoing ischemia, or stunned myocardium, but the distinction is of therapeutic significance and a dobutamine stress echocardiogram may be useful. Dobutamine has a positive

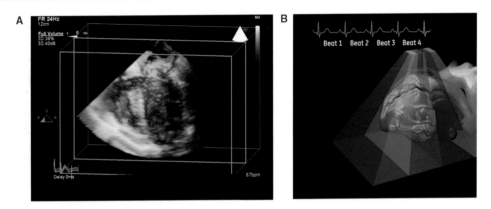

Figure 9.15 **3D evaluation of the LV.** Acquisition of a 3D dataset of the LV using (**A**) 3D transesophageal echocardiography. (**B**) Full volume acquisition by 3D transthoracic echocardiography is done with ECG gating over four cardiac cycles. *Abbreviation*: LV, left ventricle. *Source*: Photo B Courtesy of GE Healthcare.

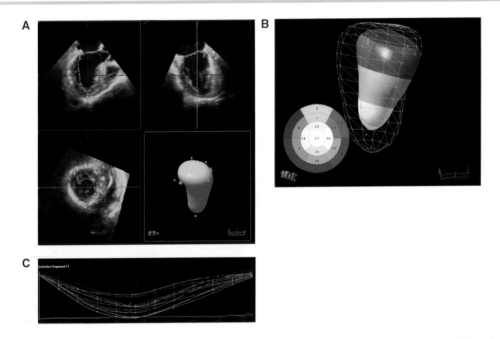

Figure 9.16 **3D model of LV function.** (**A**) The 3D full volume dataset of the LV can be processed with special analytical software to create (**B**) a dynamic seventeen segment 3D endocardial cast. (**C**) The change in volume of each of the 17 segments is plotted over time and displayed in the lower diagram. *Abbreviation*: LV, left ventricle.

inotropic effect at low doses (5–10 μg/kg/min), with additional inotropic and chronotropic effects at higher doses. The increase in systolic blood pressure (SBP) during the infusion of dobutamine can be more pronounced in hypertensive than in normotensive patients. Occasionally, a paradoxical hypotension can be observed, and this is either due to the vasodilating effect of dobutamine or transient outflow tract obstruction, but it is rarely caused by ischemia (29).

Demonstration of increased contractility in a hypokinetic or akinetic region suggests that the regional systolic function will improve either after revascularization, in the case of hibernating myocardium (30), or spontaneously after recovery from stunning (31). A biphasic response to increasing dobutamine doses, characterized by enhanced thickening at low doses (5–10 μg/kg/min) followed by deterioration of thickening at higher doses (>10 μg/kg/min), is the most accurate echocardiographic criterion to detect a viable but hypoperfused myocardium. Arnese et al. (32) found that the specificity of low-dose dobutamine echocardiography in predicting recovery of function after surgical revascularization was 95% compared with only 48% for 201-thallium single photon emission computed tomography (SPECT). The greater the number of viable myocardial segments, the greater is the probability of improvement in regional and global LV function after revascularization.

The value of low-dose dobutamine stress echocardiography for the assessment of myocardial viability has been compared with that of positron emission tomography (PET) and nuclear perfusion imaging (33). Cumulative data from multiple studies suggest that thallium SPECT images provide better sensitivity compared with dobutamine echocardiography for this indication (89% vs. 81%), but low-dose dobutamine stress echocardiography has a higher specificity (83% vs. 69%). In comparison, PET scanning has a positive predictive value of 82% and a negative predictive value of 83% for predicting recovery after revascularization, with an excellent agreement with dobutamine stress echocardiography (34).

DIASTOLIC FUNCTION

In patients with CAD, onset of ischemia rapidly results in diastolic dysfunction, even before the development of systolic dysfunction (Fig. 9.17). Two distinct patterns of abnormalities can be recognized and are associated with either impaired relaxation or compliance. An LV relaxation abnormality results in an increased delay between aortic valve closure and MV opening. This is reflected by a prolonged isovolumic relaxation time (IVRT) ≥ 100 ms, slower decay of the atrioventricular gradient in early diastole (prolonged deceleration time ≥ 270 ms), reduced rapid ventricular filling (reduced E-wave velocity) due to a reduced pressure gradient between the atrium and the ventricle after MV opening, and a greater contribution of left atrium (LA) contraction to ventricular filling (increased A-wave velocity) resulting in an E/A ratio <1 (Fig. 9.18). A mild relaxation abnormality will usually be associated with a prominent systolic component of the pulmonary venous inflow. A pseudo-normal pattern, which is associated with an elevation of the left ventricular end diastolic pressure (LVEDP), is manifested in the pulmonary veins by an increase in the maximal velocity (peak velocity ≥ 35 cm/s) and duration (at least 30 ms more than the mitral A-wave duration) of the A reversal wave during atrial contraction.

Restriction to LV filling due to abnormal compliance leads to a different Doppler pattern. The elevated atrial pressure and increased atrioventricular gradient is manifested by an increased peak E-wave velocity and a short deceleration time, as the ventricle has poor compliance and the LV and LA pressures equilibrate rapidly. The following diastasis plateau phase during which little flow occurs between the chambers is usually shortened or absent. The ensuing A-wave is decreased at the time of atrial contraction because of elevated LV diastolic pressure. In this restrictive type of diastolic dysfunction the E/A ratio is increased (>2), and the deceleration time is shortened (<150 ms) as is the IVRT (<70 ms). A pseudo-normal pattern characterized by a normal E/A ratio and normal deceleration time exists between these two opposite abnormalities, because of an increase in the left atrial pressure (LAP).

Tissue velocity Doppler imaging (TDI) is a relatively new echocardiographic method that can be used to quantify myocardial velocities. When the

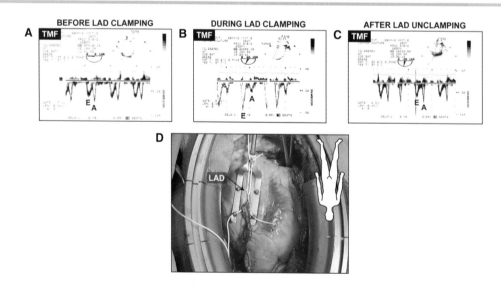

Figure 9.17   Diastolic function. (A–C) Pulsed wave Doppler of TMF velocities obtained in a 66-year-old man during off-pump bypass surgery. During the clamping of the LAD artery, the TMF pattern changed from **(A)** a predominant A wave, to **(B)** predominant E wave with short deceleration time suggesting a restrictive pattern. This reverted back to baseline after **(C)** completion of revascularization. Intraoperative aspect of the **(D)** LAD anastomosis is shown. *Abbreviations*: A, peak late diastolic TMF velocity; E, peak early diastolic TMF velocity; LAD, left anterior descending; TMF, transmitral flow. *Source*: Photo D courtesy of Dr. Raymond Cartier.

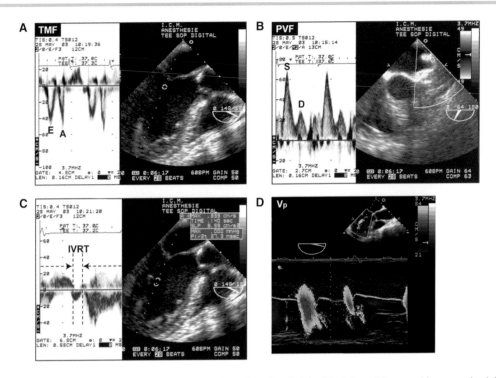

Figure 9.18 Diastolic dysfunction. Impaired left ventricular relaxation is identified in a 66-year-old man scheduled for coronary revascularization and aortic valve replacement. The predominant *A* wave on (**A**) the pulsed wave Doppler TMF, increased *S* wave on (**B**) the PVF, prolonged (**C**) IVRT of 140 ms (**C**) and reduced Vp on (**D**) color M-mode are consistent with grade 1/4 diastolic dysfunction. *Abbreviations*: A, peak late diastolic TMF velocity; D, peak diastolic PVF velocity; E, peak early diastolic TMF velocity; IVRT, isovolumic relaxation time; PVF, pulmonary venous flow; S, peak systolic PVF velocity; TMF, transmitral flow; Vp velocity of propagation.

pulsed wave Doppler sample volume is positioned on the myocardium at the annulus level, early and late diastolic motion is detected and a E_m/A_m *(or* E'/A' *or e/a)* ratio can be generated. This ratio, similar to the mitral inflow velocity *(E/A)* ratio, decreases with aging and ischemic heart disease (see Fig. 10.17). Studies in patients with ischemic heart disease have demonstrated that E_m is often reduced, the E_m/A_m ratio is <1, and IVRT is prolonged in patients when LV segmental dysfunction is present (17) (Fig. 9.18). In patients with acute myocardial infarction, Alam et al. (35) determined the systolic and diastolic velocities at four different sites on the mitral annulus (septal, anterior, lateral, and inferior sites). Interestingly, the early diastolic velocities were particularly affected above the site of infarction (E-wave 0.67 m/s at the anterior site compared with 0.82 m/s at the inferior site in anterior myocardial infarction, and 0.64 m/s at the inferior site compared with 0.95 m/s at the anterior site in inferior myocardial infarction ($p < 0.001$). Garcia-Fernandez et al. (36) also observed a reduced E_m and E_m/A_m ratio in patients with significant CAD, but normal segmental LV function.

COMPLICATIONS AND ASSOCIATED FINDINGS

In a cardiac emergency, the cause of abnormalities such as a new murmur on physical examination, EKG changes, a rise in myocardial enzymes, pulmonary

edema, and hemodynamic instability, must be rapidly established. These critically ill patients are often on mechanical respiratory and/or hemodynamic support. In this context, TEE is well tolerated, rapid, and provides additional information. It is particularly useful in excluding cardiac tamponade and aortic dissection (see Chapters 12 and 23) and in diagnosing the complications of acute myocardial infarction such as papillary muscle rupture or dysfunction, ventricular septal defect (VSD), ventricular aneurysm and/or pseudoaneurysm, severe LV dysfunction, right ventricular (RV) infarction, and ventricular free wall rupture. Assessment of mitral regurgitation (MR) is another indication for TEE, as this approach allows better visualization of the mitral apparatus and provides important information about both the severity and the mechanism of the regurgitation before surgery.

Ventricular Septal Defect

A VSD is a well-recognized complication of either anterior or inferior wall infarction, occurring in 1% to 2% of patients within the first week after infarction. The combination of a first transmural infarction in a territory supplied by a single diseased coronary vessel and the absence of collaterals contributes to increased shear stress between the necrotic tissue and the non-infarcted myocardium, where the rupture typically occurs (37). Clinically, the patient presents with a new holosystolic murmur (which may be absent in extreme shock) and worsening heart failure. Prompt diagnosis is essential because deterioration may be rapid and the presence of shock is associated with an increased risk of a fatal outcome.

The VSD usually appears on echocardiography as a single perforation that varies between one to several centimeters in diameter. It is often described as a "through and through" hole, but the VSD is usually irregularly shaped and serpiginous. The appearance of the defect may be preceded by formation of a septal aneurysm with thinning, which may be seen to bulge into the RV during systole. Defects with a serpentine course are more difficult to visualize.

When complicating an anterior infarction, the VSD is usually located near the apex in association with anterior akinesis (Figs. 9.19–9.22). When a VSD occurs after an inferior infarction, the apex is generally spared and the defect is in the basal septum, usually associated with an extensive area of inferior wall dyskinesis. Systolic flow can be identified by PW Doppler, but color flow Doppler imaging allows demonstration of the defect site, with a left-to-right mosaic signal indicating turbulence, which is best seen in the RV (Fig. 9.20). The right ventricular systolic pressure (RVSP) can be estimated from the difference between the systolic arterial pressure obtained by the cuff method or the arterial line, and the peak transventricular systolic

gradient obtained by CW Doppler (see Fig. 5.28). Accurate assessment of RV function is also critical, as this is a major predictor of outcome.

In general, patients with a large acute VSD do poorly with conservative management, dying from multiorgan failure as a result of systemic hypoperfusion. Therefore, surgery is warranted in almost all cases in which significant left to right shunting is present (Q_p:Q_s > 2:1), unless the patient is already moribund. The timing of surgery is crucial. In general, when a patient is deemed a candidate for surgery, an emergency operation is undertaken to prevent further hemodynamic deterioration. In a few patients with a small VSD and less significant shunting, conservative management for a period of 10 to 14 days may be warranted to permit the friable infarct to become more fibrous and facilitate subsequent surgery.

In some centers, an approach combining early percutaneous closure with delayed surgery has been implemented (see Chapter 29). However, percutaneous closure of the VSD may not be possible when there is a very large defect, or multiple defects. There have also been a few reports of the use of a ventricular assist device to bridge a patient to a delayed operative repair.

Intraoperative TEE permits detection of any residual shunt as well as assessment of regional and global ventricular function after weaning from cardiopulmonary bypass (CPB). The operative mortality for emergency repair of post-infarction VSDs ranges from 19% to more than 50%, and is predicted by patient age, preoperative shock, and RV function.

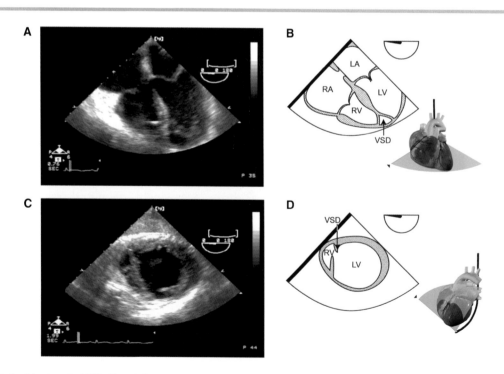

Figure 9.19 Apical ischemic VSD. Post-infarct apical VSD in a 56-year-old man with a recent anterior myocardial infarction. The VSD is located at the LV apex as seen in the (**A,B**) mid-esophageal four-chamber and (**C,D**) transgastric apical short-axis views. *Abbreviations*: LA, left atrium; LV, left ventricle; RA, right atrium; RV, right ventricle; VSD, ventricular septal defect.

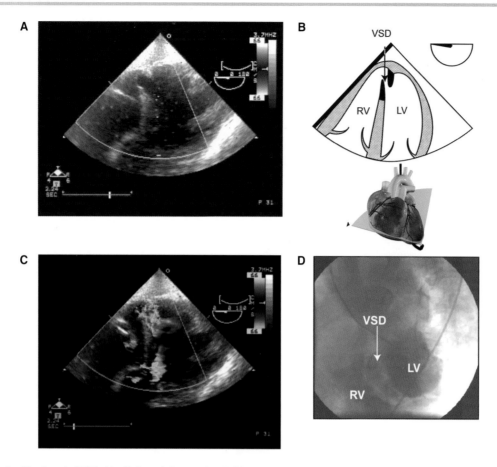

Figure 9.20   Apical ischemic VSD. (A–C) Post-infarct apical VSD in a 60-year-old man with anterior myocardial infarction using a deep transgastric long-axis view. The color Doppler localizes the VSD at the apex. **(D)** Left ventriculography demonstrates passage of contrast media from the LV to the RV through the serpiginous VSD. *Abbreviations*: LV, left ventricle; RV, right ventricle; VSD, ventricular septal defect. *Source*: Photo D courtesy of Dr. Philippe L. L'Allier.

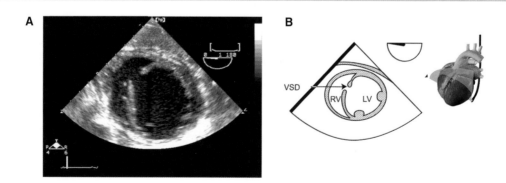

Figure 9.21   Ischemic VSD. Post-infarct VSD in a 62-year-old man. **(A,B)** Transgastric mid short-axis view of the VSD located in the mid-portion of the ventricular septum. *Abbreviations*: LV, left ventricle; RV, right ventricle; VSD, ventricular septal defect.

Papillary Muscle Dysfunction or Injury and Evaluation of Mitral Regurgitation

Dysfunction of the MV and support apparatus can occur in patients with myocardial infarction and lead to severe heart failure (Fig. 9.23). With acute partial or complete rupture of a papillary muscle (1% of myocardial infarctions), severe MR may occur suddenly and require prompt surgical correction. More commonly, the papillary muscle dysfunction will result from ischemia and segmental wall dysfunction, and be less severe. Because of its single blood supply from

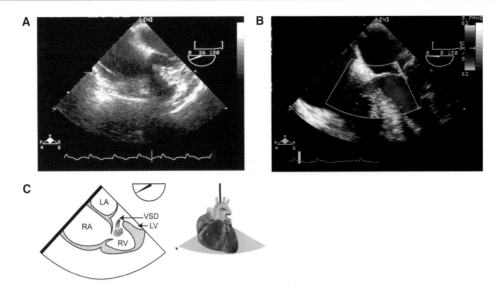

Figure 9.22   Ischemic VSD. New VSD in a 71-year-old man after inferior myocardial infarction. The mid-esophageal four-chamber view (**A,C**) with color Doppler (**B**) shows the acquired VSD in the basal septum. *Abbreviations*: LA, left atrium; LV, left ventricle; RA, right atrium; RV, right ventricle; VSD, ventricular septal defect.

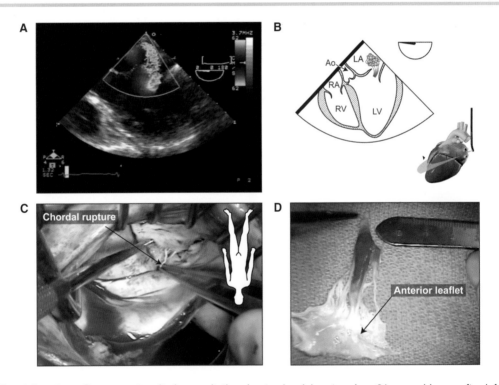

Figure 9.23   Chordal rupture. Severe acute mitral regurgitation due to chordal rupture in a 61-year-old man after inferior myocardial infarction. (**A,B**) Mid-esophageal color Doppler view with flail anterior (A3) leaflet and severe mitral regurgitation. The ruptured chorda (**C**) is seen at the time of surgery and after resection of the ischemic postero-medial papillary muscle (**D**). *Abbreviations*: Ao, aorta; LA, left atrium; LV, left ventricle; RA, right atrium; RV, right ventricle. *Source*: Photos C and D courtesy of Dr. Michel Pellerin.

the RCA, the posteromedial papillary muscle is the most often affected, usually in the setting of an acute inferior wall infarction (Fig. 9.24). In contrast, the anterolateral papillary muscle is rarely affected as it has a dual blood supply from the diagonal branches of the LAD artery and the circumflex artery (Fig. 9.24).

The diagnosis requires a high index of suspicion as the systolic murmur heard in patients with acute

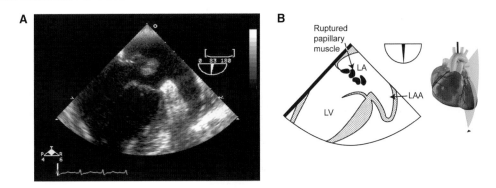

Figure 9.24 Ruptured papillary muscle. (A,B) Mid-esophageal two-chamber view shows a flail posterior mitral leaflet caused by acute postero-medial papillary muscle rupture following an inferior myocardial infarction. *Abbreviations*: LA, left atrium; LAA, left atrial appendage; LV, left ventricle.

severe MR may not be impressive because of near equalization of LV and LAP, and systemic hypotension. Because TTE has a high specificity but a low sensitivity in detecting papillary-muscle rupture, TEE is helpful when the TTE is nondiagnostic. Papillary muscle rupture is obvious when the head of the papillary muscle prolapses into the LA during systole (Fig. 9.24). A discrete mass can be seen attached to the prolapsing anterior or posterior leaflet. The longitudinal views may show the ruptured head of the papillary muscle moving back and forth between the LV and LA. A flail mitral leaflet, defined as an upturning of the leaflet toward the LA in systole, is often noted.

Mitral leaflet morphology will otherwise be normal in the setting of ischemic MR. When severe flail of one leaflet is present, the regurgitant orifice will be large and the mitral regurgitant flow will be less turbulent. As color Doppler techniques can be less reliable in such cases, PW Doppler interrogation of the pulmonary veins, easily visualized with TEE, is an important aspect of the evaluation of the severity of MR (see Chapter 17 section on ischemic mitral valve). Systolic reversal of pulmonary venous flow indicates severe MR. Because the characteristics of MR may change as a consequence of alterations in loading conditions, it is preferable to perform the TEE examination before the induction of general anesthesia.

Hemodynamic support with an intra-aortic balloon pump (IABP) will help augment forward flow during systole. Immediate operative intervention, prior to further clinical deterioration, is generally indicated. MV replacement, rather than an attempt at repair, is usually performed, as fixation of the ruptured papillary muscle head is ineffective. Coronary artery bypass grafting is performed concomitantly unless the distal coronary arteries are ungraftable. Intraoperative TEE permits assessment of the mitral prosthesis, as well as ventricular function. The mortality of the procedure is predicted by patient age, cardiogenic shock, and the extent of LV dysfunction.

Left Ventricular Thrombus

Left ventricular thrombus formation was a relatively frequent complication of acute myocardial infarction before the era of thrombolytic therapy. Thrombus is most often found after large anterior wall infarcts particularly when a ventricular aneurysm is present (Fig. 9.25). Although the superiority of TEE over TTE for the detection of atrial thrombi is undisputed, the situation is not as clear for the detection of ventricular thrombi. This has been attributed to difficulty in visualizing the LV apex from the esophagus because of limited resolution at increased depths. With the help of TEE, Chen et al. (38) examined the nature of equivocal echodense structures found with TTE in the LV apical region. Left ventricular thrombus was identified with certainty by TEE in 53% of their patients, and the investigators concluded that TTE and TEE can be complementary for this indication.

Particular attention should be paid to the detection of an LV thrombus in the presence of a recent or old anterior infarct, when there is a wall motion abnormality in the apical region, or when a cardiac source of embolus is suspected. The deep transgastric or transgastric two-chamber views are the most useful for its detection. It may occasionally be helpful to acquire a series of intermediate planes at the same level when doubt remains about a possible mass in the apical region (Fig. 9.26).

While the presence of an LV thrombus is not in itself an indication for operation, it is not uncommon for patients undergoing cardiac surgery to have a diagnosis of a possible or definite LV thrombus. Because of the risk of embolization during intraoperative cardiac manipulation, exploration of the LV cavity is warranted. In patients with an anteroapical infarct, this may be accomplished via a ventriculotomy through the scar. Alternatively, the LV cavity may be inspected by thoracoscopy through the aortic valve. Removal of the thrombus requires painstaking debridement but will prevent subsequent embolization.

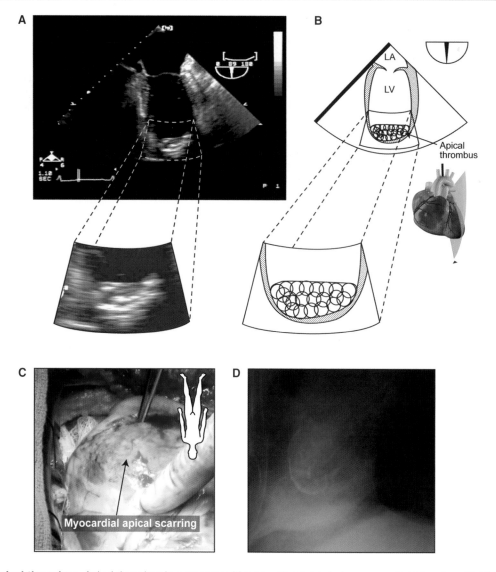

Figure 9.25   Apical thrombus. Apical thrombus in a 79-year-old man with prior anterior myocardial infarction. **(A,B)** Mid-esophageal two-chamber view with close-up view of the calcifed thrombus. **(C)** In the operating room, the thrombus was felt under the calcified scar. **(D)** Lateral chest X-ray shows the calcified aneurysm. *Abbreviations*: LA, left atrium; LV, left ventricle. *Source*: Photo C courtesy of Dr. Raymond Cartier.

Right Ventricular Infarction

Occasionally, an inferior myocardial infarction may extend into the RV free wall and compromise RV function. Because its management differs substantially from that of LV infarction, early and accurate diagnosis of RV infarction is imperative (39).

Echocardiography can be very helpful in the diagnosis of RV infarction (Fig. 9.27). Findings include RV regional hypokinesis or akinesis or global RV dysfunction (40). Left ventricular inferior wall involvement is usually present. Because infarction of the RV may sometimes be revealed only by dysfunction of its inferior wall, attention should be paid to this region in optimized transgastric SAX views. The SAX view has

been shown to have the highest sensitivity (82%), with a specificity ranging from 62% to 93% for hemodynamically significant RV infarction (41).

Right ventricular dilatation, abnormal interventricular septal motion, tricuspid regurgitation (TR), reduced systolic excursion of the tricuspid annulus, and dilatation of the inferior vena cava (IVC) can also point toward the correct diagnosis.

Interatrial septal bowing toward the LA, indicating an increased right to left atrial pressure gradient, is a prognostic marker in RV infarction as patients with this finding have a higher incidence of hypotension and heart block, resulting in a higher mortality (42). Pharmacologic and physiologic support of the RV after infarction is usually sufficient to allow recovery after

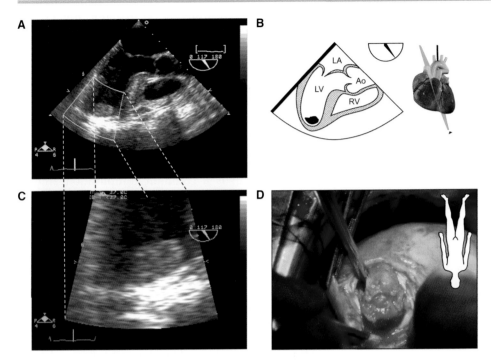

Figure 9.26   Apical thrombus. (A, B) LV apical ball thrombus is seen in a mid-esophageal long-axis view in a 68-year-old woman before thrombectomy. **(C)** Zooming is useful to confirm the observation. **(D)** Intraoperative findings are shown. *Abbreviations*: Ao, aorta; LA, left atrium; LV, left ventricle; RV, right ventricle. *Source*: Photo D courtesy of Dr. Michel Carrier. 🖱

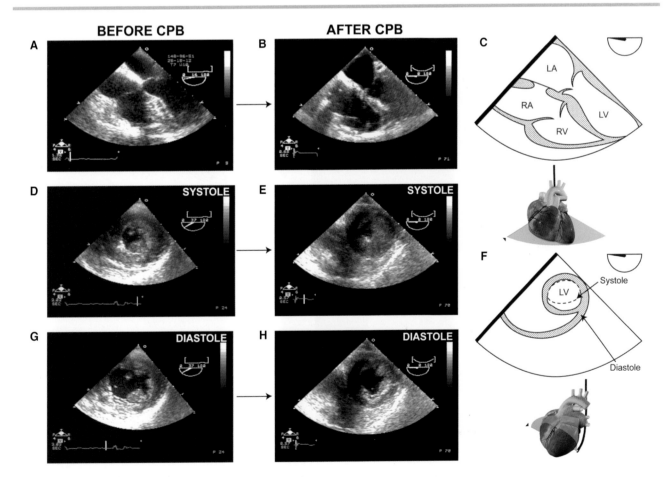

Figure 9.27   RV ischemia. Severe acute RV ischemic dysfunction is seen in a 71-year-old woman after CPB. The mid-esophageal four-chamber views demonstrate **(A–C)** the new appearance of acute RV dilatation, and LV inferior wall akinesis is indicated by **(D–H)** the dotted line on the transgastric mid short-axis views. *Abbreviations*: CPB, cardiopulmonary bypass; LA, left atrium; RA, right atrium; RV, right ventricle. 🖱

several days to a week, but in rare cases, temporary mechanical circulatory support with a right ventricular assist device (RVAD) may be required (43).

Ventricular Dilatation

Infarct expansion, defined as a disproportionate dilation of the infarct segment with stretching and thinning of the infarct zone, contributes to global cardiac enlargement with marked augmentation of left ventricular end-diastolic volume (LVEDV) within 48 hours. This in turn may be a harbinger of myocardial wall rupture and eventual LV aneurysm formation.

Two-dimensional echocardiography is ideally suited for assessing dynamic changes in LV shape and allows detection of infarct expansion. Echocardiographic features in LV dilatation include abrupt angulation in the contour of the proximal anteroseptal wall in the LAX view and a segmental dilation in the transgastric mid SAX view. At this level, direct measurement of the segment length is possible, the papillary muscles serving as internal landmark to divide the ventricle into anterior and posterior segments. While in the first few days after a transmural infarction, ventricular dilatation mostly involves the infarcted segment, remodeling of the entire LV cavity involving adjacent and nonischemic regions will be observed later.

Surgical intervention for global ventricular dilatation and dysfunction is usually limited to cardiac transplantation and implantation of ventricular assist devices. However, passive ventricular restraint devices have recently undergone clinical trials with promising results. Intraoperative TEE is a critical modality for assessment of all of these interventions.

Left Ventricular Aneurysm

A LV aneurysm is a common complication among survivors of nonreperfused transmural myocardial infarctions. Aneurysms occur four times more often at the apex and at the anterior wall than at the inferobasal wall (Fig. 9.28). True aneurysms result from expansion of the infarcted area and thinning of the myocardium. All three layers of the ventricular wall are preserved. The aneurysm may cause angina, heart failure, or ventricular arrhythmias.

Echocardiographically, the aneurysmal segments are dyskinetic or akinetic, and the distortion of the LV shape consists of an outpouching of ventricular myocardium with well defined borders (Figs. 9.29 and 9.30) and a wide neck persisting in diastole. However, differentiating a true aneurysm from a pseudoaneurysm may sometimes be difficult.

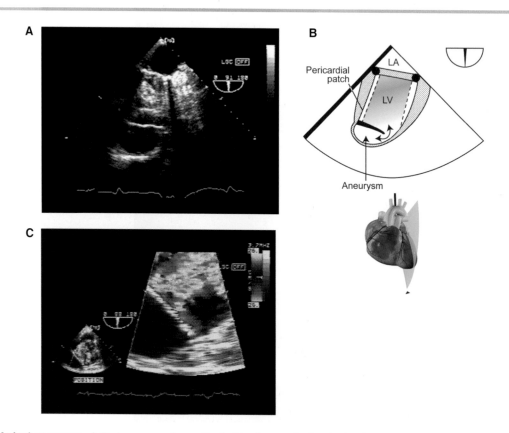

Figure 9.28 Apical aneurysm. Apical aneurysm in a patient with prior prosthetic mitral valve replacement and left ventricular aneurysm repair with a pericardial patch. **(A,B)** Mid-esophageal two-chamber view shows the dysfunctional pericardial patch above the apical aneurysm. **(C)** Zoomed color Doppler view of the patch confirms flow between the LV and the aneurysm. *Abbreviations*: LA, left atrium; LV, left ventricle.

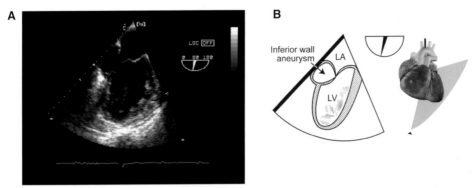

Cardiac index: 1.6 liter/min/m²

Figure 9.29 Inferior LV aneurysm. Large inferior basal left ventricular aneurysm in a 57-year-old man. (**A,B**) Mid-esophageal two-chamber view: presence of spontaneous contrast in the LV. The cardiac index was 1.6 L/min/m². *Abbreviations*: LA, left atrium; LV, left ventricle.

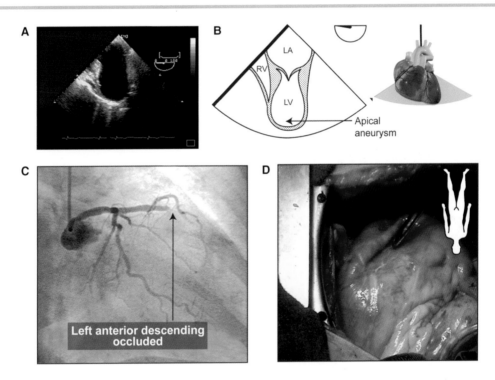

Figure 9.30 Apical LV aneurysm. Apical left ventricular aneurysm in a 71-year-old man. (**A,B**) Mid-esophageal four-chamber view. (**C**) Coronary angiography confirms complete obstruction of the left anterior descending artery. (**D**) Intraoperative findings include LV wall thinning. *Abbreviations*: LA, left atrium; LV, left ventricle; RV, right ventricle. *Source*: Photo D courtesy of Drs. Nicolas Noiseux and Michel Carrier.

A pseudoaneurysm, or false aneurysm, is a relatively rare complication of myocardial infarction, trauma, laceration or abscess. It results from the rupture of the ventricular free wall with a localized hemopericardium contained by adherent fibrous parietal pericardium (Fig. 9.31). Echocardiographically, this shows as an outpouching connected to the LV cavity by a narrow neck with an abrupt discontinuity (rupture) of the myocardial wall echoes, as opposed to the gradual thinning of the wall into a true aneurysm. Color flow imaging will also show bidirectional to-and-fro flow into the pseudoaneurysmal sac which may be partially filled with thrombus. During systole, expansion of the LV pseudoaneurysm contrasts with the LV cavity getting smaller. Figure 9.32 illustrates the difference in dimensions between a pseudo- and a true aneurysm.

A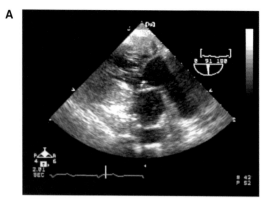

B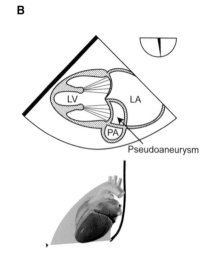

Pseudoaneurysm

C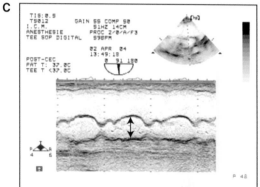

Figure 9.31 Pseudoaneurysm. (A,B) Transgastric two-chamber view of a 71-year-old man shows an unsuspected antero-basal LV pseudoaneurysm located near the LA. He had sustained a thoracic trauma 10 years ago. (C) The systolic expansion (arrow) and diastolic emptying of the pseudoaneurysm is shown on M-mode. *Abbreviations*: LA, left atrium; LV, left ventricle; PA, pulmonary artery.

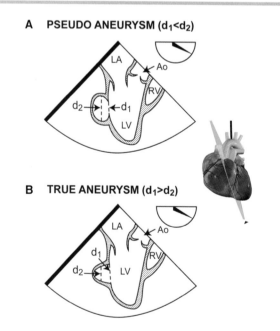

A   PSEUDO ANEURYSM (d₁<d₂)

B   TRUE ANEURYSM (d₁>d₂)

Figure 9.32 Pseudoaneurysm and true aneurysm. The differences between a pseudo and a true aneurysm are illustrated. (A) In a pseudoaneurysm, the diameter of the orifice (d1) is smaller than the diameter of the aneurysm (d2). (B) The opposite is found in a true aneurysm. *Abbreviations*: Ao, aorta; LA, left atrium; LV, left ventricle; RV, right ventricle.

Surgery for an LV true aneurysm involves resection of a portion of the aneurysmal segment and reconstruction of the defect by endoventricular aneurysmorrhaphy, a Dor approach, or a modified linear closure. Visually directed endocardial resection is often carried out when this substrate has resulted in significant ventricular arrhythmias. Ventricular aneurysm resection can result in dramatic improvements in ventricular geometry, wall stress, and oxygen demand, leading to symptomatic benefit. Mortality in elective procedures is low. In contrast, surgery for false aneurysms is usually required on an urgent or emergent basis and carries a much more substantial risk. As a ventricular pseudoaneurysm is a contained rupture, mortality with nonoperative management is high, and immediate surgery is warranted as soon as the diagnosis is made. Endoventricular patch repair of the ruptured transmural infarct is the theoretically ideal approach, but a variety of adjunctive techniques including glue and fixation have also been reported.

Myocardial Rupture

Rupture of the LV free wall is usually a sudden event that accounts for 8% to 17% of all in-hospital deaths in the postinfarction period. It generally occurs in elderly hypertensive patients with Q-wave infarcts. The sites of myocardial rupture are equally distributed between the anterior, posterior, and lateral walls. Usually, there is an acute clinical deterioration with recurrent chest pain, massive hemopericardium, hemodynamic deterioration, electromechanical dissociation, and sudden death within minutes. A subacute form has been recognized with ongoing chest pain, hemodynamic deterioration, and signs of pericardial tamponade. In this form, a very high index of suspicion, together with urgent echocardiographic examination, is crucial.

Two-dimensional echocardiography, the most sensitive and expeditious diagnostic modality for detecting subacute free wall rupture, shows a pericardial effusion and the presence of echogenic pericardial thrombus (44). The associated findings of regional dilatation and decreased wall thickness may increase the specificity of echocardiography for rupture. The sensitivity and specificity of echocardiographic criteria for the diagnosis of rupture were investigated prospectively by Lopez-Sendon et al. (45). The presence of cardiac tamponade, a pericardial effusion >5 mm, and high density intrapericardial echoes suggestive of thrombus have a diagnostic sensitivity of 70% and more and specificity more than 90% for the diagnosis of myocardial rupture. Direct identification of the myocardial tear with TTE is difficult and TEE may be useful in these unstable patients.

Uncontained rupture of the LV free wall precludes surgical intervention. A contained rupture that is not immediately fatal is treated as described earlier for a pseudoaneurysm.

CORONARY ARTERY IMAGING AND ASSESSMENT OF CORONARY VASODILATOR RESERVE

Although visualization rates of 58% to 90% have been described for the left main coronary artery with TTE, the right coronary and circumflex arteries are visualized only in 40% and 30% of cases, respectively. The superior resolution offered by the high frequency transducers (5–7 MHz) and the proximity of the coronary arteries to the esophagus account for improved coronary imaging with TEE. The numerous imaging planes provided by multiplane TEE allow enhanced visualization of extended lengths of the coronary arteries and provide a more reliable appraisal of any given abnormality (Figs. 9.2 and 9.3).

A stenosis is defined as an area of apparent luminal narrowing with high-intensity echoes followed by normal lumen. Color flow imaging helps to identify and follow the course of each coronary artery, a mosaic flow pattern often being present in the areas of suspected stenosis. Tardif et al. (46) reported a sensitivity and specificity of 100% for detection of left main coronary artery narrowing when compared with angiography. In addition, the proximal segments of the LAD, circumflex, and right coronary arteries were visualized in 84%, 80%, and 62% of patients, respectively. The sensitivity and specificity for detection of proximal stenosis were 80% and 100% for the LAD artery, 89% and 100% for the circumflex artery, and 82% and 100% for the RCA, respectively.

It is also possible to evaluate the coronary flow vasodilator reserve with TEE to determine the functional significance of a coronary stenosis (47). The coronary vasodilator reserve is defined as the ratio between the maximal (hyperemic) and baseline flows, and its assessment requires the use of a physiologic stimulus (coronary occlusion) or vasorelaxant drugs (adenosine, dipyridamole, papaverine). The coronary hyperemic response is impaired, not only in patients with a significant epicardial coronary stenosis but also in those with systemic hypertension, diabetes mellitus, hypertrophic cardiomyopathy, or syndrome X who can have microvascular disease. Using color Doppler flow and adjusting the PW Doppler sample window as parallel as possible to the coronary flow, baseline velocities are measured. A vasodilator drug is then administered and coronary blood flow velocity is measured again.

Iliceto et al. (48) studied LAD coronary artery velocities in 15 patients and observed that the flow reserve was 2.94 in normal patients and 1.46 in those with significant stenoses. A good correlation was found between coronary flow reserve as measured by TEE and directly by an intracoronary Doppler catheter (49). Redberg et al. (50) reported that a coronary flow reserve value greater than 2.1, as determined by TEE, had a sensitivity of 86%, a specificity of 79%, and positive and negative predictive values of 46% and 96%, respectively, in predicting the absence of a critical coronary artery narrowing, compared with quantitative coronary angiography.

CONCLUSION

TEE is a sensitive tool in the perioperative setting for detecting segmental myocardial ischemia and for assessing its impact on regional and global systolic functions and on diastolic function. In addition, mechanical complications of an acute myocardial infarction can be detected and evaluated thoroughly using the transesophageal approach.

REFERENCES

1. Daniel WG, Mugge A. Transesophageal echocardiography. N Engl J Med 1995; 332:1268–1279.
2. Cerqueira MD, Weissman NJ, Dilsizian V, et al. Standardized myocardial segmentation and nomenclature for tomographic imaging of the heart: a statement for healthcare professionals from the Cardiac Imaging Committee of the Council on Clinical Cardiology of the American Heart Association. Circulation 2002; 105:539–542.
3. Smith JS, Cahalan MK, Benefiel DJ, et al. Intraoperative detection of myocardial ischemia in high-risk patients: electrocardiography versus two-dimensional transesophageal echocardiography. Circulation 1985; 72:1015–1021.
4. Gallagher KP, Kumada T, Koziol JA, et al. Significance of regional wall thickening abnormalities relative to transmural myocardial perfusion in anesthetized dogs. Circulation 1980; 62:1266–1274.
5. Shah PM, Kyo S, Matsumura M, et al. Utility of biplane transesophageal echocardiography in left ventricular wall motion analysis. J Cardiothorac Vasc Anesth 1991; 5:316–319.

6. Rouine-Rapp K, Ionescu P, Balea M, et al. Detection of intraoperative segmental wall-motion abnormalities by transesophageal echocardiography: the incremental value of additional cross sections in the transverse and longitudinal planes. Anesth Analg 1996; 83:1141–1148.

7. van Daele ME, Sutherland GR, Mitchell MM, et al. Do changes in pulmonary capillary wedge pressure adequately reflect myocardial ischemia during anesthesia? A correlative preoperative hemodynamic, electrocardiographic, and transesophageal echocardiographic study. Circulation 1990; 81:865–871.

8. Leung JM, O'Kelly B, Browner WS, et al. Prognostic importance of postbypass regional wall-motion abnormalities in patients undergoing coronary artery bypass graft surgery. SPI Research Group. Anesthesiology 1989; 71:16–25.

9. Sheehan FH, Bolson EL, Dodge HT, et al. Advantages and applications of the centerline method for characterizing regional ventricular function. Circulation 1986; 74:293–305.

10. Shapiro E, Marier DL, St John Sutton MG, et al. Regional non-uniformity of wall dynamics in normal left ventricle. Br Heart J 1981; 45:264–270.

11. Force T, Kemper A, Perkins L, et al. Overestimation of infarct size by quantitative two-dimensional echocardiography: the role of tethering and of analytic procedures. Circulation 1986; 73:1360–1368.

12. Lang RM, Bierig M, Devereux RB, et al. Recommendations for chamber quantification: a report from the American Society of Echocardiography's Guidelines and Standards Committee and the Chamber Quantification Writing Group, developed in conjunction with the European Association of Echocardiography, a branch of the European Society of Cardiology. J Am Soc Echocardiogr 2005; 18: 1440–1463.

13. Berning J, Steensgaard-Hansen F. Early estimation of risk by echocardiographic determination of wall motion index in an unselected population with acute myocardial infarction. Am J Cardiol 1990; 65:567–576.

14. Kan G, Visser CA, Koolen JJ, et al. Short and long term predictive value of admission wall motion score in acute myocardial infarction. A cross sectional echocardiographic study of 345 patients. Br Heart J 1986; 56:422–427.

15. Maclaren G, Kluger R, Prior D, et al. Tissue Doppler, strain, and strain rate echocardiography: principles and potential perioperative applications. J Cardiothorac Vasc Anesth 2006; 20:583–593.

16. Bach DS, Armstrong WF, Donovan CL, et al. Quantitative Doppler tissue imaging for assessment of regional myocardial velocities during transient ischemia and reperfusion. Am Heart J 1996; 132:721–725.

17. Derumeaux G, Ovize M, Loufoua J, et al. Doppler tissue imaging quantitates regional wall motion during myocardial ischemia and reperfusion. Circulation 1998; 97:1970–1977.

18. Edvardsen T, Aakhus S, Endresen K, et al. Acute regional myocardial ischemia identified by 2-dimensional multiregion tissue Doppler imaging technique. J Am Soc Echocardiogr 2000; 13:986–994.

19. Palka P, Lange A, Donnelly JE, et al. Differentiation between restrictive cardiomyopathy and constrictive pericarditis by early diastolic doppler myocardial velocity gradient at the posterior wall. Circulation 2000; 102:655–662.

20. Abraham TP, Nishimura RA, Holmes DR Jr, et al. Strain rate imaging for assessment of regional myocardial function: results from a clinical model of septal ablation. Circulation 2002; 105:1403–1406.

21. Pislaru C, Abraham TP, Belohlavek M. Strain and strain rate echocardiography. Curr Opin Cardiol 2002; 17:443–454.

22. Yip G, Abraham T, Belohlavek M, et al. Clinical applications of strain rate imaging. J Am Soc Echocardiogr 2003; 16:1334–1342.

23. Sutherland GR, Di Salvo G, Claus P, et al. Strain and strain rate imaging: a new clinical approach to quantifying regional myocardial function. J Am Soc Echocardiogr 2004; 17:788–802.

24. Skulstad H, Urheim S, Edvardsen T, et al. Grading of myocardial dysfunction by tissue Doppler echocardiography: a comparison between velocity, displacement, and strain imaging in acute ischemia. J Am Coll Cardiol 2006; 47:1672–1682.

25. Leitman M, Lysyansky P, Sidenko S, et al. Two-dimensional strain-a novel software for real-time quantitative echocardiographic assessment of myocardial function. J Am Soc Echocardiogr 2004; 17:1021–1029.

26. Becker M, Hoffmann R, Kuhl HP, et al. Analysis of myocardial deformation based on ultrasonic pixel tracking to determine transmurality in chronic myocardial infarction. Eur Heart J 2006; 27:2560–2566.

27. Amundsen BH, Helle-Valle T, Edvardsen T, et al. Noninvasive myocardial strain measurement by speckle tracking echocardiography: validation against sonomicrometry and tagged magnetic resonance imaging. J Am Coll Cardiol 2006; 47:789–793.

28. Monaghan MJ. Role of real time 3D echocardiography in evaluating the left ventricle. Heart 2006; 92:131–136.

29. Marcovitz PA, Bach DS, Mathias W, et al. Paradoxic hypotension during dobutamine stress echocardiography: clinical and diagnostic implications. J Am Coll Cardiol 1993; 21:1080–1086.

30. Cigarroa CG, deFilippi CR, Brickner ME, et al. Dobutamine stress echocardiography identifies hibernating myocardium and predicts recovery of left ventricular function after coronary revascularization. Circulation 1993; 88:430–436.

31. Smart SC, Sawada S, Ryan T, et al. Low-dose dobutamine echocardiography detects reversible dysfunction after thrombolytic therapy of acute myocardial infarction. Circulation 1993; 88:405–415.

32. Arnese M, Cornel JH, Salustri A, et al. Prediction of improvement of regional left ventricular function after surgical revascularization. A comparison of low-dose dobutamine echocardiography with 201Tl single-photon emission computed tomography. Circulation 1995; 91:2748–2752.

33. Perrone-Filardi P, Pace L, Prastaro M, et al. Assessment of myocardial viability in patients with chronic coronary artery disease. Rest-4-hour-24-hour 201Tl tomography versus dobutamine echocardiography. Circulation 1996; 94: 2712–2719.

34. Bonow RO. Identification of viable myocardium. Circulation 1996; 94:2674–2680.

35. Alam M, Wardell J, Andersson E, et al. Effects of first myocardial infarction on left ventricular systolic and diastolic function with the use of mitral annular velocity determined by pulsed wave doppler tissue imaging. J Am Soc Echocardiogr 2000; 13:343–352.

36. Garcia-Fernandez MA, Azevedo J, Moreno M, et al. Regional diastolic function in ischaemic heart disease using pulsed wave Doppler tissue imaging. Eur Heart J 1999; 20:496–505.

37. Hill JD, Stiles QR. Acute ischemic ventricular septal defect. Circulation 1989; 79:I112–I115.

38. Chen C, Koschyk D, Hamm C, et al. Usefulness of transesophageal echocardiography in identifying small left ventricular apical thrombus. J Am Coll Cardiol 1993; 21:208–215.

39. Kinch JW, Ryan TJ. Right ventricular infarction. N Engl J Med 1994; 330:1211–1217.

40. Haddad F, Couture P, Tousignant C, et al. The right ventricle in cardiac surgery, a perioperative perspective. I. Anatomy, physiology, and assessment. Anesth Analg 2009; 108:407–421.

41. Lopez-Sendon J, Garcia-Fernandez MA, Coma-Canella I, et al. Segmental right ventricular function after acute myocardial infarction: two-dimensional echocardiographic study in 63 patients. Am J Cardiol 1983; 51:390–396.

42. Lopez-Sendon J, Lopez de SE, Roldan I, et al. Inversion of the normal interatrial septum convexity in acute myocardial infarction: incidence, clinical relevance and prognostic significance. J Am Coll Cardiol 1990; 15:801–805.

43. Haddad F, Couture P, Tousignant C, et al. The right ventricle in cardiac surgery, a perioperative perspective. II. Pathophysiology, clinical importance, and management. Anesth Analg 2009; 108:422–433.

44. Hermoni Y, Engel PJ. Two-dimensional echocardiography in cardiac rupture. Am J Cardiol 1986; 57:180–181.

45. Lopez-Sendon J, Gonzalez A, Lopez de SE, et al. Diagnosis of subacute ventricular wall rupture after acute myocardial infarction: sensitivity and specificity of clinical, hemodynamic and echocardiographic criteria. J Am Coll Cardiol 1992; 19:1145–1153.

46. Tardif JC, Vannan MA, Taylor K, et al. Delineation of extended lengths of coronary arteries by multiplane transesophageal echocardiography. J Am Coll Cardiol 1994; 24:909–919.

47. Wilson RF, Marcus ML, White CW. Prediction of the physiologic significance of coronary arterial lesions by quantitative lesion geometry in patients with limited coronary artery disease. Circulation 1987; 75:723–732.

48. Iliceto S, Marangelli V, Memmola C, et al. Transesophageal Doppler echocardiography evaluation of coronary blood flow velocity in baseline conditions and during dipyridamole-induced coronary vasodilation. Circulation 1991; 83:61–69.

49. Zehetgruber M, Porenta G, Mundigler G, et al. Transesophageal versus intracoronary Doppler measurements for calculation of coronary flow reserve. Cardiovasc Res 1997; 36:21–27.

50. Redberg RF, Sobol Y, Chou TM, et al. Adenosine-induced coronary vasodilation during transesophageal Doppler echocardiography. Rapid and safe measurement of coronary flow reserve ratio can predict significant left anterior descending coronary stenosis. Circulation 1995; 92:190–196.

10

Global Ventricular Function and Hemodynamics

André Y. Denault and Pierre Couture
Université de Montréal, Montreal, Quebec, Canada

Jean Buithieu
McGill University, Montreal, Quebec, Canada

Annette Vegas
University of Toronto, Toronto, Ontario, Canada

INTRODUCTION

An important role of perioperative transesophageal echocardiography (TEE) includes the determination of baseline systolic and diastolic function of the right ventricle (RV) and left ventricle (LV) before a surgical procedure. Changes in ventricular function during cardiac and noncardiac procedures in some cases may lead to severe hemodynamic instability, which is considered a category 1 indication for the use of TEE when unresponsive to therapy (1).

NORMAL RIGHT AND LEFT VENTRICULAR MORPHOLOGY

The normal ventricular morphology and quantitative evaluation of ventricular size and function are also described in Chapters 4 and 5 and in the American Society of Echocardiography (ASE) guidelines (2,3).

NORMAL RIGHT AND LEFT VENTRICULAR PHYSIOLOGY

Descent of the Base, Segmental Contraction, and Septal Curvature

Several points should be emphasized in the evaluation of ventricular function. Systolic contraction of myocardial fibers results in an increase of LV wall thickness and a decrease in wall diameter and length. There are normal regional variations in the thickening of ventricular segments with increasing contractility from the base to the apex. Normal LV function is associated with both radial shortening and longitudinal 15–20 mm displacement of the base toward the apex, which can be quantified using M-mode (4) or tissue Doppler imaging (5), and correlates with ejection fraction (Fig. 10.1). There is a normal rightward ventricular septal curvature because normal LV pressure is superior to RV pressure.

The physiology of the RV is distinctly different from that of the LV (Table 10.1) (6). The output of the RV must match that of the LV. It does this, however, with one-fourth to one-fifth of the stroke work. This particular arrangement is heavily dependent on the low vascular resistance of the pulmonary bed. The RV is, therefore, exquisitely afterload-sensitive and is prone to failure if there are acute changes. Both the RV and the LV are arranged in series and, therefore, the output of one must necessarily influence the output of the other. Because both are in close proximity and are contained within the pericardium, there is the possibility of direct interaction through the interventricular septum (IVS). Furthermore, the superficial muscle fibers of the RV are shared with the LV. Up to 50% of RV work can be generated by the LV. In fact, in experiments where the LV and RV were electrically isolated, pacing the LV resulted in the generation of a normal RV pressure trace while pacing the RV did not result in any significant RV pressure development. The IVS is also important to RV function. Inactivation of the septum can result in a significant decline in RV pressure development. Furthermore, large increases in RV size and septal shifting result in a decrease in LV output.

Pressure-Volume Relationship

The relationship between ventricular function and hemodynamics is best described using pressure-volume curves. These curves allow the graphical description of ventricular function by displaying the volume of a single cardiac cycle against pressure over time (Fig. 10.2). This includes seven time-related events. Diastole starts with isovolumic relaxation (phase 4), continues with the opening of the mitral valve (MV) and early LV filling, diastasis and atrial systole (phases 5–7) and ends with MV closure prior to isovolumic contraction (phase 1). Systole begins with the isovolumic contraction (phase 1), proceeds with the opening of the aortic valve (AoV) and ejection of

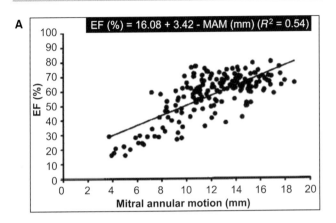

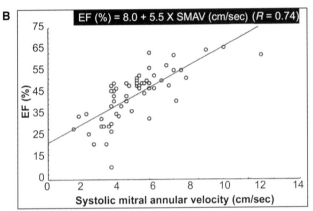

Figure 10.1 Annular motion and EF. Compare the relationship between EF and MAM in 182 patients (**A**) and SMAV by tissue Doppler in 60 patients (**B**). *Abbreviations*: EF, ejection fraction; MAM, mitral annular motion; SMAV, systolic mitral annular velocity. *Source*: Adapted with permission from Refs. 4 and 5.

the stroke volume (SV) (phases 2 and 3). The pressure-volume diagram can be obtained through continuous pressure and volume measurement but is rarely done in clinical practice.

Individual determinants of the pressure-volume curve may be obtained using TEE to assess volumes, and estimation of pressures using a pulmonary artery catheter and a systemic arterial pressure catheter

(Fig. 10.3). The left ventricular end-diastolic pressure (LVEDP) is estimated by the pulmonary artery occlusion pressure (Paop) or pulmonary capillary wedge pressure (PCWP) at end diastole, in the absence of any obstruction between the pulmonary capillary bed and the LV such as mitral stenosis. Systolic arterial pressure (SAP) estimates left ventricular end-systolic pressure (LVESP) if aortic valvular obstruction is absent (7,8). The left ventricular end-systolic area (LVESA) and left ventricular end-diastolic area (LVEDA) obtained from TEE transgastric (TG) short-axis (SAX) views approximate the left ventricular end-systolic volume (LVESV) and left ventricular end-diastolic volume (LVEDV). The SV is calculated from the ratio of the thermodilution-derived cardiac output (CO) to the heart rate (HR) or through Doppler measurement (see Chapter 5, equation 5.30). The area within the left ventricular pressure-volume curve is the left ventricular stroke work [LVSW = SV × (mean arterial pressure, or MAP-Paop) × 0.0136], and this value is obtained through automated calculation of the cardiopulmonary profile.

The RV pressure-volume loop, on the other hand, is more trapezoidal or triangular shaped (Fig. 10.4). There is a very small isovolumic phase as the RV must overcome only the low pressure system of the pulmonary vasculature. The ejection phase begins early and the RV continues to eject well beyond the establishment of peak RV pressure during systole. This is possible because of the low impedance of the lung vasculature and a low pulmonary artery pressure. There then follows a short isovolumic relaxation phase. If the pulmonary vascular resistance rises, the RV pressure-volume loop may assume a more square shape.

Preload, afterload, and contractility, the determinants of cardiac function, are easily plotted on the LV pressure-volume curves (Fig. 10.5). Each change in these determinants will affect the pressure-volume relationship differently. In the following discussion, when possible, the effects of changes in cardiac function and their determinants will be explained by using the pressure-volume relationship.

Preload

A decrease in preload is associated with a fall in LVEDV and LVEDP resulting in a leftward and downward shift

Table 10.1 Characteristics of Right and Left Ventricle

Characteristics	Right ventricle	Left ventricle
Structure	Inflow region, trabeculated myocardium, infundibulum	No infundibulum, mitro-aortic continuity
Shape	From the side: triangular; cross section; crescentic	Elliptic
Volume (end diastolic)	49–101 mL/m^2	44–89 mL/m^2
Mass (g/m^2)	<35 g/m^2 ≈ 1/6 LV mass	<130 g/m^2 (men); <100 g/m^2 (women)
Ejection fraction	40–68% >45%[a]	57–74% >50%[a]
Ventricular elastance (mmHg/mL)	1.30 ± 0.84	5.48 ± 1.23
Ventricular compliance	Higher compliance than LV	5.0 ± 0.52 × 10^{-2}
Adaptation to disease	Better adaptation to volume overload states	Better adaptation to pressure overload states

Normal parameters of the right compared with the left ventricle. [a]Range of normal values depends on method of acquisition.
Source: With permission from Ref. 6.

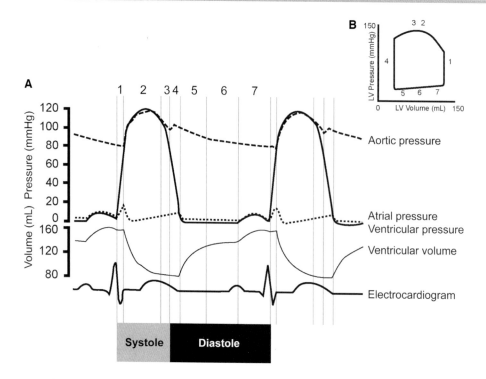

Figure 10.2 Pressure and volume during a cardiac cycle. (**A**) Changes in aortic, atrial and ventricular pressures, and ventricular volume in relation to the electrocardiogram are presented. LV pressure and volume over time during a cardiac cycle is characterized by seven time-related events. Isovolumic contraction (1) is followed by early (2) and late (3) ejection. Diastole starts with isovolumic relaxation (4) followed by the early filling phase after the opening of the mitral valve (5), diastasis (6), and atrial contraction (7). (**B**) The corresponding LV pressure-volume relationship during one cardiac cycle is shown. *Abbreviation*: LV, left ventricle.

of the pressure-volume curve (Fig. 10.5A). It is difficult, clinically, to differentiate between hypovolemia and reduced systemic vascular resistance (SVR) using TEE because both conditions will lead to reduction in preload. Both two-dimensional (2D) and Doppler indices have been used, and validated, to estimate LV filling pressure and volume. Clinically useful echocardiographic 2D images for the diagnosis of reduced preload are the progressive reduction in LVEDA, LV end-systolic cavity obliteration (Fig. 10.6), interatrial septal displacement (Fig. 10.7), and both inferior (Fig. 10.8) and superior vena cava collapsibility (10) (Fig. 10.9). These indices will be discussed in more detail in section "Fluid Responsiveness."

Afterload

In the preoperative clinical setting, echocardiographic indices of afterload are not routinely measured. Afterload can, however, be estimated using the arterial elastance, that is, the ratio of LVESP over the LVESV (11), or by estimating the LV end-systolic wall stress, which combines M-mode or 2D measurements with pressure data (see equations 10.11 and 10.12). An increase in afterload is associated with an increase in the LVESP necessary to open the AoV and, consequently, an increase in LVESV (Fig. 10.5B), while the

slope of the relationship or the elastance remains unchanged. An often unrecognized important clinical scenario leading to an increase in afterload is seen with the systolic anterior motion (SAM) of the MV and its associated left ventricular outflow tract (LVOT) obstruction which results in mosaic flow due to aliasing on color imaging of the LVOT (Fig. 10.10).

Contractility and Ventricular Performance

Changes in preload and afterload displaces the pressure-volume loops along a line called maximal elastance. Decreasing (or increasing) contractility is associated with a downward (or upward) shift of the elastance and a displacement of the pressure-volume relationship toward the right (or the left). In Figure 10.5C, for example, the decrease in contractility (dotted loop) results in a greater LVESV for the same LVESP. The concept of elastance is important to understand because this measure is considered relatively independent of changes in preload and afterload. Measurements such as ejection fraction and CO are not pure indices of contractility but rather markers of ventricular performance. Consequently, changes in preload or afterload may affect the ejection fraction but no changes in elastance will be observed. A study with patients undergoing coronary artery bypass also

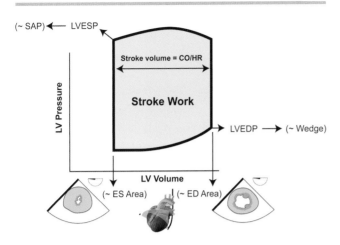

Figure 10.3 LV pressure-volume loop. The LV pressure-volume relationship during one cardiac cycle is shown. The LVESP can be estimated using SAP and the LVEDP can be estimated with the pulmonary artery-derived "wedge" pressure at end-diastole. Using echocardiography, the LV ES volume can be estimated with the ES area and the LV ED volume can be estimated with the ED area. The stroke volume, which is the difference between the ED volume and the ES volume, can be calculated from the ratio of the CO obtained by Doppler or thermodilution divided by HR. The LV stroke work corresponds to the area of the LV pressure-volume diagram (gray area). Changes in LV compliance can explain why filling pressure does not always correlate with ventricular size. *Abbreviations*: CO, cardiac output; ED, end-diastolic; ES, end-systolic; HR, heart rate; LV, left ventricle; LVED, left ventricular end-diastolic; LVEDP, LV end-diastolic pressure; LVES, left ventricular end-systolic; LVESP, LV end-systolic pressure; SAP, systolic arterial pressure.

documented the fact that despite the absence of significant postoperative change in SV, fractional area change (FAC) and CO, the elastance index suggested a reduction in contractility after the surgical procedure (Fig. 10.11) (12). In clinical practice, elastance is rarely obtained because artificial preload alteration is required to calculate the slope of the pressure-volume relationship.

The most commonly used echocardiographic evaluation of ventricular performance includes measurements of FAC, ejection fraction, and CO. FAC provides an estimation of ejection fraction and is usually obtained from a TG view (Fig. 10.6).

ASSESSMENT OF GLOBAL LEFT VENTRICULAR SYSTOLIC FUNCTION

Several indices of LV global systolic function can be derived from simple linear and area LV measurements and calculation of LV volume. Single measurements used to assess LV function are less accurate in the presence of regional wall motion abnormalities involving the other ventricular segments. It is important to note that some indices assess LV systolic performance, and these should not be confused with measurements of ejection fraction. Ejection fraction calculation can be obtained through the measurement of ventricular volumes from the four- and two-chamber views using one of several formulas (see Fig. 5.22) available for volume measurements (3). The SV and CO can be calculated from either 2D volume end-diastolic and end-systolic measurements or volumetric Doppler-derived results. Other indirect echocardiographic signs useful in the identification of reduced left ventricular systolic function include the presence of intracavitary spontaneous echo contrast, increased anterior MV leaflet septal distance (see Fig. 11.19), reduced mitral annular displacement (13), and an abnormal myocardial performance index (MPI) (14).

Stroke Volume, Cardiac Output, and Cardiac Index

The SV is the blood volume ejected from the LV during each systole and can be calculated from the difference between the LVEDV and LVESV obtained

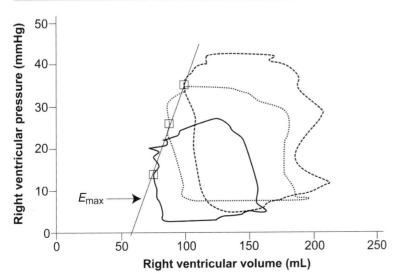

Figure 10.4 RV pressure-volume loop. The RV pressure-volume loops are shown under different loading conditions. The slope of maximum time varying elastance (E_{max}) is displayed on the graph. *Abbreviation*: RV, right ventricle. *Source*: With permission from Ref. 6 and adapted from Ref. 9.

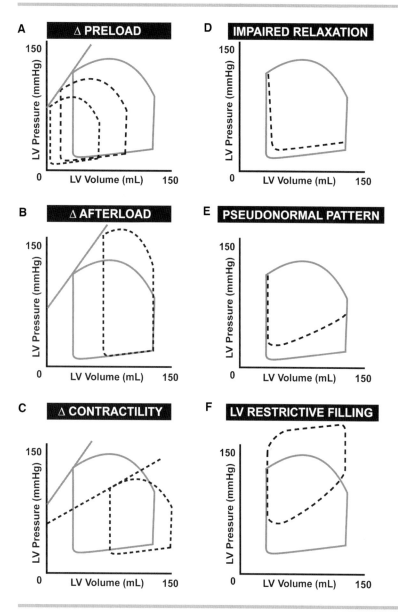

Figure 10.5   Pressure volume relationship. LV pressure-volume relationship with changes in preload, afterload, contractility, and diastolic function is shown. (**A–C**) Changes in systolic function. (**A**) Decrease in preload: leftward and downward shift of the LV pressure-volume relationship with a reduction in EDP and in EDV. The elastance (left upper line) connects all the end-systolic points through which the pressure-volume diagram moves. (**B**) Increase in afterload: rightward and upward shift of the pressure-volume relationship with an increase in end-systolic pressure and in end-systolic volume. (**C**) Reduction in contractility: downward shift of the elastance with rightward displacement of the pressure-volume diagram. (**D–F**) Changes in diastolic function: with increasing severity, higher EDP is observed for the same EDV. (**D**) Stage I diastolic dysfunction: delayed LV relaxation. (**E**) Stage II diastolic dysfunction: pseudonormal filling pattern. (**F**) Stage III diastolic dysfunction: restrictive filling. *Abbreviations*: EDP, end-diastolic pressure; EDV, end-diastolic volume; LV, left ventricle.

by the previously described M-mode or 2D echocardiographic methods (Fig. 10.12). Alternatively, the SV can be calculated by the Doppler volumetric method (see equation 5.30).

The CO is the amount of blood pumped by the heart per minute and most commonly reported in liters per minute:

$$SV = LVEDV - LVESV \qquad (10.1)$$

$$CO = SV \times HR \times 0.001 \qquad (10.2)$$

where CO is the cardiac output (L/min), SV is the stroke volume (mL), and HR is the heart rate (bpm).

The CO is often indexed to the patient's body size to facilitate comparison with reference values. The cardiac index (CI) is obtained by the equation:

$$CI = \frac{CO}{BSA} \qquad (10.3)$$

where CI is the cardiac index (in L/min/m^2) and BSA is the body surface area (m^2).

Ejection Fraction

The left ventricular ejection fraction (LVEF) is defined as the percentage (or fraction) of the LVEDV which is ejected with each systole, that is, the ratio of the SV to the LVEDV (Fig. 10.12). The LVEF (in %) can be expressed by the equation:

$$LVEF = \frac{SV}{LVEDV} \times 100 \qquad (10.4)$$

$$= \frac{LVEDV - LVESV}{LVEDV} \times 100$$

where LVEF is the left ventricular ejection fraction (%), SV is the stroke volume (mL), LVEDV is the left ventricular end-diastolic volume (mL), and LVESV is

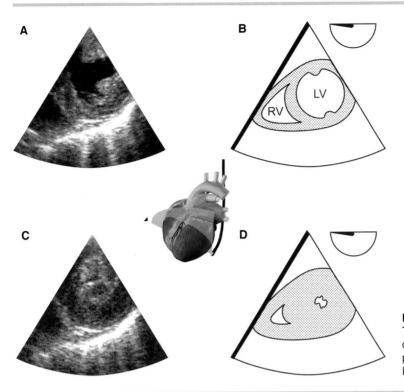

Figure 10.6 LV end-systolic cavity obliteration.
Transgastric mid short-axis views of the LV during diastole (**A,B**) and systole (**C,D**) in a hypovolemic patient demonstrates cavity obliteration. *Abbreviations*: LV, left ventricle; RV, right ventricle.

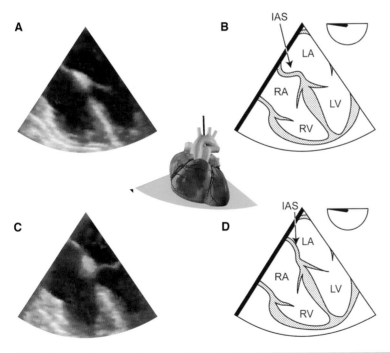

Figure 10.7 Interatrial septal displacement. The use of IAS displacement for the assessment of filling pressure is seen from the mid-esophageal four-chamber view in a patient following cardiopulmonary bypass. (**A,B**) The IAS is deviated to the right implying the atrial pressure is higher on the left than on the right. The pulmonary artery occlusion pressure or "wedge" was 17 mmHg. (**C,D**) Following vasodilator therapy, the "wedge" pressure dropped to 7 mmHg and now the IAS is displaced toward the left. This is consistent with the left atrial pressure being lower than the right. *Abbreviations*: IAS, interatrial septum; LA, left atrium; LV, left ventricle; RA, right atrium; RV, right ventricle.

the left ventricular end-systolic volume (mL). The normal LVEF is 55% to 75%.

Ejection fraction is a measure of myocardial performance and represents the efficiency of the global cardiac pump to eject part of its end-diastolic volume. Estimation of LVEF is affected by cardiac preload, afterload, and myocardial contractility, as discussed previously. Ejection fraction does not

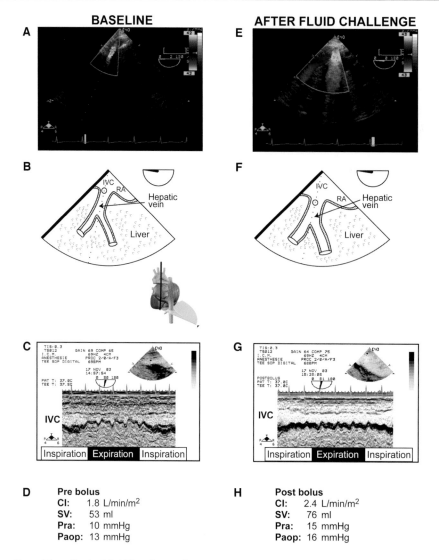

BASELINE

AFTER FLUID CHALLENGE

D **Pre bolus**
CI: 1.8 L/min/m²
SV: 53 ml
Pra: 10 mmHg
Paop: 13 mmHg

H **Post bolus**
CI: 2.4 L/min/m²
SV: 76 ml
Pra: 15 mmHg
Paop: 16 mmHg

Figure 10.8   Fluid loading. The effect of fluid loading on hemodynamic and echocardiographic parameters in a 62-year-old man on mechanical ventilation is shown. **(A,B)** At baseline, the diameter of the IVC and hepatic veins is small. **(C)** Using M-mode, the IVC collapses during the lowest intrathoracic pressure period, the expiration phase of positive-pressure ventilation. **(D)** The cardiac index CI is 1.8 L/min/m². **(E–G)** After a fluid challenge, the diameter of the IVC and hepatic veins has enlarged without significant IVC collapse. **(H)** The CI and filling pressure increased. *Abbreviations*: CI, cardiac index; IVC, inferior vena cava; Paop, pulmonary artery occlusion pressure; Pra, right atrial pressure; RA, right atrium; SV, stroke volume.

necessarily mirror CO. A patient may have a high ejection fraction but a small SV (and CO), as occurs in hypovolemia. In addition, for the same SV or CO, LVEF can be significantly different (15) (Fig. 10.13).

Linear Measurements

Simple linear measurements can be used in different formulas to assess global LV systolic performance. The ASE no longer recommends the use of linear measurements to assess ejection fraction (3).

Fractional Shortening

Left ventricular fractional shortening (FS) is defined as the percentage of change (shortening) of the LV cavity dimension with each systole (Fig. 10.14). The FS (%) is expressed by the equation:

$$FS = \frac{LVEDD - LVESD}{LVEDD} \times 100 \qquad (10.5)$$

where FS is the fractional shortening (%), LVEDD is the left ventricular end-diastolic dimension (cm), and LVESD is the left ventricular end-systolic

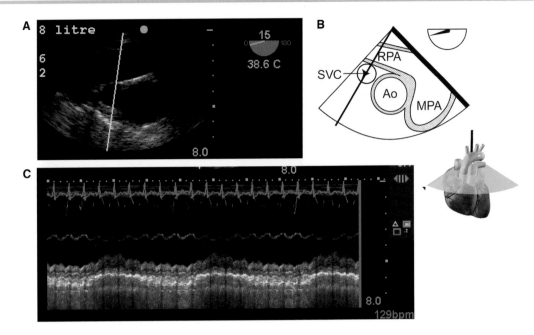

Figure 10.9 Respiratory variation of the SVC. (A,B) Mid-esophageal ascending Ao short-axis view in a 76-year-old man in the intensive care unit after removal of 1.8 liters with dialysis is shown. **(C)** Using M-mode, significant respiratory variation of the diameter of the SVC was present. *Abbreviations*: Ao, aorta; MPA, main pulmonary artery; RPA, right pulmonary artery; SVC, superior vena cava.

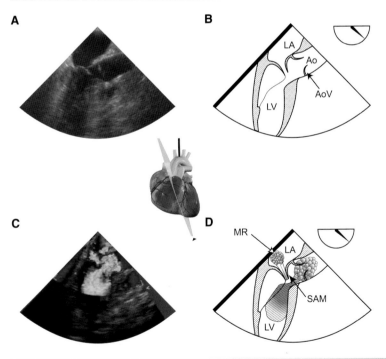

Figure 10.10 Dynamic LVOT obstruction. (A–D) Mid-esophageal long-axis views in a 38-year-old man with septic shock and hemodynamic instability are shown. Part of the anterior mitral valve leaflet is obstructing the LVOT **(A,B)** associated with MR seen with color Doppler **(C,D)**. His hemodynamic condition improved with fluid and ß-blockade. *Abbreviations*: Ao, aorta; AoV, aortic valve; LA, left atrium; LV, left ventricle; LVOT, left ventricular outflow tract; MR, mitral regurgitation; SAM, systolic anterior motion.

dimension (cm). The normal FS is 26% to 45% (16,17). In patients with LV concentric hypertrophy, midwall fractional shortening is preferred and can be computed from linear measurements of cavity size (3,18,19).

Ejection Fraction by Quinones Method

The LVEF can be determined from estimation of the end-diastolic and end-systolic volumes derived from

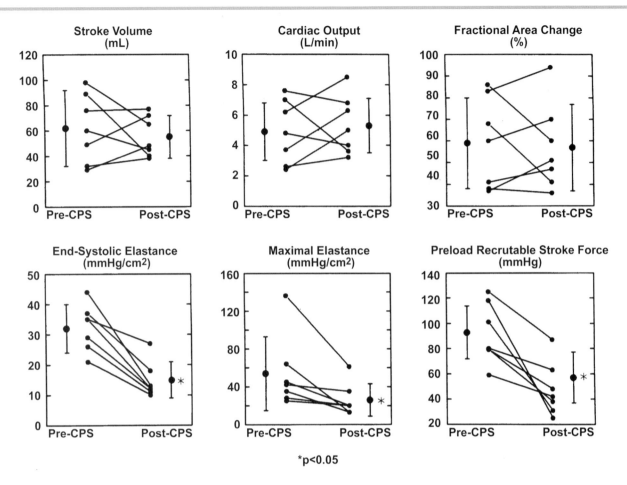

Figure 10.11 Pressure-volume related indices. Changes in SV, CO, FAC, end-systolic elastance, maximal elastance, and preload recruitable stroke force in seven patients before and after CPS. No significant changes were observed in SV, CO and FAC. However the indices based on the pressure-volume relationship were lower after CPS. *Abbreviations*: CO, cardiac output; CPS, cardiopulmonary bypass surgery; FAC, fractional area change; SV, stroke volume. *Source*: With permission from Ref. 12.

standard M-mode measurements of the LV cavity dimension (Fig. 10.14). The uncorrected LVEF (%) is calculated from the equation:

$$LVEF = \frac{LVEDD^2 - LVESD^2}{LVEDD^2} \times 100 \qquad (10.6)$$

where LVEF is the left ventricular ejection fraction (%), LVEDD is the left ventricular end-diastolic dimension (cm), and LVESD is the left ventricular end-systolic dimension (cm). A correction factor (K) can be added for contraction at the LV apex, which is +10% for normal apex, +5% for hypokinetic apex, 0% for akinetic apex, −5% for dyskinetic apex, or −10% for apical aneurysm (20). This method bases its estimate of the LVEF only on the change of the LV minor axis.

An alternate estimation of the corrected LVEF, as described by Quinones and colleagues (21), accounts for the change in both the minor and major axis during systole.

$$LVEF = \%\Delta D^2 + \left[(1 - \%\Delta D^2)(\%\Delta L)\right] \qquad (10.7)$$

where

$$\%\Delta D^2 = \frac{LVEDD^2 - LVESD^2}{LVEDD^2} \times 100$$

where $\%\Delta D^2$ is the uncorrected LVEF, LVEF is the left ventricular ejection fraction (%), LVEDD is the left ventricular end-diastolic dimension (cm), LVESD is the left ventricular end-systolic dimension (cm), and L is a correction for apical contraction.

$$\%\Delta L = +15\% \text{ if normal apex}$$
$$= +5\% \text{ if hypokinetic apex}$$
$$= 0\% \text{ if akinetic apex}$$
$$= -5\% \text{ if lightly dyskinetic apex}$$
$$= -10\% \text{ if frankly dyskinetic apex}$$

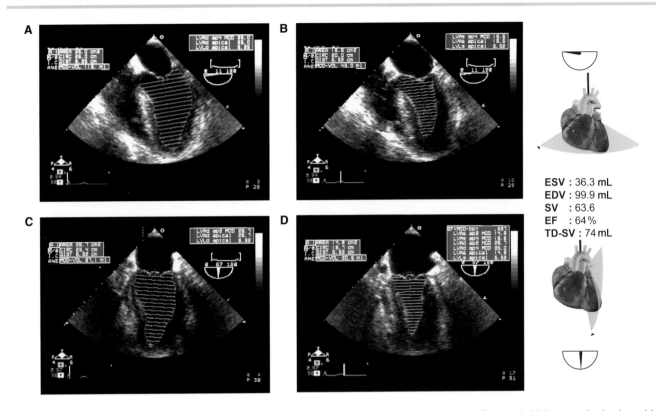

ESV : 36.3 mL
EDV : 99.9 mL
SV : 63.6
EF : 64%
TD-SV : 74 mL

Figure 10.12 Simpson's method of discs. Measurement of left ventricular volumes by modified Simpson's biplane method using mid-esophageal four-chamber (**A,B**) and two-chamber (**C,D**) views. The calculated SV based on echocardiography was slightly different from the SV measured with TD. *Abbreviations*: EDV, end-diastolic volume; EF, ejection fraction; ESV, end systolic volume; SV, stroke volume; TD, thermodilution.

Area Measurements

Fractional Area Change

The FAC can be used for the estimation of LV systolic performance. The FAC (%) is expressed by the equation:

$$FAC = \frac{EDA - ESA}{EDA} \times 100 \qquad (10.8)$$

where FAC is the fractional area change (%), EDA is the end-diastolic area (cm^2), and ESA is the end-systolic area (cm^2).

The LV areas are obtained by tracing the inner edge of the endocardium, excluding the papillary muscles, in the TG SAX views (Fig. 10.15). The normal FAC values range from 36% to 64%, depending on the level where it is measured: 40% for the base, 50% at the mid-papillary muscle, and 60% at the apical levels (2). Though not specifically measuring LVEF, studies have shown good correlation between the FAC and the LVEF measured by both radionuclide and contrast biplane ventriculography (22). By tracking the endocardial border automatically, using integrated back-scatter, attempts were made to obtain real-time end-diastolic and end-systolic areas, and hence online real-time FAC measurements. However, compared with manual tracing by experienced operators, the automated border detection system tended to overestimate the ESA and underestimate the EDA, resulting in an unacceptably low FAC estimate (23). These errors were, in part, due to inadequate tracking influenced by critical time-gain compensation settings, myocardial dropout (anisotropy), and moving of the region of interest.

Systolic Time Intervals

Left ventricular systolic performance can also be evaluated by measuring several systolic time intervals, particularly the pre-ejection period and left ventricular ejection time (LVET). The left ventricular pre-ejection period (LVPEP) is measured from the onset of the QRS to the opening of the AoV. The LVET, or period, encompasses the time between the AoV opening and closure, and can be measured using TEE (24) (Fig. 10.16). Both parameters decrease with increasing HR, though the LVPEP/LVET ratio is less affected by HR. Furthermore, with worsening systolic function, the ratio changes to a greater extent than its component as the LVPEP increases while the LVET decreases. The LVPEP/LVET ratio is normally less than 0.35 (or 35%)

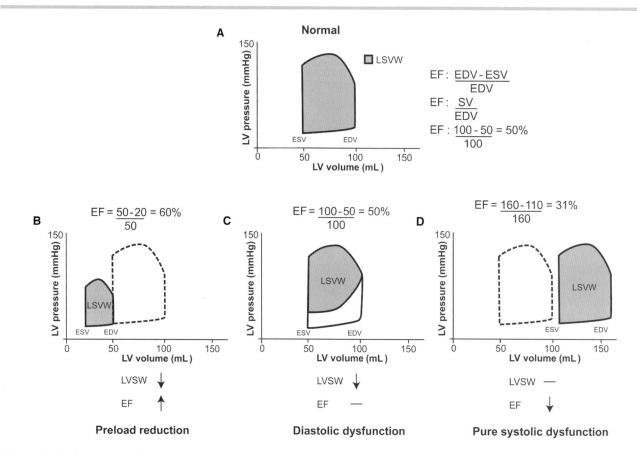

Figure 10.13 Pressure-volume relationship. (**A**) Normal pressure-volume relationship with LV pressure on the y-axis and LV volume on the x-axis. The EF is equal to SV divided by EDV. Three scenarios are presented to explain discrepancy between changes in LVSW and EF. (**B**) Acute preload reduction is associated with a leftward displacement of the pressure-volume relationship. This results in a reduction of LVSW and an increase in EF. (**C**) Diastolic dysfunction is associated with an up-sloping of the pressure-volume relationship. This results in a reduction in LVSW but no change in EF. (**D**) Finally, pure systolic dysfunction was associated with a rightward displacement of the pressure-volume relationship. In this condition, LVSW will be unchanged, but EF will be reduced. *Abbreviations*: EDV, end-diastolic volume; EF, ejection fraction; ESV, end-systolic volume; LV, left ventricle; LVSV, stroke volume; LVSW, left ventricular stroke work. *Source*: Adapted with permission from Ref. 15.

and, in a small study, has shown good correlation with LVEF measured by contrast left ventriculography (26).

Mitral Annulus Motion

The motion of the mitral annulus toward the apex can also be used as an indirect measure of LV systolic function. It is usually measured in the apical four-chamber view, where the movement of the mitral annulus is parallel to the ultrasound beam and is normally 12 ± 2 mm. A motion of <8 mm in a four-chamber view has been reported to have a sensitivity of 98% and a specificity of 82% in the identification of an ejection fraction less than 50% (13). Pai et al. (27) examined the mitral annular systolic excursion in 57 patients with a wide range of LV ejection fraction (13–84%) and found a good correlation ($r = 0.95$, $p < 0.001$) between the mitral annulus motion and the ejection fraction, as measured by the radionuclide approach (Fig. 10.17).

Myocardial Performance Index

The right and left ventricular MPI incorporates both systolic and diastolic time intervals, measured by Doppler, to assess systolic and diastolic function. The MPI is described by the equation:

$$\text{MPI} = \frac{\text{IVCT} + \text{IVRT}}{\text{ET}} \qquad (10.9)$$

where IVCT is the isovolumic contraction time, IVRT is the isovolumic relaxation time, and ET is the ejection time (Fig. 10.18). A normal LV MPI is 0.39 ± 0.05. Systolic dysfunction manifests as an increased IVCT, increased IVRT, and decreased ET, resulting in an MPI > 0.50 (28,29).

dP/dt

In the presence of mitral regurgitation (MR), the rate of change of the regurgitant jet velocity in early systole

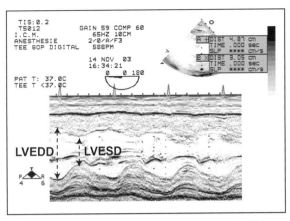

$$FS: \frac{LVEDD - LVESD}{LVEDD} \qquad EF: \frac{LVEDD^2 - LVESD^2}{LVEDD^2}$$

$$FS: \frac{4.8 - 3.0}{4.8} = 37.5\% \qquad EF: \frac{(4.8)^2 - (3.0)^2}{(4.8)^2} = 61\%$$

$$FS: (normal = 28\text{-}45\%) \qquad EF: (normal = 55\text{-}75\%)$$

Figure 10.14 Fractional shortening. Calculation of FS and EF uses the LVEDD and LVESD in a 64-year-old man before coronary revascularization. *Abbreviations*: EF, ejection fraction; FS, fractional shortening; LVEDD, left ventricular end-diastolic diameter; LVESD, left ventricular end-systolic diameter.

allows calculation of *dP/dt*, the maximum slope of pressure rise in the LV. The time required for the MR velocity to rise from 1 to 3 m/s is then determined. According to the modified Bernoulli equation, and assuming a normal left atrial pressure (LAP), the LV pressure will have increased by 32 mmHg (from 4 to 36 mmHg) in that time. The normal rate of pressure change is >1200 mmHg/s. In contrast, it will be decreased below 1000 mmHg/s in the presence of poor LV systolic function (Fig. 10.19). A good correlation has been reported between invasively measured *dP/dt* and that measured by Doppler echocardiography (30). When MR is mild, a left-sided contrast agent may be used to enhance the regurgitant Doppler signal.

Circumferential Fiber Shortening

Circumferential fiber shortening is a different index of systolic function. As circumference and diameter are directly related by π, circumference change can be converted from diameter reduction. Furthermore, by dividing the extent of shortening over the LVET, this index reflects the mean velocity of ventricular circumferential shortening of the minor axis of the LV (mean Vcf), as illustrated by the following equation:

$$MeanVcf = \frac{FS}{LVET} = \frac{LVEDD - LVESD}{LVEDD \times LVET} \quad (10.10)$$

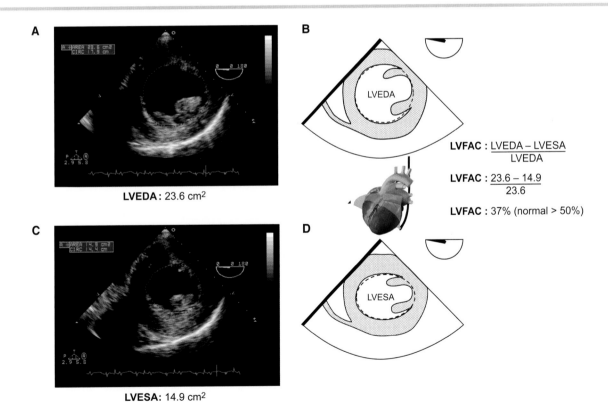

$$LVFAC: \frac{LVEDA - LVESA}{LVEDA}$$

$$LVFAC: \frac{23.6 - 14.9}{23.6}$$

$$LVFAC: 37\% \text{ (normal} > 50\%)$$

LVEDA: 23.6 cm²

LVESA: 14.9 cm²

Figure 10.15 Fractional area change. A 75-year-old man with unstable angina is undergoing emergency revascularization. Transgastric mid short-axis views of the LV in diastole (**A,B**) and in systole (**C,D**) provide the measurements to calculate the FAC which was 37%. Note exclusion of the papillary muscles during tracing of the areas. *Abbreviations*: EDA, end-diastolic area; ESA, end-systolic area; FAC, fractional area change; LV, left ventricle.

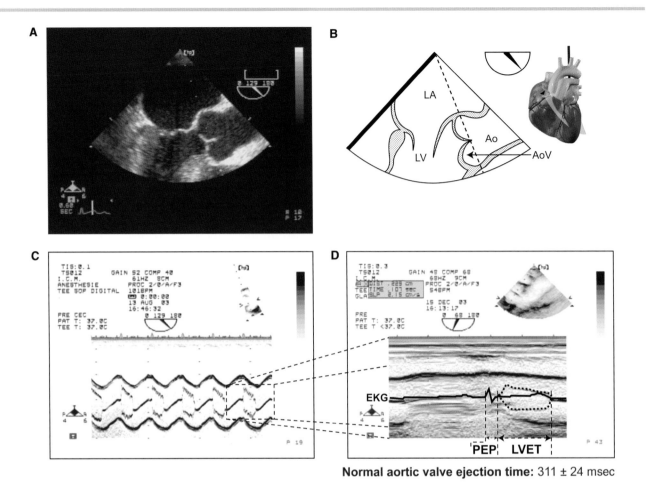

Figure 10.16 LV time indices. Mid-esophageal AoV long-axis view (**A,B**) with M-mode (**C**) on the AoV at a sweep speed of 25mm/s. (**D**) M-mode at a sweep speed of 100mm/s with the EKG tracing positioned in the M-mode. The LV PEP is measured from the onset of the QRS to the opening of the AoV. The LVET corresponds to the duration of AoV opening. Normal values are those obtained from healthy adults. *Abbreviations*: Ao, aorta; AoV, aortic valve; EKG, electrocardiogram; LA, left atrium; LV, left ventricle; LVET, left ventricular ejection time; PEP, pre-ejection period. *Source*: from Ref. 25.

where Mean Vcf is the mean rate of circumferential fiber shortening (in units of circumferences per second, or circ/s), LVEDD is the left ventricular end-diastolic dimension (cm), LVESD is the left ventricular end-systolic dimension (cm), LVET is the left ventricular ejection time or period (seconds), and FS is the left ventricular fractional shortening (in fraction, not %). The normal Vcf is 1.09 ± 0.3 circ/s (31).

Wall Stress

Finally, evaluation of LV wall stress provides an index of systolic function believed to be less dependent on loading conditions. Usually measured in systole, it requires measurement of the LV cavity dimension, the wall thickness (measured in the posterior wall), and the systolic blood pressure (sBP).

The left ventricular meridian wall stress is calculated according to the equation:

$$LVWS_{meridian} = 0.334 \frac{sBP \times LVESD}{PWT[1+(PWT/LVESD)]} \quad (10.11)$$

where LVWS is the left ventricular wall stress (dynes/cm^2), sBP is the systolic blood pressure (mmHg), LVESD is the left ventricular end-systolic diameter (cm), and PWT is the posterior wall thickness (cm).

As peak wall stress occurs during the isovolumetric contraction, the LV dimension can be obtained at end diastole. Therefore, LV meridian wall stress can be obtained from the following simplified equation:

$$LVWS_{meridian} = \frac{sBP \times LVEDD}{PWT} \quad (10.12)$$

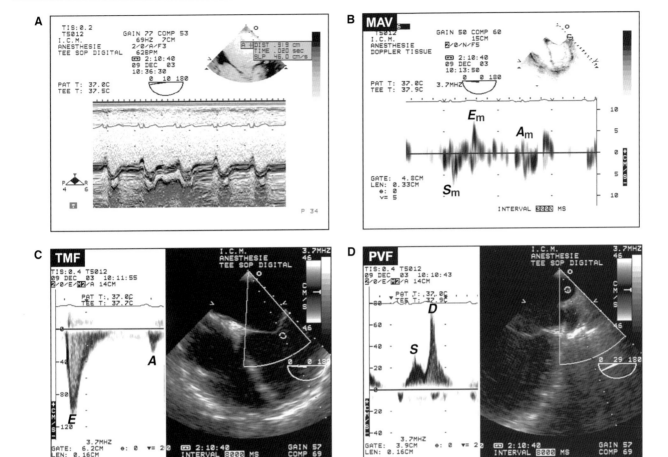

Figure 10.17 Restrictive LV filling. A 56-year-old woman has ischemic dilated cardiomyopathy and an ejection fraction of 20% before LV remodeling procedure. **(A)** M-mode of the lateral mitral annulus shows a decreased displacement of 9 mm. **(B)** Tissue Doppler of the lateral mitral annulus shows reduced MAV. **(C)** Pulsed wave Doppler of TMF with high E/A ratio. **(D)** Pulsed wave Doppler of PVF with decreased systolic fraction and S/D ratio. These features are consistent with restrictive LV filling. *Abbreviations: A*, A, peak late diastolic TMF velocity; A_m, Am, peak late diastolic MAV; *D*, D, peak diastolic PVF velocity; *E*, E, peak early diastolic TMF velocity; E_m, Em, peak early diastolic MAV; LV, left ventricle; MAV, mitral annular velocity; PVF, pulmonary venous flow; *S*, S, peak systolic PVF velocity; S_m, systolic MAV; TMF, transmitral flow.

Three-Dimensional Echocardiography

Three-dimensional (3D) echocardiography offers rapid acquisition of quantitative and qualitative anatomic data independent of mathematical assumptions, even in the presence of complex distortions of LV shape. It, therefore, provides a unique technique to evaluate LV function in a 3D format that allows more reliable, accurate, and reproducible measurement of LV volume, mass, and ejection fraction compared with biplane 2D echocardiography (32) (Fig. 10.20).

ASSESSMENT OF GLOBAL RIGHT VENTRICULAR SYSTOLIC FUNCTION

Quantitative Right Ventricular Function

The RV shape does not easily lend itself to mathematical modeling. Its shape approximates that of a half bullet minus a ¼ ellipsoid (½ bullet with a concave medial border or a crescent). The best models, which predict RV volume, include the modified biplane pyramidal ($^2/_3 A_{4ch} L_s$) and the monoplane ellipsoid ($^3/_8 \pi (A_{4ch})^2 L_{4ch}$). The RV is a crescent and this is not well accounted for in the modeling and does not maintain its shape throughout the cardiac cycle (6). Geometric models underestimate right ventricular ejection fraction (RVEF) when compared with magnetic resonance imaging (MRI) methods. However, when the RV increases in size and volume, the RVEF estimate improves as the RV assumes a more consistent ellipsoid shape throughout the cardiac cycle. Finally, the endocardial border is often poorly defined where proper, accurate tracings of the RV area in the four-chamber view are not possible. Because of its complex geometry, no quantitative method to assess RV volume has been officially endorsed by the ASE. In the 2005 ASE guidelines, normal values for RV dimensions and function were proposed (3).

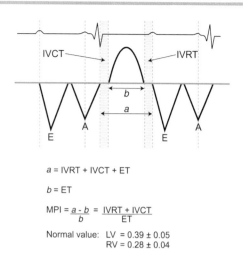

a = IVRT + IVCT + ET

b = ET

$$MPI = \frac{a - b}{b} = \frac{IVRT + IVCT}{ET}$$

Normal value: LV = 0.39 ± 0.05
RV = 0.28 ± 0.04

Figure 10.18 Myocardial performance index. To calculate the MPI or Tei index of the LV, the transmitral flow is used for measurement of the duration "a" from the end of atrial contraction (A-wave) to the beginning of LV filling (E-wave). The ET or "b" is measured from a deep transgastric long-axis view Doppler interrogation of the left ventricular outflow tract. The MPI of the RV is similarly obtained using the transtricuspid flow and the mid-esophageal ascending aorta short-axis view for the right ventricular outflow tract. *Abbreviations*: A, peak late diastolic TMF velocity; E, peak early diastolic TMF velocity; ET, ejection time; IVCT, isovolumic contraction time; IVRT, isovolumic relaxation time; LV, left ventricle; MPI, myocardial performance index; RV, right ventricle. *Source*: from Ref. 28.

An eccentricity index has been described as where the two minor axes of the LV are measured in the TG SAX views; L1, infero-anterior and L2, septal to lateral (Fig. 10.21). The L1/L2 ratio is normally 1.0 and describes a circular LV TG SAX geometry at both end systole (ES) and end diastole (ED) (33). In patients with pulmonary hypertension, the ES and ED ratios were found to be 1.44 ± 0.16 and 1.26 ± 0.11. In RV volume overload, the ES index did not deviate significantly from 1.0 but the ED index measured 1.26 ± 0.12 (34). The visual aspect of these ratios, however, is readily apparent to the moderately trained eye in the clinical setting. The RV size is, therefore, often qualitatively assessed. In the mid-esophageal four-chamber view, it is normally no more than two-third the size of the LV and does not share its apex.

Myocardial Performance Index

The MPI, also known as the Tei index (for Dr Tei), is described by the following relationship: (IVCT + IVRT)/RVET, which is the sum of the isovolumic contraction and relaxation times divided by the right ventricular ejection time (Fig. 10.18). It can be measured using Doppler techniques. It is meant to represent a global index of RV performance. A normal value is approximately 0.28. Increasing values represent a reduction in myocardial performance.

The RV MPI has been validated in several disease states, congenital heart disease, primary pulmonary hypertension, myocardial infarction, and chronic

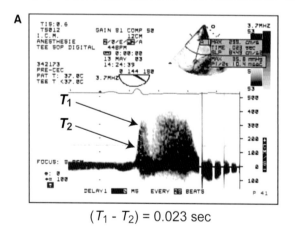

$(T_1 - T_2)$ = 0.023 sec

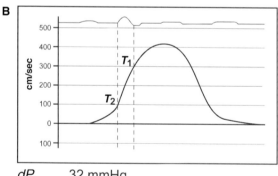

$$\frac{dP}{dt} = \frac{32 \text{ mmHg}}{(T_1 - T_2) \text{ sec}}$$
(normal > 1200 mmHg/sec)

T_1 : time at 300 cm/sec on the CW velocity profile which correspond to 36 mmHg pressure gradient

T_2 : time at 100 cm/sec on the CW velocity profile which correspond to 4 mmHg pressure gradient

Figure 10.19 Left ventricular *dP/dt*. (A,B) Measurement of left ventricular change in pressure over time (d*P*/d*t*) using CW Doppler of the mitral regurgitant flow in a 58-year-old man demonstrates the d*P*/d*t* was 32 mmHg per 0.023 seconds or 1391 mmHg/s before surgery. *Abbreviation*: CW, continuous wave.

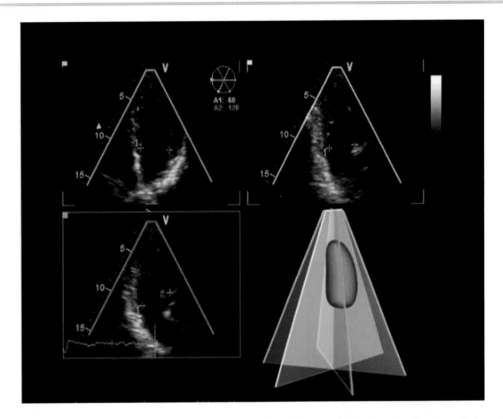

Figure 10.20 3D echocardiography. Transthoracic apical four-chamber view acquisition for 3D estimation of left ventricular function. *Source*: Courtesy of GE Healthcare.

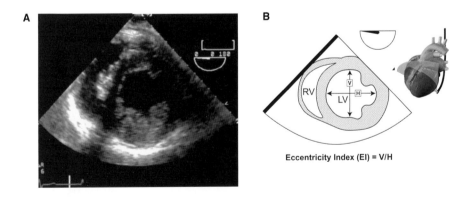

Figure 10.21 Eccentricity index. (A,B) Using the transgastric mid short-axis view of the LV and RV, the EI corresponds to the ratio of the vertical (V)/horizontal (H) diameter of the LV. *Abbreviations*: EI, eccentricity index; LV, left ventricle; RV, right ventricle. *Source*: Adapted with permission from Ref. 6.

respiratory disease (35–38). A small prospective study has suggested that RV MPI may be useful in stratifying patients undergoing high-risk valvular surgery (39). The index is meant to be independent of HR and loading conditions. However, as the RV fails, an increase in preload would tend to shorten the IVRT and normalize the index. This has been reported in acute, severe RV myocardial infarction (38). The RV MPI is also less reliable in the presence of arrhythmias or high-grade atrioventricular block.

Tricuspid Annular Plane Excursion

This measurement is usually taken using M-mode. It measures the maximum distance the tricuspid annulus descends in systole. This value has been correlated with RV ejection fraction. An excursion of 20 mm correlates with an RVEF of 50% and an excursion inferior to 5 mm correlates with an RVEF of 20%. Again, this measurement is impractical using TEE, as lining up the annular motion, with either Doppler or M-mode, can be quite difficult in several views except the deep TG view or with the use of anatomic M-mode (Fig. 10.22). Furthermore, tethering, rotation, and translation can add motion unrelated to annular excursion and lead to erroneous measurements.

Recent studies cast doubts on TAPSE's (tricuspid annular plane excursion) specificity (40), particularly in critically ill patients (41).

Tricuspid Annular Velocity

The tricuspid annulus descends toward the apex in systole. The tricuspid annular velocity (TAV) measures longitudinal function and is a gross representation of global systolic and diastolic function. Tricuspid systolic velocity is higher than that of the MV. In transthoracic echocardiography (TTE), the apical four-chamber view allows for adequate alignment of the ultrasound beam with annular motion. In TEE,

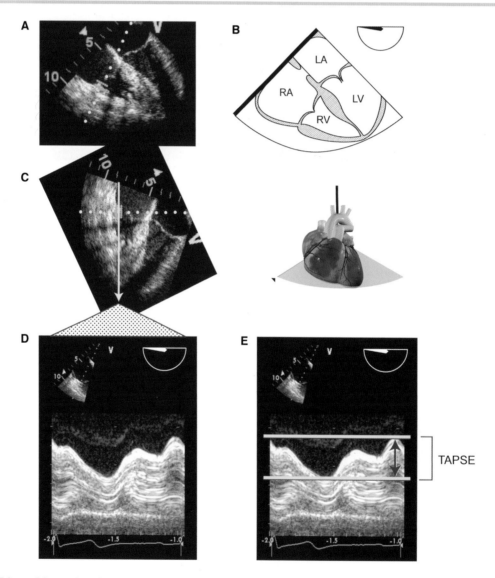

Figure 10.22   Tricuspid annular plane systolic excursion. (A–E) Steps in the measurement of the TAPSE using anatomic M-mode are shown. First a mid-esophageal four-chamber view (**A,B**) is acquired and the M-mode cursor is positioned along the plane of the TAPSE motion (**C**) to obtain the M-mode figure of this displacement (**D**). The lower point corresponds to the maximal systolic excursion and the upper point is the atrial contraction. (**E**) The TAPSE is equal to the total systolic displacement of the tricuspid annulus which is normally 20–25 mm. *Abbreviations*: LA, left atrium; LV, left ventricle; RA, right atrium; RV, right ventricle; TAPSE, tricuspid annular plane systolic excursion. *Source*: Adapted with permission from Ref. 6.

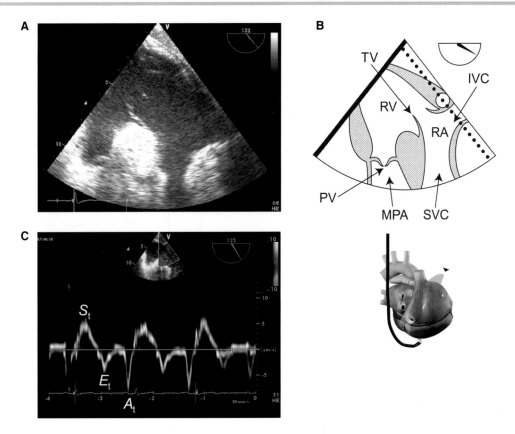

Figure 10.23 TDI for RV function. (A,B) Deep transgastric RV inflow/outflow long-axis view allows the evaluation of both the pulsed wave Doppler interrogation of the TV and TDI of the tricuspid annulus along the dotted line. **(C)** Tissue Doppler signal obtained at the base of the tricuspid annulus. *Abbreviations*: A_t, peak late diastolic TAV; E_t, peak early diastolic TAV; IVC, inferior vena cava; MPA, main pulmonary artery; PV, pulmonic valve; RA, right atrium; RV, right ventricle; S_t, tricuspid systolic tissue Doppler velocity; SVC, superior vena cava; TAV, tricuspid annular velocity; TDI, tissue Doppler imaging; TV, tricuspid valve: *Source*: Adapted with permission from Ref. 6.

however, novel approaches must be used as the four-chamber view does not allow proper alignment (Fig. 10.23). In this case, the TG RV inflow view can be adjusted to align for annular motion. Using spectral Doppler, peak annular velocities are measured (Fig. 10.23). Normal peak systolic TAV is 14 to 16 cm/s, and a TAV inferior to 12 cm/s has been associated with reduced RVEF.

With quantitative off-line analysis performed on stored color tissue Doppler imaging data using specialized software, four distinct waves (Fig. 10.23) are identified: isovolumic (IV), systolic ejection (S), the E and A waves in diastole. Velocities measured using this method are "average" over the size of the sample volume and cannot be compared with the spectral pulsed wave (PW) Doppler method. Using TEE under general anesthesia, the S-wave velocity is 5.2 cm/s, and in TTE at the lateral annulus, the S-wave velocity is normally 7.6 cm/s. With the color tissue Doppler method, isovolumic acceleration, a load independent index of contractility can be measured (Fig. 10.24) (42). Under general anesthesia and using TEE, its normal value is 1.7 m/s^2.

LEFT VENTRICULAR DYSFUNCTION

Acute Vs. Chronic Etiology

Acute LV dysfunction can be either systolic or diastolic in origin. It is typically associated with both increased wall motion score index (see Chapter 9) and moderate to severe diastolic dysfunction. Severe LV systolic dysfunction will sometimes be accompanied by pulsus alternans, where the LV stroke volume and sBP will be decreased on every alternate beat (Fig. 10.25). Left ventricular diastolic dysfunction is commonly seen in unstable patients after cardiac surgery, even in patients with normal systolic function (43). Chronic LV systolic dysfunction is associated with ventricular dilatation and diastolic dysfunction, which can range in severity from mildly delayed relaxation to restrictive filling pattern (see section "Diastolic Dysfunction"). Atrial dilatation is more common in chronic conditions but can also be observed in the acute setting and often correlates with the degree of diastolic dysfunction. This can be associated with mitral annular dilatation, MR, and atrial fibrillation.

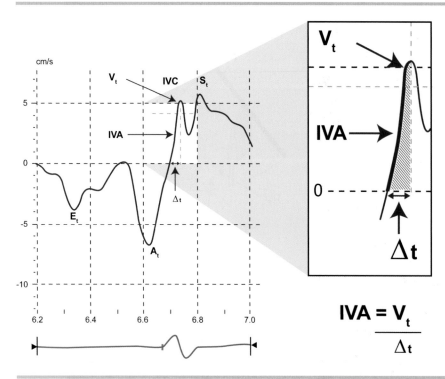

Figure 10.24 Isovolumic acceleration. Mean tissue color Doppler velocities of the basal tricuspid annulus during a cardiac cycle. The dominant slope is used to measure the IVA. *Abbreviations*: A_t, peak late diastolic TAV; E_t, peak early diastolic TAV; IVA, isovolumic acceleration; IVC, isovolumic contraction; S_t, tricuspid systolic tissue Doppler velocity; t, time; TAV, tricuspid annular velocity; V_t, tissue Doppler velocity during IVC. *Source*: Adapted with permission from Ref. 6.

$$IVA = \frac{V_t}{\Delta t}$$

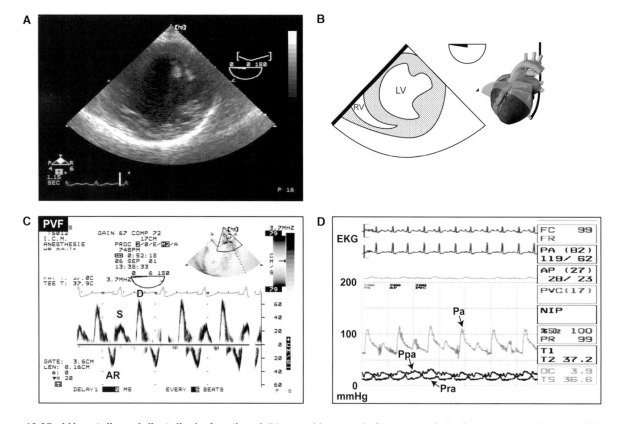

Figure 10.25   LV systolic and diastolic dysfunction. A 71-year-old woman before revascularization presents with severe LV systolic and diastolic dysfunction. **(A,B)** The transgastric mid short-axis view demonstrates a dilated LV with severe systolic dysfunction. **(C)** PVF shows diastolic predominance (S < D) consistent with moderate to severe diastolic dysfunction. **(D)** Pulsus alternans on the Pa tracing was present. *Abbreviations*: AR, peak atrial reversal PVF velocity; D, peak diastolic PVF velocity; EKG, electrocardiogram; Pa, arterial pressure; Ppa, pulmonary artery pressure; Pra, right atrial pressure; PVF, pulmonary venous flow; RV, right ventricle; S, *S*, peak systolic PVF velocity.

Problems Confounding Diagnosis

In the evaluation of LV function, several errors can be made in the measurement of LV dimensions. In the mid-esophageal four-chamber view, the apex of the LV can be foreshortened leading to underestimation of ventricular volume. Further retroflexion of the probe tip may reduce the impact of this problem. A TG SAX view with an oblique cross section leads not only to faulty measurements of LV dimensions, but also to misinterpretation of regional wall motion. Moderate to severe MR or ventricular septal defect (VSD) may result in a LVEF that overestimates intrinsic myocardial contractility. The presence of MR allows the measurement of LV dP/dt, a different index of LV contractility and function (Fig. 10.19) that can be used to predict ejection fraction postoperatively (44). Finally, the estimation of LVEF may vary according to the site of measurement as one moves from the ventricular apex (75%) to the mid SAX (65%) to the base of the heart (50%). Longitudinal contraction [shortening of the LV long axis (LAX)] contributes 10% to 15% of the ejection fraction.

Transesophageal Echocardiographic Evaluation

Figures 10.26 to 10.29 summarize our simplified approach to the evaluation of ventricular function using four specific TEE views. These TEE views allow the evaluation of both left and right ventricular systolic and diastolic dysfunction and also mitral, aortic, and tricuspid valvular function.

Dynamic Left Ventricular Outflow Tract Obstruction

Dynamic left ventricular outflow tract obstruction (LVOTO) is a well-known complication in surgical patients (Fig. 10.30) following MV repair (45,46) with or without asymmetric LV hypertrophy (47), post AoV replacement (48), and during lung transplantation (49). It is also increasingly recognized in conditions associated with severe preload reduction without significant cardiac disease (Fig. 10.10). The presence of dynamic LVOTO has been reported in 5% to 10% of hemodynamically unstable patients in the intensive care unit (ICU) (50,51). Dynamic LVOTO has been

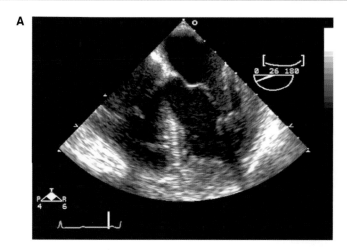

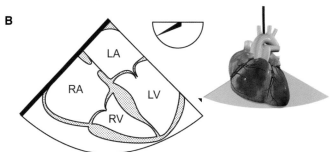

2D:
Atrial and ventricular chamber size
Mitral and tricuspid annular motion
LV and RV wall motion score
Mitral annular diameter

PW Doppler:
Transmitral and transtricuspid signal
Pulmonary vein

Color Flow Imaging:
Mitral and tricuspid valve interrogation

Tissue Doppler:
Lateral mitral annulus velocity

Figure 10.26 Mid-esophageal four-chamber view for biventricular function evaluation. (A,B) Right and left atrial and ventricular dimensions are evaluated as well as regional contractility and mitral annular motion with this view. Volumetric stroke volume through the mitral valve is measured from the mitral annulus diameter and mitral inflow modal VTI obtained by PW Doppler at the annulus level. Both the transmitral and transtricuspid PW Doppler inflow signal correct alignment for Doppler measurement should be verified by color Doppler imaging. The lateral mitral annular plane is optimized for tissue Doppler imaging by left-sided rotation and pullback. The left upper pulmonary vein can also be interrogated with PW Doppler. *Abbreviations*: 2D, two-dimensional; LA, left atrium; LV, left ventricle; PW, pulsed wave; RA, right atrium; RV, right ventricle; VTI, velocity-time integral.

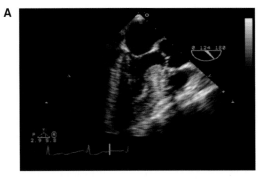

PW Doppler:
Transmitral Doppler signal

IVRT:
Transmitral Doppler signal at annulus
(for CO calculation)

Color Flow Imaging:
Mitral and aortic valve interrogation

Tissue Doppler:
Mitral annulus interrogation

Color M-mode:
Mitral inflow Vp measurement

Figure 10.27   Mid-esophageal long-axis view for LV function evaluation. (A,B) This view is ideal to quickly screen for both mitral and aortic regurgitation with color Doppler. The transmitral PW Doppler signal is often of higher quality than at 0°. IVRT, tissue Doppler interrogation of the mitral annulus and color M-mode Vp are easily obtained. CO of the LV can be obtained using mitral annulus diameter and PW Doppler interrogation of the mitral valve at the same level. *Abbreviations*: Ao, aorta; CO, cardiac output; IVRT, isovolumic relaxation time; LA, left atrium; LV, left ventricle; PW, pulsed wave; RV, right ventricle; Vp, velocity of propagation. 🖱

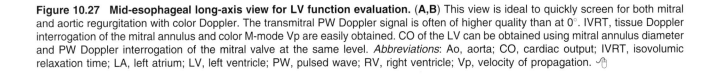

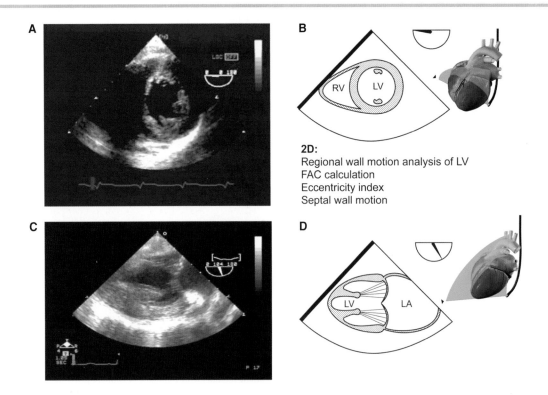

2D:
Regional wall motion analysis of LV
FAC calculation
Eccentricity index
Septal wall motion

Figure 10.28   Transgastric view for biventricular function evaluation. (A,B) The transgastric mid short-axis view is used to obtain the FAC, wall motion score and eccentricity indices to evaluate LV systolic function. Attention is paid to septal wall motion which can be altered with RV dysfunction. **(C,D)** A two-chamber view is obtained to ensure that the mid short-axis view is perpendicular to the ventricular axis and to complete the basal and apical wall motion score evaluation of the mid-esophageal four-chamber. *Abbreviations*: 2D, two-dimensional; FAC, fractional area change; LA, left atrium; LV, left ventricle; RV, right ventricle. 🖱

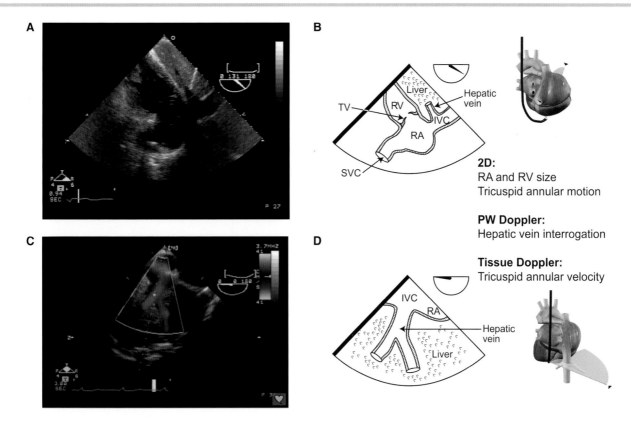

Figure 10.29 Transgastric views for RV function evaluation. (A,B) Transgastric RV long-axis view evaluates right sided chamber size, PW Doppler interrogation of the hepatic vein and tissue Doppler evaluation of the tricuspid annulus. **(C,D)** Transgastric IVC view at 0° with rightward rotation is used to perform PW Doppler interrogation of the HV. *Abbreviations*: IVC, inferior vena cava; PW, pulsed wave; RA, right atrium; RV, right ventricle; SVC, superior vena cava; TV, tricuspid valve.

described in a variety of clinical situations such as postoperative hemorrhage (52), myocardial infarction (53), intra-aortic balloon pump use (54), cardiac tamponade (55), apical ballooning syndrome (56), sepsis (57), severe pancreatitis (58), dobutamine stress echocardiography (59), and pheochromocytoma (60).

The pressure-volume relationship associated with dynamic LVOTO shows the effect of an increased afterload (Fig. 10.5B). In susceptible patients, decreased preload and afterload, and increased contractility states can lead to the appearance or the worsening of dynamic LVOTO. In patients with dynamic LVOTO, the mitral-septal contact from SAM of the MV leaflets is displaced into the outflow tract and is associated with MR. Distinguishing LVOT obstruction from pure MR, as a cause of hemodynamic instability associated with a "V" wave, is critical (Fig. 10.30) as the treatment of these two conditions is quite different: afterload reduction, inotropic support, and increase in HR are recommended for MR but would be deleterious for LVOT obstruction.

Dynamic LVOTO can be suspected by the presence of flow acceleration on color Doppler (see Fig. 30.10A). A characteristic systolic late-peaking, dagger-shaped flow profile can be demonstrated on continuous wave (CW) Doppler (see Fig. 30.10C). While SAM is the most frequent causative factor of dynamic

LVOTO in patients with hypertrophic cardiomyopathy or after MV repair, systolic mid-ventricular cavity obliteration is usually responsible for the obstruction in patients after AoV replacement (48,60). Determining the correct mechanism of dynamic LVOTO is important as it ensures the appropriateness and the extent of the surgical intervention when medical management fails.

RIGHT VENTRICULAR DYSFUNCTION

Importance

Right ventricular systolic dysfunction is associated with high morbidity after cardiac surgery (61,62), chest trauma (63), and sepsis (64) and can be difficult to diagnose with conventional hemodynamic criteria (43). Davila-Roman et al. observed that RV dysfunction cannot be differentiated from LV dysfunction using pulmonary artery catheter derived variables in the postbypass period (65). This stresses the importance of the echocardiographic assessment of RV function.

Transesophageal Echocardiography Findings

Echocardiographic evaluation of RV function includes measurements of chamber size, evaluation of regional wall motion, ventricular septal motion, tricuspid

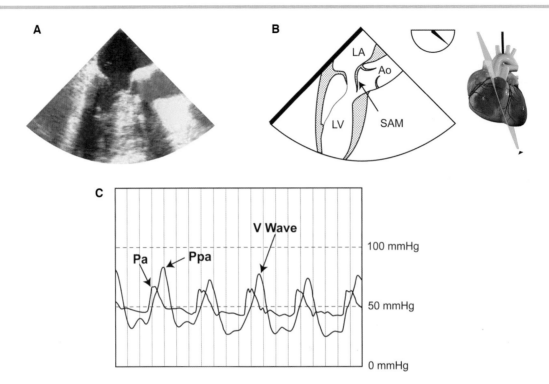

Figure 10.30 LVOT obstruction. (A,B) The mid-esophageal long-axis view shows LVOT obstruction secondary to LV septal hypertrophy in a 53-year-old man after aortic valve replacement. **(C)** Systemic hypotension was associated with the appearance of a giant "V" wave on the wedged Ppa tracing as the patient was weaned from cardiopulmonary bypass. The "V" wave was secondary to mitral regurgitation from abnormal SAM. This patient did not respond to medical therapy and underwent mitral valve replacement. *Abbreviations*: Ao, aorta; LA, left atrium; LV, left ventricle; LVOT, left ventricular outflow tract; Pa, arterial pressure; Ppa, pulmonary artery pressure; SAM, systolic anterior motion.

annular displacement, and vena cava size (6). Evaluation can be complemented with PW Doppler interrogation of the pulmonary outflow tract, tricuspid inflow, and hepatic venous flow and tissue Doppler interrogation of the tricuspid annulus. These measurements can be obtained using the mid-esophageal four-chamber view (Fig. 10.26), the TG SAX (Fig. 10.28) and LAX views (Fig. 10.29) of the RV.

Echocardiographic manifestations of RV failure are RV hypokinesis, RV and RA dilatation, reduction in annular tricuspid displacement (Fig. 10.31), IVC plethora and abnormal Doppler profile of the hepatic veins (66). Right ventricular dilatation is considered mild, moderate, or severe when the right ventricular end-diastolic area (RVEDA) measured from a four-chamber view is smaller, equal, or greater than LVEDA (normal < 0.6). The mid-esophageal four-chamber view (Fig. 10.32) will also show loss of the typical RV triangular shape and can be used to calculate RV FAC (Fig. 10.33) and measure tricuspid annular motion (Fig. 10.22).

With RV volume overload, the RV will be dilated and the ventricular septum, normally convex toward the RV, will be flattened or even convex toward the LV during diastole only, showing a diastolic "D" shaped septum (Fig. 10.33), with associated paradoxical motion during systole. With RV pressure overload, flattening of the ventricular septum occurs during both systole and diastole. When RV failure is secondary to increased afterload, TEE signs include paradoxical septal motion (Fig. 10.34), shortened pulmonary flow acceleration time, biphasic pulmonary flow (Fig. 10.35) in the presence of pulmonary hypertension, and increased tricuspid regurgitation (TR) jet velocity.

Dynamic Right Ventricular Outflow Tract Obstruction

Right ventricular outflow tract (RVOT) obstruction can be extrinsic or intrinsic. Extrinsic compression can occur, for instance, from an aortic (67) or pulmonary artery aneurysm (68), mediastinal hematoma (69), or from direct surgical compression during off-pump surgery. Intrinsic compression can be seen in congenital heart disease (70), congenital surgery (71), septal patch repair (72), and lung transplantation (70).

It is typically classified as subvalvular, valvular, or supravalvular. The dynamic form of RVOT obstruction occurs in a setting of reduced preload and hypertrophied RV, exacerbated by inotropic drugs (73). It

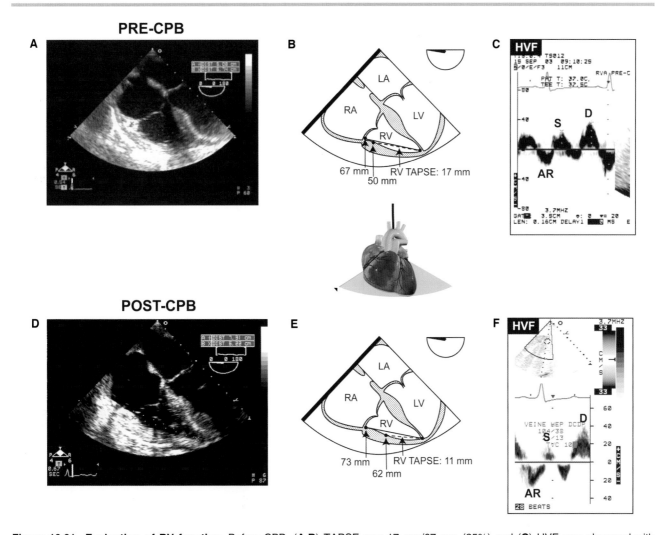

Figure 10.31 Evaluation of RV function. Before CPB, (**A,B**) TAPSE was 17 mm/67 mm (25%) and (**C**) HVF was abnormal with systolic attenuation consistent with abnormal RV diastolic function. After CPB, (**D,E**) TAPSE was 11 mm/73 mm (15%) with (**F**) more pronounced HVF systolic attenuation consistent with worsened systolic function. *Abbreviations*: AR, peak atrial reversal HVF velocity; CPB, cardiopulmonary bypass; D, peak diastolic HVF velocity; HVF, hepatic venous flow; LA, left atrium; LV, left ventricle; RA, right atrium; RV, right ventricle; S, peak systolic HVF velocity; TAPSE, tricuspid annular plane systolic excursion.

has been observed in biventricular hypertrophic cardiomyopathy (74) and after lung transplantation (75). Gradients of 25 mmHg or more in the RVOT have been detected in 4% in a series of 800 consecutive patients undergoing cardiac surgery (76). The diagnosis can be established by RV catheterization and by TEE (75) (Figs. 10.36–10.38). Color M-mode should allow simultaneous visualization of RVOT collapse and associated flow acceleration (74,76,77).

DIASTOLIC DYSFUNCTION

Left Ventricular Diastolic Dysfunction

Diastolic function should be an integral part of the evaluation of cardiac function. Indeed, LV diastolic dysfunction is as good a predictor of difficult weaning

from cardiopulmonary bypass (CPB) as systolic dysfunction (78). Diastolic dysfunction can be isolated or associated with systolic dysfunction or pericardial disease. Echocardiographically, LV diastolic dysfunction has been classified as mild (impaired LV relaxation), moderate (pseudonormal pattern), and severe (LV restrictive filling) with increasing LV filling pressures.

We use a combination of Doppler-derived variables in the diagnosis of LV diastolic dysfunction (Fig. 10.39) (79) and a diagnostic algorithm (Fig. 10.40) (80).

Diastolic dysfunction alters the pressure-volume relationship (Fig. 10.5D–F) and could explain some of the observed changes between filling pressure and ventricular volume observed after CPB. Impaired or delayed relaxation (mild diastolic dysfunction) results in decreased LV pressure decay during diastole and prolonged IVRT. This will be reflected with higher

PRE-CPB

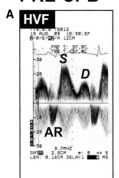

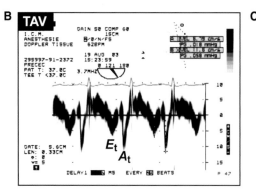

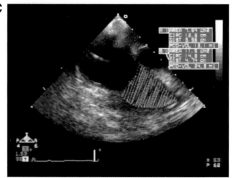

	EDA	ESA	FAC
Pre-CPB:	11.6 cm²	7.6 cm²	34 %
Post-CPB:	16.2 cm²	8.4 cm²	48 %

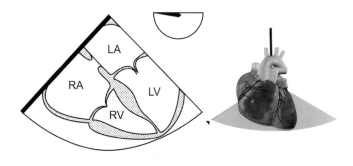

POST-CPB

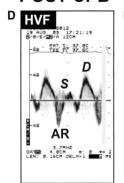

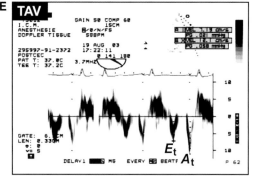

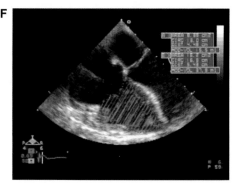

Figure 10.32 RV systolic and diastolic function. A 65-year-old man with previous inferior myocardial infarction is scheduled for coronary revascularization. (**A–C**) Before CPB the ejection fraction of the LV is 20% with a low cardiac index of 1.5 L/min/m². (**A**) Pulsed wave Doppler HVF shows systolic flow predominance. (**B**) TAV by tissue Doppler shows E_t/A_t ratio < 1 ($E_t = 5.7$ and $A_t = 11.5$ cm/s). Both suggest mild RV diastolic dysfunction. (**C**) The FAC of the RV is 34%. (**D–F**) Post-CPB. (**D**) The HVF showed new blunting of the systolic flow. (**E**) TAV is increased with a similar ratio ($E_t = 7.1$ and $A_t = 12.1$ cm/s) suggesting decreased RV compliance. (**F**) RV FAC increased to 48% consistent with the surgeon's visual appreciation of improved RV function. Upon arrival to the intensive care unit, the cardiac index was 3.0 L/min/m². *Abbreviations*: A_t, peak late diastolic TAV; AR, peak atrial reversal HVF velocity; CPB, cardiopulmonary bypass; D, peak diastolic HVF velocity; EDA, end-diastolic area; ESA, end-systolic area; E_t, peak early diastolic TAV; FAC, fractional area change; HVF, hepatic venous flow; LA, left atrium; LV, left ventricle; RA, right atrium; RV, right ventricle; S, peak systolic HVF velocity; TAV, tricuspid annular velocity.

diastolic filling pressure for the same LV volume (Fig. 10.5D).

Echocardiographic evaluation of abnormal relaxation using PW Doppler interrogation of the MV will demonstrate prolonged IVRT, prolonged E-wave deceleration time, and a reduction of the E/A ratio. The pulmonary vein PW Doppler signal will show an increased S/D ratio. Tissue Doppler of the mitral annulus will demonstrate an E_m/A_m ratio <1 while

on color M-mode, V_p will be decreased (Fig. 10.41). The delayed relaxation abnormality is the most common form of diastolic dysfunction (64% in our practice) (80). It is commonly associated with LV hypertrophy either due to hypertension or aortic stenosis (AS).

Left ventricular restrictive filling abnormality represents a more severe degree of diastolic dysfunction. This is associated with an upward shift of the diastolic pressure-volume curve (Fig. 10.5F). In these

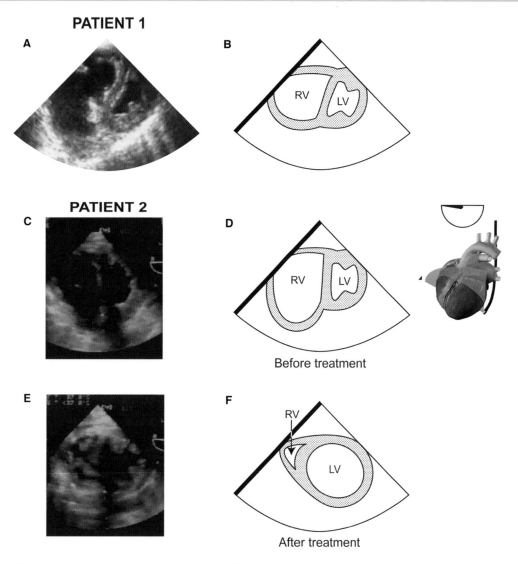

Figure 10.33 RV systolic dysfunction. (A,B) TG mid SAX view of a 50-year-old woman with severe pulmonary hypertension associated with scleroderma shows the RV is dilated with a D-shaped LV and systolic septal flattening. **(C–F)** RV dysfunction from fluid overload in another patient before **(C,D)** and after **(E,F)** vasodilator therapy. Note the reduction in RV size and change in septal curvature after treatment in these TG mid SAX views. *Abbreviations*: LV, left ventricle; RV, right ventricle; SAX, short axis; TG, transgastric.

patients the following echocardiographic findings are observed: PW Doppler of the mitral inflow reveals shortened IVRT and E-wave deceleration time, a high E/A ratio >2; PW Doppler interrogation of the pulmonary vein shows predominant diastolic flow, while tissue Doppler imaging of the mitral annulus demonstrates reduced E_m velocity and decreased color M-mode propagation velocity. This type of abnormality is commonly seen in hemodynamically unstable patients before or after cardiac surgery (Fig. 10.42).

Finally, in patients with relaxation abnormalities and increased filling pressure, a moderate or intermediate form of diastolic dysfunction called the pseudonormal pattern is seen. The expression "pseudonormal" is a consequence of the normal looking PW Doppler mitral inflow signal while the pulmonary venous flow (PVF) pattern is clearly abnormal ($S/D < 1$). With a pseudonormal pattern, the pressure-volume diagram will demonstrate moderate upward elevation of the diastolic waveform (Fig. 10.5E). Echocardiographically, it is characterized by reduced IVRT, a pseudonormal E/A ratio and deceleration time, PVF with inverted S/D ratio < 1 and atrial reversal wave velocity exceeding 40 cm/s, abnormal tissue Doppler of the mitral annulus with a reduced E_m/A_m ratio and abnormally low color M-mode propagation velocity (Fig. 10.43) (79).

A   PEEP 0

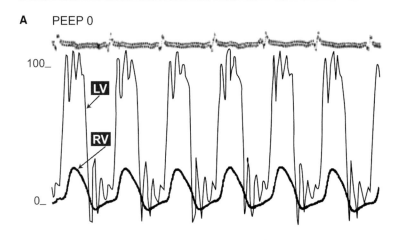

B   PEEP 20

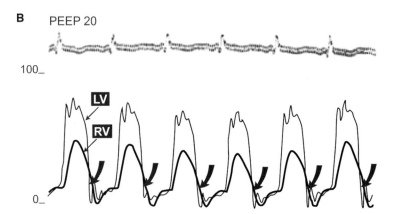

Figure 10.34 Paradoxical septal motion. (**A**) As shown on these simultaneous left and right intraventricular pressure tracings, LV ejection outlasts RV ejection duration during ventilation without PEEP. (**B**) After application of 20 cm H_2O of PEEP, the increased RV afterload results in RV ejection outlasting LV ejection duration. This transiently results in a RV pressure greater than LV pressure (arrow) during the late systolic/early diastolic period. This is responsible for the abnormal septal curvature and motion seen at this time in some patients with acute cor pulmonale. *Abbreviations*: LV, left ventricle; PEEP, positive end-expiratory pressure; RV, right ventricle. *Source*: Courtesy of Drs. Girard and Vieillard-Baron.

PULMONARY HYPERTENSION

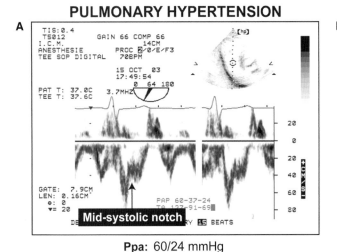

Ppa: 60/24 mmHg

NORMAL PATIENT

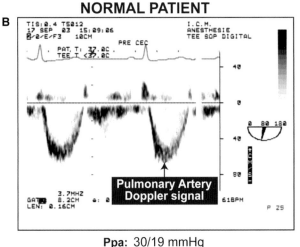

Ppa: 30/19 mmHg

Figure 10.35 Mid-systolic notch in pulmonary hypertension. (**A**) Pulmonary hypertension in a hemodynamically unstable 70-year-old man with a Ppa of 60/24 mmHg shows a mid-systolic notch in the signal. (**B**) For comparison, a normal pulmonary artery Doppler signal is shown from a 64-year-old woman before coronary revascularization with a Ppa of 30/19 mmHg. *Abbreviation*: Ppa, pulmonary artery pressure.

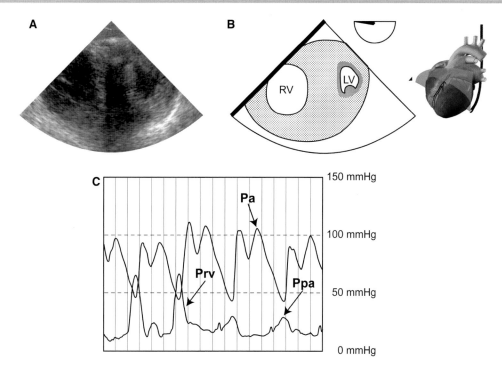

Figure 10.36 RVOT obstruction. A 75-year-old man developed RVOT obstruction after coronary revascularization and aortic valve replacement. The procedure was complicated by two failed attempts of weaning from cardiopulmonary bypass requiring intra-aortic balloon counterpulsation. **(A,B)** Transgastric mid short-axis view revealed a dilated and hypertrophied RV. Unexplained acute right heart failure was present without pulmonary hypertension. **(C)** Ppa was 34/22 mmHg and right atrial pressure 20 mmHg. However, a significant systolic pressure gradient between the Prv and the pulmonary artery was present. *Abbreviations*: LV, left ventricle; Pa, arterial pressure; Ppa, pulmonary artery pressure; Prv, right ventricular pressure; RV, right ventricle; RVOT, right ventricular outflow tract.

These abnormalities represent a spectrum of disease severity ranging from the milder form of diastolic dysfunction, shown by impaired relaxation abnormalities, to the more severe form such as the restrictive filling pattern. In the perioperative monitoring of cardiac function, particularly in the postbypass setting, changes in diastolic function commonly occur irrespective of those in systolic function. Worsening of diastolic function tends to correlate with subsequent deterioration of the hemodynamic function.

Right Ventricular Diastolic Dysfunction

Right ventricular dysfunction in patients undergoing cardiac surgery is also associated with difficult weaning from CPB and hemodynamic instability (43,80).

PW Doppler interrogation of the tricuspid valve (TV) inflow (81) (Fig. 10.44), hepatic veins (66) (Figs. 10.31, 10.32, and 10.45), and tissue Doppler of the tricuspid annulus (82) (Figs. 10.23, 10.32, and 10.44) allow assessment of RV diastolic function. An algorithm in the diagnosis of RV diastolic dysfunction has been developed and used in our practice (Fig. 10.46) (80) using a combination of Doppler parameters.

When invasive hemodynamic tracings are available through a pulmonary artery catheter, we have also observed a correlation between the RV diastolic pressure tracing and RV diastolic dysfunction (Figs. 10.44 and 10.45).

The diastolic assessment of the RV cannot be equated with that of the LV as the RV is not necessarily a closed system in diastole. The constraints imposed by the pulmonary vascular impedance and the pulmonary artery diastolic pressure can be exceeded by the right atrial systolic pressure. This diastolic ejection becomes more important in certain disease states. Furthermore, the RV is more adaptable to volume changes than the LV. Its compliance is maintained throughout a broad range of volume changes resulting in negligible increases in RV end-diastolic pressure. Generally speaking, *E* velocity is lower in the RV than the LV. The deceleration time is longer in the RV. There is, however, large variability due to the effect of respiration but not in age.

Transtricuspid flow can be an unreliable measure of RV diastolic function. Under certain conditions, the RV may become more like a passive conduit (RV infarct, constrictive/restrictive disease of the RV). If the pulmonary artery pressures (PAP) remain low,

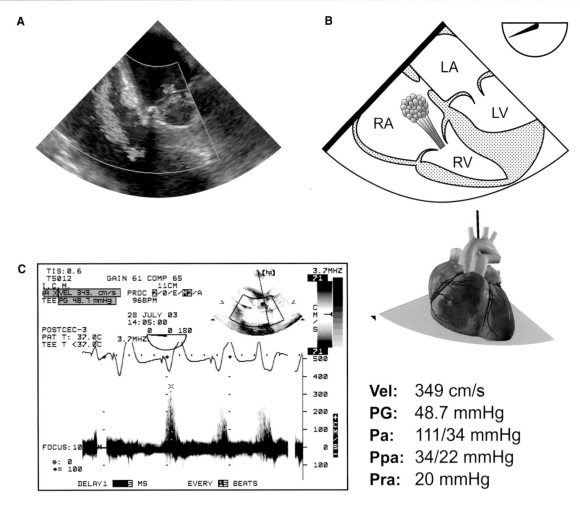

Figure 10.37   RVOT obstruction. The same patient as in Fig. 10.36 is shown. **(A,B)** The right ventricular systolic pressure is estimated at 68.7 mmHg based on a Pra of 20 mmHg and a RV to RA pressure gradient of 48.7 mmHg from a tricuspid regurgitant velocity of 349 cm/s **(C)**. Ppa was directly measured at 34/22 mmHg. This would yield an outflow tract dynamic obstruction PG of 34.7 mmHg confirmed by directed RV pressure tracing (see previous figure). The obstruction was exacerbated by intravenous milrinone and dopamine which were promptly discontinued. Weaning from cardiopulmonary bypass was then successful. The next day, all vasoactive medications were stopped and no residual RV to Ppa gradient was present. *Abbreviations*: LA, left atrium; LV, left ventricle; Pa, arterial pressure; PG, pressure gradient; Ppa, pulmonary artery pressure; Pra, right atrial pressure; RA, right atrium; RV, right ventricle; RVOT, right ventricular outflow tract; Vel, velocity.

tricuspid late (A) and possibly early (E) phases result in ejection through the pulmonic valve (PV). In this case, the A wave will not equate with filling; however, there might be increased retrograde A-wave flow in the hepatic vein. It follows that the height of the E wave may not reflect the transtricuspid pressure gradient as ejection may also occur during this phase. In volume overload, the E velocity will rise late in a disease due to the capacity of the RV to accommodate large amount of volume.

As a general rule, if restriction occurs in the face of increased PAP, inflow parameters will be similar to those of the LV. If restriction occurs in the face of normal PAP, the E velocity will be lower with an E/A

ratio that may be normal due to ejection during both E and A waves. As discussed earlier, in the absence of restriction, E velocity may not increase in the face of larger volumes due to the ability of the RV to maintain compliance. There will only be a rise in E velocity later in disease.

FLUID RESPONSIVENESS

Intravenous fluid administration is one of the most commonly performed therapies in the operating room and the ICU. Yet, surprisingly little data is available to guide its proper use. While earlier studies and classic teaching have mainly advocated the use of fixed

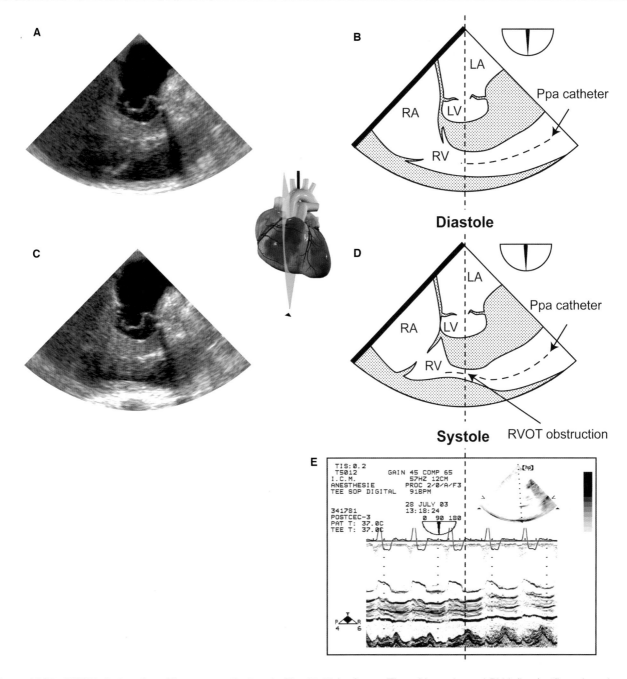

Figure 10.38 RVOT obstruction. The same patient as in Fig. 10.36 is shown. The mid-esophageal RV inflow/outflow view showed dynamic RVOT obstruction during systole in 2D (**A–D**) and M-mode (**E**). *Abbreviations*: LA, left atrium; LV, left ventricle; Ppa, pulmonary artery pressure; RA, right atrium; RV, right ventricle; RVOT, right ventricular outflow tract.

volume regimens, interest in assessing fluid responsiveness has increased as recent literature suggests that early individualized goal-directed fluid administration is associated with a better outcome (83,84).

A monitoring tool with good sensitivity and specificity to assess the fluid-responsiveness status of patients is, therefore, highly desirable. While this section will focus on echocardiographic parameters of fluid responsiveness, other indices, such as variation in arterial pressure and esophageal Doppler-derived dynamic indices, can be useful in the operating room (85) and in the ICU (86). Table 10.2 summarizes the studies evaluating various echocardiographic criteria of fluid responsiveness (87).

Table 10.2 Summary of Studies Evaluating Echocardiographic Criteria of Fluid Responsiveness

Echographic parameter	Studied population	Cutoff for positive response to fluid	Sensitivity (%)	Specificity (%)	ROC AUC	Potential pitfalls	Reference
Static volumetric indices							
LVEDA	21 Post-op CABG 20 Mixed ICU	Could not define	–	–	–	LVEDA(I) is an approximation of LVEDV, which is not valid in all circumstances	88
	19 CABG	Could not define	–	–	–		89
	33 CABG; 3 AVR	Could not define	–	–	0.58	Probably involves a different cutoff if baseline dilatation	90
	19 OPCAB	Could not define	–	–	–		91
LVEDAI	15 Septic patients	<9 cm²/m²	–	–	0.77	Preload is not a good marker of preload responsiveness	92
	19 Septic patients	Could not define	–	–	–		93
	26 Post-op CABG	LVEF <35% <26.5 cm²/m²	64	90	0.78		94
		LVEF >50% <16.7 cm²/m²	60	61	0.73		
	35 OPCAB	Could not define	–	–	0.64		95
	18 CABG	<9.05 cm²/m²	63	69	0.71		96
	21 SICU patients	<11.3 cm²/m²	89	58	0.76		97
	8 Hepatectomies	<10.5 cm²/m²	–	–	0.70		98
	24 MICU patients	Could not define	–	–	0.58		99
LVEDV	19 OPCAB	Could not define	–	–	–		91
Doppler Indices							
Mitral *E/A*	33 CABG; 3 AVR	<1.26	75	60	0.71	Affected by baseline and changes (e.g., ischemia, sepsis) in diastolic function	90
	8 Hepatectomies	<1.84	–	–	0.62		98
Systolic fraction	8 Hepatectomies	Could not define	–	–	0.42		98
Mitral deceleration time	8 Hepatectomies	>234 ms	–	–	0.68	Preload is not a good marker of preload responsiveness	98
Mitral *E/E*$_a$	24 MICU patients	Could not define	–	–	0.65	Preload is not a good marker of preload responsiveness	99

Index	Patients	Threshold				Comments	Ref
Indices of cardiorespiratory interactions							
ΔV_{peak}	19 Septic patients	>12%	100	89	—	Requires sinus rhythm	93
	20 CABG	Could not define	—	—	—	Requires sedated patient with no respiratory effort	100
	19 OPCAB	Could not define	—	—	—		91
$\%VTI_{Ao}$	21 SICU patients	>20.4%	78	92	0.87	Influenced by tidal volume. Can have false positives with RV failure	97
ΔIVC	39 Septic patients	≥12%[a]	88	95	—	Only studied in patients with sinus rhythm	101
	20 Septic patients	>18%[a]	90	90	0.91	Requires sedated patient with no respiratory effort	102
ΔSVC	66 Septic patients	>36%	90	100	0.99	Influenced by tidal volume and probably by intra-abdominal pressure	103
Indices obtained after passive leg raising							
$\%VTI_{Ao}$	34 MICU patients	>12%[b]	69	89	0.90	Not possible in all circumstances (e.g., OR)	104
	24 MICU patients	≥12.5%	77	100	0.96	Need to ensure increase in preload during maneuver. Cannot be automated	99

[a] Different calculation methods used in the two studies.

[b] ΔSV actually studied. However, since $SV = VTI_{Ao} \times$ aortic area (assumed constant), ΔSV equals $\%VTI_{Ao}$ when expressed as percent change from baseline.

Abbreviations: A, atrial TMF; AVR, aortic valve replacement; CABG, coronary artery bypass grafting; E, early TMV; Ea, atrial MAV; IVC, inferior vena cava; LVEDA, left ventricular end-diastolic area; LVEDV, left ventricular end-diastolic volume; LVEF, left ventricular ejection fraction; MAV, mitral annular velocity; MICU, medical intensive care unit; OPCAB, off-pump coronary artery bypass; OR, odds ratio; ROC AUC, area under receiver operating characteristic curve; SV, stroke volume; SVC, superior vena cava; SICU, surgical intensive care unit; TMV, transmitral flow; V_{peak}, peak velocity; VTI_{Ao}, aortic velocity time integral.

Source: Courtesy of F. Girard and A. Vieillard-Baron.

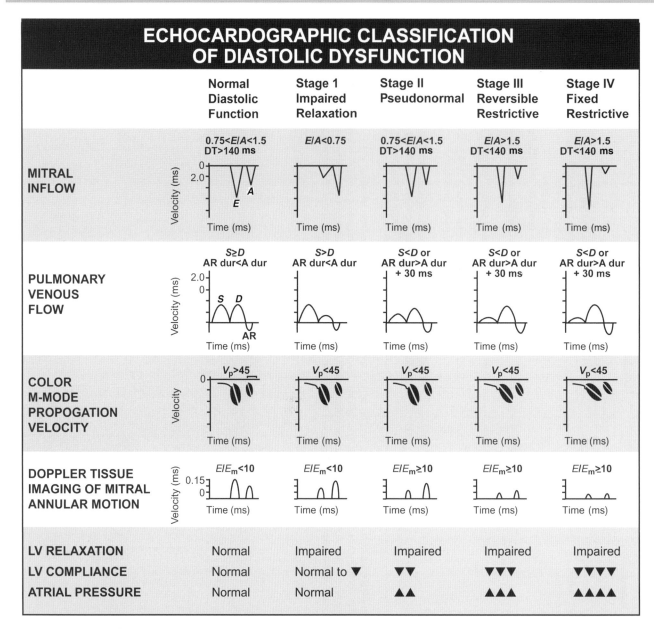

Figure 10.39   Diastolic function classification. Echocardiographic classification of diastolic dysfunction adapted for transesophageal echocardiography is shown. *Abbreviations*: A, peak late diastolic transmitral flow velocity; A dur, duration of mitral inflow A-wave; AR dur, peak pulmonary venous atrial reversal flow velocity duration; D, peak diastolic pulmonary venous flow velocity; DT, deceleration time; *E*, peak early diastolic transmitral flow velocity; *E*m, peak early diastolic myocardial velocity; LV, left ventricle; S, peak systolic pulmonary venous flow velocity; Vp, flow propagation velocity. *Source*: Adapted from Ref. 79.

Static Volumetric Indices

Volumetric indices allow a much better estimation of LV preload than pressure-based indices (105). Changes in LVEDA closely track changes in effective circulating blood volume (106) and, in the right clinical context, a fall in LVEDA from a known baseline likely indicates volume responsiveness. Single values of LVEDA have not been found to be useful in predicting a patient's response to volume administration. However, clinically useful information can probably be obtained in extreme cases.

Left ventricular end-systolic cavity obliteration is likely to be a reliable sign of volume responsiveness (107) (Fig. 10.6), while a RVEDA/LVEDA ≥ 1 indicating RV failure will conversely predict a lack of response to fluids (108). Left ventricular end-systolic cavity obliteration and its relationship to hypovolemia

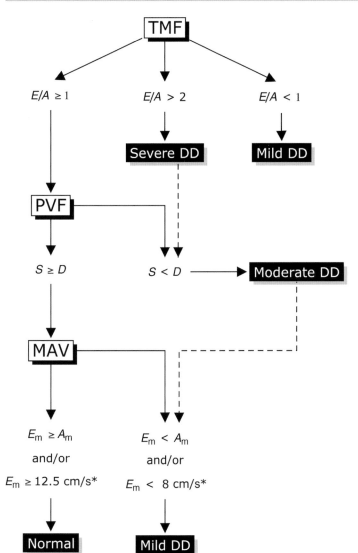

Figure 10.40 LV diastolic dysfunction algorithm. LV diastolic function is classified using pulsed wave Doppler of the TMF, PVF and tissue Doppler examination of MAV. Patients with a pacemaker, atrial fibrillation, non-sinus rhythm, mitral stenosis, severe mitral and aortic regurgitation are excluded from analysis. *Normal E_m is within an 8–12.5 cm/s interval. *Abbreviations*: A, peak late diastolic TMF velocity; A_m, peak late diastolic MAV; D, peak diastolic PVF velocity; DD, diastolic dysfunction; E, peak early diastolic TMF velocity; E_m, peak early diastolic MAV; LV, left ventricle; MAV, mitral annular velocity; PVF, pulmonary venous flow; S, peak systolic PVF velocity; TMF, transmitral flow. *Source*: With permission from Ref. 80.

was studied by Leung and Levine (107) in 139 patients undergoing cardiac surgery who were monitored continuously with TEE using the TG mid-papillary view. Hypovolemia, defined as a 10% reduction in LVEDA, was present in 80% of the observations of LV end-systolic cavity obliteration. Consequently, this sign can occur in patients with increased ventricular performance, where a reduction in LVESV may be observed, without necessarily a reduction in LVEDV.

Furthermore, the use of LVEDA as a predictor of responsiveness to increasing preload has been shown to be limited (88,92,93). It should be emphasized that, although LVEDA is a very good marker of preload, preload is not preload responsiveness. Depending on the systolic and diastolic ventricular function, many different Frank–Starling curves are possible, and it is impossible to predict whether a given preload will fall on the steep (preload-responsive) or flat (preload-unresponsive) part of the curve (Fig. 10.47).

Secondly, studying only LV preload is inadequate for effective administration of intravenous fluids as both ventricles need to be preload responsive. Also, as demonstrated by Reuter et al. (94), baseline LV dilatation thwarts any attempt at defining a single cutoff value. Finally, not all the evidence supports the use of LVEDA as a surrogate for LVEDV (109).

Kusumoto et al. (110) studied atrial septal displacement as an index of reduced preload. Normally LAP is superior to right atrial pressure (RAP), causing the interatrial septum to bulge toward the right, convexity toward the RA, during most of the cardiac cycle (Fig. 10.7). In patients with mechanical ventilation, the authors observed that mid-systolic reversal of the interatrial septal normal convexity occurred during expiration in 64 of 72 episodes when the wedge pressure was <15 mmHg and only two of 40 episodes when it was >15 mmHg. If the mid-systolic reversal of the atrial septum occurred during both inspiration and expiration, the wedge would usually be <10 mmHg.

Doppler Indices

Doppler indices used to estimate LV filling pressure include PW Doppler interrogation of MV inflow, PVF, tissue Doppler interrogation of the MV annulus, and a combination.

Mitral Inflow

The E/A ratio of the MV inflow signal correlates with LV filling pressure (111,112) and PCWP (113). Acute preload reduction is associated with a reduction of the E/A ratio of the MV inflow signal. Lattik et al. (90) observed that patients with normal, or mildly abnormal, diastolic function and a low to normal E/A ratio respond to a fluid bolus by increasing their CO and SV as opposed to patients with elevated E/A ratio (Fig. 10.48). The MV E/A ratio was superior to LV filling pressure and 2D echocardiographic area measurements in predicting the response to volume infusion (90).

While Doppler indices of mitral flow have been found to vary with changing preload (Fig. 10.49), they have not been found to be good markers of fluid responsiveness. The wide variety of baseline diastolic function makes defining a precise cutoff a difficult task. However, it is probably fair to assume that a restrictive pattern is associated with a lack of response to volume.

Pulmonary Venous Flow

The difference between the duration of the atrial reversal wave in the pulmonary veins and that of the mitral A-wave is a useful variable for the estimation of LVEDP (114). As downstream LV filling pressure is increased, the duration of the atrial reversal in the pulmonary veins increases and exceeds the duration of the mitral A-wave. The PVF flow pattern has also been studied as an index of preload. Kuecherer et al. (115) reported the inverse relationship between the PVF ratio of the systolic to diastolic (S/D) velocity-time integral and the left atrial filling pressure. Girard et al. (116) demonstrated a greater respiratory variation of the systolic component (S) with PCWP <18 mmHg.

Tissue Doppler, Color M-Mode, and Combined Indices

Recently, the E/e ratio of the MV inflow E velocity to the MV annulus e (also labeled E_a or E_m) has been demonstrated to be a good surrogate for the assessment of filling pressures in both spontaneously breathing (117) and ventilated (118) patients. The E/e ratio ≥ 9 best identifies patients with LVEDP > 12 mmHg (119,120). The velocity of propagation (V_p) of the E-wave, assessed by color M-mode and tissue Doppler imaging of the MV annulus, has been used in the estimation of LV filling pressure. An E/V_p ratio of the MV inflow E velocity to the color M-mode V_p with a value >1.5 best identifies patients with PCWP >

Table 10.3 Summary of the Doppler Indices in the Evaluation of Hypovolemia

	Decrease in filling pressure	Increase in filling pressure
MV inflow PW Doppler		
• E velocity	↓	↑
• A velocity	↑	↓
• E/A ratio	↓	↑
• Deceleration time	↑	↓
Pulmonary veins PW Doppler		
• S velocity	↑	↓
• D velocity	↓	↑
• AR velocity	↓	↑
• AR duration	↓	↑
• S/D VTI ratio	↑	↓
• Respiratory variations	↑	↓
MV annulus tissue Doppler		
• e velocity	↓	↑
• a velocity	↑	↓
• e/a	↓	↑
Color M-mode		
• Velocity of propagation (V_p) of the E	↓	↑
Derived indices		
• Duration (MV A wave) minus (PV AR wave)	↓	↑
• E/e	↓	↑
• E/V_p	↓	↑

Abbreviations: a, atrial MAV; A, atrial TMF; AR, atrial reversal PVF; D, diastolic PVF; e, early MAV; E, early TMF; MAV, mitral annular velocity; MV, mitral valve; PW, pulsed wave; PV, pulmonic valve; PVF, pulmonic venous flow; S, systolic PVF; TMF, transmitral flow; V_p, velocity of propagation; VTI, velocity time integral.

12 mmHg (121,122). Both E/e and E/V_p ratios have been shown to correlate well with LV filling pressure independently of ventricular function. Like the direct measurement of filling pressures, these indices are not good markers of fluid responsiveness.

However, given limitations of fluid-responsiveness indices, some guidelines recommend the use of fluid challenges (123). To prevent development of pulmonary edema from a fluid challenge, assessment of filling pressures using the E/e index during fluid infusion may be a less invasive alternative to the currently suggested central venous pressure (CVP) or Paop (124). Table 10.3 summarizes the effect of a reduction, or an increase, in preload on these Doppler parameters.

Indices of Cardiorespiratory Interactions

Rising intrathoracic pressure from tidal volume insufflation causes a decrease in venous return leading to a marked fall in RV SV in patients on the steep part of their Frank–Starling curve. The ensuing lower LV preload will lead to a lower LV SV, the importance of which will depend on the LV's own Frank–Starling curve. The magnitude of the decrease of LV SV, as assessed by the change in peak aortic velocity

TISSUE DOPPLER: $E_m < A_m$

VELOCITY OF PROPAGATION

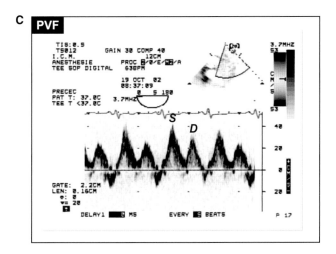

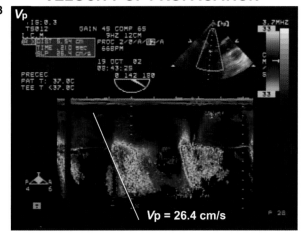

Figure 10.41 Stage 1 diastolic dysfunction (impaired relaxation). A 72-year-old woman undergoing coronary revascularization before cardiopulmonary bypass shows (**A**) tissue Doppler of the lateral MAV $E_m < A_m$ velocity, (**B**) color M-mode Vp E-wave of 26.4 cm/s and (**C**) normal S and D waves on PVF. *Abbreviations*: A_m, peak late diastolic MAV; D, peak diastolic PVF velocity; E_m, peak early diastolic MAV; MAV, mitral annular velocity; PVF, pulmonary venous flow; S, peak systolic PVF velocity; Vp, propagation velocity.

(ΔV_{peak}), or in aortic flow velocity time integral (VTI or %VTI$_{Ao}$), will suggest both the LV and RV's ability to respond to volume (Fig. 10.50). Such indices have proven to be very reliable although some conflicting evidence exists for ΔV_{peak} (91,100). However, these techniques require a regular cardiac rhythm and the complete lack of respiratory drive. The use of tidal volumes <7 cc/kg have been shown to increase the incidence of false negatives in some settings (125), and false positives have been described in cases of RV failure (103).

Vieillard-Baron et al. (10) observed that the presence of superior vena cava (SVC) diameter collapse during positive-pressure ventilation correlated with a significant reduction in preload measured using Doppler velocities in the pulmonary artery. They defined a collapsibility index, as the maximal expiratory SVC diameter minus the minimal inspiratory SVC diame-

ter divided by the maximal SVC diameter on expiration. Patients with an index >60% had an inspiratory decrease in RV outflow velocity close to 70%, as opposed to patients with a collapsibility index of <30%, who had a decrease in RV outflow velocities only to 30%. Fluid challenge reduced the variation in the diameter of the SVC through a change in caval zone condition in a similar fashion to the West zones conditions (Fig. 10.9).

The indices of the collapsibility of the SVC (ΔSVC) and of the distention of the inferior vena cava (IVC or ΔIVC) have shown to be useful in the assessment of fluid responsiveness. Briefly, a lack of respiratory variation in the diameter of the SVC or the IVC will be a marker of either a failing RV or a fluid-replete state (126). The more accurate of the two indices, ΔSVC > 36%, has a sensitivity of 90% and a specificity of 100% for predicting an increase

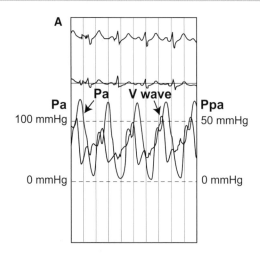

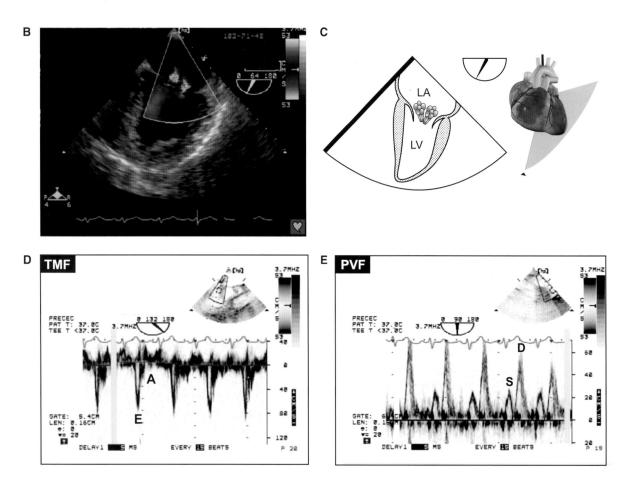

Figure 10.42   Stage III LV diastolic dysfunction (restrictive filling). A 61-year-old woman with cardiogenic shock is brought to the operating room for emergency coronary revascularization. (**A**) She was hemodynamically unstable on an intra-aortic balloon pump and vasoactive support. A 50 mmHg "V" wave on the wedged pulmonary artery catheter tracing was seen without any significant mitral regurgitation on color flow imaging (**B,C**). (**D**) TMF showed an E/A ratio >2 with a deceleration time <60 ms and isovolumic relaxation time of 40 ms. (**E**) The left upper PVF showed an abnormal *S/D* ratio with *S* wave blunting. *Abbreviations: A*, peak late diastolic TMF velocity; *D*, peak diastolic PVF velocity; *E*, peak early diastolic TMF velocity; LA, left atrium; LV, left ventricle; Pa, arterial pressure; Ppa, pulmonary arterial pressure; PVF, pulmonary venous flow; *S*, peak systolic PVF velocity; TMF, transmitral flow.

BEGINNING OF PROCEDURE

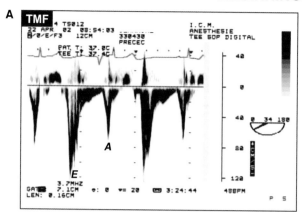

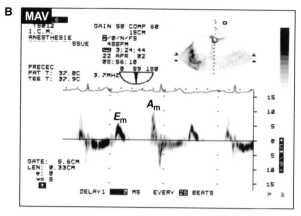

END OF PROCEDURE

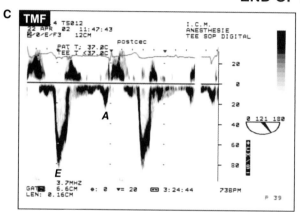

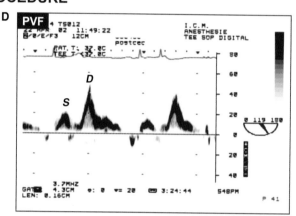

Figure 10.43 **Stage II and III LV diastolic dysfunction.** At the beginning of off-pump bypass surgery in a 73-year-old woman, the TMF demonstrates *E/A* ratio >1 (**A**) with a tissue Doppler MAV *E*m/*A*m ratio <1 (**B**) consistent with at least moderate diastolic dysfunction (pseudonormal pattern). Following revascularization, a higher *E/A* ratio (**C**) with left upper PVF blunted *S*-wave (**D**) suggests worsening diastolic function and higher operating filling pressures. This was associated with significant hemodynamic instability requiring vasoactive support. *Abbreviations*: A, peak late diastolic TMF velocity; A_m, peak late diastolic MAV; D, peak diastolic PVF velocity; E, peak early diastolic TMF velocity; E_m, peak early diastolic MAV; LV, left ventricle; MAV, mitral annular velocity; PVF, pulmonary venous flow; S, peak systolic PVF velocity; TMF, transmitral flow.

in CI (103). Complete absence of respiratory effort is required and, although untested, a low tidal volume probably also decreases sensitivity. When the above conditions are not met, measurement of the IVC's diameter (<12 mm) indicates a fluid responsive state, while a dilated IVC (>20 mm) indicates a fluid replete state (127). Finally, studies have not included patients with intra-abdominal hypertension, an open thorax, or an open abdomen, all factors which may affect the precision of ΔSVC and ΔIVC.

Indices Obtained After Passive Leg Raising

As a way to circumvent the limitations of cardiorespiratory interactions, the passive leg raising (PLR) maneuver has been advocated as a way to generate increased preload transiently and evaluate its effect on CO. Early results studying the effect of PLR on changes in aortic VTI (%VTI$_{Ao}$) are very encouraging. A significant increase of aortic VTI following PLR has been shown to predict an increase in CO following intravenous fluid administration. Notably, these studies included patients who were spontaneously breathing (104) or who had atrial fibrillation (99). The use of automated beds makes this technique relatively simple to perform (128). Preload (e.g., LVEDA) should be monitored to ensure that sufficient volume is recruited by PLR. Unfortunately, by its very nature, PLR-guided assessment of fluid responsiveness cannot be automated or be continuously available. Finally, it won't be possible to implement the PLR maneuver in a number of clinical settings, including most situations in the operating room.

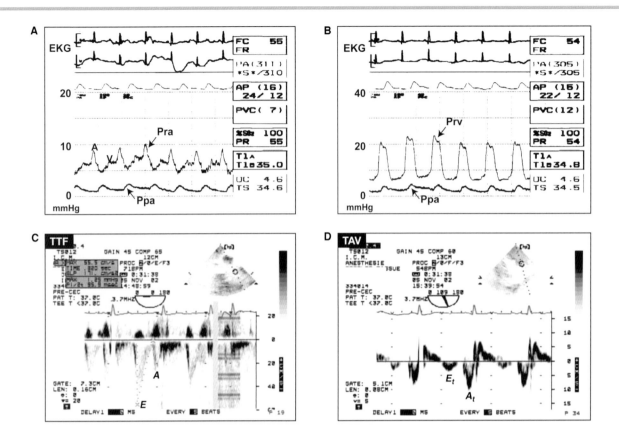

Figure 10.44 RV diastolic dysfunction. A 70-year-old man before cardiac revascularization presents with mild RV diastolic dysfunction. The Pra waveform (**A**) demonstrates a predominant "A" wave and the Prv waveform (**B**) a normal relatively flat diastolic tracing. (**C**) The pulsed wave Doppler TTF tracing shows a predominant E-wave with a prolonged deceleration time (320 ms). (**D**) TAV present an E_t/A_t ratio consistent with mild RV diastolic dysfunction. The hepatic venous flow was normal (not shown). The atrial kick can be seen on the beating heart. The Pra, Prv, and Ppa are on a 0–20, 0–40, and 0–200 mmHg scale respectively. *Abbreviations*: A, peak late diastolic TTF velocity; A_t, peak late diastolic TAV; E, peak early diastolic TTF velocity; E_t, peak early diastolic TAV; EKG, electrocardiogram; Ppa, pulmonary artery pressure; Pra, right atrial pressure; Prv, right ventricular pressure; RV, right ventricle; TAV, tricuspid annular velocity; TTF, transtricuspid flow.

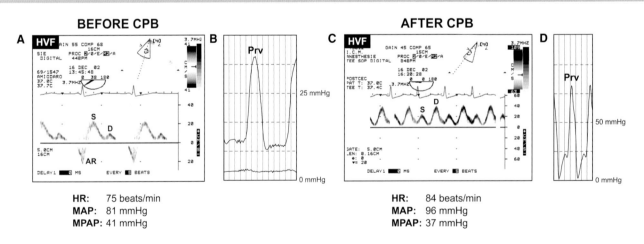

Figure 10.45 RV diastolic dysfunction. A 56-year-old man scheduled for aortic valve replacement presents with RV diastolic dysfunction. (**A**) HVF Doppler before CPB showed a normal S/D ratio >1 but with an increased AR wave. (**B**) He had a normal Prv waveform despite preoperative pulmonary hypertension with a MPAP of 41 mmHg. (**C**) After CPB, the S/D ratio is <1 with predominant D-wave. (**D**) This was associated with a change in the slope of the Prv in diastole from a flat to a steep diastolic waveform. Weaning from CPB was difficult requiring 17.5 µg/min of noradrenaline and 0.4 µg/kg/min of nitroglycerin. The abnormal RV filling can be appreciated visually. *Abbreviations*: AR, peak atrial reversal HVF velocity; CPB, cardiopulmonary bypass; D, peak diastolic HVF velocity; HR, heart rate; HVF, hepatic venous flow; MAP, mean arterial pressure; MPAP, mean pulmonary artery pressure; Prv, right ventricular pressure; RV, right ventricle; S, peak systolic HVF velocity.

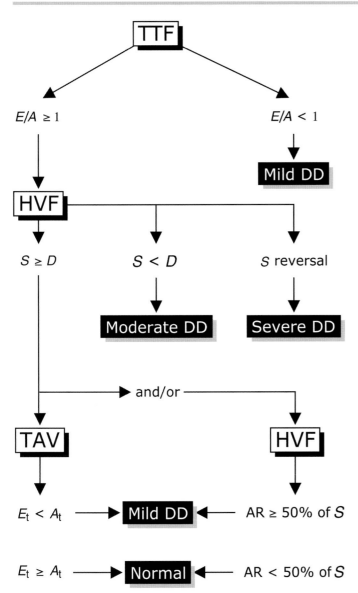

Figure 10.46 RV diastolic dysfunction algorithm. Diastolic function is classified by pulsed wave Doppler of the TTF, HVF and tissue Doppler imaging of the TAV. Patients with a pacemaker, atrial fibrillation, non-sinus rhythm, moderate to severe tricuspid regurgitation and tricuspid annuloplasty are excluded from analysis. *Abbreviations*: *A*, peak late diastolic TTF velocity; AR, peak atrial reversal HVF velocity; A_t, peak late diastolic TAV; DD, diastolic dysfunction; *D*, peak diastolic HVF velocity; *E*, peak early diastolic TTF velocity; E_t, peak early diastolic TAV; HVF, hepatic venous flow; RV, right ventricle; *S*, peak systolic HVF velocity; TAV, tricuspid annular velocity; TTF, transtricuspid flow. *Source*: With permission from Ref. 78.

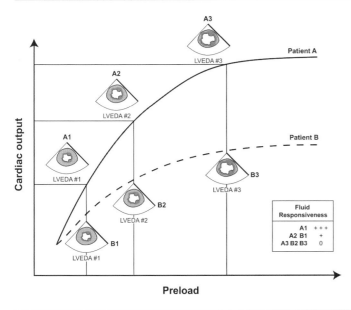

Figure 10.47 Fluid responsiveness, preload and cardiac function. The relation between cardiac output and preload, estimated using LVEDA, in two different patients (A and B) with different ventricular function is shown. For the same LVEDA the response to fluid will be different depending on the position where the actual LVEDA lies in the ventricular function curve. Therefore, patient A1 will respond to volume more than patient B1. Patient A3 and patient B2 and B3 will respond poorly to volume. This illustrates why absolute LVEDA does not necessarily correlate with volume responsiveness. *Abbreviation*: LVEDA, left ventricular end-diastolic area. *Source*: Adapted from Ref. 87.

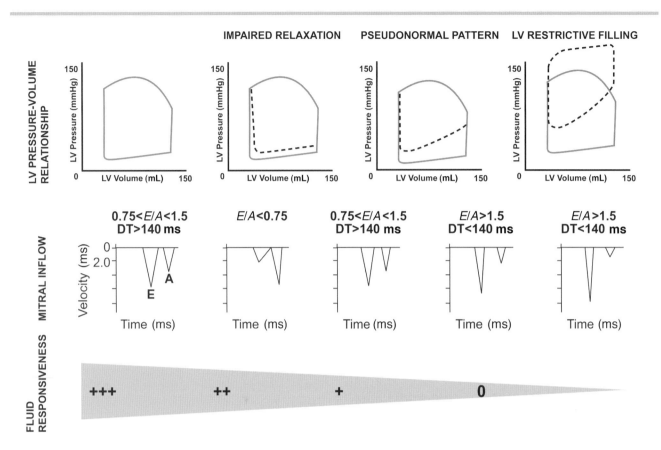

IMPAIRED RELAXATION   PSEUDONORMAL PATTERN   LV RESTRICTIVE FILLING

Figure 10.48   Fluid responsiveness and diastolic function. LV pressure-volume relationship in diastolic dysfunction and corresponding TMF demonstrates as diastolic function deteriorates, fluid responsiveness decreases. *Abbreviations*: A, peak late diastolic TMF velocity; DT, deceleration time; E, peak early diastolic TMF velocity; LV, left ventricular; TMF, transmitral flow.

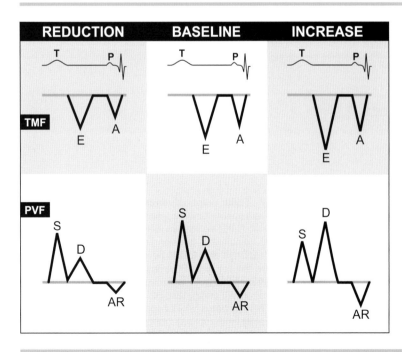

Figure 10.49   Effect of preload on Doppler velocities. The effect of changes in preload on the pulsed wave Doppler interrogation of TMF and PVF is shown. With reduction in preload, both the early diastolic TMF E wave and the diastolic D wave of the PVF are reduced. With an increase in preload, the TMF E wave and PVF D wave are increased. *Abbreviations*: A, peak late diastolic TMF velocity; AR, peak atrial reversal PVF velocity; D, peak diastolic PVF velocity; E, peak early diastolic TMF velocity; PVF, pulmonary venous flow; S, peak systolic PVF velocity; TMF, transmitral valve flow.

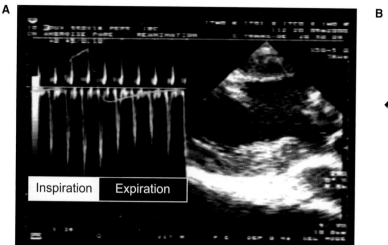
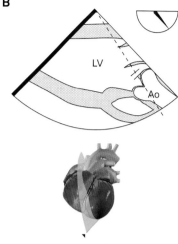

Figure 10.50 Respiratory variations of Doppler velocities. (A,B) Fluid responsiveness can be assessed by measuring respiratory variations in either LVOT or aortic peak velocity (ΔVpeak) or flow velocity-time integral (%VTI). In this patient, a pulsed wave Doppler positioned in the LVOT showed marked respiratory variations in both ΔVpeak and %VTI$_{LVOT}$. This correctly identified occult hypovolemia. Correction of this volume deficit with administration of intravenous fluids led to an increased cardiac output. To be accurate, these indices require that patients be mechanically ventilated and without any spontaneous breathing activity. *Abbreviations*: Ao, aorta; LV, left ventricle; LVOT, left ventricular outflow tract. *Source*: Courtesy of Drs. Girard and Vieillard-Baron.

CONCLUSION

In summary, TEE is an important tool for evaluation of global LV and RV systolic and diastolic function. It provides a unique and rapid diagnostic tool that has been, so far, unsurpassed in the setting of hemodynamic instability.

REFERENCES

1. Douglas PS, Khandheria B, Stainback RF, et al. ACCF/ASE/ACEP/ASNC/SCAI/SCCT/SCMR 2007 appropriateness criteria for transthoracic and transesophageal echocardiography: a report of the American College of Cardiology Foundation Quality Strategic Directions Committee Appropriateness Criteria Working Group, American Society of Echocardiography, American College of Emergency Physicians, American Society of Nuclear Cardiology, Society for Cardiovascular Angiography and Interventions, Society of Cardiovascular Computed Tomography, and the Society for Cardiovascular Magnetic Resonance endorsed by the American College of Chest Physicians and the Society of Critical Care Medicine. J Am Coll Cardiol 2007; 50:187–204.
2. Schiller NB, Shah PM, Crawford M, et al. Recommendations for quantitation of the left ventricle by two-dimensional echocardiography. American Society of Echocardiography Committee on Standards, Subcommittee on Quantitation of Two-Dimensional Echocardiograms. J Am Soc Echocardiogr 1989; 2:358–367.
3. Lang RM, Bierig M, Devereux RB, et al. Recommendations for chamber quantification: a report from the American Society of Echocardiography's Guidelines and Standards Committee and the Chamber Quantification Writing Group, developed in conjunction with the European Association of Echocardiography, a branch of the European Society of Cardiology. J Am Soc Echocardiogr 2005; 18:1440–1463.
4. Emilsson K, Alam M, Wandt B. The relation between mitral annulus motion and ejection fraction: a nonlinear function. J Am Soc Echocardiogr 2000; 13:896–901.
5. Alam M, Wardell J, Andersson E, et al. Effects of first myocardial infarction on left ventricular systolic and diastolic function with the use of mitral annular velocity determined by pulsed wave Doppler tissue imaging. J Am Soc Echocardiogr 2000; 13:343–352.
6. Haddad F, Couture P, Tousignant C, et al. The right ventricle in cardiac surgery, a perioperative perspective: I. Anatomy, physiology, and assessment. Anesth Analg 2009; 108:407–421.
7. Gorcsan J, III, Denault AY, Gasior TA, et al. Rapid estimation of left ventricular contractility from end-systolic relations by echocardiographic automated border detection and femoral arterial pressure. Anesthesiology 1994; 81:553–562.
8. Denault AY, Gorcsan J III, Mandarino WA, et al. Left ventricular performance assessed by echocardiographic automated border detection and arterial pressure. Am J Physiol 1997; 272:H138–H147.
9. Dell'Italia LJ, Walsh RA. Application of a time varying elastance model to right ventricular performance in man. Cardiovasc Res 1988; 22:864–874.
10. Vieillard-Baron A, Augarde R, Prin S, et al. Influence of superior vena caval zone condition on cyclic changes in right ventricular outflow during respiratory support. Anesthesiology 2001; 95:1083–1088.
11. Sunagawa K, Maughan WL, Sagawa K. Optimal arterial resistance for the maximal stroke work studied in isolated canine left ventricle. Circ Res 1985; 56:586–595.
12. Gorcsan J III, Gasior TA, Mandarino WA, et al. Assessment of the immediate effects of cardiopulmonary bypass

on left ventricular performance by on-line pressure-area relations. Circulation 1994; 89:180–190.

13. Simonson JS, Schiller NB. Descent of the base of the left ventricle: an echocardiographic index of left ventricular function. J Am Soc Echocardiogr 1989; 2:25–35.

14. Tei C, Dujardin KS, Hodge DO, et al. Doppler index combining systolic and diastolic myocardial performance: clinical value in cardiac amyloidosis. J Am Coll Cardiol 1996; 28:658–664.

15. Bouchard MJ, Denault AY, Couture P, et al. Poor correlation between hemodynamic and echocardiographic indexes of left ventricular performance in the operating room and intensive care unit. Crit Care Med 2004; 32:644–648.

16. Drexler M, Erbel R, Muller U, et al. Measurement of intracardiac dimensions and structures in normal young adult subjects by transesophageal echocardiography. Am J Cardiol 1990; 65:1491–1496.

17. Colan SD, Parness IA, Spevak PJ, et al. Developmental modulation of myocardial mechanics: age- and growth-related alterations in afterload and contractility. J Am Coll Cardiol 1992; 19:619–629.

18. de Simone G, Devereux RB, Roman MJ, et al. Assessment of left ventricular function by the midwall fractional shortening/end-systolic stress relation in human hypertension. J Am Coll Cardiol 1994; 23:1444–1451.

19. Aurigemma GP, Silver KH, Priest MA, et al. Geometric changes allow normal ejection fraction despite depressed myocardial shortening in hypertensive left ventricular hypertrophy. J Am Coll Cardiol 1995; 26:195–202.

20. Weyman AE. Principles and Practice of Echocardiography. 2nd ed. Philadelphia: Lea & Febiger, 1994.

21. Quinones MA, Waggoner AD, Reduto LA, et al. A new, simplified and accurate method for determining ejection fraction with two-dimensional echocardiography. Circulation 1981; 64:744–753.

22. Rich S, Sheikh A, Gallastegui J, et al. Determination of left ventricular ejection fraction by visual estimation during real-time two-dimensional echocardiography. Am Heart J 1982; 104:603–606.

23. Cahalan MK, Ionescu P, Melton HE Jr., et al. Automated real-time analysis of intraoperative transesophageal echocardiograms. Anesthesiology 1993; 78:477–485.

24. Swaminathan M, Phillips-Bute BG, Mathew JP. An assessment of two different methods of left ventricular ejection time measurement by transesophageal echocardiography. Anesth Analg 2003; 97:642–647.

25. Kupari M, Koskinen P. Systolic flow velocity profile in the left ventricular outflow tract in persons free of heart disease. Am J Cardiol 1993; 72:1172–1178.

26. Garrard CL Jr., Weissler AM, Dodge HT. The relationship of alterations in systolic time intervals to ejection fraction in patients with cardiac disease. Circulation 1970; 42:455–462.

27. Pai RG, Bodenheimer MM, Pai SM, et al. Usefulness of systolic excursion of the mitral annulus as an index of left ventricular systolic function. Am J Cardiol 1991; 67:222–224.

28. Eidem BW, O'Leary PW, Tei C, et al. Usefulness of the myocardial performance index for assessing right ventricular function in congenital heart disease. Am J Cardiol 2000; 86:654–658.

29. Moller JE, Sondergaard E, Poulsen SH, et al. Serial Doppler echocardiographic assessment of left and right ventricular performance after a first myocardial infarction. J Am Soc Echocardiogr 2001; 14:249–255.

30. Chen C, Rodriguez L, Lethor JP, et al. Continuous wave Doppler echocardiography for noninvasive assessment of left ventricular dP/dt and relaxation time constant from

mitral regurgitant spectra in patients. J Am Coll Cardiol 1994; 23:970–976.

31. Colan SD, Borow KM, Neumann A. Left ventricular end-systolic wall stress-velocity of fiber shortening relation: a load-independent index of myocardial contractility. J Am Coll Cardiol 1984; 4:715–724.

32. Jacobs LD, Salgo IS, Goonewardena S, et al. Rapid online quantification of left ventricular volume from real-time three-dimensional echocardiographic data. Eur Heart J 2006; 27:460–468.

33. Davlouros PA, Niwa K, Webb G, et al. The right ventricle in congenital heart disease. Heart 2006; 92(suppl 1):i27–i38.

34. Ryan T, Petrovic O, Dillon JC, et al. An echocardiographic index for separation of right ventricular volume and pressure overload. J Am Coll Cardiol 1985; 5:918–927.

35. Eidem BW, Tei C, O'Leary PW, et al. Nongeometric quantitative assessment of right and left ventricular function: myocardial performance index in normal children and patients with Ebstein anomaly. J Am Soc Echocardiogr 1998; 11:849–856.

36. Yamaguchi K, Miyahara Y, Yakabe K, et al. Right ventricular impairment in patients with chronic respiratory failure on home oxygen therapy–non-invasive assessment using a new Doppler index. J Int Med Res 1998; 26:239–247.

37. Yeo TC, Dujardin KS, Tei C, et al. Value of a Doppler-derived index combining systolic and diastolic time intervals in predicting outcome in primary pulmonary hypertension. Am J Cardiol 1998; 81:1157–1161.

38. Yoshifuku S, Otsuji Y, Takasaki K, et al. Pseudonormalized Doppler total ejection isovolume (Tei) index in patients with right ventricular acute myocardial infarction. Am J Cardiol 2003; 91:527–531.

39. Haddad F, Denault AY, Couture P, et al. Right ventricular myocardial performance index predicts perioperative mortality or circulatory failure in high-risk valvular surgery. J Am Soc Echocardiogr 2007; 20:1065–1072.

40. Lopez-Candales A, Rajagopalan N, Saxena N, et al. Right ventricular systolic function is not the sole determinant of tricuspid annular motion. Am J Cardiol 2006; 98:973–977.

41. Lamia B, Teboul JL, Monnet X, et al. Relationship between the tricuspid annular plane systolic excursion and right and left ventricular function in critically ill patients. Intensive Care Med 2007; 33:2143–2149.

42. Tousignant CP, Bowry R, Levesque S, et al. Regional differences in color tissue Doppler-derived measures of longitudinal right ventricular function using transesophageal echocardiography and transthoracic echocardiography. J Cardiothorac Vasc Anesth 2008; 22(3):400–405.

43. Costachescu T, Denault AY, Guimond JG, et al. The hemodynamically unstable patient in the intensive care unit: hemodynamic vs. transesophageal echocardiographic monitoring. Crit Care Med 2002; 30:1214–1223.

44. Pai RG, Bansal RC, Shah PM. Doppler-derived rate of left ventricular pressure rise. Its correlation with the postoperative left ventricular function in mitral regurgitation. Circulation 1990; 82:514–520.

45. Freeman WK, Schaff HV, Khandheria BK, et al. Intraoperative evaluation of mitral valve regurgitation and repair by transesophageal echocardiography: incidence and significance of systolic anterior motion. J Am Coll Cardiol 1992; 20:599–609.

46. Jebara VA, Mihaileanu S, Acar C, et al. Left ventricular outflow tract obstruction after mitral valve repair. Results of the sliding leaflet technique. Circulation 1993; 88:II30–II34.

47. Brown ML, Abel MD, Click RL, et al. Systolic anterior motion after mitral valve repair: is surgical intervention necessary? J Thorac Cardiovasc Surg 2007; 133:136–143.

48. Bartunek J, Sys SU, Rodrigues AC, et al. Abnormal systolic intraventricular flow velocities after valve replacement for aortic stenosis. Mechanisms, predictive factors, and prognostic significance. Circulation 1996; 93:712–719.

49. Murtha W, Guenther C. Dynamic left ventricular outflow tract obstruction complicating bilateral lung transplantation. Anesth Analg 2002; 94:558–559.

50. Heidenreich PA, Stainback RF, Redberg RF, et al. Transesophageal echocardiography predicts mortality in critically ill patients with unexplained hypotension. J Am Coll Cardiol 1995; 26:152–158.

51. Gouello JP, Bouachour G, Vincent JF, et al. [Detection of left cardiopathy using echocardiography during acute respiratory failure in chronic respiratory insufficiency]. Rev Mal Respir 1995; 12:145–150.

52. Kirschner E, Berger M, Goldberg E. Hypertrophic obstructive cardiomyopathy presenting with profound hypotension. Role of two-dimensional and Doppler echocardiography in diagnosis and management. Chest 1992; 101:711–714.

53. Di Chiara A., Plewka M, Fioretti PM. Systolic anterior movement of mitral valve during acute apical myocardial infarction: An unusual mechanism of acute mitral regurgitation. J Am Soc Echocardiogr 1999; 12:1117–1121.

54. Morewood GH, Weiss SJ. Intra-aortic balloon pump associated with dynamic left ventricular outflow tract obstruction after valve replacement for aortic stenosis. J Am Soc Echocardiogr 2000; 13:229–231.

55. Deligonul U, Uppstrom E, Penick D, et al. Dynamic left ventricular outflow tract obstruction induced by pericardial tamponade during acute anterior myocardial infarction. Am Heart J 1991; 121:190–194.

56. Yoshioka T, Hashimoto A, Tsuchihashi K, et al. Clinical implications of midventricular obstruction and intravenous propranolol use in transient left ventricular apical ballooning (Tako-tsubo cardiomyopathy). Am Heart J 2008; 155:526–527.

57. Mingo S, Benedicto A, Jimenez MC et al. Dynamic left ventricular outflow tract obstruction secondary to catecholamine excess in a normal ventricle. Int J Cardiol 2006; 112:393–396.

58. Auer J, Berent R, Weber T, et al. Catecholamine therapy inducing dynamic left ventricular outflow tract obstruction. Int J Cardiol 2005; 101:325–328.

59. Pellikka PA, Oh JK, Bailey KR, et al. Dynamic intraventricular obstruction during dobutamine stress echocardiography. A new observation. Circulation 1992; 86:1429–1432.

60. Golbasi Z, Sakalli M, Cicek D, et al. Dynamic left ventricular outflow tract obstruction in a patient with pheochromocytoma. Jpn Heart J 1999; 40:831–835.

61. Reichert CL, Visser CA, van den Brink RB, et al. Prognostic value of biventricular function in hypotensive patients after cardiac surgery as assessed by transesophageal echocardiography. J Cardiothorac Vasc Anesth 1992; 6:429–432.

62. Maslow AD, Regan MM, Panzica P, et al. Precardiopulmonary bypass right ventricular function is associated with poor outcome after coronary artery bypass grafting in patients with severe left ventricular systolic dysfunction. Anesth Analg 2002; 95:1507–1518.

63. Eddy AC, Rice CL, Anardi DM. Right ventricular dysfunction in multiple trauma victims. Am J Surg 1988; 155:712–715.

64. Mitsuo T, Shimazaki S, Matsuda H. Right ventricular dysfunction in septic patients. Crit Care Med 1992; 20:630–634.

65. Davila-Roman VG, Waggoner AD, Hopkins WE, et al. Right ventricular dysfunction in low output syndrome after cardiac operations: assessment by transesophageal echocardiography. Ann Thorac Surg 1995; 60:1081–1086.

66. Pinto FJ, Wranne B, St Goar FG, et al. Hepatic venous flow assessed by transesophageal echocardiography. J Am Coll Cardiol 1991; 17:1493–1498.

67. Doshi SN, Kim MC, Sharma SK, et al. Images in cardiovascular medicine. Right and left ventricular outflow tract obstruction in hypertrophic cardiomyopathy. Circulation 2002; 106:e3–e4.

68. Agarwal S, Choudhary S, Saxena A, et al. Giant pulmonary artery aneurysm with right ventricular outflow tract obstruction. Indian Heart J 2002; 54:77–79.

69. Tardif JC, Taylor K, Pandian NG, et al. Right ventricular outflow tract and pulmonary artery obstruction by postoperative mediastinal hematoma: delineation by multiplane transesophageal echocardiography. J Am Soc Echocardiogr 1994; 7:400–404.

70. Dall'Agata A, Cromme-Dijkhuis AH, Meijboom FJ, et al. Use of three-dimensional echocardiography for analysis of outflow obstruction in congenital heart disease. Am J Cardiol 1999; 83:921–925.

71. Bennink GB, Hitchcock FJ, Molenschot M, et al. Aneurysmal pericardial patch producing right ventricular inflow obstruction. Ann Thorac Surg 2001; 71:1346–1347.

72. Basaria S, Denktas AE, Ghani M, et al. Ventricular septal defect patch causing right ventricular inflow tract obstruction. Circulation 1999; 100:e12–e13.

73. Kirshbom PM, Tapson VF, Harrison JK, et al. Delayed right heart failure following lung transplantation. Chest 1996; 109:575–577.

74. Stierle U, Sheikhzadeh A, Shakibi JG, et al. Right ventricular obstruction in various types of hypertrophic cardiomyopathy. Jpn Heart J 1987; 28:115–125.

75. Gorcsan J, III, Reddy SC, Armitage JM, et al. Acquired right ventricular outflow tract obstruction after lung transplantation: diagnosis by transesophageal echocardiography. J Am Soc Echocardiogr 1993; 6:324–326.

76. Denault AY, Chaput M, Couture P, et al. Dynamic right ventricular outflow tract obstruction in cardiac surgery. J Thorac Cardiovasc Surg 2006; 132:43–49.

77. Ritchie ME, Davila-Roman VG, Barzilai B. Dynamic right ventricular outflow obstruction after single-lung transplantation. Biplane transesophageal echocardiographic findings. Chest 1994; 105:610–611.

78. Bernard F, Denault AY, Babin D, et al. Diastolic dysfunction is predictive of difficult weaning from cardiopulmonary bypass. Anesth Analg 2001; 92:291–298.

79. Khouri SJ, Maly GT, Suh DD, et al. A practical approach to the echocardiographic evaluation of diastolic function. J Am Soc Echocardiogr 2004; 17:290–297.

80. Denault AY, Couture P, Buithieu J, et al. Left and right ventricular diastolic dysfunction as predictors of difficult separation from cardiopulmonary bypass. Can J Anaesth 2006; 53:1020–1029.

81. Ozer N, Tokgozoglu L, Coplu L, et al. Echocardiographic evaluation of left and right ventricular diastolic function in patients with chronic obstructive pulmonary disease. J Am Soc Echocardiogr 2001; 14:557–561.

82. Caso P, Galderisi M, Cicala S, et al. Association between myocardial right ventricular relaxation time and pulmonary arterial pressure in chronic obstructive lung disease: analysis by pulsed Doppler tissue imaging. J Am Soc Echocardiogr 2001; 14:970–977.

83. Noblett SE, Snowden CP, Shenton BK, et al. Randomized clinical trial assessing the effect of Doppler-optimized fluid management on outcome after elective colorectal resection. Br J Surg 2006; 93:1069–1076.

84. Bundgaard-Nielsen M, Holte K, Secher NH, et al. Monitoring of peri-operative fluid administration by individualized

goal-directed therapy. Acta Anaesthesiol Scand 2007; 51:331–340.

85. Grocott MP, Mythen MG, Gan TJ. Perioperative fluid management and clinical outcomes in adults. Anesth Analg 2005; 100:1093–1106.

86. Monnet X, Teboul JL. Volume responsiveness. Curr Opin Crit Care 2007; 13:549–553.

87. Vignon P, Cholley B, Slama M, et al. Échocardiographie Doppler chez le patient en état critique. Issy-les-Moulineaux: Elsevier, 2008.

88. Tousignant CP, Walsh F, Mazer CD. The use of transesophageal echocardiography for preload assessment in critically ill patients. Anesth Analg 2000; 90:351–355.

89. Bennett-Guerrero E, Kahn RA, Moskowitz DM, et al. Comparison of arterial systolic pressure variation with other clinical parameters to predict the response to fluid challenges during cardiac surgery. Mt Sinai J Med 2002; 69:96–100.

90. Lattik R, Couture P, Denault AY, et al. Mitral Doppler indices are superior to two-dimensional echocardiographic and hemodynamic variables in predicting responsiveness of cardiac output to a rapid intravenous infusion of colloid. Anesth Analg 2002; 94:1092–1099.

91. Belloni L, Pisano A, Natale A, et al. Assessment of fluid-responsiveness parameters for off-pump coronary artery bypass surgery: a comparison among LiDCO, transesophageal echocardiography, and pulmonary artery catheter. J Cardiothorac Vasc Anesth 2008; 22:243–248.

92. Tavernier B, Makhotine O, Lebuffe G, et al. Systolic pressure variation as a guide to fluid therapy in patients with sepsis-induced hypotension. Anesthesiology 1998; 89:1313–1321.

93. Feissel M, Michard F, Mangin I, et al. Respiratory changes in aortic blood velocity as an indicator of fluid responsiveness in ventilated patients with septic shock. Chest 2001; 119:867–873.

94. Reuter DA, Kirchner A, Felbinger TW, et al. Usefulness of left ventricular stroke volume variation to assess fluid responsiveness in patients with reduced cardiac function. Crit Care Med 2003; 31:1399–1404.

95. Hofer CK, Muller SM, Furrer L, et al. Stroke volume and pulse pressure variation for prediction of fluid responsiveness in patients undergoing off-pump coronary artery bypass grafting. Chest 2005; 128:848–854.

96. Preisman S, Kogan S, Berkenstadt H, et al. Predicting fluid responsiveness in patients undergoing cardiac surgery: functional haemodynamic parameters including the Respiratory Systolic Variation Test and static preload indicators. Br J Anaesth 2005; 95:746–755.

97. Charron C, Fessenmeyer C, Cosson C, et al. The influence of tidal volume on the dynamic variables of fluid responsiveness in critically ill patients. Anesth Analg 2006; 102:1511–1517.

98. Solus-Biguenet H, Fleyfel M, Tavernier B, et al. Non-invasive prediction of fluid responsiveness during major hepatic surgery. Br J Anaesth 2006; 97:808–816.

99. Lamia B, Ochagavia A, Monnet X, et al. Echocardiographic prediction of volume responsiveness in critically ill patients with spontaneously breathing activity. Intensive Care Med 2007; 33:1125–1132.

100. Wiesenack C, Fiegl C, Keyser A, et al. Assessment of fluid responsiveness in mechanically ventilated cardiac surgical patients. Eur J Anaesthesiol 2005; 22:658–665.

101. Feissel M, Michard F, Faller JP, et al. The respiratory variation in inferior vena cava diameter as a guide to fluid therapy. Intensive Care Med 2004; 30:1834–1837.

102. Barbier C, Loubieres Y, Schmit C, et al. Respiratory changes in inferior vena cava diameter are helpful in predicting fluid responsiveness in ventilated septic patients. Intensive Care Med 2004; 30:1740–1746.

103. Vieillard-Baron A, Chergui K, Rabiller A, et al. Superior vena caval collapsibility as a gauge of volume status in ventilated septic patients. Intensive Care Med 2004; 30:1734–1739.

104. Maizel J, Airapetian N, Lorne E, et al. Diagnosis of central hypovolemia by using passive leg raising. Intensive Care Med 2007; 33:1133–1138.

105. Kumar A, Anel R, Bunnell E, et al. Pulmonary artery occlusion pressure and central venous pressure fail to predict ventricular filling volume, cardiac performance, or the response to volume infusion in normal subjects. Crit Care Med 2004; 32:691–699.

106. Cheung AT, Savino JS, Weiss SJ, et al. Echocardiographic and hemodynamic indexes of left ventricular preload in patients with normal and abnormal ventricular function. Anesthesiology 1994; 81:376–387.

107. Leung JM, Levine EH. Left ventricular end-systolic cavity obliteration as an estimate of intraoperative hypovolemia. Anesthesiology 1994; 81:1102–1109.

108. Schneider AJ, Teule GJ, Groeneveld AB, et al. Biventricular performance during volume loading in patients with early septic shock, with emphasis on the right ventricle: a combined hemodynamic and radionuclide study. Am Heart J 1988; 116:103–112.

109. Urbanowicz JH, Shaaban MJ, Cohen NH, et al. Comparison of transesophageal echocardiographic and scintigraphic estimates of left ventricular end-diastolic volume index and ejection fraction in patients following coronary artery bypass grafting. Anesthesiology 1990; 72:607–612.

110. Kusumoto FM, Muhiudeen IA, Kuecherer HF, et al. Response of the interatrial septum to transatrial pressure gradients and its potential for predicting pulmonary capillary wedge pressure: an intraoperative study using transesophageal echocardiography in patients during mechanical ventilation. J Am Coll Cardiol 1993; 21:721–728.

111. Mulvagh S, Quinones MA, Kleiman NS, et al. Estimation of left ventricular end-diastolic pressure from Doppler transmitral flow velocity in cardiac patients independent of systolic performance. J Am Coll Cardiol 1992; 20:112–119.

112. Nomura M, Hillel Z, Shih H, et al. The association between Doppler transmitral flow variables measured by transesophageal echocardiography and pulmonary capillary wedge pressure. Anesth Analg 1997; 84:491–496.

113. Appleton CP, Galloway JM, Gonzalez MS, et al. Estimation of left ventricular filling pressures using two-dimensional and Doppler echocardiography in adult patients with cardiac disease. Additional value of analyzing left atrial size, left atrial ejection fraction and the difference in duration of pulmonary venous and mitral flow velocity at atrial contraction. J Am Coll Cardiol 1993; 22:1972–1982.

114. Kimura K, Murata K, Tanaka N, et al. The importance of pulmonary venous flow measurement for evaluating left ventricular end-diastolic pressure in patients with coronary artery disease in the early stage of diastolic dysfunction. J Am Soc Echocardiogr 2001; 14:987–993.

115. Kuecherer HF, Muhiudeen IA, Kusumoto FM, et al. Estimation of mean left atrial pressure from transesophageal pulsed Doppler echocardiography of pulmonary venous flow. Circulation 1990; 82:1127–1139.

116. Girard F, Couture P, Boudreault D, et al. Estimation of the pulmonary capillary wedge pressure from transesophageal pulsed Doppler echocardiography of pulmonary venous flow: influence of the respiratory cycle during mechanical ventilation. J Cardiothorac Vasc Anesth 1998; 12:16–21.

117. Arques S, Roux E, Luccioni R. Current clinical applications of spectral tissue Doppler echocardiography (E/E′ ratio) as a noninvasive surrogate for left ventricular

diastolic pressures in the diagnosis of heart failure with preserved left ventricular systolic function. Cardiovasc Ultrasound 2007; 5:16.

118. Combes A, Arnoult F, Trouillet JL. Tissue Doppler imaging estimation of pulmonary artery occlusion pressure in ICU patients. Intensive Care Med 2004; 30:75–81.

119. Nagueh SF, Middleton KJ, Kopelen HA, et al. Doppler tissue imaging: a noninvasive technique for evaluation of left ventricular relaxation and estimation of filling pressures. J Am Coll Cardiol 1997; 30:1527–1533.

120. Kim YJ, Sohn DW. Mitral annulus velocity in the estimation of left ventricular filling pressure: prospective study in 200 patients. J Am Soc Echocardiogr 2000; 13:980–985.

121. Garcia MJ, Ares MA, Asher C, et al. An index of early left ventricular filling that combined with pulsed Doppler peak E velocity may estimate capillary wedge pressure. J Am Coll Cardiol 1997; 29:448–454.

122. Firstenberg MS, Levine BD, Garcia MJ, et al. Relationship of echocardiographic indices to pulmonary capillary wedge pressures in healthy volunteers. J Am Coll Cardiol 2000; 36:1664–1669.

123. Antonelli M, Levy M, Andrews PJ, et al. Hemodynamic monitoring in shock and implications for management. International Consensus Conference, Paris, France, 27–28 April 2006. Intensive Care Med 2007; 33:575–590.

124. Vincent JL, Weil MH. Fluid challenge revisited. Crit Care Med 2006; 34:1333–1337.

125. De Backer D, Heenen S, Piagnerelli M, et al. Pulse pressure variations to predict fluid responsiveness: influence of tidal volume. Intensive Care Med 2005; 31:517–523.

126. Jardin F, Vieillard-Baron A. Ultrasonographic examination of the venae cavae. Intensive Care Med 2006; 32:203–206.

127. Teboul JL. SRLF experts recommendations: indicators of volume resuscitation during circulatory failure. Ann Fr Anesth Reanim 2005; 24:568–576.

128. Monnet X, Teboul JL. Passive leg raising. Intensive Care Med 2008; 34:659–663.

11

Cardiomyopathy

Miguel A. Barrero Garcia
*Centre Hospitalier Régional de Trois-Rivières Affiliated to the
Université de Montréal, Montreal, Quebec, Canada*

Anthony Ralph-Edwards and George Djaiani
Toronto General Hospital, Toronto, Ontario, Canada

Philippe L.-L'Allier and Anique Ducharme
Université de Montréal, Montreal, Quebec, Canada

INTRODUCTION

Cardiomyopathy comprises a heterogeneous group of diseases that directly involve the heart muscle resulting in an abnormally thickened, enlarged, or stiff heart. Recent classifications (1) are based on ongoing developments in understanding the underlying mechanisms. Figure 11.1 summarizes the classification of the cardiomyopathies. This chapter will review the typical cardiomyopathies; dilated, hypertrophied, and restrictive as well as the atypical, apical, and non-compaction.

HYPERTROPHIC CARDIOMYOPATHY

Epidemiology

Hypertrophic cardiomyopathy (HCM) is defined morphologically by a hypertrophied, nondilated left ventricle (LV) without an obvious cause such as systemic or cardiac diseases known to produce wall thickening (2). This disorder is transmitted as an autosomal dominant trait in about half of patients, amid identification of more than 200 mutations on at least 11 different genes (3). Most of these mutations encode for sarcomeric proteins (such as myosin heavy chain and tropomyosin), resulting in myofibrillar disarray and dysfunctional myocytes, which in turn triggers reactional hypertrophy. The multitude of genetic defects and their variable penetrance accounts for the clinical heterogeneity of this disease, even within the same family. The cause of HCM in the remainder of patients is unknown.

This disorder has an estimated prevalence of 1/500 individuals in the general population (4), though can be found in 0.5% of the patients referred for an echocardiogram. It is a common cause of sudden death in the young, particularly athletes, and an important substrate for heart failure disability at any age (2).

Clinical Features

The clinical manifestations are quite diverse. Patients with HCM can be completely asymptomatic or present with heart failure, exertional dyspnea, angina, postexertional syncope, or life-threatening arrhythmias. The estimated annual mortality rate is 1% to 2% with sudden death, the first manifestation in as many as 10%. It is of clinical importance to distinguish between the obstructive and nonobstructive forms of HCM as management strategies are usually tailored to the hemodynamic status. A common characteristic feature of HCM (obstructive and nonobstructive) is diastolic dysfunction (5). Diastolic dysfunction from excessive wall thickness results in abnormal LV relaxation causing impaired ventricular filling, increased LV end-diastolic pressure (LVEDP), and consequently, pulmonary congestion and dyspnea, which can be potentiated by LV outflow tract (LVOT) obstruction.

Angina occurs without epicardial coronary stenosis as a result of multiple mechanisms: inadequate capillary density, impaired coronary flow (from high LV diastolic pressure or myocardial muscle bridges), or small vessel disease with exacerbation of O_2 demand during LVOT obstruction. Exertional syncope may be due to hypotension, caused by the inability to increase cardiac output because of the obstruction, together with inappropriate vasodilatation or arrhythmia. Sudden death usually results from arrhythmogenic substrate that predisposes to malignant ventricular arrhythmias, with a variable role from triggers such as hypotension, ischemia, or supraventricular arrhythmias (6).

Anatomical Features

The anatomic hallmark of HCM is ventricular hypertrophy with increased myocardial mass, small LV cavity size, and dilated left atrium (LA) due to high LVEDP (5). The increased wall thickness varies in

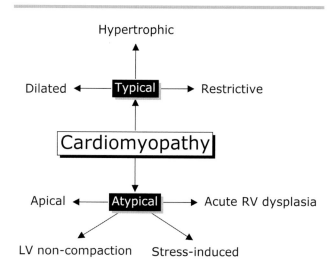

Hypertrophic

Dilated ← **Typical** → Restrictive

Cardiomyopathy

Apical ← **Atypical** → Acute RV dysplasia

LV non-compaction   Stress-induced

Figure 11.1 Classification of cardiomyopathies. Cardiomyopathies can be considered to fall into 2 categories: typical and atypical. *Abbreviations*: LV, left ventricular; RV, right ventricular.

(1–7%). The mitral valve (MV) may be intrinsically abnormal: the papillary muscles can be displaced anteriorly and the leaflets elongated. These abnormalities, associated with a hypertrophied bulging basal septum, will maximally reduce the LVOT diameter, providing a substrate for dynamic subaortic obstruction. Mid-cavitary obstruction may also occur from anomalous papillary muscle insertion, preferential mid-ventricular or papillary muscle hypertrophy and malalignment.

The LV function is usually hyperdynamic. However, longstanding HCM might evolve, and the hypertrophic segments could be replaced by thinner, dysfunctional fibrotic wall with dilated LV systolic and diastolic dimensions. This end-stage HCM is indistinguishable from dilated cardiomyopathy (DCM) and occurs in ∼10% to 20% of patients.

Pathophysiology of Outflow Tract Obstruction

Almost a quarter of the patients with septal hypertrophy will have significant resting LVOT obstruction. In the others, the obstruction may be absent at rest but revealed by provocative maneuvers or changes in hemodynamic conditions. There is a general consensus that a true mechanical impediment to the LV ejection exists resulting from the MV and its apparatus moving anteriorly, termed systolic anterior motion (SAM).

severity and distribution; the "classic" asymmetric hypertrophy of the septal wall represents 70% to 75% of cases (Fig. 11.2), followed by basal septal location (10–15%), concentric symmetrical (5%), apical (5%), and isolated hypertrophy of the lateral wall

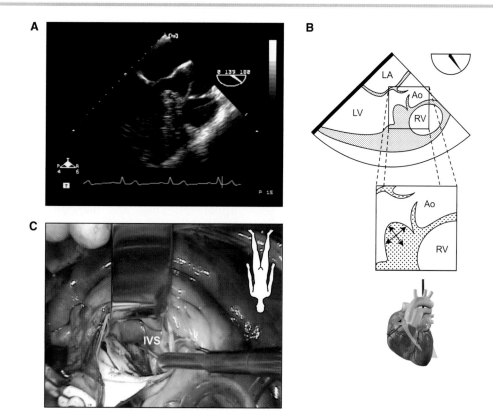

Figure 11.2 Hypertrophic septal cardiomyopathy. (A,B) Mid-esophageal long-axis view of a 26-year-old man with hypertrophic septal cardiomyopathy shows the septal thickness is 26.6 mm. The septal measurements that the surgeon requires for septal myectomy are shown in the zoomed box. **(C)** Intraoperative view of the IVS before septal myectomy. *Abbreviations*: Ao, aorta; IVS, interventricular septum; LA, left atrium; LV, left ventricle; RV, right ventricle. *Source*: Photo C courtesy of Dr. Nancy Poirier.

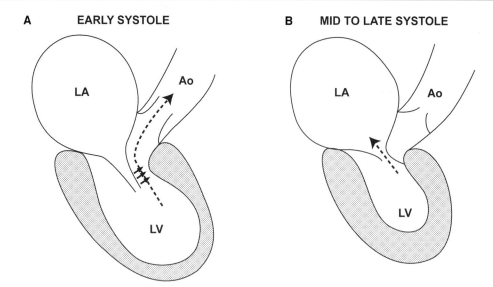

A   EARLY SYSTOLE

B   MID TO LATE SYSTOLE

Figure 11.3   Mechanism of SAM. (A) In early systole, septal hypertrophy causes the narrowed LVOT to be closer to the mitral valve. **(B)** The resulting Venturi forces drag the AMVL and apparatus toward the septum, causing leaflet-septal contact in mid-systole, LVOT obstruction and mitral regurgitation. *Abbreviations*: AMVL, anterior mitral valve leaflet; Ao, aorta; LA, left atrium; LV, left ventricle; LVOT, left ventricular ouflow tract; SAM, systolic anterior motion. *Source*: Adapted from Ref. 66.

Rapid LV ejection from the hypertrophied LV will increase the velocity of blood flow across the narrowed LVOT, producing a *Venturi effect*. These forces will drag the abnormal mitral leaflets and support apparatus toward the septum (7), creating a defect in MV closure; the point of coaptation will occur in the body of the elongated leaflets instead of at their tips. The portion of the anterior leaflet distal from the coaptation point is then free to move within the subaortic flow (anteriorly and superiorly), leading to mitral leaflet-septum contact causing further LVOT narrowing (Fig. 11.3). Another proposed mechanism of SAM is the drag effect (10). The midseptal bulge redirects outflow direction so that it comes from a lateral and posterior direction. The abnormally directed outflow gets behind and lateral to the enlarged MV, catches it, and pushes it into the septum. In both mechanisms, the severity and duration of the SAM is highly related to the extent of the subaortic obstruction (7). The SAM also creates a gap between the mitral leaflets, in which mitral regurgitation (MR) can develop. MR occurs predominantly in mid-to-late systole, reflecting the dynamic nature of this insufficiency. The jet of MR is usually directed posteriorly (59%), but central (38%) and anterior jets (3%) can also be found, owing to concurrent prolapse of the posterior leaflet (11,12). This sequence of events follows the "eject-obstruct-leak" pattern described in earlier angiographic studies. The amount of MR is related to the degree of LVOT obstruction and is usually moderate in severity. Other factors influencing MR severity includes MV prolapse, annular calcification, and leaflet damage from repeated trauma.

Latent obstruction is associated with localized subaortic hypertrophy (in 53% of cases) or with hypertrophy involving the basal 2/3 of the septum (in 35%). Right ventricular (RV) outflow tract obstruction may also be present, owing to RV hypertrophy with dynamic reduction in RV outflow tract size (13). Left ventricular outflow tract obstruction does not develop in patients with isolated apical, lateral, or free wall hypertrophy. In the nonobstructive forms of the disease, no significant pressure gradient is present either at rest or with provocative maneuvers.

An important characteristic of the subaortic obstruction is its dynamic nature. Any hemodynamic conditions reducing ventricular volume (e.g., hypovolemia) will accentuate the apposition of the elongated MV leaflets against the septum of the smaller cavity, thus increasing the outflow gradient. Enhanced contractility (e.g., due to increased levels of endogenous or exogenous catecholamines) will also increase the flow velocity, and therefore the dragging force on the mitral apparatus. Thus, any maneuvers that decrease the preload and afterload or increase the inotropic state would exacerbate or even provoke an LVOT obstruction. A physiological example of this phenomena is the postextrasystolic potentiation. Normally, the compensatory pause following a ventricular extrasystole leads to (*i*) an increase in the LV diastolic volume, stretching the ventricular fibers; (*ii*) increased calcium reuptake; and (*iii*) reduced afterload, due to lower aortic end-diastolic pressure. All these phenomena promote increased contractility of the next beat, resulting in a higher aortic pulse pressure. In hypertrophic obstructive cardiomyopathy (HOCM), this phenomenon increases the gradient between the LV and the aortic pressure and leads to a paradoxically smaller aortic systolic pressure than on the previous beats: this constitutes the Braunwald–Brockenbrough sign (Fig. 11.4).

Many drugs can have deleterious hemodynamic effects in patients with HOCM. Those with vasodilatory or positive inotropic properties are known to increase the LVOT gradient. In contrast, negative

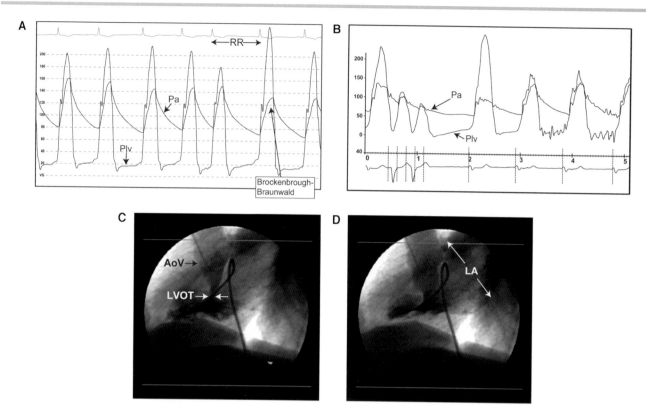

Figure 11.4 Brockenbrough-Braunwald phenomenon. Two examples of this phenomenon on Plv and Pa hemodynamic tracings are shown. **(A,B)** In HOCM, postextrasystolic potentiation of LV contraction results in a higher gradient between the LV and the aorta and a decreased aortic pulse pressure than on the previous beats. **(C,D)** Left ventriculography in a patient with HOCM and LVOT obstruction. Note the "hurricane tail" appearance of the LVOT during systole from systolic anterior displacement of the MV in the LVOT. **(D)** The LA is dilated from the incompetent MV leading to mitral regurgitation. See text for details. *Abbreviations*: AoV, aortic valve; HOCM, hypertrophic obstructive cardiomyopathy; LA, left atrium; LV, left ventricle; LVOT, left ventricular outflow tract; MV, mitral valve; Pa, arterial pressure; Plv, left ventricular pressure.

inotropic (β-blockers and calcium antagonists) or pure vasopressive drugs can have beneficial effects. Knowledge of all the conditions that modulates this dynamic process is essential when caring for patients with HOCM. The Valsalva maneuver is a useful tool at the bedside to unmask or increase an LVOT gradient. By lowering the preload, this maneuver increases the dynamic obstruction and the intensity of the cardiac systolic murmur, a useful sign to differentiate it from that of fixed aortic valvular stenosis.

Echocardiographic Features

Echocardiography is an indispensable tool in the diagnosis and follow-up of HCM patients. It permits the evaluation of the extent and severity of the hypertrophy, LVOT obstruction, and degree of MR.

M-Mode and Two-Dimensional Imaging

Hypertrophy and systolic function. The most striking feature is LV hypertrophy, which is often asymmetrical (Fig. 11.2). Hypertrophy is defined as an increased LV mass, indexed to the body surface area (BSA). Methods to calculate LV mass have been validated

mainly with transthoracic echocardiography (TTE), by measuring mid-ventricular LV cavity dimension and the ventricular septal and posterior wall thickness at end-diastole (see Fig. 5.23). Real-time three dimensional echocardiography has been utilized to measure LV mass in an attempt to overcome the limitations of conventional methods (mainly due to the variability in wall thickness and dimensions throughout the LV), but data confirming its utility are still lacking. The upper limit of normal for wall thickness in diastole is 9 mm for women and 10 mm for men (14). Hypertrophy is considered asymmetrical if the ratio of septal wall thickness to posterior wall exceeds 1.3 (15).

With transesophageal echocardiography (TEE), it is recommended to measure the wall thickness by M-mode in the transgastric mid-papillary short axis (SAX) view at 0°, paying particular attention to avoid oblique measurements and ensuring correct alignment by obtaining a circular left ventricular cavity. Precise measurements are essential since the severity of the hypertrophy carries an important prognostic value, being highly correlated with the risk of sudden death, independently of LVOT obstruction (16). A wall thickness of more than 30 mm triples the risk of sudden death and is one of the major risk factors for the implantation of a cardiac defibrillator for primary prevention of sudden cardiac death. Hence, given the asymmetrical nature of the disease, one must be cautious and use multiple views when evaluating the extent and severity of HCM. The long axis (LAX) (120°) and four-chamber (0°) mid-esophageal views are useful to visualize the entire septum, particularly the more frequently involved basal part.

Earlier studies have described changes in the acoustic texture of the affected myocardium, with a ground-glass appearance of the hypertrophied muscle. This was thought to represent abnormal cells architecture and myocardial fibrosis. This finding is neither sensitive nor specific for the diagnosis of HCM and can be present in other conditions (amyloidosis, hypertensive disease with renal insufficiency, and glycogen storage disease), or be absent in affected individuals. Nevertheless, hyperechogenic (fibrotic) lesions are often seen in the septum at the level of the mitral-septal contact.

The systolic function is usually well preserved in HCM, until late in the course of the disease. The ejection fraction is usually supranormal because the presence of a small ventricular cavity size, and increased wall thickness results in reduced wall stress.

Consequently, the hypertrophied ventricle will contract forcefully in face of a reduced afterload.

MV apparatus. In addition to the abnormally large and elongated mitral leaflets, other MV abnormalities can be found. Ruptured chordae, anomalous papillary muscles insertion, leaflet(s) prolapse, or degenerative changes from repeated septal contact have all been described in association with HOCM and can result in severe MR. The direction of the MR jet is an important clue for the underlying mechanism, because an anterior or central jet cannot be exclusively related to dynamic obstruction but is due to concomitant disease, often a primary leaflet pathology (17). Calcification of the mitral annulus is a frequent finding and, occasionally, the only hint to the potential for dynamic LVOT obstruction. Special attention should be taken to identify these MV abnormalities preoperatively, since they will need to be addressed separately to ensure complete correction of the MR.

Systolic anterior motion of the mitral valve. The SAM of the MV and its contact with the septum is best evaluated in the mid-esophageal five chamber (0°) or LAX views (120°). The extent and duration of the mitral-septal contact can also be appreciated using M-mode of the LV in the same views (Fig. 11.5).

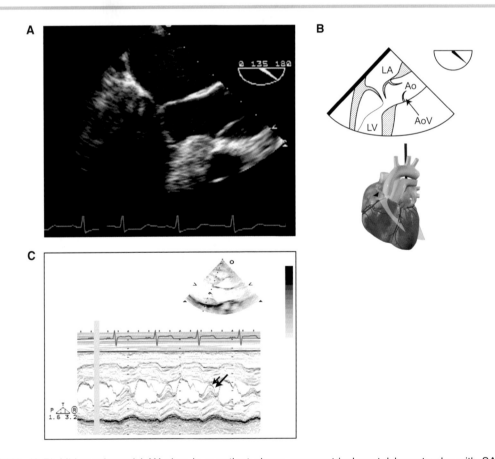

Figure 11.5 SAM. (A,B) Mid-esophageal LAX view in a patient shows asymmetrical septal hypertrophy with SAM and dynamic obstruction of the LVOT. **(C)** Transthoracic M-mode echocardiography of the mitral valve in a LAX view, demonstrating SAM of the mitral leaflets toward the septum wall (arrow). *Abbreviations*: Ao, aorta; AoV, aortic valve; LA, left atrium; LAX, long-axis; LV, left ventricle; LVOT, left ventricular outflow tract; RA, right atrium; RV, right ventricle; SAM, systolic anterior motion.

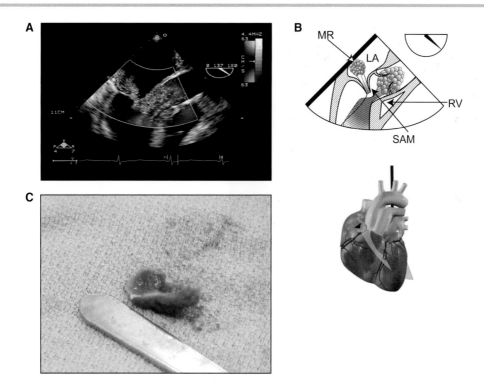

Figure 11.6 MR in hypertrophic cardiomyopathy. The preoperative transesophageal echocardiographic exam of a 26-year-old man with hypertrophic cardiomyopathy and refractory symptoms despite optimal medical therapy is shown. (**A,B**) Mid-esophageal long-axis view with color Doppler shows flow acceleration in the subaortic region and posteriorly directed MR. (**C**) The resected basal septum specimen is shown. *Abbreviations*: LA, left atrium; MR, mitral regurgitation; RV, right ventricle; SAM, systolic anterior motion. *Source*: Photo C courtesy of Dr. Nancy Poirier.

Significant LVOT obstruction is present when the septal contact lasts at least 30% of the systole duration, giving the highest SAM severity grade of 4+. The transgastric (TG) LAX view at 120° and the deep TG view at 0° both display the LVOT but the latter is the optimal view to assess the LVOT gradient by TEE.

Other findings. First, the LA is often dilated because of associated MR (Fig. 11.6), chronically increased LV diastolic pressure, and the presence of atrial fibrillation, which is a frequent complication of HCM. Second, as the LVOT obstruction begins in mid- or late systole, the aortic cusps may close prematurely as a result of the reduced flow in the later half of the ejection period. This mid-systolic closure is best appreciated using M-mode of the aortic valve (AoV) at the mid-esophageal LAX (120°) view (Fig. 11.7). Finally, the right ventricle and the right ventricular outflow (RVOT) must also be carefully inspected, as they too can occasionally be involved (13).

Doppler and Color Flow Imaging

Color flow Doppler. Color flow imaging (CFI) is essential to localize the obstruction at the LVOT level; the turbulent color flow acceleration is seen below the AoV that differentiates it from true valvular aortic stenosis (AS). This can be demonstrated using the mid-esophageal LAX view at 135° (Fig. 11.2). Alternatively,

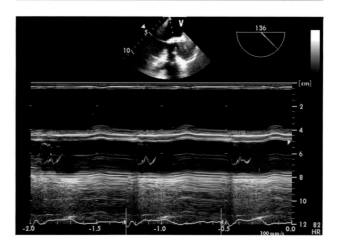

Figure 11.7 Mid-systolic closure of the AoV. Mid-esophageal AoV long-axis M-mode view through the AoV in a 69-year-old woman shows mid-systolic closure from systolic anterior motion of the mitral valve after AoV replacement. *Abbreviation*: AoV, aortic valve.

TG LAX or deep TG views (Fig. 11.8) with CFI can also display the flow acceleration, although less precisely because of the farther position of the LVOT in the scanned field. The SAM of the MV distorts the

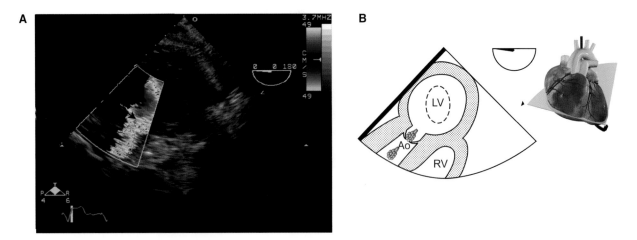

Figure 11.8 LVOT obstruction. (A,B) Color Doppler transgastric view shows color flow acceleration in the LVOT. This is a good interrogation angle for pulsed or continuous wave Doppler. *Abbreviations*: Ao, aorta; LV, left ventricle; LVOT, left ventricular outflow tract; RV, right ventricle.

coaptation point of the leaflets, resulting in a posterior jet of MR (Fig. 11.6). Therefore, variable degree of MR almost always accompanies the obstructive form of HCM. The severity of MR should be quantified as usual, but can greatly fluctuate over time given the dynamic nature of the SAM; this phenomenon may be particularly important in the operating room (OR) where under general anesthesia, the LVOT obstruction may partially or completely disappear.

Pulsed wave Doppler. The pulsed wave (PW) Doppler is useful for precisely identifying the level of the obstruction, particularly in the mid-ventricle. The PW Doppler sample volume is advanced progressively

from the apex to the LVOT in an LAX view (ideally through the deep transgastric views) until a rapid increase in flow velocity is encountered, locating the obstruction. However, the PW Doppler is of limited value to evaluate severe obstruction or gradients in series (e.g., valvular and subvalvular), as the V_1 velocity proximal to the stenosis exceeds the Nyquist limit and is therefore already aliasing. By definition, continuous wave (CW) Doppler will yield the sum of all gradients, as it measures the highest velocity in the LV-aorta axis (Fig. 11.9). Planimetry of the AoV in a SAX view can help sort out the severity of concomitant valvular stenosis.

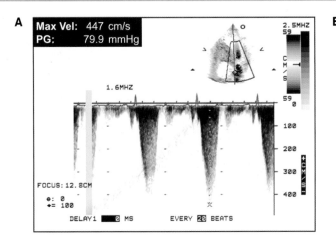
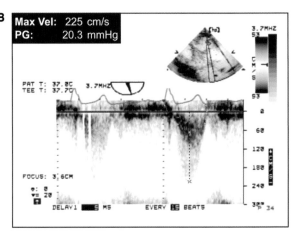

Figure 11.9 Pressure gradient in LVOT obstruction. Measurement of the LVOT PG in two patients with HOCM is shown. **(A)** In the first patient, a maximal instantaneous systolic PG of 79.9 mmHg is obtained from a transthoracic exam. Note the dagger shape of the Doppler signal. **(B)** In the second patient, a 26-year-old man with asymmetrical septal HOCM, the peak systolic PG obtained from a transgastric long-axis view is measured at 20.3 mmHg after induction of general anesthesia. The gradient was however much higher (56 mmHg) in the awake state. *Abbreviations*: HOCM, hypertrophic obstructive cardiomyopathy; LVOT, left ventricular outflow tract; Max Vel, maximum velocity; PG, pressure gradient.

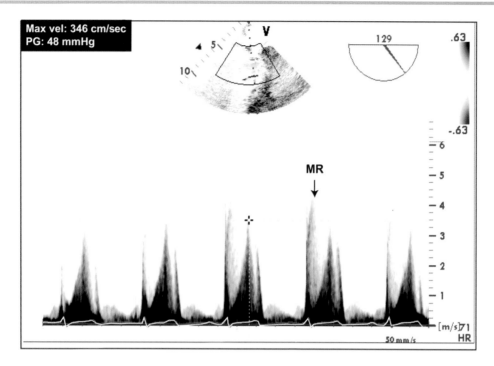

Figure 11.10 Dagger shape CW Doppler signal. A 60-year-old man with aortic stenosis and septal hypertrophy after aortic valve replacement demonstrates acquired LVOT obstruction. CW Doppler of the LVOT obtained in a mid-esophageal long-axis view has a dagger shape, which begins simultaneously or after the QRS, with a 48 mmHg PG. Also present in the CW Doppler signal is MR. The MR occurs before isovolumic contraction, in the CW signal it begins before the QRS of the electrocardiogram. *Abbreviations*: CW, continuous wave; LVOT, left ventricular outflow tract; MR, mitral regurgitation; PG, pressure gradient; Vel, velocity.

Continuous wave Doppler. The severity of LVOT obstruction is assessed with CW Doppler. Increased flow velocity can be detected by positioning the Doppler beam through the LVOT, parallel to the flow acceleration, guided by CFI as needed, using the deep TG views or TG LAX view at 110° to 120°. The LVOT obstructive dynamic gradient is late peaking and significantly rises in mid- to late systole. The CW Doppler velocity profile takes a characteristic *dagger* shape (Fig. 11.10), in contrast to the more symmetrical shape of a fixed valvular stenosis or a regurgitant jet of MR. Maneuvers to modify the loading condition should unmask latent LVOT or midventricular obstructions. Performing a Valsalva maneuver or inhalation of amyl nitrite is often impractical in sedated patients; instead intravenous or sublingual nitroglycerin administration can be used to decrease preload and, to a lesser extent, afterload to provoke or enhance the obstruction. There is no additional diagnostic benefit to enhance an already severe dynamic obstruction in a given patient.

The Doppler signal of the LVOT obstruction is occasionally confused with the signal of MR, particularly when the jet is directed anteriorly toward the subaortic atrial wall. The timing and duration of the velocity profile might help differentiate the two (Fig. 11.10). The typical MR Doppler signal is usually of a longer duration and begins sooner, as it includes the isovolumetric contraction and relaxation times. However, when MR is entirely due to SAM of the MV, it begins after the onset of the LVOT obstruction.

Hence, the velocity profile starts later in systole and usually terminates with MV opening. In LVOT dynamic obstruction, the signal ends with AoV closure. The PW Doppler signal with the sample volume located in the LVOT also helps identifying the true origin of the velocity signal obtained.

The MR peak velocity should be higher than the obstruction velocity and can even be used to estimate the LVOT gradient. For example, an MR peak velocity of 6 m/s corresponds to an instantaneous left atrial-left ventricular systolic gradient of 144 mmHg from the simplified Bernoulli equation. The ventricular systolic pressure can then be calculated by adding the LA pressure (estimated by the wedge pressure from a pulmonary artery catheter); if the LA pressure is 20 mmHg, the LV peak systolic pressure is estimated at 164 mmHg (see Fig. 5.32). The peak LVOT gradient can be easily estimated by subtracting the systemic systolic blood pressure from the estimated systolic LV pressure, hence, 164 mmHg − 120 mmHg = 44 mmHg. This way of approximating the LVOT gradient can be useful when the Doppler tracing quality is unsatisfactory. However, care must be taken to ensure that the MR Doppler signal is complete and taken parallel to the regurgitant jet.

Diastolic Function

Systolic function is usually normal, but abnormal diastolic function can be found in approximately 80% of HCM patients, whether or not a subaortic gradient is present. Ventricular hypertrophy and fibrosis lead to abnormal chamber stiffness and delayed ventricular relaxation, the commonest diastolic pattern. Interestingly, there seems to be little correlation between the severity of diastolic dysfunction and the extent of hypertrophy (6). The increased role of the atrial contraction in LV filling helps understand the dramatic clinical deterioration of HCM patients when they develop atrial fibrillation. More severe patterns of diastolic function also occur. As the left atrial pressure increases, either by reduced LV compliance or by MR, the driving pressure for early filling increases resulting in a restrictive filling pattern. The combination of tissue Doppler imaging (TDI) with transmitral flow analysis provides reliable predictions of LV filling pressures (18). Mitral annulus velocity (*e*, also designated by E_a, E_m, or E') is decreased in most patients, even those with positive genotype and no phenotypical changes. The E/e ratio may also be more reliable for estimating pulmonary capillary wedge pressure (PCWP) than mitral inflow velocity variables alone; studies have demonstrated that PCWP is higher than 20 mmHg when E/e is more than 10 (using the lateral annulus *e*) (19) or 15 (using the septal annulus *e*) (20).

Conditions Simulating HCM

Hypertrophy

The differential diagnosis of HOCM consists of a number of conditions producing either LV hypertrophy (either symmetrical or asymmetrical) or SAM with LVOT obstruction. Aortic stenosis, systemic hypertension, metabolic disorders, and amyloidosis can all lead to increased symmetrical wall thickness. Asymmetrical hypertrophy has been described in isolated RV hypertrophy caused by pressure overload, which produces a disproportional increase in septal wall thickness relative to the normal left ventricular posterior wall (21). Also a patient with concentric left ventricular hypertrophy (LVH) that has sustained a posterior myocardial infarction (MI) can exhibit asymmetrical hypertrophy from thinning and fibrosis of the infarcted region. Amyloidosis, Freidriech's ataxia, myxedema, and D-transposition have all been associated with a disproportionate increase in septal wall thickness. Older people are sometimes found to have sigmoid-shape LV with a prominent basal septum that bulges in the LVOT. This finding is probably due to a more acute angle between the septal bulge and the aortic root and is not considered a pathological state.

SAM and Left Ventricular Outflow Tract Obstruction

Systolic anterior motion of the MV and subsequent LVOT obstruction can theoretically happen whenever predisposing conditions occur (see Fig. 30.10). The highest incidence of spontaneously occurring SAM outside HCM is D-transposition of the great vessels where it has been noted after an atrial switch operation or in patients without corrective surgery (22). Systolic anterior motion and LVOT obstruction have also been precipitated by hypovolemia in hypertensive older

individuals with LVH (see Fig. 10.10). Systolic anterior motion can also be seen in cases of significant posterior mitral annulus calcification, anomalous papillary muscle, and in patients post acute MI with apical dysfunction and hyperdynamic basal function.

Two post-operative conditions may be complicated by SAM and, hence, deserve special attention. Significant SAM can develop in a patient with preexisting LVH from AS following AoV replacement (Figs. 11.7 and 11.10). This results from the acute reduction in afterload, which allows increased LV ejection in a small LVOT, thereby producing subvalvular stenosis or mid-ventricular obstruction. This is usually transient and responds well to volume loading and cessation of inotropic drugs, but in certain cases, surgical correction may be required (Fig. 10.30) (23). The complication of SAM after MV repair for prolapse varies from 2% to 14% (24) and is more frequent in patients with bileaflet myxomatous disease. The underlying mechanisms include anterior displacement of the coaptation point, a longer and redundant posterior leaflet (with or without a more acute mitroaortic angle), causing the MV apparatus to be displaced toward the LVOT and be dragged by the outflow. Preoperatively, a longer posterior leaflet relatively to the anterior (anterior/posterior length ratio ≤1.3) and a shorter distance (≤2.5 cm) between the coaptation point and the septum are predictors of SAM development post repair (Fig. 11.11) (25). For some patients the problem can be alleviated by increasing left ventricular filling or by reducing inotropic support. However, other patients require MV replacement or subsequent repair. The sliding technique has been developed to decrease the incidence of this complication by reducing the posterior leaflet redundancy (Fig. 11.12) (26).

Monitoring Therapy

Intensive Care Unit and Noncardiac Surgery

The HOCM patient can benefit from TEE as a hemodynamic monitor, particularly in clinical situations with rapidly changing loading conditions in the intensive care unit (ICU) or the OR.

Noncardiac surgery is a stressful event for an HOCM patient and may be associated with significant adverse cardiac events in 40% of patients (27). Surgery is often associated with rapid shift of blood and volume, and anesthetic drugs frequently reduce vascular systemic resistance, worsening LVOT obstruction. To that effect, TEE will have an increasing role in the future to guide fluid and drug administration in different surgical settings (28).

Caring for an HOCM patient in the ICU can be challenging as inotropes and vasodilators can paradoxically decrease cardiac output by increasing LVOT obstruction. Invasive hemodynamic monitoring with Swan-Ganz catheter demonstrates elevated filling pressures that are difficult to interpret with significant diastolic dysfunction. Transesophageal echocardiography is particularly useful in providing direct evaluation of LVOT obstruction, SAM, and

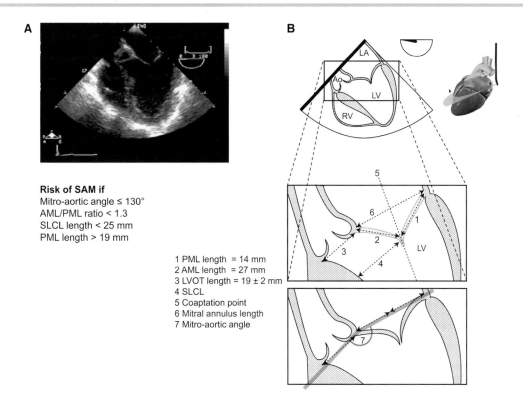

Risk of SAM if
Mitro-aortic angle ≤ 130°
AML/PML ratio < 1.3
SLCL length < 25 mm
PML length > 19 mm

1 PML length = 14 mm
2 AML length = 27 mm
3 LVOT length = 19 ± 2 mm
4 SLCL
5 Coaptation point
6 Mitral annulus length
7 Mitro-aortic angle

Figure 11.11 Risk factors of SAM. (A,B) Measurements used to assess the risk for postoperative systolic anterior motion after septal resection from a mid-esophageal four-chamber view. *Abbreviations*: AML, anterior mitral valve leaflet; Ao, aorta; LA, left atrium; LV, left ventricle; LVOT, left ventricular outflow tract; PML, posterior mitral valve leaflet; RA, right atrium; RV, right ventricle; SLCL, septum to leaflet coaptation length.

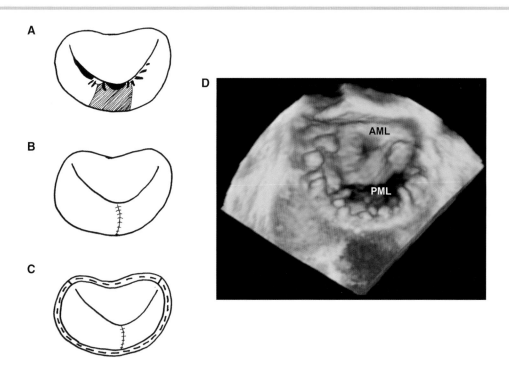

Figure 11.12 Sliding technique. (A–C) The Carpentier sliding leaflet technique for preventing SAM of the mitral leaflets is illustrated. **(A)** In the case of excess PML tissue the quadrangular resection is completed by two triangular resections. **(B)** The PML remnants are translated medially to close the gap. **(C)** The repair is completed and an annuloplasty ring is implanted to reinforce the repair. **(D)** A real-time 3D transesophageal image viewed from the left atrial side shows the details of the repair. *Abbreviations*: AML, anterior mitral valve leaflet; PML, posterior mitral valve leaflet; SAM, systolic anterior motion.

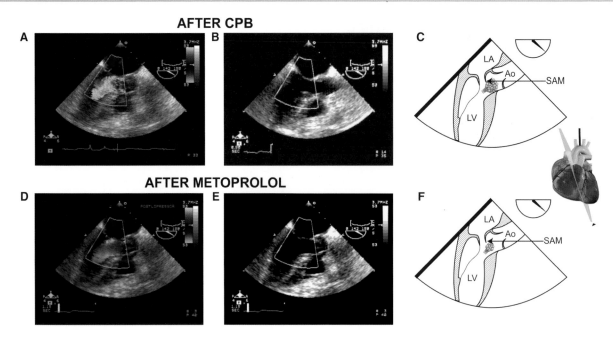

Figure 11.13   Metoprolol and LVOT obstruction. (**A–C**) Mid-esophageal long axis views show flow acceleration in the LVOT in a 63-year-old hemodynamically unstable woman immediately after CPB for coronary revascularization. (**D–F**) There was clinical improvement after administration of an intravenous bolus of metoprolol. *Abbreviations*: Ao, aorta; CPB, cardiopulmonary bypass; LA, left atrium; LV, left ventricle; LVOT, left ventricular outflow tract; SAM, systolic anterior motion.

degree of MR. By integrating hemodynamic and echo-cardiographic monitoring data, it is easier to administer the ideal amount of fluid properly or to introduce and titrate drugs that reduce the inotropic state (calcium channel blockers, β-blockers) (Fig. 11.13) and adjust mechanical circulatory assistance (see Fig. 21.6) or selectively increase systemic vascular resistance (vaso-pressors) to minimize LVOT obstruction (28).

Nonsurgical Septal Ablation

Symptomatic HOCM patients are initially managed with negative inotropic drugs (β-blockers, calcium channel blockers, disopyramide). Rarely, dual chambers pacemakers can be implanted to improve symptoms, presumably by reducing the LVOT gradient. However, for those who remain symptomatic despite maximal medical therapy, mechanical relief of the obstruction should be considered. Surgical myomectomy is the traditional treatment of choice (Fig. 11.6), but catheter-based septal ablation has evolved into an acceptable alternative in selected patients with isolated subaortic obstruction (29). Both techniques reduce LVOT obstruction and symptoms, possibly to a lesser extent with the percutaneous approach (29). Echocardiography is an essential tool to assist the operators for both interventions.

The first case of septal ablation with coronary ethanol injection was described in 1995 (30). Selective injection of alcohol in one or two septal branches of the left anterior descending (LAD) artery is performed to induce a localized septal MI at the site of the SAM-septal contact. The proximal septal branch is

selectively cannulated, and an angioplasty balloon is initially positioned and inflated; angiographic contrast media is then injected through the distal lumen to identify unwanted potential of spillage back into the LAD or in another coronary bed by way of collaterals, before the definitive ethanol injection. At our institution, myocardial contrast echocardiography is routinely used before definitive alcohol injection to define the distribution of each potential septal branch and appropriately select the one(s) supplying the target myocardium (Fig. 11.14). This method minimizes the risk of major complications, such as papillary muscle, anterior or inferior wall extension of the infarct zone, and maximizes the success rate.

Echocardiography (TTE or TEE) together with continuous hemodynamic monitoring (aortic and apical left ventricular catheters) is used to monitor the acute changes in LVOT gradient. An immediate drop in the LVOT systolic pressure gradient is typically obtained (Fig. 11.15), together with an acute decrease in MR severity. Procedural success is usually defined as a 50% reduction in resting LVOT gradient or abolishment of provocable gradient (Fig. 11.15) (29). There is 90% success in carefully selected patients (LVOT obstruction with SAM without structural MV anomaly and septal thickness ≥16 mm). Further improvement in LVOT gradient is expected during 6- to 12-month follow-up, as septal thinning and fibrosis supervenes. Complications of septal ablation include complete atrioventricular block (5–15%, as high as 50%) and ventricular septal defect that is unreported if the initial septal thickness is more than 18 mm.

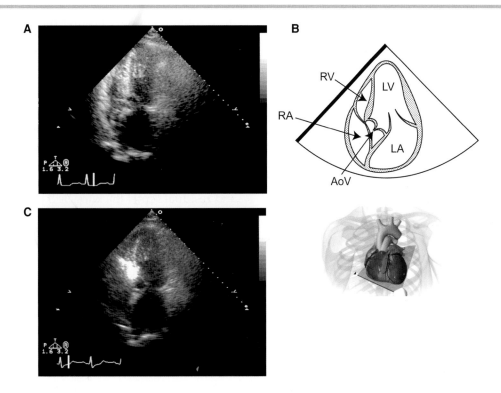

Figure 11.14 Percutaneous alcohol septal ablation. (A,B) Transthoracic apical five-chamber view before the procedure is shown. **(C)** Myocardial contrast enhancement of the brightened septal area confirms that the septal branch to be injected is indeed the one providing the vascular supply to the SAM septal contact region. *Abbreviations*: AoV, aortic valve; LA, left atrium; LV, left ventricle; RA, right atrium; RV, right ventricle; SAM, systolic anterior motion.

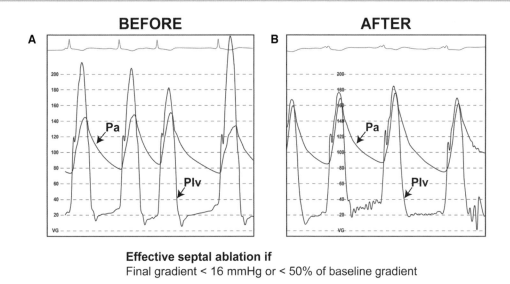

Effective septal ablation if
Final gradient < 16 mmHg or < 50% of baseline gradient

Figure 11.15 Percutaneous septal ablation. Left ventricular (Plv) and aortic (Pa) pressure hemodynamic tracings before **(A)** and immediately after **(B)** percutaneous alcohol septal ablation show a greatly improved resting systolic pressure gradient.

Surgical Septal Myectomy

The surgical septal myectomy, first described by Brock in 1957, is still in use today. The procedure involves the removal of a rectangular portion of the hypertrophied septum by a transaortic approach. The surgery is very effective in relieving the obstruction and reducing the symptoms (29) with a less than 2% mortality rate in experienced centers (6). Accepted indications for surgery include symptomatic patients with resting LVOT gradients of more than 50 mmHg with symptoms unrelieved or intolerant of medication and some high-risk groups, such as young patients with a very thick septum or a strong family history of sudden death.

The success of the procedure depends on excising the appropriate amount of septum to significantly enlarge the LVOT; thus reducing the flow acceleration in the LVOT, alleviating the concomitant SAM with obstruction and possibly the MR (6). Intraoperative TEE is now an invaluable tool to assist the surgeon in this task: the septum can be measured precisely (Fig. 11.2), and the extent and level of obstruction (usually the region of the septal-mitral contact, but not always) can be identified to guide the septal myectomy procedure (9). Important measurements obtained by TEE include the septal thickness, length of hypertrophied septum, and distance of the SAM-septal contact point to base of the right coronary cusp measured at end-diastole and the risk factors for SAM (Fig. 11.11). The presence of a mid-ventricular obstruction, which can be masked by the outlet obstruction, may require a longer resection.

A meticulous examination of the mitral apparatus is warranted to define the amount and mechanism of the MR. In a study by Yu et al. (31) all patients free of anatomic MV abnormality exhibit significant reduction of the MR by septal myectomy alone. None needed MV surgery postoperatively. In contrast, half of the patients with superimposed mitral pathology needed valve surgery in addition to their septal myectomy procedure. Interestingly, 97% of the "pure" HOCM-related MR is directed posteriorly as compared with none in those with additional causes of MR. Thus, an MR jet directed posteriorly seems to predict a good response to surgery. In addition, every patient who is considered for surgery should have a coronary angiogram to document the presence or absence of coronary artery disease (CAD), coronary anomalies, and myocardial bridges.

Myectomy is performed using cardiopulmonary bypass (CPB) with single right atrial cannulation and venting of the LV. The septal resection is done through a transverse aortotomy. Care is taken not to disrupt the sinotubular junction as this may result in postoperative aortic insufficiency.

The myectomy resection involves three separate incisions in the septum. The initial septal subaortic incision is made with a #11 scalpel blade and starts 2 mm below the AoV right cusp. The depth of this initial incision depends on the septal thickness estimate, by TEE and palpation. The depth should leave a residual septal thickness of 8 mm, similar to the LV free wall below the septum. The direction of the initial incision is toward the apex and parallel with the LVOT. The length of the initial incision depends on the extent of the hypertrophy, but generally is 35 to 50 mm long; it is most important that the resection is carried at least 1 cm below the SAM-septal contact point. For patients with mid-ventricular obstruction, the incision should extend at least to the level of the anteroseptal papillary muscle head. The second incision is made parallel to the first, and 2 mm to the right of the MV insertion.

The third incision begins 2 mm below and parallel to the aortic annulus connecting the proximal extent of the first and second incisions. The depth of this incision is only 2 mm because a deeper incision would become too shallow. Once the septum is exposed with this incision, it allows a second cut, also 2 mm deep in a more anterior direction. A third 2 mm incision may be required to establish the depth of the resection, guided by transmural palpation and the depth of the first and second incisions. Once the appropriate depth of the third incision is established, the block of muscle to be excised is dissected distally toward the apex, confirming by repeated palpation that the direction and residual septal thickness is 5 to 8 mm. The area of the specimen resected should approximate the AoV area, on average measuring 25 mm wide, 45 mm in length, and 15 mm in depth.

After separation from CPB, the adequacy of the myectomy is checked by TEE. In a mid-esophageal LAX view, the LVOT should be a normal diameter, SAM and MR should be abolished, allowing the MV to close in a normal plane of apposition. On Doppler interrogation, the MR should be considerably less or absent, and the LVOT gradient less than 10 mmHg, with minimal or no increase in gradient after an induced extrasystole or isoproterenol (Fig. 11.16). A suboptimal surgical result may require reinstitution of CPB in as many as 20% of patients to correct a residual gradient, SAM, or moderate MR (32).

Excessive muscle resection can create complete AV block (7% of cases) (29) or a ventricular septal defect, either acutely or during the healing period (Fig. 11.17).

DILATED CARDIOMYOPATHY

Epidemiology

Dilated cardiomyopathy is characterized by ventricular chamber enlargement and systolic dysfunction with normal LV wall thickness (2). Its estimated prevalence is 1:2500 and represents the most frequent indication for cardiac transplantation (2). Dilated cardiomyopathy may be primary or originate from secondary causes. A complete review of its causes is beyond the scope of this chapter and can be found in the 2008 Canadian heart failure guidelines (33). Familial cause constitutes 20% to 35% of cases, predominantly transmitted in an autosomal dominant fashion (although with incomplete and age-dependent penetrance). The diagnosis of *idiopathic* DCM should be reserved for patient in whom no other etiologic factor can be found after a thorough evaluation. Unfortunately, the echocardiographic features provide little insight in the underlying cause, and DCM represents usually a final common pathway for different disorders.

Clinical Features

Dyspnea, fatigue, and edema are the most frequent symptoms of DCM, with 95% of the patients having symptomatic manifestations of heart failure during

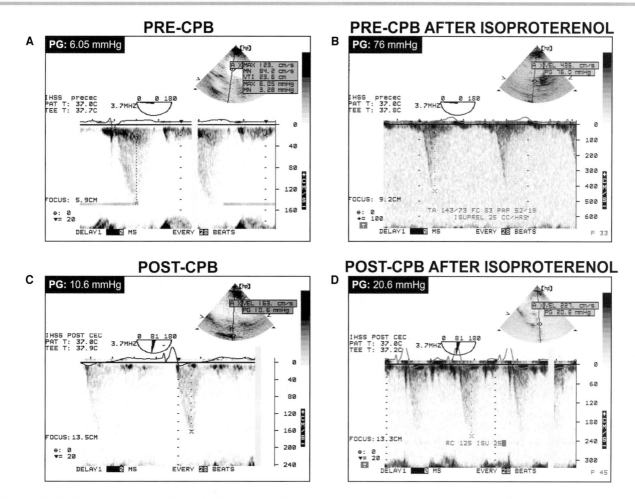

Figure 11.16 Isoproterenol testing. (**A–D**) Aortic outflow spectral Doppler traces from a 46-year-old man with hypertrophic cardiomyopathy are shown. (**A,B**) The pre-CPB maximum PG (**A**) before (6.05 mmHg) and (**B**) after (76 mmHg) isoproterenol at 1.6 mg/min are shown. (**C,D**) Following septal myectomy there was a less pronounced increase in the PG from 10.6 mmHg to 20.6 mmHg after the use of isoproterenol. *Abbreviations*: CPB, cardiopulmonary bypass; PG, pressure gradient.

the course of their illness. Some will complain of exertional chest pain indistinguishable from angina, even in the absence of epicardial coronary stenosis. This is believed to be secondary to increased wall stress with reduced coronary flow reserve. Ventricular or supraventricular arrhythmias are frequent in DCM, but sudden death is unusual at initial presentation, although it is the mode of death in 12% of these patients during the course of their disease (34). The risk of thromboembolic events in clinically stable patients is low (1–3% per year), even in those with echocardiographic evidence of intracardiac thrombi (35). These thrombi may originate from the ventricles or atria, the latter being usually associated with atrial fibrillation.

Echocardiographic Features

Chambers Dilatation

The hallmark of DCM is left, and to a variable degree, RV dilatation. Systolic (>50 mm) and diastolic (>70 mm) LV dimensions and volumes are increased (14). Changes

in the LV geometry occur along with gradual dilatation, preferentially in the SAX; hence, the LV cavity becomes more spherical. This is measured by the sphericity index (diastolic LAX dimension/SAX dimension), approaching 1.0 in severe DCM (normal is ≥1.5) (36). As stated previously, it is recommended that the dimension of the LV be measured using M-mode in the transgastric SAX view at the level of the papillary muscles (Fig. 11.18). The ventricular volumes can be estimated with the Simpson's method of disks (see Fig. 5.22), but with caution, since it often underestimates the true volumes due to the foreshortening of the apex with TEE. Ventricular mass is also increased in DCM, principally from eccentric hypertrophy secondary to increased LV dimensions and variable degree of increased wall thickness. This compensatory hypertrophy seems to identify patients with a better prognosis (37).

Right ventricular involvement is variable and usually parallels LV dilatation but its presence carries independant prognostic information. Right ventricular involvement may also be secondary to pulmonary hypertension or tricuspid regurgitation (TR).

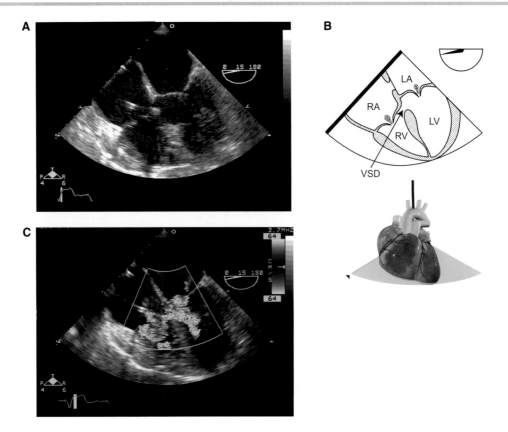

Figure 11.17 VSD after surgical myectomy. A VSD occurring 2 weeks after surgical septal myectomy is shown. (**A,B**) The mid-esophageal four-chamber view demonstrates the VSD at the previous myectomy site. (**C**) Color Doppler depicts flow going across the interventricular septum with an important left-to-right shunt through the VSD. *Abbreviations*: LA, left atrium; LV, left ventricle; RA, right atrium; RV, right ventricle; VSD, ventricular septal defect.

Occasionally, the RV is spared by the disease process, in which case an ischemic etiology should be suspected, particularly if regional wall motion abnormalities are present. Right and left atrial dilatation is common in DCM as a result of chronically elevated filling pressure and/or atrial fibrillation.

Ventricular Systolic Dysfunction

Reduced contractility is characteristic of DCM. Evaluation of global and segmental wall motion should be done using multiple windows; the TG SAX views at 0° are particularly useful for this purpose (Fig. 11.18). The decrease in systolic function is typically diffuse, but regional wall motion abnormalities can be present, suggesting an underlying ischemic etiology. However, this finding is neither sensitive nor specific for CAD, as regional wall motion abnormalities have been described in DCM in the absence of coronary lesion.

Many techniques have been described to quantify systolic function (see Chapters 5 and 10): "E" point-septal separation (Fig. 11.19), volumetric-based measurements, Doppler-derived stroke volume quantification, dP/dt evaluation, myocardial performance index calculation, or simple global visual estimation. The ejection fraction correlates inversely but imperfectly to the prognosis.

Diastolic Dysfunction and LV Dyssynchrony

Patients with DCM can exhibit all the different patterns of diastolic dysfunction, from abnormal relaxation to a restrictive filling pattern or the intermediate pseudonormal profile. Interestingly, the severity of diastolic dysfunction carries independent prognostic implication in addition to left ventricular ejection fraction (LVEF), RV function and clinical status using the New York Heart Association (NYHA) classification. Patients with severe diastolic dysfunction and restrictive filling pattern have a worse prognosis in terms of need for transplantation or death (38). Moreover, patients who revert to a milder degree of diastolic dysfunction with medical treatment have a better prognosis than those who persistently exhibit a restrictive filling pattern despite optimal therapy (39). Furthermore, attenuation of the systolic flow in the pulmonary veins reflects increased left-sided filling pressures and has also been shown to be an independent predictor of adverse events (Fig. 11.20) (40).

Mitral annular TDI provides additional information to that obtained with PW Doppler. For instance a small e (<7 cm/s) has a good correlation with more severe diastolic dysfunction and a high E/e ratio (>15) reliably indicates a higher PWCP (>20 mmHg) and, therefore, a worse prognosis (19,20). Furthermore, TDI

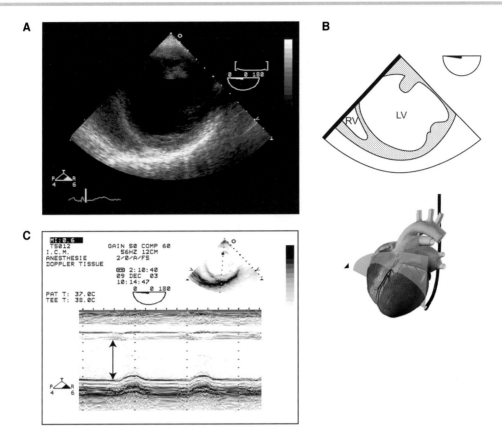

Figure 11.18 Dilated cardiomyopathy. (A,B) Transgastric mid short-axis view in a 56-year-old woman with dilated ischemic cardiomyopathy with M-mode (**C**) shows akinesis of the inferior wall and hypokinesis of the anterior wall. The LV end-diastolic diameter (arrow) is dilated at 7.1 cm (normal 5.5 cm). *Abbreviations*: LV, left ventricle; RV, right ventricle.

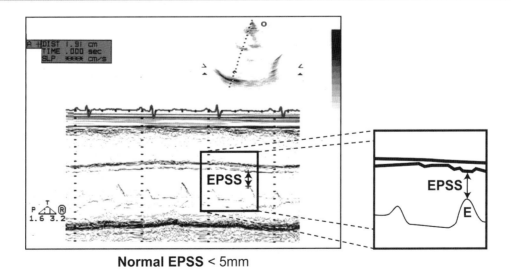

Normal EPSS < 5mm

Figure 11.19 E point septal separation (EPSS). Transthoracic parasternal long-axis view shows an increased EPSS on an M-mode tracing of a patient with dilated cardiomyopathy.

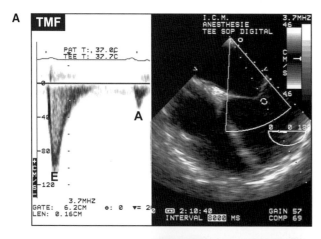

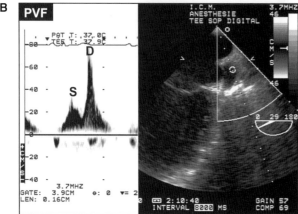

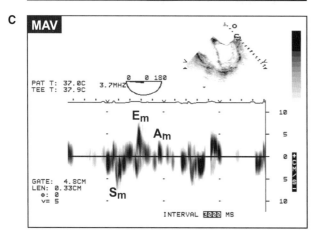

Figure 11.20   Diastolic function in dilated ischemic cardiomyopathy. Stage III diastolic dysfunction (restrictive left ventricular filling) in a 56-year-old woman with dilated ischemic cardiomyopathy demonstrated by pulsed wave Doppler interrogation of the (**A**) TMF, (**B**) PVF and (**C**) tissue Doppler examination of the lateral mitral annulus. *Abbreviations*: A, peak late diastolic TMF velocity; Am, peak late diastolic MAV; D, peak diastolic PVF velocity; Em, peak early diastolic MAV; MAV, mitral annular velocity; PVF, pulmonary venous flow; S, peak systolic PVF velocity; Sm, systolic MAV; TMF, transmitral flow.

is being increasingly used for LV dyssynchrony assessment and consideration for cardiac resynchronization therapy (CRT). TDI, by enabling measurement of peak systolic velocities in different regions of the myocar

dium and the time intervals between electrical (QRS) and mechanical activities (regional S wave by TDI), may help to predict which patients will have a good response to CRT (see Chapter 29). Many parameters have been suggested; among them, intraventricular mechanical dyssynchrony (defined as ≥65 ms difference in time-to-peak TDI systolic velocity between lateral and septal segments) seems to be predictive of both clinical response and LV reverse remodeling (41).

Other Findings: Mitral and TR or Thrombus

Mitral regurgitation is frequently present with DCM, resulting from incomplete coaptation of the leaflets, with two underlying mechanisms: (*i*) alteration in the geometry of the subvalvular and valvular apparatus and/or (*ii*) dilatation of the annulus. Because of the ventricular dilatation, apical displacement of the papillary muscles occurs, creating traction on the leaflets and displacing their coaptation point apically. This impairs the ability of the leaflets to coapt normally, their closing point occurring only at their tips, and therefore incompletely. Annular dilatation can exacerbate this already incomplete coaptation by modifying the geometry of the MV annulus (from a saddle-shaped oval to a more circular shape), thus increasing the valve area that needs to be sealed. The resulting central MR jet could be semiquantified by color flow Doppler and other adjunct methods (Fig. 11.21). Of note, severe MR with secondary left ventricular dilatation and dysfunction can sometimes be confused with a primary cardiomyopathic process with secondary MR. Careful examination of the mitral apparatus and the regurgitant jet will usually determine the initial underlying mechanism.

Tricuspid regurgitation can be secondary to RV dilatation (and annular dilatation) or from pulmonary hypertension. In the absence of RVOT obstruction, the maximum TR velocity can be used to estimate the pulmonary artery systolic pressure, although the angle of Doppler interrogation may not be ideal in TEE (Fig. 11.22).

Ventricular thrombi may also be associated with DCM, usually found at the apex of the LV; they are believed to result from blood stasis caused by the low flow velocity. The adjacent LV wall is usually akinetic or even aneurysmal. The thrombus' echogenicity is usually different from the underlying myocardium, helping to differentiate between the two. Multiple views should confirm their presence and help to differentiate a thrombus from prominent LV trabeculations or false tendon and aberrant chords. Round and protruding thrombi are easy to demonstrate; in contrast, laminated thrombi (Fig. 11.23) may be more difficult to diagnose and must be suspected whenever the apical cavity has an unusually round appearance, or if akinetic apical walls exhibit increased or even normal thickness. The propensity of such thrombus to cause embolic event is variable. It is probably higher in the month following an MI, or with mobile or protruding thrombus in the LV cavity. Anticoagulation is clinically recommended whenever an LV thrombus is found.

Left atrial thrombus, usually located in the left atrial appendage, can be demonstrated in patients with

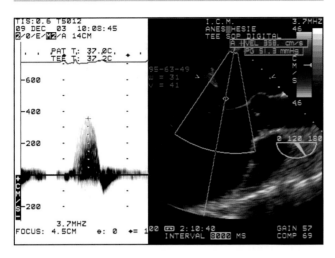

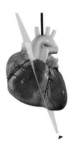

Measured values

Vel	: 358 cm/s
Mitral PG	: 51 mmHg
Systolic Pa	: 95 mmHg
Paop V wave	: 41 mmHg

Doppler estimated LAP

= Systolic Pa - Mitral PG

= 95 mmHg - 51 mmHg

= 44 mmHg

Figure 11.21 MR in dilated cardiomyopathy. LAP can be estimated from the MR signal in a 56-year-old woman with dilated ischemic cardiomyopathy prior to coronary revascularization, surgical ventricular remodeling and mitral valve repair. The maximal PG between the LV and LA was 51 mmHg. If we assume that the systolic arterial pressure (Pa = 95 mmHg) is equal to the LV systolic pressure, the estimated maximal LAP is (95 mmHg − PG) equal to 44 mmHg. The Paop showed a "V" wave of 41 mmHg. *Abbreviations*: LA, left atrium; LAP, left atrial pressure; LV, left ventricle; MR, mitral regurgitation; Paop, pulmonary artery occlusion pressure; PG, pressure gradient; Vel, velocity.

DCM and may be a source of embolism (Fig. 11.24). This finding is usually encountered in the presence of atrial fibrillation. Spontaneous swirling echo contrast can also be demonstrated and has been associated with an increased incidence of thromboembolic events.

RESTRICTIVE AND INFILTRATIVE CARDIOMYOPATHY

Definition

Restrictive cardiomyopathy (RCM) is characterized by a myocardial process that restricts ventricular filling, resulting in elevated ventricular diastolic pressures, typically with normal or slightly decreased systolic function, usually with normal ventricular size; it can affect the LV or both ventricles. Etiologies are numerous and include storage diseases, infiltrative disorders, myocardial noninfiltrative process, endomyocardial diseases and are idiopathic (Fig. 11.25). Taken together, RCM are much less frequently encountered than their dilated or hypertrophic counterparts. In contrast to DCM with their common final findings, the unique features of the different restrictive conditions warrant separate considerations. We will briefly review the typical findings of RCM and then discuss more specifically the features of amyloidosis, sarcoidosis, hemochromatosis, and carcinoid heart disease.

Clinical Findings

Restrictive LV filling with elevated diastolic pressures is the hallmark of RCM leading to dyspnea, exercise intolerance, and orthopnea. Right ventricular involvement is suggested by the presence of congestive peripheral manifestations such as elevated jugular venous pressure, peripheral edema, and ascites. In the absence of cardiomegaly, these clinical findings should raise the suspicion of either RCM or constrictive pericarditis. The differentiation between the two is important since surgical resection of the pericardium could cure the latter. A search for involvement of other organs is essential in the diagnosis, as it can help identify an underlying systemic disease responsible for the cardiac manifestations which could, although rarely, respond to a specific treatment.

Echocardiographic Features

Ventricular dimensions and systolic function are usually normal in RCM. Wall thickness, although typically normal in the idiopathic form, can be increased in infiltrative disorders like amyloidosis. In contrast, the left and right atria are markedly enlarged because of chronically elevated filling pressures. The presence of a large LA size (>60 mm) is an independent predictor of mortality in patients with idiopathic RCM (42).

The demonstration of abnormal filling patterns of both ventricles is necessary for the diagnosis of RCM. Typically, a restrictive filling pattern is encountered, with elevated early E wave velocity, short mitral deceleration time (DT), and increased E/A ratio (>2). Elevated left atrial pressure causes early MV opening, shortening the isovolumic relaxation time (IVRT) and producing an increased early diastolic E wave velocity. The LV diastolic pressure rises rapidly during atrial emptying and LV filling because of ventricular stiffness, leading to an abrupt ending of the early diastolic filling with a short DT. This is the equivalent of the square root sign seen on the pressure curves of the LV or RV. The atrial contribution to ventricular filling is reduced by the elevated diastolic pressure resulting in a smaller A wave velocity in the mitral inflow patterns and an increased atrial reversal flow velocity and duration in the pulmonary and hepatic venous flows. There is reduced systolic component of the venous flow, producing diastolic flow velocity predominance with S/D ratio <1.

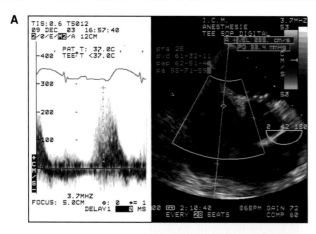

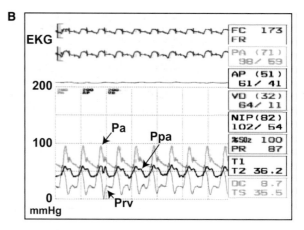

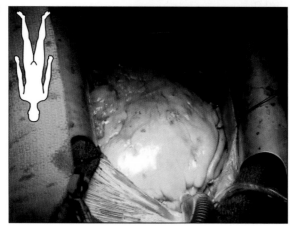

Measured values

Vel	: 289 cm/s
Tricuspid PG	: 33 mmHg
Systolic Prv	: 64 mmHg
Systolic Ppa	: 61 mmHg
Pra	: 25 mmHg

Doppler estimated systolic Prv

= Tricuspid PG + Pra

= 33 mmHg + 25 mmHg

= 58.4 mmHg

Figure 11.22   TR in dilated cardiomyopathy. Acute TR associated with RV dysfunction occurred in a 56-year-old woman with dilated ischemic cardiomyopathy after revascularization, surgical ventricular remodeling and mitral annuloplasty. (**A**) The TR maximum PG was 33.4 mmHg and the estimated systolic Prv was 58 mmHg. (**B**) This estimation was close to the measured Ppa value of 61 mmHg. Note the square root appearance of the Prv waveform associated with RV dysfunction. (**C**) Intraoperative aspect of the dilated RV after the procedure. *Abbreviations*: EKG, electrocardiogram; Pa, arterial pressure; PG, pressure gradient; Ppa, pulmonary artery pressure; Pra, right atrial pressure; Prv, right ventricular pressure; RV, right ventricle; TR, tricuspid regurgitation; Vel, velocity. *Source*: Photo C courtesy of Dr. Pierre Pagé.

The restrictive filling pattern is the classic diastolic profile encountered in RCM and sinus rhythm, particularly when symptoms are overt (Fig. 11.25). Interestingly enough, less severe forms can be found earlier in the course of the disease or after aggressive treatment of reversible etiologies (33). Alternatively, restrictive filling pattern can also be demonstrated in severe DCM, severe aortic regurgitation (AR), or significant hypertrophy.

Difference Between RCM and Constrictive Pericarditis

It is critical to distinguish the clinically similar RCM from constrictive pericarditis, as the latter can be cured with surgical removal of the diseased pericardium. Some echocardiographic characteristics, in particular ventricular interdependence, help to differentiate the two conditions.

In constrictive pericarditis, because of the fixed volume caused by the rigid pericardium, ventricular volume respiratory variation in one cavity is associated with reciprocal change in the opposite one. In the presence of pericardial constriction, during inspiration, the RV enlarges from increased venous return and the LV will become smaller. This can be demonstrated by 2D or best by M-mode examination of transgastric SAX views. Doppler respiratory variations will exhibit reciprocal and exaggerated changes (>25%) of the mitral and tricuspid inflow velocities as well as systolic pulmonary venous flow blunting or reversal, which resolves after pericardiectomy.

Newer techniques like TDI of the mitral annular motion or color M-mode seems promising in discriminating the two pathologies (see Fig. 12.23). In RCM, the mitral annular *e* velocity is decreased while in restrictive pericarditis *e* is usually ≥8 cm/s; with color M-mode, mitral flow propagation velocity is

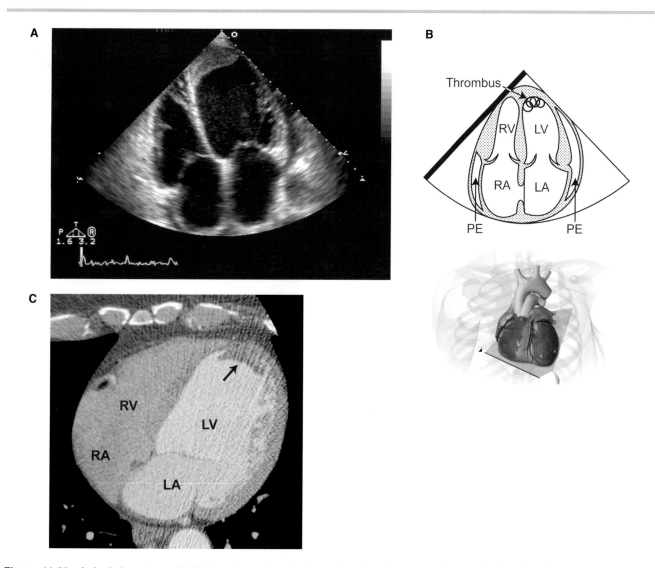

Figure 11.23 Apical thrombus. (A,B) Transthoracic apical four-chamber view in a patient with dilated cardiomyopathy shows a laminated LV apical thrombus. **(C)** Axial 16-DCT image in a 63-year-old man showing LV dilatation with apical thinning and a small curvilinear noncalcified thrombus at the apex of the LV. *Abbreviations*: LA, left atrium; LV, left ventricle; PE, pericardial effusion; RA, right atrium; RV, right ventricle.

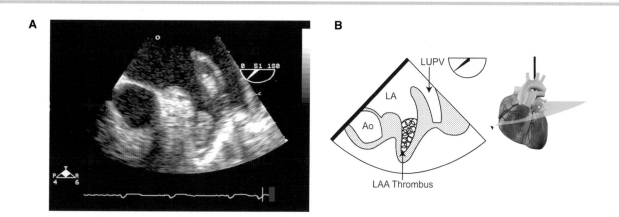

Figure 11.24 LAA thrombus. (A,B) Mid-esophageal LAA view at 51° of a patient in atrial fibrillation with dilated cardiomyopathy shows a thrombus in the LAA. *Abbreviations*: Ao, aorta; LA, left atrium; LAA, left atrial appendage; LUPV, left upper pulmonary vein.

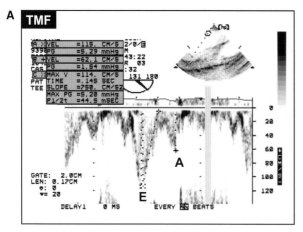

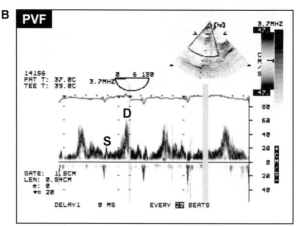

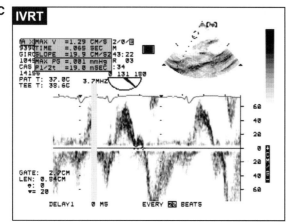

Figure 11.25 Restrictive cardiomyopathy in Duchenne dystrophy. Stage III diastolic dysfunction (restrictive diastolic filling pattern) in a 36-year-old ventilator-dependent patient. A restrictive diastolic filling pattern was confirmed using (**A**) pulsed wave Doppler interrogation of TMF with an E/A ratio of 1.85 and a deceleration time of 145 ms. (**B**) Pulsed wave Doppler interrogation of PVF with an S/D ratio of less than 1. (**C**) Measurement of the IVRT from the mid-esophageal PW Doppler at 131° sampled at the junction of the tip of the mitral valve and left ventricular outflow tract. The IVRT was shortened at 65 ms. The patient died shortly after hospitalization. *Abbreviations*: A, peak late diastolic TMF velocity; D, peak diastolic PVF velocity; E, peak early diastolic TMF velocity; IVRT, isovolumic relaxation time; PVF, pulmonary venous flow; PW, pulsed wave; S, peak systolic PVF velocity; TMF, transmitral flow.

<45 cm/s in RCM, while it is ≥45 cm/s in restrictive pericarditis. Some other but less specific findings such as elevated pulmonary pressures, more than moderate MR (or TR) or increased wall thickness may all suggest the presence of RCM. In contrast, finding a thickened or calcified pericardium rather suggests constrictive pericarditis.

An integrated approach using other diagnostic tools helps identify the correct diagnosis: hemodynamic pressure tracings from left and right heart catheterization, clinical clues, thoracic imaging (MRI, CT), and endomyocardial biopsy.

Amyloidosis

Cardiac amyloidosis, the commonest RCM, is caused by amyloid fibrils deposition in the myocardium, valve tissue, atrial septum, pericardium, and conduction system. Cardiac involvement is usually associated with the primary and the senile forms of amyloidosis.

Echocardiographic features (Fig. 11.26) include a progressive increase in RV and LV wall thickness, typically symmetrical with a characteristic "speckled" appearance and normal-sized or even small ventricular cavities. The severity of the wall thickening is a prognostic marker. Systolic function is preserved until late in the course of the disease. Small to moderate pericardial effusion is also commonly encountered. Of note, SAM and LVOT obstruction can sometimes coexist and be confused with HCM (43). A thickened atrial septum with multivalvular involvement (usually mild to moderate regurgitation) with low QRS voltage on the ECG are useful clues to the diagnosis of amyloidosis.

Although a restrictive filling pattern is typically encountered in advanced disease, observational studies have shown that in some patients the degree of diastolic dysfunction, which parallels disease progression, may evolve in time. The patients initially exhibit a delayed relaxation pattern (E/A < 1, prolonged DT),

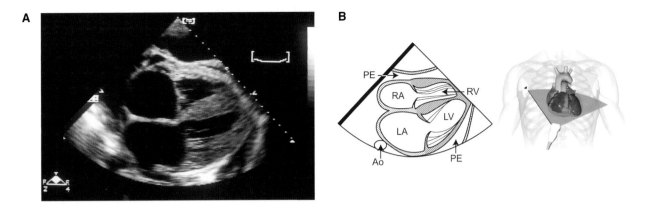

Figure 11.26 Amyloidosis. (A,B) Transthoracic subcostal view in a patient with amyloidosis shows biatrial enlargement, increased ventricular wall thickness with characteristic sparkling appearance and a small circumferential PE. *Abbreviations*: Ao, aorta; LA, left atrium; LV, left ventricle; PE, pericardial effusion; RA, right atrium; RV, right ventricle.

progressing to a pseudonormal and finally to the typical restrictive filling profile. The severity of diastolic dysfunction encountered is highly correlated to the prognosis: the shorter the DT, the worse the survival rate (44).

Sarcoidosis

Sarcoidosis is a granulomatous disorder of unknown etiology involving multiple systems. The lungs and mediastinal lymph nodes are the most commonly involved structures by noncaseating granulomas, although virtually any organ can be infiltrated by these. Heart involvement is clinically present in approximately 5% to 10% of patients, but reaches 25% in autopsy series, suggesting that a high degree of suspicion is necessary in these patients. Cardiac sarcoidosis may affect the ventricular septum with secondary conduction abnomalities, the papillary muscle with associated MR, or the pericardium. Even more troublesome is the fact that sudden death can be the first cardiac manifestation of the disease (45).

Myocardial sarcoidosis leads to fibrosis, resulting in increased stiffness, like RCM, but with earlier decrease in systolic function and ventricular dilatation as a rule. Regional wall motion abnormalities, from patchy granuloma involvement, are common even in the absence of CAD and tend to involve the basal and mid-ventricular segments. Ventricular aneurysm can also be found. Severe pulmonary sarcoidosis can also lead to pulmonary hypertension and secondary RV hypertrophy with variable degree of dysfunction, without myocardial involvement per se.

Hemochromatosis

Hemochromatosis is an autosomal recessive disease that causes iron deposition in tissues, resulting in heart failure, hepatic cirrhosis, diabetes, as well as pituitary, skin, and gonadal involvement. A clinical picture indistinguishable from the primary form can be seen with iron overload secondary to multiple transfusions for the treatment of severe anemia. Cardiac involvement is the initial presentation for 15% of patients and is the cause of death in 30% of untreated patients. Early diagnosis is important, since the heart disease can be reversed with phlebotomy, at least initially.

The echocardiographic features of symptomatic cardiac hemochromatosis are dilatation of the LV or both ventricles with reduced systolic function, which can mimic DCM (46). Wall thickness can be slightly increased, particularly in the earlier stage of the disease when the LV diameters and function are still normal. The valves appeared to be spared by the process. Echocardiography is also a useful tool in the evaluation of response to treatment.

Carcinoid Heart Disease

Carcinoid tumors are rare neuroendocrine malignancies, with approximately 90% located in the gastrointestinal system. The most malignant tumors are located in the ileum and must be invasive or metastasize to produce the carcinoid syndrome characterized by facial flushing, intractable secretory diarrhea and bronchoconstriction. The incidence of carcinoid tumors is 1:75,000 of which 50% develop carcinoid syndrome and of those 50% have carcinoid heart disease. Carcinoid heart disease is mostly due to the paraneoplastic effects of vasoactive substances released by the malignant cells rather than direct metastatic effect on the heart (47). There is preferential right heart involvement, with signs of heart failure secondary to severe dysfunction of tricuspid and pulmonary valves (regurgitation, stenosis, or both).

Echocardiography shows right atrial and ventricular dilatation in up to 90% of cases, with ventricular septal wall motion abnormalities in almost half of the cases (46). The right heart valve leaflets and subvalvular structures are usually thickened, shortened, and retracted, leading to incomplete coaptation and secondary significant regurgitation and less commonly stenosis (see Fig. 18.21). Interestingly, calcification of affected valves is rare and may be considered a notable negative echocardiographic feature of carcinoid heart disease (47).

ATYPICAL CARDIOMYOPATHIES

Apical Cardiomyopathy

The unusual form of apical hypertrophy can be missed if a meticulous examination is not performed, because LV wall thickness is usually not increased at the basal and mid levels. As a general rule, the apex is often foreshortened in TEE but can be imaged at the mid-esophageal level by retroflexing the probe or in transgastric view by pushing the probe further than the SAX mid-papillary level. Furthermore, differentiation between apical hypertrophy and apical thrombus may be difficult, but apical wall motion is usually abnormal in the latter.

Noncompacted Left Ventricle

In humans, the LV is less trabeculated than the RV, and it is unusual to find more than three prominent trabeculations in the LV. Left ventricular myocardial noncompaction (LVNC) is a recently recognized primary congenital cardiomyopathy characterized by a distinctive spongy morphological appearance of the LV myocardium, resulting from an arrest in the normal embryogenesis. Left ventricular myocardial noncompaction predominantly involves the distal (apical or lateral) portion of the LV walls, presenting with deep intertrabecular recesses (also called sinusoids) that are in communication with the ventricular cavity (2). Many cases of LVNC have been primarily misdiagnosed as HCM (49), DCM (50), RCM (51), apical hypertrophy (52), endocardial fibroelastosis (53), or endomyocardial fibrosis (54). Recent developments in echocardiography with second harmonic imagings permits a better visualization of the LV apical regions, including detection of trabeculations and recesses and suggest that LVNC has a higher prevalence than previously thought.

Epidemiology

The prevalence of LVNC varies from 0.05% to 0.24%/year in echocardiographic studies, probably reflecting both ethnic differences and increasing awareness of this abnormality in certain centers. Both familial and nonfamilial cases have been described. Men represent two-thirds of cases, because of possible X-linked recessive inheritance with heterogeneity (55). Several genetic mutations have been described, including genes encoding for dystrophin or α-dystrobrevin (in LVNC associated with congenital heart disease), but also genes for transcription factors limited to the heart and mitochondrial mutations (56), usually leading to isolated forms of LVNC.

Clinical Features

Heart failure symptoms are predominant, being present in 52% of the patients, usually associated with LV systolic dysfunction, followed by palpitations or syncope (16%) (57). Prognosis is poor with premature death by either end-stage heart failure or sudden death (58). The electrocardiogram is abnormal in 94% of the patients, with signs of LV hypertrophy and ST-T changes, Wolff-Parkinson-White syndrome, ventricular tachycardia, abnormalities in the cardiac conduction system, and atrial fibrillation have also been reported (57). The pathophysiologic mechanisms of heart failure, systolic dysfunction, and arrhythmia in LVNC are unknown, but myocardial ischemia may play a role. In addition, LVNC is believed to be associated with embolic events, 24% as an initial presentation (58), but the majority of reported cases also presented other risk factors for increased embolic risk (59). Thus, it is currently uncertain whether LVNC with its intramyocardial recesses is a source of cardiac embolism or whether associated abnormalities are responsible for the embolic events.

Anatomical Features

The intramyocardial recesses are usually located at the LV apex and its adjacent parts of the lateral and inferior walls, probably due to regional nonuniformity, in which the thickest part of the LV wall is basal and the myocardium becomes thinner toward the apex. Three different morphology of LVNC has been described: (*i*) extensive spongy transformation of the myocardium, similar to a hemangioma, and frequently associated with other cardiac morphologic abnormalities (53); (*ii*) prominent coarse trabeculations of the ventricular wall and deep recesses of the ventricular cavity, covered with endocardium, not communicating with the coronary arteries and usually not associated with other cardiac morphologic abnormalities (50); and (*iii*) a dysplastic appearance of the myocardium with thinned myocardium and excessive trabeculations, not associated with other cardiac morphologic abnormalities (60). Currently, it is uncertain whether these different morphologies represent different diseases or diverse stages of the same disease process.

At least five pathogenetic concepts have been suggested to explain the occurrence of LVNC. Complete description is beyond the scope of this chapter and can be found elsewhere (57). A high incidence of LV hypertrabeculation has been found in patients with secondary cardiomyopathies due to neuromuscular disorders, partially resembling LVNC but not fulfilling noncompaction criteria (59). Until further is known, it has been suggested that LVNC and left ventricular hypertrabeculation not be used as interchangeable terms.

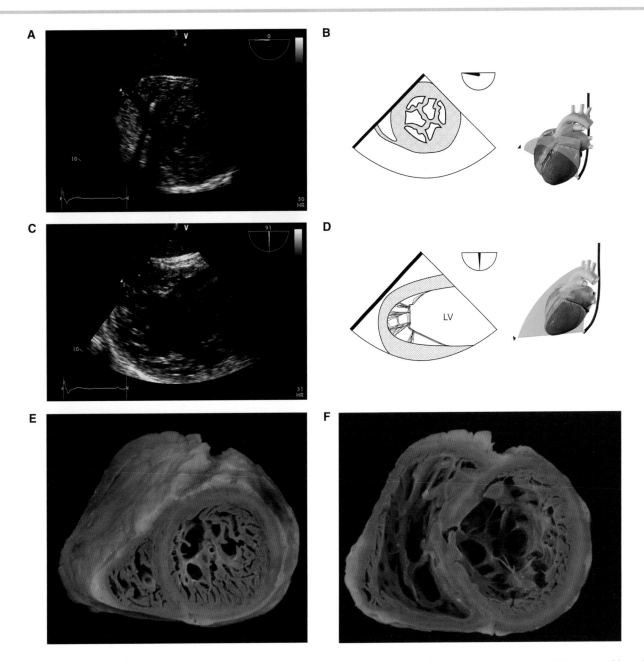

Figure 11.27 Noncompacted LV. Transgastric mid short-axis (**A,B**) and two-chamber (**C,D**) views in a 43-year-old woman with end-stage heart failure just before cardiac transplantation. Note the apical deep recess typically filled with blood. (**E,F**) Aspect of the heart removed after cardiac transplantation. Ventricular septal defect can be associated with this type of cardiomyopathy. *Abbreviation*: LV, left ventricle. *Source*: Courtesy of Dr Philippe Romero.

Echocardiographic Features

The typical echocardiographic image of noncompacted myocardium is characterized by an altered structure of the LV myocardium with extremely thickened, hypokinetic ventricular segments consisting of two layers. There is a thin epicardial compacted zone and a thicker noncompacted endocardial zone, with deep recesses filled with blood from the LV cavity (Fig. 11.27) (57). Proposed echocardiographic

criteria, recently validated (61) are: (*i*) absence of coexistent cardiac anomalies, (*ii*) the presence of a two-layer structural and segmental LV wall thickening with an end-systolic ratio of noncompacted to compacted layers ≥2:1 (100% of cases), (*iii*) Doppler color imaging evidence of flow within the intertrabecular recesses (95% of patients), and (*iv*) hypokinetic noncompacted segments predominantly located in the apical, mid-lateral and mid-inferior regions of

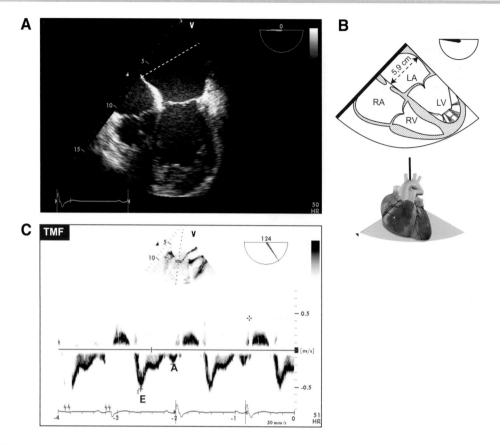

Figure 11.28   Noncompacted LV. (A,B) Mid-esophageal four-chamber view in a 43-year-old woman with end-stage heart failure just before cardiac transplantation shows a dilated LA and deep LV apical recess. **(C)** TMF shows an elevated E (54 cm/s) to A (20 cm/s) wave ratio. *Abbreviations*: A, peak late diastolic TMF velocity; E, peak early diastolic TMF velocity; RA, right atrium; RV, right ventricle; LA, left atrium; LV, left ventricle; TMF, transmitral flow.

the LV (89% of patients). Additional echocardiographic findings include reduced systolic function (82%), enlarged left ventricular end-diastolic dimension (67%), variable degrees of LV diastolic dysfunction (Fig. 11.28), and LV thrombi (10%) (58). Contrast echocardiography may help in patients with suggestive findings but nondiagnostic echocardiographic exam.

Arrythmogenic RV Dysplasia

Right ventricular dysplasia is a rare clinical entity with a prevalence of 1:1000 that represents a specific ventricular pathology associated with ventricular arrhythmias and sudden cardiac death (62). The ventricular abnormality is secondary to fatty infiltration of the RV free wall resulting in regional wall motion abnormality progressing to RV dilatation. A task force from the European Society of Cardiology and the International Society and Federation of Cardiology (63) proposed diagnostic criteria based on six elements: family history, conduction disease, repolarization abnormalities and arrhythmias on ECG, tissue characterization of myocardial wall on biopsy and using diagnostic modalities such as echocardiogra-

phy. The echocardiographic features reported by Nava et al. (64) and Yoerger et al. (65) include RV dilatation particularly in the RV outflow tract and reduced RV fractional area change with variable regional wall motion abnormalities. Small saccular aneurysms of the right ventricle have also been described in this condition (66).

Stress-Induced Cardiomyopathy

See Chapter 30.

NONTRANSPLANT SURGERY

With the increasing prevalence of heart failure and the limited organ supply for transplant, new surgical therapies have emerged to help patients with end-stage heart failure. Partial left ventriculotomy (Batista procedure), dynamic cardiomyoplasty, patch ventriculoplasty or isolated MV repair are procedures designed to unload the LV, reduce the wall stress to increase heart performance, and alleviate symptoms (Fig. 11.29). The role of TEE in these settings is evolving.

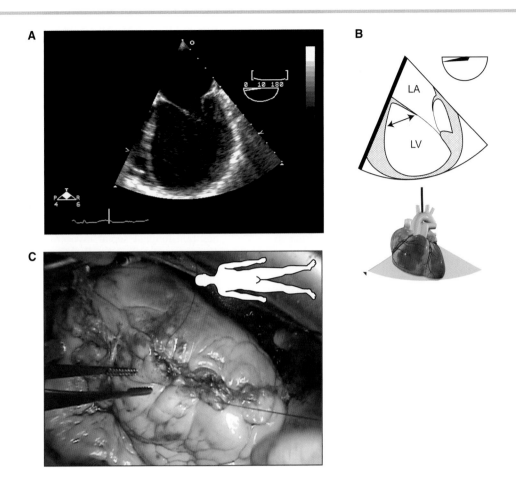

Figure 11.29 Ventricular remodeling. (A,B) Mid-esophageal four-chamber view in a 56-year-old woman with dilated ischemic cardiomyopathy before coronary revascularization, surgical ventricular remodeling and mitral valve repair shows increased septal to anterior mitral leaflet separation (arrow). **(C)** Surgical aspect of the heart after remodeling. *Abbreviations*: LA, left atrium; LV, left ventricle. *Source*: Photo C courtesy of Dr. Pierre Pagé.

CONCLUSION

Echocardiography is an essential diagnostic tool for differentiating the categories of cardiomyopathy; it also helps in the identification of the associated abnormalities that can be encountered in specific diseases and can markedly influence the treatment of a given patient. Moreover, it can also be useful in the evaluation of the response of an individual to a specific treatment. Finally, TEE is an invaluable tool in the monitoring of these same patients when undergoing noncardiac surgery or when they suffered from superimposed acute illnesses.

REFERENCES

1. Elliott P, Andersson B, Arbustini E, et al. Classification of the cardiomyopathies: a position statement from the European Society Of Cardiology Working Group on Myocardial and Pericardial Diseases. Eur Heart J 2008; 29:270–276.
2. Maron BJ, Towbin JA, Thiene G, et al. Contemporary definitions and classification of the cardiomyopathies: an American Heart Association Scientific Statement from the Council on Clinical Cardiology, Heart Failure and Transplantation Committee; Quality of Care and Outcomes Research and Functional Genomics and Translational Biology Interdisciplinary Working Groups; and Council on Epidemiology and Prevention. Circulation 2006; 113: 1807–1816.
3. Marian AJ, Salek L, Lutucuta S. Molecular genetics and pathogenesis of hypertrophic cardiomyopathy. Minerva Med 2001; 92:435–451.
4. Maron BJ, Gardin JM, Flack JM, et al. Prevalence of hypertrophic cardiomyopathy in a general population of young adults. Echocardiographic analysis of 4111 subjects in the CARDIA Study. Coronary Artery Risk Development in (Young) Adults. Circulation 1995; 92:785–789.
5. Braunwald E. Hypertrophic cardiomyopathy—continued progress. N Engl J Med 1989; 320:800–802.
6. Spirito P, Seidman CE, McKenna WJ, et al. The management of hypertrophic cardiomyopathy. N Engl J Med 1997; 336:775–785.
7. Pollick C, Morgan CD, Gilbert BW, et al. Muscular subaortic stenosis: the temporal relationship between systolic anterior motion of the anterior mitral leaflet and the pressure gradient. Circulation 1982; 66:1087–1094.
8. Sherrid MV, Gunsburg DZ, Moldenhauer S, et al. Systolic anterior motion begins at low left ventricular outflow tract velocity in obstructive hypertrophic cardiomyopathy. J Am Coll Cardiol 2000; 36:1344–1354.

9. Braunwald E. Heart disease a textbook of cardiovascular medicine. 5th ed. Philadelphia: Saunders, 1997.

10. Sherrid MV, Chaudhry FA, Swistel DG. Obstructive hypertrophic cardiomyopathy: echocardiography, pathophysiology, and the continuing evolution of surgery for obstruction. Ann Thorac Surg 2003; 75:620–632.

11. Grigg LE, Wigle ED, Williams WG, et al. Transesophageal Doppler echocardiography in obstructive hypertrophic cardiomyopathy: clarification of pathophysiology and importance in intraoperative decision making. J Am Coll Cardiol 1992; 20:42–52.

12. Schwammenthal E, Nakatani S, He S, et al. Mechanism of mitral regurgitation in hypertrophic cardiomyopathy: mismatch of posterior to anterior leaflet length and mobility. Circulation 1998; 98:856–865.

13. Doshi SN, Kim MC, Sharma SK, et al. Images in cardiovascular medicine. Right and left ventricular outflow tract obstruction in hypertrophic cardiomyopathy. Circulation 2002; 106:e3–e4.

14. Lang RM, Bierig M, Devereux RB, et al. Recommendations for chamber quantification: a report from the American Society of Echocardiography's Guidelines and Standards Committee and the Chamber Quantification Writing Group, developed in conjunction with the European Association of Echocardiography, a branch of the European Society of Cardiology. J Am Soc Echocardiogr 2005; 18:1440–1463.

15. Henry WL, Clark CE, Epstein SE. Asymmetric septal hypertrophy. Echocardiographic identification of the pathognomonic anatomic abnormality of IHSS. Circulation 1973; 47:225–233.

16. Spirito P, Maron BJ. Relation between extent of left ventricular hypertrophy and diastolic filling abnormalities in hypertrophic cardiomyopathy. J Am Coll Cardiol 1990; 15:808–813.

17. Nagueh SF, Mahmarian JJ. Noninvasive cardiac imaging in patients with hypertrophic cardiomyopathy. J Am Coll Cardiol 2006; 48:2410–2422.

18. Nagueh SF, Lakkis NM, Middleton KJ, et al. Doppler estimation of left ventricular filling pressures in patients with hypertrophic cardiomyopathy. Circulation 1999; 99:254–261.

19. Nagueh SF, Middleton KJ, Kopelen HA, et al. Doppler tissue imaging: a noninvasive technique for evaluation of left ventricular relaxation and estimation of filling pressures. J Am Coll Cardiol 1997; 30:1527–1533.

20. Ommen SR, Nishimura RA, Appleton CP, et al. Clinical utility of Doppler echocardiography and tissue Doppler imaging in the estimation of left ventricular filling pressures: A comparative simultaneous Doppler-catheterization study. Circulation 2000; 102:1788–1794.

21. Maron BJ, Clark CE, Henry WL et al. Prevalence and characteristics of disproportionate ventricular septal thickening in patients with acquired or congenital heart diseases: echocardiographic and morphologic findings. Circulation 1977; 55:489–496.

22. Maron BJ, Gottdiener JS, Perry LW. Specificity of systolic anterior motion of anterior mitral leaflet for hypertrophic cardiomyopathy. Prevalence in large population of patients with other cardiac diseases. Br Heart J 1981; 45:206–212.

23. Schwinger ME, O'Brien F, Freedberg RS, et al. Dynamic left ventricular outflow obstruction after aortic valve replacement: a Doppler echocardiographic study. J Am Soc Echocardiogr 1990; 3:205–208.

24. Lee KS, Stewart WJ, Lever HM, et al. Mechanism of outflow tract obstruction causing failed mitral valve repair. Anterior displacement of leaflet coaptation. Circulation 1993; 88:II24–II29.

25. Maslow AD, Regan MM, Haering JM, et al. Echocardiographic predictors of left ventricular outflow tract obstruction and systolic anterior motion of the mitral valve after mitral valve reconstruction for myxomatous valve disease. J Am Coll Cardiol 1999; 34:2096–2104.

26. Jebara VA, Mihaileanu S, Acar C, et al. Left ventricular outflow tract obstruction after mitral valve repair. Results of the sliding leaflet technique. Circulation 1993; 88:II30–II34.

27. Haering JM, Comunale ME, Parker RA, et al. Cardiac risk of noncardiac surgery in patients with asymmetric septal hypertrophy. Anesthesiology 1996; 85:254–259.

28. Nam E, Toque Y, Quintard JM, et al. Use of transesophageal echocardiography to guide the anesthetic management of cesarean section in a patient with hypertrophic cardiomyopathy. J Cardiothorac Vasc Anesth 1999; 13:72–74.

29. Qin JX, Shiota T, Lever HM, et al. Outcome of patients with hypertrophic obstructive cardiomyopathy after percutaneous transluminal septal myocardial ablation and septal myectomy surgery. J Am Coll Cardiol 2001; 38:1994–2000.

30. Sigwart U. Non-surgical myocardial reduction for hypertrophic obstructive cardiomyopathy. Lancet 1995; 346:211–214.

31. Yu EH, Omran AS, Wigle ED, et al. Mitral regurgitation in hypertrophic obstructive cardiomyopathy: relationship to obstruction and relief with myectomy. J Am Coll Cardiol 2000; 36:2219–2225.

32. Marwick TH, Stewart WJ, Lever HM, et al. Benefits of intraoperative echocardiography in the surgical management of hypertrophic cardiomyopathy. J Am Coll Cardiol 1992; 20:1066–1072.

33. Malcom J, Arnold O, Howlett JG, et al. Canadian Cardiovascular Society Consensus Conference guidelines on heart failure—2008 update: best practices for the transition of care of heart failure patients, and the recognition, investigation and treatment of cardiomyopathies. Can J Cardiol 2008; 24:21–40.

34. Dec GW, Fuster V. Idiopathic dilated cardiomyopathy. N Engl J Med 1994; 331:1564–1575.

35. Hunt SA, Abraham WT, Chin MH, et al. ACC/AHA 2005 guideline update for the diagnosis and management of chronic heart failure in the adult: a report from the American College of Cardiology/American Heart Association Task Force on Practice Guidelines (Writing Committee to Update the 2001 Guidelines for the Evaluation and Management of Heart Failure): developed in collaboration with the American College of Chest Physicians and the International Society for Heart and Lung Transplantation: endorsed by the Heart Rhythm Society. Circulation 2005; 112:e154–e235.

36. Di Donato M, Dabic P, Castelvecchio S, et al. Left ventricular geometry in normal and post-anterior myocardial infarction patients: sphericity index and 'new' conicity index comparisons. Eur J Cardiothorac Surg 2006; 29 suppl 1:S225–S230.

37. Feild BJ, Baxley WA, Russell RO Jr, et al. Left ventricular function and hypertrophy in cardiomyopathy with depressed ejection fraction. Circulation 1973; 47:1022–1031.

38. Xie GY, Berk MR, Smith MD et al. Prognostic value of Doppler transmitral flow patterns in patients with congestive heart failure. J Am Coll Cardiol 1994; 24:132–139.

39. Pinamonti B, Zecchin M, Di Lenarda A, et al. Persistence of restrictive left ventricular filling pattern in dilated cardiomyopathy: an ominous prognostic sign. J Am Coll Cardiol 1997; 29:604–612.

40. Dini FL, Dell'Anna R, Micheli A, et al. Impact of blunted pulmonary venous flow on the outcome of patients with left ventricular systolic dysfunction secondary to either ischemic or idiopathic dilated cardiomyopathy. Am J Cardiol 2000; 85:1455–1460.

41. Bax JJ, Bleeker GB, Marwick TH, et al. Left ventricular dyssynchrony predicts response and prognosis after cardiac

resynchronization therapy. J Am Coll Cardiol 2004; 44: 1834–1840.

42. Ammash NM, Seward JB, Bailey KR, et al. Clinical profile and outcome of idiopathic restrictive cardiomyopathy. Circulation 2000; 101:2490–2496.

43. Oh JK, Tajik AJ, Edwards WD, et al. Dynamic left ventricular outflow tract obstruction in cardiac amyloidosis detected by continuous-wave Doppler echocardiography. Am J Cardiol 1987; 59:1008–1010.

44. Klein AL, Hatle LK, Taliercio CP, et al. Serial Doppler echocardiographic follow-up of left ventricular diastolic function in cardiac amyloidosis. J Am Coll Cardiol 1990; 16:1135–1141.

45. Newman LS, Rose CS, Maier LA. Sarcoidosis. N Engl J Med 1997; 336:1224–1234.

46. Olson LJ, Baldus WP, Tajik AJ. Echocardiographic features of idiopathic hemochromatosis. Am J Cardiol 1987; 60:885–889.

47. Fox DJ, Khattar RS. Carcinoid heart disease: presentation, diagnosis, and management. Heart 2004; 90:1224–1228.

48. Pellikka PA, Tajik AJ, Khandheria BK, et al. Carcinoid heart disease. Clinical and echocardiographic spectrum in 74 patients. Circulation 1993; 87:1188–1196.

49. Agmon Y, Connolly HM, Olson LJ, et al. Noncompaction of the ventricular myocardium. J Am Soc Echocardiogr 1999; 12:859–863.

50. Angelini A, Melacini P, Barbero F, et al. Evolutionary persistence of spongy myocardium in humans. Circulation 1999; 99:2475.

51. Hamamichi Y, Ichida F, Hashimoto I, et al. Isolated noncompaction of the ventricular myocardium: ultrafast computed tomography and magnetic resonance imaging. Int J Cardiovasc Imaging 2001; 17:305–314.

52. Sakamoto T. Apical hypertrophic cardiomyopathy (apical hypertrophy): an overview. J Cardiol 2001; 37 Suppl 1: 161–178.

53. Allenby PA, Gould NS, Schwartz MF, et al. Dysplastic cardiac development presenting as cardiomyopathy. Arch Pathol Lab Med 1988; 112:1255–1258.

54. Mousseaux E, Hernigou A, Azencot M, et al. Endomyocardial fibrosis: electron-beam CT features. Radiology 1996; 198:755–760.

55. Bleyl SB, Mumford BR, Brown-Harrison MC, et al. Xq28-linked noncompaction of the left ventricular myocardium: prenatal diagnosis and pathologic analysis of affected individuals. Am J Med Genet 1997; 72:257–265.

56. Stollberger C, Finsterer J, Valentin A, et al. Isolated left ventricular abnormal trabeculation in adults is associated with neuromuscular disorders. Clin Cardiol 1999; 22: 119–123.

57. Stollberger C, Finsterer J. Left ventricular hypertrabeculation/noncompaction. J Am Soc Echocardiogr 2004; 17:91–100.

58. Oechslin EN, Attenhofer Jost CH, Rojas JR, et al. Long-term follow-up of 34 adults with isolated left ventricular noncompaction: a distinct cardiomyopathy with poor prognosis. J Am Coll Cardiol 2000; 36:493–500.

59. Stollberger C, Finsterer J, Blazek G. Left ventricular hypertrabeculation/noncompaction and association with additional cardiac abnormalities and neuromuscular disorders. Am J Cardiol 2002; 90:899–902.

60. Duru F, Candinas R. Noncompaction of ventricular myocardium and arrhythmias. J Cardiovasc Electrophysiol 2000; 11:493.

61. Frischknecht BS, Attenhofer Jost CH, Oechslin EN, et al. Validation of noncompaction criteria in dilated cardiomyopathy, and valvular and hypertensive heart disease. J Am Soc Echocardiogr 2005; 18:865–872.

62. Gemayel C, Pelliccia A, Thompson PD. Arrhythmogenic right ventricular cardiomyopathy. J Am Coll Cardiol 2001; 38:1773–1781.

63. McKenna WJ, Thiene G, Nava A, et al. Diagnosis of arrhythmogenic right ventricular dysplasia/cardiomyopathy. Task Force of the Working Group Myocardial and Pericardial Disease of the European Society of Cardiology and of the Scientific Council on Cardiomyopathies of the International Society and Federation of Cardiology. Br Heart J 1994; 71:215–218.

64. Nava A, Bauce B, Basso C, et al. Clinical profile and long-term follow-up of 37 families with arrhythmogenic right ventricular cardiomyopathy. J Am Coll Cardiol 2000; 36:2226–2233.

65. Yoerger DM, Marcus F, Sherrill D, et al. Echocardiographic findings in patients meeting task force criteria for arrhythmogenic right ventricular dysplasia: new insights from the multidisciplinary study of right ventricular dysplasia. J Am Coll Cardiol 2005; 45:860–865.

66. Baran A, Nanda NC, Falkoff M, et al. Two-dimensional echocardiographic detection of arrhythmogenic right ventricular dysplasia. Am Heart J 1982; 103:1066–1067.

12

Pericardium

Yan-Fen Shi, André Y. Denault, Yoan Lamarche, and Jean-Claude Tardif
Université de Montréal, Montreal, Canada

Massimiliano Meineri
University of Toronto, Toronto, Canada

INTRODUCTION

Echocardiography is used widely to assess the peri-cardium and extracardiac anatomical structures for evaluation of conditions such as pericardial effusion (PE). Spectral Doppler evaluation, in relation to respiratory changes, has given useful insights into the physiological consequences of these abnormalities and helped to confirm the presence of cardiac tamponade or differentiate between pericardial constriction and restrictive cardiomyopathy (RCMP). Finally, echocardiography has become extremely useful in aiding diagnostic pericardiocentesis and catheter drainage as well as in evaluating the results of surgical drainage and pericardectomy.

NORMAL PERICARDIUM

The pericardium prevents unrestrained wide displacement of the heart in the thoracic cavity during body motion.

The outer pericardial layer is fibrous and lined with a serous surface (the parietal pericardium) that is reflected over the epicardium (as the visceral pericardium) (Fig. 12.1). Those two layers delineate a virtual space, the pericardial cavity, which completely surrounds the heart with the exception of areas located posteriorly near the origin of the great vessels. The areas where the parietal and visceral layers of the pericardium meet constitute pericardial reflections. As a result of these, the pericardial sac behind the heart forms two blind pockets: the transverse sinus is small, horizontal and located under the ascending aorta (Ao) and pulmonary artery trunk (Figs. 12.2 and 12.3); the oblique sinus is relatively larger, vertically oriented and interposed between the pulmonary veins (Fig. 12.3). The pericardial space normally contains a small amount of serous liquid (20–50 mL), lubricating heart movements (rotation and translation) during the cardiac cycle.

PERICARDIAL EFFUSION AND CARDIAC TAMPONADE

The amount of serous liquid in the pericardial sac can increase due to increased production or decreased resorption from inflammation, myocardial infarction, infection, neoplasia, or intracardiac-pericardial communication. As a result, the larger collection of pericardial fluid separates the visceral pericardium from the parietal layer. When pericardial pressure exceeds intracardiac pressure, the PE causes cardiac tamponade. Even with the recent advances in medical imaging, echocardiography remains the gold standard for the evaluation of PE and cardiac tamponade.

Pericardial Effusion

Location, Volume, and Nature of PE

A PE is recognized on echocardiography as an echo-free space in the pericardial sac adjacent to the cardiac structures. Two types of effusion may be observed: free effusions, where the pericardial fluid is able to move within the pericardial sac without limitations, and loculated effusions, where the pericardial fluid is compartmentalized in the pericardial sac (Figs. 12.4 and 12.5). With the patient recumbent, or in left lateral decubitus, excess pericardial fluid tends to move posteriorly and laterally, being characteristically less prominent at the apex than at the base of the heart. With greater fluid collection, the echo-free space extends up to the posterior atrioventricular groove, and behind the left atrium (LA), in the oblique sinus, with decreasing amount of fluid from the left ventricle (LV) to the LA. The transthoracic echocardiographic (TTE) subcostal view can demonstrate fluid between the diaphragm and the right ventricle (RV). On transesophageal echocardiography (TEE), pericardial fluid will be noticeable in the transverse sinus (Figs. 12.2, 12.4, and 12.5) between the ascending Ao and the right pulmonary artery. Moreover, it can accumulate in front of the left atrial appendage (LAA) next to the LV (Fig. 12.4).

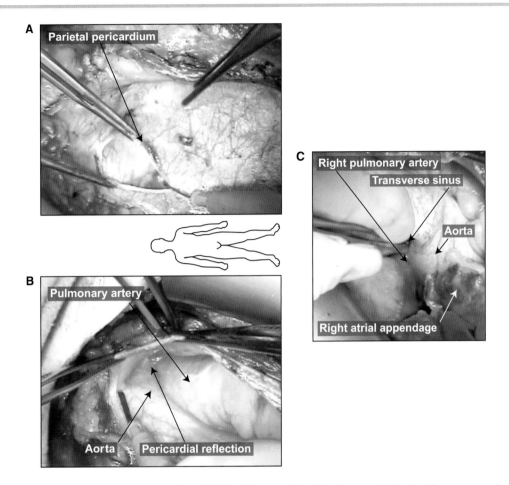

Figure 12.1   Intraoperative views of the pericardium. (A) The fibrous pericardium is opened showing the serous pericardium which is divided into two layers: parietal and visceral. The parietal pericardium is fused to the fibrous pericardium and the visceral pericardium is over the heart. **(B)** A pericardial reflection is seen close to the ascending aorta and pulmonary artery. **(C)** The transverse sinus is seen behind the ascending aorta in front of the right pulmonary artery. *Source*: Courtesy of Dr. Michel Pellerin.

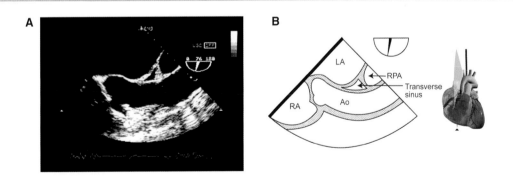

Figure 12.2   Transverse pericardial sinus. (A,B) Modified mid-esophageal ascending Ao long-axis view at 76° demonstrates pericardial fluid in the transverse sinus. *Abbreviations*: Ao, aorta; LA, left atrium; RA, right atrium; RPA, right pulmonary artery.

In long-standing inflammatory PEs, a web of adherences between the visceral and parietal pericardium may stretch as the gradually accumulating fluid separates the two layers. If fibrous bridges rupture, echogenic fibrous strands may become visible in the effusion and on the epicardial surface (Fig. 12.4). Depending on their distribution, PEs can become loculated between adherences.

Assessment of the volume of free PEs is, at best, semiquantitative and based on the size of the heart

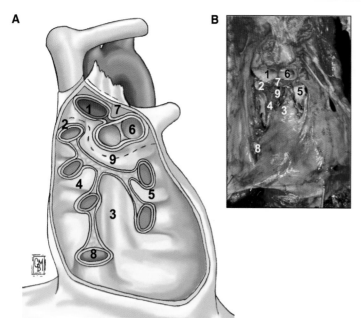

1 Ascending aorta
2 Superior vena cava
3 Oblique sinus
4 Right pulmonary veins
5 Left pulmonary veins
6 Pulmonary artery
7 Ligamentum arteriosum
8 Inferior vena cava
9 Transverse sinus

Figure 12.3 Pericardial sac. Pericardial sac with the heart removed in an anatomical drawing (**A**) and autopsy specimen (**B**). The oblique pericardial sinus is mostly posterior to the left atrium and left ventricle. The transverse sinus is bounded by the great vessels. *Sources*: Diagram A courtesy of Gian-Marco Busato and Photo B courtesy of Dr. Nicolas Dürrleman.

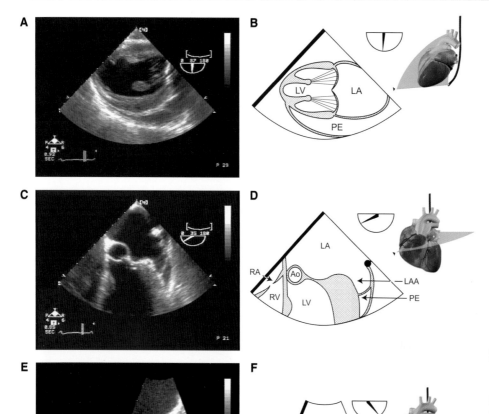

Figure 12.4 Pericardial effusion. A 67-year-old man with a renal transplant undergoing coronary revascularization presents with a PE. (**A,B**) Transgastric two-chamber view: the PE was seen anterior to the LV. (**C,D**) Mid-esophageal view: the PE is visible next (anterior) to the LAA. (**E,F**) Fibrin clot is seen in the transverse sinus. *Abbreviations*: Ao, aorta; LA, left atrium; LAA, left atrial appendage; LV, left ventricle; PA, pulmonary artery; PE, pericardial effusion; RA, right atrium; RV right ventricle.

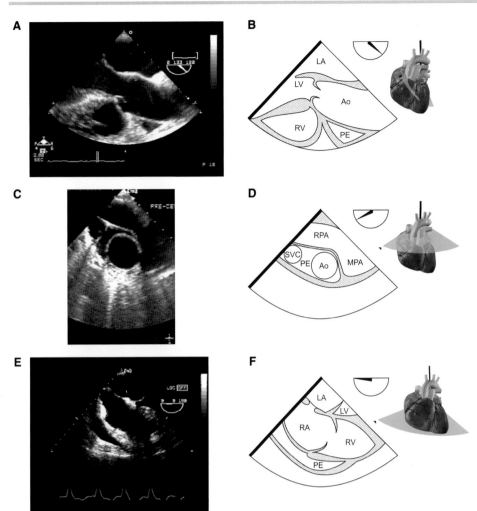

Figure 12.5 Pericardial effusion. (**A,B**) Mid-esophageal aortic valve long-axis view: PE is anterior to the ascending Ao and communicates with the transverse sinus. (**C,D**) Mid-esophageal ascending Ao short-axis view: PE present between the Ao and the SVC. (**E,F**) Mid-esophageal four-chamber view: PE is seen anterior to the RV and RA. *Abbreviations*: Ao, aorta; LA, left atrium; LV, left ventricle; ME, mid-esophageal; MPA, main pulmonary artery; PE, pericardial effusion; RPA, right pulmonary artery; RA, right atrium; RV, right ventricle; SVC, superior vena cava.

and the distribution of fluid around it. The following estimations of PEs may be used: a PE less than 50 mL may not be reliably detected. Small effusions (<200 mL) are usually only detectable posteriorly. Moderate effusions (200–500 mL) are generally present both posteriorly and anteriorly and can have a thickness of up to ~1.5 cm. Large (>500 mL) PEs are most often circumferential (1). Other authors suggest that the size of a PE should be considered small when the separation between parietal and visceral pericardium is less than 0.5 cm, moderate when it is between 0.5 and 2 cm, and large when it is more than 2 cm (2).

Assessment of the echotexture of the PE is also important. A highly echogenic effusion suggests the presence of blood while fibrin strands are often associated with chronicity. Echo-free effusion can be either a transudate or an exudate. The presence of an echogenic pericardial mass raises the possibility of neoplasia.

Differentiating PE from Epicardial Fat, Pleural Fluid

Epicardial fat can be mistaken for pericardial fluid. Typically, epicardial fat is mildly echogenic and

seen anterior to the heart but is absent posteriorly (Fig. 12.6). A retrocardiac left pleural effusion is the most common posterior finding mistaken for a PE. The differentiating points include: (*i*) a retrocardiac left pleural effusion presenting as a large posterior effusion in the absence of any anterior effusion; (*ii*) a pleural effusion lacking the characteristic decrease in echo-free space width from LV to LA seen with a PE; and (*iii*) the echo-free space being posterior to the descending thoracic Ao in the case of a pleural effusion but anterior to the descending Ao (i.e., between the descending Ao and the posterior LV wall) with a PE (Fig. 12.7). In the mid-esophageal four-chamber view, an isolated echo-free space superior to the right atrium (RA) most likely represents pleural fluid.

Pericardial and pleural effusions may coexist in the same patient. They can be recognized by locating the position of the descending thoracic Ao and by identifying the pericardium as the membrane separating the two echo-free spaces. Indeed the presence of a small PE often aids in the accurate identification of a pleural effusion (Fig. 12.8).

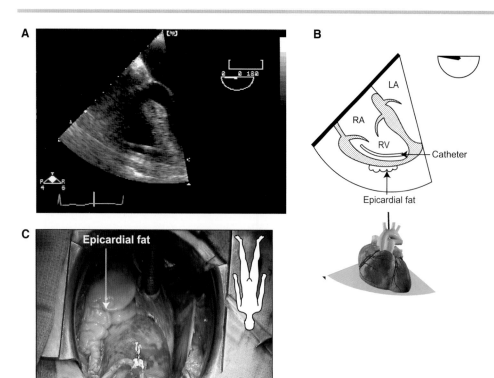

Figure 12.6 Epicardial fat. Mid-esophageal four-chamber view (**A,B**) shows epicardial fat in a 67-year-old man before aortic surgery correlating with the intraoperative findings (**C**). *Abbreviations*: LA, left atrium; RA, right atrium; RV, right ventricle. *Source*: Intraoperative clip courtesy of Dr Michel Pellerin.

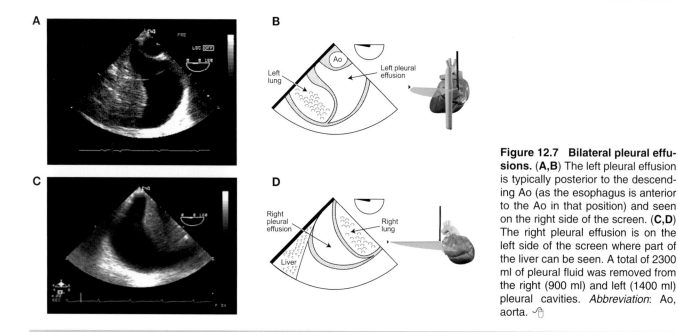

Figure 12.7 Bilateral pleural effusions. (**A,B**) The left pleural effusion is typically posterior to the descending Ao (as the esophagus is anterior to the Ao in that position) and seen on the right side of the screen. (**C,D**) The right pleural effusion is on the left side of the screen where part of the liver can be seen. A total of 2300 ml of pleural fluid was removed from the right (900 ml) and left (1400 ml) pleural cavities. *Abbreviation*: Ao, aorta.

Cardiac Tamponade

Cardiac tamponade is a clinical diagnosis that occurs when a PE causes the pericardial pressure to exceed the intracardiac pressure, resulting in impaired cardiac filling. The amount of fluid alone is of less importance than the rapidity of fluid accumulation for the occurrence of tamponade. A slowly expanding PE can become quite large (up to 1000 mL) with little increase in pericardial pressure, while rapid accumulation of fluid, with a volume as small as 100 mL, may be sufficient to increase the pericardial

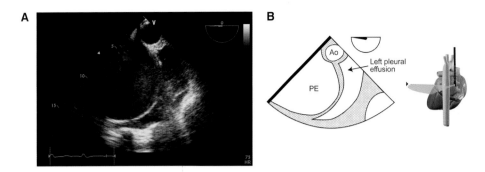

Figure 12.8   Pleural and pericardial effusion. (A,B) Descending Ao short-axis view in a 77-year-old man diagnosed with tamponade shows both pericardial and pleural effusions. Note that the left pleural effusion is posterior to the descending Ao. *Abbreviation*: Ao, aorta.

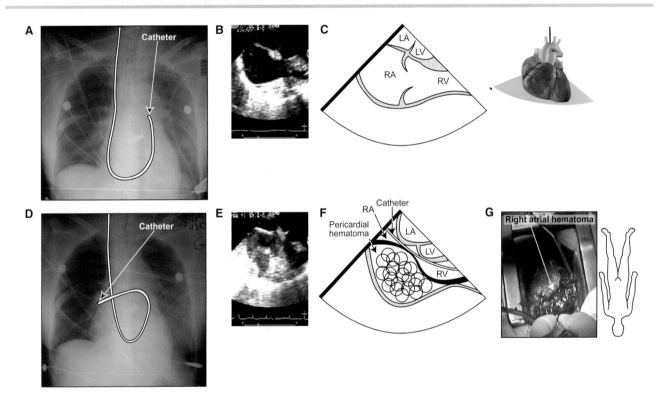

Figure 12.9   Cardiac tamponade. A 29-year-old woman became hemodynamically unstable after aortic valve surgery. Cardiac tamponade was suspected from serial chest X-rays (**A–D**): the pulmonary artery catheter tip had moved from its initial medial position (**A**) to a more distal position (**D**) due to the displacement of the right-sided cardiac chambers by the suspected pericardial process. (**E,F**) Diagnosis by repeat TEE: a new pericardial thrombus compresses the right heart chambers, compared with the intraoperative mid-esophageal four-chamber view (**B,C**). (**G**) Diagnosis confirmation at surgical reexploration. *Abbreviations*: LA, left atrium; LV, left ventricle; RA, right atrium; RV, right ventricle.

pressure markedly and cause cardiac tamponade. This J-shaped curve indicates that a sudden increase in the volume of pericardial fluid can slightly stretch the pericardium, and thus an increase of as little as 100 or 200 mL may elevate pericardial pressure from its normal ambient, or slightly sub-ambient value, to 30 mmHg or more, defining severe cardiac tamponade

(3). It is important to remember that tamponade after cardiac surgery will often be due to a localized PE (Figs. 12.9–12.11). In contemporary practice, echocardiography, combined with clinical features, has become a gold standard for diagnosing cardiac tamponade and has proven useful for directing the treatment.

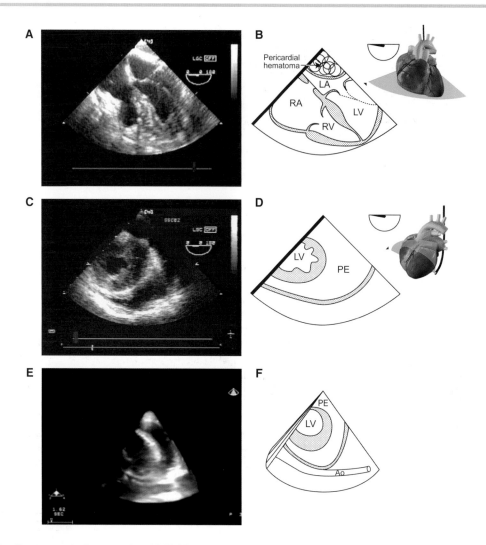

Figure 12.10   Cardiac tamponade examples. (A,B) Mid-esophageal four-chamber view with left atrial compression, which was missed on transthoracic echocardiography. **(C,D)** Transgastric mid short-axis view with left ventricular compression in two hemodynamically unstable patients after cardiac surgery. **(E,F)** Transthoracic three-dimensional echo of a large circumferential pericardial effusion. *Abbreviations*: Ao, aorta; LA, left atrium; LV, left ventricle; PE, pericardial effusion; RA, right atrium; RV right ventricle; TTE, transthoracic echocardiography.

Two-Dimensional Echocardiographic Features of Cardiac Tamponade

Cardiac tamponade is suspected, clinically, in the presence of hypotension, tachycardia, pulsus paradoxus, and distended jugular veins. Two-dimensional (2D) echocardiography helps confirm the diagnosis when the following signs are present: (*i*) moderate to large PE; (*ii*) RA systolic collapse that lasts for more than one-third of systole; (*iii*) RV diastolic collapse; (*iv*) reciprocal changes in RV and LV volumes during respiration; and (*v*) inferior vena cava (IVC) plethora.

Right atrial systolic collapse. Right atrial systolic collapse is believed to be an early sign of cardiac tamponade because this chamber has the lowest intracavitary pressure. When intrapericardial pressure

exceeds right atrial systolic pressure, inversion or collapse of the right atrial free wall occurs. Relative to the cardiac cycle, the longer the duration of right atrial free wall inversion, the higher the intrapericardial pressure is in relation to the right atrial pressure (RAP) and the greater is the likelihood of cardiac tamponade. Right atrial systolic inversion duration longer than 30% of the cardiac cycle has been considered a sensitive indicator for the diagnosis of tamponade (2). Right atrial systolic collapse is best sought in the mid-esophageal four-chamber view but may be seen wherever the RA can be well visualized (Fig. 12.11). Of note, if the pericardial reflection in the oblique sinus behind the LA is sufficiently high to allow fluid accumulation, the LA may also demonstrate systolic collapse.

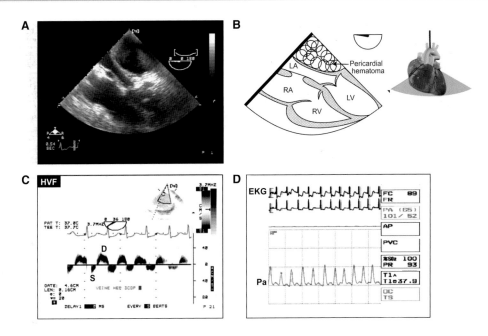

Figure 12.11 Loculated hematoma. Localized tamponade in a 74-year-old woman after mitral valve repair is present. **(A,B)** Mid-esophageal four-chamber view: a pericardial hematoma in the oblique sinus is compressing the LA. **(C)** The HVF Doppler signal showed an S wave reversal. This persisted despite evacuation of the pericardial hematoma, suggesting instead residual right ventricular diastolic dysfunction. **(D)** No significant pulsus paradoxus was seen. *Abbreviations*: D, peak diastolic HVF velocity; EKG, electrocardiogram; HVF, hepatic venous flow; LA, left atrium; LV, left ventricle; Pa, arterial pressure; RA, right atrium; RV, right ventricle; S, peak systolic HVF velocity.

Right ventricular diastolic collapse. Right ventricular diastolic collapse is a more specific, but less sensitive, sign than right atrial collapse for the diagnosis of cardiac tamponade. This sign occurs when intrapericardial pressure exceeds RV diastolic pressure. Right ventricular diastolic collapse can be seen in the mid-esophageal four-chamber view or in the RV inflow-outflow view at the level of the aortic valve (AoV).

Right and left ventricular dimension changes with respiration. Right ventricular dimension and volume normally increase with spontaneous inspiration and decrease during expiration; opposite changes are observed with positive-pressure ventilation. These respiratory variations are exaggerated in the presence of cardiac tamponade and are accompanied by exaggerated reciprocal changes in LV dimension and volume (4). Exaggerated reciprocal respiratory variations in RV and LV dimensions and volumes are best demonstrated with simultaneous recording of the respiratory cycle (Fig. 12.12). On 2D imaging the reciprocal variation in ventricular volumes is also recognized by the abnormal ventricular septal motion toward the LV in diastole during spontaneous inspiration that normalizes during spontaneous expiration (Fig. 12.13).

Inferior vena cava plethora. The IVC can be visualized from both esophageal and transgastric views (Fig. 12.14). The normal decrease in IVC diameter (measured near its junction with the RA) during inspiration is more than 50% in spontaneously breathing patients and is inversely related to central venous pressure. Thus, IVC plethora is defined as a dilated IVC with less than 50% reduction in diameter with spontaneous inspiration (5). As elevated right-sided pressures are part of tamponade physiology, the absence of IVC plethora strongly argues against global cardiac tamponade. Although sensitive, IVC plethora is not a specific indicator of tamponade as it only reflects elevated RAP.

Doppler Features in Cardiac Tamponade

With normal physiology, small increases (<15%) in tricuspid and pulmonic peak flow velocities and RV stroke volume (SV) and corresponding decreases (<10%) in left-sided parameters are seen during inspiration (Fig. 12.15). These respiratory variations are markedly increased in tamponade. Both tricuspid and pulmonic valve (TV, PV) peak velocities nearly double with spontaneous inspiration, while both mitral (E velocity) and aortic valve (MV, AoV) velocities are decreased by more than 25% (Fig. 12.15) (6). In cardiac tamponade, the greatest respiratory variations are observed on the first beat after the beginning of inspiration. Similar changes are observed in patients with significant chronic obstructive pulmonary disease (COPD) due to wide intrathoracic

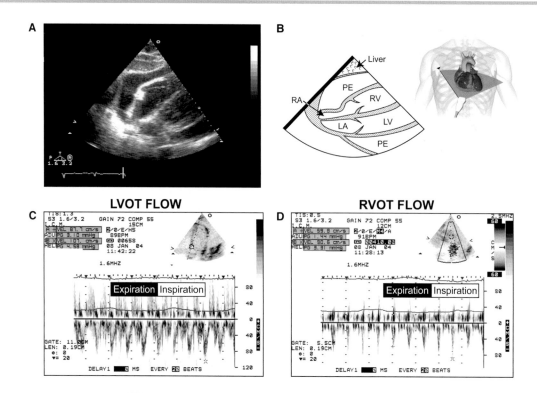

LVOT FLOW

RVOT FLOW

Figure 12.12 Cardiac tamponade. Cardiac tamponade in a 53-year-old woman treated for pericarditis. (**A,B**) Transthoracic subcostal view with right atrial collapse. (**C,D**) Pulsed wave Doppler examination: note that the RVOT velocities increase with spontaneous inspiration with opposite respiratory changes in the LVOT velocities. *Abbreviations*: LA, left atrium; LV, left ventricle; LVOT, left ventricular outflow tract; PE, pericardial effusion; RA, right atrium; RV, right ventricle; RVOT, right ventricular outflow tract. *Source*: Courtesy of Drs. François Haddad and François Marcotte.

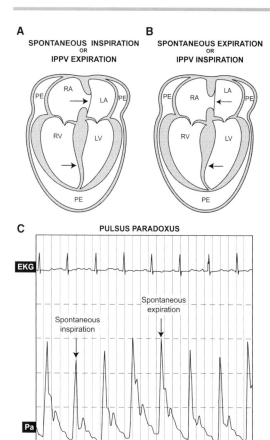

Figure 12.13 Tamponade physiology. Ventricular changes with respiration in tamponade are presented. (**A**) During spontaneous inspiration with more negative intrathoracic pressure, an increase in venous return results in higher right-sided pressures causing a leftward shift in the interatrial and interventricular septum. During intermittent positive-pressure ventilation (IPPV), this occurs during the expiration phase instead, with the passive decrease of positive pressure. (**B**) The opposite changes occur in spontaneous expiration or IPPV inspiration. (**C**) These changes manifest as pulsus paradoxus on the Pa trace. *Abbreviations*: EKG, electrocardiogram; IPPV, intermittent positive-pressure ventilation; LA, left atrium; LV, left ventricle; Pa, arterial pressure; PE, pericardial effusion; RA, right atrium; RV, right ventricle.

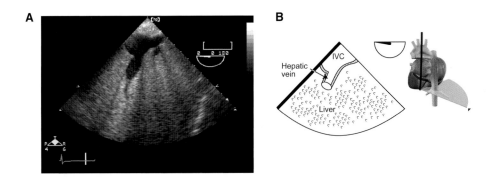

Figure 12.14 Hepatic vein and IVC. (A,B) Transgastric IVC long-axis view shows dilatation of both the IVC and hepatic vein in this mechanically ventilated 49-year-old woman with tamponade. *Abbreviation*: IVC, inferior vena cava.

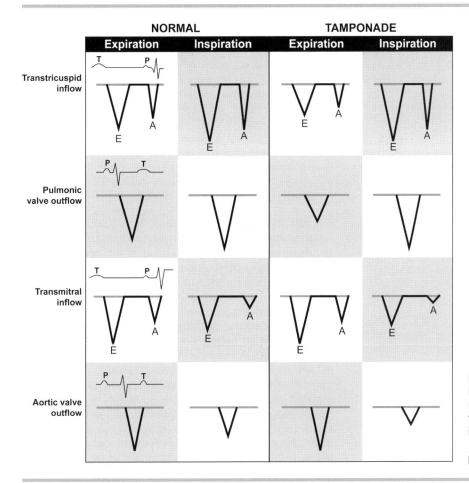

Figure 12.15 Normal and tamponade Doppler profiles. This diagram compares respiratory changes in various Doppler flows during normal and tamponade physiology with spontaneous breathing. *Abbreviations*: A, peak late diastolic velocity; E, peak early diastolic velocity.

pressure changes, but, in contrast, the velocity changes are more gradual and the largest variation does not appear in the first cardiac beat to occur during inspiration. Further, respiratory variations in conjunction with a reciprocal expiratory decrease of more than 25% in the late diastolic hepatic venous flow (HVF) velocity (or even diastolic flow reversal) strongly suggests cardiac tamponade (Fig. 12.16).

The increase in right venous return observed during normal spontaneous inspiration occurs instead during the expiration phase with positive-pressure mechanical ventilation, when the intrathoracic pressure passively decreases. Thus, the classic diagnostic Doppler changes described in cardiac tamponade during spontaneous breathing are opposite when patients are under positive-pressure mechanical ventilation.

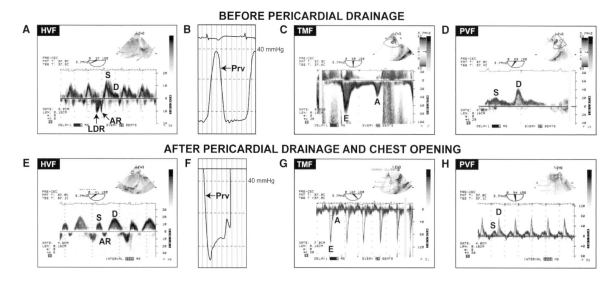

Figure 12.16 Drainage of pericardial effusion. (A–H) Spectral Doppler profiles in a 50-year-old woman scheduled for coronary revascularization with a pericardial effusion. (**A**) The HVF showed intermittent LDR with normal S/D ratio >1. (**B**) Note the flat diastolic portion of the Prv curve. (**C**) The E/A ratio was > 1 on the TMF and S/D ratio < 1 on the PVF. (**D**) Following pericardial drainage of 200 mL after chest opening, the HVF S/D ratio became < 1 with disappearance of the LDR (**E**), the diastolic slope of the Prv increased (**F**) and both the E/A ratio of the TMF (**G**) and the S/D ratio of the PVF (**H**) became more pronounced. These observations are consistent with a deterioration of both right and left ventricular diastolic function. *Abbreviations*: A, peak late diastolic TMF velocity; AR, peak atrial reversal HVF velocity; D, peak diastolic HVF or PVF velocity; E, peak early diastolic TMF velocity; HVF, hepatic venous flow; LDR, late diastolic reversal HVF velocity; Pra, right atrial pressure; Prv, right ventricular pressure; PVF, pulmonary venous flow; S, peak systolic HVF or PVF velocity; TMF, transmitral flow.

Also, drainage of PE in patients under positive-pressure ventilation can be associated with deterioration of RV diastolic function secondary to the sudden increase in venous return (Fig. 12.16).

Localized Chamber Compression from Hematoma

Regional PEs are common after cardiac surgery, due to localized bleeding and thrombus formation, and may cause tamponade from compression of the lower pressure RA and LA (7). A mid-esophageal four-chamber view can show a pericardial hematoma compressing the right atrial free wall resulting in a slit-like appearance of the right atrial cavity (Fig. 12.9). The RV, LA, and LV can also be compressed (Figs. 12.10 and 12.11). In the postoperative cardiac patient with often limited windows because of surgical wounds and drains, TEE is superior to TTE in diagnosing localized tamponade and differentiating it from other causes of hemodynamic instability (see Fig. 21.11). The classical respiratory changes in the Doppler signals and hemodynamic parameters are less evident with localized effusions (Fig. 12.11) (8). However, abnormal right-sided diastolic patterns suggestive of restrictive ventricular filling are commonly seen (Fig. 12.11).

Pericardiocentesis and Surgical Drainage Assessment

Two-dimensional echocardiography is extremely valuable in assisting pericardiocentesis. Echocardiography not only confirms the presence of pericardial fluid but also confirms whether it is loculated. It can also identify the optimal approach for pericardiocentesis, by defining the area of largest fluid accumulation most easily reached percutaneously, while avoiding vital organs and abnormal structures. Injection of an ultrasound contrast agent through the pericardiocentesis needle may help to ensure that it is located in the pericardial cavity. Similarly, ultrasound contrast injection through an intravenous line may help to localize the origin of pericardial fluid by demonstrating its escape from one of the cardiac chambers.

In adult patients, pericardiocentesis is most often assisted using TTE imaging guidance. However, TEE monitoring during pericardiocentesis has the advantages of allowing better imaging of the PE without interfering with the sterile procedure field and helping to monitor fluid disappearance during pericardiocentesis drainage. When using TEE, it may be easier to detect the guide-wire then the needle tip (Fig. 12.17).

CONSTRICTIVE PERICARDITIS

Echocardiographic Findings in Constrictive Pericarditis

Constrictive pericarditis (CP) is characterized by impaired diastolic cardiac filling due to the abnormal pericardium constraining the cardiac structures like a rigid shell, separating the intrathoracic pressure changes from the intracardiac pressure (Fig. 12.18).

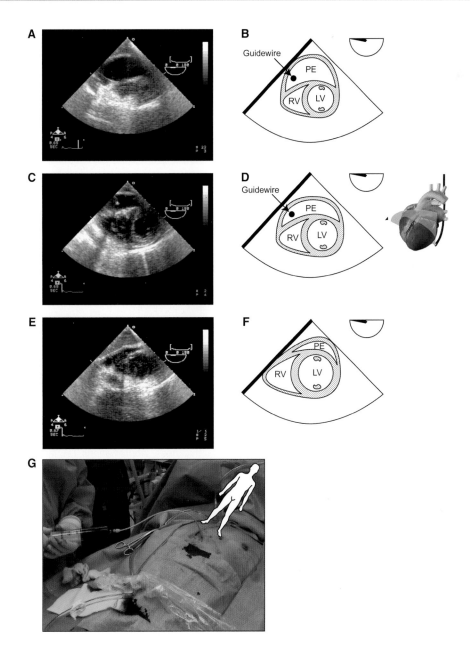

Figure 12.17   Pericardial drainage. (A–G) Percutaneous pericardial drainage of pericardial fluid assisted with transesophageal echocardiography in the operating room. The guidewire is seen behind the ventricles in these transgastric short-axis views. A total of 900 ml of fluid was removed. *Abbreviations*: LV, left ventricle; PE, pericardial effusion; RV, right ventricle. *Source*: Photo G courtesy of Dr. Raymond Cartier.

Echocardiographic findings in CP include:

1. Thickened pericardium (>3 mm), which may be difficult to demonstrate (9).
2. Abnormal septal motion (Fig. 12.19), with exaggerated inspiratory leftward movement of both the atrial and ventricular septa, and abnormal bouncing of the interventricular septum due to ventricular interdependence.

3. Restrictive filling pattern (Fig. 12.20) on pulsed wave (PW) Doppler examination of atrioventricular inflow, showing high E and small A velocities (E/A ratio > 1.5), short E wave deceleration time (<160 ms), and isovolumetric relaxation time (IVRT < 70 ms). This is consistent with increased LV and RV filling pressures and similar to patients with RCMP.

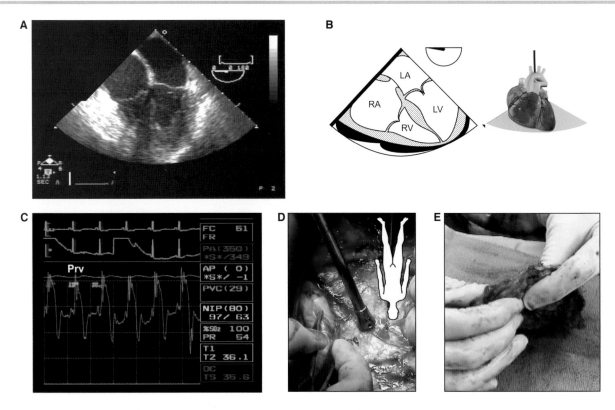

Figure 12.18   Pericardectomy. A 69-year-old man is undergoing pericardectomy for constrictive pericarditis. (**A,B**) A mid-esophageal four-chamber view shows a dilated RA and LA with deviation of the atrial and ventricular septa toward the left, suggesting significantly increased right sided pressure. (**C**) Prv tracing shows typical diastolic square root sign consistent with restrictive filling. (**D,E**) Upon opening of the chest cavity, the fibrinous pericardium is seen with abnormal thickness. *Abbreviations*: LA, left atrium; LV, left ventricle; Prv, right ventricular pressure; RA, right atrium; RV, right ventricle. *Source*: Courtesy of Dr. Raymond Cartier.

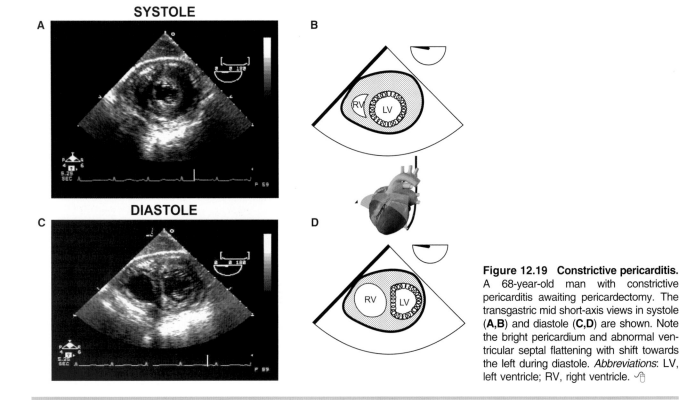

Figure 12.19   Constrictive pericarditis. A 68-year-old man with constrictive pericarditis awaiting pericardectomy. The transgastric mid short-axis views in systole (**A,B**) and diastole (**C,D**) are shown. Note the bright pericardium and abnormal ventricular septal flattening with shift towards the left during diastole. *Abbreviations*: LV, left ventricle; RV, right ventricle.

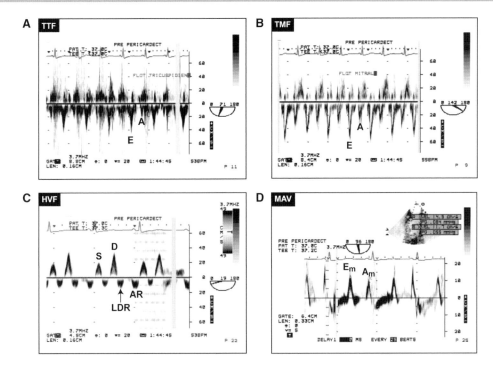

Figure 12.20 Constrictive pericarditis. A mechanically ventilated 68-year-old man with constrictive pericarditis is scheduled for pericardectomy. Both the Doppler (**A**) TTF and (**B**) TMF demonstrate predominance of the early E diastolic velocity with respiratory variation. (**C**) HVF Doppler tracing shows abnormal S blunting with D flow predominance and even LDR. (**D**) MAV shows normal Em velocity which argues against the presence of restrictive cardiomyopathy. *Abbreviations*: A, peak late diastolic TMF or TTF velocity; Am, peak late diastolic MAV; AR, peak atrial reversal HVF velocity; D, peak diastolic HVF velocity; E, peak early diastolic TMF or TTF velocity; Em, peak early diastolic MAV; HVF, hepatic venous flow; LDR, late diastolic reversal HVF velocity; MAV, mitral annular velocity; S, peak systolic HVF velocity; TMF, transmitral flow; TTF, transtricuspid flow.

4. Respiratory variation of the mitral inflow and pulmonary venous flow velocities is present.

Doppler echocardiography performed simultaneously with respirometry is a useful method to diagnose CP, as marked respiratory changes in ventricular filling and central venous flow velocities result from a thickened pericardial shell that shields the heart from the variation in intrathoracic pressure (Fig. 12.21) (10). The change in intrathoracic pressure is not transmitted to the cardiac chambers because of the rigid pericardium; the pulmonary venous pressure decreases to a greater degree than the left atrial and LV pressure. The decreased pressure gradient responsible for LV filling results in decreased LV output with inspiration. In the right-sided cavities, during spontaneous inspiration, the intrathoracic pressure drop leads to increased venous return to the RA and increased RV filling. As the total cardiac volume is fixed by the constraining pericardium, a decrease in LV volume is consequently accompanied by a reciprocal increase in RV volume, characteristic of ventricular interdependence. This is reflected by a leftward shift, or bulging of the septum, which further contributes to decreased LV compliance.

Pulsed wave Doppler examination during spontaneous inspiration shows a characteristic decrease more than 25% of the mitral inflow E velocity and pulmonary venous flow D wave velocity with a concomitant increase more than 40% to 50% in tricuspid inflow E velocity, while HVF diastolic velocity will typically decrease and, in some patients, reverse during the opposite expiratory phase (Fig. 12.21).

Positive-pressure inspiration decreases systemic venous return that is followed by reduced LV output. In the early phase, however, LV stroke volume increases because the increased intrathoracic pressure compresses the LV and increases the pressure gradient between intra- and extrathoracic vascular beds. Hence, positive-pressure mechanical ventilation will display an inverted pattern of respiratory variations in the Doppler mitral inflow and pulmonary venous flow tracing in patients with CP. Thus, positive-pressure inspiration causes an increase (instead of the usual decrease) in the mitral inflow and pulmonary venous flow Doppler velocities, with reciprocal changes in the tricuspid inflow and HVF. The percentage of change in the peak

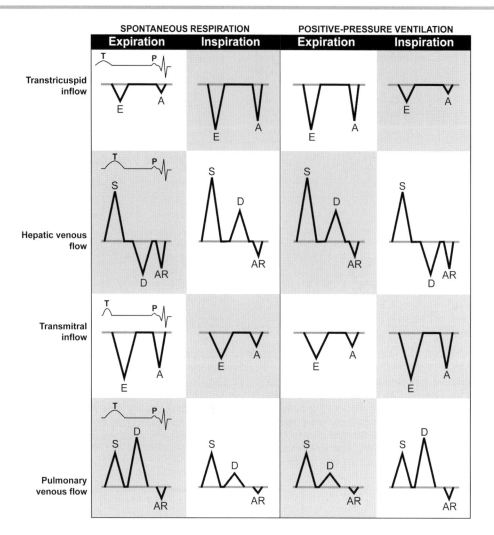

Figure 12.21 Constrictive pericarditis. Doppler changes in transtricuspid flow, hepatic venous flow, transmitral inflow and pulmonary venous flow during spontaneous respiration and positive pressure ventilation in constrictive pericarditis. *Abbreviations*: A, peak late diastolic TMF or TTF velocity; AR, peak atrial reversal HVF or PVF velocity; D, peak diastolic HVF or PVF velocity; E, peak early diastolic TMF or TTF velocity; HVF, hepatic venous flow; PVF, pulmonary venous flow; S, peak systolic HVF or PVF velocity; TMF, transmitral flow; TTF, transtricuspid flow. *Source*: Adapted from Ref. 10.

velocities, induced by positive-pressure ventilation, is in the same range as reported during spontaneous breathing (Fig. 12.21).

5. Pulsed wave tissue Doppler Imaging (TDI) in CP shows normal or elevated mitral annular early E_m velocity (also known as e, E' or E_a) as opposed to the reduced E_m velocity in RCMP (11).

6. Extracardiac abnormalities include dilated IVC and hepatic veins, with peritoneal fluid in patients with chronic right-sided failure. Pericardial calcifications are more easily seen on the chest X-Ray, computed tomography (CT), or magnetic resonance imaging (MRI) (Fig. 12.22).

Differentiating CP from RCMP

Restrictive cardiomyopathy is an uncommon disease characterized by normal-sized ventricles with dia-

stolic dysfunction (see Chapter 11). The differential diagnosis between RCMP and CP is challenging, because the two entities share many hemodynamic features. The main differences between RCMP and CP are as follows:

1. Atrial enlargement: bi-atrial enlargement is generally more marked in RCMP than CP.

2. Pulmonary artery pressure: patients with RCMP typically have moderate to severe pulmonary hypertension, while those with CP have only mild elevations in pulmonary arterial pressure. Estimation of pulmonary pressure can be performed from tricuspid and pulmonic regurgitation jet velocity.

3. Doppler respiratory variations: in CP, the mitral inflow E and pulmonary venous peak diastolic (D) velocity will typically vary by more than 25% between expiration and inspiration. In contrast,

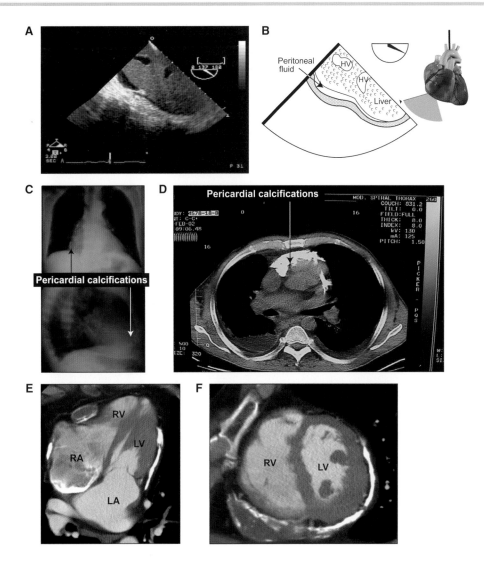

Figure 12.22 Constrictive pericarditis. Associated findings in constrictive pericarditis from a 66-year-old man scheduled for pericardectomy. (**A,B**) Peritoneal fluid from right-sided failure. Note the dilated hepatic veins. Pericardial calcifications seen as bright linear opacities on the chest X-ray (**C**) and on the chest computed tomography anteriorly (**D**), around the right atrium (**E**). *Abbreviations*: HV, hepatic vein; LA, left atrium; LV, left ventricle; RA, right atrium; RV, right ventricle.

the respiration variation of the mitral inflow E velocity will be less than 10% with RCMP.

4. Tissue Doppler imaging: TDI interrogation of the lateral MV annulus in RCMP will typically reveal decreased early peak E_m velocity of longitudinal expansion to less than 8.0 cm/s while it will be preserved (>8.0 cm/s) in CP (Fig. 12.20). The Doppler myocardial velocity gradient (MVG) from the LV posterior wall also helps to differentiate between RCMP and CP. The MVG corresponds to the slope of linear regression of the myocardial velocity estimates along each M-mode scan line throughout the thickness of the myocardium. Indeed, the MVG measured during early ejection and during rapid ventricular filling is decreased in RCMP patients compared with both normal and CP patients during ventricular ejection and rapid ventricular filling (12). In addition, during isovolumic relaxation, the MVG is positive in RCMP and negative in both normal and CP patients.

5. Color M-mode flow propagation of LV filling: a slope ≥100 cm/s for the first aliasing contour in color M-mode flow propagation of LV filling can predict patients with CP, while it is typically reduced less than 45 cm/s in RCMP (13).

An algorithm that incorporates mitral inflow Doppler signal and tissue Doppler has been proposed to differentiate constriction from restrictive cardiomyopathy and normal physiology (Fig. 12.23) (14). The sensitivity and specificity of the different Doppler criteria for CP are shown in Table 12.1 (13).

Constrictive Pericarditis vs. Restrictive Cardiomyopathy

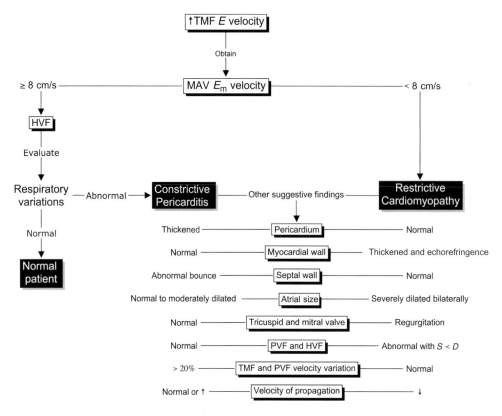

Figure 12.23 Constrictive pericarditis. Algorithm to differentiate constrictive pericarditis from restrictive cardiomyopathy. *Abbreviations*: HVF, hepatic venous flow; LV, left ventricle; MAV, mitral annular velocity; PVF, pulmonary venous flow; TMF, transmitral flow. *Source*: Adapted from Ref. 14.

Table 12.1   Useful Doppler Criteria Favoring Constrictive Pericarditis over Restrictive Cardiomyopathy

Method	Variable	Criteria for CP	Specificity (%)	Sensitivity (%)
Mitral Doppler	Resp. variation in peak E	≥10%	84	91
Pulmonary vein Doppler	Resp. variation in peak D	≥18%	79	91
Tissue Doppler	Peak E_m	≥8 cm/s	89	100
Color M-mode	Slope of first alias	≥100 cm/s	74	91

Abbreviations: CP, constrictive pericarditis; Resp., respiratory.
Source: Adapted from Ref. 13.

Pericardectomy

The treatment for pericardial constriction is pericardectomy. The indications, surgical techniques, key monitoring features, and possible complications will be described briefly. Pericardectomy should be considered after the diagnosis of CP, before the onset of class IV heart failure, to limit the operative mortality (15). When operated early, survival is similar to general population after an initial 1% to 10% operative mortality.

Pericardectomy is usually done through a median sternotomy without heparinization or cardiopulmonary bypass (CPB) support. Alternative approaches, such as dual thoracotomies or left anterolateral thoracotomy, can be used in patients with posteriorly localized pericardial thickening.

After sternotomy, a plane of dissection between the pericardium and epicardium is developed and, traditionally, the LV is progressively freed first to avoid RV dilatation. The pericardium is excised from the anterior surface of the heart, from the right to the left phrenic nerve. The diaphragmatic pericardium is usually left in place except for the region of the IVC, which can also be restricted and can account for residual symptoms. The pericardium is then removed from

Table 12.2 Echocardiographic and Hemodynamic Signs of Adverse Events During Pericardectomy

Complications during pericardectomy	Echocardiographic and hemodynamic signs
Residual left ventricular constriction	Right ventricular distention
Coronary injury	Wall motion abnormality
Heart chamber injury	Hypovolemia, low cardiac output
Persistent bleeding	Hypovolemia, low cardiac output
Hypothermia	Arythmogenicity

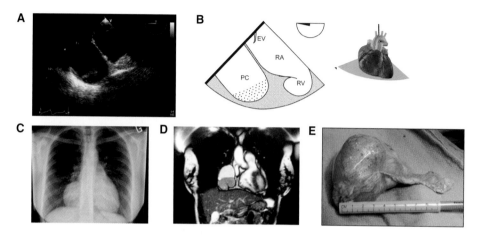

Figure 12.24 Pericardial cyst. (A,B) Mid-esophageal views at 0° with right sided rotation in a 28-year-old woman show an echolucent cavity consistent with a pericardial cyst adjacent to the RA and LA. Compare with chest X-ray (**C**) magnetic resonance imaging coronal view (**D**) and pathological specimen (**E**). *Abbreviations*: EV, Eustachian valve; PC, pericardial cyst; RV, right ventricle. *Source*: Photo E courtesy of Dr. Michel Pellerin.

the atrial surface and superior vena cava (SVC) if constriction is still present. The objective of the pericardiectomy is to restore normal ventricular pressure-volume relationships and free the inflows of the RV and LV (16).

A careful examination of the systolic and diastolic profiles of the LV and RV is of paramount importance, as well as the evaluation of high velocity flows in the SVC, IVC, and pulmonary veins, which can suggest residual constriction.

The potential intraoperative complications of pericardectomy are significant bleeding, coronary injury, heart chamber injury, RV distention, and hypothermia. Echocardiographic and hemodynamic signs of these complications are illustrated in Table 12.2. In patients with class IV heart failure, perioperative mortality can be as high as 46%, most frequently from persistent low cardiac output (CO) (15). Normalization of the diastolic profile has been associated with good symptomatic relief in the postoperative follow-up (17).

PERICARDIAL CYST

Pericardial cysts are uncommon intrathoracic lesions and typically located in the right cardiophrenic angles on chest X-Ray. Transthoracic echocardiography will reveal a spherical cystic echo-free space contiguous to the heart. Usually, they are associated with an excel-

lent long-term prognosis and are often detected incidentally. Complicated clinical courses, including sudden death, have been reported (18), especially when pericardial cysts cause compression of cardiac structures and hemodynamic changes. Transesophageal echocardiography can help to recognize malignant cardiac-compressing pericardial cysts in life-threatening conditions (Fig. 12.24) (19).

CONGENITAL ABSENCE OF THE PERICARDIUM

Congenital absence of the pericardium (CAP) is a rare clinical entity whose features may range from a small or partial defect in the pericardium to a complete absence of the entire pericardium. The condition is often asymptomatic and found incidentally on postmortem examination, during intrathoracic surgery, or suspected from abnormal chest X-ray findings. These include levoposition of the heart, loss of the right heart border, abnormal left heart border with herniated left atrial appendage, prominence of a pulmonary artery segment, and interposition of lung between the aorta or the main pulmonary trunk or between the left hemidiaphragm and the inferior border of the heart. Chest X-ray combined with MRI usually establish the diagnosis, while echocardiography is useful to exclude other cardiac disease. Transthoracic examination usually requires a more lateral apical window because of the marked displacement of the apex near the mid-to-posterior axillary line. Cardiac hypermobility, downward displacement of the heart (cardioptosis), abnormal ventricular septal motion, and RV dilatation are among the echocardiographic features so far reported (20,21). The differential diagnosis of these findings from other causes of RV enlargement and volume overload may prove difficult by echocardiography alone and might benefit from complementary TEE examination (22). In the presence of debilitating symptoms or herniation and/or incarceration of cardiac structure(s), surgical procedures have been tried, including pericardioplasty, extension of partial pericardial defect or pericardiectomy, left atrial appendectomy, and lysis of adherences.

CONCLUSION

In summary, TEE is a powerful tool in the diagnosis of pericardial disorders. The 2010 guidelines support the use of TEE in all cardiac or thoracic aortic surgery patients (see Chapter 31) (23).

REFERENCES

1. Chuttani K, Pandian NG, Mohanty PK, et al. Left ventricular diastolic collapse. An echocardiographic sign of regional cardiac tamponade. Circulation 1991; 83:1999–2006.
2. Spodick DH. Acute cardiac tamponade. N Engl J Med 2003; 349:684–690.
3. Shabetai R. Pericardial effusion: haemodynamic spectrum. Heart 2004; 90:255–256.
4. Gerber TC, Safford RE. Intrapericardial Doppler flow signals in cardiac tamponade. Clin Cardiol 1999; 22:231–232.
5. Himelman RB, Kircher B, Rockey DC, et al. Inferior vena cava plethora with blunted respiratory response: a sensitive echocardiographic sign of cardiac tamponade. J Am Coll Cardiol 1988; 12:1470–1477.
6. Merce J, Sagrista-Sauleda J, Permanyer-Miralda G, et al. Correlation between clinical and Doppler echocardiographic findings in patients with moderate and large pericardial effusion: implications for the diagnosis of cardiac tamponade. Am Heart J 1999; 138:759–764.
7. Pepi M, Muratori M, Barbier P, et al. Pericardial effusion after cardiac surgery: incidence, site, size, and haemodynamic consequences. Br Heart J 1994; 72:327–331.
8. Larose E, Ducharme A, Mercier LA, et al. Prolonged distress and clinical deterioration before pericardial drainage in patients with cardiac tamponade. Can J Cardiol 2000; 16:331–336.
9. Ling LH, Oh JK, Tei C, et al. Pericardial thickness measured with transesophageal echocardiography: feasibility and potential clinical usefulness. J Am Coll Cardiol 1997; 29:1317–1323.
10. Klein AL, Cohen GI. Doppler echocardiographic assessment of constrictive pericarditis, cardiac amyloidosis, and cardiac tamponade. Cleve Clin J Med 1992; 59:278–290.
11. Oki T, Tabata T, Yamada H, et al. Right and left ventricular wall motion velocities as diagnostic indicators of constrictive pericarditis. Am J Cardiol 1998; 81:465–470.
12. Palka P, Lange A, Donnelly JE, et al. Differentiation between restrictive cardiomyopathy and constrictive pericarditis by early diastolic doppler myocardial velocity gradient at the posterior wall. Circulation 2000; 102:655–662.
13. Rajagopalan N, Garcia MJ, Rodriguez L, et al. Comparison of new Doppler echocardiographic methods to differentiate constrictive pericardial heart disease and restrictive cardiomyopathy. Am J Cardiol 2001; 87:86–94.
14. Ha JW, Oh JK, Ommen SR, et al. Diagnostic value of mitral annular velocity for constrictive pericarditis in the absence of respiratory variation in mitral inflow velocity. J Am Soc Echocardiogr 2002; 15:1468–1471.
15. McCaughan BC, Schaff HV, Piehler JM, et al. Early and late results of pericardiectomy for constrictive pericarditis. J Thorac Cardiovasc Surg 1985; 89:340–350.
16. Kasravi B, Ng D, Chandraratna PA. Continuous intraoperative transesophageal echocardiography during pericardiectomy for constrictive pericarditis revealing dynamic change in chamber size. Echocardiography 2005; 22:431–433.
17. Senni M, Redfield MM, Ling LH, et al. Left ventricular systolic and diastolic function after pericardiectomy in patients with constrictive pericarditis: Doppler echocardiographic findings and correlation with clinical status. J Am Coll Cardiol 1999; 33:1182–1188.
18. Fredman CS, Parsons SR, Aquino TI, et al. Sudden death after a stress test in a patient with a large pericardial cyst. Am Heart J 1994; 127:946–950.
19. Antonini-Canterin F, Piazza R, Ascione L, et al. Value of transesophageal echocardiography in the diagnosis of compressive, atypically located pericardial cysts. J Am Soc Echocardiogr 2002; 15:192–194.
20. Connolly HM, Click RL, Schattenberg TT, et al. Congenital absence of the pericardium: echocardiography as a diagnostic tool. J Am Soc Echocardiogr 1995; 8:87–92.
21. Gatzoulis MA, Munk MD, Merchant N, et al. Isolated congenital absence of the pericardium: clinical presentation, diagnosis, and management. Ann Thorac Surg 2000; 69:1209–1215.
22. Fukuda N, Oki T, Iuchi A, et al. Pulmonary and systemic venous flow patterns assessed by transesophageal Doppler echocardiography in congenital absence of the pericardium. Am J Cardiol 1995; 75:1286–1288.
23. Practice guidelines for perioperative transesophageal echocardiography: an updated report by the American Society of Anesthesiologists and the Society of Cardiovascular Anesthesiologists Task Force on Transesophageal Echocardiography. Anesthesiology 2010; 112:1084–1096.

13

Echocardiography During Cardiac Surgery

Pierre Couture, André Y. Denault, and Raymond Cartier

Université de Montréal, Montreal, Quebec, Canada

INTRODUCTION

Several indications for perioperative transesophageal echocardiography (TEE) have become well-established in cardiac surgery (1). The 2010 guidelines support the use of TEE in all cardiac or thoracic aortic surgery patients (see Chapter 31). However, many other indications for the use of TEE remain controversial. As more experience is acquired with the use of perioperative TEE, the favorable impact of routine use of TEE in pediatric and adult cardiac surgery has been documented (2–17). The objective of the present chapter is to review some of the general applications of TEE during cardiac surgery. Monitoring of segmental and global myocardial function, assessment of valvular function, and aortic pathology will also be discussed, although briefly, as they have been reviewed in more detail in other chapters.

DEVICES USED DURING CARDIOPULMONARY BYPASS

Many devices are used during cardiopulmonary bypass (CPB). In cardiac surgery, TEE can be used to assist in the insertion and to ensure the proper functioning and location of the various catheters.

Central Venous and Intracardiac Catheters

The use of surface ultrasound techniques to assist the insertion of central venous catheters has been described (18). While TEE is less helpful for this purpose, it has been used to guide central venous catheter placement in children and adults with congenital heart disease. In these patients, correct placement of a catheter in the superior vena cava (SVC) [at 10 mm from the junction of the SVC with the right atrium (RA)] was achieved in 100% of cases guided by TEE compared with 86% in the control group (19). Thus, TEE may be particularly useful in this population, as external topographical landmarks and withdrawn blood color are less reliable to confirm proper vessel cannulation.

The mid-esophageal (ME) bicaval view at ~90–130° (Fig. 13.1) may be helpful to confirm proper guidewire position prior to introduction of the introducer sheath into the jugular vein, especially when difficulty in passing the guidewire is encountered (20). Improper intra-arterial insertion of a central venous catheter can be detected by TEE, particularly when the subclavian vein approach is used (21). Other authors have suggested using TEE during pulmonary artery catheter insertion after tricuspid valve (TV) surgery to avoid damage to the tricuspid annuloplasty ring (22).

Finally, in the course of difficult catheter insertion, TEE may disclose a persistent left SVC known to be present in 0.5% of adults and 1% of children. This is usually connected to the RA via a dilated coronary sinus (CS), but may sometimes open into the left atrium (LA), resulting in a right-to-left shunt. Catheter tip placement in the CS via a persistent left SVC may lead to arrhythmias or angina (23) and preclude the insertion of a retrograde cardioplegia catheter. The diagnosis of persistent left SVC is confirmed when ultrasound contrast injection through a left-sided vein appears in the dilated CS before the RA as seen in an ME four-chamber view (Fig. 13.2).

Mediastinal Catheter for Pleural Fluid Drainage

The detection of pleural effusions using TEE was first reported in the early years after its introduction (24). Pleural effusions are visualized as crescent-shaped, echo-free areas and are seen by rotating the transducer shaft clockwise from the ME four-chamber view to image the right pleural space and counterclockwise from the LA toward the left pleural space (see Fig. 12.7). With the patient in the supine position, the fluid on the dorsal side of the pleural space is observed between the lung and the aorta (Ao) on the left side, and the lung and esophagus on the right side. The Ao appears to be helpful in visualizing the fluid located in the most dorsal portion of the left pleural space because it acts as an acoustic window. The lung parenchyma, adjacent to the pleural effusion, is commonly atelectatic and appears echogenic, consistent with minimal attenuation of ultrasound echoes due to the absence of normal air. On the right side, it may be more difficult to detect pleural fluid because there is no acoustic window (25). Suction catheters appear as an echogenic structure with acoustic shadowing in the

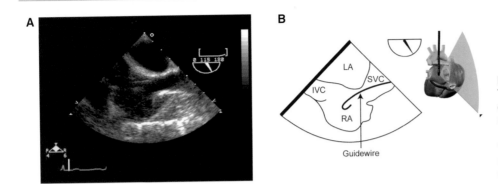

Figure 13.1 Guidewire. (A,B) The J-shaped guidewire is seen originating from the SVC in this mid-esophageal bicaval view at 115°. *Abbreviations*: IVC, inferior vena cava; LA, left atrium; RA, right atrium; SVC, superior vena cava.

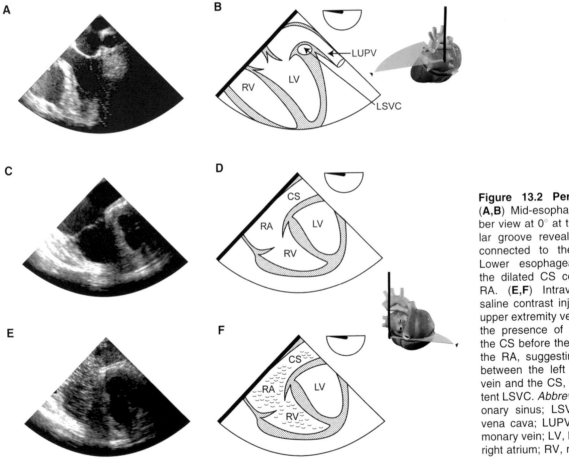

Figure 13.2 Persistent LSVC. (A,B) Mid-esophageal four-chamber view at 0° at the atrioventricular groove reveals a dilated CS connected to the LSVC. **(C,D)** Lower esophageal view shows the dilated CS coursing into the RA. **(E,F)** Intravenous agitated saline contrast injected in the left upper extremity vein demonstrates the presence of microbubbles in the CS before their appearance in the RA, suggesting a connection between the left upper extremity vein and the CS, that is, a persistent LSVC. *Abbreviations*: CS, coronary sinus; LSVC, left superior vena cava; LUPV, left upper pulmonary vein; LV, left ventricle; RA, right atrium; RV, right ventricle.

clear echo-free space, while larger chest tubes appear as double parallel linear echodensities. The volume of pleural fluid can be estimated by measuring the maximal cross-sectional area (CSA max) and axial length (AL) (pleural fluid volume = CSA max X AL (25,26). Pleural fluid volume calculated by this formula correlated strongly with actual pleural fluid volume in cardiac surgical patients (25). Transesophageal echocardiography can detect small volumes of pleural fluid on both sides of the chest: median detection volume (range) was 125 mL (50–200) on the left and 225 mL (150–300) on the right side (25). Using TEE, the drainage of pleural fluid can be monitored by the shrinking and ultimate disappearance of the echo-free space. Large pleural fluid effusions have also been associated with the syndrome of cardiac tamponade with small pericardial effusion (27). In these patients, large pleural effusions and small to moderate pericardial effusions were observed with echocardiographic signs of cardiac tamponade that resolved completely after pleural tap (27).

Vascular Clamp Placement and Aortic Cannulation

Perioperative cerebrovascular events may occur in up to 6% of patients undergoing coronary revascularization (28). Complications include stroke, prolonged encephalopathy, stupor, or seizures, and these adverse neurologic events are associated with a 10-fold increase in mortality rate from 2% to 21% and prolonged hospitalization from 10 to 25 days (29). The presence of severe atherosclerosis in the ascending and transverse Ao increases exponentially with age and has been associated with the risk of embolic complications and stroke. Patients with documented aortic arch atheroma had a significantly higher incidence of intraoperative stroke than those without (15% vs. 2%) (30). Multiple classification systems are currently used to grade the severity of atherosclerotic disease (see example in Fig. 23.13) (31). Grades IV and V atheromas, found frequently to represent superimposed thrombi on ulcerated atherosclerotic plaques, have the highest potential for embolization. Noncalcified, hypoechoic plaques, believed to be rich in lipidic material and thus less stable, are also believed at risk of embolization, irrespective of their morphology (32).

The topography of aortic atherosclerosis enhances its precision as a predictor of stroke in patients undergoing coronary surgery (33). In this study, the presence of ascending aortic atheroma (defined as intimal thickening >0.5 mm) in more than 50% of the ascending Ao was associated with a fourfold increase in early postoperative stroke (<30 days). In addition, ascending aortic atheromas were associated with reduced rated of five-year stroke-free survival. There is also a strong association between the presence of severe aortic stenosis (AS) and severity of aortic atheromas, suggesting that AS might be a manifestation of the atherosclerotic process (34).

Disruption of atherosclerotic plaques or thrombi and dissection may occur during aortic manipulation with cannulation, cross-clamping, side-clamping, and clamp removal (Fig. 13.3). Studies using TEE and detection of cerebral embolization with transcranial Doppler have shown that approximately 50% of the emboli occur during instrumentation of the heart and great vessels and 50% occur randomly while on CPB (35).

Identification of atherosclerotic lesions by TEE may be limited by incomplete visualization of the ascending thoracic Ao (36). The mid and distal ascending and transverse Ao where cannulation and clamping are performed may frequently be obscured by shadowing from the air in the trachea and the right mainstem bronchus. A study using biplane TEE found that as much as 42% of the ascending Ao (or a length of 4.5 cm) was not visualized with TEE (37). In

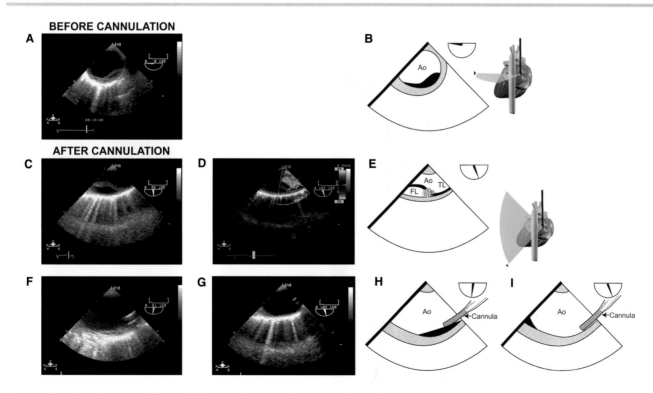

Figure 13.3 Aortic cannulation. A 60-year-old man with a thoracic aortic aneurysm is scheduled for a Bentall procedure. (**A,B**) Examination of the descending Ao before cannulation revealed the presence of thickened intima compatible with an intramural hematoma. (**C–E**) Shortly after the onset of flow in the aortic cannula, a new dissecting flap associated with a FL was seen. (**F–I**) The cannula positioned close to the hematoma was then pulled back. *Abbreviations*: Ao, aorta; FL, false lumen; TL, true lumen.

addition, TEE failed to identify the aortic cannula in 26 of the 27 patients studied and epiaortic scanning identified severe atheroma in five patients (37). Manual palpation may also be attempted to detect significant atheromas but this misses severe disease in 50% to 70% of patients, as only large calcified plaques are identified by this approach (36).

Epiaortic ultrasonographic (EAU) imaging has, therefore, become the gold standard in the intraoperative assessment of the thoracic Ao (31). Indeed, moderate to severe atheromas in the descending thoracic Ao detected by TEE have a 34% positive predictive value but a 100% negative predictive value for concomitant lesions in the ascending Ao, when compared with EAU (38). This would suggest that EAU need not be performed if TEE screening of the descending Ao is negative, but this has not yet been tested prospectively. Other authors have advocated performing EAU in patients with a history of transient ischemic attacks, stroke, severe peripheral vascular disease, palpable calcifications in the ascending Ao, calcified aortic knob on chest X-ray, and in those older than 60 years (36). In a large-scale patient population undergoing cardiac surgery, Rosenberger et al. recently found that epiaortic ultrasonography to detect ascending aortic atheroma has a significant impact on surgical decision making in more than 4% of cardiac surgical patients, and might result in improved perioperative neurologic outcome (39).

Focal areas of moderate to severe atheromas, with thickness more than 3 mm, located in the surgical field, warrant a change in operative technique to avoid manipulation and disruption of these lesions (see Figs. 23.13 and 23.14). More aggressive management of severe extensive disease, especially protruding plaques, is more controversial because the changes in technique often involve deep hypothermic circulatory arrest and atherectomy or aortic replacement (see Fig. 23.38) (36).

Transesophageal echocardiography can also be used for detection and monitoring of complications associated with femoral or axillary arterial cannulation for surgical repair of aortic dissection (40). Malperfusion can occur in either femoral or axillary perfusion; the incidence was as high as 10.2% versus 3.4% in one series (40). Malperfusion is suspected when systemic hypotension occurs and TEE may show collapsed true lumen and perfusion of the false lumen. Long aortic cannulas in the aortic arch were also used during acute aortic dissection (41) (Fig. 13.4), and TEE was used to confirm adequate guidewire positioning in the true lumen during aortic dissection (Figs. 13.5 and 13.6).

Coronary Sinus Catheter

The technique for inserting the retrograde cardioplegia catheter from the internal jugular vein into the CS has been described using the Port-access system (Heartport Inc., Redwood City, California, U.S.) (see Fig. 20.10). Initially, TEE can been used to visualize the catheter entering the CS orifice followed by fluoroscopy to advance the wire and catheter to the correct depth. The longitudinal view of the CS is imaged in a lower esophageal level at 0° (Fig. 13.7). However, catheter guidance is best performed using the bicaval view at 100° (Fig. 13.8A) while locating the orifice of

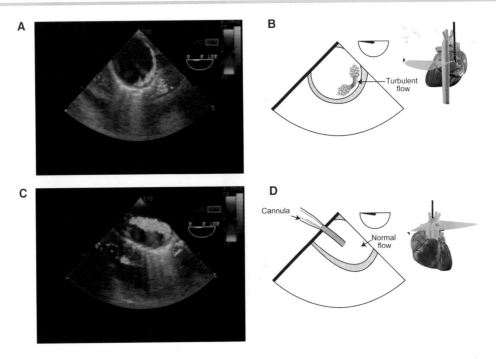

Figure 13.4 Aortic cannula. (A,B) Mid-esophageal descending aorta short-axis view shows malposition of an aortic cannula leading to turbulent flow and increased pressure in the arterial line. **(C,D)** Normal flow is restored and the arterial pressure reduced by pulling back the cannula. *Source*: Courtesy of Dr. Peter Sheridan.

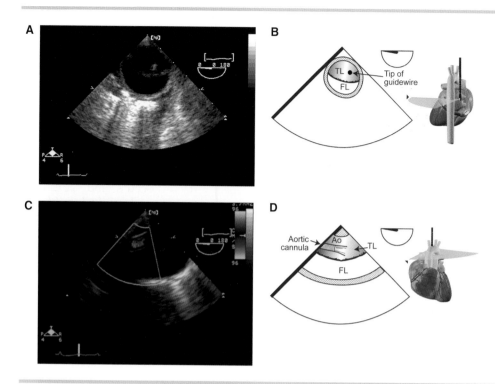

Figure 13.5 Aortic dissection. A 59-year-old woman with sudden onset of severe chest pain was transferred to the hospital where the diagnosis of aortic dissection was made. By CT scan the aortic dissection involved the proximal ascending, transverse and all the remaining distal aorta (Ao) down to the iliac arteries. (**A,B**) Mid-esophageal short-axis view of the descending thoracic Ao, showing the intimal flap separating the TL from the FL. (**C,D**) High-esophageal view of the transverse Ao: cannulation of the proximal aortic arch for cardiopulmonary bypass was performed under transesophageal echocardiography guidance to secure TL perfusion. *Abbreviations*: Ao, aorta, FL, false lumen; TL, true lumen. *Sources*: Adapted from Ref. 41 and courtesy of Drs. Nicolas Noiseux and Raymond Cartier.

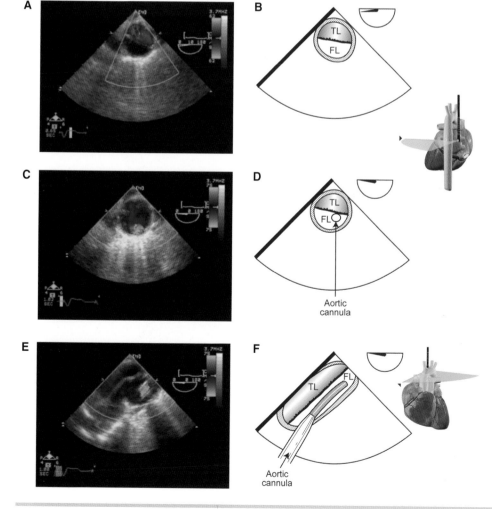

Figure 13.6 Aortic dissection. Aortic dissection involving the transverse and descending thoracic Ao. (**A,B**) Transverse view at 0° of the distal descending thoracic Ao with color Doppler imaging showing flow in the TL. (**C,D**) Proximal descending Ao and (**E,F**) distal transverse Ao: the aortic cannula is observed incorrectly positioned in the FL. *Abbreviations*: Ao, aorta; FL, false lumen; TL, true lumen.

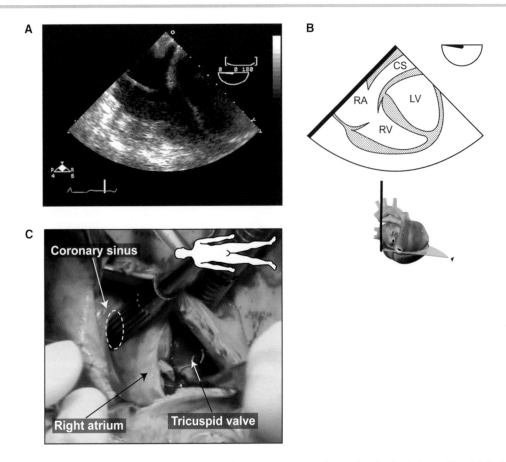

Figure 13.7   Coronary sinus visualization. (A,B) Lower esophageal view at 0° gives a longitudinal view of the CS in the left posterior atrioventricular groove near the gastroesophageal junction. **(C)** Intraoperative view of the CS in a 56-year-old woman before tricuspid annuloplasty through a right atriotomy. The suctioning device is in the CS. *Abbreviations*: CS, coronary sinus; LV, left ventricle; RA, right atrium; RV, right ventricle. *Source*: Photo C courtesy of Dr. Louis P. Perrault.

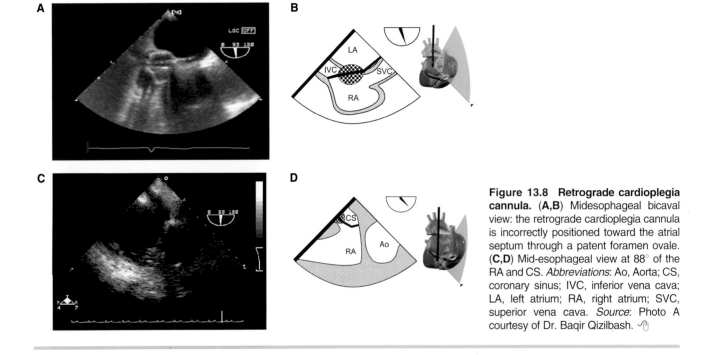

Figure 13.8   Retrograde cardioplegia cannula. (A,B) Midesophageal bicaval view: the retrograde cardioplegia cannula is incorrectly positioned toward the atrial septum through a patent foramen ovale. **(C,D)** Mid-esophageal view at 88° of the RA and CS. *Abbreviations*: Ao, Aorta; CS, coronary sinus; IVC, inferior vena cava; LA, left atrium; RA, right atrium; SVC, superior vena cava. *Source*: Photo A courtesy of Dr. Baqir Qizilbash.

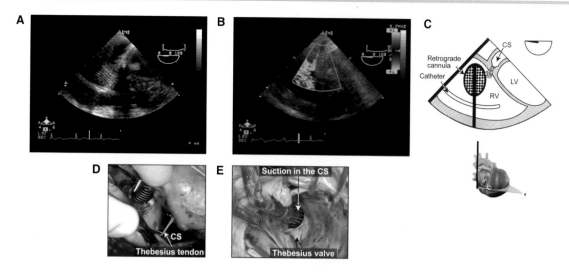

Figure 13.9 Thebesian valve. A reoperation on the mitral valve is planned for this 23-year-old man. (**A–C**) The retrograde cannula could not be inserted into the CS. This was due to an ostial stenosis of the CS, perhaps from a previous cannulation or a large Thebesian valve. The CS flow acceleration is demonstrated with color Doppler in these lower esophageal views. (**D,E**) Intraoperative aspect of two types of Thebesian valve at the ostium of the CS: (**D**) the first is a rudimentary small ligament and (**E**) the second a more developed valve. *Abbreviations*: CS, coronary sinus; LV, left ventricle; RV, right ventricle. *Source*: Photos D and E courtesy of Dr. Michel Pellerin.

the sinus from this plane: as the inferior vena cava (IVC) is visualized, the probe shaft is rotated toward the patient's left; the CS can be identified following its course in the left atrioventricular groove where it appears in cross section as a circular structure. A transgastric RV longitudinal view at 90° may also be used to visualize the CS (Fig. 13.8C). Simultaneous visualization of both SVC and CS is often facilitated by changing the viewing angle to 110° or more. The CS must be distinguished from the IVC, which is twice as broad in diameter, located to the right of the CS and leads to the liver (42).

Insertion of a CS catheter from the RA is often uncomplicated and its position easily confirmed by palpation and pressure tracing measurements. However, difficult insertion may be anticipated when ostial abnormalities, the thebesian valve and a small or stenotic sinus from previous procedures, are present (Fig. 13.9). In these circumstances, TEE can assist cannulation, and confirm and monitor adequate catheter placement (Fig. 13.10) (43). Coronary sinus injury leading to atrioventricular groove hematoma may result from high perfusion pressure, traumatic stylet guided catheter insertion, or laceration due to balloon overinflation during retrograde cardioplegia infusion and can be detected by TEE (44) (Fig. 13.11). Detailed discussion on catheter positioning in minimally invasive cardiac surgery is addressed in Chapter 20.

Vents, Venous, and Arterial Cannulation

Proper functioning of vents and the venous cannulation catheter during CPB is confirmed both by surgical palpation and on TEE by observing emptied right and left ventricular cavities (Fig. 13.12). Insertion of vent cannulas can be associated with immediate complications such as local trauma or hematomas mimicking masses (see Fig. 25.22) or late complications after removal with stenosis of the right upper pulmonary vein in aortic valve surgery (Fig. 13.13).

During double venous cannulation (Fig. 13.14), malposition of the IVC cannula in a suprahepatic vein impairs venous return to the CPB reservoir, and, when recognized, is easily corrected by repositioning the cannula under TEE guidance (Fig. 13.15). Repositioning of a venous cannula during femorofemoral CPB using TEE has also been described (24). Obstruction to IVC flow following removal of the cannula must be ruled out (Figs. 13.16 and 13.17). This would be associated with dilated IVC and reduced or absent hepatic venous flow.

The role of TEE and EAU imaging to position the aortic and femoral cannula has been discussed previously. While the frequency of intraoperative aortic dissection during cardiac surgery is infrequent at 0.16%, its mortality rises to 20% when discovered intraoperatively versus 50% for dissections diagnosed postoperatively. A rapid increase in aortic dimensions and/or a color change visually perceivable in the ascending or transverse Ao constitute a key to early diagnosis as well as a high degree of suspicion. Usually TEE can confirm the diagnosis of intraoperative aortic type A dissection, provided that the typical echocardiographic signs are present in the aortic segments accessible to TEE. An acute aortic type A dissection limited to the distal ascending Ao and/or proximal aortic arch (De-Bakey type II) can

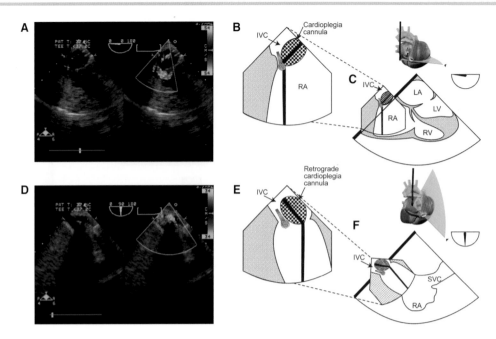

Figure 13.10 Retrograde cardioplegia cannula. Retrograde cardioplegia cannula malpositioned in the outlet of the IVC during cardiopulmonary bypass in a 64-year-old woman undergoing revascularization is shown in lower esophageal 0° (**A–C**) and 90° (**D–F**) views. *Abbreviations*: IVC, inferior vena cava; LA, left atrium; LV, left ventricle; RA, right atrium; RV, right ventricle; SVC, superior vena cava.

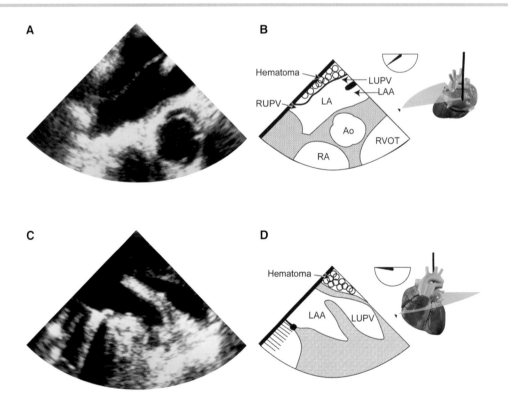

Figure 13.11 Coronary sinus hematoma. (A,B) Intraoperative mid-esophageal view: hematoma adjacent to the thin posterior wall of the LA and extending behind the RUPV in this mid-esophageal view. **(C,D)** Repeat TEE one hour later in the intensive care unit: the hematoma is now compressing the LUPV, near the LAA. *Abbreviations*: Ao, ascending aorta; LA, left atrium; LAA, left atrial appendage; LUPV, left upper pulmonary vein; RA, right atrium; RUPV, right upper pulmonary vein; RVOT, right ventricular outflow tract; TEE, transesophageal echocardiography. *Source*: Adapted from Ref. 44.

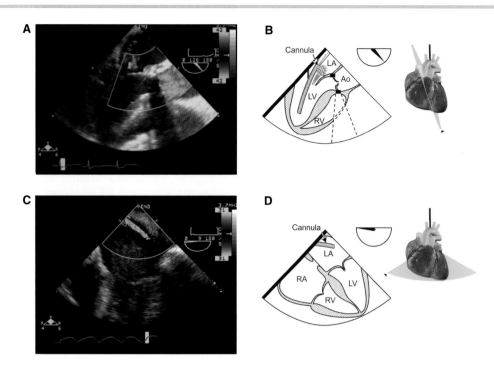

Figure 13.12 Left ventricular decompression cannula (vent). (A,B) 60-year-old man undergoing aortic valve replacement. Mid-esophageal long-axis view: a left ventricular decompression cannula is advanced through the left atrium (LA) and mitral valve (MV) from the right upper pulmonary vein. The vent causes incomplete closure of the MV, hence the presence of mitral regurgitation (MR) helps to confirm that the cannula is adequately positioned. **(C,D)** 51-year-old man operated on for aortic regurgitation secondary to aortic dissection. Mid-esophageal four-chamber view: the decompression cannula is malpositioned in the LA only and no MR is visible. *Abbreviations*: Ao, aorta; LA, left atrium; LV, left ventricle; ME, mid-esophageal; MR, mitral regurgitation; MV, mitral valve; RA, right atrium; RV, right ventricle.

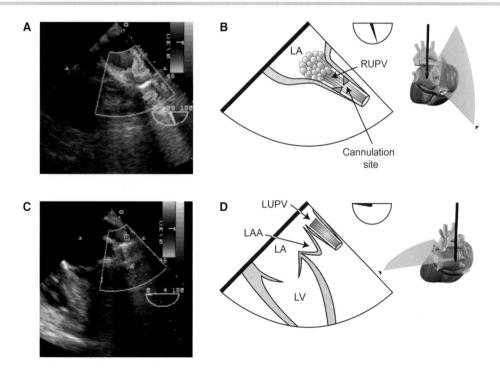

Figure 13.13 Vent complication. (A,B) Mid-esophageal modified bicaval view with color Doppler imaging shows RUPV stenosis after removal of the left atrial vent in a patient during a re-do aortic valve procedure. A peak systolic velocity of 120 cm/s is recorded with flow acceleration and aliasing in the RUPV in this modified bicaval view. **(C,D)** Mid-esophageal four-chamber view: in contrast, a velocity of 80 cm/s with no aliasing is found in the LUPV in this mid-esophageal four-chamber view. *Abbreviations*: LA, left atrium; LAA, left atrial appendage; LUPV, left upper pulmonary vein; LV, left ventricle; RUPV, right upper pulmonary vein.

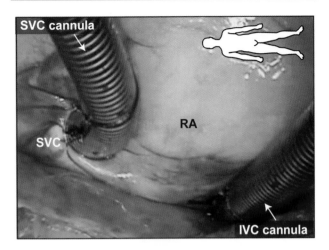

Figure 13.14 Venous cannulas. Position of both the SVC cannula inserted through the right atrial appendage and IVC cannula is shown. *Abbreviations*: IVC, inferior vena cava; RA, right atrium; SVC, superior vena cava. *Source*: Courtesy of Dr. Michel Pellerin.

be missed by TEE. Direct EAU scanning can overcome this limitation (45).

After CPB, TEE can detect aortic dissection involving the proximal aortic arch at the aortic cannulation site, which can extend distally (Fig. 13.18). Although the site of the initial intimal tear is most often located at the site of arterial cannulation, dissection can also originate distally from the trauma induced by the jet of blood from the aortic cannula to a fragile atherosclerotic Ao (46). The incidence of retrograde ilioaortic dissection may be as high as 3% with common femoral artery cannulation for standard CPB. However, a false-positive TEE diagnosis of dissection has been described with femoral CPB (see Fig. 20.16) (47). Layering of blood with crystalloid pump-prime produces a fluid interface simulating an intimal flap, with the stasis of aortic blood flow mimicking slow flow in a false lumen. This phenomenon may be present in up to 50% of femoral bypass cases and occurs as soon as 30 to 40 seconds after initiation of CPB. Retrograde arterial dissection may also result in retroperitoneal surgical dissection. This presents as an echo-free space under the liver and anterior to the kidneys (48) (Fig. 13.19).

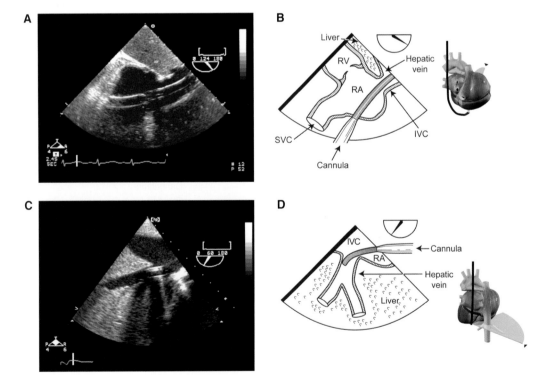

Figure 13.15 Venous cannula. (A,B) Deep transgastric longitudinal view at 120° through the RV shows the venous cannula correctly located in the IVC. **(C,D)** Transgastric IVC long-axis view at 0° shows the venous cannula incorrectly located in a hepatic vein. This explained the poor venous return to the cardiopulmonary bypass reservoir. *Abbreviations*: IVC, inferior vena cava; RA, right atrium; RV, right ventricle; SVC, superior vena cava.

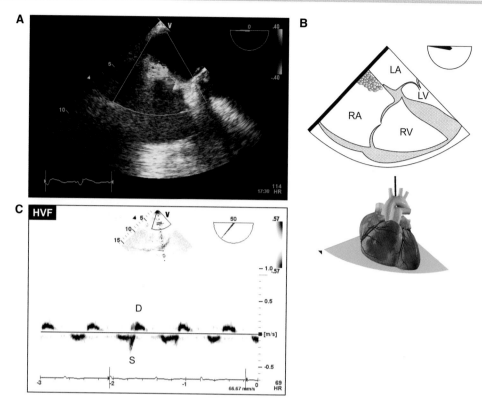

Figure 13.16 Partially occluded IVC. (A,B) Mid-esophageal RV color Doppler view in a patient after aortic valve replacement shows turbulent flow at the entrance of the IVC. This was secondary to a partial obstruction of the IVC at the site of cannulation. **(C)** There was significantly reduced HVF with systolic reversal. *Abbreviations*: D, peak diastolic HVF velocity; HVF, hepatic vein flow; IVC, inferior vena cava; LA, left atrium; LV, left ventricle; RA, right atrium; RV, right ventricle; S, peak systolic HVF velocity.

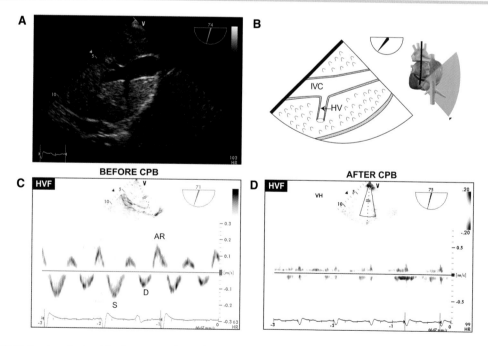

Figure 13.17 IVC occlusion during Fontan procedure. (A,B) Transgastric IVC long-axis view shows a dilated IVC following a Fontan procedure due to a partial occlusion at the level of the graft anastomosis to the IVC. **(C,D)** HVF is present before **(C)** and is almost absent after CPB **(D)**. *Abbreviations*: AR, peak atrial reversal HVF velocity; CPB, cardiopulmonary bypass; D, peak diastolic HVF velocity; HR, heart rate; HV, hepatic vein; HVF, hepatic venous flow; IVC, inferior vena cava; S, peak systolic HVF velocity.

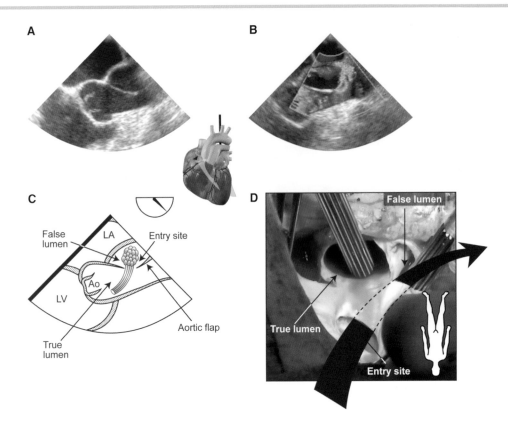

Figure 13.18   Aortic dissection. An aortic dissection involving the ascending Ao most likely from a tear in the posterior Ao at the site of previous aortic cannula insertion. (**A–C**) Mid-esophageal aortic valve long-axis views demonstrate an intimal flap extending to the sinotubular junction as well as flow from the true to the false lumen through an entry site. (**D**) Surgical findings showing the true lumen and the entry site. *Abbreviations*: Ao, aorta; LA, left atrium; LV, left ventricle. *Source*: Photo D courtesy of Dr. Michel Carrier.

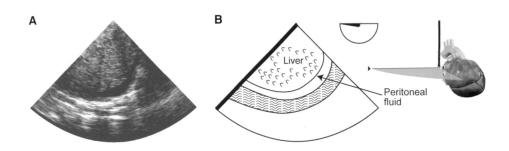

Figure 13.19   Peritoneal bleed. (A,B) Transgastric view shows a new echo-free space (blood) around the liver consistent with a new peritoneal bleeding from arterial dissection during the insertion of a femoral arterial cannula.

CARDIAC PHYSIOLOGY AND PROCEDURES BEFORE CPB

Controlled Ventilation

The hemodynamic effects of mechanical ventilation on the RV and LV function are complex and interrelated. They depend on the tidal volume, the amount of positive pressure, and the underlying baseline RV and LV function. The effects of positive-pressure ventilation (PPV) on the RV might be summarized as an increase in RV afterload relative to a reduced RV preload (49). The final result is a reduced RV stroke output resulting in decreased filling of the LV (Fig. 13.20) (50,51).

The contribution of increased RV outflow impedance to the adverse consequences of respiratory support has often been underestimated because it can be

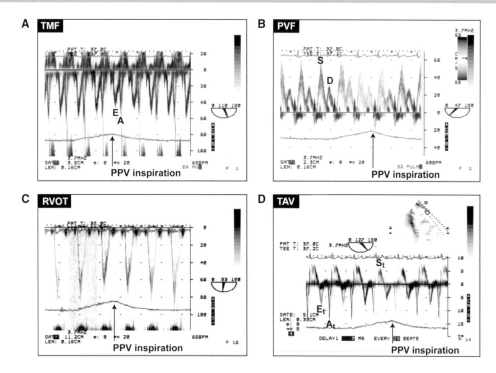

Figure 13.20 Ventilation and Doppler flow. The effect of PPV is shown on the Doppler (**A**) TMF, (**B**) PVF, (**C**) RVOT velocity and (**D**) TAV. Note the reduction in systolic velocities in all four Doppler signals with positive-pressure inspiration displayed with simultaneous respirograms. *Abbreviations*: A, peak late diastolic TMF velocity; At, peak late diastolic TAV; D, peak diastolic PVF velocity; E, peak early diastolic TMF velocity; Et, peak early diastolic TAV; PPV, positive-pressure ventilation; PVF, pulmonary venous flow; RVOT, right ventricular outflow tract; S, peak systolic PVF velocity; St, peak systolic TAV; TAV, tricuspid annular velocities; TMF, transmitral flow.

partly offset by increasing preload. In acute respiratory distress syndrome (ARDS) patients with adequate preload, intermittent PPV with a tidal volume of 8 mL/kg impaired RV systolic function by increasing RV afterload (49). Using TEE, lung inflation during PPV was shown to decrease pulmonary arterial flow velocity-time integral (VTI) from 14.2 ± 2.6 cm at end-expiration to 11.3 ± 2.1 cm at end-inspiration. This was followed (rather than preceded) by a decrease in tricuspid inflow VTI, thus confirming an increase in RV outflow impedance. This reduction in VTI occurred without concomitant decrease in RA or RV diastolic dimensions. However, an increased RV systolic dimensions was observed causing a drop in inspiratory RV ejection fraction consistent with impaired RV systolic function. In normovolemic patients, left atrial (LA) filling improved with increased LA dimensions, which indicates that blood might be squeezed from the capillary bed, as suggested by other authors (52).

Cyclical changes in RV outflow were greater in patients with partial collapse of the SVC during PPV. Patients with an SVC caval collapsibility index (defined as the difference between SVC maximal expiratory diameter and minimal inspiratory diameter over the maximal diameter) more than 60% had greater inspiratory decrease in RV outflow velocity (~70%) compared with patients with an index less than 30% (~30%) (50) (see Fig. 10.9). Thus, a specific preload limitation is added to the increase in outflow

impedance in these patients and results in suboptimal filling of the LV. The effect of PPV on RV afterload can also be demonstrated using a four-chamber view and measuring caval diameter changes (Fig. 13.21). Jet ventilation that uses a small tidal volume can improve oxygenation in certain patients and reduce the effect of PPV on RV function (see Fig. 30.15).

The negative impact of mechanical ventilation on the loading condition of both the RV and LV is worsened by the application of positive end-expiratory pressure (PEEP) that reduces preload through a decrease in systemic venous return and an increase in RV afterload (Fig. 13.22) (53). Lower levels of PEEP ($<8\,cmH_2O$) have minimal hemodynamic effects while higher levels ($\geq 16\,cmH_2O$) have been reported to cause concomitant reduction in RV and LV dimensions with displacement of the interventricular septum (IVS) toward the right (54). In contrast, following uncomplicated coronary artery bypass graft (CABG) surgery, the application of 20 cmH_2O of PEEP for 10 minutes resulted in increased RV diastolic area (27%) that coincided with a reduction of early mitral inflow E velocity of 25% and pulmonary artery flow velocity of 27% at end-expiration and 42% at end-inspiration (55). The increase in RV dimension is apparently the result of a greater impedance increase than the reduction of systemic venous return. The LV and RV function, as assessed by fractional area change (FAC) on TEE, was not affected by the application of PEEP. On the other

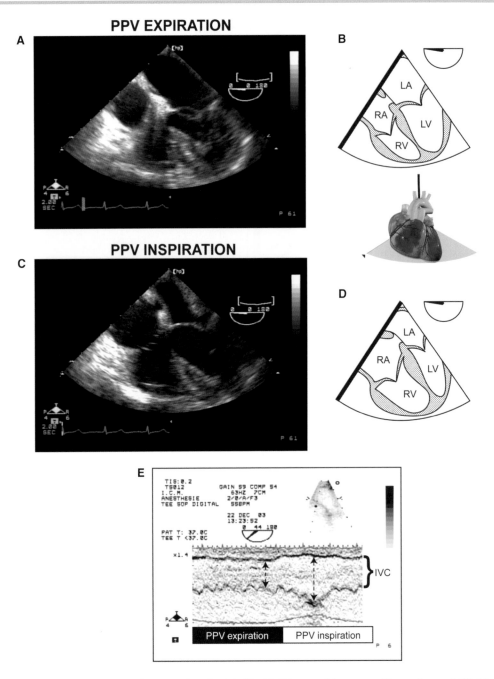

Figure 13.21   Effect of PPV. Aortic valve replacement is scheduled in this 59-year-old woman with previous mild RV dysfunction. (**A–D**) Use of PPV was associated with significant reduction in the diameter of the RA during expiration (**A,B**) compared with inspiration (**C,D**) in these mid-esophageal four-chamber views. (**E**) Changes in diameter of the IVC using M-mode at the junction of the RA occur with ventilation. Again note that during PPV-inspiration, the diameter of the IVC increases. *Abbreviations*: IVC, inferior vena cava; LA, left atrium; LV, left ventricle; PPV, positive-pressure ventilation; RA, right atrium; RV, right ventricle.

hand, open lung ventilation does not increase right ventricular outflow impedance following elective cardiac surgery even if the PEEP level was higher than conventional ventilation (56). In that study, open lung ventilation (recruitment maneuvers followed by low tidal volume and elevated level of PEEP) was used. Despite the use of high level of PEEP (14.4 cmH$_2$O $\pm$ 4 vs. 5 cmH$_2$O), open lung ventilation does not change right ventricular outflow impedance during expiration

and decreases right ventricular outflow impedance during inspiration. Recruitment maneuvers followed by elevated PEEP avoid atelectasis that decreases hypoxic pulmonary vasoconstriction in nonaerated lung areas and overdistention in aerated areas, explaining the fact that RV outflow impedance did not increase despite elevated level of PEEP (56).

The effect of PEEP (20 cmH$_2$O) on left atrial inflow assessed by pulmonary venous flow (PVF) decreased

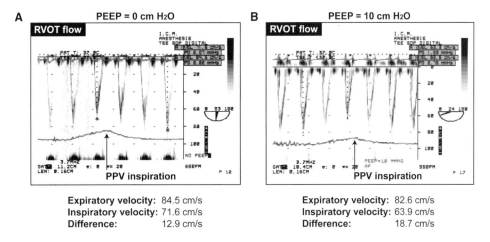

Expiratory velocity: 84.5 cm/s
Inspiratory velocity: 71.6 cm/s
Difference: 12.9 cm/s

Expiratory velocity: 82.6 cm/s
Inspiratory velocity: 63.9 cm/s
Difference: 18.7 cm/s

Figure 13.22 PEEP. The effect of 10 cmH$_2$O PEEP on RVOT velocities obtained from a deep transgastric view: absolute velocities values were reduced and the inspiratory to expiratory gradient increased. *Abbreviations*: PEEP, positive-end expiratory pressure; PPV, positive-pressure ventilation; RVOT, right ventricular outflow tract.

the systolic component, while the early diastolic component did not change (57). Consequently, baseline systolic predominance was changed to a slight diastolic predominance at a higher level of PEEP, perhaps reflecting diminished LA compliance secondary to high intrathoracic pressures. Thus, the LA pressure rises during systole when the mitral valve (MV) is closed and the decreased pulmonary vein to left atrial gradient results in reduced left atrial inflow. The LV with thicker walls is less influenced by high intrathoracic pressure. Variations in PVF have also been described with PPV and are more important in patients with pulmonary capillary wedge pressure (PCWP) less than 18 mmHg (58).

Anesthestic Drugs

A complete review of the hemodynamic effects of anesthetic agents is beyond the scope of this chapter, but we will briefly describe the hemodynamic effects of inhalation agents and intravenous anesthetics, as they may influence cardiac function and echocardiographic measurements. For a detailed discussion the reader is referred to Estafanous et al. (59).

Reduction in myocardial contractility, induced by the administration of volatile anesthetic agents, may not be detected with the conventional ventricular performance indices such as FAC and circumferential fiber shortening. The use of pressure-dimension indices such as the end-systolic elastance and preload recruitable stroke force are more sensitive to reductions in myocardial contractility, but their measurements are considerably more complex than the traditional indices of myocardial performance (60).

Inhalation Agents

All the inhalation anesthetics produce dose-related negative inotropic effects. Enflurane and halothane depress myocardial contractility to a similar extent

(61) but more severely than isoflurane, desflurane, and sevoflurane (62). A rapid increase in desflurane concentration may however stimulate the sympathetic nervous system inducing an increase in heart rate (HR) and temporarily mask its negative inotropic effect (63). Moreover, enflurane and halothane also induce an increase in LV filling pressure. Indices of contractility appear more sensitive to a given concentration of a volatile anesthetic in abnormal hearts than in normal hearts (64). Nitrous oxide has a weak direct myocardial depressant action that may be counterbalanced by sympathetic activation (65). Xenon is a noble gas with potent anesthetic and analgesic properties. In patients without cardiac diseases, xenon did not reduced contractility (66).

There is a lack of noninvasively derived data regarding the effects of potent volatile anesthetic agents on diastolic function. Using invasive measurements of diastolic function, halothane and enflurane seem to prolong the isovolumic relaxation period and increase chamber stiffness, while isoflurane, sevoflurane, and desflurane prolong the isovolumic relaxation period but without altering invasively measured myocardial chamber stiffness (59). Little data is available in the literature regarding the effect of nitrous oxide on diastolic function.

Studies in intact animals and humans have shown a decrease in systemic vascular resistance (SVR) in a dose-dependant fashion by isoflurane, enflurane, sevoflurane, and desflurane, while halothane has minimal direct effect (67). Potent inhalation anesthetics can also reduce preload through direct (vascular smooth muscle dilatation) and indirect (sympathetic nervous system) mechanisms. Nitrous oxide raises central venous pressure (CVP) by increasing both venous tone and SVR and by possibly decreasing LV contractility (65).

Finally, volatile anesthetics have been found to be cardioprotective in many studies of myocardial ischemia and reperfusion. In contrast, nitrous oxide appears to be detrimental. The mechanisms of cardioprotection are largely unknown, although potential mechanisms include favorable alteration of the determinants of myocardial oxygen supply and demand, preservation of high energy phosphates, modification of intracellular calcium handling, and activation of adenosine triphosphate-regulated potassium channels (68).

Intravenous Anesthetic Agents on Systolic Function

Opioids. Most evidence indicates that fentanyl produces little or no direct change in myocardial contractility and that opioids have depression-sparing actions when combined with a potent inhaled agent. Maintaining preload is essential to promote hemodynamic stability and preserve adequate cardiac function. Opioids can decrease preload through direct sympatholytic and vagotonic actions (69).

Benzodiazepines. Benzodiazepines by themselves produce only a mild decrease in myocardial contractility. Nevertheless, ventricular filling pressures can decrease after the induction of anesthesia with benzodiazepines, particularly during hypovolemia. The SVR may also decrease, resulting in lowering of systemic blood pressure by up to 20% (70,71).

Propofol. More often than not, propofol has been shown to be a direct myocardial depressant in animals and humans. Using arterial systolic blood pressure (SBP) and TEE LV short axis (SAX) measurements to evaluate the end-systolic pressure-volume relationship in humans, propofol has dose-dependent, negative inotropic properties (72). Furthermore, the negative inotropic properties of propofol are greater than those of equipotent doses of thiopental in both intensity and duration (Fig. 13.23). Milder sedative concentrations of propofol (0.65–2.6 µg/mL) produce significant vasodilatation but no direct negative inotropic effects (73). Venodilatation and reduction in preload, as well as dose-related arterial vasodilatation and afterload reduction, have been demonstrated to be important effects of propofol administration. These phenomena affect the systemic circulation to a greater degree than the pulmonary circulation.

Barbiturates. Myocardial contractility is decreased with barbiturates, through mechanisms involving calcium transport and its interaction with myofibrils. Its negative inotropic action is greater than that produced by benzodiazepines, etomidate, or ketamine, but probably not as large as the one produced by potent inhaled anesthetics (74).

Ketamine. Induction doses of ketamine increase HR, cardiac output (CO), pulmonary and systemic blood pressure, as well as pulmonary and SVR. Effects on pulmonary arterial pressure (Ppa) may be greater than on systemic arterial pressure. Higher doses can result in paradoxical effects, with predominant hemodynamic depression instead of stimulation (75).

Etomidate. Etomidate produces the fewest hemodynamic changes among the sedative-hypnotic agents. The inotropic effects of etomidate are mild. Dose-dependent decreases in sympathetic tone, venous return, preload, and cardiac contractility can occur with etomidate but are typically less obvious than with thiopenthal. Arterial blood pressure usually remains stable (76).

Effect of Intravenous Anesthetic Agents on Diastolic Function

Little data is available on the effect of intravenous anesthetic agents on diastolic function. Gare et al. (77) studied the effects of sedative doses of midazolam and propofol in patients with normal and mild diastolic dysfunction (relaxation abnormalities), using transthoracic mitral inflow pulsed wave (PW) Doppler and annular tissue Doppler imaging. Their results suggest that sedation with midazolam or propofol does not affect the indices of LV diastolic performance in the two groups.

Couture et al. studied the effect of induction of general anesthesia on biventricular diastolic filling pattern in patients with diastolic dysfunction undergoing coronary artery bypass grafting surgery (78). Using a diastolic function algorithm (79) they found that biventricular filling patterns are significantly altered after

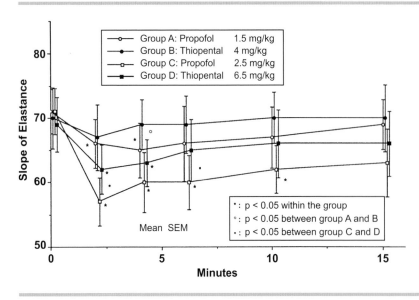

Figure 13.23 Elastance. Changes in left ventricular elastance (mmHg/ml) as a parameter of contractility after successive single-bolus intravenous injections of thiopental (4.0 and 6.5 mg/kg) and propofol (1.5 and 2.5 mg/kg) are shown. *Abbreviations*: SEM, standard error of the mean. *Source*: Reproduced with permission from Ref. 72.

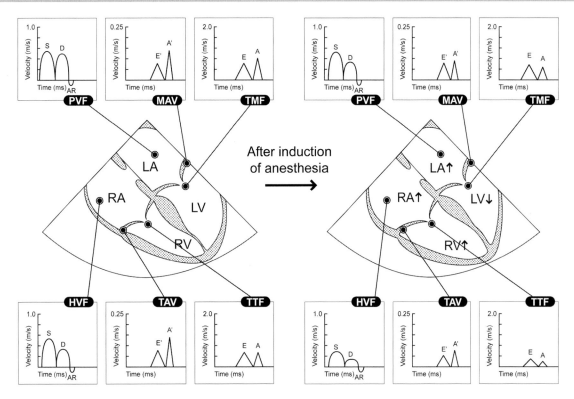

Figure 13.24 Effect of the induction of anesthesia on cardiac function. Summary of the changes in cardiac dimensions and bi-ventricular filling patterns after the induction of anesthesia is presented. Peak early (E) and peak late (A) diastolic flow velocities were measured for TMF and TTF. Peak S, D, and AR flow velocities were measured for velocity HVF and PVF. Peak early (E') and peak late (A') diastolic velocities were measured for MAV and TAV. *Abbreviations*: AR, peak atrial reversal velocity; D, peak diastolic velocity; HVF, hepatic venous flow; LA, left atrium; LV, left ventricle; MAV, mitral annulus velocity; PVF, pulmonary venous flow; RA, right atrium; RV, right ventricle; S, peak systolic velocity; TAV, tricuspid annulus velocity; TMF, transmitral flow; TTF, transtricuspid flow. *Source*: With permission from Ref. 78.

induction of general anesthesia, as reflected by a decrease in left ventricular dimension, an increase in bi-atrial diameters and right ventricular dimensions, and a decrease in Doppler velocities with a greater decrease in atrial components. These changes can be explained to some extent by a reduction in venous return resulting in a decrease in LV end-diastolic area, alterations in left and right atrial function, and increase in pulmonary vascular resistance with PPV. Although an improvement in LV diastolic function score after the anesthetic induction was noted, it was difficult to dissociate the effect of diastolic function from the loading conditions. Consequently, the real incidence and severity of LV diastolic dysfunction may be underestimated if assessed after the induction of anesthesia (Fig. 13.24).

Nonanesthetic Drugs Commonly Used During Cardiac Surgery

Positive Inotropic Drugs

Endogenous Catecholamines

Epinephrine. Epinephrine is a potent α- and β-adrenoreceptor agonist. In the heart, epinephrine is a potent stimulant of myocardial inotropy, has significant arrhythmogenic potential, and increases stroke volume

(SV), coronary blood flow, and HR. β-Agonist effects predominate at low doses of 0.01 to 0.03 μg/kg/min and α-agonist effects causing vasoconstriction at higher doses.

Norepinephrine. Norepinephrine, predominantly, stimulates α-adreno receptors although concurrent stimulation of the myocardial β_1-adrenoreceptors occurs to a lesser extent. Thus, blood pressure rises as a result of increased SVR; this in turn tends to decrease the HR because of vagal reflex pathways that overcome the direct stimulation of myocardial β_1-adrenergic receptors. Norepinephrine is considered a positive inotropic agent particularly at low doses where the β_1 effects predominate over the peripheral α effect. The overall cardiac effects of norepinephrine include increased SV, coronary blood flow, and arrhythmogenic potential while there is minimal change in CO and a potential decrease in HR.

Dopamine. The cardiovascular effects of dopamine are dose dependent. At low doses (1–3 μg/kg/min), dopamine predominantly stimulates dopaminergic receptors. At moderate doses (3–10 μg/kg/min), dopamine directly stimulates β_1- and β_2-receptors, explaining its positive inotropic effects. At high intravenous doses (10–15 μg/kg/min), α-stimulation predominates and causes vasoconstriction.

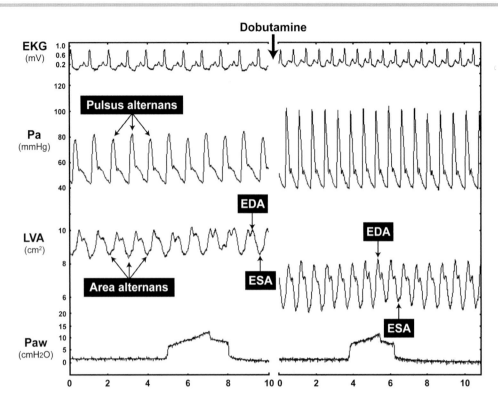

Figure 13.25 Dobutamine. Effect of dobutamine on hemodynamic and echocardiographic parameters. Dobutamine induces an increase in heart rate and Pa, a decrease EDA and ESA with a significant increase in SA (SA = EDA − ESA) and in FAC (FAC = EDA − ESA/EDA). Note that pulsus alternans and area alternans disappear after the use of dobutamine. The continuous LVA tracing was obtained by automated border detection through acoustic quantification. *Abbreviations*: EDA, end-diastolic area; EKG, electrocardiogram; ESA, end-systolic area; FAC, fractional area change; LVA, left ventricular area; Pa, arterial pressure; Paw, airway pressure; SA stroke area. *Source*: Courtesy of Dr. Michael R. Pinsky.

Synthetic Catecholamines

Dobutamine.   Dobutamine is primarily a direct β-agonist, relatively selective for the β$_1$-receptor subtype and also has peripheral α$_1$-receptor effects. In clinical doses (2–15 μg/kg/min), it is a positive inotrope, with modest increase in HR and minimal change in SVR due to offsetting peripheral α and β$_2$ effects. Dobutamine administration in patients with RV failure also has positive inotropic effects. After CPB in patients undergoing CABG, dobutamine improves LV performance by a dose-dependent increase in HR, as SV decreased with higher dobutamine doses (80). This was indicated by an increase in cardiac index (CI), decreased PCWP, decreased end-diastolic (EDA) and end-systolic areas (ESA) (Fig. 13.25), and increased FAC as seen by TEE.

A low dose of dobutamine has also been used intraoperatively to predict improvement in regional myocardial function after CABG (81). Indeed, using TEE to assess regional wall motion, a positive response to low-dose dobutamine (5 μg/kg/min) before CPB could predict improved regional contractility with a positive predictive value of 0.88 early after weaning from CPB and a value of 0.94 30 minutes after the administration of protamine. On the other side, the lack of improvement with dobutamine was less predictive. The same group of investigators (82) later reported a positive predictive value of 0.81 to predict improved regional contractility at one year. Again, regional contractility evolution could not be predicted in the case of failure to improve with low-dose dobutamine before revascularization with a negative predictive value of 0.34.

Phosphodiesterase Inhibitors

Phosphodiesterase inhibitors prevent the breakdown of cyclic adenosine monophosphate (AMP), prolonging its effectiveness and augmenting its physiologic response. In addition to positive inotropic properties, phosphodiesterase inhibitors cause vasodilatation. The bypiridines (formerly amrinone) and milrinone are two drugs of this class commonly used during cardiac surgery. In cardiac surgical patients, a milrinone-loading dose of 50 μg/kg followed by a continuous infusion of 0.5 μg/kg/min, resulted in a plasma concentration in excess of 100 ng/mL, producing a substantial hemodynamic effect (83).

Milrinone administered after separation from CPB improves LV function as measured by an increase in CI and SVI, decrease in SVR and minimal change in HR, mean arterial pressure (MAP), PCWP, and CVP as well as EDA measured by TEE (84).

Velocity of circumferential shortening corrected for HR, an index of cardiac performance not affected by preload, significantly increased (84). Tissue Doppler indices of left and right ventricular function are also improved by milrinone (85). Amrinone and milrinone were found to have similar hemodynamic effects in patients undergoing elective cardiac surgery (86).

Milrinone also improves diastolic parameters in patients with heart failure, reducing diastolic pressure at any given volume while elevating the maximum rate of rise of LV pressure (18%) and decreasing the mean aortic pressure. The peak LV-filling rate increased by 42% and the PCWP decreased (87). In cardiac surgery, CPB is associated with a 20% decrease in LV compliance as measured by change in left ventricular end-diastolic area (LVEDA) in relation to the left atrial pressure (LAP). Administration of milrinone after CPB was associated with a partial return of LV compliance to pre-CPB values (88). However, in patients with preoperative diastolic dysfunction, milrinone did not improve post-operative filling properties (85) nor at six-month follow-up (89) (Fig. 13.26).

Phosphodiesterase inhibitors can also improve RV function and reduce RV afterload after cardiac surgery. The administration of amrinone in the post-operative period improves RV contractility, as reflected by an increase in end-systolic elastance obtained by TEE (90).

Despite the favorable effects on biventricular function, administration of phosphodiesterase inhibitors may cause a decrease in preload and afterload, which could require substantial volume loading (guided by TEE) and administration of vasoactive agents like phenylephrine, norepinephrine, and dopamine. Administration of milrinone through inhalation has been proposed as an alternative to avoid systemic hypotension (91).

Other Vasoactive Agents

Levosimendan. Levosimendan is a new inodilator that exerts its inotropic effect by interacting with troponin C (the binding protein for calcium) to enhance the calcium sensitivity of cardiac cardiomyocytes and induces peripheral and coronary vasodilation by opening ATP-sensitive channels. In addition to its inotropic effects, levosimendan exerts a direct positive lusitropic effect in patients with left ventricular hypertrophy. Jörgensen et al. showed that levosimendan shortens the isovolumic relaxation time and improved LV filling early after aortic valve replacement, while the loading conditions and HR were kept constant (92). The mechanism for the positive lusitropic effects can be attributed to phosphodiesterase III inhibition at higher concentration (93).

Phenylephrine. Phenylephrine, an α_1-adrenergic agonist, is frequently administered to increase arterial pressure during anesthesia. In patients with coronary artery disease, an intravenous bolus may cause a transient increase in the LV wall stress with an impairment of LV global function, as suggested by the observed decrease in FAC (Fig. 13.27) and velocity

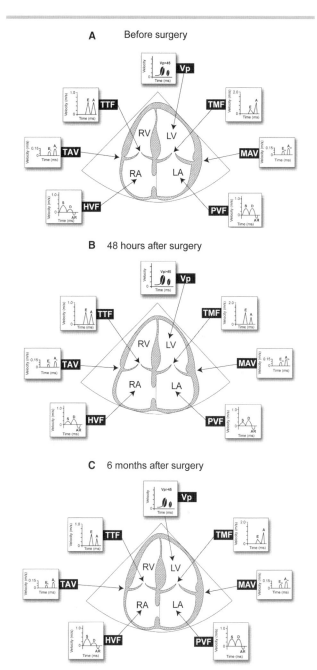

Figure 13.26 Milrinone and diastolic function. Effect of milrinone on cardiac dimensions and diastolic function Doppler profiles using an apical four-chamber view from trans-thoracic echocardiography. (**A**) Baseline before surgery. (**B**) Changes at 48 hours after coronary revascularization: increase in both left and right atrial size is observed. This is associated with deterioration in both left and right ventricular diastolic parameters. (**C**) Changes at six months after surgery: no significant difference is seen compared with the preoperative echocardiographic parameters. No difference was observed between the control and the milrinone group. *Abbreviations*: A, peak late diastolic velocity; Am, peak late diastolic MAV; AR, peak atrial reversal velocity; At, peak late diastolic TAV; D, peak diastolic velocity; HVF, hepatic venous flow; LA, left atrium; LV, left ventricle; MAV, mitral annular velocities; PVF, pulmonary venous flow; RA, right atrium; RV, right ventricle; S, peak systolic velocity; TAV, tricuspid annular velocity; TMF, transmitral flow; TTF, trans-tricuspid flow; Vp, velocity of propagation. *Source*: With permission from Ref. 89.

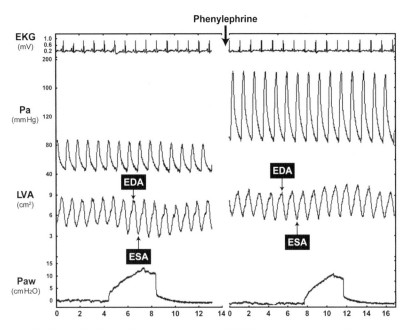

Figure 13.27 Phenylephrine. Effect of phenylephrine on hemodynamic and echocardiographic parameters. Phenylephrine did not change heart rate, induced an increase in Pa, EDA and ESA with no significant change in SA (SA = EDA − ESA) and in FAC (FAC = EDA − ESA/EDA). The continuous LVA tracing was obtained by automated border detection through acoustic quantification. *Abbreviations*: EDA, end-diastolic area; EKG, electrocardiogram; ESA, end-systolic area; FAC, fractional area change; LVA, left ventricular area; Pa, arterial pressure; Paw, airway pressure; SA, stroke area. *Source*: Courtesy of Dr. Michael R. Pinsky.

of circumferential shortening. As these indices of LV global function are afterload dependent, the impairment of LV function with phenylephrine most likely reflects the increase in LV wall stress rather than altered intrinsic myocardial contractility.

Phenylephrine given to patients with valvular AS did not exhibit any negative effect on ventricular performance, as ventricular afterload in this group of patients is mainly dependent on the pressure gradient across the aortic valve (AoV) rather than on the SVR (94).

Internal Mammary Dissection

During this period, TEE may be used to monitor the global and segmental ventricular functions (see Chapters 9 and 10) and to detect the occurrence of pneumothorax and hemothorax.

CARDIAC PHYSIOLOGY AND PROCEDURES DURING CPB

Hypothermia, Hemodilution, and Nonpulsatile Flow

The period on CPB can indirectly affect cardiac physiology through general effects including hypothermia, hemodilution, and nonpulsatile flow.

The adverse effects of hypothermia on myocardial performance are illustrated by studies demonstrating a decreased incidence of low-output syndrome and lower cardiac isoenzyme fractions elevation in the group kept warm (95).

To decrease viscosity and increase tissue perfusion, hemodilution is used with CPB, particularly during hypothermia. In patients with a normal heart, acute normovolemic hemodilution to 80 g/L of hemoglobin caused a decrease in SVR and an increase in CO pro-

portional to the hemodilution, whereas systemic pressure and HR remained unchanged (96). Using TEE, they also observed that the FAC increased from 44 ± 7% to 60 ± 9% as a result of increased LVEDA and reduced left ventricular end systolic area (LVESA) while diastolic function was unchanged.

Finally, although organ perfusion seems better maintained with pulsatile than nonpulsatile perfusion, in fact little is known about its real effect on cardiac function.

Myocardial Perfusion and Cardioplegia

For a detailed review of myocardial intraoperative perfusion echocardiography, the reader is referred to a comprehensive review by Aronson and Wiencek (97). One application of contrast echocardiography is the evaluation of cardioplegia delivery. Homogenous delivery of cardioplegia is an important component of myocardial protection. Poorly protected myocardial segments may have decreased contractility following ischemia. Cardioplegic solutions can be delivered via the aortic root (antegrade) or through the CS (retrograde).

Although coronary stenosis may impede the uniform distribution of cardioplegic solutions, myocardial protection may also be impaired by noncoronary causes. For instance, antegrade cardioplegia administered through the aortic root may be incompletely delivered to the coronary arteries during transient aortic regurgitation (AR) inadvertently induced by aortic cross-clamping (Fig. 13.28). Using intraoperative contrast TEE, in patients with a normal AoV, antegrade administration of cardioplegia was associated with AR in 25% of the cases (98). Significant AR during antegrade cardioplegia distends the heart and is easily identified by the surgeon. Gentle cardiac

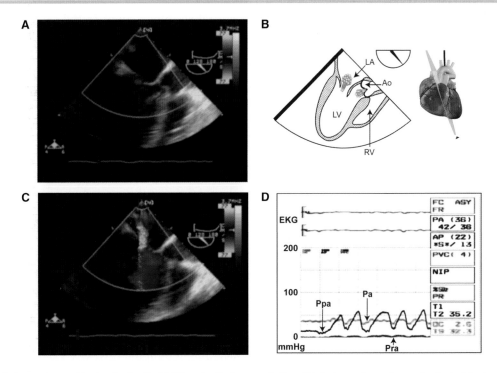

Figure 13.28 Antegrade cardioplegia. Aortic (**A,B**) and mitral regurgitation (**C**) during antegrade cardioplegia infusion in a 75-year-old woman undergoing revascularization is shown in these mid-esophageal long-axis views. (**D**) New waves were seen on the Ppa tracing secondary to mitral regurgitation. This confirms that the LV vent is well positioned. *Abbreviations*: Ao, aorta; EKG, electrocardiogram; LA, left atrium; LV, left ventricle; Pa, arterial pressure; Ppa, pulmonary artery pressure; Pra, right atrial pressure; RV, right ventricle.

compression can be performed to avoid ventricular overdistension and myocardial ischemia. The delivery of cardioplegia as assessed by myocardial opacification with concomitant contrast injection was decreased in patients with severe AR compared with patients without AR (98). Regurgitation of cardioplegic solution into the LV may also lead to LV dilatation and mitral regurgitation (MR) easily diagnosed with TEE and the pulmonary artery catheter (Fig. 13.28).

Because antegrade delivery of cardioplegia may result in inhomogeneous perfusion of myocardium in patients with occluded or severely stenotic coronary arteries, retrograde cardioplegia via the CS has been proposed to provide better myocardial protection. Using myocardial contrast TEE in patients with significant coronary artery disease and good collateral circulation to the LV, warm antegrade cardioplegia was found to provide better LV myocardial perfusion than retrograde cardioplegia (99). Several explanations are proposed: (*i*) retrograde perfusion may provide reduced perfusion because the cardioplegia catheter may be positioned too distally, causing the occlusion of veins that drain into the distal portion of the CS, especially the middle and small cardiac veins; (*ii*) veins draining in the CS may have a uni- or bicuspid valve at their origin, impeding retrograde progression of the cardioplegic solution; (*iii*) retrograde delivery may be limited by the presence of widespread venovenous anastomoses. Shunting of retrograde perfusion into both LV and RV cavities

via the thebesian channels could be visualized (99). Right ventricular perfusion was poor with both techniques before coronary revascularization (25% vs. 7% of visualized segments for antegrade vs. retrograde cardioplegia), a finding that was confirmed by other authors (100).

Reduced RV perfusion with antegrade delivery may be explained by the lack of collateral circulation in patients with occluded or severely stenotic right coronary artery (RCA). Cardioplegic perfusion of the right coronary bypass graft early after cardioplegic arrest may improve RV protection. Evaluation of myocardial perfusion would allow surgeons to assess both the patency of bypass grafts and the regional distribution of myocardial flow subserved by each graft. Using TEE and sonicated Renografin-76 injected in the aortic root after the completion of CABG, Aronson et al. (101) found that areas with perfusion defects after revascularization but before separation from CPB correlated with regional wall motion abnormalities after separation from CPB.

Spontaneous Echo Contrast

At the beginning of CPB, intracardiac blood flow decreases and spontaneous echo contrast may be observed, particularly in the LA, even in normal hearts. The significance of spontaneous echo contrast in pathologic hearts has been discussed in previous chapters (see Chapter 11 and Fig. 25.25).

CHANGES IN CARDIAC PHYSIOLOGY DURING WEANING FROM CPB

The termination of CPB presents a challenging task to the anesthesiologist. The myocardium is often compromised by acute dysfunction from the residual effects of cardioplegia, iatrogenic ischemia, and hyperkalemia superimposed on chronic abnormalities in ventricular performance. Although it is usually not critical to successful weaning from CPB, TEE monitoring has several advantages over conventional hemodynamic monitoring during this period.

Assessment of Regional Left Ventricular Function

The reader is referred to Chapter 9 for a more detailed discussion on the value and limitations of myocardial ischemia monitoring with TEE. Transesophageal echocardiography can detect myocardial ischemia more reliably than electrocardiography in cardiac surgery. Importantly, there is a correlation between ischemic episodes detected by TEE and adverse outcomes in cardiac surgery. In patients having elective coronary revascularization, 33% of patients with postbypass wall-motion abnormalities had a myocardial infarction compared with none in patients without wall motion abnormalities (102). Myocardial infarction occurs five times more often in patients displaying ischemia on electrocardiogram (EKG) and TEE compared with patients without ischemia (103).

However, the main interest of intraoperative TEE is focused on the period after reperfusion (104,105). Detection of persistent systolic wall motion abnormalities is associated with postoperative cardiac systolic wall motion abnormalities, more myocardial necrosis as evidenced by higher elevation of cardiac enzyme levels, and more subsequent clinical events such as pulmonary edema and atrial fibrillation (106). Thus, persistent regional wall motion abnormalities in revascularized areas after reperfusion should lead the surgeon to reassess the adequacy of the coronary bypass graft. Indeed, Swaminathan et al. (107) found that deterioration of regional wall motion immediately after coronary artery bypass graft surgery is associated with a doubling of major adverse cardiac events (death, myocardial infarction, or myocardial revascularization) up to two years after the procedure.

Assessment of Global Left Ventricular Function

In patients difficult to wean from CPB, TEE is useful to determine the etiology of hemodynamic instability, to monitor cardiac function while therapy is initiated, and to assess global and regional LV function after termination of CPB.

Intraoperatively, global LV function is most frequently assessed by estimating the FAC of the LV (see Chapter 5). This measurement is readily obtained by imaging the heart in the transgastric SAX view at the mid-papillary level of the LV. The FAC overestimates LV function if regional wall motion abnormalities exist at the base or apex of the LV, because they are not taken into account in the calculation. Moreover, the measurement of FAC is a load-dependent index of LV performance (108) and loading conditions must be considered in its interpretation. The end-systolic pressure-volume relationship is a relatively load-independent measure of LV contractility (termed elastance) that can be measured using both continuous TEE-automated border detection and femoral arterial pressure measurements. This index has been shown to decrease after CPB (109) (Fig. 13.29). Even if the end-systolic pressure-volume relationship may appear to be a better parameter of LV function, the FAC can still be used to guide clinical decision making. For example, in an unstable patient with hyperdynamic LV function and a small LVEDA, hypovolemia is the most likely cause of hemodynamic compromise. On the other hand, if the FAC is decreased with increased LVEDA, the most likely cause of instability is decreased LV contractility, suggesting that inotropic therapy would be helpful.

The circumferential velocity of shortening is another index of contractility that incorporates a time-related element and seems to be less preload-dependent than the FAC (see Chapter 10). Its value in normal individuals is 1.09 ± 0.3 circumferences per second (110).

Preload Assessment

Preload is an important determinant of cardiac function, which is traditionally measured in clinical settings by the PCWP as an estimate of left ventricular end-diastolic pressure (LVEDP). The relationship between LVEDP and LV diastolic volume is altered by several variables, including myocardial ischemia, afterload reduction, the use of vasopressors, and ventricular interaction.

Preload can be assessed by TEE through direct measurement of cavity dimensions as an estimate of left ventricular end-diastolic volume (LVEDV). Left ventricular end-diastolic area more accurately reflects LV preload than PCWP (111). It is measured from the SAX transgastric view at the mid-papillary muscle. A LVEDA of ≤ 5.5 cm^2/m^2 reflects hypovolemia, but can also be present in the hyperdynamic heart. In severe hypovolemia, near-obliteration of the LV cavity in systole usually accompanies the decrease in LVEDA (see Chapter 10). In a cardiac surgical group, there is no threshold of LVEDA below which a large proportion of patients increase their CO after volume administration, with the responders being unfortunately distributed over a wide range of LVEDA (112). The analysis of mitral inflow Doppler filling pattern may suggest the patient's location on the diastolic pressure-volume relationship (see Fig. 10.48) and predict the improvement in CO after intravascular fluid challenge in patients undergoing CABG (113).

Measuring volume responsiveness seems to be an interesting concept to optimize preload. Fluid responsiveness means that a significant volume expansion should induce a significant increase in CO, reflecting the fact that the heart is on the steep

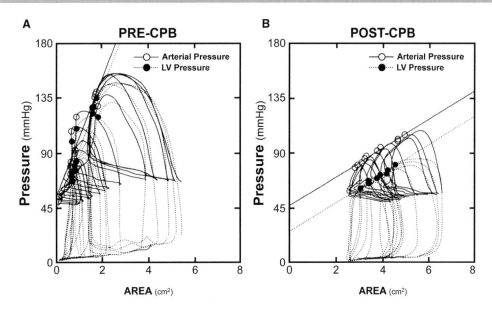

Figure 13.29 **Pressure-area loops.** Simultaneous arterial pressure-area loops (solid lines) and LV pressure-area loops (dashed lines) before (**A**) and after (**B**) CPB. The LV pressure end-systolic elastance (E'es) decreased from 49 to12 mmHg/cm^2 with similar change in arterial E'es from 50 to12 mmHg/cm^2. The LV area is used to estimate LV volume. *Abbreviations*: CPB, cardiopulmonary bypass; LV, left ventricle. *Source*: Reproduced with permission from Ref. 109.

part of the Frank-Starling curve (114). Echocardiographic parameters can be related to respiratory variations in the vena cava diameters and respiratory variations in the left ventricular SV.

Respiratory variations in the vena cava diameters can be used to predict preload responsiveness. The IVC ends at the floor of the RA, just after crossing the diaphragm. It carries about 80% of the venous return to the RA. Its route is intra-abdominal and is subject to intra-abdominal pressure. It can be visualized in mechanically ventilated patients using a transthoracic subxiphoid approach (see Fig. 6.5). The maximal diameter of the vessel is observed during inflation and the minimal during expiration. In mechanically ventilated patients, the plot of IVC diameter has two portions, the first steep portion, where any slight increase in CVP induces a marked increase in IVC diameter, reflects a compliant vessel with a preload reserve and the second flat portion, where even a marked increase in CVP is unable to dilate the vessel further, reflects a poorly compliant vessel without preload reserve (114). In mechanically septic patients, the respiratory variations in IVC diameter can be used to predict fluid responsiveness (115). The distensibility index of the IVC (dIVC) was calculated as the ratio of IVC diameter change (D_{max} at end-inspiration minus D_{min} at end-expiration) over the D_{min}, expressed as a percentage. Patients were separated into responders (increase in CI > 15%) and nonresponders (increase in CI < 15%). Using a threshold dIVC of 18% responders and nonresponders were discriminated with 90% sensitivity and 90% specificity (114). These respiratory variations were

studied in patients with normal intra-abdominal pressure.

On the other hand, the SVC ends at the top of the RA and its route is purely intrathoracic. It carries about 20% of the venous return to the RA. It can be visualized by TEE. Cyclic increase in intrathoracic pressure can induce partial or complete collapse of the vessel. Akin to the distensibility index of the IVC, the SVC collapsibility index is calculated as the ratio of SVC diameter change (D_{max} at end-expiration minus D_{min} at end-inspiration) over D_{max}. Patients with an SVC caval collapsibility index above 36% predicted an increase in CI after volume expansion of more than 11%, with a specificity of 100% and a sensitivity of 90% (114).

Pulse pressure variations can be used in clinical practice to predict fluid responsiveness. Because pulse pressure is directly dependent on left ventricular (LV) stroke volume, LV stroke volume variations can also be used to predict fluid responsiveness. Animal study suggests correlation between amplitude of the variation of the VTI of the aortic flow and hypovolemia (116). Change in descending aortic blood velocity, as an estimation of SV, can also be monitored using esophageal Doppler. A threshold of 17% discriminates responders and nonresponders with a sensitivity of 83% and a specificity of 76% (117). Feissel et al. (118) assessed the respiratory variations in maximal velocity of the aortic flow in patients with septic shock. They found that respiratory changes in maximal velocity were a good predictor of fluid responsiveness (a threshold of 12% discriminates responders and nonresponders with a sensitivity of 100% and a specificity of 89%) (see Chapter 30).

Left atrial pressure can also be inferred from the PVF pattern as measured by PW Doppler examination. In normal hearts, the PVF has a systolic and diastolic forward phase followed by an atrial reversal phase corresponding to the atrial contraction (see Fig. 4.25). When LAP is less than 15 mmHg, the PVF shows systolic flow predominance and elevation of LAP more than 15 mmHg results in diastolic flow predominance. The ratio of systolic to total PVF VTI is negatively correlated with LAP (119). However, PVF pattern is also modified by other factors, including age, HR, CO, LV systolic and diastolic function, and LA function. Other studies have found a correlation between the atrial reversal velocity (120) or the relative duration of the mitral inflow and the PVF A-wave and the LVEDP (121).

Mitral inflow pattern is not only affected by preload but also by the state of LV relaxation, compliance, and systolic function as well as LA compliance (122). There are significant correlations between PCWP (<10 mmHg) and the mitral deceleration time ($\geq$150 ms) or slope in patients with decreased LV systolic function (EF < 35%) undergoing CABG with sensitivity (93.3%), specificity (100%), and positive predictive value (100%) (123). Mitral E velocity, corrected for the influence of left ventricular relaxation relates also well to mean PCWP and may be used to estimate LV filling pressure (124). An E/e (or E/E', E/E_m, E/E_a) ratio >10 detected a mean PCWP >15 mmHg, with a sensitivity of 97% and specificity of 78%.

Finally, the PCWP can be estimated by observing the behavior of the atrial septal motion during PPV. At normal levels of preload, the increase in right-sided venous return relative to that on the left side with passive mechanical expiration will cause a midsystolic reversal in the septal convexity toward the left. The presence of expiratory midsystolic reversal is associated with a PCWP less than 15 mmHg with a positive predictive value of 0.97. When mid-systolic reversal is present during all ventilatory phases, the PCWP is probably less than 10 mmHg (positive predictive value = 0.85) (125) (see Fig. 10.7). These findings should, however, be interpreted with caution in patients displaying severe mitral or tricuspid regurgitation. In addition as discussed in Chapter 10, end-diastolic area and filling pressures per se are not necessarily indicative of fluid responsiveness (see Fig. 10.47).

Assessment of Right Ventricular Function

Assessment of the RV function is reviewed in Chapter 10 (51). Right ventricular dysfunction may present the following features on TEE examination: right atrial and ventricular dilatation, decreased tricuspid annular longitudinal motion, regional wall motion abnormalities, shift of the atrial and the ventricular septum toward the left, tricuspid regurgitation, and plethora of the IVC. In addition, on hepatic venous flow PW Doppler interrogation, increased atrial reversal velocity can be present in mild RV dysfunction, while systolic attenuation or reversal will be observed in more severe cases (see Fig. 10.45).

Acute RV failure after cardiac surgery may result from pulmonary embolism, RV infarction, poor RV preservation by cardioplegia during CPB, air embolism to the RCA, significant pulmonary hypertension, or RV dysfunction secondary to LV dysfunction.

The diagnosis of RV dysfunction before (126,127) or after (128) CPB has prognostic and therapeutic implications (129). Although not systematically assessed in cardiac surgical patients, RV dysfunction is associated with higher mortality in patients with hypotension despite inotropic therapy. Hospital mortality is as high as 86% compared with 30% to 40% for patients with moderately impaired or normal RV function with severe LV systolic dysfunction and only 15% for those with normal RV and LV systolic function (128). The presence of pre-CPB RV dysfunction defined as an RV FAC less than 35% predicted a poor outcome after CABG in patients with severe LV systolic dysfunction (126). Patients with poor RV FAC required a longer duration of mechanical ventilatory support (12 vs. 1 day, $p < 0.01$), a longer intensive care unit (ICU) stay (14 vs. 2 days, $p < 0.01$), and hospital stay (14 vs. 7 days, $p = 0.02$); LV diastolic dysfunction was more frequent and severe in these patients, while improvement in LV ejection fraction immediately after CPB was decreased (4.1 $\pm$ 8.3% vs. 12.5 $\pm$ 9.2%, $p = 0.03$). Finally, all patients with poor RV function died within two years of surgery, while 94% of patients with preserved RV function survived beyond that period.

Assessment of Diastolic Function

For a complete discussion of diastolic function, the reader is referred to Chapter 10. Left ventricular diastolic dysfunction is encountered in 30% to 80% of patients undergoing cardiac surgery (79,130). Their presence before CPB predicts difficult weaning, the need for inotropic support at the end of the procedure, and mortality (79,130–133).

The clear effect of CPB, transient global ischemia, CABG, and cardioplegic solutions on the LV diastolic function is controversial. Indeed, while myocardial revascularization improves LV diastolic stiffness and Doppler indices of ventricular relaxation when evaluated weeks to months after surgery (134), only a few studies have documented the effects of CABG on LV diastolic function in the early postoperative period. The potential improvement in diastolic function by revascularization could be offset by global ischemia during the cardioplegic arrest. If changes in the mitral inflow Doppler profile suggesting diastolic dysfunction are described post CPB, no clear change in ventricular relaxation could be demonstrated after statistical correction for the effect of HR on the mitral indices (135). In fact, Humphrey et al. (136) have reported an improvement in diastolic relaxation after CABG and CPB using LV intracavitary pressure and dimension measurements. More recently, Shi et al. (89) using newer echocardiographic modalities and the recommended classification of the American Society of Echocardiography

(137,138) studied the short- and long-term evolution of biventricular diastolic performance in patients with left diastolic dysfunction undergoing coronary artery bypass surgery. Moderate and severe left ventricular diastolic dysfunction increased from 2.0% preoperatively to 9.7% two days postoperatively. The patterns at six months were similar to those observed preoperatively. Similar evolution over time was found for right ventricular diastolic function (89) (Fig. 13.26).

Air Detection

During valvular heart surgery, and occasionally during CABG, when veins are anastomosed to the ascending Ao, air is introduced into the heart cavities and may lead to coronary and cerebral embolism. Transesophageal echocardiography is useful to detect the presence of intracardiac air and to assess the efficacy of the measures to eliminate it. Intracardiac air can be present as:

1. Air bubbles: these present as highly mobile, strongly echogenic dots, often accompanied by side lobe and reverberation artifacts with acoustic shadowing. Because of their buoyancy, bubbles will gather in the superior aspects of cardiac chambers (Fig. 13.30). Dynamic tearing away of small air bubbles from the surface of an air pocket into the cardiac chambers can also be observed and is known as the popcorn sign.

2. Pooled air: this is depicted as a highly mobile, strongly echogenic line or area adjacent to the wall at the highest level in each chamber and also accompanied by side lobe and reverberation artifacts with acoustic shadowing.

The most frequent location of intracardiac air in patients undergoing left cardiotomy is the right upper pulmonary vein (RUPV), followed by the LV, the LA, and the right sinus of Valsalva (140). All patients undergoing right cardiotomy displayed air trapping in the main and the right pulmonary arteries. Air in the pulmonary arteries is stopped by the lungs that act as filters. Air in the RUPV is visualized near their junction to the LA. Pooled air is also found in the superior aspect of the LA near the atrial septum as well as in the apex of the left atrial appendage (LAA). Intracardiac air may also accumulate along the anterior mitral leaflet and in the apex of the LV near the ventricular septum. Bubbles in the right sinus of Valsalva are easily mobilized and expelled within several beats of LV contraction (Fig. 13.30).

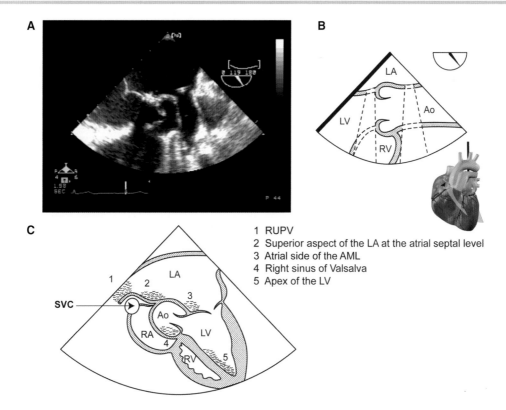

1 RUPV
2 Superior aspect of the LA at the atrial septal level
3 Atrial side of the AML
4 Right sinus of Valsalva
5 Apex of the LV

Figure 13.30 Intracardiac air. (A,B) Mid-esophageal long-axis view in a 78-year-old woman after mitral valve replacement shows residual air localized in the LA associated with acoustic shadowing. **(C)** Most frequent sites of retained air after cardiopulmonary bypass are shown. *Abbreviations*: AML, anterior mitral valve leaflet; Ao, aorta; LA, left atrium; LV, left ventricle; RA, right atrium; RV, right ventricle; RUPV, right upper pulmonary vein; SVC, superior vena cava. *Source*: Diagram C adapted with permission from Ref. 139.

When TEE still reveals the persistence of air in the cardiac chambers, other procedures to remove it are suggested:

1. Filling the cardiac chambers with blood during suturing with concomitant application of suction to the LV or aortic root vent
2. Venting through a balloon inserted into the LV in patients undergoing MV valve surgery
3. Allowing the air to flow out of the ascending Ao through a cardioplegic needle with the patient's head down
4. Applying hyperinflation of the lungs
5. Aspirating air through fine needles located in the LA or the LV apex
6. Expelling air out of the LV by agitation
7. Administrating cardioplegia into the LV vent

CHANGES IN CARDIAC PHYSIOLOGY AFTER CPB

Protamine

After CPB, protamine sulfate administration may have a hypotensive effect partly by decreasing SVR. Additional human data also suggest that protamine sulfate may have cardiovascular depressant properties that become apparent in patients with impaired LV function (141).

Right and Left Ventricular Contractile Function and Valve Function

Reevaluation of right and left ventricular systolic and diastolic function can be performed as previously described, as well as valvular assessment as described in Chapters 14 to 18.

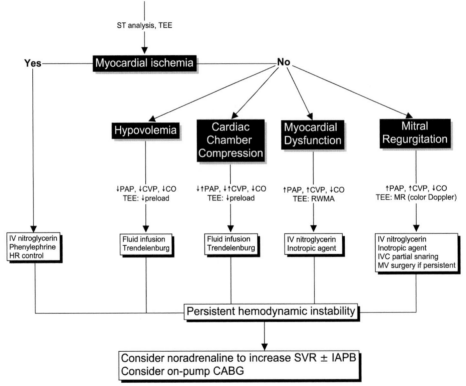

Figure 13.31   Hemodynamic instability during off-pump CABG surgery. An approach to the hemodynamically unstable patient with reduced CO during off-pump CABG is presented. The first step is to rule out ischemia. If ischemia is absent, four diagnoses can be encountered based on combined hemodynamic data and TEE. In hypovolemia, PAP, CVP, and the left and right ventricle cavity size will be decreased. The same observation can be made during cardiac compression, however PAP and CVP can also increase from the extrinsic compression. Elevated filling pressure with regional wall motion abnormalities will be present during myocardial dysfunction. This condition can lead to acute mitral regurgitation. A therapeutic strategy is suggested for each of these conditions. *Abbreviations*: CABG, coronary artery bypass graft; CVP, central venous pressure; CO, cardiac output; HR, heart rate; IABP, intra-aortic balloon pump; IV, intravenous; IVC, inferior vena cava; MR, mitral regurgitation; MV, mitral valve; PAP, pulmonary artery pressure; RWMA, regional wall motion abnormality; SVR, systemic vascular resistance; TEE, transesophageal echocardiography. *Source*: Adapted from Ref. 106.

HEMODYNAMIC CHANGES DURING OFF-PUMP CORONARY ARTERY BYPASS SURGERY

Hemodymanic variations in off-pump coronary artery bypass grafting (OP-CABG) may be due to mobilization and stabilization of the heart, or myocardial ischemia during coronary occlusion. Each type of stabilization device can also produce its own related hemodynamic effects (106). Hemodynamic instability during OP-CABG can be secondary to ischemia, reduced preload, cardiac compression, myocardial dysfunction, mitral regurgitation, or a combination of these causes (Fig. 13.31).

Myocardial Ischemia

During OP-CABG, all the monitoring methods have limitations. TEE is most useful during cardiac manipulations when hypotension is associated with increased filling pressure. In this situation, TEE can help to differentiate between cardiac dysfunction secondary to myocardial ischemia, in which regional wall motion abnormalities will be present from a much more common scenario where the increase in filling pressure is secondary to extracardiac compression. The two-dimensional transesophageal four- and two-chamber view are the most useful, since the transgastric SAX view may be difficult to obtain, particularly during circumflex and right coronary anastomosis.

Reduced Preload

Hypotension secondary to hypovolemia is usually associated with a decrease in pulmonary artery pressure (PAP) and CVP. Fluid loading and Trendelenburg position restore CO by increasing venous hydrostatic pressure and, subsequently, left ventricular preload. If these maneuvers are ineffective, vasopressors are considered. TEE can be useful to confirm hypovolemia and fluid responsiveness if the patient remains hypotensive.

Myocardial Dysfunction

Systolic Function

Hemodynamic instability related to severe systolic dysfunction is characterized by an increase in PAP and CVP, along with a decrease in CO. Transesophageal echocardiography monitoring is particularly helpful to differentiate between systolic dysfunction associated with regional wall motion abnormalities from cardiac compression where the increase in filling pressure is secondary to cardiac compression (Fig. 13.32). Transesophageal echocardiography may be considered in patients with known preoperative systolic function or in patients who remain hypotensive despite IV nitroglycerine and inotropic support. During off-pump beating heart CABG, most of the

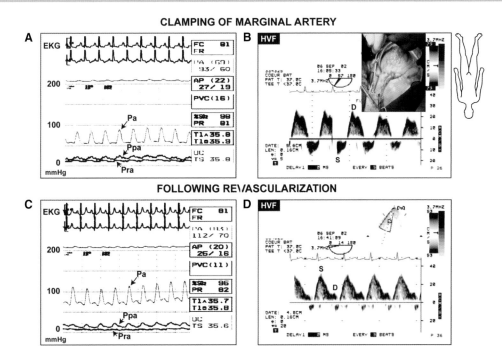

Figure 13.32 RV diastolic dysfunction. Transient severe RV diastolic dysfunction is present in a 72-year-old patient undergoing off-pump coronary artery bypass surgery. During clamping of the left obtuse marginal artery, the patient became hemodynamically unstable. **(A)** This was associated with a reduction in systolic and diastolic systemic Pa down to 93/60 mmHg, a slight increase in systolic and diastolic Ppa to 27/19 mm Hg and an increase in Pra of 16 mmHg. **(B)** Systolic flow reversal in the HVF was present. **(C,D)** These abnormalities normalized after revascularization was completed. *Abbreviations*: D, peak diastolic HVF velocity; EKG, electrocardiogram; HVF, hepatic venous flow; Pa, arterial blood pressure; Ppa, pulmonary artery pressure; Pra, right atrial pressure; RV, right ventricle; S, peak systolic HVF velocity. *Source*: Photo B courtesy of Dr. Raymond Cartier.

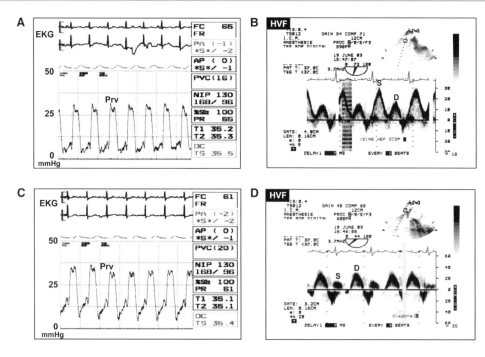

Figure 13.33 RV diastolic dysfunction. Occurrence of right ventricular diastolic dysfunction during off-pump bypass surgery in a 67-year-old man. (**A,B**) Baseline: Prv tracing and HVF profile with normal systolic flow predominance. (**C,D**) Hemodynamic instability during clamping of the left diagonal coronary artery: note the steeper diastolic slope on the Prv tracing with diastolic flow predominance on the HVF Doppler profile and inversion of the S/D ratio. *Abbreviations*: D, peak diastolic HVF velocity; EKG, electrocardiogram; HVF, hepatic venous flow; Prv, right ventricular pressure; RV, right ventricle; S, peak systolic HVF velocity.

new wall motion abnormalities resolve within a few minutes after revascularization (106).

Diastolic Dysfunction

The role of diastolic function during OP-CABG surgery is not reported in the literature. While changes in diastolic function may occur, it is difficult to differentiate the effects of cardiac compression, myocardial ischemia, or loading conditions (Fig. 13.33).

Cardiac Compression

During positioning and stabilization of the left anterior descending and diagonal arteries for OPCABG, the compression type stabilizer device must be applied with minimal pressure to avoid direct compression of the left ventricular outflow tract, which could cause abnormal diastolic expansion. On the other side, with the Medtronic Octopus® system (vacuum suction type stabilizer), the main causes of hemodynamic disturbance during positioning are thought to be decreased right ventricular filling and, to a lesser extent, left ventricular filling, by direct ventricular compression. Volume loading, Trendelenburg position, and vasopressor infusion usually correct these derangements. Transesophageal echocardiography is indicated in patients who are not responsive to the above treatment and helps to differentiate between extracardiac compression and

cardiac systolic and diastolic dysfunction (Figs. 13.33 and 13.34).

Mitral Regurgitation

In occasional cases, significant acute MV dysfunction can precipitate hemodynamic instability following heart positioning or coronary artery clamping. Patients who are most at risk to develop severe MV regurgitation are those with preexisting myocardial dysfunction or mild to moderate mitral regurgitation. When increases in PAP and CVP are observed, color Doppler TEE of the MV can make the diagnosis. Nitroglycerin and inotropic agents may be considered. Further preload reduction with IVC clamping has been used to control an acute increase in PAP unresponsive to usual treatment (142). MV repair or replacement may be considered if persistent after revascularization.

CONCLUSION

In conclusion, the role of TEE during cardiac surgery has shifted from a diagnostic tool to a complete monitoring and a diagnostic device. This allows the cardiac anesthesiologist to follow each step of the surgical procedure and to provide continuous feedback to the surgeon (Table 13.1). This requires both knowledge in TEE and in the surgical procedure and good communication skills.

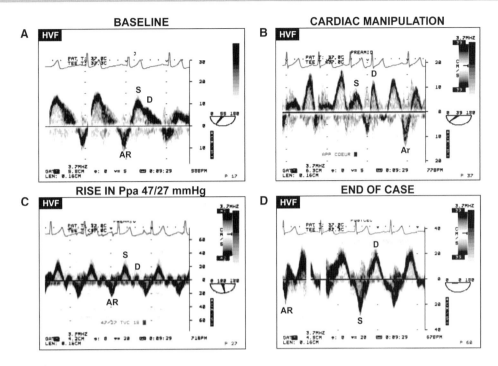

Figure 13.34 RV diastolic dysfunction. Worsening right ventricular diastolic function parameters on HVF Doppler examination during mitral valve repair in a 69-year old man. (**A**) Baseline: Normal systolic (S) flow predominance. (**B**) During manual cardiac manipulations of the heart, the S velocity is reduced. (**C**) With further elevation of the Ppa to 47/27, the AR velocity increases in relation to the S-wave. (**D**) Finally at the end of the procedure, systolic flow reversal is observed. *Abbreviations*: AR, peak atrial reversal HVF velocity; D, peak diastolic HVF velocity; HVF, hepatic venous flow; Ppa, pulmonary pressure; RV, right ventricle; S, peak systolic HVF velocity.

Table 13.1 Summary of the Role of TEE in Patients Undergoing Cardiac Surgery

	Importance
Before the procedure	
• Left and right ventricular function	Loading condition and need for postoperative inotropic and/or mechanical support
• Aortic, mitral, tricuspid, and pulmonic valve competency	Detect unrecognized valvular disease
PFO	Risk of hypoxia by left-to-right shunt if right ventricular dysfunction
• Aortic atheromatosis (epiaortic)	Grade 4 or 5 could complicate cannula insertion
• Detection of pleural effusion	Optimization of oxygenation and ventilation
• Monitor the insertion of devices: PA catheter, CPB and cardioplegias cannulas, and intra-aortic balloon counterpulsation	Early detection and correction of devices misplacement
During CPB	
• Monitor the position of CPB and cardioplegias cannulas	Early detection and correction of cannula displacement
• De-airing process	Air removed before weaning from CPB
After CPB	
• Reevaluate left and right ventricular function	Loading condition and need for postoperative inotropic and/or mechanical support
• Reevaluate valvular function	New onset regurgitation, LVOT and RVOT dynamic obstruction could complicate weaning from CPB
• Reevaluate aorta	Rule out new iatrogenic aortic dissection
• Reevaluate inferior vena cava	Rule out new iatrogenic obstruction
• Rule out significant pleural effusion	Optimize chest tube drainage
In the intensive care unit	
• Rule out specific complications if hemodynamically unstable	Tamponade, ventricular dysfunction, valvular insufficiency, LVOT and RVOT dynamic obstruction, hypovolemia, shunting through a PFO, intracavitary thrombus, peritoneal bleeding

Abbreviations: CPB, cardiopulmonary bypass; LVOT, left ventricular outflow tract; PA, pulmonary artery; PFO, patent foramen ovale; RVOT, right ventricular outflow tract; TEE, transesophageal echocardiography.

REFERENCES

1. Practice Guidelines for Perioperative Transesophageal Echocardiography: An Updated Report by the American Society of Anesthesiologists and the Society of Cardiovascular Anesthesiologists Task Force on Transesophageal Echocardiography. Anesthesiology 2010; 112:1–13.
2. Deutsch HJ, Curtius JM, Leischik R, et al. Diagnostic value of transesophageal echocardiography in cardiac surgery. Thorac Cardiovasc Surg 1991; 39:199–204.
3. Kato M, Nakashima Y, Levine J, et al. Does transesophageal echocardiography improve postoperative outcome in patients undergoing coronary artery bypass surgery? J Cardiothorac Vasc Anesth 1993; 7:285–289.
4. Bryan AJ, Barzilai B, Kouchoukos NT. Transesophageal echocardiography and adult cardiac operations. Ann Thorac Surg 1995; 59:773–779.
5. Ungerleider RM, Kisslo JA, Greeley WJ, et al. Intraoperative echocardiography during congenital heart operations: experience from 1,000 cases. Ann Thorac Surg 1995; 60:S539–S542.
6. Stevenson JG. Role of intraoperative transesophageal echocardiography during repair of congenital cardiac defects. Acta Paediatr Suppl 1995; 410:23–33.
7. Bergquist BD, Bellows WH, Leung JM. Transesophageal echocardiography in myocardial revascularization: II. Influence on intraoperative decision making. Anesth Analg 1996; 82:1139–1145.
8. Sutton DC, Kluger R. Intraoperative transoesophageal echocardiography: impact on adult cardiac surgery. Anaesth Intensive Care 1998; 26:287–293.
9. Rosenfeld HM, Gentles TL, Wernovsky G, et al. Utility of intraoperative transesophageal echocardiography in the assessment of residual cardiac defects. Pediatr Cardiol 1998; 19:346–351.
10. Mishra M, Chauhan R, Sharma KK, et al. Real-time intraoperative transesophageal echocardiography—how useful? Experience of 5,016 cases. J Cardiothorac Vasc Anesth 1998; 12:625–632.
11. Sheil ML, Baines DB. Intraoperative transoesophageal echocardiography for paediatric cardiac surgery—an audit of 200 cases. Anaesth Intensive Care 1999; 27:591–595.
12. Michel-Cherqui M, Ceddaha A, Liu N, et al. Assessment of systematic use of intraoperative transesophageal echocardiography during cardiac surgery in adults: a prospective study of 203 patients. J Cardiothorac Vasc Anesth 2000; 14:45–50.
13. Click RL, Abel MD, Schaff HV. Intraoperative transesophageal echocardiography: 5-year prospective review of impact on surgical management. Mayo Clin Proc 2000; 75:241–247.
14. Couture P, Denault AY, McKenty S, et al. Impact of routine use of intraoperative transesophageal echocardiography during cardiac surgery. Can J Anaesth 2000; 47:20–26.
15. Sloth E, Pedersen J, Olsen KH, et al. Transoesophageal echocardiographic monitoring during paediatric cardiac surgery: obtainable information and feasibility in 532 children. Paediatr Anaesth 2001; 11:657–662.
16. Schmidlin D, Schuepbach R, Bernard E, et al. Indications and impact of postoperative transesophageal echocardiography in cardiac surgical patients. Crit Care Med 2001; 29:2143–2148.
17. Eltzschig HK, Rosenberger P, Loffler M, et al. Impact of intraoperative transesophageal echocardiography on surgical decisions in 12,566 patients undergoing cardiac surgery. Ann Thorac Surg 2008; 85:845–852.
18. Troianos CA, Savino JS. Internal jugular vein cannulation guided by echocardiography. Anesthesiology 1991; 74:787–789.
19. Andropoulos DB, Stayer SA, Bent ST, et al. A controlled study of transesophageal echocardiography to guide central venous catheter placement in congenital heart surgery patients. Anesth Analg 1999; 89:65–70.
20. Sawchuk C, Fayad A. Confirmation of internal jugular guide wire position utilizing transesophageal echocardiography. Can J Anaesth 2001; 48:688–690.
21. Nelson JE, Croft LB, Nahar T, et al. Evaluation of subclavian catheter position. J Cardiothorac Vasc Anesth 1999; 13:359–361.
22. Zimmermann P, Steinhubel B, Greim CA. Facilitation of pulmonary artery catheter placement by transesophageal echocardiography after tricuspid valve surgery. Anesth Analg 2001; 93:242–243.
23. Catoire P, Beydon L, Delaunay L, et al. Persistent left superior vena cava diagnosed by transesophageal echocardiography. J Cardiothorac Vasc Anesth 1993; 7:375–379.
24. Orihashi K, Hong YW, Chung G, et al. New applications of two-dimensional transesophageal echocardiography in cardiac surgery. J Cardiothorac Vasc Anesth 1991; 5:33–39.
25. Capper SJ, Ross JJ, Sandstrom E, et al. Transoesophageal echocardiography for the detection and quantification of pleural fluid in cardiac surgical patients. Br J Anaesth 2007; 98:442–446.
26. Swenson JD, Bull DA. Intraoperative diagnosis and treatment of pleural effusion based on transesophageal echocardiographic findings. Anesth Analg 1999; 89:309–310.
27. Saito Y, Donohue A, Attai S, et al. The syndrome of cardiac tamponade with "small" pericardial effusion. Echocardiography 2008; 25:321–327.
28. Wareing TH, Davila-Roman VG, Daily BB, et al. Strategy for the reduction of stroke incidence in cardiac surgical patients. Ann Thorac Surg 1993; 55:1400–1407.
29. Roach GW, Kanchuger M, Mangano CM, et al. Adverse cerebral outcomes after coronary bypass surgery. Multicenter Study of Perioperative Ischemia Research Group and the Ischemia Research and Education Foundation Investigators. N Engl J Med 1996; 335:1857–1863.
30. Katz ES, Tunick PA, Rusinek H, et al. Protruding aortic atheromas predict stroke in elderly patients undergoing cardiopulmonary bypass: experience with intraoperative transesophageal echocardiography. J Am Coll Cardiol 1992; 20:70–77.
31. Glas KE, Swaminathan M, Reeves ST, et al. Guidelines for the performance of a comprehensive intraoperative epiaortic ultrasonographic examination: recommendations of the American Society of Echocardiography and the Society of Cardiovascular Anesthesiologists; endorsed by the Society of Thoracic Surgeons. Anesth Analg 2008; 106:1376–1384.
32. Tunick PA, Kronzon I. Atheromas of the thoracic aorta: clinical and therapeutic update. J Am Coll Cardiol 2000; 35:545–554.
33. Van der Linden J, Bergman P, Hadjinikolaou L. The topography of aortic atherosclerosis enhances its precision as a predictor of stroke. Ann Thorac Surg 2007; 83:2087–2092.
34. Weisenberg D, Sahar Y, Sahar G, et al. Atherosclerosis of the aorta is common in patients with severe aortic stenosis: an intraoperative transesophageal echocardiographic study. J Thorac Cardiovasc Surg 2005; 130:29–32.
35. Murkin JM. Etiology and incidence of brain dysfunction after cardiac surgery. J Cardiothorac Vasc Anesth 1999; 13:12–17.

36. Beique FA, Joffe D, Tousignant G, et al. Echocardiography-based assessment and management of atherosclerotic disease of the thoracic aorta. J Cardiothorac Vasc Anesth 1998; 12:206–220.

37. Konstadt SN, Reich DL, Quintana C, et al. The ascending aorta: how much does transesophageal echocardiography see? Anesth Analg 1994; 78:240–244.

38. Konstadt SN, Reich DL, Kahn R, et al. Transesophageal echocardiography can be used to screen for ascending aortic atherosclerosis. Anesth Analg 1995; 81:225–228.

39. Rosenberger P, Shernan SK, Loffler M, et al. The influence of epiaortic ultrasonography on intraoperative surgical management in 6051 cardiac surgical patients. Ann Thorac Surg 2008; 85:548–553.

40. Orihashi K, Sueda T, Okada K, et al. Detection and monitoring of complications associated with femoral or axillary arterial cannulation for surgical repair of aortic dissection. J Cardiothorac Vasc Anesth 2006; 20:20–25.

41. Noiseux N, Couture P, Sheridan P, et al. Aortic cannulation for type A dissection: guidance by transesophageal echocardiography. Interact CardioVasc Thorac Surg 2003; 2:178–180.

42. Clements F, Wright SJ, de Bruijn N. Coronary sinus catheterization made easy for Port-Access miimally invasive cardiac surgery. J Cardiothorac Vasc Anesth 1998; 12:96–101.

43. Akhtar S. Off-axis view using a multiplane transesophageal echocardiography probe facilitates cannulation of the coronary sinus. J Cardiothorac Vasc Anesth 1998; 12:374–375.

44. Poirier NC, Ugolini P, Pellerin M, et al. Transesophageal echocardiographic evaluation of perioperative coronary sinus trauma. Ann Thorac Surg 1998; 66:573–575.

45. Demertzis S, Casso G, Torre T, et al. Direct epiaortic ultrasound scanning for the rapid confirmation of intraoperative aortic dissection. Interact Cardiovasc Thorac Surg 2008; 7:725–726.

46. Varghese D, Riedel BJ, Fletcher SN, et al. Successful repair of intraoperative aortic dissection detected by transesophageal echocardiography. Ann Thorac Surg 2002; 73:953–955.

47. Watke CM, Clements F, Glower DD, et al. False-positive diagnosis of aortic dissection associated with femoral cardiopulmonary bypass. Anesthesiology 1998; 88:1119–1121.

48. Yamaura K, Okamoto H, Maekawa T, et al. Detection of retroperitoneal hemorrhage by transesophageal echocardiography during cardiac surgery. Can J Anaesth 1999; 46:169–172.

49. Vieillard-Baron A, Loubieres Y, Schmitt JM, et al. Cyclic changes in right ventricular output impedance during mechanical ventilation. J Appl Physiol 1999; 87:1644–1650.

50. Vieillard-Baron A, Augarde R, Prin S, et al. Influence of superior vena caval zone condition on cyclic changes in right ventricular outflow during respiratory support. Anesthesiology 2001; 95:1083–1088.

51. Haddad F, Couture P, Tousignant C, et al. The right ventricle in cardiac surgery, a perioperative perspective: I. Anatomy, physiology, and assessment. Anesth Analg 2009; 108:407–421.

52. Brower R, Wise RA, Hassapoyannes C, et al. Effect of lung inflation on lung blood volume and pulmonary venous flow. J Appl Physiol 1985; 58:954–963.

53. Fellahi JL, Valtier B, Beauchet A, et al. Does positive end-expiratory pressure ventilation improve left ventricular function? A comparative study by transesophageal echocardiography in cardiac and noncardiac patients. Chest 1998; 114:556–562.

54. Schuster S, Erbel R, Weilemann LS, et al. Hemodynamics during PEEP ventilation in patients with severe left ventricular failure studied by transesophageal echocardiography. Chest 1990; 97:1181–1189.

55. Poelaert JI, Reichert CL, Koolen JJ, et al. Transesophageal Echo-doppler evaluation of the hemodynamic effects of positive-pressure ventilation after coronary artery surgery. J Cardiothorac Vasc Anesth 1992; 6:438–443.

56. Reis MD, Klompe L, Mekel J, et al. Open lung ventilation does not increase right ventricular outflow impedance: An echo-Doppler study. Crit Care Med 2006; 34:2555–2560.

57. Meijburg HW, Visser CA, Wesenhagen H, et al. Transesophageal pulsed-Doppler echocardiographic evaluation of transmitral and pulmonary venous flow during ventilation with positive end-expiratory pressure. J Cardiothorac Vasc Anesth 1994; 8:386–391.

58. Girard F, Couture P, Boudreault D, et al. Estimation of the pulmonary capillary wedge pressure from transesophageal pulsed Doppler echocardiography of pulmonary venous flow: influence of the respiratory cycle during mechanical ventilation. J Cardiothorac Vasc Anesth 1998; 12:16–21.

59. Estafanous FG, Barash PG, Reves JG. Cardiac Anesthesia: Principles and Clinical Practice. 2nd ed. Philadelphia: Lippincott Williams & Wilkins, 2001.

60. Declerck C, Hillel Z, Shih H, et al. A comparison of left ventricular performance indices measured by transesophageal echocardiography with automated border detection. Anesthesiology 1998; 89:341–349.

61. Van Trigt P, Christian CC, Fagraeus L, et al. The mechanism of halothane-induced myocardial depression. Altered diastolic mechanics versus impaired contractility. J Thorac Cardiovasc Surg 1983; 85:832–838.

62. Eger EI. New inhaled anesthetics. Anesthesiology 1994; 80:906–922.

63. Weiskopf RB, Moore MA, Eger EI, et al. Rapid increase in desflurane concentration is associated with greater transient cardiovascular stimulation than with rapid increase in isoflurane concentration in humans. Anesthesiology 1994; 80:1035–1045.

64. Kemmotsu O, Hashimoto Y, Shimosato S. Inotropic effects of isoflurane on mechanics of contraction in isolated cat papillary muscles from normal and failing hearts. Anesthesiology 1973; 39:470–477.

65. Pagel PS, Kampine JP, Schmeling WT, et al. Effects of nitrous oxide on myocardial contractility as evaluated by the preload recruitable stroke work relationship in chronically instrumented dogs. Anesthesiology 1990; 73:1148–1157.

66. Wappler F, Rossaint R, Baumert J, et al. Multicenter randomized comparison of xenon and isoflurane on left ventricular function in patients undergoing elective surgery. Anesthesiology 2007; 106:463–471.

67. Lerman J, Oyston JP, Gallagher TM, et al. The minimum alveolar concentration (MAC) and hemodynamic effects of halothane, isoflurane, and sevoflurane in newborn swine. Anesthesiology 1990; 73:717–721.

68. Cope DK, Impastato WK, Cohen MV, et al. Volatile anesthetics protect the ischemic rabbit myocardium from infarction. Anesthesiology 1997; 86:699–709.

69. Stanley TH, Webster LR. Anesthetic requirements and cardiovascular effects of fentanyl-oxygen and fentanyl-diazepam-oxygen anesthesia in man. Anesth Analg 1978; 57:411–416.

70. Cote P, Gueret P, Bourassa MG. Systemic and coronary hemodynamic effects of diazepam in patients with normal and diseased coronary arteries. Circulation 1974; 50:1210–1216.

71. Nakae Y, Kanaya N, Namiki A. The direct effects of diazepam and midazolam on myocardial depression in cultured rat ventricular myocytes. Anesth Analg 1997; 85:729–733.

72. Mulier JP, Wouters PF, Van AH, et al. Cardiodynamic effects of propofol in comparison with thiopental: assessment with a transesophageal echocardiographic approach. Anesth Analg 1991; 72:28–35.

73. Schmidt C, Roosens C, Struys M, et al. Contractility in humans after coronary artery surgery. Anesthesiology 1999; 91:58–70.

74. Gelissen HP, Epema AH, Henning RH, et al. Inotropic effects of propofol, thiopental, midazolam, etomidate, and ketamine on isolated human atrial muscle. Anesthesiology 1996; 84:397–403.

75. Jackson AP, Dhadphale PR, Callaghan ML, et al. Haemodynamic studies during induction of anaesthesia for open-heart surgery using diazepam and ketamine. Br J Anaesth 1978; 50:375–378.

76. Gooding JM, Corssen G. Effect of etomidate on the cardiovascular system. Anesth Analg 1977; 56:717–719.

77. Gare M, Parail A, Milosavljevic D, et al. Conscious sedation with midazolam or propofol does not alter left ventricular diastolic performance in patients with pre-existing diastolic dysfunction: a transmitral and tissue Doppler transthoracic echocardiography study. Anesth Analg 2001; 93:865–871.

78. Couture P, Denault AY, Shi Y, et al. Effects of anesthetic induction in patients with diastolic dysfunction. Can J Anaesth 2009; 56:357–365.

79. Denault AY, Couture P, Buithieu J, et al. Left and right ventricular diastolic dysfunction as predictors of difficult separation from cardiopulmonary bypass. Can J Anaesth 2006; 53:1020–1029.

80. Romson JL, Leung JM, Bellows WH, et al. Effects of dobutamine on hemodynamics and left ventricular performance after cardiopulmonary bypass in cardiac surgical patients. Anesthesiology 1999; 91:1318–1328.

81. Aronson S, Dupont F, Savage R, et al. Changes in regional myocardial function after coronary artery bypass graft surgery are predicted by intraoperative low-dose dobutamine echocardiography. Anesthesiology 2000; 93:685–692.

82. Dupont FW, Lang RM, Drum ML, et al. Is there a long-term predictive value of intraoperative low-dose dobutamine echocardiography in patients who have coronary artery bypass graft surgery with cardiopulmonary bypass? Anesth Analg 2002; 95:517–523.

83. Levy JH, Bailey JM, Deeb GM. Intravenous milrinone in cardiac surgery. Ann Thorac Surg 2002; 73:325–330.

84. Kikura M, Levy JH, Michelsen LG, et al. The effect of milrinone on hemodynamics and left ventricular function after emergence from cardiopulmonary bypass. Anesth Analg 1997; 85:16–22.

85. Couture P, Denault AY, Pellerin M, et al. Milrinone enhances systolic, but not diastolic function during coronary artery bypass grafting surgery. Can J Anaesth 2007; 54:509–522.

86. Rathmell JP, Prielipp RC, Butterworth JF, et al. A multi-center, randomized, blind comparison of amrinone with milrinone after elective cardiac surgery. Anesth Analg 1998; 86:683–690.

87. Monrad ES, McKay RG, Baim DS, et al. Improvement in indexes of diastolic performance in patients with congestive heart failure treated with milrinone. Circulation 1984; 70:1030–1037.

88. Lobato EB, Gravenstein N, Martin TD. Milrinone, not epinephrine, improves left ventricular compliance after cardiopulmonary bypass. J Cardiothorac Vasc Anesth 2000; 14:374–377.

89. Shi Y, Denault AY, Couture P, et al. Biventricular diastolic filling patterns after coronary artery bypass graft surgery. J Thorac Cardiovasc Surg 2006; 131:1080–1086.

90. Ochiai Y, Morita S, Tanoue Y, et al. Effects of amrinone, a phosphodiesterase inhibitor, on right ventricular/arterial coupling immediately after cardiac operations. J Thorac Cardiovasc Surg 1998; 116:139–147.

91. Denault AY, Lamarche Y, Couture P, et al. Inhaled milrinone: a new alternative in cardiac surgery? Semin Cardiothorac Vasc Anesth 2006; 10:346–360.

92. Jörgensen K, Bech-Hanssen O, Houltz E, et al. Effects of levosimendan on left ventricular relaxation and early filling at maintained preload and afterload conditions after aortic valve replacement for aortic stenosis. Circulation 2008; 117:1075–1081.

93. Raja SG, Rayen BS. Levosimendan in cardiac surgery: current best available evidence. Ann Thorac Surg 2006; 81:1536–1546.

94. Goertz AW, Seeling W, Heinrich H, et al. Effect of phenylephrine bolus administration on left ventricular function during high thoracic and lumbar epidural anesthesia combined with general anesthesia. Anesth Analg 1993; 76:541–545.

95. Lichtenstein SV, Ashe KA, el Dalati H, et al. Warm heart surgery. J Thorac Cardiovasc Surg 1991; 101:269–274.

96. Bak Z, Abildgard L, Lisander B, et al. Transesophageal echocardiographic hemodynamic monitoring during preoperative acute normovolemic hemodilution. Anesthesiology 2000; 92:1250–1256.

97. Aronson S, Wiencek JG. Intraoperative perfusion echocardiography. J Cardiothorac Vasc Anesth 1994; 8:97–107.

98. Voci P, Bilotta F, Caretta Q, et al. Mechanisms of incomplete cardioplegia distribution during coronary artery surgery. An intraoperative transesophageal contrast echocardiography study. Anesthesiology 1993; 79:904–912.

99. Borger MA, Wei KS, Weisel RD, et al. Myocardial perfusion during warm antegrade and retrograde cardioplegia: a contrast echo study. Ann Thorac Surg 1999; 68:955–961.

100. Aronson S, Jacobsohn E, Savage R, et al. The influence of collateral flow on the antegrade and retrograde distribution of cardioplegia in patients with an occluded right coronary artery. Anesthesiology 1998; 89:1099–1107.

101. Aronson S, Lee BK, Wiencek JG, et al. Assessment of myocardial perfusion during CABG surgery with two-dimensional transesophageal contrast echocardiography. Anesthesiology 1991; 75:433–440.

102. Leung JM, O'Kelly B, Browner WS, et al. Prognostic importance of postbypass regional wall-motion abnormalities in patients undergoing coronary artery bypass graft surgery. SPI Research Group. Anesthesiology 1989; 71:16–25.

103. Comunale ME, Body SC, Ley C, et al. The concordance of intraoperative left ventricular wall-motion abnormalities and electrocardiographic S-T segment changes: association with outcome after coronary revascularization. Multicenter Study of Perioperative Ischemia (McSPI) Research Group. Anesthesiology 1998; 88:945–954.

104. Kotoh K, Watanabe G, Ueyama K, et al. On-line assessment of regional ventricular wall motion by transesophageal echocardiography with color kinesis during minimally invasive coronary artery bypass grafting. J Thorac Cardiovasc Surg 1999; 117:912–917.

105. Malkowski MJ, Kramer CM, Parvizi ST, et al. Transient ischemia does not limit subsequent ischemic regional dysfunction in humans: a transesophageal echocardiographic study during minimally invasive coronary artery bypass surgery. J Am Coll Cardiol 1998; 31:1035–1039.

106. Couture P, Denault AY, Limoges P, et al. Mechanisms of hemodynamic changes during off-pump coronary artery bypass surgery. Can J Anaesth 2002; 49:835–849.

107. Swaminathan M, Morris RW, De Meyts DD, et al. Deterioration of regional wall motion immediately after coronary artery bypass graft surgery is associated with long-term major adverse cardiac events. Anesthesiology 2007; 107:739–745.

108. Robotham JL, Takata M, Berman M, et al. Ejection fraction revisited. Anesthesiology 1991; 74:172–183.

109. Gorcsan J III, Denault AY, Gasior TA, et al. Rapid estimation of left ventricular contractility from end-systolic relations by echocardiographic automated border detection and femoral arterial pressure. Anesthesiology 1994; 81:553–562.

110. Colan SD, Borow KM, Neumann A. Left ventricular end-systolic wall stress-velocity of fiber shortening relation: a load-independent index of myocardial contractility. J Am Coll Cardiol 1984; 4:715–724.

111. Thys DM, Hillel Z, Goldman ME, et al. A comparison of hemodynamic indices derived by invasive monitoring and two-dimensional echocardiography. Anesthesiology 1987; 67:630–634.

112. Tousignant CP, Walsh F, Mazer CD. The use of transesophageal echocardiography for preload assessment in critically ill patients. Anesth Analg 2000; 90:351–355.

113. Lattik R, Couture P, Denault AY, et al. Mitral Doppler indices are superior to two-dimensional echocardiographic and hemodynamic variables in predicting responsiveness of cardiac output to a rapid intravenous infusion of colloid. Anesth Analg 2002; 94:1092–1099.

114. Charron C, Caille V, Jardin F, et al. Echocardiographic measurement of fluid responsiveness. Curr Opin Crit Care 2006; 12:249–254.

115. Barbier C, Loubieres Y, Schmit C, et al. Respiratory changes in inferior vena cava diameter are helpful in predicting fluid responsiveness in ventilated septic patients. Intensive Care Med 2004; 30:1740–1746.

116. Slama M, Masson H, Teboul JL, et al. Respiratory variations of aortic VTI: a new index of hypovolemia and fluid responsiveness. Am J Physiol Heart Circ Physiol 2002; 283:H1729–H1733.

117. Monnet X, Rienzo M, Osman D, et al. Esophageal Doppler monitoring predicts fluid responsiveness in critically ill ventilated patients. Intensive Care Med 2005; 31:1195–1201.

118. Feissel M, Michard F, Mangin I, et al. Respiratory changes in aortic blood velocity as an indicator of fluid responsiveness in ventilated patients with septic shock. Chest 2001; 119:867–873.

119. Kuecherer HF, Muhiudeen IA, Kusumoto FM, et al. Estimation of mean left atrial pressure from transesophageal pulsed Doppler echocardiography of pulmonary venous flow. Circulation 1990; 82:1127–1139.

120. Nishimura RA, Abel MD, Hatle LK, et al. Relation of pulmonary vein to mitral flow velocities by transesophageal Doppler echocardiography. Effect of different loading conditions. Circulation 1990; 81:1488–1497.

121. Appleton CP, Galloway JM, Gonzalez MS, et al. Estimation of left ventricular filling pressures using two-dimensional and Doppler echocardiography in adult patients with cardiac disease. Additional value of analyzing left atrial size, left atrial ejection fraction and the difference in duration of pulmonary venous and mitral flow velocity at atrial contraction. J Am Coll Cardiol 1993; 22:1972–1982.

122. Yamamoto K, Nishimura RA, Chaliki HP, et al. Determination of left ventricular filling pressure by Doppler echocardiography in patients with coronary artery disease: critical role of left ventricular systolic function. J Am Coll Cardiol 1997; 30:1819–1826.

123. Nomura M, Hillel Z, Shih H, et al. The association between Doppler transmitral flow variables measured by transesophageal echocardiography and pulmonary capillary wedge pressure. Anesth Analg 1997; 84:491–496.

124. Nagueh SF, Middleton KJ, Kopelen HA, et al. Doppler tissue imaging: a noninvasive technique for evaluation of left ventricular relaxation and estimation of filling pressures. J Am Coll Cardiol 1997; 30:1527–1533.

125. Kusumoto FM, Muhiudeen IA, Kuecherer HF, et al. Response of the interatrial septum to transatrial pressure gradients and its potential for predicting pulmonary capillary wedge pressure: an intraoperative study using transesophageal echocardiography in patients during mechanical ventilation. J Am Coll Cardiol 1993; 21:721–728.

126. Maslow AD, Regan MM, Panzica P, et al. Precardiopulmonary bypass right ventricular function is associated with poor outcome after coronary artery bypass grafting in patients with severe left ventricular systolic dysfunction. Anesth Analg 2002; 95:1507–1518.

127. Haddad F, Denault AY, Couture P, et al. Right ventricular myocardial performance index predicts perioperative mortality or circulatory failure in high-risk valvular surgery. J Am Soc Echocardiogr 2007; 20:1065–1072.

128. Reichert CL, Visser CA, van den Brink RB, et al. Prognostic value of biventricular function in hypotensive patients after cardiac surgery as assessed by transesophageal echocardiography. J Cardiothorac Vasc Anesth 1992; 6:429–432.

129. Haddad F, Doyle R, Murphy DJ, et al. Right ventricular function in cardiovascular disease, part II: Pathophysiology, clinical importance, and management of right ventricular failure. Circulation 2008; 117:1717–1731.

130. Bernard F, Denault AY, Babin D, et al. Diastolic dysfunction is predictive of difficult weaning from cardiopulmonary bypass. Anesth Analg 2001; 92:291–298.

131. Vaskelyte J, Stoskute N, Kinduris S, et al. Coronary artery bypass grafting in patients with severe left ventricular dysfunction: predictive significance of left ventricular diastolic filling pattern. Eur J Echocardiogr 2001; 2:62–67.

132. Liu J, Tanaka N, Murata K, et al. Prognostic value of pseudonormal and restrictive filling patterns on left ventricular remodeling and cardiac events after coronary artery bypass grafting. Am J Cardiol 2003; 91:550–554.

133. Merello L, Riesle E, Alburquerque J, et al. Risk scores do not predict high mortality after coronary artery bypass surgery in the presence of diastolic dysfunction. Ann Thorac Surg 2008; 85:1247–1255.

134. Lawson WE, Seifert F, Anagnostopoulos C, et al. Effect of coronary artery bypass grafting on left ventricular diastolic function. Am J Cardiol 1988; 61:283–287.

135. Houltz E, Hellstrom A, Ricksten SE, et al. Early effects of coronary artery bypass surgery and cold cardioplegic ischemia on left ventricular diastolic function: evaluation by computer-assisted transesophageal echocardiography. J Cardiothorac Vasc Anesth 1996; 10:728–733.

136. Humphrey LS, Topol EJ, Rosenfeld GI, et al. Immediate enhancement of left ventricular relaxation by coronary artery bypass grafting: intraoperative assessment. Circulation 1988; 77:886–896.

137. Khouri SJ, Maly GT, Suh DD, et al. A practical approach to the echocardiographic evaluation of diastolic function. J Am Soc Echocardiogr 2004; 17:290–297.

138. Nagueh SF, Appleton CP, Gillebert TC, et al. Recommendations for the evaluation of left ventricular diastolic function by echocardiography. J Am Soc Echocardiogr 2009; 22:107–133.

139. Bettex D, Chassot PD. Échocardiographie transoesophagienne en anesthésie-réanimation. Paris: Ed. Pradel, 1997:329.

140. Orihashi K, Matsuura Y, Hamanaka Y, et al. Retained intracardiac air in open heart operations examined by transesophageal echocardiography. Ann Thorac Surg 1993; 55:1467–1471.

141. Del Re MR, Ayd JD, Schultheis LW, et al. Protamine and left ventricular function: a transesophageal echocardiography study. Anesth Analg 1993; 77:1098–1103.

142. Couture P, Denault AY, Sheridan P, et al. Partial inferior vena cava snaring to control ischemic left ventricular dysfunction. Can J Anaesth 2003; 50:404–410.

14

Native Aortic Valve

François A. Béïque
McGill University, Montreal, Quebec, Canada

Christine Watremez
Cliniques universitaires Saint-Luc, Brussels, Belgium

INTRODUCTION

The aortic valve (AoV) is part of the aortic root. Pathology involving the AoV can originate from, or be caused by, its intimacy with surrounding structures. Echocardiography has become the standard tool to diagnose and evaluate AoV pathology. This chapter will review the echocardiographic features related to normal and pathological findings associated with aortic stenosis (AS) and aortic regurgitation (AR).

ANATOMY OF THE AORTIC VALVE

Normal AoV Anatomy

The ascending aorta (Ao) is approximately 5-cm long and has two distinct segments. The proximal segment is the aortic root which extends from the aortoventricular junction (AVJ) inferiorly to the sinotubular junction (STJ) beyond which is the distal segment, the tubular ascending Ao. The aortic root is comprised of the AoV cusps, the AoV annulus, the STJ, the sinuses of Valsalva, and the coronary ostia. Above the AoV, an outpouching of the aortic wall forms the sinuses of Valsalva, which represent the widest portion of the aortic root and contain the coronary ostia (Fig. 14.1).

The AoV has three distinct symmetrical cusps: right coronary, left coronary, and noncoronary (Fig. 14.2). Each coronary cusp attaches to the aortic wall in a curvilinear fashion, forming a crown-shaped aortic annulus with three tips located at the STJ (Fig. 14.3). Measurement of the aortic root at the STJ is generally 10% to 15% larger than at the left ventricular outflow tract (LVOT) (Fig. 14.1). The right and left coronary cusps are associated with the origin of the coronary artery that bears the same name. The noncoronary cusp, located posteriorly, is not associated with a coronary ostium and is in proximity to the atrial septum. The height of the aortic cusps is slightly less than half the length of its free margin. The free edge of each cusp is concave, and there is a large contact zone between the cusps, which creates a visible zone of redundancy, the lunula, above the closure line (Fig. 14.3). On the ventricular surface of each aortic cusp, the nodule of Arantius is located in the center of the free edge at the point of coaptation (Fig. 14.3).

Lambl's excrescences are thin mobile filamentous strands on the AoV commonly observed in increasing incidence with age. They are variable in number; appear near the closure line, measuring 1 mm in thickness and up to 1 cm in length. They contain a fibroelastic core covered by a thin layer of endothelial cells and may originate from small endothelial tears on the AoV surface. These strands are not pathological and should not be mistaken for AoV pathology or endocarditis (see Chapter 25, Fig. 25.7).

The relationship of the AoV to structures within or near the base of the heart is important in understanding pathological echocardiographic findings. The AoV is part of the fibroskeleton at the base of the heart. The left and noncoronary cusps are in fibrous continuity with the anterior leaflet of the mitral valve (MV) (Fig. 14.4). This fibrous continuity is the subaortic curtain or mitral-aortic intervalvular fibrosa. It is located between the two fibrous trigones that are the strongest components of the cardiac fibroskeleton. The left trigone is in proximity to the posterior aspect of the left coronary cusp, while the right fibrous trigone is opposite the noncoronary cusp (Fig. 14.4). The conduction system is located near the posterior noncoronary cusp and may be injured during AoV surgery or involved by endocarditis. The membranous septum immediately below the AoV is divided by the attachment of the tricuspid valve (TV) into an interventricular and an atrioventricular component (Fig. 14.4). The AoV is also in proximity to other heart valves and to both the left and right atria (LA, RA).

Congenital Anomalies of the AoV

Congenital anomalies of the AoV include bicuspid, unicuspid, and quadricuspid valves. Pentacuspid AoVs have also been described. The commonest congenital anomaly is a bicuspid AoV with an occurrence of 1% to 2% in the general population.

A bicuspid AoV may have two equal cusps without a raphe and a unicommissural opening that

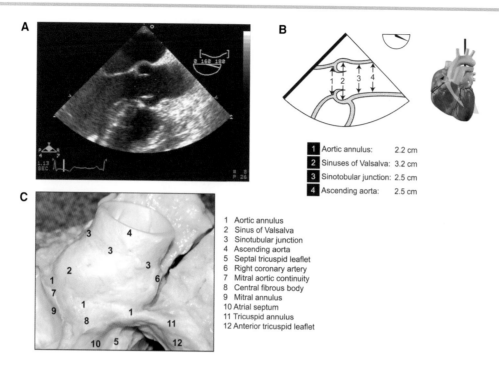

Figure 14.1   Aortic root anatomy. Mid-esophageal aortic valve long-axis view (**A,B**) of the aortic root with measurements obtained during systole compared with the anatomic specimen (**C**). *Source*: Photo C courtesy of Nicolas Dürrleman.

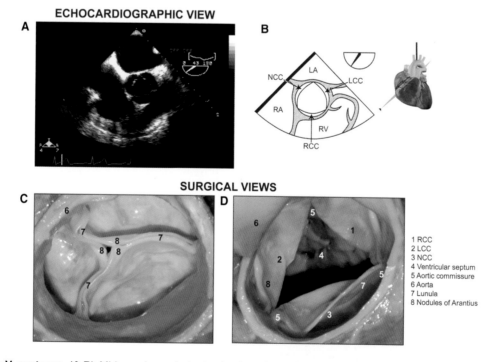

Figure 14.2   AoV anatomy. (A,B) Mid-esophageal short-axis view shows the AoV in systole compared with the anatomic view in diastole (**C**) and in systole (**D**). *Abbreviations*: AoV, aortic valve; LA, left atrium; LCC, left coronary cusp; NCC noncoronary cusp; RA, right atrium; RCC, right coronary cusp; RV, right ventricle. *Source*: Photos C and D courtesy of Nicolas Dürrleman.

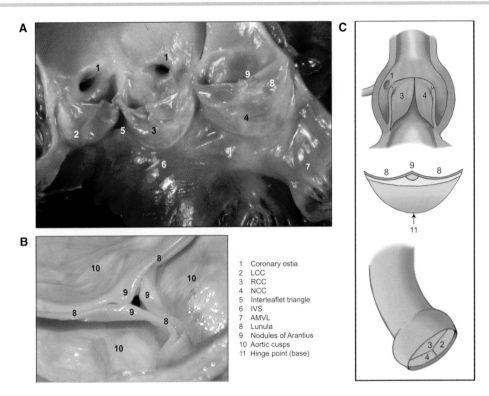

Figure 14.3   AoV anatomy. (A) Open view of the aortic root shows the aortic-mitral curtain which represents the fibrous continuity (intervalvular fibrosa) between the aortic root and the AMVL. **(B)** Anatomical aspect of the AoV shows the curvilinear attachment of each aortic cusp (10), the lunula (8), and the location of the nodules of Arantius (9) near the middle portion of each cusp edge. **(C)** Schematic representation of the AoV anatomy. *Abbreviations*: AMVL, anterior mitral valve leaflet; AoV, aortic valve; IVS, interventricular septum; LCC, left coronary cusp; NCC, noncoronary cusp; RCC, right coronary cusp. *Source*: Photo B courtesy of Nicolas Dürrleman and illustration C with permission, copyright Gian-Marco Busato.

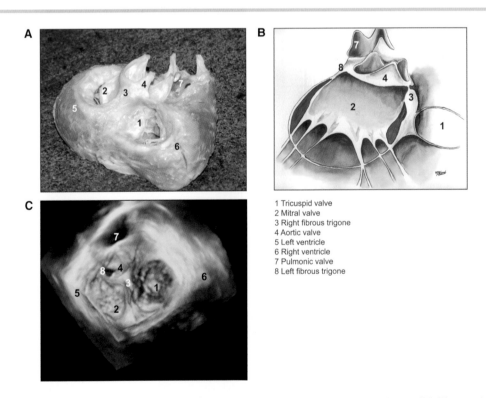

Figure 14.4   Fibrous skeleton. (A) Anatomic specimen showing the fibrous skeleton of the heart. **(B)** The aortic-mitral curtain is located between the right and left fibrous trigone. **(C)** Full volume 3D transesophageal echocardiographic image of the base of the heart shown from the atrial side. *Source*: Photo A courtesy of Dr Nicolas Dürrleman.

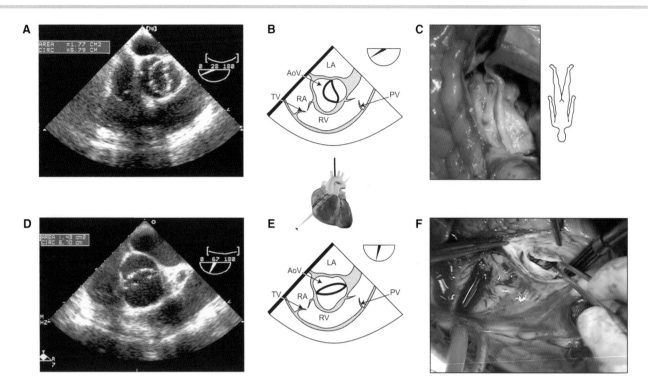

Figure 14.5 Bicuspid AoV. Mid-esophageal AoV short-axis views (**A,B,D,E**) and surgical examples (**C,F**), demonstrating an oval-shaped orifice orientated either vertically (**A–C**) or horizontally (**D–F**). *Abbreviations*: AoV, aortic valve; LA, left atrium; PV, pulmonic valve; RA, right atrium; RV, right ventricle; TV, tricuspid valve.

may be oriented in either a vertical or a horizontal position (Fig. 14.5). More commonly, a bicuspid valve will have one small cusp and a larger one with a raphe resulting from the failure of separation of two cusps. In approximately 80% of cases, the raphe will be observed between the right and the left coronary cusps, resulting in a smaller posterior and larger anterior cusp (Fig. 14.6). Fusion of the left and noncoronary cusps is rare. The rudimentary raphe observed in a bicuspid AoV predisposes the larger leaflet to restricted leaflet motion and premature calcification. In a short-axis (SAX) view, a bicuspid valve with a raphe between two cusps will have an eccentric opening in systole (nearer one of the aortic walls), while in diastole the valve may appear to have normal tricuspid morphology (Fig. 14.6). Therefore, echocardiographic evaluation of the AoV should be done in systole and in diastole. In a long-axis (LAX) view, a bicuspid AoV will have an asymmetric closure line and systolic doming may be observed. Systolic doming occurs when the AoV does not fully open and is most commonly associated with bicuspid AoVs but may also be observed with commissural fusion in rheumatic heart disease. A bicuspid AoV is bicommissural when the patient has three cusps, but two of them are fused with a raphe. When two equal cusps are seen without a raphe, the bicuspid valve is also described as unicommissural (Fig. 14.7). A unicuspid AoV may be acommissural or unicommissural: the latter has one commissure with only one attachment

point next to the aortic wall. The orifice is eccentric and usually tear-drop shaped, and although a raphe may be observed, the opening does not extend to the opposite aortic wall (Fig. 14.7). Quadricuspid AoVs occur in approximately 0.01% of the population and usually have four equal cusps symmetrically separated by an X-shaped commissure in diastole, but may also have asymmetric leaflets (Fig. 14.8). Unlike bicuspid and unicuspid AoVs where stenosis is the predominant pathology, quadricuspid AoVs tend to be associated with AR.

Echocardiographic Imaging of the AoV

The AoV can be imaged by inserting the transesophageal echocardiography (TEE) probe to a depth of approximately 35 cm from the upper incisors at the mid-esophageal level. With the transducer at 0°, a slightly off-axis longitudinal view of the AoV in a five-chamber view, at 45° (±15°) the AoV is in its SAX, and at 135° (±15°) the LAX views of the AoV will be obtained (Fig. 14.9).

The five-chamber view at 0° is not included in the American Society of Echocardiography/Society of Cardiovascular Anesthesiologists (ASE/SCA) comprehensive Perioperative TEE Assessment Guidelines but may occasionally prove useful in assessing AoV pathology. At 0°, the right and the noncoronary cusps of the AoV are usually imaged, but sometimes part of the left coronary cusp may be seen off-axis,

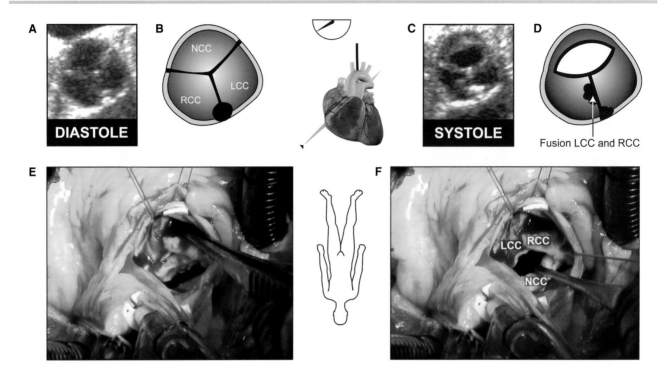

Figure 14.6 Bicuspid AoV. (**A–D**) Zoom of mid-esophageal AoV short-axis views of a bicuspid bi-commissural AoV with a raphe between the LCC and RCC. Note that in diastole (**A,B**) the raphe gives the impression that the AoV has three normal cusps. (**E,F**) In the surgical aortotomy view, the NCC is located posteriorly in the lower part, as opposed to the transesophageal echocardiographic view where it is seen on the upper part of the screen. *Abbreviations*: AoV, aortic valve; LCC, left coronary cusp, NCC, non-coronary cusp; RCC, right coronary cusp. *Source*: Photos E and F courtesy of Dr. Denis Bouchard.

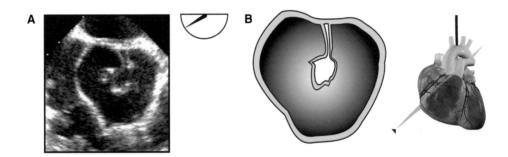

Figure 14.7 Unicuspid unicommissural AoV. (**A,B**) Mid-esophageal AoV short-axis view: the unicuspid AoV appearance has been likened to a shirt collar, toilet seat or tear drop. *Abbreviation*: AoV, aortic valve.

giving the appearance of a pseudomass in the LVOT (Fig. 14.10).

In the LAX view at 135°, the cusp furthest from the transducer next to the right ventricle (RV) is the right cusp, while the cusp closest to the transducer is either the left or the noncoronary cusp. Leftward (counterclockwise) rotation of the probe shaft in the LAX view will image the right ventricular outflow tract (RVOT), pulmonary artery (PA), left main coronary artery, and the left coronary cusp. Rightward (clockwise) rotation of the probe will bring the non-coronary cusp in view.

These three mid-esophageal TEE views can be used to assess the coaptation and the excursion of each cusp and to rule out the presence of either prolapse or decreased cusp mobility. The SAX view of the AoV is most useful to assess the morphology and can also be used for measuring the aortic valve area (AVA) by planimetry. Mid-esophageal views are particularly important to assess valvular, subvalvular, or aortic root pathology by two-dimensional (2D), M-mode, and color Doppler imaging. However, these views are not ideally suited for spectral pulsed wave (PW) or continuous wave (CW) Doppler interrogation

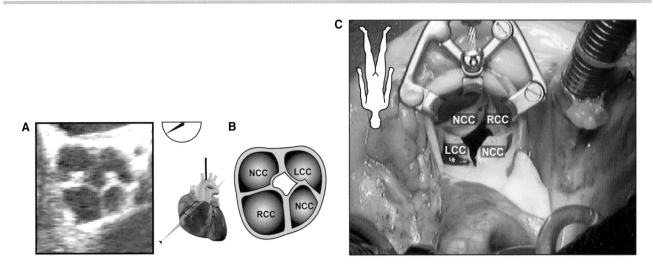

Figure 14.8 Quadracuspid AoV. (A,B) Zoomed mid-esophageal AoV short-axis view shows the lack of central coaptation of the quadracuspid AoV which results in a diamond shaped regurgitant orifice. **(C)** Intraoperative finding through the corresponding surgical aortotomy view. *Abbreviations*: AoV, aortic valve; LCC, left coronary cusp; NCC, non-coronary cusp; RCC, right coronary cusp. *Source*: Photo C courtesy of Raymond Cartier.

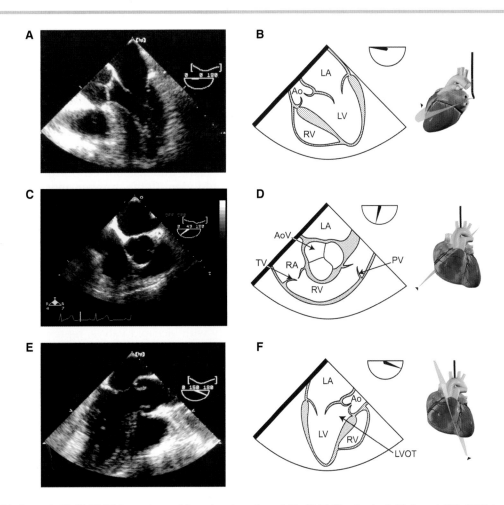

Figure 14.9 ME views AoV. (A,B) Mid-esophageal five-chamber view at 0°. **(C,D)** Short-axis AoV view at 45°. **(E,F)** Long-axis view at 135°. *Abbreviations*: Ao, aorta; AoV, aortic valve; LA, left atrium; LV, left ventricle; LVOT, left ventricular outflow tract; ME, mid-esophageal; PV, pulmonic valve; RA, right atrium; RV, right ventricle; TV, tricuspid valve.

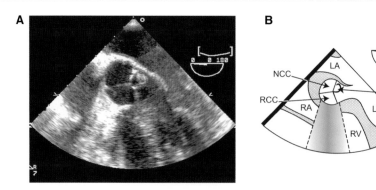

Figure 14.10 Five-chamber view. The off-axis five-chamber view at 0° of the aortic valve shows an oblique view of the LCC giving the appearance of a pseudomass in the left ventricular outflow tract. *Abbreviations*: LA, left atrium; LCC, left coronary cusp; LV, left ventricle; NCC, non-coronary cusp; RCC, right coronary cusp; RA, right atrium; RV, right ventricle.

of the AoV because the ultrasound beam is misaligned with the direction of aortic blood flow.

Transgastric imaging of the AoV provides complementary views to optimize spectral Doppler alignment (Fig. 14.11). With the probe positioned at the transgastric mid-papillary level, the transducer can be rotated from 0° to a LAX view of the AoV at 120° (±15°). A deeper transgastric view at 0°, with marked anteflexion of the TEE probe or light anteflexion from a more basal view at 0°, may also allow optimal spectral Doppler interrogation of the LVOT and AoV. The accuracy of Doppler flow velocity measurements will reach 94% if the angle between the direction of flow and the ultrasound beam does not exceed 20°.

AORTIC STENOSIS

Etiology of AS

Congenital and Acquired AoV Stenosis

The etiology of AS is either acquired or congenital. The most common etiology of congenital AS is a bicuspid AoV. Unicuspid and quadricuspid valves can also lead to AS. Most patients born with a bicuspid AoV will have a normal life span without pathological valvular deterioration, but symptomatic severe degenerative calcific AS usually occurs around 50 years of age.

Rheumatic and calcific degeneration are acquired etiologies of AS. Rheumatic involvement is characterized by thickening or fibrocalcification of the cusp edges, restricted mobility, and commissural fusion, resulting in a triangular systolic orifice (Fig. 14.12). The MV is frequently involved in rheumatic heart disease such that isolated rheumatic AoV disease is rare. Nonrheumatic AoV calcific degeneration is the commonest cause of AS in older adults as its incidence increases with age. It is characterized by calcification that usually starts from the annulus and extends into the body of the aortic cusps reducing cusp. Leaflet mobility becomes reduced, but there is usually no commissural fusion and the opening is stellate shaped as opposed to the elliptical opening observed with bicuspid AoV pathology (Fig. 14.12).

Patients with a three-cusped AoV will more often develop symptoms from severe AS around 70 years of age. Once moderate aortic stenosis is present, the average rate of progression is an increase in the mean pressure gradient of 7 mmHg per year, an increase in the jet velocity of 0.3 m/s/yr and a decrease in the AVA of 0.1 cm²/yr (1). Increased age, the presence of coronary artery disease, hypercholesterolemia, and renal disease are associated with a more rapid progression of AS. Although the progression of AS in patients with degenerative calcification tends to be faster than in rheumatic heart disease, it is difficult to predict the rate of progression in individual patients. Survival significantly decreases when left ventricular ejection fraction (LVEF) decreases to <45% to 50% or when the left ventricular end-systolic dimension (LVESD) exceeds 55 mm (1).

Two-dimensional echocardiographic evaluation should identify the number, morphology (thickening, calcification), and mobility (restriction) of the aortic cusps. Systolic doming occurs when the AoV does not fully open and is most commonly associated with bicuspid AoVs, but may also be observed with commissural fusion in rheumatic heart disease (Fig. 14.12). Senile calcification or AoV sclerosis may occur without stenosis. Indirect signs of significant AS include the presence of left ventricular (LV) hypertrophy (usually concentric). Poststenotic aortic root dilatation, particularly with bicuspid valves, represents an inherent aortopathy rather than a consequence of the altered hemodynamics from the AS (Fig. 14.13) (2,3). An association between bicuspid AoV disease and coarctation of the descending thoracic Ao has also been reported.

The continuous wave Doppler flow profile in mild AS will be characterized by an early peaking triangular-shaped velocity envelope. With more severe AS, the peak moves toward midsystole with a more rounded envelope, while in dynamic subaortic obstruction, the late peaking velocity envelope has a concave upward curve in early systole as described below (4).

Supra- and Subaortic Stenosis

Patients with a significant systolic gradient across the AoV should always be evaluated for evidence of

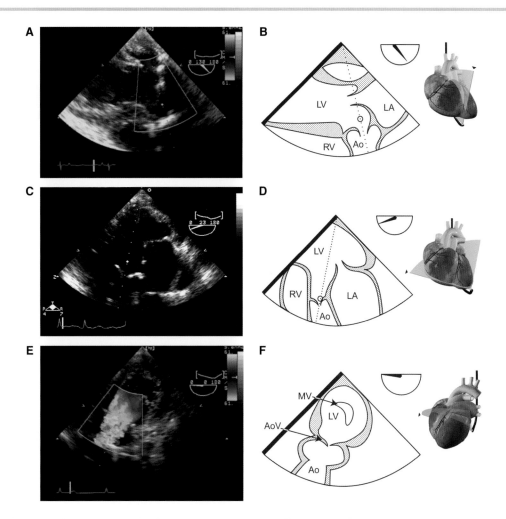

Figure 14.11 TG views of the AoV. (A,B) TG long-axis view at 130°. **(C,D)** Deep TG view at 29° with marked probe anteflexion. In those two views, note the longitudinal imaging of the MV. **(E,F)** Basal TG view of the AoV at 0° obtained by anteflexing the probe displays the MV in short axis. In all of these views, the aortic flow is aligned with the Doppler ultrasound beam. *Abbreviations*: Ao, aorta; AoV, aortic valve; LA, left atrium; LV, left ventricle; MV, mitral valve; RV, right ventricle; TG, transgastric.

supravalvular (Fig. 14.14) or subvalvular disease. While native supravalvular stenosis is uncommon, subvalvular stenosis (proximal to the AoV) may originate from dynamic obstruction or fixed structural abnormalities. Congenital causes of fixed subvalvular obstruction include the presence of a subaortic membrane (Fig. 14.15) or diaphragm and tunnel subvalvular stenosis.

Dynamic LVOT obstruction can occur with hypertrophic obstructive cardiomyopathy (HOCM), basal septal hypertrophy, and following MV repair (Fig. 14.16). In these conditions, the systolic gradient across the LVOT will increase with tachycardia, increased contractility, and decreased ventricular filling. The dynamic LVOT obstruction is associated with systolic anterior motion (SAM) of the MV, which is thought to result from either the "venturi" effect and/or drag forces (see Chapter 11). Significant septal contact of the anterior mitral leaflet indicates severe SAM (Fig. 14.16) and is usually associated with a posteriorly directed jet of mitral regurgitation (MR).

Unlike fixed AS, the peak systolic gradient occurs in late systole, giving a typical dagger-shaped appearance to the Doppler signal envelope (Fig. 14.16). As the obstruction increases in late systole, flow across the AoV decreases and premature closure of the AoV may be observed on 2D and M-mode imaging.

Quantitative Assessment of AS

Recent guidelines recommend the following primary hemodynamic parameters for clinical evaluation of AS severity: (*i*) jet velocity, (*ii*) mean transaortic gradient, and (*iii*) valve area by the continuity equation (4).

Jet Velocity

The maximum jet velocity is measured across the narrowed AoV orifice using CW Doppler alignment in the transgastric views. The gray scale is adjusted to obtain a smooth velocity curve with a dense outer edge and clear maximum velocity. In patients with an irregular rhythm,

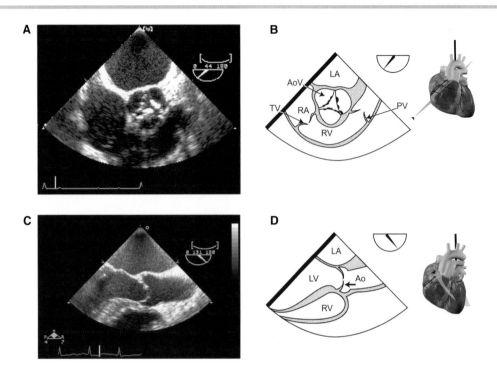

Figure 14.12   Aortic stenosis. (A,B) ME AoV short-axis view at 44° shows severe calcific non-rheumatic aortic stenosis with absence of commissural fusion of the AoV. **(C,D)** ME long-axis at 131° shows AoV systolic doming (arrow) and commissural fusion characteristic of rheumatic heart disease. *Abbreviations*: Ao, aorta; AoV, aortic valve; LA, left atrium; LV, left ventricle; ME, mid-esophageal; PV, pulmonic valve; RA, right atrium; RV, right ventricle; TV, tricuspid valve.

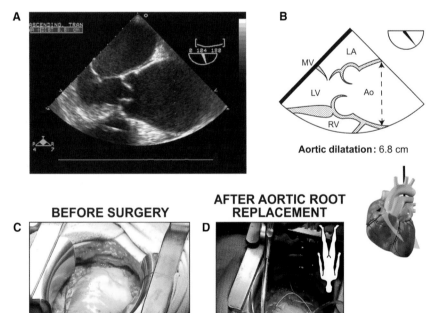

Figure 14.13   Bicuspid AoV stenosis and aortic aneurysm. (A,B) Mid-esophageal AoV long-axis view at 104° during systole shows restricted cusp opening and ascending aortic dilatation of 6.8 cm. **(C,D)** Intraoperative findings are shown before resection of the aortic aneurysm and after AoV and root replacement. *Abbreviations*: Ao, aorta; AoV, aortic valve; LA, left atrium; LV, left ventricle; MV mitral valve; RV, right ventricle. *Source*: Photos C and D courtesy of Dr. Michel Pellerin.

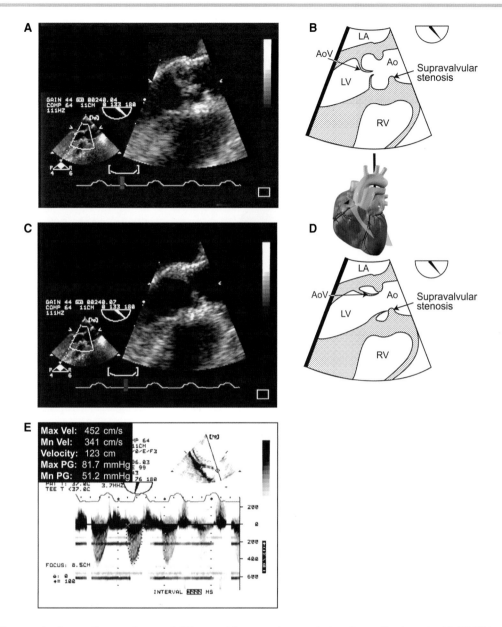

Figure 14.14   Supravalvular aortic membrane. A 25-year-old woman is operated on for aortic stenosis. (**A–D**) Mid-esophageal AoV long-axis view in diastole and systole showing normal aortic cusp opening but a stenosing membrane present 9 mm above the level of the AoV. (**E**) Continuous wave Doppler with 81.7mmHg Max and 51.2 mmHg Mn PG measured across the stenosing membrane. *Abbreviations*: Ao, aorta; AoV, aortic valve; LA, left atrium; LV, left ventricle; Max, maximal; Mn, mean; PG, pressure gradient; RV, right ventricle; Vel, velocity.

a minimum of five to eight consecutive beats should be recorded and averaged for measurement.

The flow velocity ratio (FVR), also known as the dimensionless index, is defined as follows:

$$FVR = \frac{V_{LVOT}}{V_{AoV}} \tag{14.1}$$

where V_{LVOT} is the flow velocity proximal to the stenosis in the LVOT and V_{AoV} is the maximal flow velocity distal to the obstruction in the vena contracta. The respective velocity-time integrals may alternatively be substituted for the peak velocities. The dimensionless index expresses the size of the valvular orifice area as a fraction of the LVOT area and thus removes the error related to LVOT measurement in the continuity equation. This index is less affected by variations in stroke volume and cardiac output. An FVR of ≤0.25 is consistent with severe AS and corresponds to a valve area that is 25% of normal (4). The FVR may prove particularly useful in the setting of low output–low gradient AS or AS in patients with a low ejection fraction.

Pressure Gradient

The Bernoulli equation. The measured blood flow velocity across cardiac valves can be converted

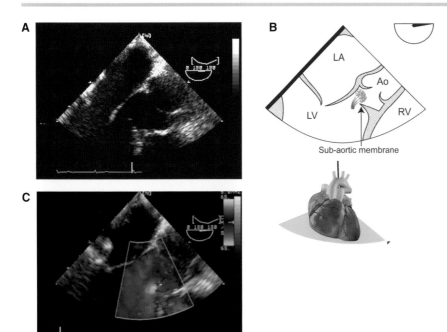

Figure 14.15 Subvalvular aortic membrane. (**A,B**) Mid-esophageal aortic valve long-axis view in a patient with a subaortic membrane is shown. (**C**) Only mild acceleration is seen at the level of the membrane. This was an incidental finding in a patient scheduled for coronary revascularization and was not associated with any significant gradient. *Abbreviations*: Ao, aorta; LA, left atrium; LV, left ventricle; RV, right ventricle.

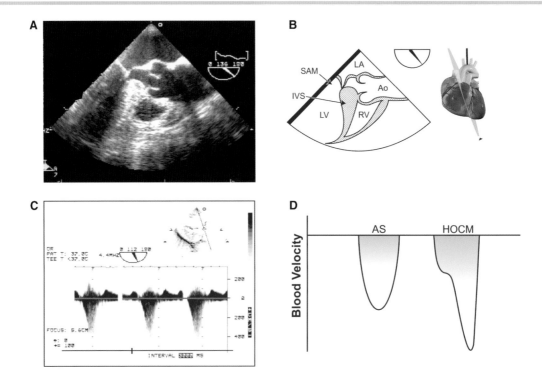

Figure 14.16   HOCM. (**A,B**) Mid-esophageal aortic valve long-axis view shows SAM and the septal contact of the anterior mitral valve leaflet in a patient with severe basal hypertrophy. SAM is often associated with a posteriorly directed jet of mitral regurgitation and significant LVOT obstruction and flow acceleration. Continuous wave Doppler interrogation of a patient with HOCM (**C**) compared with valvular AS. (**D**). Dynamic LVOT obstruction is characterized by a late peaking dagger-shaped velocity profile. *Abbreviations*: Ao, aorta; AS, aortic stenosis; HOCM, hypertrophic obstructive cardiomyopathy; IVS, interventricular septum; LA, left atrium; LV, left ventricle; LVOT, left ventricular outflow tract; RV, right ventricle; SAM, systolic anterior motion.

to a pressure gradient according to the Bernoulli equation. This equation takes into account flow acceleration, viscous friction, and convective acceleration using a complex mathematical formula (see equation 5.13). Flow acceleration and viscous friction have little impact on the pressure gradient and can be ignored in the calculations. Therefore, the modified Bernoulli equation only accounts for convective acceleration. In the modified Bernoulli equation, the pressure gradient (ΔP) measured with spectral Doppler across the AoV can be calculated as follows:

$$\Delta P = 4 \times \left(V_{AoV}^2 - V_{LVOT}^2 \right) \qquad (14.2)$$

where V_{AoV} is the maximal velocity measured by continuous wave Doppler and V_{LVOT} is the LVOT velocity measured by pulsed wave Doppler. In most cases, the square value of the V_{LVOT} velocity is insignificant compared with V_{AoV}, and the Bernoulli equation can be simplified to

$$\Delta P = 4 \times V_{AoV}^2 \qquad (14.3)$$

The ASE task force on Doppler quantifications recommends that the simplified Bernoulli equation should not be used when the LVOT velocity exceeds 1.5 m/s (11) or when the aortic velocity is <3.0 m/s (4). The aortic velocity jet that is used should be the highest velocity signal obtained from the interrogated echocar-diographic views, and lower maximum velocity signals should not be reported. Fine linear vertical noise signal artifacts at the peak of the curve should not be included in the tracing of the outer edge of the Doppler envelope (4). Note that the degree of underestimation will be 5% or less if the angle between blood flow and the ultra-sound beam is kept below 15° (4).

Doppler pressure gradient vs. cardiac catheterization. Doppler-derived measurements correspond to an instantaneous gradient, while the pull-back technique of the catheter from the Ao to the left ventricle (LV) during cardiac catheterization represents a peak-to-peak pressure difference. This explains, in part, why the measured peak-to-peak gradient in the catheterization laboratory is often lower than the instantaneous gradient obtained with Doppler echo-cardiography. However, the mean pressure gradient correctly measured by simultaneous pressure tracings from the LV, and the aortic root during cardiac catheterization, correlates well with the mean gradient obtained with Doppler echocardiography (Fig. 14.17).

Pitfalls of Pressure Gradient

Pressure recovery. Pressure recovery (PR) is the increase in pressure that occurs downstream from a stenosis due to reconversion of kinetic energy into potential energy (Fig. 14.18). Pressure recovery is an important phenomenon that may result in a measured

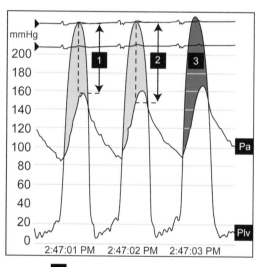

1 Peak to peak

2 Peak instantaneous

3 Mean gradient

Figure 14.17 Aortic valve gradients by catheterization. The peak-to-peak PG is measured between the peak Plv and the Pa, which may not be simultaneous in time, particularly with the delayed upstroke of the Pa (pulsus tardus). Doppler peak PG corresponds to the maximal instantaneous PG. The maximal instantaneous PG is higher than the peak-to-peak PG traditionally reported by cardiac catheterization. The Doppler mean PG corresponds to the surface between the Plv and Pa pressure (in dark grey). *Abbreviations*: Pa, arterial pressure; PG, pressure gradient; Plv, left ventricular pressure. *Source*: Courtesy of Dr. Philippe L.-L'Allier.

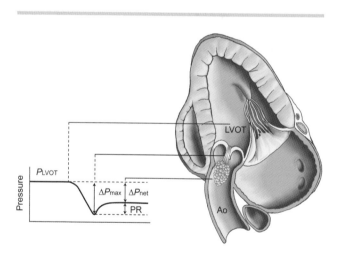

Figure 14.18 Pressure recovery. Deep-transgastric long-axis view is used to illustrate the concept of PR. Elevated pressure is recorded at the LVOT (P_{LVOT}). The pressure drops beyond the aortic stenosis. The maximal pressure difference ($\Delta Pmax$) is measured at the level of the VC and corresponds to the maximal pressure gradient measured by continuous wave Doppler. Further beyond the VC, the pressure partially increased back: if an invasive catheter pressure measurement is taken at this level, the recovered aortic pressure results in a lower measured pressure gradient compared to Doppler measurements. The pressure difference between the LVOT and the PR is the net transvalvular pressure ($\Delta Pnet$). *Abbreviations*: Ao, aorta; LVOT, left ventricular outflow tract; P, Pressure; PR, pressure recovery; VC, vena contracta. *Source*: Courtesy of Dr. Philippe Pibarot and illustration with permission, copyright Gian-Marco Busato.

Doppler mean systolic gradient that is 3 to 54 mmHg higher than the measured catheter gradient (7). Indeed, the Doppler measurement reflects the highest pressure gradient across the stenosis, or the difference between the highest proximal pressure and the lowest distal pressure, which occurs immediately downstream from the AoV at the vena contracta.

The measured Doppler gradient should correspond to the invasively measured gradient if the catheter is positioned at the level of the vena contracta. However, the catheter is frequently positioned in the ascending Ao rather than at the level of the vena contracta. This explains, in part, the discrepancy observed between Doppler- and catheter-derived pressure gradients across the AoV. The measured pressure gradient will progressively decrease over several centimeters as the catheter is withdrawn beyond the AoV and the pressure recovers in the ascending Ao. As most of the PR occurs in the first few centimeters, the catheter gradient is unlikely to be affected by PR if the downstream measurement is made at least 5 cm away from the stenotic valve in the ascending Ao.

The PR phenomenon distal to the AS is secondary to flow stream deceleration, with reduction in kinetic energy and conversion to potential energy (5). In severe aortic stenosis where there is abrupt widening from a small stenotic orifice to the larger ascending aorta, this conversion of kinetic to potential energy is less likely to occur because of unfavorable geometry and turbulence (4). Pressure recovery is greatest when there is gradual widening of a stenosis since turbulence is reduced. Therefore, PR is related to the ratio of the stenotic area to the cross-sectional area of the ascending aorta and can be calculated using the following formula (4):

$$PR = 4v^2 \times \frac{2AVA}{AoA} \times \frac{1-AVA}{AoA} \qquad (14.4)$$

where v is the velocity across the AoV, AVA is the effective orifice area of the aortic valve calculated from the continuity equation, and AoA is the cross-sectional area of the ascending aorta. At present, this correction is not used routinely in most echocardiography laboratories. Given the small EOA in AS, the PR is only clinically relevant when the diameter of the Ao is <3 cm in a patient with at least moderate AS (6–9). When the Ao is <3 cm^2, the initial Doppler measured pressure drop between the LV and vena contracta may be higher than the actual pressure drop across the stenotic valve.

In patients with an eccentric jet across a stenotic AoV, VanAuker et al. (10) have demonstrated, using a computational model, that for a constant anatomic area, the effective valve area decreased, the maximal pressure gradient increased, and the distance to complete PR increased with the degree of jet eccentricity.

Mitral regurgitation. Improper alignment of the Doppler signal may result in the inadvertent measurement of the MR pressure gradient instead of the AoV pressure gradient. This is more likely to occur when the jet of MR is directed anteriorly toward the wall of the LA beneath the Ao. It is, therefore, important to differentiate the characteristics of these two Doppler signals. The MR jet starts earlier with MV closure at the onset of the isovolumic contraction period compared with the AS signal that begins after the isovolumic contraction phase. The MR jet also lasts longer and ends later at the start of the mitral inflow early E velocity. The MR and AS signals may also be differentiated by the diastolic company they keep: the MR signal will be accompanied by a mitral inflow signal (with E and A waves), while the aortic signal may be associated with a typical AR signal (Fig. 14.19).

The presence of MV disease can be a confounding factor in the evaluation of AS. MR severity does not affect the calculation of valve area but may result in a low gradient even if severe AS is present. Similarly

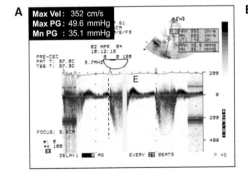
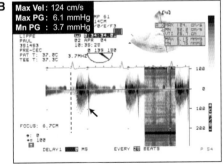

Figure 14.19 MR and aortic Doppler signal. The timing during continuous wave Doppler trace shows the difference between MR and possible aortic stenosis in a 61-year-old man. **(A)** The MR Doppler signal was obtained from a deep transgastric long-axis view and yielded a mean PG of 35.1 mmHg. The MR Doppler signal begins with the QRS of the electrocardiogram during the isovolumic contraction period. **(B)** The Doppler signal from the aortic outflow starts later after the QRS following the isovolumic contraction period. Note also the closure click observed with aortic sclerosis (arrow) in this patient. *Abbreviations*: E, peak early diastolic TMF velocity; Max, maximum; Mn, mean; MR, mitral regurgitation; PG, pressure gradient; TMF, transmitral flow; Vel, velocity.

severe mitral stenosis (MS) may be associated with a low cardiac output (CO) and low-flow gradient (4).

Pressure gradient in high- and low-output state. The measurement of aortic pressure gradient will overestimate the severity of AS in high-output states such as liver failure, anemia, hemodialysis, or sepsis. Conversely, in low-output states with cardiac decompensation, the ventricle may be unable to generate a significant gradient even if the AS is critical. Since blood flow is proportional to the square of the pressure gradient, a small increase in blood flow will translate into a more significant change in the measured pressure gradient.

Pressure gradient in patients with AR. Approximately 80% of patients with AS will also have AR. In patients with mild or moderate AR, measurement of AS severity is usually not significantly affected. However, in patients with severe AR, there will be a high transaortic volume flow; the peak and mean gradient across the AoV may, therefore, be higher than expected for a given AVA (4).

Pressure gradient in patients with LVH and hypertension. Patients with AS and hypertension will often have associated left ventricular hypertrophy (LVH). The presence of LVH may be associated with diastolic dysfunction and a small left ventricle. This may result in a smaller stroke volume (SV) with a lower than expected gradient for a given AVA. Approximately 35% to 45% of patients with AS will also have hypertension (4). An increase in LV pressure load with hypertension may result in a decreased ventricular function and blood flow across the AoV. Uncontrolled hypertension may, therefore, cause changes in flow and gradients but should not affect the measurement of the AVA (4).

Pitfall of the simplified Bernoulli equation. Software from echocardiography systems uses the simplified Bernoulli equation to measure pressure gradients and assumes V_1 (velocity in the LVOT) to be negligible in the calculation. However, when subaortic LVOT velocities are increased, this assumption is no longer valid. The ASE task force on Doppler quantifications recommends that a V_1 value >1.5 m/s must be included in the calculations for the Bernoulli equation (11). The European and ASE also recommend that V_1 should also be included when the aortic peak velocity is <3.0 m/s (4). This will usually occur in patients with subaortic obstruction as seen in HOCM, severe basal septal hypertrophy, or hyperdynamic states in the pediatric patient (e.g., sepsis, stress, severe anemia, hyperthyroidism, and so on). Finally, significant AR may also result in a large SV and increased V_1. In those situations, software from most echocardiographic systems can be reprogrammed to include V_1 in the calculation of pressure gradients.

Pressure gradient and serial stenosis. In patients with dynamic LVOT obstruction and SAM, it is difficult to determine the proportion of the pressure gradient that is attributable to the obstruction at the valvular versus the subvalvular level (e.g., HOCM). Planimetry of the AVA by 2D imaging may help identify the degree of stenosis at the valve level in this situation. Measurement of V_1 proximal to the AoV

and distal to the subvalvular obstruction may reflect turbulent flow distal to an obstruction and invalidate the Bernoulli equation.

Aortic Valve Area

Two-dimensional measurement of AVA. A normal AVA measures 3.0 to 4.0 cm^2. The AVA is commonly measured with planimetry tracing of the AoV orifice in the mid-esophageal SAX view during systole (Fig. 14.20) (12). It is important to advance and withdraw the TEE probe to identify the level with the smallest AoV opening. Overestimation of AVA can occur if planimetry tracing is performed with an oblique plane, above or below the most stenotic level of the AoV (Fig. 14.20). As stenotic valves open and close more slowly than normal valves and remain maximally opened for a shorter period of time, the maximal rather than the mean planimetered area should be used as it corresponds more closely to the mean Doppler-derived measurements (13).

The Doppler-derived EOA is smaller than the anatomic planimetered AVA. The EOA, not the anatomic AVA, is the primary predictor of clinical outcome. Planimetry may be an acceptable alternative when Doppler estimation of flow velocities is unreliable (4).

In the measurement of volumetric flow across a three-cusped nonstenotic AoV, the shape of an equilateral triangle can be used for the measurement of AVA. Although the orifice of the AoV varies throughout systole and resembles more a circle than a triangle when fully opened, the area of an isosceles triangle is considered to represent the average nonstenotic AVA during systole. The measurement of the average AVA can be used for volumetric flow calculation (Fig. 14.21). The area of an isosceles triangle can easily be calculated by measuring the distance between two commissures (L) and applying the following formula:

$$\text{Area} = 0.433 \times L^2 \tag{14.5}$$

Doppler-derived measurement of AVA: the continuity equation. Doppler-derived measurements of the AVA are usually performed using the continuity equation. This is based on the principle that flow across the LVOT must equal flow across the AoV. The ASE task force on Doppler quantification recommends that the measurement of blood flow velocity in the LVOT should be performed with the PW Doppler sample volume positioned approximately 5 mm beneath the AoV (11). However, in patients with aortic stenosis, it is recommended to initially position the sample volume 1 cm proximal to the aortic valve and to gradually move the sample volume toward the aortic valve until spectral broadening. Once spectral broadening occurs, the sample volume is moved back until a narrow band of velocities is obtained (4). Maximum blood flow velocity across the AoV can then be obtained with CW Doppler.

Measurement of the AVA using the continuity equation and peak velocities is obtained through the following formulas:

$$\text{Flow} = \text{area}(\text{cm}^2) \times \text{velocity}(\text{cm/s}) = \text{cm}^3/\text{s}$$

$$\text{Flow LVOT} = \text{Flow AoV} \tag{14.6}$$

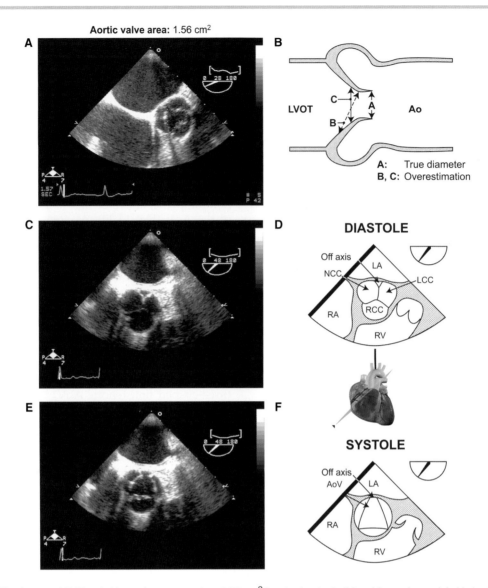

Aortic valve area: 1.56 cm^2

A: True diameter
B, C: Overestimation

Figure 14.20 Planimetry. (A) The AoV area is measured as 1.56 cm^2 by planimetry in this mid-esophageal AoV short-axis view at 28°. **(B)** In aortic stenosis overestimation of the AoV area can occur if the measurement plane is below or oblique to the most stenotic portion of the valve. **(C–F)** In another patient there is separation at the base of the commissure (12 o'clock) between the LCC and the NCC, indicating the imaging plane is suboptimally aligned with the true short axis of the AoV. Planimetry of the orifice during systole from this view would overestimate the AoV area. *Abbreviations*: Ao, aorta; AoV, aortic valve; LA, left atrium; LCC, left coronary cusp; LVOT, left ventricular outflow tract; NCC, non-coronary cusp; RA, right atrium; RCC, right coronary cusp; RV, right ventricle.

$$\text{Area}_{\text{LVOT}} \times V_{\text{LVOT}} = \text{Area}_{\text{AoV}} \times V_{\text{AoV}}$$

$$\text{AVA} = \text{Area}_{\text{LVOT}} \times \frac{V_{\text{LVOT}}}{V_{\text{AoV}}}$$

$$= \frac{\pi r^2 \times V_{\text{LVOT}}}{V_{\text{AoV}}}$$

$$= \frac{\pi (d_{\text{LVOT}}^2 / 4) \times V_{\text{LVOT}}}{V_{\text{AoV}}}$$

$$\text{AVA} = \frac{0.785\, d_{\text{LVOT}}^2 \times V_{\text{LVOT}}}{V_{\text{AoV}}} \qquad (14.7)$$

Measurement of the AVA can also be performed using the volumetric principle in the continuity equation by substituting the velocity measurement (cm/s) with the measurement of the velocity-time integral (VTI):

$$\text{Area}_{\text{LVOT}} \times \text{VTI}_{\text{LVOT}} = \text{Area}_{\text{AoV}} \times V_{\text{AoV}}$$

$$\text{AVA} = \frac{0.785\, d_{\text{LVOT}}^2 \times \text{VTI}_{\text{LVOT}}}{\text{VTI}_{\text{AoV}}} \qquad (14.8)$$

A difference of 0.2 cm^2 in the measurement of the AVA using either technique is not uncommon.

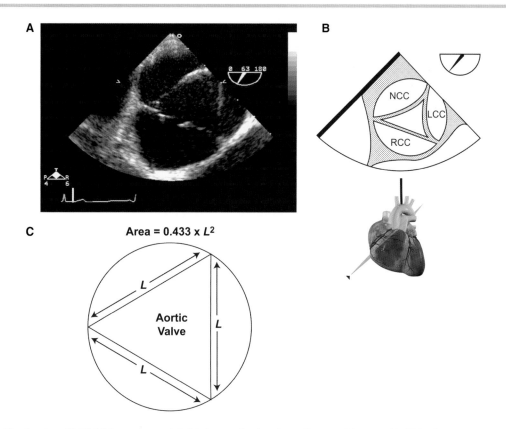

Figure 14.21 Planimetry. (A,B) Mid-esophageal AoV short-axis view in a 42-year-old man with Ehler-Danlos disease shown during systole; the area of the equilateral triangle (**C**) represents the average AoV area. *Abbreviations*: AoV, aortic valve; L, length; LCC, left coronary cusp; NCC, non-coronary cusp; RCC, right coronary cusp.

A rapid way to estimate the AVA in the operating room in a patient with a pulmonary catheter is to use the calculated thermodilution-derived SV instead of the LVOT-derived SV (Fig. 14.22). However, this introduces two additional potential sources of error. First, it uses a different algorithm and timing than the Doppler-derived measurement of SV. Moreover, Doppler insonation angulation errors would normally affect measurements of V (or TVI) of both LVOT and AoV rather similarly. When using the thermodilution-derived SV, the Doppler insonation angulation errors of the AoV would not be offset by that of the LVOT (replaced by the thermodilution value), adding another source of variability in the calculation of AVA.

Despite these limitations, the use of the thermodilution-derived SV in the continuity equation remains useful to validate the calculated AVA obtained by Doppler-derived measurement of SV across the LVOT (14). A significant discrepancy between the two AVA measurements may reveal mismeasurement of thermodilution-derived SV or the LVOT diameter, as well as misalignment of the ultrasound beam or malposition of the Doppler sample volume in the LVOT. The presence of spectral broadening may indicate that the sample volume is positioned too close to the AoV in the area of proximal acceleration. In this scenario, measurement of V_1 will be overestimated. Conversely, V_1 will be underestimated if the Doppler sample volume is positioned too far from the AoV.

The European Association of Echocardiography and the ASE recommend that the LVOT measurement in the continuity equation should be made in the location where PW Doppler sampling is obtained and not immediately below the AoV as described below for sizing of prosthesis (4). Measurement of the LVOT should be performed in an LAX view from the inner edge of the anterior mitral leaflet to the inner edge of the septal endocardium in mid-systole in a plane that is parallel to the AoV and within 0.5 to 1.0 cm of the AoV orifice (Fig. 14.1). It should be remembered that the LVOT becomes more elliptical in many patients, which may underestimate the CSA of the LVOT (4). It is also important to ensure that the measurement of the LVOT is perpendicular and not oblique. Adequate visualization of symmetrical leaflet separation and symmetrical sinuses of Valsalva in a longitudinal view of the AoV should improve the accuracy of the LVOT measurement. Diameter measurements are also more likely to be accurate in the zoom function and may decrease measurement variability.

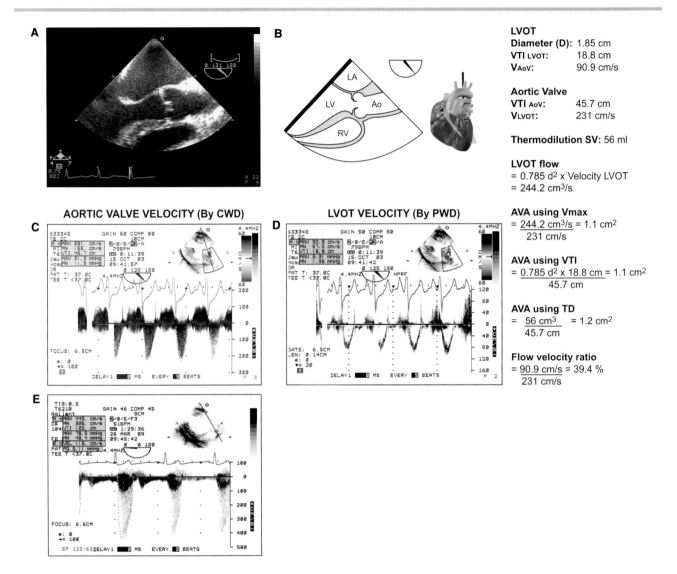

LVOT
Diameter (D): 1.85 cm
VTI LVOT: 18.8 cm
V AoV: 90.9 cm/s

Aortic Valve
VTI AoV: 45.7 cm
V LVOT: 231 cm/s

Thermodilution SV: 56 ml

LVOT flow
= 0.785 d² x Velocity LVOT
= 244.2 cm³/s

AVA using Vmax
$$= \frac{244.2 \text{ cm}^3/s}{231 \text{ cm/s}} = 1.1 \text{ cm}^2$$

AVA using VTI
$$= \frac{0.785 \text{ d}^2 \times 18.8 \text{ cm}}{45.7 \text{ cm}} = 1.1 \text{ cm}^2$$

AVA using TD
$$= \frac{56 \text{ cm}^3}{45.7 \text{ cm}} = 1.2 \text{ cm}^2$$

Flow velocity ratio
$$= \frac{90.9 \text{ cm/s}}{231 \text{ cm/s}} = 39.4 \text{ \%}$$

AORTIC VALVE VELOCITY (By CWD)

LVOT VELOCITY (By PWD)

Figure 14.22 Various methods for calculation of AVA. (A,B) Mid-esophageal AoV long-axis view of the LVOT in a 71-year-old woman with aortic stenosis. **(C)** Max aortic velocity across the AoV, obtained by CWD **(D)** LVOT velocity obtained by PWD. On the right, the AVA is calculated using either the LVOT flow velocity, TVI or the stroke volume derived from TD. **(E)** Example of CWD double envelope technique in a patient with severe aortic stenosis: the darker lower-velocity envelope is used for LVOT and the fainter higher-velocity envelope is used for AoV velocity. The flow velocity (dimensionless) ratio is 25.5%, consistent with severe aortic stenosis. *Abbreviations*: Ao, aorta; AoV, aortic valve; AS, aortic stenosis; AVA, aortic valve area; CWD, continuous wave Doppler; d, diameter; LA, left atrium; LV, left ventricle; LVOT, left ventricular outflow tract; Max, maximum; PWD, pulsed wave Doppler; RV, right ventricle; SV, stroke volume; TD, thermodilution; V_{max}, maximum velocity; VTI, velocity-time integral.

In the measurement of LVOT diameter for selecting the size of a homograft or prosthesis, the use of an LAX view is often preferred. Extreme care must be taken to ensure that the measurement of the LVOT diameter is made from the base of the right cusp insertion to the base of the opposite cusp insertion. The measurement is from the base of the right cusp insertion on interventricular septum to the base of the opposite cusp insertion at the junction of the anterior MV leaflet (4). Adequate visualization of both symmetrical leaflet separation and sinuses of Valsalva in this view should improve the accuracy of the LVOT measurement.

As this measurement is squared, a small error will be magnified in the calculation of the AVA. In a study by Harpaz et al. (15), the end-diastolic measurement of the LVOT was a more accurate predictor of AoV prosthetic size than the end-systolic measurement (16). However, the author believes that either the end-diastolic or the early systolic measurement (Fig. 14.23) correlates well with the intraoperative surgical measurement of the LVOT.

AVA and the double envelope technique. Flow velocity in the LVOT and across the AoV are both represented with CW Doppler when the spectral Doppler tracing depicts, simultaneously, two distinct

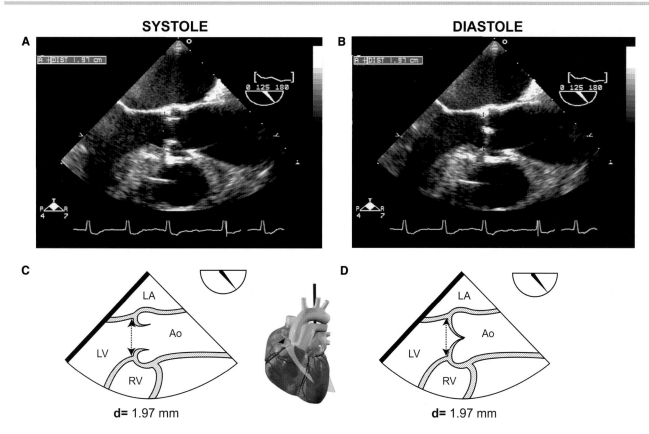

Figure 14.23   LVOT diameter. Measurement of LVOT diameter (d) at the aortic annulus in early systole (**A,B**) and end-diastole (**C,D**) is shown in these mid-esophageal aortic valve long-axis views at 125°. No significant difference is noted. By convention it is measured at end-diastole. *Abbreviations*: Ao, aorta; LA, left atrium; LV, left ventricle; LVOT, left ventricular outflow tract; RV, right ventricle.

and superimposed Doppler signals (double envelope) (17,18). The lower-velocity envelope represents flow in the LVOT, and the "lighter" high-velocity envelope represents flow across the AoV. Either velocity or VTI can be used for each of the two envelopes in the calculation of AVA in the continuity equation. The double envelope is not always visible, but when present, it is an accurate and rapid method to measure flow in the LVOT and across a stenotic AoV. The double envelope technique is especially useful when the hemodynamic conditions fluctuate because of arrhythmias, or during surgical manipulation of the heart, as it ensures that the measurement of flow across the LVOT and AoV is obtained simultaneously with the same SV volume.

AVA: planimetry vs. the continuity equation. Measurement of the AVA using the Gorlin formula during cardiac catheterization correlates well with the measurements obtained with either TEE planimetry or the continuity equation by transthoracic echocardiography (TTE) (19). Although some authors have stated that these three methods may be used interchangeably, others have found that TEE planimetry overestimates the AVA measured by the other two methods (20). This apparent discrepancy may be

explained by other studies where the correlation between TEE planimetry and Doppler measurement was dependent on the amount of valvular calcification (Table 14.1). In a study by Cormier et al. (12), the hemodynamic and echocardiographic correlation in the estimation of the AVA in patients with milder grade 1 or 2 AoV calcification was good as opposed to those with more abundant grade 3 or 4 calcifications where a poor correlation between these two measurement techniques was observed.

AVA and blood flow. Changes in flow may affect the measurement of the AVA. In a study by Tardif et al. (21), patients with moderate or severe AS, acute changes in SV and CO, did not result in significant changes in the TEE measurement of AVA by planimetry. In a subsequent study, Tardif et al. (22) compared

Table 14.1   Aortic Valve Calcification

Grade 1	No calcification
Grade 2	Small isolated calcification spots
Grade 3	Multiple larger calcification spots interfering with cusp motion
Grade 4	Extensive calcifications of all cusps with restricted cusp motion

simultaneous determination of the AVA by the Gorlin formula and by TEE under different transvalvular flow conditions. While the CO increased by 42% and the mean pressure gradient across a stenotic AoV increased by 54% during dobutamine infusion, the AVA by TEE planimetry did not change. However, using the Gorlin formula, there was a difference of 0.44 cm² between calculations made under minimal flow versus maximal flow (22). This study suggests that the Gorlin calculation of the AVA has disproportionate flow dependence and that the measured increase in area with this technique does not correlate with a true widening of the orifice.

Pitfalls in the measurement of AVA.

Pseudo-AS   In patients with low CO and pressure gradient across the AoV, blood flow may be insufficient to fully mobilize and open the AoV cusps. This low-flow/low-gradient AS is defined by an LVEF <40%, a calculated AVA <1.0 cm², and a mean transvalvular pressure gradient <30 to 40 mmHg (4,23).

This dilemma can be resolved by performing repeat measurements with a higher cardiac output and stroke volume under a dobutamine intravenous infusion. Dobutamine stress hemodynamics (DSH) can help distinguish between patients with severe AS causing LV systolic function and patients with moderate AS with another cause of LV dysfunction. DSH has the potential to stratify operative risk in low-flow/low-gradient AS. Patients without contractile reserve on DSH, defined by an increase in ejection fraction or SV of <20% compared with baseline values, have a high operative mortality (32%) compared with patients with contractile reserve (5%) (24).

Several criteria have been proposed in the literature to differentiate truly severe AS from pseudo-AS. In true AS, the following would be observed: a peak DSH mean gradient >40 mmHg, a peak DSH AVA <1.0 cm², and an increase in AVA <0.3 cm² (4).

Recently Blais et al. (25) proposed the use of a new parameter, the projected EOA (EOA$_{proj}$) at normal transvalvular flow rate (250 mL/s), to better differentiate truly severe and pseudo-severe AS during dobutamine stress echocardiography. This projected EOA is obtained after plotting EOA against transvalvular flow (Q) at each dobutamine stage. Valve compliance (VC) is derived as the slope of the regression line fitted to the EOA versus Q plot. The EOA$_{proj}$ is calculated as

$$EOA_{proj} = EOA_{rest} + VC \times (250 - Q_{rest}) \qquad (14.9)$$

where EOA$_{rest}$ and Q_{rest} are the EOA and Q at rest. An indexed EOA$_{proj}$ <0.55 cm²/m² was found to be the best criterion to discriminate truly severe from pseudo-severe AS.

M-mode   Aortic stenosis is characterized by decreased aortic leaflet excursion in systole. The M-mode can be used to measure aortic cusp separation in the evaluation of AS. This measurement may, however, significantly overestimate or underestimate the severity of AS if the valve is bicuspid, or when asymmetric leaflet separation occurs (Fig. 14.24). This is, therefore, not very useful in the quantification of AS.

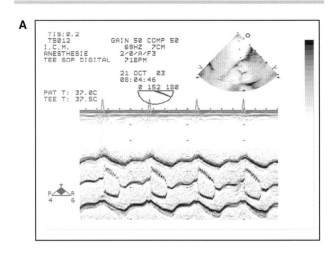

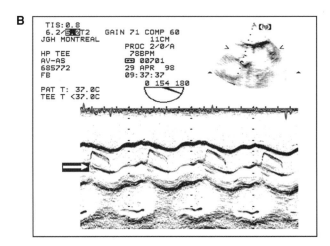

Figure 14.24   M-mode. Mid-esophageal AoV long-axis M-mode views of a normal AoV (**A**) compared to a patient with an immobile right coronary cusp (arrow) and opposing aortic cusp with preserved mobility (**B**). *Abbreviation*: AoV, aortic valve.

Grading AS

Measurement of the transvalvular gradient and the AVA (by either planimetry and/or the continuity equation) is the most commonly used and validated method to quantify the severity of AS with echocardiography. Table 14.2 summarizes the classification of AS. No single calculated number should be relied upon as many patients have a discrepancy in stenosis severity based on maximal velocity (mean gradient) and calculated valve area. To resolve any discrepancy, it is important to confirm the accurate measurements obtained and assess LV function and the presence of AR, as outlined in Table 14.3. Clinical outcome is based primarily on the use of Doppler velocity data. Therefore, cardiac catheterization is not recommended and is only indicated when there is discrepancy with clinical data or when echocardiography is nondiagnostic (4).

Table 14.2 Aortic Valve Stenosis Classification

Aortic valve	Normal	Mild stenosis	Moderate stenosis	Severe stenosis
AVA (cm^2)	3.0–4.0	>1.5	1.0–1.5	<1.0
Indexed AVA (cm^2/m^2)		>0.85	0.6–0.85	<0.6
Aortic jet velocity (m/s)	≤2.5	2.6–2.9	3.0–4.0	>4.0
Flow velocity ratio		>0.50	0.25–0.50	<0.25
Mean gradient (mmHg)		<20[a] <30[b]	20–40[a] 30–50[a]	>40[a] >50[b]

[a]American Heart Association and American College of Cardiology.
[b]European Society of Cardiology.
Abbreviation: AVA, aortic valve area.
Source: Adapted from Ref. 4.

Table 14.3 Resolution of Apparent Discrepancies in Measures of AS Severity

A. When AS velocity >4 m/s and AVA >1.0 cm^2
  1. Check LVOT diameter measurement and compare with previous studies
  2. Check LVOT velocity signal for flow acceleration
  3. Calculate indexed AVA when
     a. Height is <135 cm (5'5")
     b. BSA <1.5 m^2
     c. BMI <22 (equivalent to 55 kg or 120 lb at this height)
  4. Evaluate AR severity
  5. Evaluate for high cardiac output
     a. LVOT stroke volume
     b. 2D LV EF and stroke volume
Likely causes: high-output state, moderate-to-severe AR, large body size

B. AS velocity ≤4 m/s and AVA ≤1.0 cm^2
  1. Check LVOT diameter measurement and compare with previous studies[a]
  2. Check LVOT velocity signal for distance from valve
  3. Calculate indexed AVA when
     a. Height is <135 cm (5'5")
     b. BSA <1.5 m^2
     c. BMI <22 (equivalent to 55 kg or 120 lb at this height)
  4. Evaluate for low transaortic flow volume
     a. LVOT stroke volume
     b. 2D LV EF and stroke volume
     c. MR severity
     d. Mitral stenosis
  5. When EF <55%
     a. Assess degree of valve calcification
     b. Consider dobutamine stress echocardiography
Likely causes: low cardiac output, small body size, severe MR

Abbreviations: AR, aortic regurgitation; AS, aortic stenosis; AVA, aortic valve area; BMI, body mass index; BSA, body surface area; EF, ejection fraction; LV, left ventricular; LVOT, left ventricular outflow tract; MR, mitral regurgitation.
Source: Adapted from Ref. 4.

AORTIC REGURGITATION

Etiology of AR

Aortic regurgitation may be caused by aortic root dilatation, dissection, or intrinsic cusp pathology. Recently, El Khoury et al. (26,27) described a functional classification of AR (Table 14.4) that addresses most of the pathological aspects of leaking AoVs (Fig. 14.25). Like Carpentier's classification of MV diseases, this AR functional classification primarily focuses on the mech-

Table 14.4 Surgical and TEE Classification of Aortic Regurgitant Lesion

Type 1	Enlargement of the aortic root with normal cusps
Type 2	Cusp prolapse or fenestration
Type 3	Poor cusp tissue quality or quantity

Abbreviation: TEE, transesophageal echocardiography.
Source: Adapted from Refs. 26,27.

anisms of valve dysfunction and helps the surgeon in choosing the most appropriate surgical technique to restore normal valve physiology. Furthermore, the functional anatomy of AR, defined by TEE, is strongly and independently predictive of valve repairability and postoperative outcome (27). In this classification, the AoV is no longer considered isolated but is a part of a functional entity that comprises the sinuses of Valsalva, the AoV cusps, the commissures, and the interleaflet triangles (28).

Type 1 dysfunction is identified as dilatation of any components of the aortic root, including the AoV annulus, the sinuses of Valsalva, and the STJ, typically with normal AoV cusps. Type 1a AR occurs in patients with a dilated ascending Ao when enlargement of the STJ causes outward displacement of the commissures (Fig. 14.26). Isolated dilatation of the ascending Ao not involving the aortic root is not considered as a plausible mechanism of AR. In type 1b (Fig. 14.25) AR is associated with aortic root dilation. Aortic root disease leading to dilatation and AoV regurgitation includes Marfan's syndrome, Ehlers–Danlos' syndrome (Fig. 14.27), and aortitis. Patients with a bicuspid AoV also have abnormal elastic properties in the Ao leading to dilatation of the aortic root even if there is no AS and the AR is only mild or trivial. Type 1c is associated with isolated dilatation of the functional aortic annulus (FAA), which includes superiorly the STJ and inferiorly the aorto-ventricular junction (AVJ). Type 1c is usually present in association with other pathologies. Type 1d is observed when dilation of the FAA is associated with leaflet perforation. In type 1 AR, TEE analysis in the LAX view shows reduced coaptation length and central AR parallel to the LVOT (Fig. 14.26).

Type 2 dysfunction occurs in the presence of an eccentric AR jet from either a cusp prolapse or a cusp fenestration. Fenestration of a cusp-free edge occurs in the presence of an eccentric AR jet but no definite evidence of cusp prolapse (Fig. 14.28). Careful inspection

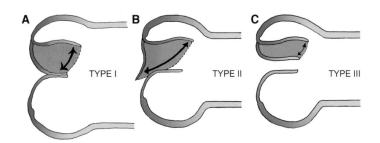

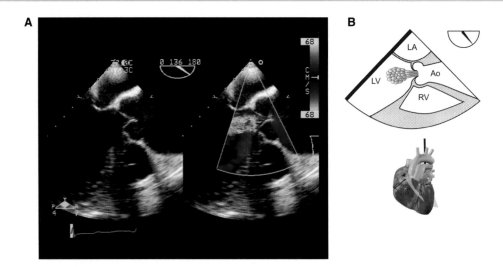

EL KHOURY FUNCTIONAL CLASSIFICATION			
	TYPE I (a-d)	TYPE II	TYPE III
Cusp Motion	Normal	Excessive	Restricted
AR Direction	Central	Eccentric	Central or Eccentric
Etiology	a) Dilated ascending aorta and STJ b) Dilated aotic root c) Dilated aortic annulus d) Dilated aortic annulus and cusp perforation	a) Prolapse b) Flail c) Fenestration	a) Commissural fusion b) Calcification

Figure 14.25 El Khoury's functional classification of AR. This classification is based on the opening and closing motion of the aortic cusps. (**A**) Type 1 has normal cusp motion and AR is on the basis of cusp perforation or annular dilatation. (**B**) In type II dysfunction (excessive cusp motion) the free edge of the cusp travels below the plane of the aortic annulus during diastole. (**C**) Type III dysfunction implies restricted cusp opening during systole and diastole. *Abbreviations*: Ao, aorta; AR, aortic regurgitation; STJ, sinotubular junction. *Sources*: Adapted from Ref. 26. Illustrations courtesy of Gian-Marco Busato.

Figure 14.26 Type I AR: dilated ascending Ao and STJ. (A,B) Mid-esophageal aortic valve long-axis view at 136°: the STJ and ascending Ao are enlarged. *Abbreviations*: Ao, aorta; AR, aortic regurgitation; LA, left atrium; LV, left ventricle; RV, right ventricle; STJ, sinotubular junction. ⌐

of LAX gray scale and color Doppler images usually allow identification of small defects near the free edge of the affected cusp. Cusp prolapse is present whenever the free edge of one or more AoV cusps overrides the plane of the aortic annulus. As in MV prolapse, the resulting regurgitant jet is eccentric and directed in the opposite direction to the pathological cusp: a prolapse of the right coronary cusp will give rise to a jet directed posteriorly (Fig. 14.29), while a prolapse of any of the posterior cusps will cause a jet directed anteriorly (Fig. 14.30). In this case, the SAX analysis of the AV will help distinguish between a prolapse of either the left or the noncoronary cusp (Fig. 14.30).

Cusp prolapse can be categorized into three subtypes: cusp flail, partial cusp prolapse, and whole cusp prolapse. Cusp flail is defined as the complete eversion

of a cusp into the LVOT and is best imaged in a LAX view (Fig. 14.29). Partial cusp prolapse is considered whenever the distal part of a cusp prolapses into the LVOT. This is usually associated with a clear bending of the cusp body visible both in the LAX and SAX views (Fig. 14.32), and with the presence of a small circular or oval structure near the cusp free edge on SAX view. Whole cusp prolapse is considered each time the free edge of a cusp clearly overrides the plane of the aortic annulus, the entire body of the cusp billowing into the LVOT. This billowing can be appreciated as a circular structure in the SAX view of the LVOT, immediately below the valve (Fig. 14.31). Partial cusp prolapse is more subtle and often presents as a bend in the cusp causing malcoaptation (Fig. 14.32).

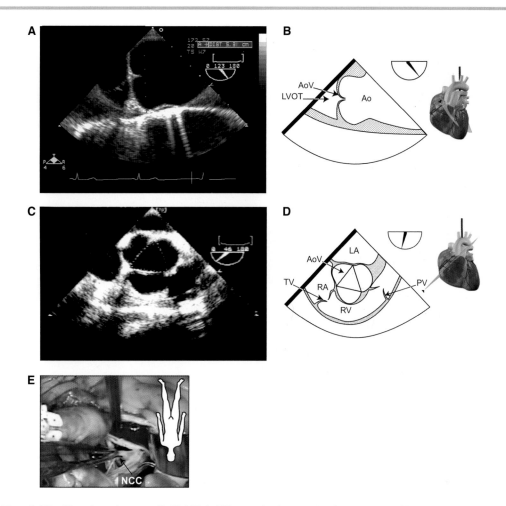

Figure 14.27   Type I AR: dilated aortic root. (A,B) ME AoV long-axis view at 123° in a 42-year-old man with Ehler-Danlos disease: the aortic root measures 53 mm at the level of the sinuses of Valsalva. **(C,D)** ME AoV short-axis view at 46° in a patient shows a dilated aortic root from enlarged sinuses of Valsalva: the aortic cusps are stretched, with decreased central coaptation. Any further dilatation would result in increased AR. **(E)** Intraoperative finding in a 70-year-old man with the same pathology and a NCC fenestration. *Abbreviations*: Ao, aorta; AoV, aortic valve; AR, aortic regurgitation. LA, left atrium; LVOT, left ventricular outflow tract; ME, mid-esophageal; NCC, non-coronary cusp; PV, pulmonic valve; RA, right atrium; RV, right ventricle; TV, tricuspid valve. *Source*: Photo E courtesy of Dr. Michel Pellerin.

The type 3 AR is defined by poor cusp tissue quality with decreased cusp mobility, resulting in poor coaptation. Intrinsic cusp pathology is either congenital or can be acquired with connective tissue disorders, rheumatic heart disease, degenerative calcification, or infective endocarditis. Type 3 AR is usually central and, because the valve is stiffer, originates higher in the sinuses of Valsalva. The valve is thickened, more echogenic (Fig. 14.33), sometimes presenting calcifications and fused commissures. Reduced valve opening with cusp doming can be present as curving toward the midline of the Ao during systole. Subacute bacterial endocarditis may cause cusp destruction, perforation, or tear causing various degrees of AR (Fig. 14.34). Periaortic abscess must be excluded in these patients (Fig. 14.35). In such complex cases, the new technology of live 3D TEE may help localize the exact abnormalities (Fig. 14.34).

As AR may result from multiple causes, it is essential to perform a complete and systematic TEE examination of the AoV and ascending Ao. Moreover, a precise echocardiographic analysis of the cusps is important to determine valve reparability. Some authors have proposed a grading of aortic calcifications (29) (Table 14.1). AoV repair often seems more feasible in moderately calcified valves (< grade 3) and when calcifications are confined to the free margins instead of involving the cusp body. Some TEE factors associated with better chance of bicuspid AoV repair are the presence of an eccentric jet (type II, cusp prolapse) and the absence of cusp thickening, calcification, or commissural thickening (30,31). All types of AR mechanisms can be observed when dealing with bicuspid AoVs.

The AR seen during aortic dissection may have been preexisting if previous annuloaortic ectasia and/or dilatation of the STJ were present (see Chapter 23). However, AR during aortic dissection most often results from disruption of the cusp geometry when the intimal flap itself prolapses across the AoV or when the cusp insertion between the

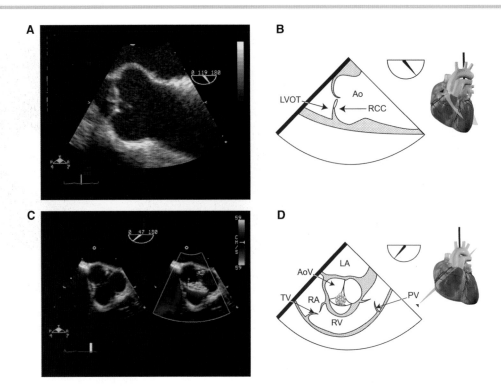

Figure 14.28   Type II AR: AoV fenestration. A patient with a fenestration near the free edge of the RCC is seen in the mid-esophageal AoV long-axis view at 119° (**A,B**) and short-axis view at 47° (**C,D**). *Abbreviations*: Ao, aorta; AoV, aortic valve; AR, aortic regurgitation; LA, left atrium; LVOT, left ventricular outflow tract; PV, pulmonic valve; RA, right atrium; RCC, right coronary cusp; RV, right ventricle; TV, tricuspid valve.

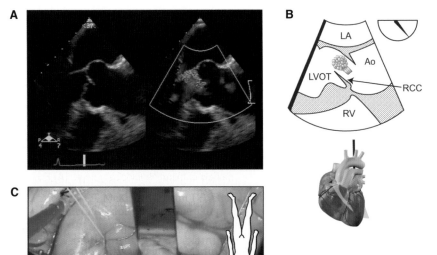

Figure 14.29   Type II AR: AoV flail. (A,B) Mid-esophageal AoV long-axis view: the AR jet is eccentric and directed toward the anterior mitral valve leaflet. (**C**) Intraoperative findings. *Abbreviations*: Ao, aorta; AoV, aortic valve; AR, aortic regurgitation; LA, left atrium; LVOT, left ventricular outflow tract; NCC, noncoronary cusp; RCC, right coronary cusp; RV, right ventricle. *Source*: Photo C courtesy of Dr. Pierre Pagé.

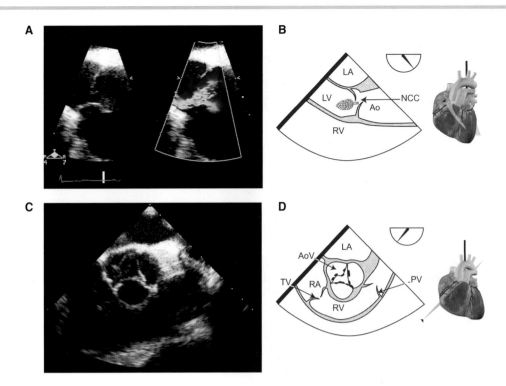

Figure 14.30 **Type II AR: AoV prolapse. (A,B)** ME AoV long-axis view in a man with a whole cusp prolapse of one of the posterior AoV cusps; the AR jet is directed towards the ventricular septum. **(C,D)** In this case the ME AoV short-axis view is necessary to see that the diseased cusp is the NCC. *Abbreviations*: Ao, aorta; AoV, aortic valve; AR, aortic regurgitation; LA, left atrium; LV, left ventricle; ME, mid-esophageal; NCC, non-coronary; PV, pulmonic valve; RA, right atrium; RV, right ventricle; TV, tricuspid valve.

STJ and the aortic annulus is involved by the dissection (32).

When the AR jet is eccentrically directed toward the base of the anterior mitral leaflet, diastolic fluttering of the anterior mitral leaflet may be seen on 2D imaging or with M-mode (Fig. 14.36). When it is directed toward the ventricular septum, it may cause aneurysmal lesions of this wall (Fig. 14.37). Significant AR can cause relative MS in late diastole corresponding clinically to the Austin–Flint murmur. Other clues suggesting significant AR include increased aortic systolic expansion (Corrigan pulse), a restrictive mitral inflow pattern, a left ventricular end-systolic diameter >55 mm, and reverse diastolic doming of the MV. In patients with severely elevated left ventricular end-diastolic pressure (LVEDP), diastolic MR, premature closure of the MV, and early AoV opening may be observed. Late diastolic MR is a better predictor of severe AR than either M-mode demonstration of premature MV closure or early AoV opening.

Quantification of AR

Jet Height/LVOT Height

Color Doppler imaging can be used to quantify the severity of AR. The ratio of jet height to LVOT diameter measured immediately below the cusps in the TEE LAX view at 120° to 150° (or five-chamber view at 0°) correlates well with the severity of AR and is a good predictor of the angiographic grade. In mild AR, the jet height is less than one-third of the LVOT diameter, while this ratio exceeds two-thirds in severe AR (Fig. 14.38) (33,34). Occasionally, this method may overestimate the true severity of AR when the imaging plane happens to be aligned with a narrow jet of AR, spanning most of the commissural closure line as may be observed in the bicuspid AoV with a vertical commissure. Likewise, the severity of AR could be underestimated if the imaging plane is tangential to a narrow regurgitant jet. In patients with an eccentric regurgitant jet, the measurement of jet height should be done perpendicular to the axis of the jet direction. In a TTE study by Evangelista et al. (35), jet eccentricity decreased correlation with angiographic grade by underestimating the severity of AR. The jet width (height) was defined as the smallest diameter of the jet at the junction of the LVOT and the aortic annulus in the parasternal LAX view. In that study, the jet width corresponded better with the angiographic grade of AR than the ratio of jet height to LVOT height. However, in several echocardiography laboratories, the ratio of jet height to LVOT diameter remains one of the most commonly used measurements to assess the severity of AR in spite of its limitations.

SAX Jet Area/LVOT Area

The ratio of the regurgitant jet area to the LVOT area in the SAX view immediately below the AoV can be used to estimate the severity of AR with color Doppler

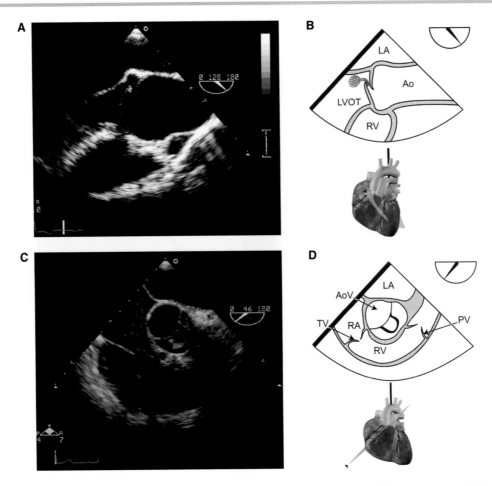

Figure 14.31   Type II AR: AoV prolapse. Prolapse of a whole cusp in a bicuspid AoV. **(A,B)** Mid-esophageal AoV long-axis view: the free edge of the anterior cusp overrides the plane of the aortic annulus with the entire body of the cusp billowing into the LVOT. **(C,D)** Mid-esophageal AoV SAX view: The billowing appears as a circular structure. *Abbreviations*: Ao, aorta; AoV, aortic valve; AR, aortic regurgitation; LA, left atrium; LV, left ventricle; LVOT, left ventricular outflow tract; PV, pulmonic valve; RA, right atrium; RV, right ventricle; SAX, short-axis; TV, tricuspid valve.

imaging. It is essential that this measurement is made high in the LVOT, where part of the AoV is still visualized to ensure that the jet is truly measured at its origin. This measurement was slightly more predictive of AR severity by angiography than jet height to LVOT height (35). It is, however, the opinion of the author that this measurement often underestimates the severity of AR.

Flow Reversal

On PW Doppler examination of the proximal descending thoracic Ao, mild early diastolic flow reversal is often observed in normal patients but this flow reversal usually has a low velocity and a short duration. However, the presence of holodiastolic flow reversal on PW Doppler examination of the descending thoracic Ao is indicative of severe AR (Fig. 14.39) (36). This finding proves particularly useful in assessing AR when the regurgitant jet is eccentric and more difficult to quantify at the valve level. Some authors recommend measuring flow reversal in the proximal aortic arch using an upper esophageal aortic arch LAX view. Although Doppler alignment will be relatively parallel to blood

flow in this view, measurement of diastolic flow reversal is more commonly performed in the descending thoracic aorta with TTE and should be more indicative of significant AR because Doppler sampling is positioned further downstream from the AoV. The further flow reversal is detected in the descending thoracic aorta or in the abdominal aorta, the more severe the AI. Intraoperative TEE measurement of flow reversal in the proximal descending thoracic aorta can be easily obtained with TEE. Although the Doppler angle obtained with TEE will be closer to 45° in the descending thoracic aorta, the VTI ratio of forward flow to diastolic flow reversal should remain constant because the effect of angulation will affect forward and reverse flow equally. As AI severity increases, the ratio of diastolic flow to forward flow will increase. During TTE assessment of diastolic flow reversal in the descending thoracic aorta, an initial velocity ≥0.6 m/s and an end diastolic velocity ≥0.2 m/s is indicative of severe AR (36). Flow reversal VTI >20 cm is also associated with severe AR. Color M-mode Doppler interrogation of the proximal descending thoracic Ao

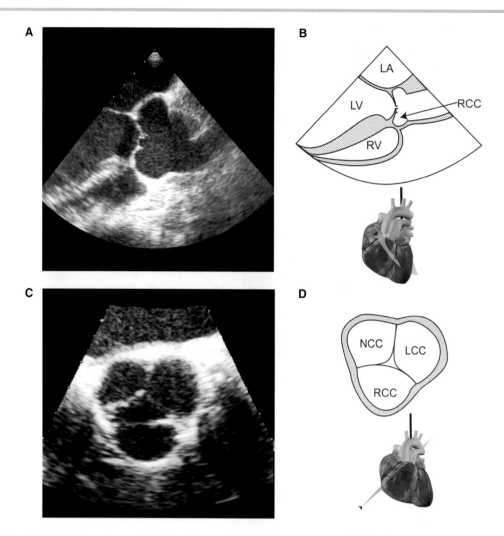

Figure 14.32 Type II AR: AoV prolapse. Partial prolapse of the right coronary cusp (RCC) observed on a mid-esophageal AoV long-axis (**A,B**) and short-axis (**C,D**) views. *Abbreviations*: AoV, aortic valve; AR, aortic regurgitation; LCC, left coronary cusp; LA, left atrium; LV, left ventricle; NCC, non-coronary cusp; RCC, right coronary cusp; RV, right ventricle.

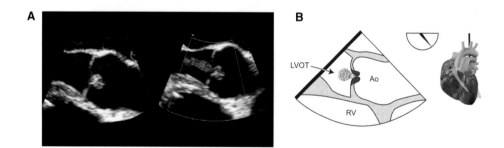

Figure 14.33 Type III AR. (**A,B**) Mid-esophageal long-axis view. The cusps are thickened and more echogenic without calcification. *Abbreviations*: AR, aortic regurgitation; LVOT, left ventricular outflow tract; RV, right ventricle.

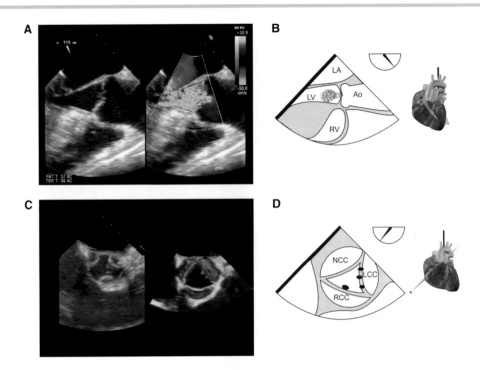

Figure 14.34 Type III aortic regurgitation from endocarditis. (A,B) Mid-esophageal AoV long-axis view. **(C,D)** 2D and 3D AoV short-axis views of a destroyed LCC due to endocarditis. *Abbreviations*: Ao, aorta; AoV, aortic valve; LA, left atrium; LV, left ventricle; LCC, left coronary cusp; NCC, non-coronary cusp; RCC, right coronary cusp; RV, right ventricle.

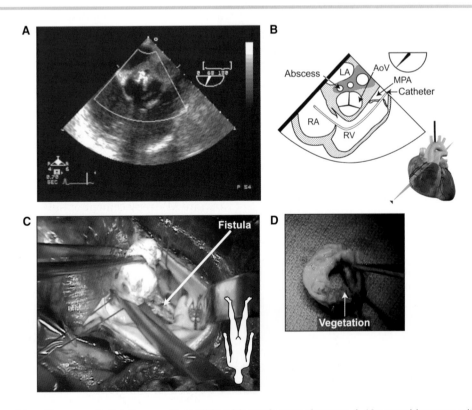

Figure 14.35 Type III aortic regurgitation from endocarditis with aortic root abscess. A 46-year-old woman with a bicuspid AoV is diagnosed with endocarditis. A posterior abscess with a fistula was diagnosed from this mid-esophageal AoV short-axis view **(A,B)** and confirmed intraoperatively **(C,D)**. *Abbreviations*: AoV, aortic valve; LA, left atrium; MPA, main pulmonary artery; RA, right atrium; RV, right ventricle. *Source*: Photos C and D courtesy of Dr Michel Pellerin.

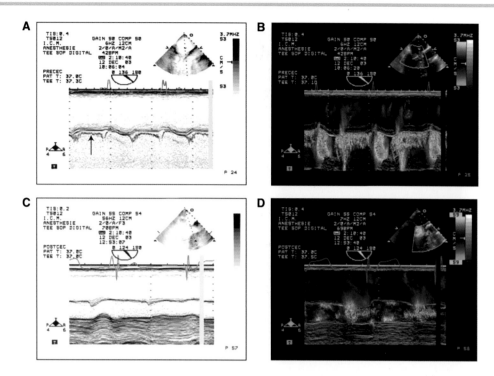

Figure 14.36 MV fluttering from AR. Severe AR with anterior mitral valve leaflet fluttering in a 56-year-old man. (**A,C**) M-mode from a mid-esophageal aortic valve long-axis view before (**A**) and after AVR (**C**). Note the disappearance of the anterior leaflet fluttering (arrow) after intervention. (**B,D**) Corresponding color M-mode with significant AR before (**B**) and trivial AR (**D**) after AVR. *Abbreviations*: Ao, aorta; AR, aortic regurgitation; AVR, aortic valve replacement; MV, mitral valve.

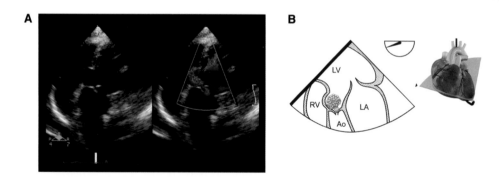

Figure 14.37 IVS pseudoaneurysm. IVS pseudoaneurysm as a secondary lesion from an eccentric regurgitant jet in a patient with a bicuspid aortic valve and posterior cusp prolapse. (**A,B**) Deep transgastric long-axis view. *Abbreviations*: Ao, aorta; IVS, interventricular septum; LA, left atrium; LV, left ventricle; RV, right ventricle.

can also be used to assess pandiastolic flow reversal as seen in Figure 14.39.

Regurgitant Fraction

The measured flow across a regurgitant cardiac valve is increased as it includes not only the effective forward SV but also the regurgitant volume. Thus, the difference in measured SV across a competent valve (the effective forward flow) and the SV across the incompetent valve represents the regurgitant volume (see Fig. 5.36). The regurgitant fraction (RF) is the ratio of the regurgitant volume over the SV across the regurgitant valve. For AR, the forward flow across the AoV is compared with the diastolic volumetric flow across the MV, provided the MV is competent.

$$\text{Ao regurgitant volume} = \text{SV}_{\text{LVOT}} - \text{SV}_{\text{MV}}$$

$$\text{Ao regurgitant fraction} = \frac{\text{SV}_{\text{LVOT}} - \text{SV}_{\text{MV}}}{\text{SV}_{\text{LVOT}}}$$

$$(14.10)$$

The stroke volume across the LVOT (SV_{LVOT}) is measured by Doppler volumetric method (Fig. 14.12) and

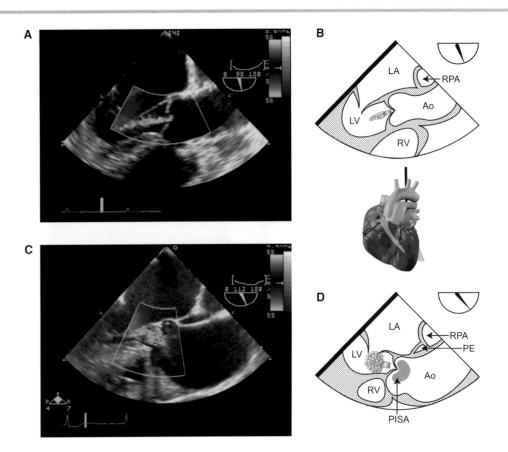

Figure 14.38   Aortic regurgitation. (A,B) Color Doppler mid-esophageal AoV long-axis view at 98° in a patient with mild AR: the width of the regurgitant jet immediately below the AoV is less then one-third of the LVOT diameter. **(C,D)** Same view at 112° in a different patient: the width of the AR jet is as wide as the LVOT diameter, consistent with severe AR. Note also the hemisphere of PISA on the aortic side of the anatomic regurgitant orifice and the dilated ascending Ao. *Abbreviations*: Ao, aorta; AoV, aortic valve; AR, aortic regurgitation; LA, left atrium; LV, left ventricle; LVOT, left ventricular outflow tract; PE, pericardial effusion; PISA, proximal isovelocity surface area; RPA, right pulmonary artery; RV, right ventricle.

the stroke volume across the competent mitral valve (SV_{MV}) is obtained with the same Doppler volumetric method with the following particularities. First, the mitral annular cross-sectional area (CSA) requires the measurement of the diameter at the annulus in both the mid-esophageal four- and two-chamber views (d_{4ch} and d_{2ch}) using the formula of an ellipse:

$$\text{MV annular CSA} = \frac{\pi(d_{4ch} \times d_{2ch})}{4} \qquad (14.11)$$

The volumetric flow across the MV is then obtained by positioning the PW Doppler sample volume at the level of the mitral annulus (not at the tip of the leaflets, as seen in the assessment of diastolic function) and tracing the VTI by using the modal velocity, that is, the brightest signal of the envelope (rather than the maximal velocity at the outer edge of the envelope). The product of mitral inflow VTI (cm) and mitral annular area (cm²) yields the mitral diastolic SV (cm³ or mL) (see equation 5.46). Alternatively, flow across any other competent valve could also be used, although it is more difficult to align the spectral

Doppler ultrasound beam properly with the direction of tricuspid or pulmonic flow by TEE.

Pitfalls of RF. The measurement of RF is not usually done by anesthesiologists in the operating room because it is time consuming and may distract from patient care and monitoring. Moreover, the measurement of the SV across the MV and the AoV should be done under the same hemodynamic conditions. Therefore, as these measurements are obtained sequentially rather than simultaneously, rapid transient changes occurring during anesthesia and/or surgery may affect the validity of the obtained RF.

Another important source of error originates from the measurement of the mitral annulus and LVOT diameter. A small error in the measurement of these diameters is magnified to its square value in the calculation of the CSA for the measurement of the volumetric flow rate.

Measurement of the aortic regurgitant volume is also critically influenced by misalignment of the PW Doppler sample volume. Doppler angulation exceeding 20° between the ultrasound beam and the direction of flow will yield a value lower than the true forward aortic SV and consequently a lower aortic

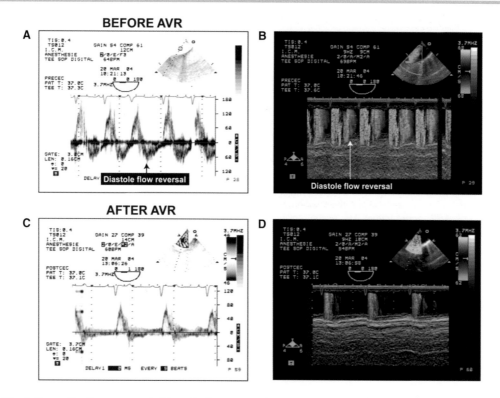

Figure 14.39 Diastolic aortic flow reversal. Diastolic flow reversal in the distal ascending aorta in a 78-year-old man with severe aortic regurgitation due to endocarditis. Diastolic flow reversal is shown using pulsed wave Doppler (**A**) and color M-mode (**B**) interrogation of the ascending aorta prior to surgery which disappears after AVR (**C,D**). *Abbreviation*: AVR, aortic valve replacement.

regurgitant volume. Overestimation of the effective forward SV at the MV will also result in a smaller aortic regurgitant volume. This may occur when the sample volume is located at the tip of the mitral leaflets rather than at the level of the mitral annulus. Sampling at the leaflet tips may also incur contamination of the mitral inflow signal with the AR jet, which would further underestimate the aortic RF. Conversely, the aortic forward SV and corresponding aortic regurgitant volume will be overestimated if the sampling volume is positioned too close to the AoV in the flow acceleration zone. Even with careful attention to these pitfalls, an RF of 20% has been calculated in normal subjects, making this measurement less reliable than it may appear to be (11,34).

Effective Regurgitant Orifice

The effective regurgitant orifice (ERO) area provides a quantitative assessment of the severity of AR. The following methods can be used to calculate the ERO.

ERO measurement with 2D planimetry. Planimetry of the end-diastolic gap between the aortic cusps with TEE measures the anatomic regurgitant orifice area that has been shown to correlate with TTE measurements and angiographic grading of the AR (Fig. 14.40) (37).

ERO measurement with the PISA method. The proximal isovelocity surface area (PISA) method is based on the principle of conservation of mass (see Chapter 5). Although it is more commonly used in the

quantification of MR, it has also been validated in the assessment of the AR (38). From the transgastric views (Fig. 14.41), the AR jet is directed toward the transducer during diastole, forming hemispheric shells of isovelocity above the valve, coded in progressively lighter shades of red until the velocity exceeds the Nyquist limit and changes to shades of blue. The aliasing velocity of the hemispheric shell where the color switches from red to blue is given by the Nyquist limit, indicated on the color scale (38 cm/s in Fig. 14.41). The surface of the hemispheric shell is calculated from its radius with the formula $2\pi r^2$. The aliasing velocity at the radius of the hemispheric shell (v_r) and its surface area are used to calculate the flow rate of the regurgitant lesion. By continuity equation, this is equal to the flow rate at the minimal regurgitant orifice, where the aortic regurgitant velocity reaches its maximum velocity $(V_{AR\,max})$ during early diastole and can be measured by CW Doppler across the AoV (Fig. 14.41). Thus, the continuity equation using PISA and ERO flow rate will give an estimate of the aortic regurgitation (AR) area as follows:

$$\text{Flow} = \text{area}(\text{cm}^2) \times \text{velocity}(\text{cm/s}) = \text{cm}^3/\text{s}$$

$$\text{AR flow rate} = \text{PISA flow rate}$$

$$\text{ERO}_{AR} \times V_{AR\,max} = \text{PISA} \times V_r \tag{14.12}$$

$$\text{ERO}_{AR} = \frac{2\pi r^2 \times V_r}{V_{AR\,max}} \tag{14.13}$$

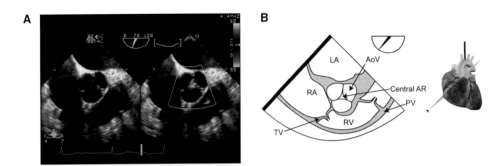

Figure 14.40 ERO area. ERO assessment by 2D planimetry in a patient with central AR. (**A,B**) Mid-esophageal AoV short-axis view at 70°. The anatomical ERO area is seen on two-dimensional imaging (left split screen) and with color flow imaging (right split screen). *Abbreviations*: Ao, aorta; AoV, aortic valve; AR, aortic regurgitation; ERO, effective regurgitant orifice; LA, left atrium; PV, pulmonic valve; RA, right atrium; RV, right ventricle; TV, tricuspid valve.

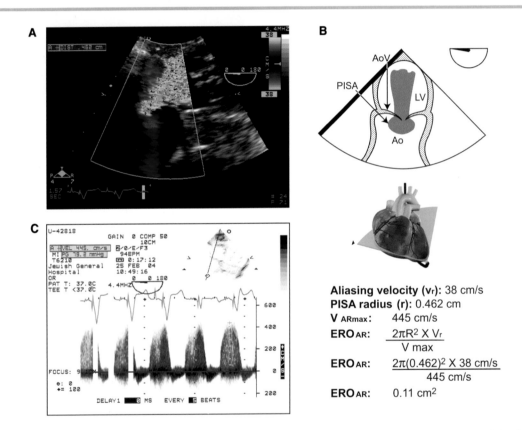

Aliasing velocity (v$_r$): 38 cm/s
PISA radius (r): 0.462 cm
V$_{ARmax}$:   445 cm/s
ERO$_{AR}$: $\dfrac{2\pi R^2 \times V_r}{V\,max}$
ERO$_{AR}$: $\dfrac{2\pi(0.462)^2 \times 38\ cm/s}{445\ cm/s}$
ERO$_{AR}$:   0.11 cm^2

Figure 14.41 PISA. ERO calculation by PISA method. (**A,B**) Color Doppler basal transgastric longitudinal view of the AoV shows the PISA on the aortic side of the AoV with the aliasing velocity (v$_r$) set at 38 cm/s (Nyquist limit). (**C**) Continuous wave Doppler tracing of the aortic regurgitant jet: the maximal aortic regurgitant velocity (V$_{AR\ max}$) was 445 cm/s. This corresponds to a peak transvalvular gradient of 79 mmHg during early diastole. The ERO can be calculated from these values and is consistent with mild-to-moderate. *Abbreviations*: Ao, aorta; AoV, aortic valve; AR, aortic regurgitation; ERO, effective regurgitant orifice; LV, left ventricle; PISA, proximal isovelocity surface area; V$_{max}$, maximal velocity.

The radius of the hemisphere is easier to measure using a magnified view and a lower Nyquist limit to create a larger hemisphere. In the measurement of the PISA radius, initial caliper position at the edge of the hemispheric PISA is easily done using color Doppler followed by color suppress to position the caliper at

the level of the regurgitant orifice of the AR jet. The PISA method for the measurement of ERO has also been validated with TTE in patients with an eccentric jet of AR (39). Technical difficulties in imaging proximal flow acceleration at the level of the AoV with TEE may limit the applicability of this technique.

ERO measurement with 2D imaging and quantitative Doppler. The total left ventricular stroke volume (LVSV) can be calculated as the difference between the left ventricular end-systolic volume (LVESV) and left ventricular end-diastolic volume (LVEDV), which can be measured from 2D images by several methods, including the Simpson's method of discs (see Chapter 5). The difference between the LVSV obtained by 2D echocardiography and the SV measured by PW Doppler across a competent valve yields the aortic regurgitant volume.

The MV is most often used as the competent valve for the measurement of SV with PW Doppler as shown in the following equations:

$$SV_{Ao} = LVEDV - LVESV$$

$$SV_{MV} = MV \text{ annular CSA} \times VTI_{MV \text{ annulus}}$$

$$AR \text{ Volume} = SV_{Ao} - SV_{MV}$$

$$ERO_{AR} (cm^2) = \frac{AR \text{ Volume } (cm^3)}{VTI_{AR}(cm)}$$

$$ERO_{AR}(cm^2) = \frac{SV_{Ao} - SV_{MV}}{VTI_{AR}} \qquad (14.14)$$

The aortic regurgitant VTI (cm) is obtained by tracing the AR spectral Doppler envelope obtained with CW Doppler across the AoV during diastole.

ERO measurement with quantitative Doppler echocardiography. The regurgitant volume can also be calculated by measuring the difference between the forward SV across the LVOT and the SV across the MV by Doppler volumetric method.

$$AR \text{ volume} = SV_{Ao} - SV_{MV}$$

$$SV_{Ao} = 0.785(d_{LVOT})^2 \times VTI_{LVOT}$$

$$SV_{MV} = 0.785(d_{4ch} \times d_{2ch}) \times VTI_{MV \text{ annulus}}$$

$$ERO_{AR}(cm^2) = \frac{AR \text{ volume } (cm^3)}{VTI_{AR} (cm)}$$

$$= \frac{SV_{Ao} - SV_{MV}}{VTI_{AR}} \qquad (14.15)$$

In a study by Kim et al. (40) in sheep, the ERO area did not change with loading conditions.

ERO measurement with color Doppler imaging of the vena contracta. The vena contracta (VC) is the narrowest point of a regurgitant jet and occurs slightly downstream of the regurgitant orifice. In AR, the vena contracta will be imaged below the AoV within the LVOT (41). Assuming a spherical regurgitant orifice, the ERO area can be calculated using the maximal vena contracta width in early diastole using the following formula:

$$ERO_{AR} = \pi \times \left(\frac{VC \text{ width}}{2}\right)^2 \qquad (14.16)$$

This technique has been validated in sheep studies. In patients, a vena contracta of >6 mm has been shown to correlate with severe AR (11,42–44) and using the equation above corresponds to an ERO of $\geq .28$ cm^2.

Vena Contracta

The vena contracta is the narrowest portion of the AR jet and occurs in the LVOT immediately below the AoV. This measurement does not appear to vary with afterload manipulation (43). As indicated previously, a vena contracta of >6 mm is indicative of severe AR. This criterion has also been validated in eccentric jets of AR (42). In those patients, measurement of the vena contracta should be performed perpendicular to the LAX of the eccentric jet.

CW Doppler and Pressure Half-Time

The intensity of the CW Doppler signal is determined by the number of red blood cells reflecting the incident ultrasound beam. Therefore, a very dense regurgitant flow signal is suggestive of a large regurgitant volume. Severe AR also results in rapid equilibration of pressures between the Ao and the LV. Thus, a rapid decay of the Ao-LV pressure gradient in diastole is also seen in severe AR. This can be assessed by the measurement of aortic regurgitant flow velocity during diastole, which reflects the instantaneous pressure gradient between the Ao and the LV from the simplified Bernoulli equation. The decay of the Ao-LV pressure gradient is estimated from the slope of the aortic regurgitant velocity and the regurgitant pressure half-time (RHT), which is defined as the time needed for the pressure gradient to fall to half of its initial value during diastole (Fig. 14.42). From the manipulations shown below, the RHT also corresponds to the time needed for the maximum velocity to decrease by 70% of its initial value.

Bernoulli equation:

$$P_{max} = 4(V_{max})^2$$

$$P_{T_{1/2}} = 4(V_{T_{1/2}})^2$$

Regurgitant pressure half-time (RHT):

$$P_{T_{1/2}} = \frac{1}{2}(P_{max})$$

Therefore,

$$4(V_{T_{1/2}})^2 = \frac{1}{2}4(V_{max})^2$$

$$V_{T_{1/2}}^2 = \frac{1}{2}V_{max}^2$$

$$V_{T_{1/2}} = \frac{V_{max}}{\sqrt{2}} \qquad (14.17)$$

$$V_{T_{1/2}} = 0.7 V_{max}$$

A deceleration slope >3 m/s^2 or a RHT <200 ms suggests either a rapidly decreasing aortic pressure or a rapidly increasing LV pressure, both suggesting the presence of severe AR (Fig. 14.42). The RHT should

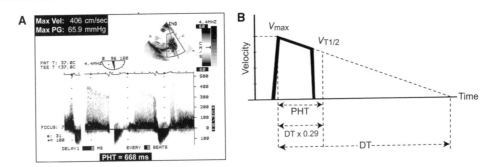

Figure 14.42 Pressure half-time. (A) Continuous wave Doppler interrogation across the regurgitant AoV from a transgastric window. The regurgitant PHT is measured at 668 ms, consistent with mild aortic regurgitation. **(B)** The relationship between the PHT and blood flow velocity across the AoV in diastole is illustrated. *Abbreviations*: AoV, aortic valve; DT, deceleration time; Max, maximum; PG, pressure gradient; PHT, pressure half-time; Vel, velocity; Vmax, maximal velocity; Vpeak, peak velocity; $V_{t1/2}$, velocity at the PHT point.

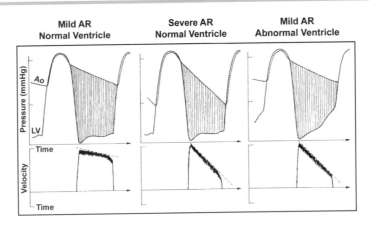

Figure 14.43 Pressure half-time. Determinants of regurgitant PHT in AR are shown. Upper panels: invasively obtained pressure tracings in the Ao and the LV. Lower panels: continuous wave Doppler tracings across the AoV during diastole. The slope of the blood flow velocity corresponds to the fall in the measured pressure gradient between the Ao and LV. The calculation of PHT with Doppler echocardiography is derived from the rate of decrease in blood flow velocity across the AoV in patients with AR. *Abbreviations*: Ao, aorta; AoV, aortic valve; AR, aortic regurgitation; LV, left ventricle; PHT, pressure half-time. *Source*: Reproduced with permission from Ref. 46.

ideally be measured on the slope of beats with longer duration. From a technical standpoint, the initial peak velocity represents the pressure gradient between the Ao and the LV during early diastole (Fig. 14.43). As this gradient should be at least 40 mmHg, an initial peak velocity <300 cm/s usually indicates improper alignment of the ultrasound beam with the regurgitant jet.

Pitfalls of RHT. Several factors must be considered in the interpretation of this quantitative measurement of AR. In certain conditions, a short RHT may not necessarily indicate severe AR: changes in LV compliance will influence the rate of pressure equilibration between the Ao and the LV. A noncompliant LV is associated with a faster LV pressure rise, causing a steeper AR slope and shorter RHT. Also, patients with chronic AR tend to have a more dilated and compliant LV, which can accommodate a greater volume of regurgitant blood. Therefore, for the same regurgitant volume, acute AR will have a

steeper AR slope and a shorter RHT compared with chronic AR (Fig. 14.43). Other conditions leading to rapidly rising LV pressure during diastole will also shorten the RHT as in restrictive cardiomyopathy or severe MR.

Grading AR

Quantification of AR remains a diagnostic challenge in some patients. In the quantification of AR, measurement of flow reversal in the descending thoracic Ao, regurgitant deceleration slope, and RHT are useful parameters. Newer approaches, including ERO measurement, vena contracta, and PISA, although promising, are not yet routinely used in clinical practice. A combination of techniques remains the most reasonable approach considering the limitations inherent in each method. The ASE has published guidelines on the evaluation of AR (45). They are summarized in Tables 14.5 to 14.7.

Table 14.5 Qualitative and Quantitative Parameters Useful in Grading Aortic Regurgitation Severity

	Mild	Moderate		Severe
Structural parameters				
LV size	Normal[a]	Normal or dilated		Usually dilated[b]
Aortic leaflets	Normal or abnormal	Normal or abnormal		Abnormal/flail or wide coaptation defect
Doppler parameters				
Jet width in LVOT–color flow[c]	Small in central jets	Intermediate		Large in central jets; variable in eccentric jets
Jet density–CW	Incomplete or faint	Dense		Dense
Diastolic flow reversal in descending aorta–PW	Brief, early diastolic reversal	Intermediate		Prominent holodiastolic reversal
Quantitative parameters[e]				
Regurgitant half-time–CW (RHT, ms)[d]	Slow >500	Medium 500–200		Steep <200
VC width (cm)[c]	<0.3	0.3–0.60		>0.6
Jet width/LVOT width (%)[c]	<25	25–45	46–64	≥65
Jet CSA/LVOT CSA (%)[c]	<5	5–20	21–59	≥60
Regurgitant volume (mL/beat)	<30	30–44	45–59	≥60
Regurgitant fraction (%)	<30	30–39	40–49	≥50
ERO$_{AR}$ (cm^2)	<0.10	0.10–0.19	0.20–0.29	≥0.30

[a]Unless there are other reasons for LV dilation. Normal 2D measurements: LV minor axis ≤2.8 cm/m^2, LV end-diastolic volume ≤82 mL/m^2 (2).
[b]Exception: would be acute AR, in which chambers have not had time to dilate.
[c]At a Nyquist limit of 50 to 60 cm/s.
[d]PHT is shortened with increasing LV diastolic pressure and vasodilator therapy and may be lengthened in chronic adaptation to severe AR.
[e]Quantitative parameters can subclassify the moderate regurgitation group into mild-to-moderate and moderate-to-severe regurgitation as shown.
Abbreviations: AR, aortic regurgitation; CSA, cross-sectional area; CW, continuous wave Doppler; ERO$_{AR}$, effective regurgitant orifice area; LV, left ventricle; LVOT, left ventricular outflow tract; RHT, regurgitant pressure half-time; PW, pulsed wave Doppler; VC, vena contracta.
Source: Adapted from Ref. 45.

Table 14.6 Echocardiographic and Doppler Parameters Used in the Evaluation of Aortic Regurgitation Severity: Utility, Advantages, and Limitations

	Utility/Advantages	Limitations
Structural parameters		
LV size	Enlargement sensitive for chronic significant AR, important for outcomes. Normal size virtually excludes significant chronic AR.	Enlargement seen in other conditions. May be normal in acute significant AR.
Aortic cusp alterations	Simple, usually abnormal in severe AR; flail valve denotes severe AR	Poor accuracy may grossly underestimate or overestimate the defect.
Doppler parameters		
Jet width or jet CSA in LVOT–color flow	Simple, very sensitive, quick screen for AR	Expands unpredictably below the orifice. Inaccurate for eccentric jets.
VC width	Simple, quantitative, good at identifying mild or severe AR	Not useful for multiple AR jets. Small values; thus small error leads to large % error.
PISA method	Quantitative. Provides both lesion severity (ERO$_{AR}$) and volume overload (Regurg. volume)	Feasibility limited by AoV calcifications. Not valid for multiple jets. Less accurate in eccentric jets. Provides peak flow and maximal ERO$_{AR}$. Possible underestimation with aortic aneurysms. Limited experience.
Flow quantitation by PW	Quantitative. Valid with multiple jets and eccentric jets. Provides both lesion severity (ERO$_{AR}$, regurg. valve fraction) and volume overload (Regurg. volume).	Not valid for combined MR and AR, unless PV is used as the competent valve.
Jet density–CW	Simple. Faint or incomplete jet compatible with mild AR	Qualitative. Overlap between moderate and severe AR. Complementary data only.
Regurgitant half-time by CW (RHT)	Simple	Qualitative; affected by changes in LV and aortic diastolic pressures.
Diastolic flow reversal in descending aorta–PW	Simple	Depends on rigidity of aorta. Brief velocity reversal is normal.

Abbreviations: AoV, aortic valve; AR, aortic regurgitation; CSA, cross-sectional area; CW, continuous wave Doppler; ERO$_{AR}$, effective regurgitant orifice area; LV, left ventricle; LVOT, left ventricular outflow tract; MR, mitral regurgitation; PISA, proximal isovelocity surface area; PV, pulmonic valve; PW, pulsed wave Doppler; regurg., regurgitant; RHT, regurgitant pressure half-time; VC, vena contracta.
Source: Adapted from Ref. 45.

Table 14.7 Application of Specific and Supportive Signs and Quantitative Parameters in the Grading of Aortic Regurgitation Severity

	Mild	Moderate	Severe
Specific signs for AR severity	Jet width <25% of LVOT[a] VC <0.3 cm[a] No or brief early diastolic flow reversal in desc Ao	Signs of AR >mild present but no criteria for severe AR	Jet width ≥65% of LVOT[a] VC >0.6 cm[a]
Supportive signs	RHT >500 ms Normal LV size[b]	Intermediate values	RHT <200 ms Holodiastolic flow reversal in desc Ao ≥Moderate LV dilatation[c]
Quantitative parameters[d]			
Regurg. volume (mL)	<30	30–44 45–59	≥60
Regurgitant fraction (%)	<30	30–39 40–49	≥50
ERO$_{AR}$ (cm^2)	<0.10	0.10–0.19 0.20–0.29	≥0.30

[a]At a Nyquist limit of 50 to 60 cm/s.
[b]LV size applied only to chronic lesions. Normal 2D measurements: LV minor-axis ≤2.8 cm/m^2, LV end-diastolic volume ≤82 mL/m^2 (2).
[c]In the absence of other etiologies of LV dilatation.
[d]Quantitative parameters can help subclassify the moderate regurgitation group into mild-to-moderate and moderate-to-severe regurgitation as shown.
Abbreviations: AR, aortic regurgitation; desc Ao, descending aorta; ERO$_{AR}$, effective regurgitant orifice area; LV, left ventricle; LVOT, left ventricular outflow tract; RHT, regurgitant pressure half-time; VC, vena contracta.
Source: Adapted from Ref. 45.

CONCLUSION

In the assessment of valvular heart disease, there are several different methods that are used to quantify and/or qualify the severity of a stenotic or regurgitant valve. There is no single golden echocardiographic measurement in the evaluation of valvular heart disease. Multiple techniques and views should be used to obtain a composite assessment of severity. Accurate echocardiographic evaluation and quantification of AoV pathology are crucial in determining whether a patient will have to undergo a surgical intervention. Detailed knowledge of the aortic root anatomy not only allows the physician to understand pathological echocardiographic findings but also provides crucial information in the planning of the surgical procedure for the patient.

ACKNOWLEDGMENTS

Special thanks to Dr Lawrence Rudski for reviewing this chapter and for his expert advice.

REFERENCES

1. Bonow RO, Carabello BA, Kanu C, et al. ACC/AHA 2006 guidelines for the management of patients with valvular heart disease: a report of the American College of Cardiology/American Heart Association Task Force on Practice Guidelines (writing committee to revise the 1998 Guidelines for the Management of Patients With Valvular Heart Disease): developed in collaboration with the Society of Cardiovascular Anesthesiologists: endorsed by the Society for Cardiovascular Angiography and Interventions and the Society of Thoracic Surgeons. Circulation 2006; 114: e84–e231.
2. Keane MG, Wiegers SE, Plappert T, et al. Bicuspid aortic valves are associated with aortic dilatation out of proportion to coexistent valvular lesions. Circulation 2000; 102: III35–III39.
3. Nistri S, Sorbo MD, Basso C, et al. Bicuspid aortic valve: abnormal aortic elastic properties. J Heart Valve Dis 2002; 11:369–373.
4. Baumgartner H, Hung J, Bermejo J, et al. Echocardiographic assessment of valve stenosis: EAE/ASE recommendations for clinical practice. J Am Soc Echocardiogr 2009; 22:1–23.
5. Otto CM. Valvular aortic stenosis: disease severity and timing of intervention. J Am Coll Cardiol 2006; 47:2141–2151.
6. Laskey WK, Kussmaul WG. Pressure recovery in aortic valve stenosis. Circulation 1994; 89:116–121.
7. Baumgartner H, Stefenelli T, Niederberger J, et al. "Overestimation" of catheter gradients by Doppler ultrasound in patients with aortic stenosis: a predictable manifestation of pressure recovery. J Am Coll Cardiol 1999; 33:1655–1661.
8. Garcia D, Dumesnil JG, Durand LG, et al. Discrepancies between catheter and Doppler estimates of valve effective orifice area can be predicted from the pressure recovery phenomenon: practical implications with regard to quantification of aortic stenosis severity. J Am Coll Cardiol 2003; 41:435–442.
9. Levine RA, Schwammenthal E. Stenosis is in the eye of the observer: impact of pressure recovery on assessing aortic valve area. J Am Coll Cardiol 2003; 41:443–445.
10. VanAuker MD, Chandra M, Shirani J, et al. Jet eccentricity: a misleading source of agreement between Doppler/catheter pressure gradients in aortic stenosis. J Am Soc Echocardiogr 2001; 14:853–862.
11. Quinones MA, Otto CM, Stoddard M, et al. Recommendations for quantification of Doppler echocardiography: a report from the Doppler Quantification Task Force of the Nomenclature and Standards Committee of the American Society of Echocardiography. J Am Soc Echocardiogr 2002; 15:167–184.
12. Cormier B, Iung B, Porte JM, et al. Value of multiplane transesophageal echocardiography in determining aortic valve area in aortic stenosis. Am J Cardiol 1996; 77:882–885.
13. Arsenault M, Masani N, Magni G, et al. Variation of anatomic valve area during ejection in patients with valvular aortic stenosis evaluated by two-dimensional echocardiographic planimetry: comparison with traditional Doppler data. J Am Coll Cardiol 1998; 32:1931–1937.

14. Perrino AC Jr., Harris SN, Luther MA. Intraoperative determination of cardiac output using multiplane transesophageal echocardiography: a comparison to thermodilution. Anesthesiology 1998; 89:350–357.

15. Harpaz D, Shah P, Bezante G, et al. Transthoracic and transesophageal echocardiographic sizing of the aortic annulus to determine prosthesis size. Am J Cardiol 1993; 72:1411–1417.

16. Reisner SA, Harpaz D, Skulski R, et al. Hemodynamic performance of four mechanical bileaflet prosthetic valves in the mitral position: an echocardiographic study. Eur J Ultrasound 1998; 8:193–200.

17. Maslow AD, Haering JM, Heindel S, et al. An evaluation of prosthetic aortic valves using transesophageal echocardiography: the double-envelope technique. Anesth Analg 2000; 91:509–516.

18. Maslow AD, Mashikian J, Haering JM, et al. Transesophageal echocardiographic evaluation of native aortic valve area: utility of the double-envelope technique. J Cardiothorac Vasc Anesth 2001; 15:293–299.

19. Kim CJ, Berglund H, Nishioka T, et al. Correspondence of aortic valve area determination from transesophageal echocardiography, transthoracic echocardiography, and cardiac catheterization. Am Heart J 1996; 132:1163–1172.

20. Bernard Y, Meneveau N, Vuillemenot A, et al. Planimetry of aortic valve area using multiplane transoesophageal echocardiography is not a reliable method for assessing severity of aortic stenosis. Heart 1997; 78:68–73.

21. Tardif JC, Miller DS, Pandian NG, et al. Effects of variations in flow on aortic valve area in aortic stenosis based on in vivo planimetry of aortic valve area by multiplane transesophageal echocardiography. Am J Cardiol 1995; 76:193–198.

22. Tardif JC, Rodrigues AG, Hardy JF, et al. Simultaneous determination of aortic valve area by the Gorlin formula and by transesophageal echocardiography under different transvalvular flow conditions. Evidence that anatomic aortic valve area does not change with variations in flow in aortic stenosis. J Am Coll Cardiol 1997; 29:1296–1302.

23. Nishimura RA, Grantham JA, Connolly HM, et al. Low-output, low-gradient aortic stenosis in patients with depressed left ventricular systolic function: the clinical utility of the dobutamine challenge in the catheterization laboratory. Circulation 2002; 106:809–813.

24. Monin JL, Quere JP, Monchi M, et al. Low-gradient aortic stenosis: operative risk stratification and predictors for long-term outcome: a multicenter study using dobutamine stress hemodynamics. Circulation 2003; 108:319–324.

25. Blais C, Burwash IG, Mundigler G, et al. Projected valve area at normal flow rate improves the assessment of stenosis severity in patients with low-flow, low-gradient aortic stenosis: the multicenter TOPAS (Truly or Pseudo-Severe Aortic Stenosis) study. Circulation 2006; 113:711–721.

26. El Khoury G, Glineur D, Rubay J, et al. Functional classification of aortic root/valve abnormalities and their correlation with etiologies and surgical procedures. Curr Opin Cardiol 2005; 20:115–121.

27. de Waroux JB, Pouleur AC, Goffinet C, et al. Functional anatomy of aortic regurgitation: accuracy, prediction of surgical repairability, and outcome implications of transesophageal echocardiography. Circulation 2007; 116:I264–I269.

28. Underwood MJ, El Khoury G, Deronck D, et al. The aortic root: structure, function, and surgical reconstruction. Heart 2000; 83:376–380.

29. Rosenhek R, Binder T, Porenta G, et al. Predictors of outcome in severe, asymptomatic aortic stenosis. N Engl J Med 2000; 343:611–617.

30. Nash PJ, Vitvitsky E, Li J, et al. Feasibility of valve repair for regurgitant bicuspid aortic valves—an echocardiographic study. Ann Thorac Surg 2005; 79:1473–1479.

31. Pettersson GB, Crucean AC, Savage R, et al. Toward predictable repair of regurgitant aortic valves: a systematic morphology-directed approach to bicommissural repair. J Am Coll Cardiol 2008; 52:40–49.

32. Movsowitz HD, Levine RA, Hilgenberg AD, et al. Transesophageal echocardiographic description of the mechanisms of aortic regurgitation in acute type A aortic dissection: implications for aortic valve repair. J Am Coll Cardiol 2000; 36:884–890.

33. Perry GJ, Helmcke F, Nanda NC, et al. Evaluation of aortic insufficiency by Doppler color flow mapping. J Am Coll Cardiol 1987; 9:952–959.

34. Oh JK, Seward JB, Tajik AJ. The Echo Manual. 2nd ed. Philadelphia: Lippincott Williams & Wilkins, 1999.

35. Evangelista A, del Castillo HG, Calvo F, et al. Strategy for optimal aortic regurgitation quantification by Doppler echocardiography: agreement among different methods. Am Heart J 2000; 139:773–781.

36. Kerut EK, McIlwain EF, Plotnick GD. Handbook of Echo-Doppler Interpretation. Armonk, NY: Futura Publishing Company, Inc., 1996.

37. Ozkan M, Ozdemir N, Kaymaz C, et al. Measurement of aortic valve anatomic regurgitant area using transesophageal echocardiography: implications for the quantitation of aortic regurgitation. J Am Soc Echocardiogr 2002; 15: 1170–1174.

38. Tribouilloy CM, Enriquez-Sarano M, Fett SL, et al. Application of the proximal flow convergence method to calculate the effective regurgitant orifice area in aortic regurgitation. J Am Coll Cardiol 1998; 32:1032–1039.

39. Sato Y, Kawazoe K, Nasu M, et al. Clinical usefulness of the proximal isovelocity surface area method using echocardiography in patients with eccentric aortic regurgitation. J Heart Valve Dis 1999; 8:104–111.

40. Kim YJ, Jones M, Shiota T, et al. Effect of load alterations on the effective regurgitant orifice area in chronic aortic regurgitation. Heart 2002; 88:397–400.

41. Ishii M, Jones M, Shiota T, et al. Quantifying aortic regurgitation by using the color Doppler-imaged vena contracta: a chronic animal model study. Circulation 1997; 96: 2009–2015.

42. Tribouilloy CM, Enriquez-Sarano M, Bailey KR, et al. Assessment of severity of aortic regurgitation using the width of the vena contracta: A clinical color Doppler imaging study. Circulation 2000; 102:558–564.

43. Willett DL, Hall SA, Jessen ME, et al. Assessment of aortic regurgitation by transesophageal color Doppler imaging of the vena contracta: validation against an intraoperative aortic flow probe. J Am Coll Cardiol 2001; 37:1450–1455.

44. Eren M, Eksik A, Gorgulu S, et al. Determination of vena contracta and its value in evaluating severity of aortic regurgitation. J Heart Valve Dis 2002; 11:567–575.

45. Zoghbi WA, Enriquez-Sarano M, Foster E, et al. Recommendations for evaluation of the severity of native valvular regurgitation with two-dimensional and Doppler echocardiography. J Am Soc Echocardiogr 2003; 16:777–802.

46. Obeid AI. Echocardiography in Clinical Practice. Philadelphia: Lippincott, 1992.

15

Perioperative Evaluation of Aortic Valve Surgery

Jean G. Dumesnil, Philippe Pibarot, and Patrick Mathieu
Université Laval, Quebec City, Quebec, Canada

Michel Van Dyck
Université Catholique de Louvain, Brussels, Belgium

SURGICAL INDICATIONS FOR AORTIC VALVE SURGERY

The American College of Cardiology (ACC) and the American Heart Association (AHA) have established guidelines for the management of patients with valvular heart disease (1). Three categories were established to indicate the weight of evidence, supporting the current recommendations. This chapter will review current indications and assessment for patients with aortic stenosis (AS) and/or aortic regurgitation (AR) undergoing an aortic valve (AoV) or aortic root procedure.

Surgical Indications for AoV Stenosis

Asymptomatic Patients

Asymptomatic patients with severe valvular AS have a 2% to 3% per year incidence of serious complications compared with an ~1% per year mortality rate related to aortic prosthesis. However, when the operative morbidity and mortality are combined with the late complication rate of prosthetic AoV replacement (AVR), there is no benefit in survival or outcome. The current recommendations are, therefore, to delay surgery in patients with severe asymptomatic AS until they develop symptoms or left ventricular (LV) systolic dysfunction. An abnormal response to exercise (e.g., exercise-limiting symptoms, hypotension) or an AoV area (AVA) <0.6 cm^2 are weaker indications for proceeding with AVR (Table 15.1). Exercise testing is increasingly utilized to elicit symptoms in patients with severe asymptomatic AS. Indeed, underestimation of symptoms by both patient and physician is common in the elderly who progressively decrease their activity level without realizing their significantly impaired functional capacity (2–4).

The Doppler echocardiographic criteria presently used to define severe valvular AS are an AVA <1.0 cm^2, an indexed AVA <0.6 cm^2/m^2, a mean gradient >40 mmHg, a maximal velocity >4.0 m/s (i.e., a maximal gradient >65 mmHg) (1), and a velocity ratio <0.25 (5). However, it should be emphasized that severe stenosis may be present with a lower transvalvular gradient and velocity in patients with a low cardiac output (CO) or even in patients with a preserved LV ejection fraction. An estimated 35% of patients with severe AS may have paradoxically low flow (stroke volume index <35 mL/m^2) and gradient despite a normal LV ejection fraction (4). When compared with normal-flow patients, such individuals have markedly increased global LV afterload, smaller LV cavities, greater concentric remodeling, decreased mid-wall radius shortening consistent with intrinsic myocardial dysfunction, and much poorer prognosis if treated medically. Yet, only 50% of these patients undergo surgery likely due to the fact that disease severity is underestimated because of the lower gradients and velocity.

Patients with severe valvular AS are at risk of rapid progression when the valve is moderately to severely calcified, and there is a >0.3 m/s increase in maximal velocity per year (6). In such cases, the chance of undergoing valve replacement or dying within four years is $>80\%$, so consideration may be given for early valve replacement in this subgroup of patients even if they are still asymptomatic (Fig. 15.1).

Symptomatic Patients

In the absence of serious comorbid disease, patients with severe AS and concomitant angina, syncope, congestive heart failure, or dyspnea should undergo AVR (1). Survival is improved by surgery even in patients with severe LV dysfunction and low-gradient severe AS, unless the LV dysfunction is irreversible (Table 15.2).

Patients Undergoing Cardiac Surgery

Patients with severe AS undergoing other cardiac surgery (revascularization) should also have an AVR even if they are asymptomatic for AS and have no LV dysfunction. The evidence also favors proceeding with AVR in patients with moderate AS (AVA of 1.0–1.5 cm^2) who are scheduled to have cardiac surgery for other pathology (1). The AVA, indexed to the body surface area (BSA), may help the decision in borderline cases involving larger or smaller than average patients (Table 15.3).

Table 15.1 Surgical Indications for AVR in Patients with AS

Class I	1. AVR is indicated for symptomatic patients with severe AS.[a] (Level of Evidence: B)
	2. AVR is indicated for patients with severe AS[a] undergoing CABG surgery. (Level of Evidence: C)
	3. AVR is indicated for patients with severe AS[a] undergoing surgery on the aorta or other heart valves. (Level of Evidence: C)
	4. AVR is recommended for patients with severe AS[a] and LV systolic dysfunction (ejection fraction less than 0.50). (Level of Evidence: C)
Class IIa	AVR is reasonable for patients with moderate AS[a] undergoing CABG or surgery on the aorta or other heart valves. (Level of Evidence: B)
Class IIb	1. AVR may be considered for asymptomatic patients with severe AS[a] and abnormal response to exercise (e.g., development of symptoms or asymptomatic hypotension). (Level of Evidence: C)
	2. AVR may be considered for adults with severe asymptomatic AS[a] if there is a high likelihood of rapid progression (age, calcification, and CAD) or if surgery might be delayed at the time of symptom onset. (Level of Evidence: C)
	3. AVR may be considered in patients undergoing CABG who have mild AS[a] when there is evidence, such as moderate-to-severe valve calcification, that progression may be rapid. (Level of Evidence: C)
	4. AVR may be considered for asymptomatic patients with extremely severe AS (aortic valve area less than 0.6 cm^2, mean gradient greater than 60 mmHg, and jet velocity greater than 5.0 m/s) when the patient's expected operative mortality is 1.0% or less. (Level of Evidence: C)
Class III	AVR is not useful for the prevention of sudden death in asymptomatic patients with AS who have none of the findings listed under the class IIa/IIb recommendations. (Level of Evidence: B)

[a]See Table 14.2.

Abbreviations: AVR, aortic valve replacement; AS, aortic stenosis; CABG, coronary artery bypass graft; CAD, coronary artery disease; LV, left ventricular.

Source: Adapted from Ref. 1.

Surgical Indications for AR

The ACC and AHA recommendations (1) for surgical indications in patients with chronic isolated AR are summarized in Table 15.4 and are based on severity of AR, presence of symptoms, LV dysfunction, or severe LV dilatation (Fig. 15.2). Close follow-up is crucial as more than 25% of patients with severe AR develop LV dysfunction or die before the onset of warning symptoms. Appropriate timing of AoV surgery is difficult, but in symptomatic patients with severe AR, the mortality rate approaches 10% per year and these patients should undergo surgery, even in the absence of LV dysfunction or significant LV dilatation. In asymptomatic patients, the discovery of LV dysfunction (ejection fraction <0.50) is a class I indication for AVR, whereas significant LV dilatation [defined as a left ventricular end-diastolic dimension (LVEDD) >75 mm and/or a left ventricular end-systolic dimension (LVESD) >55 mm] is a class IIa indication (1). Fortunately, LV systolic dysfunction is initially a reversible phenomenon, and full recovery of LV function and size following AVR is possible if surgery is performed within the first 12 months.

TYPE OF OPERATION

AoV Replacement

Choosing the correct prosthetic valve for each patient is a difficult but essential process to optimize the outcome of patients undergoing valve replacement (Table 15.5). The first step in selecting a particular prosthesis model for a patient is to choose between a mechanical and a bioprosthetic valve. The most important factors to be considered in this first step are the patient's age, life expectancy, preference, the indication/contraindication for warfarin therapy, and any comorbidities. In the recent ACC/AHA guidelines, the weight given to the patient's age has been substantially dampened, whereas much greater importance is now given to the preference of the patient (1).

Criteria that favor utilization of a mechanical valve are (i) desire of the informed patient and absence of contraindication for long-term anticoagulation; (ii) patient already on anticoagulation (mechanical prosthesis in another position or at high risk for thromboembolism); (iii) patient at risk of accelerated bioprosthesis structural deterioration (young age, hyperparathyroidism, renal insufficiency); and (iv) age <65 (AVR) or <70 years [mitral valve replacement (MVR)] and long life expectancy.

However, a bioprosthesis may be preferred in the following situations: (i) desire of the informed patient; (ii) unavailability of good-quality anticoagulation (contraindication or high risk, compliance problems, lifestyle); (iii) age ≥65 years or limited life expectancy; and (iv) woman of childbearing age desiring pregnancy with the knowledge of a strong likelihood that the bioprosthesis will eventually have to be replaced.

Our knowledge regarding the performance and durability of prostheses is continually evolving. On the other hand, it has been demonstrated that pulmonary autografts have an excellent performance rate and very long durability and, up until recently, notwithstanding the availability of the pulmonary homograft necessary for the performance of the Ross procedure; it was almost considered the ideal operation. However, initial

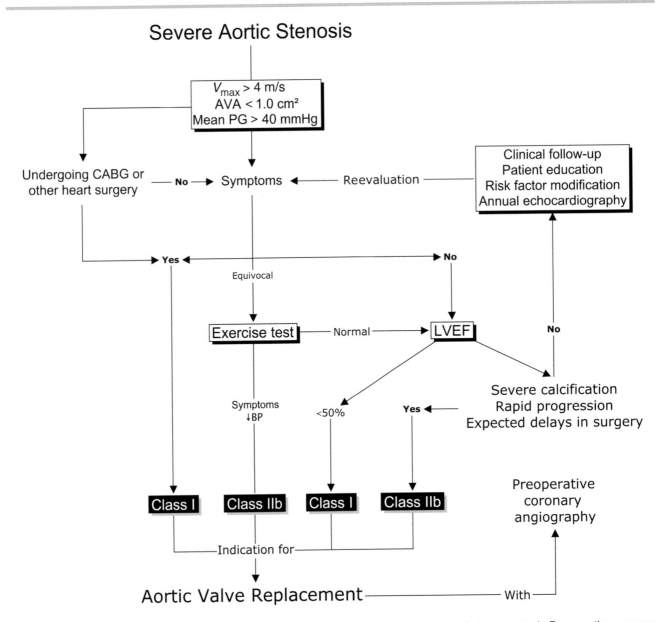

Figure 15.1 AVR indications in AS. Management strategy for patients with severe AS is presented. Preoperative coronary angiography should be performed routinely as determined by age, symptoms, and coronary risk factors. Cardiac catheterization may also be helpful when there is discordance between clinical findings and echocardiography. *Abbreviations*: AS, aortic stenosis; AVA, aortic valve area; AVR, aortic valve area; BP, blood pressure; CABG, coronary artery bypass graft surgery; echo, echocardiography; LV, left ventricular; LVEF, left ventricular ejection fraction; PG, pressure gradient; V_{max}, maximal velocity across aortic valve by Doppler echocardiography. *Source*: Adapted with permission from Ref. 1.

Table 15.2 Treatment of Coronary Artery Disease at the Time of AVR

Class I	Patients undergoing AVR with significant stenoses (greater than or equal to 70% reduction in luminal diameter) in major coronary arteries should be treated with bypass grafting. (Level of Evidence: C)
Class IIa	1. In patients undergoing AVR and coronary bypass grafting, use of the left internal thoracic artery is reasonable for bypass of stenoses of the left anterior descending coronary artery greater than or equal to 50–70%. (Level of Evidence: C)
	2. For patients undergoing AVR with moderate stenosis (50–70% reduction in luminal diameter), it is reasonable to perform coronary bypass grafting in major coronary arteries. (Level of Evidence: C)

Abbreviation: AVR, aortic valve replacement.
Source: Adapted from Ref. 1.

Table 15.3 AVR in Patients Undergoing Coronary Artery Bypass Surgery

Class I	AVR is indicated in patients undergoing CABG who have severe AS who meet the criteria for valve replacement. (Level of Evidence: C)
Class IIa	AVR is reasonable in patients undergoing CABG who have moderate AS (mean gradient 30–50 mmHg or Doppler velocity 3–4 m/s). (Level of Evidence: B)
Class IIb	AVR may be considered in patients undergoing CABG who have mild AS (mean gradient less than 30 mmHg or Doppler velocity less than 3 m/s) when there is evidence, such as moderate-to-severe valve calcification, that progression may be rapid. (Level of Evidence: C)

Abbreviations: AS, aortic stenosis; AVR, aortic valve replacement; CABG, coronary artery bypass graft.
Source: Adapted from Ref. 1.

Table 15.4 Indications for AVR or Repair in AR

Class I	1. AVR is indicated for symptomatic patients with severe AR irrespective of LV systolic function. (Level of Evidence: B)
	2. AVR is indicated for asymptomatic patients with chronic severe AR and LV systolic dysfunction (ejection fraction 0.50 or less) at rest. (Level of Evidence: B)
	3. AVR is indicated for patients with chronic severe AR while undergoing CABG or surgery on the aorta or other heart valves. (Level of Evidence: C)
Class IIa	AVR is reasonable for asymptomatic patients with severe AR with normal LV systolic function (ejection fraction greater than 0.50) but with severe LV dilatation (end-diastolic dimension greater than 75 mm or end-systolic dimension greater than 55 mm).[a] (Level of Evidence: B)
Class IIb	1. AVR may be considered in patients with moderate AR while undergoing surgery on the ascending aorta. (Level of Evidence: C)
	2. AVR may be considered in patients with moderate AR while undergoing CABG. (Level of Evidence: C)
	3. AVR may be considered for asymptomatic patients with severe AR and normal LV systolic function at rest (ejection fraction greater than 0.50) when the degree of LV dilatation exceeds an end-diastolic dimension of 70 mm or end-systolic dimension of 50 mm, when there is evidence of progressive LV dilatation, declining exercise tolerance, or abnormal hemodynamic responses to exercise.[a] (Level of Evidence: C)
Class III	AVR is not indicated for asymptomatic patients with mild, moderate, or severe AR and normal LV systolic function at rest (ejection fraction greater than 0.50) when degree of dilatation is not moderate or severe (end-diastolic dimension less than 70 mm, end-systolic dimension less than 50 mm).[a] (Level of Evidence: B)

[a]Consider lower threshold values for patients of small stature of either gender.
Abbreviations: AVR, aortic valve replacement; AR, aortic regurgitation; LV, left ventricular; CABG, coronary artery bypass graft.
Source: Adapted from Ref. 1.

enthusiasm has been somewhat dampened by the recent demonstration that the pulmonary autograft can rapidly degenerate and become stenotic in up to 20% of patients who underwent this operation (8). Three different autograft implantation techniques have been described: the original subcoronary implantation, the root replacement, and the inclusion technique. Long-term results are similar in these three techniques but the causes of autograft failure differ: autograft dilation is the main cause of reoperation in root replacement technique, while autograft cusp prolapse is the main cause of failure in the inclusion group (9).

AoV Repair

In some specialized centers with surgical expertise, AoV repair can now be performed in selected patients. This mainly applies to regurgitant valves, whereas stenotic AoV are less prone to surgical repair. Indeed, the surgeon needs good-quality aortic cusp tissue for optimal repair, a condition rarely encountered in rheumatic or calcified valve diseases. Growing experience

and good mid-term results (10,11) explain the slightly increasing number of such operations being performed worldwide.

According to the ACC guidelines, indications for AoV repair in patients with AR are the same for AVR but should be considered only in surgical centers that have developed the appropriate technical expertise, gained experience in patient selection, and demonstrated outcomes equivalent to those of AVR (1). Aortic valve repair is feasible not only in bicuspid valves (12,13) where the single coaptation line renders the correction easier but also in cases of tricuspid incompetent valves.

As for the mitral valve (MV), surgical and functional classifications have been developed, linking pathologies to specific surgical procedures (14,15). Experience gained from more than 25 years of MVR is now applied to the AoV, which is no longer considered alone but as a component of the aortic root (16). Surgical repair aims to restore normal valve anatomy but, more importantly, normal root function. Keeping this in mind, it becomes clear that, in the setting of AR correction, the analysis and understanding of the cause of the regurgitation is of paramount importance and will determine if the valve cusps are to be repaired

Chronic Severe Aortic Regurgitation

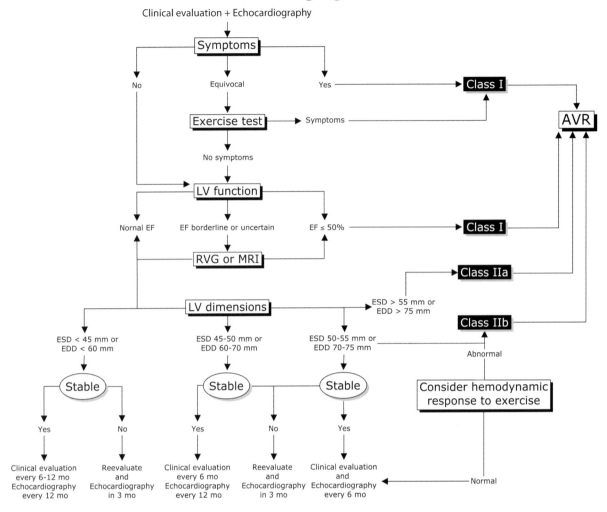

Figure 15.2 AVR indications in AR. Management strategy for patients with chronic severe AR is presented. Preoperative coronary angiography should be performed routinely as determined by age, symptoms, and coronary risk factors. Cardiac catheterization may also be helpful when there is discordance between clinical findings and echocardiography. "Stable" refers to stable echocardiographic measurements. In some centers, serial follow-up may be performed with RVG or MRI rather than echocardiography to assess LV volume and systolic function. *Abbreviations*: AR, aortic regurgitation; AVR, aortic valve replacement; EDD, end-diastolic dimension; EF, ejection fraction; ESD, end-systolic dimension; LV, left ventricle; MRI, magnetic resonance imaging; RVG, radionuclide ventriculography; SD, end-systolic dimension. *Source*: Adapted with permission from Ref. 1.

Table 15.5 Major Criteria for Aortic Valve Selection

Class I	1.	A mechanical prosthesis is recommended for AVR in patients with a mechanical valve in the mitral or tricuspid position. (Level of Evidence: C)
	2.	A bioprosthesis is recommended for AVR in patients of any age who will not take warfarin or who have major medical contraindications to warfarin therapy. (Level of Evidence: C)
Class IIa	1.	Patient preference is a reasonable consideration in the selection of aortic valve operation and valve prosthesis. A mechanical prosthesis is reasonable for AVR in patients under 65 years of age who do not have a contraindication to anticoagulation. A bioprosthesis is reasonable for AVR in patients under 65 years of age who elect to receive this valve for lifestyle considerations after detailed discussions of the risks of anticoagulation versus the likelihood that a second AVR may be necessary in the future. (Level of Evidence: C)
	2.	A bioprosthesis is reasonable for AVR in patients aged 65 years or older without risk factors for thromboembolism. (Level of Evidence: C)
	3.	Aortic valve rereplacement with a homograft is reasonable for patients with active prosthetic valve endocarditis. (Level of Evidence: C)
Class IIb		A bioprosthesis might be considered for AVR in a woman of childbearing age. (Level of Evidence: C)

Abbreviation: AVR, aortic valve replacement.
Source: Adapted from Ref. 1.

AR Class	Type I — Normal cusp motion with FAA dilatation or cusp perforation				Type II Cusp Prolapse	Type III Cusp Restriction
	IA — Dilated ascending aorta	IB — Dilated aortic root	IC — Dilated aortic annulus	ID — Fenestration		
Mechanism	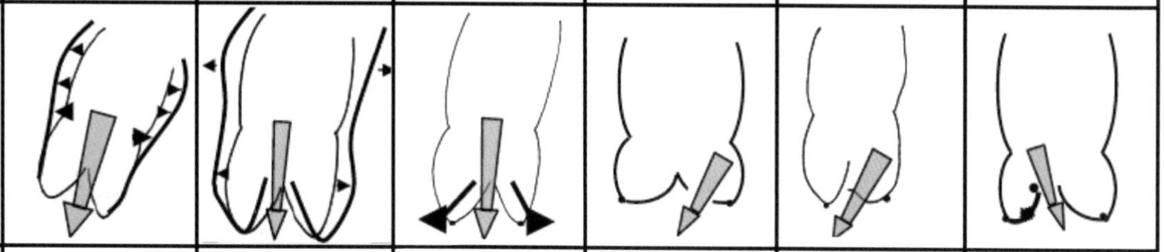					
Repair Techniques (Primary)	**STJ Remodeling** Ascending aortic graft	**Aortic Valve Sparing:** Reimplantation or Remodeling with SCA	**SCA**	**Patch Repair** Autologous or bovine pericadium	**Prolapse Repair** Plication Triangular resection Free margin Resuspension Patch	**Leaflet Repair** Shaving Decalcificatio Patch
(Secondary)	SCA		STJ Annuloplasty	SCA	SCA	SCA

Figure 15.3 Surgical repair of AR. Repair orientated functional classification of AR with description of disease mechanisms and repair techniques used. *Abbreviations*: AR, aortic regurgitation; FAA, functional aortic annulus; SCA, subcommissural annuloplasty; STJ, sinotubular junction. *Source*: Adapted with permission from Ref. 16.

alone or in conjunction with some aortic root plasty or replacement (16) (Fig. 15.3).

Valve Sparing Aortic Replacement

Type I AR can be due to cusp tethering caused by aortic root dilatation as detailed in Chapter 14. Dilatation can involve the ascending aorta (Ao) starting from the sinotubular junction (STJ) (type IA) or can present as an aneurysm of the entire aortic root with dilatation of the aortic annulus, the sinuses of Valsalva, and the STJ (type IB). Surgical treatment is different in both types. In type IA, a supracoronary tube graft is sutured above the aortic root without need for coronary artery reimplantation (Fig. 15.4). Complex cases can be present (Fig. 15.5). In type IB, the entire aortic root is replaced, and the coronary ostia reimplanted, with sparing of the native AoV, if its cusps are normal (Fig. 15.6). In such valve-sparing root replacement surgery, the diseased aortic root wall is entirely removed, only preserving the scalloped native AoV (Fig. 15.4C). Surgical techniques then differ depending on the decision to suture the valve *to* or *inside* a prosthetic tube graft.

The remodeling technique, described by Sarsam and Yacoub, consists of replacing the three sinuses of Valsalva utilizing a tailored tripartite crown-shaped Dacron tube graft (17) (Fig. 15.4D). The reimplantation technique, developed by David and Feindel, consists of suturing the scalloped native AoV inside a graft that is sutured down to the aortic annulus (10,18). This operation is claimed to offer a more stable repair without further annulus dilatation. Some surgeons also advocate the use of a more physiological Valsalva prosthesis for such root replacement (19) (Fig. 15.4E). After any reimplantation or remodeling procedure, the native AoV is inspected for the presence of iatrogenic cusp distortion or prolapse that could have resulted during the suturing of the commissures to the tube graft. Postoperative transesophageal echocardiography (TEE) will also help to verify the adequacy of cusp coaptation inside the tube graft (20).

Aortic Cusp Repair

When considering AoV repair surgery, echocardiographic assessment of the number of aortic cusps and cusp mobility is crucial. Careful preoperative echocardiographic evaluation of the opening and closure of the valve both in the long-axis (LAX) and short-axis (SAX) views can guide the surgical decision.

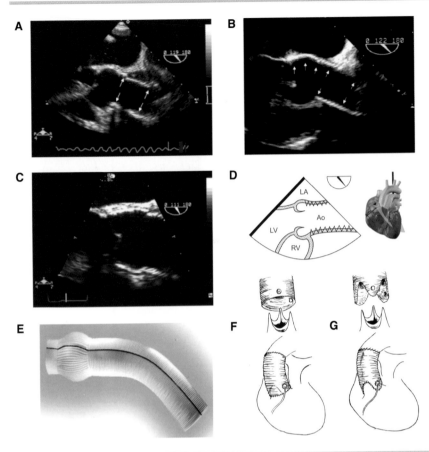

Figure 15.4 Aortic regurgitation type I repairs. (**A–D**) Mid-esophageal AoV long-axis views showing the typical aspect of the tube graft (arrows) used to replace a dilated portion of the ascending Ao. (**A**) Supracoronary graft implantation. The native AoV and sinuses of Valsalva are preserved and the prosthesis is sutured at the sinotubular junction, above the origin of the coronary arteries. (**B**) Partial remodeling procedure. The ascending Ao and the left coronary sinus are replaced with a scalloped Valsalva prosthesis. The patient's native right and non-coronary sinuses are preserved and the posterior (left) sinus is prosthetic (arrows). (**C,D**) Reimplantation procedure (Tirone David) with a Valsalva prosthesis. The native AoV has been preserved and the entire aortic root replaced with a tube graft containing neo-sinuses. (**E**) Gelweave Valsalva prosthesis is shown. (**F,G**) Schematic representation of the difference between reimplantation and remodeling is shown. *Abbreviations*: Ao, aorta; AoV aortic valve; LA, left atrium, LV, left ventricle; RV, right ventricle. *Source*: With permission, Photo E courtesy of Vascutek/Terumo, Inchinnan, Renfrewshire, Scotland.

Valve incompetence can be due to thickening, or calcifications, of the cusp free margins, to cusp retraction or commissural fusion. Such lesions are, in some cases, repairable by shaving the thickened margins, resecting the calcifications, or performing blade commissurotomy. Autologous pericardium can be used to perform cusp extension or to close cusp perforations (Fig. 15.7). However, in such repairs, the amount, quality, and suppleness of the overall cusp tissue are crucial for an optimal postoperative coaptation and ensuring intermediate and long-term results (21).

One or more aortic cusps can present with an excess of tissue or mobility, resulting in some degree of cusp prolapse (type II). Three types of cusp prolapse have been described based on the portion of the cusp overriding the plane of the aortic annulus, as described in Chapter 14. Similar to MV prolapse, aortic cusp prolapse is associated with an eccentric AR jet directed in the opposite direction. Surgical correction of a cusp prolapse usually consists of a triangular resection, or plication, of the middle portion of the prolapsing cusp (22,23), occasionally with reinforcement of the free edge by an over-and-over suture (Fig. 15.5). This is sometimes associated with a subcommissural plasty made at the level of the interleaflet triangles (Fig. 15.5H). All these surgical "gestures" can be seen echocardiographically.

AVOIDING PATIENT-PROSTHESIS MISMATCH

The anticipated hemodynamics of the prosthesis being implanted is another consideration when choosing the type of valve replacement to be performed in a given patient. Recent evidence has shown that suboptimal postoperative hemodynamics may occur in up to 70% of patients being operated on, which may have a direct impact on short- and long-term survival and improvement of functional class (24–28). Notwithstanding the rare occurrence of intrinsic prosthesis dysfunction, a suboptimal postoperative course may be due to patient-prosthesis mismatch (PPM), that is, that the effective orifice area (EOA) of the prosthesis being implanted is less than that of the normal human valve and too small to ensure optimal hemodynamics (Fig. 15.8).

Different types of prosthesis usually have different hemodynamic profiles. Prosthesis selection depends largely on the proportion of the valvular area occupied by the supporting apparatus of the prosthesis rather than by flow, and to a lesser degree, by the opening dynamics of the prosthesis. Therefore, size for size, autografts and homografts have the best hemodynamic profile as evidenced by larger postoperative EOAs and lower gradients (Fig. 15.9); they are followed in decreasing order by stentless bioprostheses, mechanical

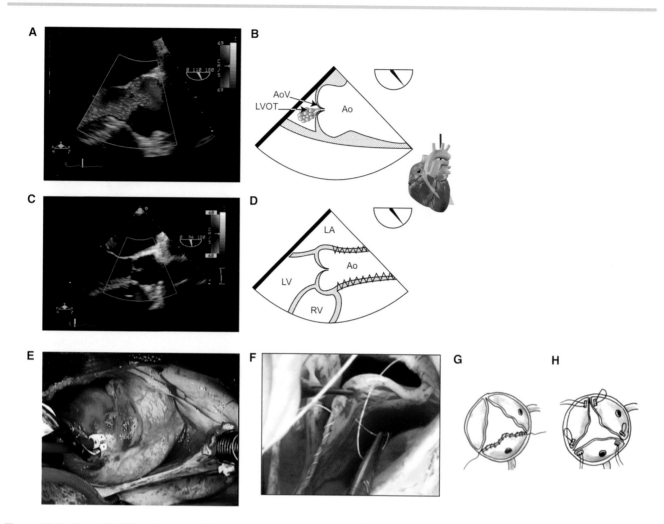

Figure 15.5 Type 1A AR and ruptured fenestration. This patient presented with a dilation of the ascending Ao starting at the STJ (type IA) and a ruptured fenestration of the RCC. (**A,B**) The mid-esophageal AoV LAX view shows the dilation of the ascending Ao starting at the STJ (diameter of 5.1 cm). Surprisingly, instead of a central jet, color Doppler interrogation shows an eccentric AR jet directed toward the anterior mitral leaflet, suggestive of a prolapse or fenestration of the RCC. Close view of the valve discloses a long mobile structure corresponding to the disrupted free margin of the cusp. (**C,D**) Mid-esophageal LAX view after repair and supracoronary tube graft replacement. (**E**) The ascending Ao is dilated with ensuing tethering of the aortic cusps. The free margin of the RCC presents with a rupture of half of its length. Because the cusp is lower than its counterparts (prolapse), surgical cusp repair will consist in a free margin placation (**F–H**), free margin resuspension, and commissural annuloplasty. The ascending Ao is then replaced with a supracoronary tube graft. *Abbreviations*: Ao, aorta; AoV, aortic valve; AR, aortic regurgitation; LA, left atrium; LAX, long axis; LV, left ventricle; LVOT, left ventricular outflow tract; RCC, right coronary cusp; RV, right ventricle; STJ, sinotubular junction. *Source*: Surgical films, courtesy of Prof. Gebrine El Khoury.

prostheses, and stented bioprostheses. There is general agreement that the postoperative indexed EOA of the prosthesis being implanted should not be <0.85 to $0.90 \text{ cm}^2/\text{m}^2$. It is suggested that the algorithm (28), described next, be followed in the operating room (OR) to achieve this goal (Fig. 15.10):

1. Calculate BSA from patient's body height and weight using the same formula as in Figure 15.10 or the charts derived from that formula.
2. Determine the minimal prosthesis EOA to avoid mismatch. This is accomplished by multiplying the desired postoperative indexed EOA (e.g.,

$0.85 \text{ cm}^2/\text{m}^2$) by the patient's BSA. Therefore, if the patient's BSA is 1.53 m^2, the minimal EOA that the prosthesis being implanted should have to avoid mismatch is 1.30 cm^2 (Fig. 15.11).

3. The prosthesis is then chosen using the published reference values of EOA for different types and sizes of prostheses (Table 15.6). To follow the above example, selecting a Carpentier–Edwards Perimount pericardial bioprosthesis, the minimal size is 21 mm to yield an EOA of 1.30 cm^2 (Fig. 15.11).
4. The aortic annulus diameter is measured at the base of the aortic cusp. Therefore, if the patient's

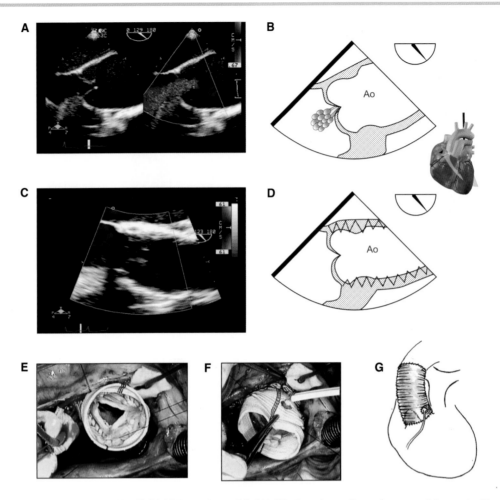

Figure 15.6   Type IB reimplantation AR. (A,B) Mid-esophageal AoV LAX view shows the aneurysm of the root with a loss of central coaptation and a central AR jet. The mid-esophageal AoV short-axis view confirms the tethering of the cusps with ensuing central AR originating at the level of the loss of coaptation. Transgastric long-axis view confirms the severity of AR (not shown). **(C,D)** Mid-esophageal AoV postreimplantation procedure showing the native AoV inside the tube graft. Coaptation is perfect without residual AR. **(E–G)** Tirone David procedure (reimplantation). The entire aortic wall is removed, only leaving the crown-shaped valve and its commissures that will be sutured inside the Dacron tube graft. Water test is perfect and the coronary arteries are reimplanted into the prosthesis. *Abbreviations*: Ao, aorta; AoV, aortic valve; AR, aortic regurgitation; LAX, long axis. *Source*: Surgical films, courtesy of Prof. Gebrine El Khoury.

annulus accepted only a size 19 mm, the available options to avoid mismatch would be either to perform an additional aortic root enlargement procedure to accommodate the 21 mm prosthesis or to use another type of prosthesis with a better hemodynamic profile (e.g., a stentless bioprosthesis or a mechanical valve) (Table 15.6).

The utilization of this strategy may help to reduce the incidence of PPM (38) without increasing operative mortality and morbidity, despite using an alternative technique to prevent PPM. Previous studies demonstrate that a prospective strategy to avoid mismatch can easily be applied with success (39). The information necessary to do the calculation is readily available as it requires only patient's height, weight, and the EOA reference values for the different types and sizes of prosthesis easily found in the literature (Table 15.6) (40).

Three caveats are worth mentioning when using these EOA values: (*i*) the values should be derived from in vivo rather than in vitro data as the latter are usually too optimistic, particularly in the case of stentless valves (41); (*ii*) values derived from geometric measurements (e.g., internal diameters or geometric areas) are totally inadequate as they do not predict postoperative gradients (28); and (*iii*) caution should, nevertheless, be exercised when new data are published.

Notwithstanding these considerations, endorsed by the Canadian Consensus Conference on Heart Valve Surgery (42) and the American Society of Echocardiography's Guidelines and Standards Committee and Task Force on Prosthetic Valves (40), the calculation of the projected indexed EOA should become an

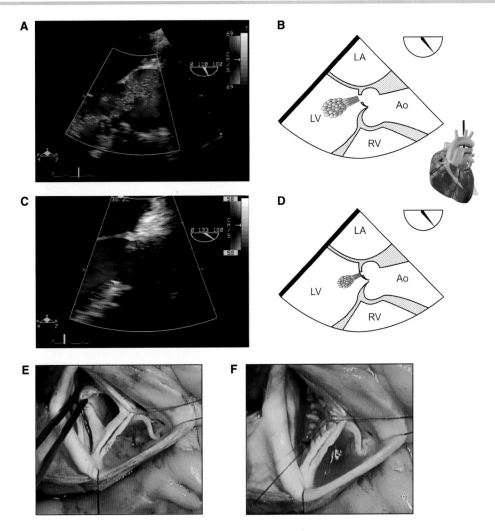

Figure 15.7 Type ID AR from perforated LCC. (A,B) Mid-esophageal aortic valve long-axis view in a patient presenting with a covered perforation of the LCC probably due to an old healed endocarditis and severe AR. **(C,D)** Same view after patch repair. Only trivial residual AR is seen. **(E,F)** Intraoperative view before and after repair with a pericardial patch. *Abbreviations*: Ao, aorta; AR, aortic regurgitation; LCC, left coronary cusp; LA, left atrium; LV, left ventricle; RV, right ventricle. *Source*: Surgical films, courtesy of Prof. Gebrine El Khoury.

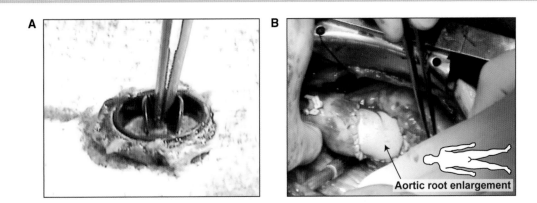

Figure 15.8 Patient-prosthesis mismatch. A 71-year-old man with a body surface area of 1.89 m² was re-operated on for symptoms of severe aortic valve stenosis. He had an AVR 4 years ago with a Carbomedics 19 mm mechanical bileaflet prosthesis (effective orifice area = 1.06 cm²). **(A)** The preoperative mean gradient was 41mmHg, although the intraoperative inspection of the prosthetic valve was completely normal. **(B)** Intraoperative view of an aortic root enlargement procedure in a 69-year-old patient with a reduced aortic diameter requiring AVR. *Abbreviation*: AVR, aortic valve replacement. *Source*: Courtesy of Dr. Michel Carrier.

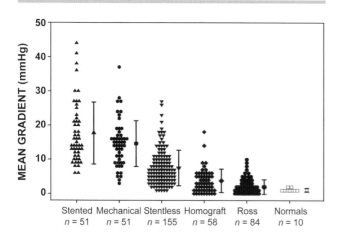

Figure 15.9 Prosthetic valve gradients. Comparison between mean gradients and type of valve prosthesis used for aortic valve replacement is shown.

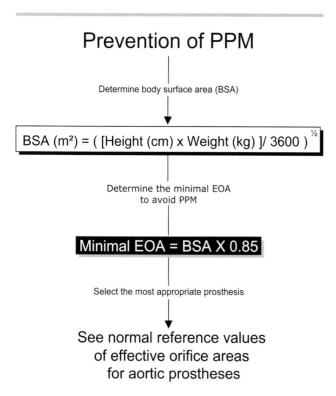

Prevention of PPM

Determine body surface area (BSA)

BSA (m²) = ([Height (cm) x Weight (kg)]/ 3600)^½

Determine the minimal EOA
to avoid PPM

Minimal EOA = BSA X 0.85

Select the most appropriate prosthesis

See normal reference values
of effective orifice areas
for aortic prostheses

Figure 15.10 Prevention of PPM. An algorithm to avoid PPM involves three easy steps. The BSA calculation is based on the Mosteller formula (29). *Abbreviations*: EOA, effective orifice area; PPM, patient-prosthetic mismatch. *Source*: Adapted from Ref. 28.

integral part of the decision process, leading to the choice of a particular type and size of prosthesis.

In this context, it should ideally be performed in the OR as it is only at that time that the aortic annulus diameter can best be measured accurately in the majority of cases. As stated, the ideal objective is that the prosthesis has an indexed EOA > 0.85 cm^2/m^2 after

operation but lower values may be acceptable in a less-active and/or older population with normal LV function.

CHOICE OF OPERATION IN PATIENTS WITH LV DYSFUNCTION

Recent evidence suggests that prosthesis size and the avoidance of PPM is an even greater consideration in patients with LV dysfunction as these factors may increase perioperative mortality. Operative mortality in patients with severe AS and low ejection fraction ($<35\%$) was 47% receiving a small size prosthesis (≤ 21 mm) compared with 15% with a larger size (>21 mm) prosthesis (43). Likewise, in a series of 1266 consecutive patients undergoing AVR, we observed a perioperative mortality of 67% in patients with severe PPM and an ejection fraction $<40\%$ compared with 3% in patients with no PPM and ejection fraction $>40\%$, intermediate mortality rates were observed in the other subgroups (Fig. 15.12) (26). There is also a strong interaction between PPM and depressed LV function to heart failure, and LV mass regression (44). Pathophysiologically, these patients appear to have a decreased ventricular reserve and are more vulnerable to the different degrees of mismatch, particularly in the critical perioperative period.

ECHOCARDIOGRAPHY IN THE OR

Before Operation

Before cardiopulmonary bypass (CPB), intraoperative TEE can be used to confirm the diagnosis as well as to establish the status of LV function. It should not, however, be seen as a substitute for a good preoperative transthoracic echocardiographic examination. Relevant preoperative information includes measurements of the AoV and aorta (see Fig. 23.1) and the mechanism of AR, the evaluation of systolic and diastolic LV function (45) (see Chapter 10), the evaluation of the presence of fistulas in patients with endocarditis (Fig. 15.13), right ventricular (RV) function in patients with pulmonary hypertension (46), and the exclusion of conditions such as mitral regurgitation (MR) (Fig. 15.14) and patent foramen ovale that could complicate the postoperative course. A significant intraoperative decrease in ventricular function should be worrisome even if it was preoperatively evaluated as being adequate. Indeed, deterioration in the intervening period may be the first manifestation of an LV myocardium with limited reserve.

During Cardiopulmonary Bypass

Details of echocardiography during CBP are given in Chapter 13.

After Cardiopulmonary Bypass

The first concern is to monitor the ventricular function to ensure that the myocardium is recuperating

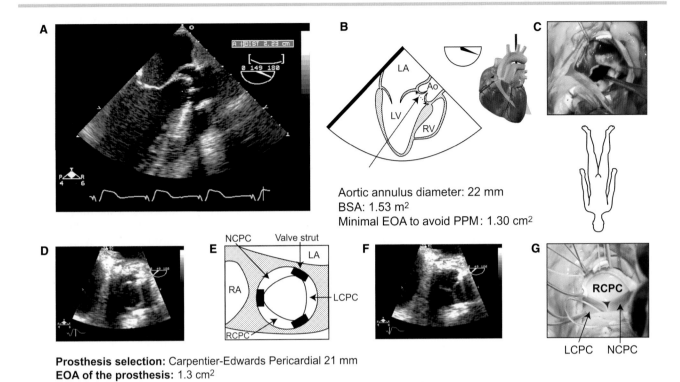

Aortic annulus diameter: 22 mm
BSA: 1.53 m^2
Minimal EOA to avoid PPM: 1.30 cm^2

Prosthesis selection: Carpentier-Edwards Pericardial 21 mm
EOA of the prosthesis: 1.3 cm^2

Figure 15.11   Aortic valve prosthesis selection. A 70-year-old man with a BSA of 1.53 m^2 is scheduled for AVR. **(A,B)** The aortic annulus measures 22 mm in the mid-esophageal AoV long-axis view. The minimal EOA required to avoid PPM should be higher than 1.53 m^2 × 0.85 cm^2/m^2 or 1.30 cm^2. **(C)** The intraoperative aspect of the native AoV is shown. **(D–F)** The selected prosthesis was a Carpentier–Edwards Perimount 21 mm with an EOA of 1.30 cm^2. **(G)** Intraoperative aspect of the bioprosthesis with the prosthetic valve cusps positioned similarly to the native AoV. *Abbreviations:* Ao, aorta; AoV, aortic valve; AVR, aortic valve replacement; BSA, body surface area; EOA, effective orifice area; LA, left atrium; LCPC, left coronary prosthetic cusp; NCPC, non-coronary prosthetic cusp; PPM, patient–prosthesis mismatch; RCPC, right coronary prosthetic cusp; RA, right atrium; RV, right ventricle. *Source:* Photos C and G courtesy of Dr. Denis Bouchard.

Table 15.6   Normal Reference Values of Effective Orifice Areas for the Aortic Prostheses

Prosthetic valve size (mm)	19	21	23	25	27	29	Reference
Aortic stented bioprostheses							
• Mosaic	1.1 ± 0.2	1.2 ± 0.3	1.4 ± 0.3	1.7 ± 0.4	1.8 ± 0.4	2.0 ± 0.4	24
• Hancock II	–	1.2 ± 0.1	1.3 ± 0.2	1.5 ± 0.2	1.6 ± 0.2	1.6 ± 0.2	24
• Carpentier–Edwards Perimount	1.1 ± 0.3	1.3 ± 0.4	1.50 ± 0.4	1.80 ± 0.4	2.1 ± 0.4	2.2 ± 0.4	24
• Carpentier–Edwards Magna[a]	1.3 ± 0.3	1.7 ± 0.3	2.1 ± 0.4	2.3 ± 0.5	–	–	30,31
• Biocor (Epic)[a]	–	1.3 ± 0.3	1.6 ± 0.3	1.8 ± 0.4	–	–	32
• Mitroflow[a]	1.1 ± 0.1	1.3 ± 0.1	1.5 ± 0.2	1.8 ± 0.2	–	–	33
Aortic stentless bioprostheses							
• Medtronic Freestyle	1.2 ± 0.2	1.4 ± 0.2	1.5 ± 0.3	2.0 ± 0.4	2.3 ± 0.5	–	24
• St. Jude Medical Toronto SPV	–	1.3 ± 0.3	1.5 ± 0.5	1.7 ± 0.8	2.1 ± 0.7	2.7 ± 1.0	24
• Cryolife O'Brien	–	1.2 ± 0.3	1.6 ± 0.4	1.9 ± 0.4	2.0 ± 0.2	2.2 ± 0.5	34
Aortic mechanical prostheses							
• Medtronic-Hall	1.2 ± 0.2	1.3 ± 0.2	–	–	–	–	24
• Medtronic Advantage	–	1.7 ± 0.2	2.2 ± 0.3	2.8 ± 0.6	3.3 ± 0.7	3.9 ± 0.7	35
• St. Jude Medical Standard	1.0 ± 0.2	1.4 ± 0.2	1.5 ± 0.5	2.1 ± 0.4	2.7 ± 0.6	3.2 ± 0.3	24
• St. Jude Medical Regent	1.6 ± 0.4	2.0 ± 0.7	2.2 ± 0.9	2.5 ± 0.9	3.6 ± 1.3	4.4 ± 0.6	36
• MCRI On-X	1.5 ± 0.2	1.7 ± 0.4	2.0 ± 0.6	2.4 ± 0.8	3.2 ± 0.6	3.2 ± 0.6	36
• Carbomedics Standard	1.0 ± 0.4	1.5 ± 0.3	1.7 ± 0.3	2.0 ± 0.4	2.5 ± 0.4	2.6 ± 0.4	24

[a]These results are based on a limited number of patients and thus should be interpreted with caution.
Source: From Ref. 37 (with permission of the American Heart Association).

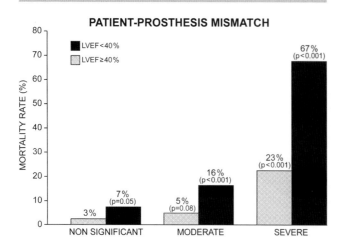

Figure 15.12   PPM and mortality. In-hospital mortality related to PPM and preoperative LVEF is shown. The p values above the bars correspond to the comparison with the group with insignificant mismatch and normal LVEF. *Abbreviations*: LVEF, left ventricular ejection fraction; PPM, patient-prosthesis mismatch. *Source*: Adapted from Ref. 26.

properly and that a satisfactory CO is generated. The next step is to examine valve morphology. Mechanical and stented bioprostheses are very echogenic, and it may be difficult to image occluders and leaflets in an SAX or LAX view.

Indirect evidence of leaflet motion in a bileaflet mechanical valve can sometimes be inferred from the reverberation artifacts associated with leaflet opening and closing. Alternatively, when one of the two leaflets is immobile, color flow Doppler may reveal an asymmetric color flow signal. The presence of an unexpectedly high gradient across an aortic mechanical prosthesis should prompt further evaluation as it may suggest a dysfunctional leaflet fixed in the closed position. Dehiscence of the prosthesis may be suggested by abnormal rocking motion of the sewing ring and significant perivalvular AR on color flow imaging.

Bioprosthetic valves can usually be imaged in the SAX view and are rarely associated with malfunction unless they are inadvertently damaged during implantation or are dysfunctional (Fig. 15.15).

Stentless prostheses and homografts have wider variation in morphology due to a lack of rigid

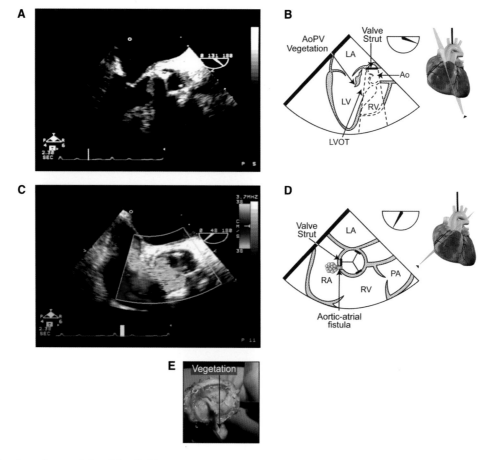

Figure 15.13   Aortic valve endocarditis. (A,B) ME long-axis view in an 83-year-old man with AoPV endocarditis shows a mobile mass. **(C,D)** Color Doppler ME AoV short-axis view demonstrates a fistula between the Ao and the RA. **(E)** Intraoperative finding was a vegetation attached to the inferior aspect of the AoPV. *Abbreviations*: Ao, aorta; AoPV, aortic prosthetic valve; AoV, aortic valve; LA, left atrium; LV, left ventricle; LVOT, left ventricular outflow tract; ME, mid-esophageal; PA, pulmonary artery; RA, right atrium; RV, right ventricle. *Source*: Photo E courtesy of Dr. Denis Bouchard.

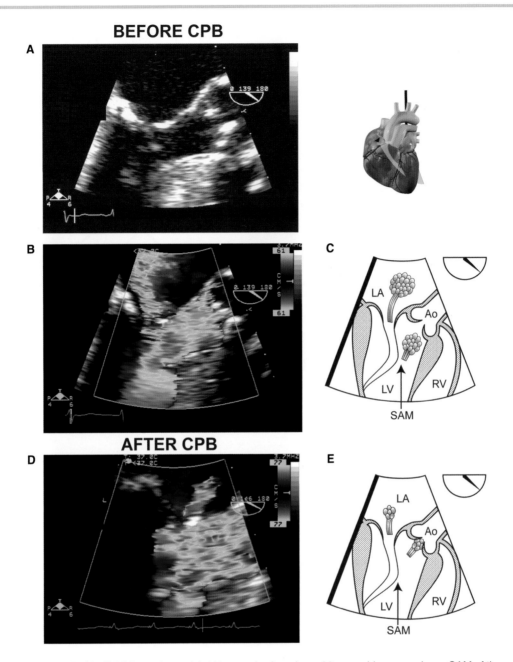

Figure 15.14   SAM with AVR. (A–C) Mid-esophageal AoV long-axis views in an 82-year-old woman shows SAM of the mitral valve and MR before AVR. **(D,E)** After AVR and septal myectomy, the SAM was still present but associated with less severe MR and a mean subvalvular gradient of 21 mmHg. *Abbreviations*: Ao, aorta; AoV, aortic valve; AVR, aortic valve replacement; CPB, cardiopulmonary bypass; LA, left atrium; LV, left ventricle; MR, mitral regurgitation; RV, right ventricle; SAM, systolic anterior motion.

support. These valvular substitutes may be implanted following a variety of techniques that, for our purposes, can be classified into two general categories:

1. The prosthesis is implanted as a root replacement, in which case the native aortic root is replaced by the porcine aortic root and requires the coronary arteries to be sectioned and reimplanted on the prosthetic root.

2. The porcine AoV and part of the porcine Ao are implanted within the patient's Ao using two suture lines, one proximal to the valve and the other one distal. There are three variations of the latter technique: complete subcoronary insertion, root inclusion, or modified subcoronary insertion (Fig. 15.16). The inclusion techniques will usually result in the formation of a virtual space between the prosthesis and the patient's Ao in which blood and/or debris may accumulate: this may appear as an echo-free

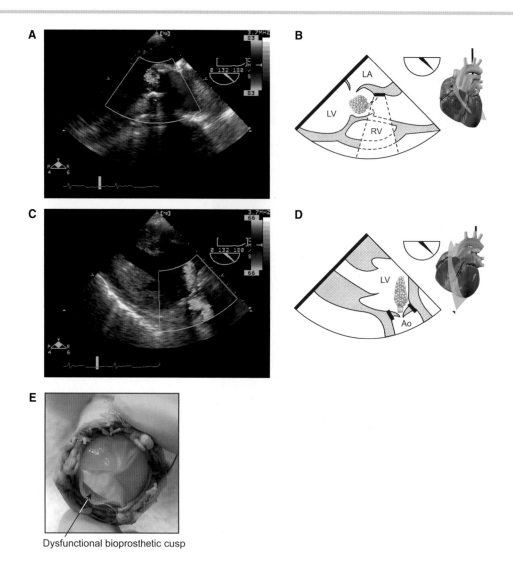

Figure 15.15 **Dysfunctional aortic valve bioprosthesis.** A 60-year-old man was reoperated on for periprosthetic AR. (**A–D**) After the procedure, abnormal significant AR is still visible on the color Doppler mid-esophageal long-axis and deep transgastric views. The new bioprosthesis was removed and replaced by another one. (**E**) Upon examination of the defective bioprosthesis, abnormal motion of one of the leaflets was noted. *Abbreviations*: Ao, aorta; AoV, aortic valve; AR, aortic regurgitation; LA, left atrium; LV, left ventricle; RV, right ventricle. *Source*: Photo E courtesy of Dr. Tack Ki Leung.

space encircling the valve (Fig. 15.17). Unless this echo-free space is very large or causes significant deformation of the valve geometry, the finding should be considered as normal, and it invariably regresses within the first few months after the operation. The regression of this perivalvular space may also explain the improvement in valve EOA and gradients observed within the first few months after operation with this type of prosthesis (8). When interpreting these images, one must, nevertheless, be attentive to a possible deformation or "crimping" of the valve, which may occur when the surgeon is overzealous in attempting to over-size the valve. If in doubt, measurement of the transvalvular velocity should be performed to

ensure the absence of abnormal obstruction to flow. In evaluating the structural integrity of stent-less prostheses, a flap corresponding to a partial dehiscence of one of the suture lines may be encountered, but this is rare.

In the case of AoV repair, the immediate post-operative result is of paramount importance. Valve repair has a good intermediate term durability that depends on the experience of the surgeon, the etiology and mechanism of AoV dysfunction, and the adequacy of the post repair cusp coaptation. In le Polain analysis of 39 patients presenting with recurrent severe AR among 251 valve repairs (47), Marfan's disease or restrictive cusp motion were more frequent

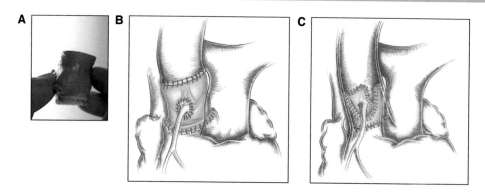

Figure 15.16 Stentless AoV. AoV replacement with a stentless Freestyle™ bioprosthesis (**A**) is shown. (**B**) Full root technique. After excising the native AoV and sinus walls, the coronary arteries are excised from the aorta and reattached to the buttonholes of the bioprosthesis. An end-to-end anastomosis attaches the bioprosthesis to the ascending aorta. (**C**) Modified subcoronary technique. The non-coronary sinus of the bioprosthesis is maintained, and right and left sinuses are scalloped. *Abbreviation*: AoV, aortic valve. *Source*: Diagrams B and C courtesy of Medtronic Inc. ⌐⊕

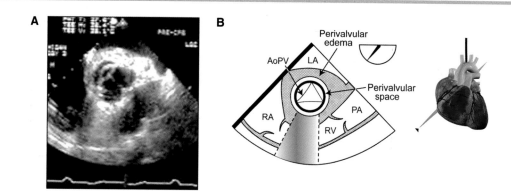

Figure 15.17 Post-operative aortic root edema. (A,B) Mid-esophageal aortic valve short-axis view shows a stentless prosthesis with a perivalvular echo-free space from an accumulation of blood and/or debris. This space usually regresses within a few months after operation. *Abbreviations*: AoPV, aortic prosthetic valve; LA, left atrium; PA, pulmonary artery; RA, right atrium; RV, right ventricle. *Source*: Courtesy of Dr. David Bach, University of Michigan. ⌐⊕

causes of unsatisfactorily attempted repair. Intraoperative TEE identified morphological and functional features associated with late repair failure, including the persistence of a residual eccentric AR jet, related to residual or newly appearing cusp prolapse, a coaptation length <5 mm, and/or cusp coaptation below the aortic annular plane and an enlarged aortic annulus. Other causes of late failure necessitating reoperation were dehiscence of valvular sutures, aortic dissection, and recurrent endocarditis (47). Causes for reoperation after repair of bicuspid AoV are symmetric cusp prolapse and an abnormally low height difference between the coaptation point of the cusps and the aortic insertion (20).

An adequate height of coaptation within the tube graft is an important factor for a favorable early result in reimplantation type of valve sparing surgery (48). The coaptation level and hence the risk for late valve incompetence seem to depend more on the fixation level of the commissures within the tube graft than on the size of the graft itself (49).

The next priority, after examining valve morphology, is to determine the presence or absence of any valvular regurgitation and its severity. In the case of mechanical prostheses, small jets of transvalvular regurgitation within the prosthesis may be normally observed: two in the case of tilting disk prostheses (e.g., Medtronic-Hall) or three in bileaflet prostheses

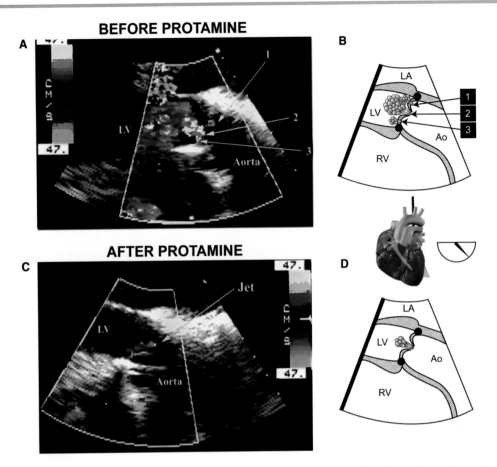

Figure 15.18 Regurgitant jets and protamine after aortic valve replacement. Color Doppler mid-esophageal long axis views at 130° of a bioprosthetic aortic valve demonstrating three regurgitant jets before (**A,B**) and one jet after protamine (**C,D**). *Abbreviations*: Ao, aorta; LA, left atrium; LV, left ventricle; RV, right ventricle. *Source*: Adapted with permission from Ref. 50.

(e.g., St-Jude or On-X). These jets, also known as closing volumes, occur as the result of the normal necessary space between the occluder(s) and the sewing ring without which jamming of these parts would occur (40). The inexperienced observer should not be alarmed by these jets, which at times may even appear moderate (2+), particularly when the jets are superimposed.

Small perivalvular jets of regurgitation may also be observed using TEE with all types of prosthesis. Some will significantly decrease after the injection of protamine (50,51) and will often disappear in the days, weeks, or months after the operation as the healing process evolves (Fig. 15.18). More severe regurgitation is rare and is most often due to a technical problem after insertion of a stentless prosthesis or a homograft. It may be either periprosthetic or centrovalvular, and more than 1+ regurgitation usually requires returning to CPB for immediate correction (Fig. 15.19). If in doubt, we use epicardial echocardiography to confirm and evaluate the severity of AR (see Chapter 6).

It is not always possible to obtain accurate measurements of intraoperative gradients. However, such measurements may become more relevant in the case of stentless prostheses, homografts, or autografts, especially if the two-dimensional (2D) images suggest some inherent technical problem (e.g., perivalvular hematoma and/or crimping of the valve).

If a high gradient is noticed in the OR, one must first determine whether it is partially, or principally, related to a high flow velocity in the left ventricular outflow tract (LVOT). In particular, relief of the valvular obstruction in patients operated on for AS may result in some remodeling and temporary narrowing of the LVOT. The administration of inotropic agents upon coming off CPB may also contribute to this phenomenon. Notwithstanding these considerations, the most frequent cause of high postoperative gradients is PPM as it may occur in up to 70% of cases (24), depending on the type of prosthesis being implanted. It is much less likely to occur if the aforementioned prospective strategy was followed (Fig. 15.10). If not, its presence may easily be

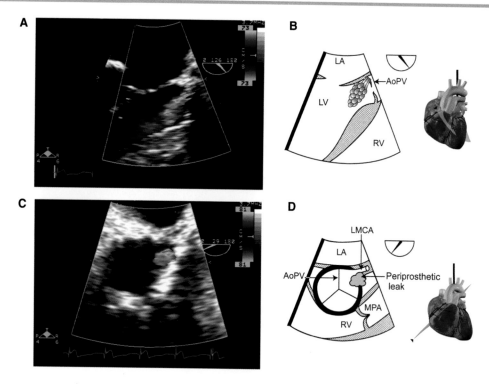

Figure 15.19 **Periprosthetic AR. (A,B)** Immediately after a bioprosthetic AVR in a 70-year-old woman, a small AR jet was seen in the color Doppler mid-esophageal AoV long-axis view. **(C,D)** In the color Doppler AoV short-axis view, it was located outside the origin of the LMCA ostium. *Abbreviations*: AoV, aortic valve; AoPV, aortic prosthetic valve; AR, aortic regurgitation; AVR, aortic valve replacement; LA, left atrium; LMCA, left main coronary artery; LV, left ventricle; MPA, main pulmonary artery; RV, right ventricle.

confirmed by going through the same algorithm after the fact, that is, dividing the reference value of the EOA of the prosthesis having been implanted by the BSA of the patient to yield the indexed EOA (Fig. 15.20). In patients with normal CO, postoperative gradients are directly related to the indexed EOA and become progressively higher as this value becomes lower. It should be emphasized that a small indexed EOA with a low systolic gradient is the worst case scenario as it is usually associated with LV dysfunction and a low CO.

An indexed EOA <0.85 cm²/m² is considered mild/moderate mismatch whereas a value <0.65 cm²/m² corresponds to severe mismatch. The latter should be considered unacceptable, whereas clinical judgment, based on patient's age, level of physical activity, and status of LV function, should be used to determine optimal conduct in patients with an indexed EOA between 0.65 and 0.85 cm²/m² (Fig. 15.20). For obvious reasons, it is clearly preferable to perform this evaluation before, rather than after, implanting the prosthesis. Reintervention to correct PPM is accomplished either by implanting another type of prosthesis with a better hemodynamic profile (e.g., stentless or mechanical) or by performing an additional aortic root enlargement procedure.

ECHOCARDIOGRAPHIC TECHNIQUE

Morphological evaluation of the AoV should be done in both the transverse and longitudinal planes (Fig. 15.21), as detailed in Chapter 14. Transvalvular gradients are best evaluated using the deep transgastric and the transgastric LAX view (Fig. 15.22). It may often be difficult to obtain satisfactory views of the AoV to obtain accurate measurements of gradients, either because the valve simply cannot be visualized in this position or the angle between the ultrasound beam and the direction of blood flow exceeds 20°, thus rendering Doppler measurements of velocities inaccurate.

An alternative approach for measuring aortic gradients in the OR is to perform epicardial measurements (see Chapter 6). A transthoracic, epiaortic probe or the TEE probe may be used for this purpose. In either case, the probe is inserted with a fair amount of gel in a sterile bag to be directly placed over the Ao by the surgeon. This approach obviously requires

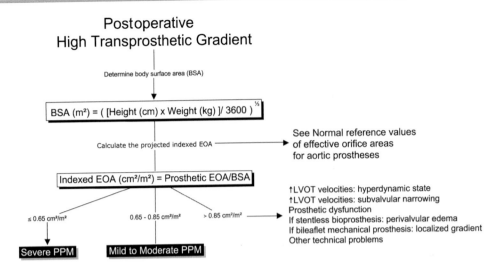

Postoperative
High Transprosthetic Gradient

Determine body surface area (BSA)

$$BSA\ (m^2) = (\ [Height\ (cm) \times Weight\ (kg)\ ]/\ 3600\ )^{\frac{1}{2}}$$

Calculate the projected indexed EOA ⟶ See Normal reference values of effective orifice areas for aortic prostheses

$$Indexed\ EOA\ (cm^2/m^2) = Prosthetic\ EOA/BSA$$

≤ 0.65 cm²/m²   0.65 - 0.85 cm²/m²   > 0.85 cm²/m²

↑LVOT velocities: hyperdynamic state
↑LVOT velocities: subvalvular narrowing
Prosthetic dysfunction
If stentless bioprosthesis: perivalvular edema
If bileaflet mechanical prosthesis: localized gradient
Other technical problems

Severe PPM   **Mild to Moderate PPM**

Figure 15.20   High transvalvular pressure gradients. An algorithm is presented for evaluating abnormally high transvalvular pressure gradients during surgery or in the immediate postoperative period. The projected indexed EOA is calculated from the normal reference value of EOA for the model and size of prosthesis implanted and patient's BSA. If the projected indexed EOA is ≤0.85 cm²/m², the abnormally high gradient is most likely due to PPM. If the projected indexed EOA is >0.85 cm²/m², several possible conditions or technical pitfalls must be ruled out before concluding the presence of an intrinsic dysfunction of the prosthesis. *Abbreviations*: BSA, body surface area; EOA, effective orifice area; LVOT, left ventricular outflow tract: PPM, patient–prosthesis mismatch.

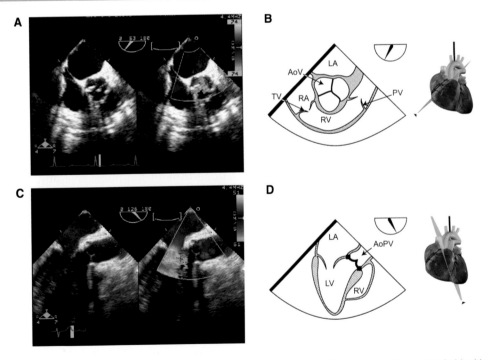

Figure 15.21   AoV replacement. (A,B) Color compare ME AoV short-axis view before surgery shows an AoV with three cusps and severe stenosis. **(C,D)** Color compare ME AoV long-axis view of the implanted stented AoPV. *Abbreviations*: AoPV, aortic prosthetic valve; AoV, aortic valve; LA, left atrium; LV, left ventricle; ME, mid-esophageal; PV, pulmonic valve; RA, right atrium; RV, right ventricle; TV, tricuspid valve.

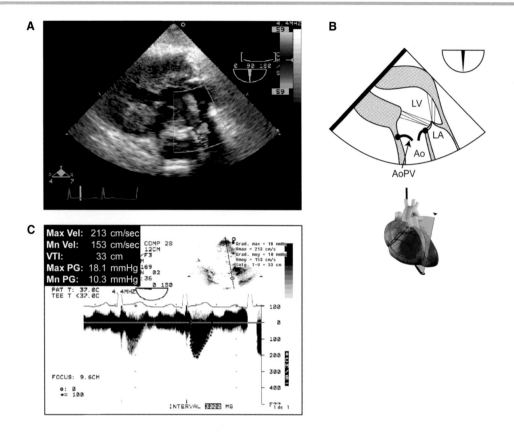

Figure 15.22 Transvalvular PG. (A,B) Transgastric view at 90° of an AoPV with mean transvalvular PG of 10.3 mmHg (**C**). *Abbreviations*: Ao, aorta; AoPV, aortic prosthetic valve; LA, left atrium; LV, left ventricle; Max, maximum; Mn, mean; PG, pressure gradient; Vel, velocity; VTI, velocity–time integral.

echocardiography-trained surgeons, but beyond this initial hurdle, we have found the rate of success in obtaining accurate measurements of gradients to be close to 100%. The use of the TEE probe is particularly convenient because it is more easily manipulated over the heart and can easily be inserted between the heart and/or great vessels and the chest wall. Other aspects of the postoperative TEE evaluation include assessment of the other valves and ruling out unexpected complications of single or complex AoV surgery (Figs. 15.22–15.25).

ECHOCARDIOGRAPHY IN THE IMMEDIATE POSTOPERATIVE PERIOD

Hemodynamic assessment of the prosthetic valve, done in the immediate postoperative period, cannot be considered as definitive because of LV remodeling, relative high-output states, and the frequent occurrence of tachycardia. The main objectives of a postoperative echocardiogram in a patient with AVR are to obtain accurate measurements of peak and mean gradients, as well as the nonindexed and indexed EOA. Echocardiograms are technically challenging because of the location of the various incisions resulting in

suboptimal images and some pitfalls associated with accurate measurements as listed here:

1. Erroneous measurement of the true diameter of the LVOT is prone to over- or underestimation from poor-quality images. Furthermore, the labeled size of the prosthetic valve sewing ring is invalidated as a substitute of the LVOT diameter by LVOT tissue protrusion or a supra-annular implantation (52).

2. High LVOT flow velocity may be abnormally increased by high CO or dynamic obstruction from temporary remodeling of the LVOT. This precludes, or limits, the validity of the simplified Bernoulli equation, which ignores the subvalvular gradient, for the estimation of transvalvular gradients or EOAs. When the subvalvular gradient is high (e.g., maximum gradient >10 mmHg), it is no longer negligible and must be subtracted from the transvalvular gradients recorded by CW Doppler to obtain the true gradient across the valve.

3. The presence of perivalvular edema or hematoma in stentless prosthesis during the immediate postoperative period may result in a lower than expected EOA during the first few months after operation.

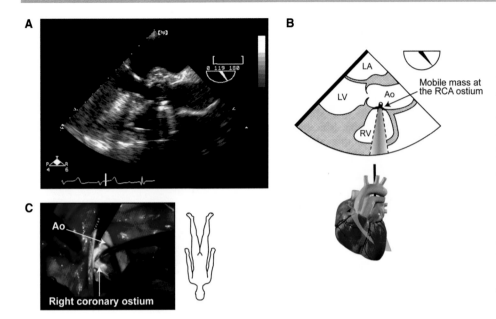

Figure 15.23   Calcium emboli. A 77-year-old woman with aortic stenosis underwent aortic valve replacement. (**A,B**) During weaning from CPB an abnormal mobile calcified mass is seen anterior to the Ao in the mid-esophageal aortic valve long-axis view. (**C**) The surgeon went back on CPB and found dislodged calcified plaques at the RCA ostium. A coronary endarterectomy was performed with an uneventful postoperative course. *Abbreviations*: Ao, aorta; CPB, cardiopulmonary bypass; LA, left atrium; LV, left ventricle; RCA, right coronary artery; RV, right ventricle. *Source*: Photo C courtesy of Dr. Raymond Cartier.

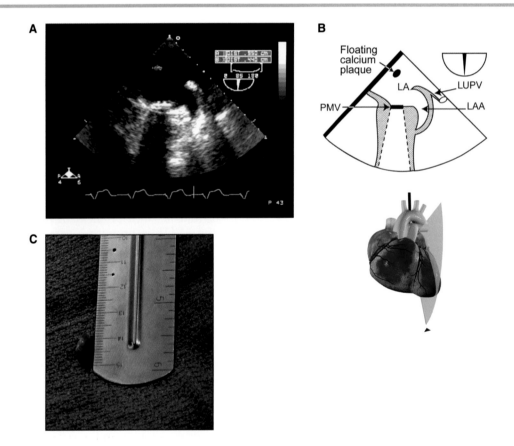

Figure 15.24   Calcium emboli. A 70-year-old man underwent coronary revascularization and combined aortic and mitral valve replacement. (**A,B**) During weaning from CPB floating material was seen in the LA in the mid-esophageal two-chamber view. The surgeon went back immediately to full CPB. (**C**) This material was a 4 × 1 mm floating calcium plaque which was removed. The patient had no postoperative neurological complications. *Abbreviations*: CPB, cardiopulmonary bypass; LAA, left atrial appendage; LA, left atrium; LUPV, left upper pulmonary vein; PMV, prosthetic mitral valve.

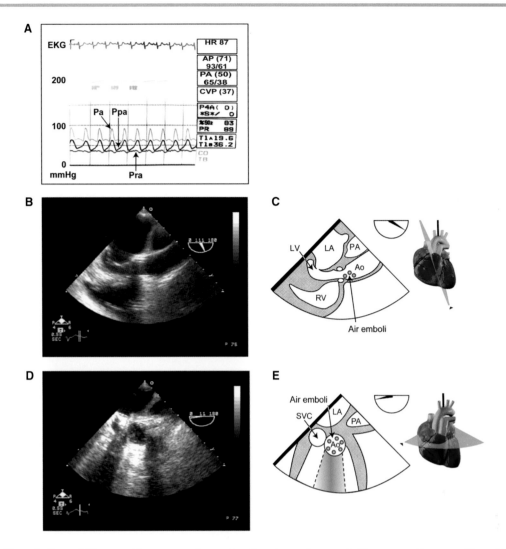

Figure 15.25 Air embolism. A 61-year-old woman underwent aortic valve replacement. She was easily weaned from CPB. As she was transferred onto the transportation bed, she developed acute pulmonary hypertension (**A**) followed by ventricular fibrillation from which she was resuscitated. (**B–E**) Mid-esophageal aortic valve long-axis and short axis views revealed strong echogenic material close to the prosthetic valve consistent with air emboli dislodged during mobilization of the patient. *Abbreviations*: Ao, aorta; CPB, cardiopulmonary bypass; EKG, electrocardiogram; LA, left atrium; LV, left ventricle; Pa, arterial pressure; PA, pulmonary artery; Ppa, pulmonary artery pressure; Pra, right atrial pressure; RV, right ventricle; SVC, superior vena cava.

For these reasons, the recording of relatively high gradients in the immediate postoperative period should not be viewed with undue concern. A simple algorithm recently described by the American Society of Echocardiography's Guidelines and Standards Committee and the Task Force on Prosthetic Valves may be used to assess abnormally high gradients in the immediate postoperative period (Fig. 15.26) (40). Given that PPM is the most frequent cause of high gradients, the first step of this algorithm is to determine if a PPM is present by calculating the projected indexed EOA rather than using the less reliable calculated EOA (see above limitations). This parameter is simply calculated by dividing the normal reference

EOA, for the model and size of prosthesis implanted (Table 15.6), by patient's BSA. If the projected indexed EOA is ≤0.85 cm²/m², the abnormally high gradient is likely due to mismatch. If the projected indexed EOA is >0.85 cm²/m², several aforementioned conditions and technical pitfalls must first be ruled out before concluding prosthesis dysfunction. In particular, an abnormally high velocity jet corresponding to a localized gradient may be recorded by CW Doppler interrogation through the smaller central slit-like orifice of bileaflet mechanical prosthesis. This is not reproduced when redirecting the ultrasound beam through either lateral major orifices. This is a limitation of the echocardiographic evaluation of bileaflet prostheses inherent

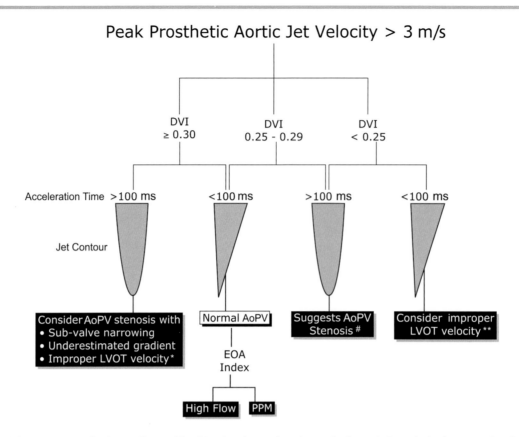

Figure 15.26 High transprosthetic gradients. Algorithm for elevated peak prosthetic aortic jet velocity incorporating the DVI, AT and jet contour. *PW Doppler sample too close to the valve (particularly when jet velocity by CW Doppler is ≥ 4 m/s). **PW Doppler sample is too far (apical) from the valve (particularly when jet velocity is 3.0–3.9 m/s). #Stenosis further substantiated by EOA derivation compared with reference values if valve type and size are known. Fluoroscopy and transesophageal echocardiography are helpful for further assessment, particularly in bileaflet valves. *Abbreviations*: AoPV, aortic prosthetic valve; fCW, continuous wave; DVI, Doppler velocity index; EOA, effective orifice area; LVOT, left ventricular outflow tract; ms, millisecond; PPM, patient-prosthesis mismatch; PW, pulsed wave. *Source*: Adapted from Ref. 40.

Table 15.7 Doppler Parameters of Prosthetic Aortic Valve Function in Mechanical and Stented Biologic Valves[a]

Parameter	Normal	Possible stenosis	Suggests significant stenosis
Peak velocity (m/s)[b]	<3	3–4	>4
Mean gradient (mmHg)[b]	<20	20–35	>35
DVI	≥0.30	0.29–0.25	<0.25
EOA (cm²)	>1.2	1.2–0.8	<0.8
Contour of the jet velocity through the PrAV	Triangular, early peaking	Triangular to intermediate	Rounded, symmetrical contour
AT (ms)	<80	80–100	>100

[a]In conditions of normal or near normal stroke volume (50–70 mL) through the aortic valve.
[b]These parameters are more affected by flow, including concomitant AR.
Abbreviations: AT, acceleration time; DVI, Doppler velocity index; EOA, effective orifice area; PrAV, prosthetic aortic valve.
Source: From Ref. 40.

in their design, which should be kept in mind when encountering a relatively high gradient in a patient with this type of mechanical prosthesis. Therefore, unless the transvalvular gradients are very high or are associated with significant symptoms or deterioration in LV function, a conservative approach with observation

and repeat assessment three to six months later is advocated.

An algorithm has also been recently proposed by the American Society of Echocardiography's Guidelines and Standards Committee and Task Force on Prosthetic Valves for evaluation of high gradients after

Table 15.8 Parameters for Evaluation of the Severity of Prosthetic Aortic Valve Regurgitation

Parameter	Mild	Moderate	Severe
Valve structure and motion			
Mechanical or bioprosthetic	Usually normal	Abnormal[a]	Abnormal[a]
Structural parameters			
LV size	Normal[b]	Normal or mildly dilated[b]	Dilated[b]
Doppler parameters (qualitative or semiquantitative)			
Jet width in central jets (% LVO diameter): color[c]	Narrow (≤25%)	Intermediate (26–64%)	Large (≥65%)
Jet density: CW Doppler	Incomplete or faint	Dense	Dense
Jet deceleration rate (PHT, ms): CW Doppler[d]	Slow (>500)	Variable (200–500)	Steep (<200)
LVO flow vs. pulmonary flow: PW Doppler	Slightly increased	Intermediate	Greatly increased
Diastolic flow reversal in the descending aorta: PW Doppler	Absent or brief early diastolic	Intermediate	Prominent, holodiastolic
Doppler parameters (quantitative)			
Regurgitant volume (mL/beat)	<30	30–59	>60
Regurgitant fraction (%)	<30	30–50	>50

[a]Abnormal mechanical valves, for example, immobile occluder (valvular regurgitation), dehiscence or rocking (paravalvular regurgitation); abnormal biologic valves, for example, leaflet thickening or prolapse (valvular), dehiscence or rocking (paravalvular regurgitation).
[b]Applies to chronic, late postoperative AR in the absence of other etiologies.
[c]Parameter applicable to central jets and is less accurate in eccentric jets; Nyquist limit of 50–60 cm/s.
[d]Influenced by LV compliance.
Abbreviations: AR, aortic regurgitation; CW, continuous wave; LV, left ventricular; LVO, left ventricular outflow; PHT, pressure half-time; PW, pulsed wave.
Source: From Ref. 40.

Table 15.9 Summary of the Role of TEE in Patients Undergoing Aortic Valve Surgery

	Importance
Before the procedure	
• See Table 13.1 for the role of TEE in cardiac surgery	
• Measurement of aortic annulus and ascending aortic dimensions	Calculation of the projected effective orifice area to prevent patient-prosthesis mismatch
	Need for concomitant aortic procedure (replacement or enlargement)
• Evaluate the severity of left ventricular septal hypertrophy	Anticipate the occurrence of dynamic LVOT obstruction and the need for septal myectomy
• Rule-out coarctation if bicuspid aortic valve disease	Concomitant repair may be considered
During CPB	
• See Table 13.1	
After CPB	
• See Table 13.1	
• Evaluate result of repair or replacement	Early detection and correction of prosthetic dysfunction or suboptimal repair
In the intensive care unit	
• See Table 13.1	

Abbreviations: CPB, cardiopulmonary bypass; LVOT, left ventricular outflow tract; TEE, transesophageal echocardiography.

AVR (Fig. 15.26). The committee has also proposed guidelines for the assessment of AoV prosthetic stenosis (Table 15.7) and regurgitation (Table 15.8). However, the difficulty of achieving accurate measurement of some Doppler-echocardiographic parameters (i.e., EOA, dimensionless velocity index, regurgitant volume, etc.) in the immediate postoperative period may limit the utilization of these algorithms and guidelines for the perioperative evaluation of prosthetic valve function.

CONCLUSION

Perioperative echocardiography may be useful to detect clinically unsuspected abnormalities that may alter, or add, operative procedures during AoV surgery (Table 15.9). Patient-prosthesis mismatch is by far the most frequent cause of high transvalvular gradients after AVR. Nevertheless, this problem can largely be avoided with the use of a prospective strategy before prosthesis implantation.

REFERENCES

1. Bonow RO, Carabello BA, Kanu C, et al. ACC/AHA 2006 guidelines for the management of patients with valvular heart disease: a report of the American College of Cardiology/American Heart Association Task Force on Practice Guidelines (writing committee to revise the 1998 Guidelines for the Management of Patients With Valvular Heart Disease): developed in collaboration with the Society of Cardiovascular Anesthesiologists: endorsed by the Society for Cardiovascular Angiography and Interventions and the Society of Thoracic Surgeons. Circulation 2006; 114: e84–e231.

2. Amato MC, Moffa PJ, Werner KE, et al. Treatment decision in asymptomatic aortic valve stenosis: role of exercise testing. Heart 2001; 86:381–386.

3. Alborino D, Hoffmann JL, Fournet PC, et al. Value of exercise testing to evaluate the indication for surgery in asymptomatic patients with valvular aortic stenosis. J Heart Valve Dis 2002; 11:204–209.

4. Hachicha Z, Dumesnil JG, Bogaty P, et al. Paradoxical low-flow, low-gradient severe aortic stenosis despite preserved ejection fraction is associated with higher afterload and reduced survival. Circulation 2007; 115:2856–2864.

5. Baumgartner H, Hung J, Bermejo J, et al. Echocardiographic assessment of valve stenosis: EAE/ASE recommendations for clinical practice. J Am Soc Echocardiogr 2009; 22:1–23.

6. Rosenhek R, Binder T, Porenta G, et al. Predictors of outcome in severe, asymptomatic aortic stenosis. N Engl J Med 2000; 343:611–617.

7. Dumesnil JG, Leblanc MH, Cartier PC, et al. Hemodynamic features of the freestyle aortic bioprosthesis compared with stented bioprosthesis. Ann Thorac Surg 1998; 66:S130–S133.

8. Briand M, Pibarot P, Dumesnil JG, et al. Midterm echocardiographic follow-up after Ross operation. Circulation 2000; 102:III10–III14.

9. de Kerchove L, Rubay J, Pasquet A, et al. Ross operation in the adult: long-term outcomes after root replacement and inclusion techniques. Ann Thorac Surg 2009; 87:95–102.

10. David TE, Feindel CM, Webb GD, et al. Long-term results of aortic valve-sparing operations for aortic root aneurysm. J Thorac Cardiovasc Surg 2006; 132:347–354.

11. Aicher D, Langer F, Lausberg H, et al. Aortic root remodeling: ten-year experience with 274 patients. J Thorac Cardiovasc Surg 2007; 134:909–915.

12. Augoustides JG, Wolfe Y, Walsh EK, et al. Recent advances in aortic valve disease: highlights from a bicuspid aortic valve to transcatheter aortic valve replacement. J Cardiothorac Vasc Anesth 2009; 23:569–576.

13. El Khoury G, Vanoverschelde JL, Glineur D, et al. Repair of bicuspid aortic valves in patients with aortic regurgitation. Circulation 2006; 114:I610–I616.

14. de Waroux JB, Pouleur AC, Goffinet C, et al. Functional anatomy of aortic regurgitation: accuracy, prediction of surgical repairability, and outcome implications of transesophageal echocardiography. Circulation 2007; 116:I264–I269.

15. El Khoury G, Glineur D, Rubay J, et al. Functional classification of aortic root/valve abnormalities and their correlation with etiologies and surgical procedures. Curr Opin Cardiol 2005; 20:115–121.

16. Boodhwani M, de Kerchove L, Glineur D, et al. Repair-oriented classification of aortic insufficiency: impact on surgical techniques and clinical outcomes. J Thorac Cardiovasc Surg 2009; 137:286–294.

17. Sarsam MA, Yacoub M. Remodeling of the aortic valve annulus. J Thorac Cardiovasc Surg 1993; 105:435–438.

18. Boodhwani M, de Kerchove L, El Khoury G. Aortic root replacement using the reimplantation technique: tips and tricks. Interact Cardiovasc Thorac Surg 2009; 8:584–586.

19. Di Bartolomeo R, Pacini D, Martin-Suarez S, et al. Valsalva prosthesis in aortic valve-sparing operations. Interact Cardiovasc Thorac Surg 2006; 5:294–298.

20. de Waroux JB, Pouleur AC, Robert A, et al. Mechanisms of recurrent aortic regurgitation after aortic valve repair: predictive value of intraoperative transesophageal echocardiography. JACC Cardiovasc Imaging 2009; 2:931–939.

21. de Kerchove L, Boodhwani M, Glineur D, et al. Effects of preoperative aortic insufficiency on outcome after aortic valve-sparing surgery. Circulation 2009; 120:S120–S126.

22. de Kerchove L, Boodhwani M, Glineur D, et al. Cusp prolapse repair in trileaflet aortic valves: free margin plication and free margin resuspension techniques. Ann Thorac Surg 2009; 88:455–461.

23. de Kerchove L, Glineur D, Poncelet A, et al. Repair of aortic leaflet prolapse: a ten-year experience. Eur J Cardiothorac Surg 2008; 34:785–791.

24. Pibarot P, Dumesnil JG. Hemodynamic and clinical impact of prosthesis-patient mismatch in the aortic valve position and its prevention. J Am Coll Cardiol 2000; 36:1131–1141.

25. Rao V, Jamieson WR, Ivanov J, et al. Prosthesis-patient mismatch affects survival after aortic valve replacement. Circulation 2000; 102:III5–III9.

26. Blais C, Dumesnil JG, Baillot R, et al. Impact of valve prosthesis-patient mismatch on short-term mortality after aortic valve replacement. Circulation 2003; 108:983–988.

27. Ruel M, Rubens FD, Masters RG, et al. Late incidence and predictors of persistent or recurrent heart failure in patients with mitral prosthetic valves. J Thorac Cardiovasc Surg 2004; 128:278–283.

28. Pibarot P, Dumesnil JG. Patient–prosthesis mismatch and the predictive use of indexed effective orifice area: is it relevant? Card Surg Today 2003; 1:43–51.

29. Mosteller RD. Simplified calculation of body-surface area. N Engl J Med 1987; 317:1098.

30. Botzenhardt F, Eichinger WB, Guenzinger R, et al. Hemodynamic performance and incidence of patient-prosthesis mismatch of the complete supraannular perimount magna bioprosthesis in the aortic position. Thorac Cardiovasc Surg 2005; 53:226–230.

31. Dalmau MJ, Maria Gonzalez-Santos J, Lopez-Rodriguez J, et al. One year hemodynamic performance of the Perimount Magna pericardial xenograft and the Medtronic Mosaic bioprosthesis in the aortic position: a prospective randomized study. Interact Cardiovasc Thorac Surg 2007; 6:345–349.

32. Dellgren G, David TE, Raanani E, et al. Late hemodynamic and clinical outcomes of aortic valve replacement with the Carpentier-Edwards Perimount pericardial bioprosthesis. J Thorac Cardiovasc Surg 2002; 124:146–154.

33. Garcia-Bengochea J, Sierra J, Gonzalez-Juanatey JR, et al. Left ventricular mass regression after aortic valve replacement with the new Mitroflow 12A pericardial bioprosthesis. J Heart Valve Dis 2006; 15:446–451.

34. Chambers JB, Rimington HM, Rajani R, et al. A randomized comparison of the Cryolife O'Brien and Toronto stentless replacement aortic valves. J Thorac Cardiovasc Surg 2007; 133:1045–1050.

35. Koertke H, Seifert D, Drewek-Platena S, et al. Hemodynamic performance of the Medtronic ADVANTAGE prosthetic heart valve in the aortic position: echocardiographic evaluation at one year. J Heart Valve Dis 2003; 12: 348–353.

36. Pibarot P, Dumesnil JG. Prosthesis-patient mismatch: definition, clinical impact, and prevention. Heart 2006; 92: 1022–1029.

37. Pibarot P, Dumesnil JG. Prosthetic heart valves: selection of the optimal prosthesis and long-term management. Circulation 2009; 119:1034–1048.

38. Bleiziffer S, Eichinger WB, Hettich I, et al Prediction of valve prosthesis-patient mismatch prior to aortic valve replacement: which is the best method? Heart 2007; 93:615–620.

39. Kulik A, Al-Saigh M, Chan V, et al Enlargement of the small aortic root during aortic valve replacement: is there a benefit? Ann Thorac Surg 2008; 85:94–100.

40. Zoghbi WA, Chambers JB, Dumesnil JG, et al Recommendations for evaluation of prosthetic valves with echocardiography and Doppler ultrasound: a report From the American Society of Echocardiography's Guidelines and Standards Committee and the Task Force on Prosthetic Valves, developed in conjunction with the American College of Cardiology Cardiovascular Imaging Committee, Cardiac Imaging Committee of the American Heart Association, the European Association of Echocardiography, a registered branch of the European Society of Cardiology, the Japanese Society of Echocardiography and the Canadian Society of Echocardiography, endorsed by the American College of Cardiology Foundation, American Heart Association, European Association of Echocardiography, a registered branch of the European Society of Cardiology, the Japanese Society of Echocardiography, and Canadian Society of Echocardiography. J Am Soc Echocardiogr 2009; 22:975–1014.

41. Bleiziffer S, Eichinger WB, Lange R. Letter by Bleiziffer et al regarding article, "Long-term outcomes after valve replacement for low-gradient aortic stenosis: impact of prosthesis-patient mismatch". Circulation 2006; 114:e627.

42. Jamieson WR, Cartier PC, Allard M, et al. Surgical management of valvular heart disease 2004. Can J Cardiol 2004; 20(suppl E):7E–120E.

43. Connolly HM, Oh JK, Schaff HV, et al. Severe aortic stenosis with low transvalvular gradient and severe left ventricular dysfunction: result of aortic valve replacement in 52 patients. Circulation 2000; 101:1940–1946.

44. Ruel M, Al Faleh H, Kulik A, et al. Prosthesis-patient mismatch after aortic valve replacement predominantly affects patients with preexisting left ventricular dysfunction: effect on survival, freedom from heart failure, and left ventricular mass regression. J Thorac Cardiovasc Surg 2006; 131:1036–1044.

45. Lund O, Flo C, Jensen FT, et al. Left ventricular systolic and diastolic function in aortic stenosis. Prognostic value after valve replacement and underlying mechanisms. Eur Heart J 1997; 18:1977–1987.

46. Malouf JF, Enriquez-Sarano M, Pellikka PA, et al. Severe pulmonary hypertension in patients with severe aortic valve stenosis: clinical profile and prognostic implications. J Am Coll Cardiol 2002; 40:789–795.

47. le Polain de Waroux J-B, Pouleur AC, Goffinet C et al. Intraoperative transoesophageal echocardiographic predictors of recurrent aortic regurgitation after aortic valve repair. Circulation 2007; 116(suppl I):I264–I269.

48. Pethig K, Milz A, Hagl C, et al. Aortic valve reimplantation in ascending aortic aneurysm: risk factors for early valve failure. Ann Thorac Surg 2002; 73:29–33.

49. Babin-Ebell J, De Vivo F, Vogt PR, et al. Impact of graft size and resuspension level of the commissures on aortic insufficiency after reimplantation of the aortic valve. Thorac Cardiovasc Surg 2007; 55:351–354.

50. Morehead AJ, Firstenberg MS, Shiota T, et al. Intraoperative echocardiographic detection of regurgitant jets after valve replacement. Ann Thorac Surg 2000; 69:135–139.

51. Lau WC, Carroll JR, Deeb GM, et al. Intraoperative transesophageal echocardiographic assessment of the effect of protamine on paraprosthetic aortic insufficiency immediately after stentless tissue aortic valve replacement. J Am Soc Echocardiogr 2002; 15:1175–1180.

52. Pibarot P, Honos GN, Durand LG, et al. Substitution of left ventricular outflow tract diameter with prosthesis size is inadequate for calculation of the aortic prosthetic valve area by the continuity equation. J Am Soc Echocardiogr 1995; 8:511–517.

16

Mitral Valve

André Saint-Pierre
Université Laval, Quebec City, Quebec, Canada

Jean Buithieu
McGill University, Montreal, Quebec, Canada

Stéphane Coutu
Université de Sherbrooke, Sherbrooke, Quebec, Canada

A. Stéphane Lambert
University of Ottawa Heart Institute, Ottawa, Ontario, Canada

INTRODUCTION

Echocardiography is the method of choice for the noninvasive assessment of the severity and mechanisms of mitral regurgitation (MR). Practice guidelines recently published by the American College of Cardiology and the American Heart Association are largely based on echocardiography evaluation (1). This chapter includes the recent recommendations of the American Society of Echocardiography (ASE) for the evaluation and assessment of the severity of native valvular regurgitation (2), with emphasis on transesophageal echocardiography (TEE) examination.

ANATOMICAL MANIFESTATIONS OF MITRAL VALVULAR LESIONS

Mitral Valve Examination

The mitral valve (MV) is a complex structure, and its functional anatomy comprises not only the valve itself with the annulus, the leaflets, the chordae tendineae, and the papillary muscles but also the fibrous skeleton, the left atrium (LA), and left ventricle (LV) (3). Dysfunction, or abnormalities, of any of these components can result in MR. The anatomical landmarks are presented on pathological specimen and corresponding echocardiographic views in Figure 16.1.

In 1999, Lambert et al. (4) published a systematic approach for the evaluation of the MV using cardiac anatomy as a reference for the description of structures, each view being used in relation to each other (Fig. 16.2A and B). Their descriptions followed the classification of Carpentier et al. (5), but they could be used with other classification systems. The description of these echocardiographic planes is depicted in Figure 16.2C–L.

The suggested anatomical two-dimensional (2D) examination is performed in a sequence of five steps.

Step 1: The mid-esophageal (ME) five-chamber view at 0° is used, initially, to evaluate the elements of the MV closer to the anterior wall, that is, the A1-A2 segments of the anterior leaflet and the P1-P2 scallops of the posterior leaflet (Fig. 16.2C and D).

Step 2: The elements of the MV near the posterior wall, A2-A3 and P2-P3 (from left to right), are then assessed by moving to an ME four-chamber view at 0° using gentle retroflexion and advancing the probe (Fig. 16.2E and F).

Step 3: From step 2, the ME two-chamber view is obtained at 90° showing orthogonal cross sections of the MV. Rotating the probe shaft clockwise completely toward the patient's right, until the commissure is no longer visible, reveals the base of the anterior leaflet and the intervalvular fibrosa (right fibrous trigone) (see Fig. 14.4). Gradual counterclockwise rotation of the probe shaft back toward the patient's left first shows the anterior cross section of the valve, with a small portion of the posterior leaflet (P3) and a large part of the anterior leaflet, A3-A2 (Fig. 16.2G and H). Continuing progressive counterclockwise rotation of the probe shaft back toward the patient's left then reaches the MV mid cross-section or mid-commissural view, where two coaptation points are visualized between P3 and A2 and between A2 and P1 (Fig. 16.2I and J). Adjusting the transducer slightly between 60° and 90° will optimize this view. As the MV orifice is C-shaped, this tomographic plane crossing the tip of the A2

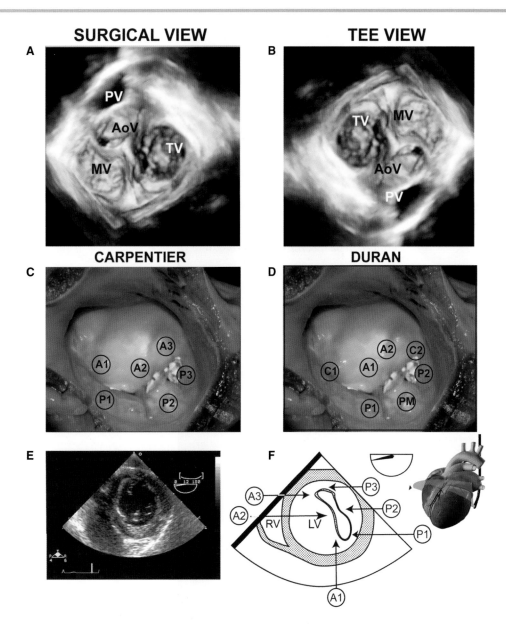

Figure 16.1 Mitral valve anatomy. (A,B) 3D TEE views in the surgical **(A)** and traditional TEE **(B)** orientations of the MV are shown. **(C)** The Carpentier classification divides both the anterior and posterior mitral leaflets into three parts: the anterior leaflet is seen above while the posterior leaflet is visible inferiorly with the lateral part of the valve (A1 and P1) oriented towards the left. **(D)** In the Duran classification, the three scallops of the posterior leaflet are named P1, P2 and Pm (*middle*). The anterior leaflet is divided in two segments, A1 and A2. The commissural areas are named C1 and C2. **(E,F)** From a transgastric basal short-axis view, the structures are visualized upside down. Indeed, the P3 segment appears at the top right of the screen, while the P1 segment is displayed to bottom. *Abbreviations*: AoV, aortic valve; MV, mitral valve; LV, left ventricle; PV, pulmonic valve; RV, right ventricle; TEE, transesophageal echocardiography; TV, tricuspid valve. *Source*: Photo B courtesy of Dr. Nicolas Dürrleman.

segment reveals coaptation points on either side of it. Thus, the apparent presence of two flow orifices should not be mistaken for a commissural point and a perforated anterior leaflet in the setting of endocarditis. Further counterclockwise rotation of the probe shaft back toward the patient's left leads to the most posterior aspect of the MV where only the P3-P2-P1 scallops are visualized (Fig. 16.2K and L).

Step 4: The probe shaft is then advanced in the stomach, where the examination moves to the transgastric basal short-axis (SAX) view at 0°. With variable anteflexion, the MV may be shown almost "en face" with a complete view of the C-shaped orifice. The use of color Doppler imaging at this level is useful to demonstrate the exact origin of the regurgitation jet(s) (Fig. 16.3). With some retroflexion, or further insertion of the probe, the subvalvular apparatus, including

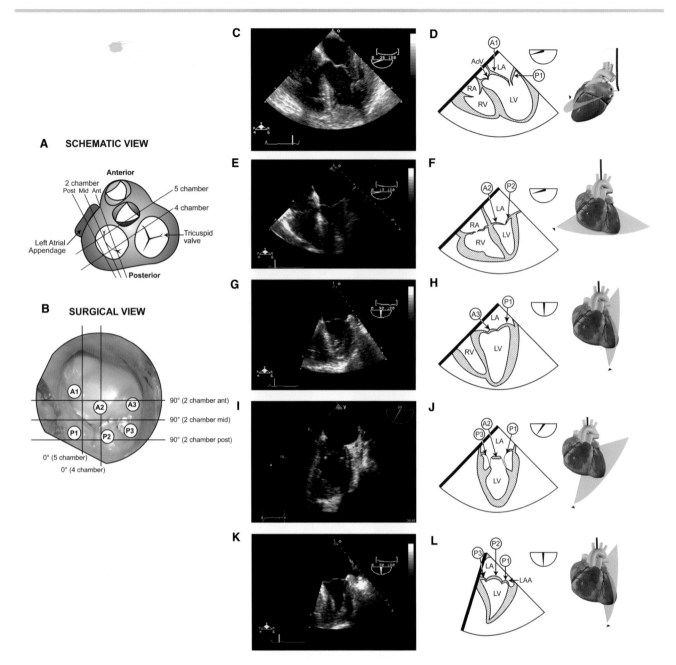

Figure 16.2   TEE assessment of MV – Mid-esophageal views. (**A**) Schematic anatomical drawing of the heart through the plane of the atrioventricular valves depicts the different planes used during a systematic TEE examination. (**B**) Corresponding surgical view of the MV from the LA. (**C,D**) ME five-chamber view of the MV at approximately 0° with slight anteflexion of the probe is shown. (**E,F**) ME four-chamber view of the MV near 0° is at a lower esophageal level than the five-chamber view. This view is thus easily obtained by either inserting the TEE probe slightly deeper and/or releasing anteflexion. (**G,H**) ME two-chamber *anterior* view at 90° is obtained with slight anterior clockwise rotation of the TEE probe shaft toward the right. Part of the RV may become visible as the field of view is progressively aimed toward the right. (**I,J**) ME two-chamber *mid* commissural view at 70° with the tip of the anterior leaflet (A2) visible in the center of the mitral annulus and the posteromedial (P3) and anterolateral (P1) scallops of the posterior leaflet attached to their respective LV wall. (**K,L**) ME two-chamber *posterior* view is obtained at 90° with slight counterclockwise posterior rotation of the TEE probe shaft toward the left. *Abbreviations*: Ant, anterior; AoV, aortic valve; LA, left atrium; LAA, left atrial appendage; LV, left ventricle; ME, mid-esophageal; Mid, middle; MV, mitral valve; Post, posterior; RA, right atrium; RV, right ventricle; TEE, transesophageal echocardiography. *Source*: Adapted with permission from Ref. 4. Photo B courtesy of Dr. Nicolas Dürrleman.

the anterolateral and posteromedial chordae and papillary muscles, may be assessed in a transverse plane at the lower right and the top of the display, respectively.

Step 5: Orthogonal views of the MV in the longitudinal plane are obtained by changing the imaging plane to 90° in the transgastric two-chamber view. This is particularly helpful to

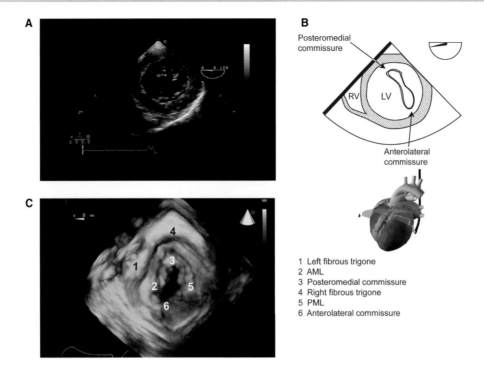

Figure 16.3 TEE Assessment of MV – Transgastric view. (**A,B**) Basal short-axis view at 0° compared with a (**C**) mid-esophageal real-time 3D view of the MV from the left atrium. Note that the TG view corresponds to the upside down rotated version of the anatomical / surgical view described in Figure 16.2. *Abbreviations*: MV, mitral valve; AML, anterior mitral leaflet; LV, left ventricle; PML, posterior mitral leaflet; RV, right ventricle; TG, transgastric.

1 Left fibrous trigone
2 AML
3 Posteromedial commissure
4 Right fibrous trigone
5 PML
6 Anterolateral commissure

evaluate the subvalvular apparatus, specifically the papillary muscles, the chordae tendineae, and their insertions on the leaflets margins (Fig. 16.4). By rotating the probe shaft counterclockwise toward the left of the patient, the anterolateral papillary muscle will be seen in the far-field near the anterior LV wall. Clockwise rotation of the probe shaft

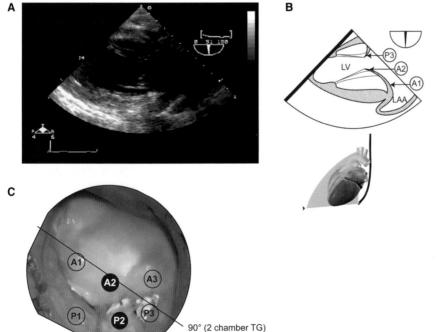

Figure 16.4 TEE Assessment of MV – Transgastric view. (**A,B**) Long-axis view at 90°, with the LAA in the far field and the (**C**) corresponding tomographic plane on the surgical view from the left atrium. *Abbreviations*: LAA, left atrial appendage; LV, left ventricle; MV, mitral valve; TG, transgastric.

toward the patient's right will bring the posteromedial papillary muscle into view in the near-field near the inferior LV wall (6).

Close inspection of the anatomical integrity of the MV by 2D examination should predict the presence of abnormal regurgitant flow, which can then be confirmed by color Doppler imaging in all the above views. The MR jet is characterized by its origin (along the mitral commissure as medial, central, or lateral or outside the commissure) and by its direction (anterior, central, posterior, or multiple). Its description should be consistent with the mechanism hypothesized from the 2D findings, such as any hyperechogenic material evoking sclerosis of the coapting surface of the leaflets, calcification in the annulus or the mitral apparatus, or hypermobile structures consistent with torn chordae tendineae or even part of the papillary muscles (7) (see Fig. 9.24).

Etiology of Mitral Regurgitation

In a review of 1000 patients undergoing MV surgery for MR, 50% had valvular degeneration, 20% rheumatic disease, 17% ischemic regurgitation, while 8% of MR originated from infectious processes, and the remaining 5% had miscellaneous causes. Identifying the causes of MR has prognostic implications for long-term survival, being 85% for floppy valve disease, 64% for organic nonfloppy valve disease, and 46% for ischemic or functional MR at six years (8).

Endocarditis

Echocardiography is an integral part of the clinical assessment of a patient with suspected endocarditis. The echocardiographic findings have been included in the Duke criteria for evidence of cardiac involvement (9) (Table 16.1).

Vegetations. The presence of vegetations constitutes a major diagnostic criterion for endocarditis in the Duke classification. Five characteristics help classify a mass as a vegetation: (*i*) a gray scale and a low level of reflectance similar to mid-myocardium; (*ii*) localization to the upstream side of the valve, for instance, on the atrial side of the MV or on the ventricular side of the aortic valve (AoV); (*iii*) localization at sites of endothelial injury from regurgitant or stenotic jet impinging on the valve or wall; (*iv*) morphologic features: mass usually lobulated, amorphous, and mobile; and (*v*) mobility of the mass may be random or appear to orbit around the valve. Fine vibratory motion may be imparted to a vegetation by the jet. Accompanying abnormalities include periannular abscess, fistulas, and severe regurgitation from disruption of the leaflet function and/or perforation.

Vegetations can also be described according to their size, density, extent, and mobility (Figs. 16.5–16.7). Complications are more likely to be associated with higher grades of mobility and lesion extent but less so with the presence of calcified elements. The size of the

Table 16.1 Duke Criteria for Endocarditis

Definite IE
Pathologic criteria
  Microorganism: demonstrated by culture or histology in a vegetation or in a vegetation that has embolized, or in an intracardiac abscess, or
  Pathologic lesions: vegetation or intracardiac abscess, confirmed by histology showing active endocarditis.

Clinical criteria[a]
  2 major criteria, or
  1 major and 3 minor criteria, or
  5 minor criteria.

Possible IE[b]
  1 major and 1 minor criterion, or 3 minor criteria.

Rejected IE
  Firm alternate diagnosis for manifestations of endocarditis, or
  Resolution of manifestations of endocarditis with antibiotic therapy for 4 days or less, or
  No pathologic evidence of infective endocarditis at surgery or autopsy after antibiotic therapy for 4 days or less
  Does not meet criteria for possible infective endocarditis, as above.

[a]Major criteria include positive blood cultures, evidence of endocardial involvement, positive echocardiogram showing a valvular vegetation or abscess, new valvular regurgitation. Minor criteria are predisposing heart condition, fever of 38° or more, vascular or immunologic manifestations, microbiologic or serologic evidence of active infection.
[b]The category of possible IE (infectious endocarditis) represents a modification from the previous published Duke criteria.
Source: Adapted from Ref. 10.

vegetation seems to be the most powerful predictor of complications. Indeed, the risk of septic emboli is increased threefold by the presence of a vegetation >10 mm (12).

When endocarditis is strongly suspected on clinical grounds and transthoracic echocardiography (TTE) does not yield positive findings, TEE is recommended (13). It has a higher sensitivity for abscess and valve perforation (14,15) and a higher diagnostic accuracy for the detection of vegetations. Its mean sensitivity for the presence of vegetations is 92%, compared with 62% for TTE.

Abscesses. An abscess is defined echocardiographically as a finite area of similar or reduced echo density within the valve annulus or an adjacent cardiac structure in the setting of a valvular infection (16). Its wall may be lined by weakened necrotizing tissue, prone to rupture with fistulization into neighboring cardiac chambers or great vessels. Abscess complicating endocarditis is encountered in up to 37% of patients and is usually associated with a complicated clinical course. The location of the abscess was identified with greater sensitivity and specificity by TEE than TTE (16). The differential diagnosis includes caseous infiltration in rheumatic disease that can mimic an MV abscess (Fig. 16.8).

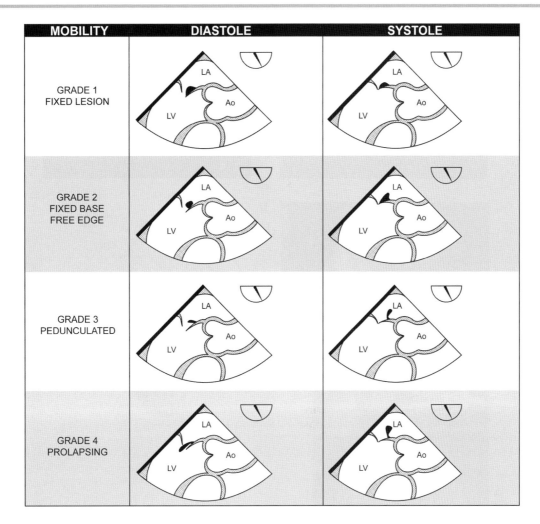

Figure 16.5 Vegetation mobility score. Schematic mid-esophageal long-axis views show the four grades of vegetation mobility in the setting of endocarditis. *Abbreviations*: Ao, aorta; LA, left atrium; LV, left ventricle. *Source*: Adapted from Ref. 11.

Rheumatic Valve Disease

Rheumatic involvement of the MV is suggested by decreased mobility of the leaflets with doming into the LV in association with valvular and subvalvular apparatus thickening, chordal shortening, fusion, and calcification.

Most patients with rheumatic MR from malcoaptation of the leaflets have some degree of concomitant stenosis, with variable involvement of the AoV and/or the tricuspid valve (TV). Mitral valve repair is not as successful for correcting MR in rheumatic valves as for other etiologies such as myxoid degeneration (17). The severity of MR also has significant bearing on the eligibility of a rheumatic mitral stenosis (MS) for treatment with percutaneous balloon valvotomy and commissurotomy, in addition to its morphology score (18,19) (see Table 16.4).

Myxomatous Degeneration

Myxomatous valve disease is characterized by thickened (>5 mm), redundant leaflets and chordae bulging into the LA during systole (20,21). In addition, the MV annulus is deemed abnormally dilated when its maximal end-diastolic annular diameter in the longitudinal or transverse plane is >34 mm (22). Regurgitation in the setting of MV myxoid degeneration and prolapse is most often associated with annular dilatation (Fig. 16.9) (23).

Myxomatous degeneration affects, preferentially, the leaflet tips that present a club-like deformity with a ground glass appearance, sometimes extending onto the inserting chordae tendineae (24). The severity of the disease may vary from minor valve billowing to severe involvement of both leaflets with frankly prolapsed or flail segments and scallops (Fig. 16.9).

On TTE, mitral valve prolapse (MVP) has traditionally been diagnosed on the basis of a posterior displacement of one or both leaflets of at least 2 mm beyond the annular plane in the parasternal long-axis (LAX) view. The same criteria have been applied to the transgastric longitudinal views, although this has not been studied extensively. The diagnosis of flail

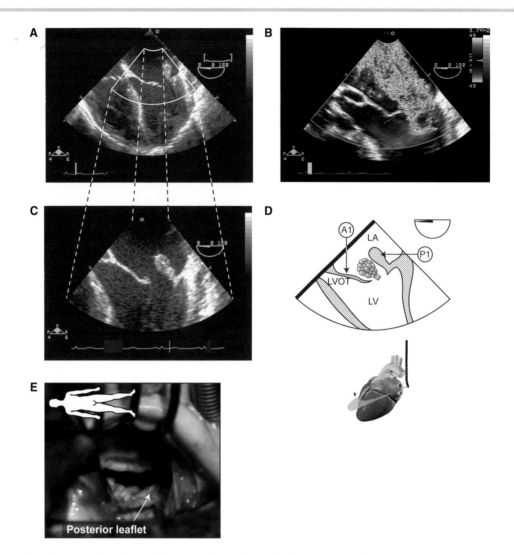

Figure 16.6 Endocarditis. Mid-esophageal four-chamber (**A,B**) and five-chamber (**C,D**) views at 0° of a 57-year-old man with endocarditis and large flail of the posterior leaflet (P1) scallop associated with severe mitral regurgitation. (**E**) Intraoperative findings confirm flail of the entire posterior leaflet. The patient underwent mitral valve replacement. *Abbreviations*: LA, Left atrium; LV, left ventricle; LVOT, left ventricular outflow tract. *Source*: Photo E courtesy of Dr. Michel Carrier.

MV by TTE is established in the presence of systolic leaflet inversion with the loss of coaptation and an associated rapidly moving linear echodensity seen in the LA, corresponding to the ruptured chordae tendineae (Figs. 16.10–16.14) (7,25).

The diagnosis of MVP by TEE may easily be missed unless one systematically examines all anterior segments and posterior scallops in multiple planes, following the method proposed by Lambert et al. (4). Using a systematic approach, Agricola et al. (26) found a 97% overall diagnostic accuracy when TEE results were compared with surgical findings. Two diagnostic pitfalls were mentioned by these authors: first, when a large P2 scallop prolapse extends over most of the posteromedial commissural area, the adjacent P3 can also, erroneously, be identified as prolapsing. As the ME four- and two-chamber views often transect the middle and lateral scallops close to P2, it

may be mistaken for either P1 or P3. This could be avoided by using the commissural and the LAX view instead. The other frequent misdiagnosis is failing to diagnose the prolapse of a scallop or a segment opposite to a more obviously prolapsing one.

Complexity of lesion and relationship to repair. Surgical correction of MR is based on dynamic TEE evaluation and static direct visual inspection of the MV. Most techniques of repair consist of a 2D geometric approach to a very complex and dynamic 3D problem. The location, direction, and mechanism of each regurgitation jet must be identified separately. Assessment of the LA diameter, LV diameter, LV segmental motion, tissue characteristics, mitral annulus diameter, height of posterior leaflet, and the length of the anterior leaflet are useful to plan the repair. The preoperative predictability of repair is a function of the complexity of the regurgitation mechanism.

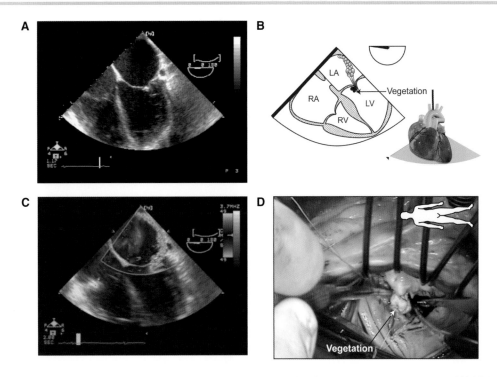

Figure 16.7 Endocarditis. A 64-year-old man with endocarditis is scheduled for mitral valve replacement. (**A**) Mid-esophageal four-chamber view shows a vegetation with a mobility score of 4 on the tip of A2 segment with (**B,C**) eccentric mitral regurgitation directed posteriorly. (**D**) Vegetation confirmed on the intraoperative findings. *Abbreviations*: LA, left atrium; LV, left ventricle; RA, right atrium; RV, right ventricle. *Source*: Photo D courtesy of Dr. Michel Pellerin.

In a report of 286 patients with MR, the feasibility of repair was found to be dependent on the mechanism, being higher in the posterior leaflet disease or flail group (88%) than the anterior leaflet disease or flail group (59%) or the severe bileaflet chordal rupture group (29%) (27). Calcifications of the annulus significantly complicates MV repair. They appear as echo-dense structures with acoustic shadowing, most commonly located in the posterior atrioventricular groove with a typical C-shape distribution between 10 and 2 o'clock in the transgastric SAX view.

Ischemic Mitral Valvular Disease

Ischemic mitral regurgitation (IMR) can be simply defined as the occurrence of MR in the clinical context of myocardial ischemia. It accounts for 13% to 30% of MV surgery and encompasses a wide range of structural and functional conditions. There are four clinical settings generally recognized for IMR: partial or complete papillary muscle rupture, acute myocardial infarction, reversible ischemia with preserved overall LV systolic function, and end-stage ischemic or non-ischemic severe LV systolic dysfunction (see Figs. 9.23 and 9.24).

Papillary muscle rupture is an example of structural MR associated with ischemia that occurs in the setting of acute myocardial infarction. Because of its dual vascular supply, the anterolateral papillary muscle is less vulnerable to coronary occlusion than the posteromedial papillary muscle so this condition is more often seen with inferior wall infarcts. The diagnosis is suspected when a new systolic murmur is heard in a previously stable patient who develops cardiogenic shock during acute myocardial infarction (Fig. 16.15). Partial rupture may also occur. Chordal rupture that is of the most common causes of flail MV can also occur in the setting of acute myocardial infarction. However, it is often associated with MVP, endocarditis, and trauma (Fig. 16.15).

Ischemic MR most often results from alterations in the LV shape due to regional wall systolic dysfunction, with preserved leaflets and annular dimensions. It is typically associated with inferior wall ischemia or infarction that involves the posteromedial papillary muscle, leading to subsequent loss of support of the middle aspects of the anterior and posterior leaflets (Fig. 16.16). In this context, the MR is often referred to as "functional" MR as the valve leaflets themselves are intact. On 2D imaging, the underlying MV apparatus is shortened, and the leaflets do not reach the level of the mitral annulus, resulting in incomplete closure and MR. The MR jet can be central, but it is often directed toward the posterolateral atrial wall.

The MR associated with end-stage ischemic heart disease and severe ventricular systolic dysfunction may arise through several mechanisms: these

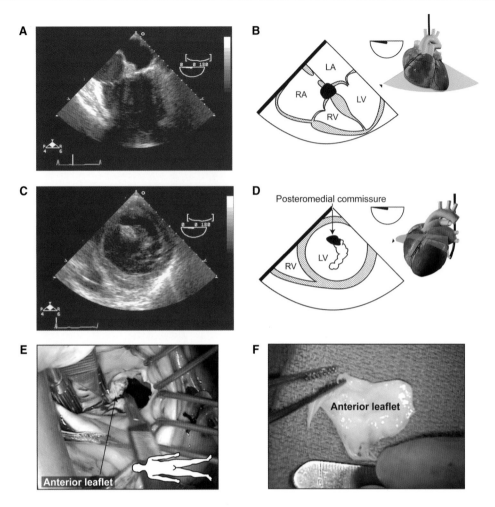

Figure 16.8   Caseous granuloma. A 63-year-old man is scheduled for aortic and MV replacement. Mitral annular and anterior leaflet thickening was seen in the mid-esophageal four-chamber (**A,B**) and transgastric basal views (**C,D**). (**E,F**) Surgical exploration of the MV disclosed the presence of material suspicious for an abscess. Pathologic examination later found it to be caseous infiltration of the MV. *Abbreviations*: LA, left atrium; LV, left ventricle; MV, mitral valve; RA, right atrium; RV, right ventricle. *Source*: Photos E and F courtesy of Dr. Michel Pellerin.

include annular dilatation, inadequate papillary muscle traction from myocardial ischemia, excessive obtuse angulation between the papillary muscle and the mitral annular plane, and significant alteration in LV geometry in association with cavity dilatation. This ventricular remodeling displaces the posterior medial papillary muscle down and away from its normal position, leading to different degrees of MR (28). The prognosis of patients with IMR is substantially worse than MR from other causes.

Traumatic MV Injury

The most frequent cardiac injury seen after blunt chest trauma is myocardial contusion. When cardiac valves are involved, the AoV is the most often damaged, followed by the MV and TV. The MV lesions may include, in order of frequency, rupture of a papillary muscle, rupture of chordae tendineae, and laceration of a leaflet. Traumatic rupture of papillary muscles is

a relatively rare cause of MR, with an occurrence of only 4% in a postmortem study of 546 patients seen for blunt chest trauma (29). The latter is frequently related to a motor vehicle accident, with injury occurring through sudden deceleration, traumatic compression of the heart, or abrupt increase in intrathoracic or intra-abdominal pressures.

A review by Simmers et al. (30) reported 25 cases of successful surgical repair of traumatic MR. The most frequent lesion observed was a tear of the anterolateral papillary muscle (32%), while other injuries included tears of the posterior leaflet (28%), the anterior leaflet (12%), and the posteromedial papillary muscle (8%). A motor vehicle accident was the origin of 60% of the cases, and the delay between the initial trauma and the surgical repair varied from a few days to 25 years.

Transesophageal echocardiography is an extremely valuable tool for excluding MV injury in the hemodynamically unstable trauma patient with pulmonary edema.

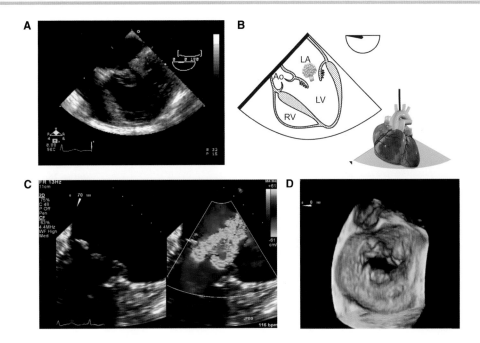

Figure 16.9   Myxomatous MV. Mid-esophageal four-chamber view (**A,B**) of a 53-year-old man with severe myxomatous thickening of both anterior and posterior MV leaflets (Barlow's disease) and central mitral regurgitation (**C**) before MV repair. (**D**) A real-time 3D zoom view of the MV seen from the LA is shown for comparison. *Abbreviations*: Ao, aorta; LA, left atrium; LV, left ventricle; MV, mitral valve; RV, right ventricle.

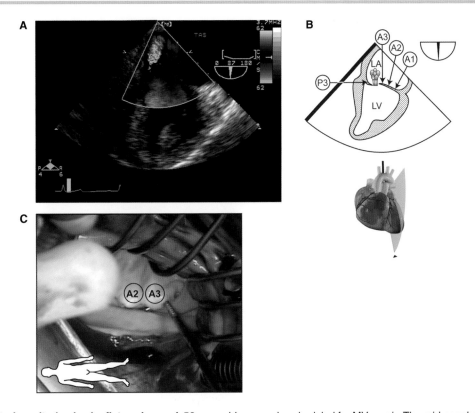

Figure 16.10   Anterior mitral valve leaflet prolapse. A 58-year-old woman is scheduled for MV repair. The mid-esophageal two-chamber view (**A,B**) shows the mitral regurgitation is secondary to a prolapsed anterior MV leaflet (A2 and A3) which is confirmed by the intraoperative findings (**C**). *Abbreviations*: LA, left atrium; LV, left ventricle; MV, mitral valve. *Source*: Photo C courtesy of Dr. Michel Pellerin.

A

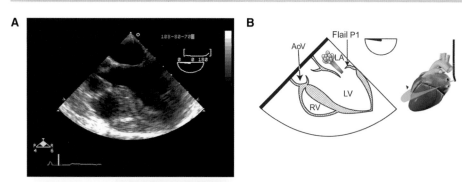

B

Figure 16.11 Posterior mitral valve leaflet prolapse. A 74-year-old woman is operated on for acute MR. (**A–C**) Mid-esophageal five-chamber view with anteflexion shows an eccentric anteriorly directed MR jet from a flail posterior leaflet (P1 scallop) which is confirmed by the intraoperative findings (**D**). *Abbreviations*: AoV, aortic valve; LA, left atrium; LV, left ventricle; MR, mitral regurgitation; MV, mitral valve; RV, right ventricle. *Source*: Photo D courtesy of Dr. Denis Bouchard.

C

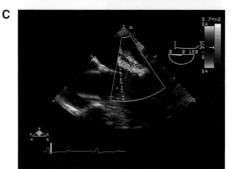

D

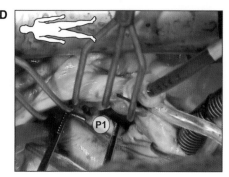

A

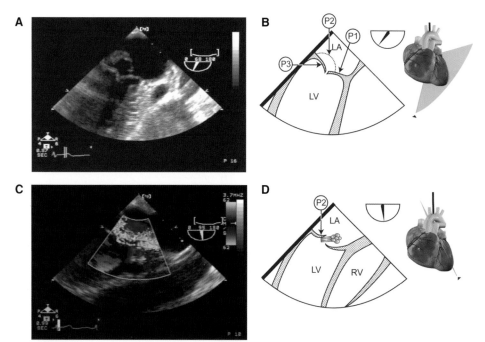

B

C

D

E

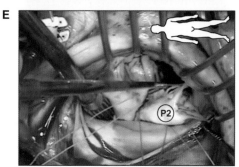

F

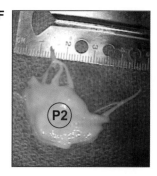

Figure 16.12 Posterior mitral valve leaflet chordal rupture. (**A,B**) ME mitral commissural view at 65° with clockwise probe rotation in a 75-year-old man shows a flail P2 scallop secondary to chordal rupture. (**C, D**) Color Doppler ME two-chamber view demonstrates an anteriorly directed mitral regurgitation jet. (**E,F**) Intraoperative findings with the excised P2 scallop are shown. *Abbreviations*: LA, left atrium; LV, left ventricle; ME, mid-esophageal; MV, mitral valve; RV, right ventricle. *Source*: Photos E and F courtesy of Dr. Michel Pellerin.

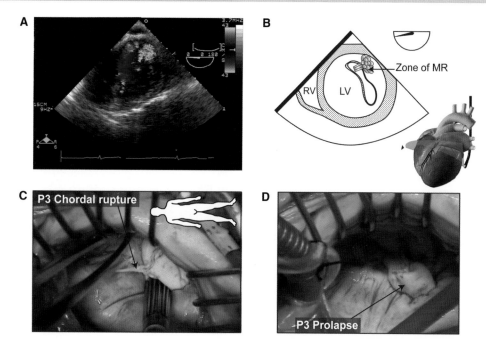

Figure 16.13 Posterior mitral valve leaflet chordal rupture. (A,B) The transgastric basal view at 0° shows an eccentric MR jet originating from the P3 area. This is due to a prolapsed P3 scallop secondary to chordal rupture in a 75-year-old man with acute MR. **(C,D)** Intraoperative findings are shown. *Abbreviations*: LV, left ventricle; MR, mitral regurgitation; MV, mitral valve; RV, right ventricle. *Source*: Photos C and D courtesy of Dr. Denis Bouchard.

FUNCTIONAL MANIFESTATIONS OF VALVE LESIONS

Two-dimensional imaging reflects the impact of volume overload from MR on the cardiac chambers. Thus, the evaluation of LA and LV size and function provides important information regarding the severity and/or chronicity of the MR, which is necessary to assess the need for, and timing of, surgery (1). Using the ASE guidelines (31), the LV end-diastolic diameter is normally <3.2 cm/m^2 (see Fig. 5.8). The LV diastolic volume is <75 mL/m^2. The normal mediolateral diameter of the LA does not exceed 2.3 cm/m^2 with a normal volume no greater than 28 mL/m^2 (see Fig. 5.10). Finally, echocardiographic signs of pulmonary hypertension and RV pressure and/or volume overload are also important clues suggesting significant MV disease.

MV Regurgitation: Mechanism and Quantification

Mitral regurgitation may be caused by one or a combination of mechanisms related to the etiologies reviewed in the preceding text. Systematic examination by 2D imaging of the valve elements and surrounding anatomical structures is aimed at assessing the quality and degree of coaptation between opposite valve surfaces and at predicting the location and severity of regurgitant jets by defining their mechanism. These findings are then confirmed by color flow imaging that should display regurgitant flow orientation and characteristics

consistent with the presumed mechanism(s) (27). The specific locations of normal and abnormal function of leaflet segments are sought, with particular attention to the leaflet motion in relation to the mitral annulus. Leaflet motion is described, using the Carpentier classification, as being excessive, normal, or restricted if a portion of the leaflet moves beyond, at, or under the annulus plane, respectively, during closure. Finally, mitral leaflet motion can be normal with associated MR (Table 16.2) (Fig. 16.17) (4,24).

Excessive leaflet mobility is a frequent mechanism of MR, and the ensuing jet is typically directed toward the contralateral side of the pathologic leaflet. Myxomatous degeneration and endocarditis are the usual culprit diseases. Regurgitation caused by papillary muscle infarction usually originates from its respective commissural area.

In contrast, restricted leaflet motion results in a jet directed toward the affected leaflet. If both leaflets are equally affected, the jet can be central. The most frequent cause of restricted leaflet motion is ischemia and less often rheumatic valve disease (32).

Finally, MR with normal leaflet motion is associated with annular dilatation, leaflet perforation (Fig. 16.18), or a congenital cleft or perforation (Fig. 16.19). The origin of the jet in the latter two conditions is frequently described as eccentric to the commissural line (27), but its direction can be central or eccentric.

The advantages and limitations of various methods to quantify MR severity (Table 16.3) will be reviewed as no single measure is foolproof.

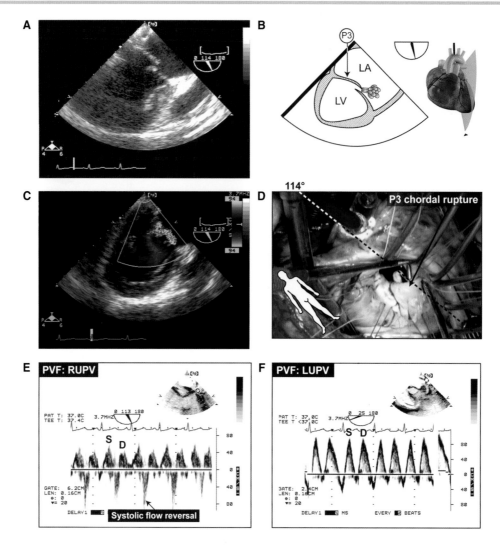

Figure 16.14 Posterior mitral valve leaflet chordal rupture. (A–C) A 64-year-old woman with acute MR due to P3 chordal rupture is seen in mid-esophageal views at 114°. The prolapsing scallop is visible with an eccentric MR jet (**C**) directed anteriorly toward the atrial wall and the RUPV. (**D**) Compare with the intraoperative findings. (**E,F**) Pulsed wave Doppler of PVF reveals the presence of systolic flow reversal in the RUPV but not in the LUPV. *Abbreviations*: D, peak diastolic PVF velocity; LA, left atrium; LUPV, left upper pulmonary vein; LV, left ventricle; MR, mitral regurgitation; MV, mitral valve; PVF, pulmonary venous flow; RUPV, right upper pulmonary vein; S, peak systolic PVF velocity. *Source*: Photo D courtesy of Dr. Michel Pellerin.

Color Flow Doppler Jet Area Mapping

This is the planimetry of the maximal color Doppler imaging area occupied by the regurgitant jet during systole. The jet area is assumed to be proportional to the regurgitant volume (33). However, the correlation between jet area and MR severity is inconsistent due to a multitude of technical and hemodynamic limitations, including LA compliance, the chronicity, and the eccentricity of the MR (2). This method, specifically, is not reliable with eccentric jets hugging LA walls because of the Coanda effect (which describe the tendency of a fluid to follow a curved surface immediately adjacent to its course). Nevertheless, small, non-eccentric jets with an area <4.0 cm² or <20% of the total LA area are usually consistent with a trivial or mild degree of MR. Of note, when using TEE, the ratio of the MR jet area to the LA area is often not entirely visualized at a given time in 64% of patients (34) due to the proximity of the transducer to the LA. In the operating room (OR), general anesthesia can reduce the area of the regurgitant jet. The use of phenylephrine to increase blood pressure will, however, improve the correlation with the measurements obtained in the awake state (Fig. 16.20) (35).

Jet Width (Vena Contracta)

This method uses the width of the regurgitant jet at its narrowest portion (vena contracta) close to its origin to evaluate lesion severity. This is best performed by obtaining high-resolution, zoomed images of the MV with color Doppler imaging in either the ME four-chamber or LAX views (34,36). The ME two-chamber

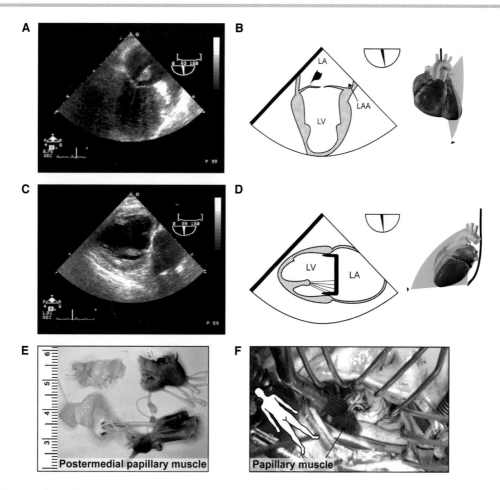

Figure 16.15 Ruptured papillary muscle. Posteromedial papillary muscle rupture resulting in acute severe MR in a 58-year-old man with acute inferior myocardial infarction. (**A,B**) The torn posteromedial papillary muscle is seen prolapsing into the LA in the mid-esophageal two-chamber view. (**C,D**) After prosthetic MVR, the subvalvular apparatus is seen from the transgastric view at 90°. (**E,F**) Pathological and intraoperative findings are shown. *Abbreviations*: LA, left atrium; LAA, left atrial appendage; LV, left ventricle; MR, mitral regurgitation; MVR, mitral valve replacement. *Source*: Photos E and F courtesy of Drs. Nicolas Noiseux and Denis Bouchard.

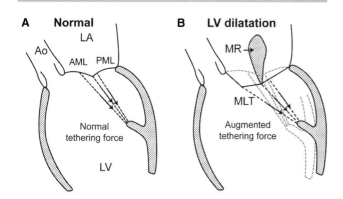

Figure 16.16 Ischemic MR. Diagram presents the leaflet tethering hypothesis for the mechanism of MLT and ischemic MR. Normal leaflet tethering (**A**) compared with leaflet tethering (**B**) caused by an apical displacement of the mitral leaflets and MR from LV dilation, systolic LV regional wall motion abnormalities, or both. *Abbreviations*: AML, anterior mitral leaflet; Ao, aorta; LA, left atrium; LV, left ventricle; MLT, mitral leaflet tenting; MR, mitral regurgitation; PML, posterior mitral leaflet.

Table 16.2 Functional Classification of Carpentier

Type I	Normal leaflet motion
Type II	Excessive leaflet motion (prolapse)
Type III	Restricted leaflet motion
	a. During systole and diastole (rheumatic)
	b. During systole (ischemic)

view is not ideally suited for this measurement as it invariably crosses through several parts of the line of leaflet coaptation and may show a wide vena contracta even in mild MR.

The correlation, reported by Hall et al. (37), between the vena contracta and the regurgitant volume or the effective regurgitant orifice area (EROA) suggests that it is reliable and efficient in predicting mild and severe MR while being less accurate for discriminating moderate degrees of MR. A vena contracta <3.0 mm usually denotes mild MR, whereas the cutoff value for severe MR has ranged between 6.0 and 8.0 mm (Fig. 16.21) (36). The size of the vena contracta is relatively independent of flow rate and driving pressure for a fixed orifice and is less sensitive

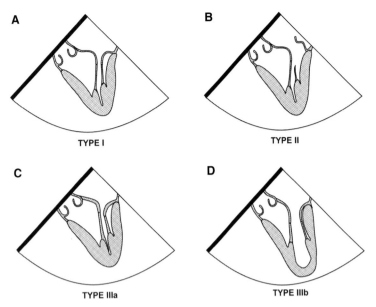

Figure 16.17 Carpentier's functional classification of mitral regurgitation. This classification is based on the opening and closing motions of the mitral leaflets. (**A**) Type 1 has normal leaflet motion and MR is on the basis of leaflet perforation or annular dilatation. (**B**) In type II dysfunction (increased leaflet motion) the leaflet free edge travels above the plane of the mitral annulus during systole due to chordal elongation or rupture. (**C**) Type IIIa dysfunction implies restricted opening leaflet motion during systole and diastole due to rheumatic changes. (**D**) Type IIIb dysfunction correlates to restricted leaflet motion during systole secondary to papillary muscle displacement and ventricular remodelling typically due to ischemia. *Abbreviation*: MR, mitral regurgitation.

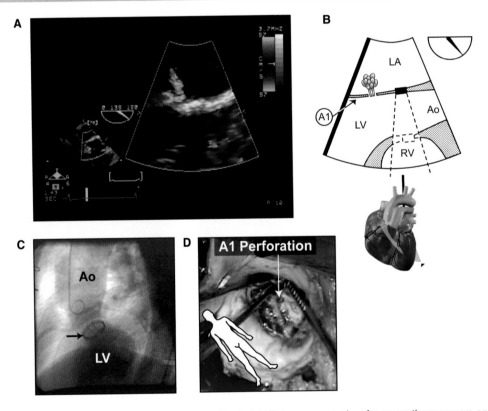

Figure 16.18 Perforated AML. A 58-year-old man with a perforated AML is re-operated on for an aortic aneurysm and severe AR after a previous AoV replacement. (**A,B**) Color Doppler mid-esophageal long-axis view shows mitral regurgitation from a perforated A1 segment. (**C**) Aortogram demonstrates the coronary arteries, aneurysmal ascending aorta and bileaflet AoV prosthesis (arrow) with severe AR opacifying the LV. (**D**) At surgery a small perforation of A1 was present just below the AoV prosthesis. *Abbreviations*: AML, anterior mitral leaflet; Ao, aorta; AoV, aortic valve; AR, aortic regurgitation; LA, left atrium; LV, left ventricle; RV, right ventricle. *Source*: Photo C courtesy of Dr. Michel Pellerin.

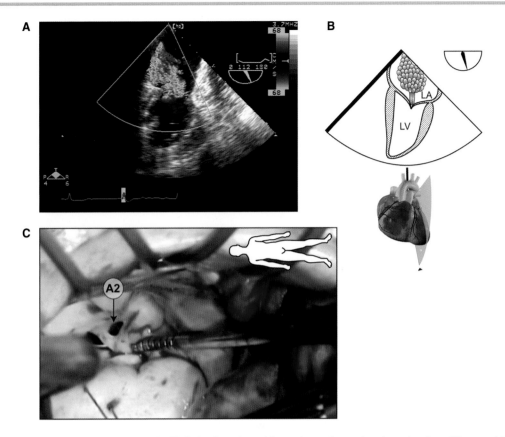

Figure 16.19 Congenital AML perforation. (A,B) Color Doppler mid-esophageal two-chamber view in a 56-year-old woman shows the new onset severe mitral regurgitation after closure of an atrial septal defect. **(C)** Exploration of the mitral valve reveals congenitally perforated A2 segment of the AML. *Abbreviations*: AML, anterior mitral leaflet; LA, left atrium; LV, left ventricle. *Source*: Photo C courtesy of Dr. Louis P. Perrault.

to hemodynamic variations (Fig. 16.22), instrument settings, orifice geometry, and interindividual interpretation (35,38). It works equally well for central and eccentric jets but is less useful in quantifying MR with multiple jets (Table 16.3).

Pulmonary Venous Flow

In normal adults, pulmonary venous flow (PVF) is characterized by predominant flow during systole (see Figs 4.25–4.28), except in younger healthy adults with good ventricular compliance. With increasing MR severity, there is systolic PVF blunting with progressive diminution of the systolic velocity. However, systolic flow blunting can also be seen in other situations such as elevated LA pressure from other etiologies like atrial fibrillation. Severe MR results in systolic flow reversal in PVF (Fig. 16.23), which is 98% specific but only 34% sensitive when compared with calculation of the effective regurgitant orifice (39). The presence of PVF systolic reversal is dependent on hemodynamic conditions (Fig. 16.24). Indeed, hypotension associated with general anesthesia may mask this reversal of systolic flow. Finally, interrogation of all pulmonary veins should be performed as an eccentric jet may be preferentially directed toward a single vein where systolic flow reversal will be found, while it may not be present in the other pulmonary veins (Fig. 16.14).

Continuous Wave Doppler

The maximal velocity of the regurgitant jet itself does not provide useful information about the severity of MR. However, the density of the continuous wave (CW) Doppler signal, which is proportional to the number of red blood cells (i.e., the regurgitant volume) reflecting the ultrasound beam, is a qualitative index of MR severity. The contour of the MR velocity profile may also provide information about MR severity: for example, a truncated, triangular jet contour with early peaking of the maximal velocity suggests elevated LA pressure or a prominent regurgitant wave in the LA.

Proximal Isovelocity Surface Area

The proximal isovelocity surface area (PISA) method is derived from the hydrodynamic principle describing flow through a narrowed orifice: as red blood cells approach the smaller orifice, their velocity gradually increases and red blood cells with similar velocity form concentric hemispheric shells with decreasing

Table 16.3 Mitral Regurgitation Severity Score

	Mild	Moderate	Severe
Structural parameters			
LA size	Normal AP diameter $\leq$2 cm/m^2 LA vol <36 mL/m^2	Normal or dilated	Usually dilated (unless acute MR)
LV size	Normal LV diameter $\leq$2.8 cm/m^2 LVEDV $\leq$82 mL/m^2	Normal or dilated	Usually dilated (unless acute MR)
MV leaflets or subvalvular apparatus	May be abnormal	May be abnormal	Dilated annulus Flail leaflet Ruptured papillary muscle
Doppler parameters			
MR jet area on CFI	<4 cm^2 <20% LA area	Variable	>10 cm^2 >40% LA area (unless wall-hugging jet)
MV inflow (PWD)	E/A <1	Variable	E >1.2 cm/s
MR jet density (CWD)	Faint	Dense	Dense
MR jet contour (CWD)	Parabolic	Parabolic	Early-peaking triangular
Pulmonary veins (PWD)	Normal systolic flow predominance	Systolic flow blunting (may also occur with high LA pressure or AF)	Systolic flow reversal
MR quantitation			
Vena contracta (cm)	<0.3	0.30–0.69		$\geq$0.70
PISA diameter (cm) at a Nyquist limit 40 cm/s	<0.4	0.4–0.89		>0.9
Regurgitant volume (mL)	<30	30–44	45–59	$\geq$60
Regurgitant fraction (%)	<30	30–39	40–49	$\geq$50
EROA (cm^2)	<0.20	0.20–0.29	0.30–0.39	$\geq$0.40

Abbreviations: A, peak late diastolic TMF velocity; AF, atrial fibrillation; AP, anteroposterior; CFI, color flow interrogation; CWD, continuous wave Doppler; E, peak early diastolic TMF velocity; EROA, effective regurgitant orifice area; LA, left atrium; LV, left ventricle; LVEDV, left ventricular end-diastolic volume; MR, mitral regurgitation; MV, mitral valve; PISA, proximal isovelocity surface area; PWD, pulsed wave Doppler; TMF, transmitral flow; vol, volume.
Source: Adapted from Ref. 2.

surface or diameter as the isovelocity increases. From this principle, the following equations are derived (see Chapter 5).

$$\mathrm{ERO} = 2\pi r^2 \frac{v_r}{V_{\mathrm{MR\,max}}} \qquad (16.1)$$

where ERO is the effective regurgitant orifice (in cm^2); r is the measured radius of the hemispheric shell of the aliased velocity; v_r is the aliased velocity at the radius r, identified as the Nyquist limit (in cm/s); and $V_{\mathrm{MR\,max}}$ is the maximal MR velocity across the orifice, obtained by CW Doppler (in cm/s).

$$\mathrm{Mitral\ regurgitant\ volume} = \mathrm{ERO}_{\mathrm{mv}} \times \mathrm{VTI}_{\mathrm{mr}} \qquad (16.2)$$

where ERO is the effective regurgitant orifice (in cm^2) and VTI$_{\mathrm{MR}}$ is the velocity-time integral (in cm) of the MR signal obtained by CW Doppler.

To calculate the ERO and the regurgitant volume, four parameters are required. The measured radius, r, of the hemispheric shell of the aliased velocity, v_r, is obtained from high-resolution, zoomed views of the MV with color Doppler imaging, carefully positioned at the center of the regurgitant jet and aligned with the jet direction. This is confirmed by the uninterrupted visualization of the hemispheric shell with the vena contracta. Failure to obtain this position will result in significant underestimation of the true radius of the hemispheric shell. Next, the v_r of the color scale is adjusted to generate a nice hemispheric shell. This is generally done by shifting the baseline of

the color scale toward the direction of the regurgitant flow or, less frequently, by changing the Nyquist limit through lowering the maximal velocity of the color scale. The range of v_r for this measurement is usually between 25 and 40 cm/s. Qualitatively, the presence of a PISA visible at a Nyquist limit of 50 to 60 cm/s should alert the existence of severe MR.

The r is measured from the edge of the hemispheric shell where the color scale changes (from one edge of the spectrum to the other) to the base of the shell at the plane of the leaflets. The latter is best visualized by intermittently turning off the color flow overlay on the freeze frame.

To complete the calculation of the ERO and the regurgitant volume, the maximal velocity, V_{MR}, and the velocity-time integral, VTI, of the regurgitant jet are measured by CW Doppler examination well aligned with the jet direction.

The PISA method is more accurate for central jets than for eccentric jets and for regurgitation with a circular orifice. It is sometimes difficult to judge the precise location of the orifice and the flow convergence shape. The r is the critical measurement as any error introduced in this parameter will be magnified to its squared value. Generally, an ERO >0.40 cm^2 is consistent with severe MR, 0.20 to 0.39 cm^2 with moderate MR, and <0.20 cm^2 with mild MR (Table 16.3). The ERO is a more robust parameter compared with color Doppler planimetry and is less altered with changing hemodynamic conditions (Fig. 16.22) (35).

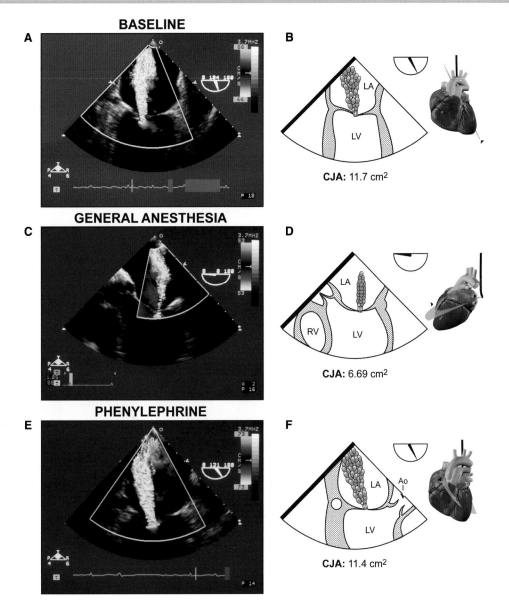

BASELINE

GENERAL ANESTHESIA

PHENYLEPHRINE

CJA: 11.7 cm²

CJA: 6.69 cm²

CJA: 11.4 cm²

Figure 16.20 Color jet area. Color jet areas are shown from different mid-esophageal views in a patient with mitral regurgitation during awake baseline state (**A,B**), after induction of general anesthesia (**C,D**) and using phenylephrine to obtain the same systolic arterial pressure (150 mmHg) as during baseline (**E,F**). Note the reduction in the jet area during general anesthesia. *Abbreviations*: Ao, aorta; CJA, color jet area; LA, left atrium; LV, left ventricle; RV, right ventricle. *Source*: Courtesy of Dr. Alexandro Gisbert and Dr. Arsène Basmadjian.

Regurgitant Volume

Determination of regurgitant volume by PISA method has been described earlier. The mitral regurgitant volume may also be obtained by the continuity equation using volumetric flow calculation (see Chapter 5) (40).

$$\text{Mitral regurgitant volume} = \text{SV}_{\text{MV}} - \text{SV}_{\text{LVOT}} \quad (16.3)$$

The stroke volume across the aortic valve (SV_{LVOT}) is given by the following equation:

$$\text{SV}_{\text{LVOT}} = 0.785 d_{\text{LVOT}}^2 \times \text{VTI}_{\text{LVOT}} \quad (16.4)$$

where d_{LVOT} is the diameter (in cm) of the left ventricular outflow tract (LVOT) and VTI_{LVOT} is the velocity-time integral (in cm) by pulsed wave (PW) Doppler.

The LVOT diameter is measured using a zoomed view of the ME AoV LAX at 135° from the base of the right coronary cusp to the base of the opposite cusp (from inner edge to inner edge). The VTI of the LVOT is best obtained by PW Doppler interrogation in the transgastric LAX view at approximately 110°, tracing the peak (outer edge of the) velocity Doppler signal envelope (41).

In the case of MR without associated significant aortic regurgitation (AR), the left ventricular total SV is given by the SV across the mitral valve (SV_{mv}):

$$\text{SV}_{\text{MV}} = 0.785 d_1 \times d_2 \times \text{VTI}_{\text{MV}} \quad (16.5)$$

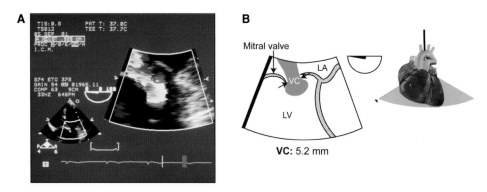

Figure 16.21 Vena contracta. Zoom of color Doppler mid-esophageal five-chamber view demonstrates moderate mitral regurgitation with a VC measured at 5.2 mm. *Abbreviations*: LA, left atrium; LV, left ventricle; VC, vena contracta. *Source*: Courtesy of Dr. Arsène Basmadjian.

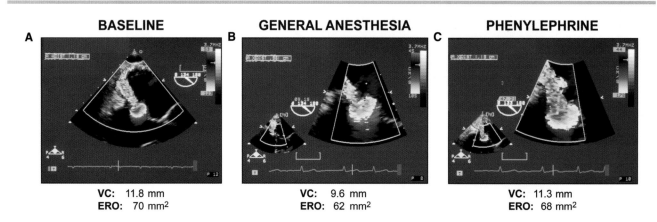

Figure 16.22 ERO area and VC. Measurement of ERO area and VC in the color Doppler mid-esophageal long-axis views show mitral regurgitation during the awake baseline state (**A**), after induction of general anesthesia (**B**) and using phenylephrine (**C**) to obtain the same arterial pressure (150 mmHg) as during baseline. Note the difference in values between the three states. *Abbreviations*: ERO, effective regurgitant orifice; VC, vena contracta. *Source*: Courtesy of Drs. Alexandro Gisbert and Arsène Basmadjian.

where d_1 is the diameter of the MV annulus in the ME four-chamber view, d_2 is the diameter of the MV annulus in the ME two-chamber view or mid-commissural, and VTI_{MV} is the velocity-time integral (in cm) measured by PW Doppler with the sample volume in the center of the MV annulus.

This equation assumes that the MV annulus has an elliptical shape and requires the measurement of the two diameters d_1 and d_2 in orthogonal views (four- and two-chamber), from inner edge to inner edge at the base of the mitral leaflets in diastole (42). The precise measurement of the VTI at the mitral annulus level requires an optimal alignment of the ultrasound beam with the direction of flow. In contrast to the LVOT, the measurement of VTI is performed at the mitral annulus tracing the modal densest velocity on the Doppler signal envelope, rather than the peak velocity (outer edge of the signal).

The reasons for this difference in how to measure the VTI come from the validation work of the Doppler volumetric method. As discussed earlier in

Chapter 5, the hydraulic equation (equation 5.26) assumes a constant mean flow velocity through a rigid circular tube of constant diameter. Several assumptions are thus made with different consequences depending on the site sampled. The original equation ideally assumes that the flow has a flat or square profile, so the sampling velocity would adequately represent average or mean flow velocity. In reality, velocity through a vessel or a cardiac orifice is not uniform. Because of friction forces, it is faster at the center of the vessel than near the edges of a cylinder, assuming a parabolic profile that is more pronounced as the vessel has a smaller diameter or a greater length. The hydraulic equation also assumes that the cross-sectional area is constant during the flow period. While the smaller and circular annulus of the semilunar aortic or pulmonic valve changes little in shape during systole, the larger and somewhat more elliptical orifice of the atrioventricular mitral valve changes in 3D-shape during the cardiac cycle. Moreover, its location changes in space relative to the Doppler

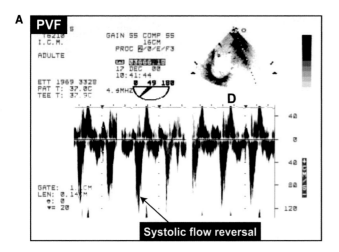

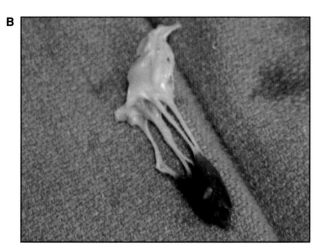

Figure 16.23 PVF systolic reversal. (A) Pulsed wave examination of the PVF shows significant systolic flow reversal (the equivalent of a "v" wave), consistent with severe MR. **(B)** Excised pathology specimen from a 61-year-old man with acute MR due to rupture of the posteromedial papillary muscle. *Abbreviations*: D, peak diastolic PVF velocity; MR, mitral regurgitation; PVF, pulmonary venous flow. *Source*: Photo A courtesy of Dr. Yves Hébert.

sample volume due to the motion of the heart base during cardiac cycle. In contradistinction to the aortic valve flow with a monophasic profile, higher velocities and relatively fixed orifice, the mitral valve flow is multiphasic (early filling, diastasis, and atrial contraction), lower velocities and an orifice in 3D that has a conical or funnel-like form from the base to the tip of the leaflets.

The validity of noninvasive echo Doppler methods of determination of stroke volume and cardiac output was thus checked against several alternate methods of cardiac output measurement, such as roller pump interposed in the vascular system, electromagnetic flow meters, or thermodilution methods. Typically, for atrioventricular valves, the VTI will be measured tracing the modal velocity, that is, along the center of the brightest velocity band on the

spectral Doppler display. Measurements obtained from outflow tracts and great vessels will use the maximal velocity, that is, the leading outer edge of the spectral Doppler display. Although the measurements of diameters for AoV and MV are the most common source of error in the calculation of volumetric flow, they were, however, found to be reproducible in an individual patient (43). In the presence of significant AR, the systemic volumetric flow can alternatively be calculated at the pulmonic valve (PV) annulus or the pulmonary artery trunk.

While the PISA method measures the ERO first and then deducts the regurgitant volume, the continuity equation yields first the regurgitant volume and then the ERO using the following equation:

$$\text{ERO}_{MV} = \frac{\text{MR Vol}}{\text{VTI}_{MR}} \qquad (16.6)$$

where ERO_{MV} is the effective regurgitant orifice of the MV (in cm^2) and VTI_{MR} is the velocity-time integral (in cm) of the mitral regurgitant signal obtained by CW Doppler, tracing the peak (outer edge) of the Doppler signal envelope.

The regurgitant fraction is given by the following equation:

$$\text{RF} = \frac{\text{Reg Vol}}{\text{SV}_{\text{Total}}} \times 100 \qquad (16.7)$$

where RF is the regurgitant fraction (in %), Reg Vol is the regurgitant volume (in mL), and SV_{Total} is the total SV (in mL) of the LV.

The regurgitant volume is obtained either by the PISA method or through the continuity equation. The total SV of the LV is obtained by volumetric measurement at the level of the MV annulus, but it can be also measured from the difference between the 2D tracing of end-diastolic and end-systolic volumes.

Determination of regurgitant volume and ERO by the continuity equation offers an advantage in the presence of very eccentric jets or multiples jets, where the PISA and vena contracta method may be more difficult to perform. On the other hand, these calculations are time consuming and require careful execution that is sometimes difficult to perform in the OR.

Integrated Approach

The ASE task force suggests a scheme of specific signs, supportive and quantitative to help grade MR (Table 16.3). The approach to the evaluation of MR severity should, ideally, integrate multiple parameters rather than depend on a single measurement. If multiple qualitative signs of MR are present, no further measurements are required. If there is discordance between these signs, or if they suggest more severe degree of MR than mild, quantitative measurements of MR through several methods should be performed.

Provocative Testing

In the OR, a change in the loading conditions is frequently observed after induction of anesthesia,

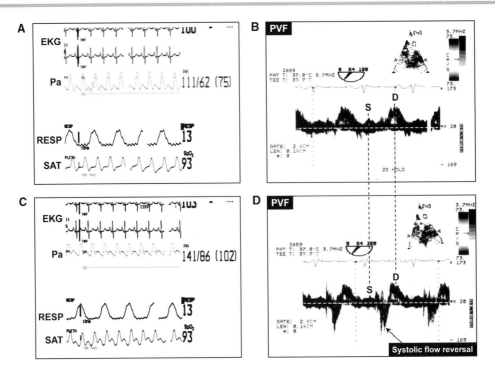

Figure 16.24   Pulmonary venous flow. The pulsed wave Doppler PVF traces are shown in response to changes loading conditions in a 54-year-old patient with MR. With a Pa of 111/62 mmHg (**A**), the PVF shows systolic blunting, with diastolic predominance (**B**). Increasing afterload by giving intravenous phenylephrine raises the Pa to 141/86 mmHg (**C**), frank systolic PVF reversal develops, consistent with severe MR (**D**). *Abbreviations*: D, peak diastolic PVF velocity; EKG, electrocardiogram; MR, mitral regurgitation; Pa, arterial pressure; PVF, pulmonary vein flow; RESP, respiration; S, peak systolic PVF velocity; SAT, saturation.

resulting in an apparent decrease in the severity of MR (Figs. 16.20 and 16.22). To reflect the state of preoperative MR correctly, dynamic reevaluation must be performed by carefully increasing systolic blood pressure using small boluses of phenylephrine (50 µg) or other vasoconstrictor agent. In a study of patients with ischemic MR, Gisbert et al. (35) reported that the severity of intraoperative MR, evaluated with phenylephrine challenge (44), was comparable with that observed, by TEE, in the awake patient. Future trend in evaluation of the potential for MR repair may include assessment of the posterior leaflet angle (45).

Patients with a preoperative posterior leaflet angle equal or greater than 45° are at very high risk for MR persistence and worse outcome when treated by restrictive annuloplasty and coronary artery bypass surgery (45).

Mitral Stenosis

The commonest etiology of MS is rheumatic heart disease. Other causes include nonrheumatic calcification or infiltration of the mitral annulus and leaflets (such as seen in chronic intoxication with ergot-derived substances), congenital lesions (parachute MV, supravalvular ring, mitral arcade), and several miscellaneous lesions (vegetation, tumor, cor triatriatum, thombi) as well as prosthetic valve dysfunction. Guidelines from the ASE and European Association of

Echocardiography for the echocardiographic assessment of valve stenosis have been proposed (46).

Echocardiographic Findings

The morphopathology of the stenotic mitral has important clinical value in the choice of advanced therapy, either percutaneous balloon valvotomy, surgical valvuloplasty, open or close commisurotomy, or prosthetic valve replacement. The typical 2D echocardiographic features of the rheumatic MV include (Fig. 16.25) (*i*) thickening and calcification of the mitral leaflets with commissural fusion; (*ii*) calcification, fusion, fibrosis, and shortening of the subvalvular apparatus; (*iii*) "hockey-stick" deformation of the anterior leaflet in diastole (described by some authors as "doming"); and (*iv*) decreased mobility of the posterior leaflet.

While a number of different scoring systems exist for describing impaired MV anatomy, none has proven to be superior, and all have limited predictive value for balloon valvuloplasty. Wilkins et al. and Abascal et al. (18,47) have proposed an echocardiographic score based on the balloon valvuloplasty registry (BVR score) for patients undergoing mitral balloon valvuloplasty based on the valve thickness, the extent of calcification, the mobility of the leaflets, and the extent of the subvalvular apparatus involvement (Table 16.4). Patients with a score under eight

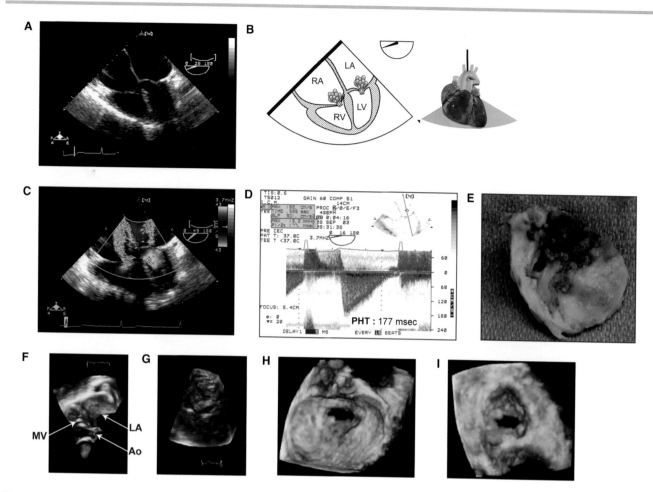

Figure 16.25 Mitral stenosis. A 51-year-old woman presents with moderate MS and MR. (**A–C**) Mitral and tricuspid regurgitation is evident on the mid-esophageal four-chamber views. (**D**) The continuous wave Doppler mean mitral diastolic gradient is measured at 4.9 mmHg with PHT of 177 ms. (**E**) Pathologic explanted stenotic MV is shown. 3D echocardiographic views of MS from an epicardial (**F,G**), transesophageal LA (**H**) and LV (**I**) orientation are shown. *Abbreviations*: Ao, aorta; LA, left atrium; LV, left ventricle; MR, mitral regurgitation; MS, mitral stenosis; MV, mitral valve; PHT, pressure half-time; RA, right atrium; RV, right ventricle. *Sources*: Photo E courtesy of Dr. Michel Pellerin. Images F and G courtesy of Philips Healthcare.

Table 16.4 Assessment of Mitral Valve Anatomy Using the BVR Score

Grade	Mobility	Subvalvular thickening	Thickening	Calcification
0	Normal mobility	No thickening	Normal leaflet thickness	No calcification
1	Highly mobile valve with only leaflets tips restricted	Minimal thickening just below the mitral leaflets	Leaflets near normal in thickness (4–5 mm)	A single area of increased echo brightness
2	Leaflet mid and base portions have normal mobility	Thickening of chordal structures extending up to one-third of the chordal length	Midleaflets normal, considerable thickening of margins (5–8 mm)	Scattered areas of brightness confined to leaflet margins
3	Valve continues to move forward in diastole, mainly from the base	Thickening extending to the distal third of the chords	Considerable thickening of all leaflet tissue (5–8 mm)	Extensive brightness extending to the mid-portion of the leaflet
4	No or minimal forward movement to the leaflets in diastole	Extensive thickening and shortening of all chordal structures extending down to the papillary muscles	Considerable thickening of all leaflet tissues (>8–10 mm)	Extensive brightness throughout much of the leaflet tissue

Each of the four characteristics is given a score from 0 to 4, and the BVR score is calculated as the sum of the four individual scores, with results ranging from 0 to 16.
Abbreviation: BVR, balloon valvuloplasty registry.
Source: Adapted from Refs. 18 and 47.

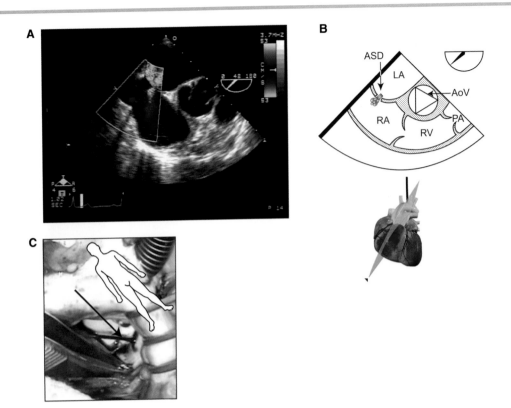

Figure 16.26 Iatrogenic ASD. An iatrogenic ASD developed following transseptal catheterization for balloon valvuloplasty in a 69-year-old man. (**A,B**) Color Doppler mid-esophageal view at 48° shows a left-to-right shunt through residual ASD. (**C**) Intraoperative findings confirm an ASD (arrow) from a LA view. *Abbreviations*: AoV, aortic valve; ASD, atrial septal defect; LA, left atrium; PA, pulmonary artery; RA, right atrium; RV, right ventricle. *Source*: Photo C courtesy of Dr. Michel Pellerin.

(8/16) fare better with a 90% chance of achieving good results. A good result is defined as a valve area >1.5 cm² or an increase of 25% of mitral valve area (MVA) above the baseline value, with a low incidence of restenosis at one year. The score is also useful in predicting the progression of the disease (48). Finally, the presence of associated moderate-to-severe MR constitutes a contraindication to percutaneous mitral valvuloplasty.

Associated Findings

Patients with rheumatic MV disease may present to valve replacement with a history of prior percutaneous balloon valvuloplasty. As the latter procedure is performed through a transseptal approach, a variable size residual atrial septal defect may, therefore, be present (Fig. 16.26).

The typical picture of severe MS includes significant LA enlargement with a normal-sized or small LV (Fig. 16.25). Left atrial thrombus should always be ruled out, especially in the presence of atrial fibrillation (Fig. 16.27). The whole LA and particularly the left atrial appendage (LAA) should be carefully scanned and examined. Spontaneous echo contrast (smoke) may be seen in the LA, particularly if the MVA is <1.4 cm². Its presence signals a very high risk for atrial thrombus (up to 60%) (49) and systemic

embolism (50). The contractility of the LAA may also be assessed by PW Doppler interrogation (Fig. 16.28) (51). When velocities are <25 cm/s, the risk of thrombosis is increased. However, when the velocities are >55 cm/s, the risk is negligible (52).

Upstream hemodynamic repercussions of MS should also be assessed. Pulmonary veins enlarge proportionately to the severity of MS. Tabata et al. (53) reported decreased peak diastolic velocities on PW Doppler examination of the PVF. More importantly, significant postcapillary pulmonary hypertension results in RV hypertrophy, dilatation, and tricuspid regurgitation (TR) (Fig. 16.25). In the transgastric mid-SAX view, flattening of the normal ventricular septal curvature is suggestive of RV pressure or volume overload (see Chapter 10). The severity of the TR must be carefully evaluated to assess the potential indication of repairing the TV at the same time of MV surgery. In the OR after induction of anesthesia and changes in loading conditions (decrease of pulmonary hypertension), a decrease in the severity of functional TR is frequently observed, so ideally TR severity is best evaluated in the awake patient before surgery.

Left ventricular systolic performance is subnormal in one-fourth of patients with MS as a result of rheumatic myocarditis. Diastolic dysfunction may also be present due to a reduction in LV compliance

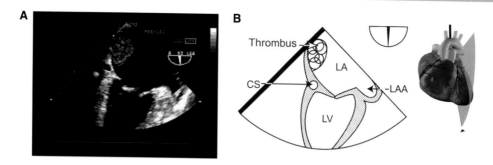

Figure 16.27   Left atrial thrombus. An elderly woman with known mitral valve stenosis is undergoing emergency surgery for acute bilateral iliac artery occlusion. (**A,B**) The mid-esophageal two-chamber view revealed a large thrombus attached to the posterior wall of the LA. *Abbreviations*: CS, coronary sinus; LA, left atrium; LAA, left atrial appendage; LV, left ventricle.

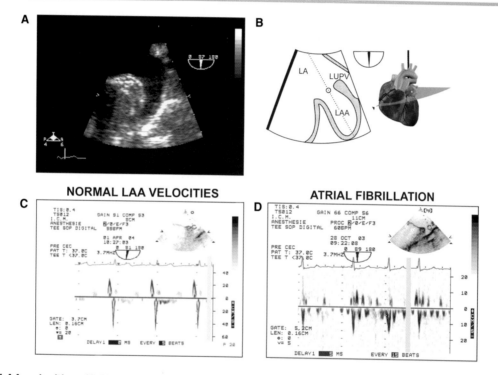

Figure 16.28   LAA velocities. (**A,B**) A 71-year-old man is undergoing aortic valve replacement. Mid-esophageal LAA view with positioning of the pulsed wave Doppler sample volume at the ostium. (**C**) Normal Doppler tracing of the LAA shows a main atrial contraction (positive) and relaxation (negative) waves, followed by much smaller secondary multiple waves. (**D**) A 52-year-old woman with mitral stenosis. The LAA Doppler tracing shows the chaotic multiple waves of variable and lower velocities (<50 cm/s) typical of atrial fibrillation. *Abbreviations*: LAA, left atrial appendage; LA, left atrium; LUPV, left upper pulmonary vein.

related to functional restriction resulting from chordal tethering and the rigid valve apparatus.

Quantitative Echocardiographic Evaluation

The severity of MS is graded on the basis of the MVA and the magnitude of the transvalvular diastolic pressure gradient (Table 16.5). As the MVA is independent of transvalvular flow, it is a more reliable measurement. The MVA can be measured by direct planimetry of the orifice in an SAX view or calculated by the pressure half-time (PHT), the continuity equation, or the proximal flow convergence methods and by the vena contracta. As patients with MS often have concomitant atrial fibrillation, measurements of Doppler signals are averaged over at least 8 to 10 cycles. Mitral inflow velocities are best obtained from the ME four-chamber and LAX views using CW Doppler.

Diastolic Pressure Gradient

The diastolic maximal and mean pressure gradient across the MV is measured from the velocities of the mitral inflow according to the modified Bernoulli

Table 16.5 Grading of Mitral Stenosis Severity

	Normal	Mild	Moderate	Severe
Mitral valve area (cm²)	4.0–5.0	1.6–2.0	1.1–1.5	<1.0
Mean diastolic gradient (mmHg)		<5	5–10	>10
Pressure half-time (ms)	60	90–150	150–220	>220
Pulmonary artery pressure (mmHg)		<30	30–50	>50

Table 16.6 Conditions Affecting MV Diastolic Pressure Gradient

Conditions	Pressure gradient
Low cardiac output	↓
High cardiac output	↑
Severe mitral regurgitation	↑
Diastolic dysfunction	↑

Abbreviation: MV, mitral valve.

equation (Fig. 16.25) using CW Doppler. Recent guidelines suggest that the mean gradient is more relevant for assessing MS than the peak gradient that is influenced by LA compliance and LV diastolic function. In addition, the mean gradient has its own prognostic value, particularly following balloon valvuloplasty (46). The ultrasound beam is optimally aligned (<20°) with the direction of the MV inflow in either the ME four-chamber or LAX views. The measurement of the pressure gradient will be influenced by two factors: the MVA and the flow through the orifice. The gradient increases with the severity of MS and the magnitude of the flow across the valve. Thus, with concomitant moderate-to-severe MR, forward flow through the mitral orifice increases. Therefore, an elevated diastolic pressure gradient may be present despite a mild degree of MS. Other conditions known to modify the pressure gradient independently of the MVA are listed in Table 16.6.

Mitral Valve Area

Planimetry

Direct planimetry of the MV orifice by TTE during mid-diastole has been well validated for determining the anatomic MVA, but requires technical expertise (54). Planimetry is considered the reference measurement of MVA (46). In TEE, the transgastric basal SAX view similarly allows direct planimetry of the MVA. As the geometry of the MV inflow resembles a funnel with the smallest cross-sectional area at the tip of the leaflets, it is important to begin scanning in 2D from the apex, slowly moving the image plane toward the base of the MV to identify the location of the smallest orifice correctly. This may be difficult to achieve as there is a tendency, with this method, to overestimate the true MVA.

An alternative method, using color Doppler imaging, was originally described for TTE (55). The smallest diameter of the stenotic mitral flow is measured in two orthogonal planes, the ME four- and two-chamber views for TEE. Using the equation for an ellipse, the MVA equals $\pi/4 \times D_{4ch} \times D_{2ch}$. This method may underestimate the true MVA.

Pressure Half-Time

The PHT is defined as the time interval in milliseconds (ms) between the maximum early diastolic transmitral pressure gradient and the time point where the pressure gradient has decreased to half its maximal initial value (see Fig. 5.34).

As the MV becomes more stenotic, the LV pressure takes more time to equalize with the LA pressure and the diastolic pressure gradient decreases more slowly. The relationship between the PHT and the MVA was determined empirically by the following equation (56)

$$MVA = \frac{220}{PHT} = \frac{759}{Mdt} \qquad (16.8)$$

where MVA is the mitral valve area (in cm²), PHT is the pressure half-time (in ms), and Mdt is the mitral deceleration time (in ms).

The severity of MS can be estimated using the PHT measured on the same CW Doppler signal previously obtained for the maximal and mean diastolic pressure gradient (Fig. 16.29).

The rate of equalization of LV and LA pressures and, therefore, the PHT may be affected by several hemodynamic factors (Table 16.7). The rate of rise of the LV diastolic pressure may be abnormally increased with significant AR or diastolic dysfunction. This results in decreased PHT, independent of the MV status, and leads to underestimation of MS severity. A concomitant eccentric AR jet may also complicate MS assessment causing a functional stenosis (the Austin–Flint phenomenon) when it prevents full diastolic excursion of the anterior mitral leaflet, and maintains it in a relatively closed position (Fig. 16.30).

The LA and LV compliance may change after valvuloplasty and cardiopulmonary bypass. For this reason, the use of PHT to determine MVA in this context may not be accurate. Moreover, the PHT equation, originally reported by Hatle et al. (56) for the native MV, has not been validated for the determination of prosthetic valve area. Nevertheless, a decrease in prosthetic valve area will be reflected by progressive lengthening of the PHT such that serial measurements of PHT are useful to follow these patients even if it cannot be used to yield the effective valve area (see Chapter 17).

Mitral valve area determination by the PHT method is also affected by declines in LA pressure due to hypovolemia or increased compliance with enlarged LA size. The decreased decay of the diastolic pressure gradient results in overestimation of the true severity of the MS. Impaired diastolic function,

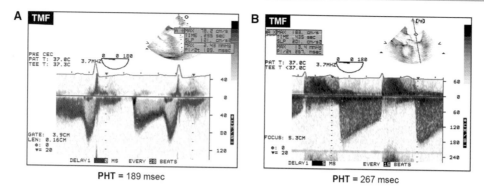

PHT = 189 msec   PHT = 267 msec

Figure 16.29 PHT in MS. Spectral continuous wave Doppler tracings of TMF. (**A**) Moderate MS in a 79-year-old patient: the PHT is 189 ms. (**B**) Severe MS in a 52-year-old woman: the PHT is 267 ms. *Abbreviations*: PHT, pressure half-time; MS, mitral stenosis; TMF, transmitral flow.

Table 16.7 Factors Affecting Pressure Half-Time (PHT)

Factors	Effect on PHT	Effect on calculated MVA by PHT method	Effect on estimation of true MS severity
↓ Ventricular compliance, aging	↓	Larger	Underestimate
Moderate-to-severe aortic regurgitation (57)	↓	Larger	Underestimate
↑ Cardiac output (58)	↓	Larger	Underestimate
Hypovolemia (58)	↑	Smaller	Overestimate
Large left atrium	↑	Smaller	Overestimate
Eccentric aortic regurgitant jet impinging on the anterior mitral leaflet opening (Austin Flint)	↑	Smaller	Overestimate

Abbreviations: MS, mitral stenosis; MVA, mitral valve area.

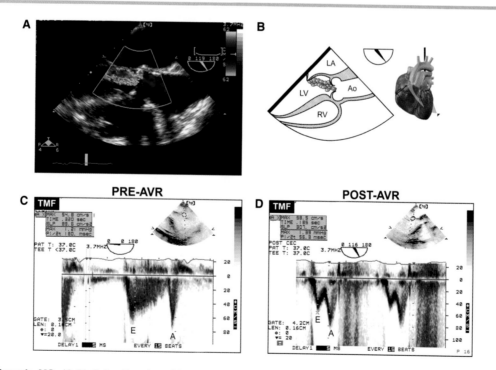

PRE-AVR   POST-AVR

Figure 16.30 Pseudo MS. (**A,B**) Color Doppler mid-esophageal long-axis view of a 78-year-old woman scheduled for AVR. (**C**) She had AR associated with a pseudo MS Doppler pattern from either restricted opening of the anterior mitral valve leaflet or contamination from the AR signal. The pressure half-time obtained from the Doppler TMF was 180 ms compared with 56 ms after AVR (**D**). *Abbreviations*: A, peak late diastolic TMF velocity; Ao, aorta; AR, aortic regurgitation; AVR, aortic valve replacement; E, peak early diastolic TMF velocity; LA, left atrium; LV, left ventricle; MS, mitral stenosis; RV, right ventricle; TMF, transmitral flow.

particularly in the elderly, can make the use of PHT in degenerative calcific MS unreliable and should be interpreted with caution and even avoided (46).

Continuity Equation

The continuity equation states that in the absence of valvular regurgitation and atrial or ventricular septal defect, the SV across the MV must equal that of other valves or subvalvular regions such as LVOT, the AoV, or PV at the same time and during hemodynamic stability.

The MVA can be obtained by applying the continuity equation: $Q_{mitral} = Q_{aortic}$, provided there is no significant MR or AR.

$$MVA = 0.785 \, d_{LVOT}^2 \, \frac{VTI_{LVOT}}{VTI_{mitral}} \qquad (16.9)$$

The VTI_{LVOT} is measured using PW Doppler examination through the transgastric LAX view at $110°$ close to the aortic annulus at the same position where the diameter of the LVOT is measured (Fig. 16.31). The VTI_{mitral} is measured by CW Doppler

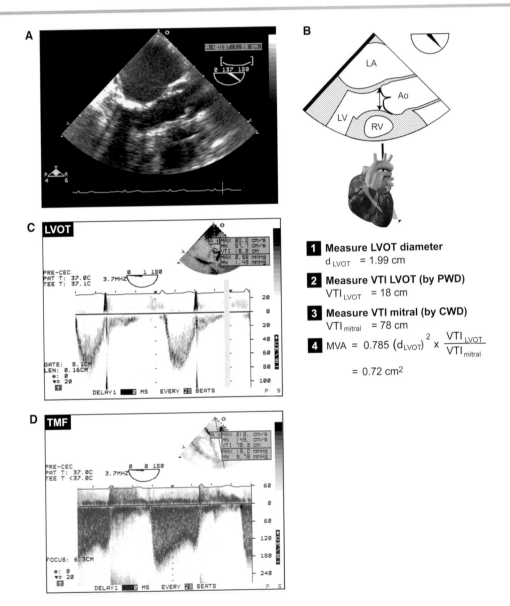

Figure 16.31 MVA continuity equation. (A,B) The LVOT diameter is measured from the mid-esophageal long-axis view at 135°. **(C)** To complete the calculation of the SV, the LVOT velocity-time integral (VTI_{LVOT}) is obtained by PW Doppler of a deep TG view at 0° (or alternatively from a TG long-axis view at 110°). The SV_{LVOT} is calculated from the product of 0.785 × (LVOT diameter)^2 and the VTI_{LVOT}. **(D)** The VTI_{mitral}, is given by CW Doppler of TMF from a mid-esophageal view. The MVA is calculated by dividing the SV_{LVOT} by the VTI_{mitral}. *Abbreviations*: Ao, aorta; CW, continuous wave; LA, left atrium; LV, left ventricle; LVOT, left ventricular outflow tract; MVA, mitral valve area; PW, pulsed wave; RV, right ventricle; SV, stroke volume; TG, transgastric; TMF, transmitral flow.

across the native or prosthetic MV from the ME four-chamber or LAX views. The continuity equation cannot be used to calculate the MS in the presence of atrial fibrillation, AR, or significant MR.

Proximal Flow Convergence

The basis of the PISA, or proximal flow convergence method, has been described earlier for MR lesions. In the case of MS, the surface surrounding the stenosed orifice is funnel-shaped rather than planar, and distorts the PISA such that a correction factor must be added in contradistinction to MR:

$$MVA = 2\pi r^2 \frac{v_r}{V_{MS\,max}} \frac{\alpha}{180} \qquad (16.10)$$

where MVA is the mitral valve area (in cm^2); r is the measured radius of the hemispheric shell of the aliased velocity; v_r is the aliased velocity at the radius r (identified as the Nyquist limit in cm/s); $V_{MS\,max}$ is the maximal velocity across the orifice, obtained by CW Doppler (in cm/s); and α is the angle measured between the two mitral leaflets.

The PISA radius is best obtained from high-resolution, zoomed ME four-chamber or LAX views. The color flow scale baseline is shifted in the direction of the flow measured, which in the case of MS is away from the transducer. In contrast to MR, Deng et al. (59) reported that an aliasing velocity of 21 cm/s is optimal for the PISA method in MS. Indeed, higher aliasing velocities may underestimate the stenotic MVA. The angle between the two mitral leaflets must also be measured for the necessary correction factor $\alpha/180$ in MS.

The PISA method appears to provide MVA estimates that are at least as accurate as the traditional echocardiographic methods with accuracy preserved in atrial fibrillation (60). Because this method applies the continuity equation with flow parameters measured on a single valve, the presence of other valve disease such as AR or MR should not affect its accuracy (61).

Vena Contracta

Measurement of vena contracta width (62) in the ME four-chamber view by color Doppler imaging can provide an accurate estimation of MVA (38). A cutoff point of ≤1 cm has a sensitivity of 88% and a specificity of 77% for the prediction of severe MS (63,64). This technique can provide an alternative to calculate the MV orifice area when the accuracy of the other methods is affected by different loading conditions (AR and MR) or difficult planimetry.

Grading MS Severity

The approach to MS is summarized in Table 16.8. In summary, MV pathology is an area where TEE plays a critical role in the evaluation of the mechanism and also the related complications that can alter most, if not all, of the other cardiac structures. The severity of MS is assessed from the mean pressure gradient and the MVA as determined by planimetry or the PHT. The severity of rheumatic MV disease relies mostly on

Table 16.8 Summary of Perioperative Evaluation of Mitral Stenosis

Global appearance of the heart chambers (large LA, small LV)
Valve morphology (BVR score)
    Presence of calcification
    Leaflet decreased mobility
    Leaflet thickening
    Involvement of subvalvular apparatus
Evaluation of associated MR
Evaluation of the severity of mitral stenosis
    Diastolic pressure gradient (maximal and mean)
    MVA by PHT method
    MVA by the continuity equation
    MVA by PISA method (better when concomitant MR or AR)
Measurement of the left atrial dimensions
Detailed examination of the left atrium and left atrial appendage to exclude atrial thrombus
Examination of the atrial septum to exclude ASD
Evaluation of RV dimensions and systolic function
Evaluation of concomitant valvular disease (aortic and tricuspid)
Quantification of tricuspid regurgitation for estimation of right-sided pressures

Abbreviations: AR, aortic regurgitation; ASD, atrial septal defect; BVR, balloon valvuloplasty registry; LA, left atrium; LV, left ventricle; MR, mitral regurgitation; MVA, mitral valve area; PHT, pressure half-time; PISA, proximal isovelocity surface area; RV, right ventricular.

MVA, while in degenerative MS, a mean gradient is more indicative of severity. The decision to intervene is based on echocardiographic assessment of severity and the presence of symptoms.

3D Evaluation of MV

There have been great improvements in MV surgery techniques in the last two decades. There is consensus on the superiority of valve repair techniques, but the feasibility of repair depends on the anatomic lesions of the valve. This underscores the importance of accurate assessment of the valve anatomy and function for clinical decision-making.

Three-dimensional TEE can provide a dynamic view of the surgical anatomy of MV valve lesions, giving the surgeon a preview of what one may encounter in the OR. It allows accurate, reliable, and reproducible assessment of the MV apparatus (65). Sophisticated 3D measurements like annular diameters, annular nonplanarity, commissural lengths, leaflet surface areas, and aortic to mitral annular orientation are possible with 3D TEE (65).

By providing accurate structural and functional information, 3D TEE echo may play an important role in the planning, optimization, and postoperative surveillance of MV repair. The surgeon could preoperatively design and customize MV repair procedure for each patient using data obtained from 3D TEE images including valve geometry, function and stress distribution, 3D-based program, and computerized virtual surgery techniques (66).

This is expected to lead to better outcome. Unfortunately, patients initially scheduled for mitral valve repair must sometimes undergo mitral valve prosthetic replacement because unforeseen abnormalities are discovered only intraoperatively and are beyond the surgeon's skills or preparation for ideal repair. Better preoperative evaluation of mitral valve disease with 3D TEE could help the early identification of complex lesions that require advanced surgical skills, planning, and/or techniques (67).

Muller et al. (68) performed 3D images reconstruction in 74 patients with MR due to Carpentier type II valve dysfunction before surgical repair. Compared with conventional TEE, 3D TEE had better sensitivity, positive and negative predictive values, and accuracy. Its greatest advantage was higher sensitivity in commissural and bileaflet defects that are difficult to evaluate by conventional TEE. The more complex the lesion, the more valuable was the information provided by 3D TEE.

Sugeng et al. (69) showed in their cohort of 211 patients that 3D TEE imaging was feasible in most patients and provided excellent imaging of native MV. In a study comparing head-to-head 3D TEE with 2D TEE in MV repair, Garcia-Orta et al. (70) concluded that 3D TEE may complement 2D study in patients with complex valve anatomy, where surgical decisions are more difficult. 3D TEE offers high accuracy in MV evaluation, and the images can be easily interpreted by professionals without a high degree of experience. Manda et al. (71) compared 3D TEE with 2D TEE in the assessment of individual MV segment/scallop prolapse and associated chordal rupture in 18 adult patients with a flail MV undergoing surgery for MR. Two-dimensional TEE was able to diagnose the prolapsing segment/scallop and associated chordal rupture correctly in only 9 of 18 patients when compared to surgery, while 3D TEE findings correlated exactly with the surgical findings in 16 of 18 patients.

There are fewer studies on MS compared to MR. They demonstrate that calculation of MVA using 3D TEE is accurate and reproducible (72,73). Xie et al. concluded in their study that 3D TEE can provide not only the anatomic structure of MV but also the smallest MV orifice and can thus accurately measure MVA (74).

In summary, the bulk of evidence shows that 3D TEE can provide important complementary information to current 2D MV assessment, thus affecting clinical decision-making and potentially the outcome.

CONCLUSION

In summary, TEE plays an outstanding role in the evaluation of MV function. Precise measurements and determination of MV lesions make this modality so far unsurpassed. The use of 3D TEE is likely to play an increasingly important role, particularly in the determination of complex mechanisms of MV pathology, and help in the context of MV repair or replacement as will be discussed in the next chapter.

REFERENCES

1. Bonow RO, Carabello BA, Kanu C, et al. ACC/AHA 2006 guidelines for the management of patients with valvular heart disease: a report of the American College of Cardiology/ American Heart Association Task Force on Practice Guidelines (writing committee to revise the 1998 Guidelines for the Management of Patients With Valvular Heart Disease): developed in collaboration with the Society of Cardiovascular Anesthesiologists: endorsed by the Society for Cardiovascular Angiography and Interventions and the Society of Thoracic Surgeons. Circulation 2006; 114:e84–e231.
2. Zoghbi WA, Enriquez-Sarano M, Foster E, et al. Recommendations for evaluation of the severity of native valvular regurgitation with two-dimensional and Doppler echocardiography. J Am Soc Echocardiogr 2003; 16: 777–802.
3. Kumar N, Kumar M, Duran CM. A revised terminology for recording surgical findings of the mitral valve. J Heart Valve Dis 1995; 4:70–75.
4. Lambert AS, Miller JP, Merrick SH, et al. Improved evaluation of the location and mechanism of mitral valve regurgitation with a systematic transesophageal echocardiography examination. Anesth Analg 1999; 88:1205–1212.
5. Carpentier AF, Lessana A, Relland JY, et al. The "physio-ring": an advanced concept in mitral valve annuloplasty. Ann Thorac Surg 1995; 60:1177–1185.
6. Poortmans G, Schupfer G, Roosens C, et al. Additional view of the mitral valve. Anesth Analg 2000; 91:494–495.
7. Mintz GS, Kotler MN, Segal BL, et al. Two-dimensional echocardiographic recognition of ruptured chordae tendineae. Circulation 1978; 57:244–250.
8. Enriquez-Sarano M, Freeman WK, Tribouilloy CM, et al. Functional anatomy of mitral regurgitation: accuracy and outcome implications of transesophageal echocardiography. J Am Coll Cardiol 1999; 34:1129–1136.
9. Durack DT, Lukes AS, Bright DK. New criteria for diagnosis of infective endocarditis: utilization of specific echocardiographic findings. Duke Endocarditis Service. Am J Med 1994; 96:200–209.
10. Li JS, Sexton DJ, Mick N, et al. Proposed modifications to the Duke criteria for the diagnosis of infective endocarditis. Clin Infect Dis 2000; 30:633–638.
11. Sanfilippo AJ, Picard MH, Newell JB, et al. Echocardiographic assessment of patients with infectious endocarditis: prediction of risk for complications. J Am Coll Cardiol 1991; 18:1191–1199.
12. Tischler MD, Vaitkus PT. The ability of vegetation size on echocardiography to predict clinical complications: a meta-analysis. J Am Soc Echocardiogr 1997; 10:562–568.
13. Khandheria BK. Suspected bacterial endocarditis: to TEE or not to TEE. J Am Coll Cardiol 1993; 21:222–224.
14. Birmingham GD, Rahko PS, Ballantyne F III. Improved detection of infective endocarditis with transesophageal echocardiography. Am Heart J 1992; 123:774–781.
15. Karalis DG, Bansal RC, Hauck AJ, et al. Transesophageal echocardiographic recognition of subaortic complications in aortic valve endocarditis. Clinical and surgical implications. Circulation 1992; 86:353–362.
16. Daniel WG, Mugge A, Martin RP, et al. Improvement in the diagnosis of abscesses associated with endocarditis by transesophageal echocardiography. N Engl J Med 1991; 324:795–800.
17. Duran CM, Gometza B, Saad E. Valve repair in rheumatic mitral disease: an unsolved problem. J Card Surg 1994; 9:282–285.
18. Wilkins GT, Weyman AE, Abascal VM, et al. Percutaneous balloon dilatation of the mitral valve: an analysis of echocardiographic variables related to outcome and the mechanism of dilatation. Br Heart J 1988; 60:299–308.
19. Marwick TH, Torelli J, Obarski T, et al. Assessment of the mitral valve splitability score by transthoracic and transesophageal echocardiography. Am J Cardiol 1991; 68:1106–1107.

20. Nishimura RA, McGoon MD, Shub C, et al. Echocardiographically documented mitral-valve prolapse. Long-term follow-up of 237 patients. N Engl J Med 1985; 313:1305–1309.

21. Grayburn PA, Berk MR, Spain MG, et al. Relation of echocardiographic morphology of the mitral apparatus to mitral regurgitation in mitral valve prolapse: assessment by Doppler color flow imaging. Am Heart J 1990; 119:1095–1102.

22. Zamorano J, Erbel R, Mackowski T, et al. Usefulness of transesophageal echocardiography for diagnosis of mitral valve prolapse. Am J Cardiol 1992; 69:419–422.

23. Pini R, Devereux RB, Greppi B, et al. Comparison of mitral valve dimensions and motion in mitral valve prolapse with severe mitral regurgitation to uncomplicated mitral valve prolapse and to mitral regurgitation without mitral valve prolapse. Am J Cardiol 1988; 62:257–263.

24. Adams DH, Filsoufi F. Another chapter in an enlarging book: repair degenerative mitral valves. J Thorac Cardiovasc Surg 2003; 125:1197–1199.

25. Cherian G, Tei C, Shah PM, et al. Diastolic prolapse in the flail mitral valve syndrome: a new observation providing differentiation from the mitral valve prolapse syndrome. Am Heart J 1982; 103:1074–1075.

26. Agricola E, Oppizzi M, De Bonis M, et al. Multiplane transesophageal echocardiography performed according to the guidelines of the American Society of Echocardiography in patients with mitral valve prolapse, flail, and endocarditis: diagnostic accuracy in the identification of mitral regurgitant defects by correlation with surgical findings. J Am Soc Echocardiogr 2003; 16:61–66.

27. Stewart WJ, Currie PJ, Salcedo EE, et al. Evaluation of mitral leaflet motion by echocardiography and jet direction by Doppler color flow mapping to determine the mechanisms of mitral regurgitation. J Am Coll Cardiol 1992; 20:1353–1361.

28. Kumanohoso T, Otsuji Y, Yoshifuku S, et al. Mechanism of higher incidence of ischemic mitral regurgitation in patients with inferior myocardial infarction: quantitative analysis of left ventricular and mitral valve geometry in 103 patients with prior myocardial infarction. J Thorac Cardiovasc Surg 2003; 125:135–143.

29. Parmley LF, Manion WC, Mattingly TW. Nonpenetrating traumatic injury of the heart. Circulation 1958; 18:371–396.

30. Simmers TA, Meijburg HW, de la Riviere AB. Traumatic papillary muscle rupture. Ann Thorac Surg 2001; 72:257–259.

31. Lang RM, Bierig M, Devereux RB, et al. Recommendations for chamber quantification: a report from the American Society of Echocardiography's Guidelines and Standards Committee and the Chamber Quantification Writing Group, developed in conjunction with the European Association of Echocardiography, a branch of the European Society of Cardiology. J Am Soc Echocardiogr 2005; 18:1440–1463.

32. Byram MT, Roberts WC. Frequency and extent of calcific deposits in purely regurgitant mitral valves: analysis of 108 operatively excised valves. Am J Cardiol 1983; 52:1059–1061.

33. Castello R, Lenzen P, Aguirre F, et al. Quantitation of mitral regurgitation by transesophageal echocardiography with Doppler color flow mapping: correlation with cardiac catheterization. J Am Coll Cardiol 1992; 19:1516–1521.

34. Kleinman JP, Czer LS, DeRobertis M, et al. A quantitative comparison of transesophageal and epicardial color Doppler echocardiography in the intraoperative assessment of mitral regurgitation. Am J Cardiol 1989; 64:1168–1172.

35. Gisbert A, Souliere V, Denault AY, et al. Dynamic quantitative echocardiographic evaluation of mitral regurgitation in the operating department. J Am Soc Echocardiogr 2006; 19:140–146.

36. Roberts BJ, Grayburn PA. Color flow imaging of the vena contracta in mitral regurgitation: technical considerations. J Am Soc Echocardiogr 2003; 16:1002–1006.

37. Hall SA, Brickner ME, Willett DL, et al. Assessment of mitral regurgitation severity by Doppler color flow mapping of the vena contracta. Circulation 1997; 95:636–642.

38. Grayburn PA, Fehske W, Omran H, et al. Multiplane transesophageal echocardiographic assessment of mitral regurgitation by Doppler color flow mapping of the vena contracta. Am J Cardiol 1994; 74:912–917.

39. Pu M, Griffin BP, Vandervoort PM, et al. The value of assessing pulmonary venous flow velocity for predicting severity of mitral regurgitation: a quantitative assessment integrating left ventricular function. J Am Soc Echocardiogr 1999; 12:736–743.

40. Stewart WJ, Jiang L, Mich R, et al. Variable effects of changes in flow rate through the aortic, pulmonary and mitral valves on valve area and flow velocity: impact on quantitative Doppler flow calculations. J Am Coll Cardiol 1985; 6:653–662.

41. Fisher DC, Sahn DJ, Friedman MJ, et al. The mitral valve orifice method for noninvasive two-dimensional echo Doppler determinations of cardiac output. Circulation 1983; 67:872–877.

42. Rokey R, Sterling LL, Zoghbi WA, et al. Determination of regurgitant fraction in isolated mitral or aortic regurgitation by pulsed Doppler two-dimensional echocardiography. J Am Coll Cardiol 1986; 7:1273–1278.

43. Lewis JF, Kuo LC, Nelson JG, et al. Pulsed Doppler echocardiographic determination of stroke volume and cardiac output: clinical validation of two new methods using the apical window. Circulation 1984; 70:425–431.

44. Konstadt SN, Louie EK, Shore-Lesserson L, et al. The effects of loading changes on intraoperative Doppler assessment of mitral regurgitation. J Cardiothorac Vasc Anesth 1994; 8:19–23.

45. Magne J, Pibarot P, Dagenais F, et al. Preoperative posterior leaflet angle accurately predicts outcome after restrictive mitral valve annuloplasty for ischemic mitral regurgitation. Circulation 2007; 115:782–791.

46. Baumgartner H, Hung J, Bermejo J, et al. Echocardiographic assessment of valve stenosis: EAE/ASE recommendations for clinical practice. J Am Soc Echocardiogr 2009; 22:1–23.

47. Abascal VM, Wilkins GT, Choong CY, et al. Echocardiographic evaluation of mitral valve structure and function in patients followed for at least 6 months after percutaneous balloon mitral valvuloplasty. J Am Coll Cardiol 1988; 12:606–615.

48. Gordon SP, Douglas PS, Come PC, et al. Two-dimensional and Doppler echocardiographic determinants of the natural history of mitral valve narrowing in patients with rheumatic mitral stenosis: implications for follow-up. J Am Coll Cardiol 1992; 19:968–973.

49. Michalis LK, Thomas MR, Smyth DW, et al. Left atrial spontaneous echo contrast assessed by TEE in patients with either native mitral valve disease or mitral valve replacement. J Am Soc Echocardiogr 1993; 6:299–307.

50. Black IW, Hopkins AP, Lee LC, et al. Left atrial spontaneous echo contrast: a clinical and echocardiographic analysis. J Am Coll Cardiol 1991; 18:398–404.

51. Mugge A, Kuhn H, Nikutta P, et al. Assessment of left atrial appendage function by biplane transesophageal echocardiography in patients with nonrheumatic atrial fibrillation: identification of a subgroup of patients at increased embolic risk. J Am Coll Cardiol 1994; 23:599–607.

52. Handke M, Harloff A, Hetzel A, et al. Left atrial appendage flow velocity as a quantitative surrogate parameter for thromboembolic risk: determinants and relationship to spontaneous echocontrast and thrombus formation—a transesophageal echocardiographic study in 500 patients

with cerebral ischemia. J Am Soc Echocardiogr 2005; 18:1366–1372.

53. Tabata T, Oki T, Fukuda N, et al. Transesophageal pulsed Doppler echocardiographic study of pulmonary venous flow in mitral stenosis. Cardiology 1996; 87:112–118.

54. Faletra F, Pezzano A Jr., Fusco R, et al. Measurement of mitral valve area in mitral stenosis: four echocardiographic methods compared with direct measurement of anatomic orifices. J Am Coll Cardiol 1996; 28:1190–1197.

55. Kawahara T, Yamagishi M, Seo H, et al. Application of Doppler color flow imaging to determine valve area in mitral stenosis. J Am Coll Cardiol 1991; 18:85–92.

56. Hatle L, Angelsen B, Tromsdal A. Noninvasive assessment of atrioventricular pressure half-time by Doppler ultrasound. Circulation 1979; 60:1096–1104.

57. Nakatani S, Masuyama T, Kodama K, et al. Value and limitations of Doppler echocardiography in the quantification of stenotic mitral valve area: comparison of the pressure half-time and the continuity equation methods. Circulation 1988; 77:78–85.

58. Firstenberg MS, Prior DL, Greenberg NL, et al. Effect of cardiac output on mitral valve area in patients with mitral stenosis: validation and pitfalls of the pressure half-time method. J Heart Valve Dis 2001; 10:49–56.

59. Deng YB, Matsumoto M, Wang XF, et al. Estimation of mitral valve area in patients with mitral stenosis by the flow convergence region method: selection of aliasing velocity. J Am Coll Cardiol 1994; 24:683–689.

60. Rifkin RD, Harper K, Tighe D. Comparison of proximal isovelocity surface area method with pressure half-time and planimetry in evaluation of mitral stenosis. J Am Coll Cardiol 1995; 26:458–465.

61. Ikawa H, Enya E, Hirano Y, et al. Can the proximal isovelocity surface area method calculate stenotic mitral valve area in patients with associated moderate to severe aortic regurgitation? Analysis using low aliasing velocity of 10% of the peak transmitral velocity. Echocardiography 2001; 18:89–95.

62. Flachskampf FA, Frieske R, Engelhard B et al. Comparison of transesophageal Doppler methods with angiography for evaluation of the severity of mitral regurgitation. J Am Soc Echocardiogr 1998; 11:882–892.

63. Abaci A, Oguzhan A, Unal S, et al. Application of the vena contracta method for the calculation of the mitral valve area in mitral stenosis. Cardiology 2002; 98:50–59.

64. Park TH, Park MA, Lee SH, et al. Measurement of vena contracta width for the assessment of severity of mitral stenosis. Heart Vessels 2006; 21:273–277.

65. Salcedo EE, Quaife RA, Seres T, et al. A framework for systematic characterization of the mitral valve by real-time three-dimensional transesophageal echocardiography. J Am Soc Echocardiogr 2009; 22:1087–1099.

66. Ryan LP, Salgo IS, Gorman RC, et al. The emerging role of three-dimensional echocardiography in mitral valve repair. Semin Thorac Cardiovasc Surg 2006; 18:126–134.

67. Adams DH, Anyanwu AC, Sugeng L, et al. Degenerative mitral valve regurgitation: surgical echocardiography. Curr Cardiol Rep 2008; 10:226–232.

68. Muller S, Muller L, Laufer G, et al. Comparison of three-dimensional imaging to transesophageal echocardiography for preoperative evaluation in mitral valve prolapse. Am J Cardiol 2006; 98:243–248.

69. Sugeng L, Shernan SK, Salgo IS, et al. Live 3-dimensional transesophageal echocardiography initial experience using the fully-sampled matrix array probe. J Am Coll Cardiol 2008; 52:446–449.

70. Garcia-Orta R, Moreno E, Vidal M, et al. Three-dimensional versus two-dimensional transesophageal echocardiography in mitral valve repair. J Am Soc Echocardiogr 2007; 20:4–12.

71. Manda J, Kesanolla SK, Hsuing MC, et al. Comparison of real time two-dimensional with live/real time three-dimensional transesophageal echocardiography in the evaluation of mitral valve prolapse and chordae rupture. Echocardiography 2008; 25:1131–1137.

72. Zamorano J, Cordeiro P, Sugeng L, et al. Real-time three-dimensional echocardiography for rheumatic mitral valve stenosis evaluation: an accurate and novel approach. J Am Coll Cardiol 2004; 43:2091–2096.

73. Binder TM, Rosenhek R, Porenta G, et al. Improved assessment of mitral valve stenosis by volumetric real-time three-dimensional echocardiography. J Am Coll Cardiol 2000; 36:1355–1361.

74. Xie MX, Wang XF, Cheng TO, et al. Comparison of accuracy of mitral valve area in mitral stenosis by real-time, three-dimensional echocardiography versus two-dimensional echocardiography versus Doppler pressure half-time. Am J Cardiol 2005; 95:1496–1499.

17

Mitral Valve Replacement and Repair

Arsène-J. Basmadjian, Christian Ayoub, and Michel Pellerin
Université de Montréal, Montreal, Quebec, Canada

TYPES OF VALVE PROSTHESES

The first successful artificial valve replacements were performed in the early 1960s (1). Prosthetic valves have a sewing ring that enables suture attachment to surrounding human tissue. They are classified according to the material (biological tissue or mechanical) and the design of the occluder. Biological tissue valves are further divided on the basis of the presence (stented) or absence (stentless) of a structural support and the tissue of origin, with homografts versus heterografts (porcine or bovine). Mechanical valves are distinguished by three main occluder designs: ball in cage, tilting disk, and bileaflet, the latter being the most commonly implanted in the mitral position.

Mechanical Valves

As a group, mechanical prosthetic valves provide long durability but with the disadvantage of requiring lifelong anticoagulation (2). The *ball-in-cage valves* were the first mechanical valves implanted. The Starr–Edwards prosthesis (Fig. 17.1) represents the typical example of this design, and has the best performance record (1). It consists of a metal cage holding a mobile silicone spherical ball with a Teflon/polypropylene sewing ring. The Beal valve is a variation of the ball-in-cage design, with the occluder consisting of a floating, mobile disc rather than a ball. While the best feature of the Starr–Edwards ball-in-cage valve was its long track record of durability, its many disadvantages included high thrombogenicity, requiring more intense anticoagulation, hemolysis, a suboptimal intrinsic hydrodynamic profile with higher transvalvular pressure gradient, and obstruction of the left ventricular outflow tract (LVOT) because of its bulky design.

Tilting or pivoting disc valves consist of a single pyrolytic or carbon-coated circular disc suspended within a metal valve-housing with either a central hole or struts that permit tilting, with a polyester or Teflon sewing ring. By design, the maximum tilting angle varies between models from 55° to 70°: consequently, in the open position, these valves have one larger (major) and one smaller (minor) orifice. Because a minimal clearance space between the moving parts is necessary to enable their unimpeded motion, small central and lateral (between the disc and the sewing

ring) transvalvular regurgitant jets may normally be demonstrated on color Doppler imaging. The Bjork–Shiley, Lillehei–Kaster, Hall–Kaster, Medtronics Hall™ (Fig. 17.1), and Omniscience represent examples of single, tilting disc prostheses.

Bileaflet valves have two semicircular discs coated with pyrolytic carbon, mounted centrally on hinges. They pivot open approximately 70° to 80° creating two equal semicircular (major) and one central slit-like (minor) orifices. As for the tilting disc valves, these prostheses normally present transvalvular converging as well as diverging regurgitant jets, at the periphery between the hemidiscs and the sewing ring, and along the central closure line between the two hemidiscs (3). The Sorin Carbomedics®, On-X® (Life Technologies, Inc., formerly MCRI), and the St. Jude Medical® valves (Fig. 17.1) are typical examples of bileaflet prostheses. The latter is the most commonly implanted bileaflet prosthetic valve worldwide.

Compared with ball-in-cage mechanical prostheses, tilting disc and bileaflet valves have an improved hydrodynamic profile as they are less bulky and also have a lower intrinsic pressure gradient and lower thrombogenicity.

Biological Tissue Valves

In the mitral position, all biological tissue prostheses are currently mounted onto a flexible or semiflexible frame with struts (i.e., stented). Heterografts (or xenografts) designate a bioprosthesis made of nonhuman tissue, either glutaraldehyde-treated porcine aortic valve (AoV) such as the Carpentier–Edwards (Fig. 17.2), Hancock, and Medtronic Intact prostheses, or reconstructed leaflets from bovine pericardium such as the Carpentier–Edwards Perimount™ (Fig. 17.2), Mitroflow, and Ionescu–Shiley valves. Homografts are made from human tissue, but they are no longer used in the mitral position because of their poor durability. While bioprostheses are advantageous as they do not require chronic anticoagulation, their lesser durability represents a significant drawback, particularly in young patients or patients with chronic renal failure (2–4). They are most commonly used in patients with contraindications to anticoagulation or in older patients. These valves comprise three leaflets that give them an interesting appearance during two-dimensional (2D)

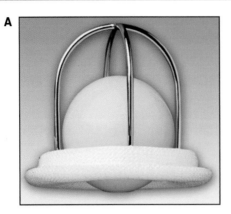

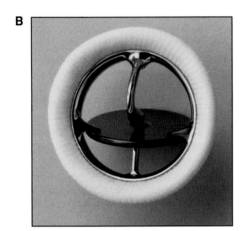

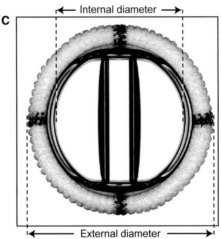

Figure 17.1 Models of mechanical valve prostheses. (**A**) Starr–Edwards (Edwards Lifesciences LLC, Irvine, California, U.S.). (**B**) Medtronic Hall (Copyright Medtronic, Inc., Minneapolis, Minnesota, U.S.). (**C**) St. Jude Medical® (Copyright St. Jude Medical, Inc., St. Paul, Minnesota, U.S.). ⌐

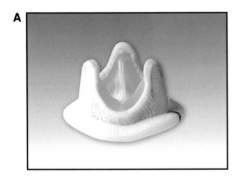

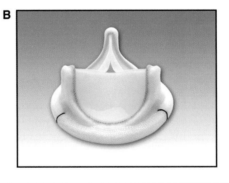

Figure 17.2 MV bioprostheses. (**A**) Carpentier–Edwards porcine. (**B**) Carpentier–Edwards Perimount™ pericardial tissue MV bioprosthesis. *Abbreviation*: MV, mitral valve. *Source*: Courtesy of Edwards Lifesciences LLC.

imaging resembling an AoV with triangular opening in the mitral position (Fig. 17.3). A functional bioprosthetic valve usually appears with thin and pliable leaflets, normal mobility, central flow, and trace or no regurgitation.

With time, biological valve leaflets and their annulus thicken and calcify, causing decreased mobility. Stenosis, regurgitation, or a combination of both, could then occur (Fig. 17.4). These can be demonstrated by 2D imaging, color Doppler imaging, and increased diastolic pressure gradient with continuous wave (CW) Doppler.

TRANSPROSTHETIC GRADIENT

All mechanical or tissue prosthetic valves are hemodynamically restrictive compared with a normal native valve. This is reflected by the transprosthetic gradient, which is routinely measured with CW Doppler across the prosthetic mitral valve (MV) during diastole. On color Doppler imaging, normal flow through tissue valves appears central; in ball-in-cage mechanical prostheses, it symmetrically curves around the ball, while in tilting disc prostheses, color flow is seen through the three orifices. 2D and

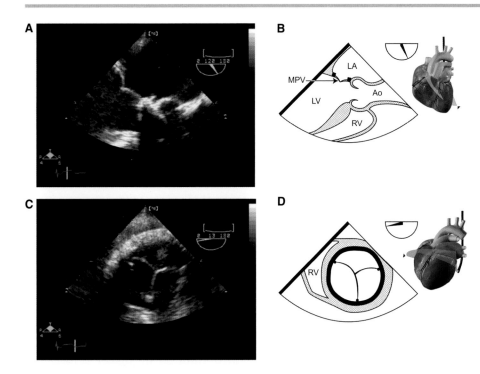

Figure 17.3 MV bioprostheses. (**A,B**) Mid-esophageal long-axis view shows the normal thickness and motion of MV bioprosthesis leaflets. (**C,D**) Transgastric view shows the three struts and three leaflets "en face" of the PMV. *Abbreviations*: Ao, aorta; LA, left atrium; LV, left ventricle; MV, mitral valve; PMV, prosthetic mitral valve; RV, right ventricle.

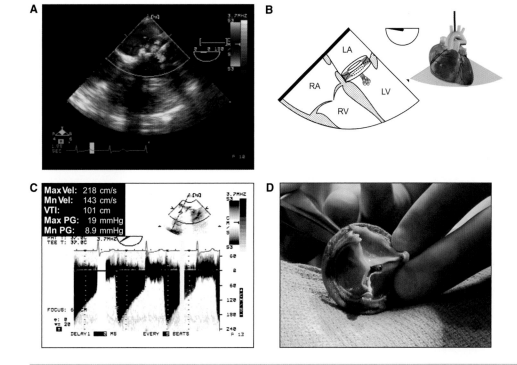

Figure 17.4 MV bioprostheses. A 79-year-old woman is undergoing reoperation for bioprosthetic MV stenosis and regurgitation. (**A,B**) Color Doppler mid-esophageal four-chamber view shows the mitral regurgitant jet and acceleration through the orifice. (**C**) An 8.9 mmHg mean PG is measured with continuous wave Doppler of transmitral flow. (**D**) Intraoperative examination of the failed MV bioprosthesis revealed severe stenosis. *Abbreviations*: LA, left atrium; LV, left ventricle; Max, maximum; Mn, mean; PG, pressure gradient; RA, right atrium; RV, right ventricle; Vel, velocity; VTI, velocity-time integral. *Source*: Photo D courtesy of Dr. Michel Pellerin.

color Doppler imaging are used to guide positioning of the CW Doppler cursor to ensure optimal alignment of the ultrasound beam with jet direction. The peak gradient is determined from the maximal Doppler flow velocity using the simplified Bernoulli equation $P = 4v^2$, where P is the pressure in mmHg and v is the velocity in m/s. As for the native MV, the mean transprosthetic gradient is obtained by tracing the diastolic CW Doppler signal (Fig. 17.5) that calculates the mean of the squared instantaneous velocities. Measurement of mean gradient is more important because it represents the gradient between the left atrium (LA) and the left ventricle (LV) throughout diastole.

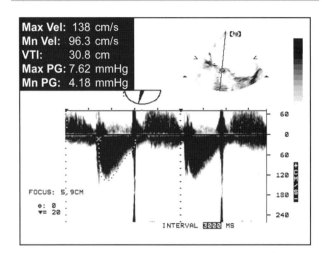

Figure 17.5 Transvalvular prosthetic PG. Measurement of the diastolic transvalvular PG with continuous-wave Doppler of transmitral flow in a functional mechanical bileaflet St. Jude PMV is shown. *Abbreviations*: Max, maximum; Mn, mean; PMV, prosthetic mitral valve; PG, pressure gradient; Vel, velocity; VTI, velocity-time integral.

The gradient evaluation must take into account the prosthetic valve type and size, as well as the heart rate and cardiac output. In the adult population, the mitral transprosthetic gradient is, however, generally less dependent on the sewing ring size than for aortic prostheses. In the mitral position at normal heart rates, the normal mean diastolic gradient of mechanical valves is 4 to 6 mmHg, and for bioprostheses, it is 3 to 5 mmHg. As with native valves, the gradient is increased with tachycardia.

Pressure recovery may also be associated with an increased gradient without intrinsic dysfunction. This is more commonly seen with AoV prostheses but can occasionally occur with mitral mechanical prostheses (5). When flow must pass through a narrowed orifice, a prosthetic orifice in this case, pressure (potential energy) is transformed into kinetic energy (i.e., velocity) then back to potential energy with some loss in the form of heat, which represents the pressure loss or gradient due to the narrowed orifice. Pressure recovery refers to the phenomenon where a certain degree of kinetic energy could return to pressure energy (see Fig. 14.18). Blood flow through the prosthesis accelerates more in the minor than in the major orifices.

Doppler gradient estimation is dependent on the maximal velocity of red blood cells, which is found at the vena contracta. Generally, when measuring the transprosthetic pressure gradient, the CW Doppler cursor is positioned through the major orifice, but inadvertent measurement through a minor orifice could result in overestimation of the true hemodynamic gradient, particularly in the smaller central slit-like minor orifice of a bileaflet mechanical prosthesis (Figs. 17.6 and 17.7) (5).

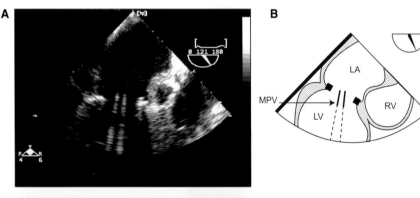

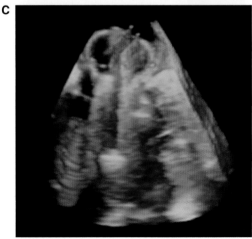

Figure 17.6 Mechanical bileaflet PMV. (A,B) Mid-esophageal long-axis view shows the normal open position of the two hemidiscs of a mechanical bileaflet St. Jude PMV. **(C)** 3D view of the mechanical bileaflet PMV in diastole from a LA orientation. *Abbreviations*: LA, left atrium; LV, left ventricle; PMV, prosthetic mitral valve; RV, right ventricle.

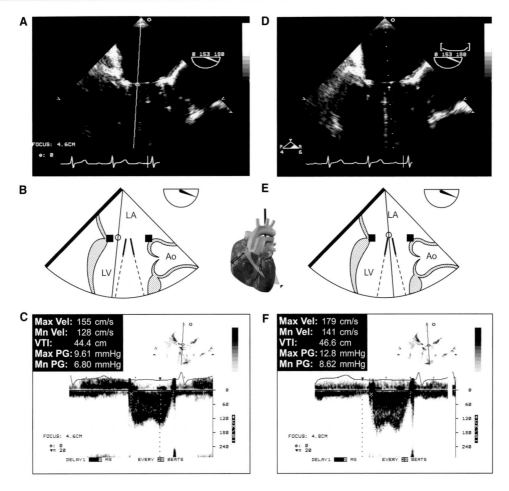

Figure 17.7 **Mechanical bileaflet PMV.** **(A,D)** Mid-esophageal long-axis views of a patient show a normal mechanical bileaflet PMV. **(C,F)** Continuous wave Doppler tracings through the prosthesis. **(C)** A 6.8 mmHg mean PG is measured when the continuous wave Doppler cursor is positioned through the lateral, major orifice **(A,B)**. In **(F)**, with the cursor sampling velocities through the central minor orifice **(D,E)**, a higher PG of 8.6 mm Hg is measured because of blood flow acceleration through this smaller slit orifice. *Abbreviations*: Ao, aorta; LA, left atrium; LV, left ventricle; Max, maximum; Mn, mean; PG, pressure gradient; PMV, prosthetic mitral valve; Vel, velocity; VTI, velocity-time integral.

PROSTHETIC VALVE AREA

Manufacturers often report prosthetic valve areas based on the anatomic inner diameter of the sewing ring or on in vitro hemodynamic data. One should be aware that these areas do not necessarily reflect the true in vivo effective orifice area of the valve, which is usually smaller. The prosthesis number usually represents the external diameter of the sewing ring (Fig. 17.1C), and the surgeon will generally try to implant the largest prosthesis for a given individual.

The pressure half-time (PHT) represents the time necessary for the maximal transvalvular gradient to reach half of its initial value during LV diastolic filling (Fig. 17.8). The PHT is equal to 0.29 × deceleration time (DT). The mitral valve area (MVA), given by the formula MVA = PHT/220, has been validated for the native MV in the absence of significant aortic regurgitation (AR) or LV dysfunction. Unfortunately, this formula has not been validated for prosthetic valves and cannot be used to estimate their effective orifice area. Nevertheless, serial measurements of the PHT in prosthetic valves is useful in detecting valvular dysfunction prospectively, as it is usually <120 ms and will increase in cases of prosthesis obstruction or thrombosis.

In the absence of significant (moderate or severe) AR or mitral regurgitation (MR), effective prosthetic MVA is calculated using the continuity equation:

$$MVA = \frac{SV_{LVOT}}{VTI_{MV}} \quad (17.1)$$

where SV_{LVOT} is the aortic stroke volume, equal to LVOT surface area × LVOT VTI (velocity-time integral), and VTI_{MV} is mitral valve diastolic velocity-time integral. These measurements are easily performed with transthoracic echocardiography (TTE) and transesophageal echocardiography (TEE). However, the measurement of LVOT VTI by TEE is occasionally technically challenging because suboptimal

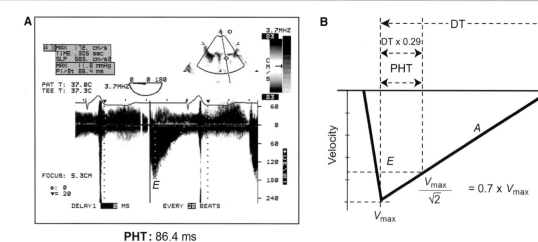

PHT: 86.4 ms

Figure 17.8 Pressure half-time. (**A**) Measurement by continuous wave Doppler of the PHT in a functional mechanical bileaflet St. Jude PMV. (**B**) The PHT corresponds to the time required for the pressure gradient to drop by half. The corresponding velocities are obtained through the simplified Bernoulli's equation. *Abbreviations*: A, peak late diastolic TMF velocity; E, peak early diastolic TMF velocity; PMV, mitral prosthetic valve; PHT, pressure half-time; Vm, mean velocity; Vmax, maximal velocity; VT1/2, velocity half-time.

transgastric windows may prevent adequate alignment of the pulsed wave (PW) Doppler with the direction of flow in the LVOT. Normal prosthetic MVAs range between 1.5 and 2.5 cm^2 (3,6).

PROSTHETIC REGURGITATION

A CW Doppler sweep of the MV prosthesis could demonstrate the presence of MR, and a strong, dense regurgitant signal suggests a more severe degree of regurgitation. However, the evaluation of transvalvular and/or periprosthetic MR is better accomplished with color Doppler imaging. The sensitivity of this modality for detecting MR is rather low with transthoracic studies because the regurgitant jets are hidden by the acoustic shadowing from the prosthetic material. A normal, or increased, mean transprosthetic pressure gradient with a large increase in maximal pressure gradient (peak pressure gradient to mean pressure gradient ratio $\geq$ 3:1), with a normal or decreased PHT, can be a clue to the presence of significant MR. Transesophageal echocardiography is ideally positioned to view regurgitant jets and has a near 100% sensitivity for MR detection as long as a systematic and meticulous evaluation is performed (7).

Prosthetic regurgitation can be divided into either "intraprosthetic" or "transprosthetic" and "paraprosthetic" or "periprosthetic." While the latter is always pathological, the former can be further divided into functional or pathological. Normally functioning prosthetic valves, particularly mechanical, have a closing volume, which is a small and short regurgitant color flow Doppler signal visible in early systole. This corresponds to the small volume of blood displaced by the occluder as it moves in closed position and does not represent true regurgitation per se.

Bioprosthetic valves (Fig. 17.3) have no, or very little, intrinsic regurgitation. Ball-in-cage models should

not have regurgitant jets, whereas tilting-disk and bileaflet valves normally have an intrinsic intraprosthetic regurgitation of a small quantity (~5–15 mL/beat), which does not represent prosthetic dysfunction. Moreover, these normal intrinsic regurgitant jets have a functional antithrombotic effect, "washing out" the prosthesis occluder edges with each systole. The specific design of each mechanical disc prosthesis shows characteristic signature intrinsic regurgitant transvalvular jets on color flow imaging. For instance, in bileaflet valves, the jets will form a converging pattern in the plane parallel to the central slit orifice as well as a diverging pattern in the plane perpendicular to it, at the periphery between discs and ring, particularly at the hinge points (Fig. 17.9) (3). The central orifice of the Medtronic Hall disc, through which it slides on the central strut, also explains its typical central regurgitant jet in addition to the jets at the periphery of the disc. Dysfunctional MR will be discussed in the following section.

MULTIPLANE TEE EVALUATION

Preoperative and immediate postoperative [pre- and post–cardiopulmonary bypass (CPB) pump] TEE evaluations require a systematic approach (7). The echocardiographic examination includes the evaluation of other (native or prosthetic) valves as well as LV size and global and regional function. Evaluation of prosthetic valve structure and function involves a full 2D imaging sweep, followed by color Doppler imaging and CW Doppler across the prosthesis and PW Doppler examination of the pulmonary veins.

2D Evaluation

Transesophageal echocardiography is the ideal tool for evaluating mitral prostheses. Rotation of the imaging angle (0–180°) at the mid-esophageal level allows

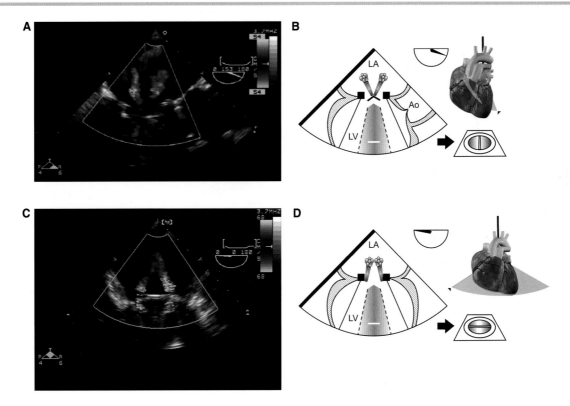

Figure 17.9 Mechanical bileaflet PMV. Color Doppler mid-esophageal long-axis and four-chamber views showing the normal signature of the diverging (**A,B**) and converging (**C,D**) regurgitant jets of a mechanical bileaflet St. Jude PMV. The diverging jets are seen when the view is perpendicular to the axis of the central slit orifice. *Abbreviations*: Ao, aorta; LA, left atrium; LV, left ventricle; PMV, prosthetic mitral valve.

identification of the optimal 2D imaging plane to observe the full motion of prosthetic valve occluders (leaflets, discs, or ball according to type). Machine settings are adjusted to optimize the image. Adequate depth is selected to visualize the prosthesis and surrounding structures to a maximum. Keeping the prosthesis in the center of the imaging display, systematic slow sweeps from one side of the sewing ring to the opposite in orthogonal views are important to detect abnormal structures or flows not present in the middle of the prosthesis. The transgastric view must also be used to complete the evaluation of the ventricular side of the prosthesis and permit visualization and evaluation of the subvalvular apparatus and the LV, which is obscured by the prosthetic material in the mid-esophageal level.

During 2D examination, a keen eye looks for reduced occluder excursion, leaflet sticking, pannus, valve rocking, abscess, foreign bodies such as thrombus or vegetation, and, particularly in the immediate post-CPB period, retained mitral valvular apparatus that could impede the free movement of the mobile components of the prosthetic valve.

During normal function, mitral bileaflet prostheses open and close symmetrically and generally in synchrony (Fig. 17.6). The poppet in the ball-in-cage prosthesis should have full to-and-fro excursion within the cage (Fig. 17.10) and not remain held in either the open or closed position. However, asyn-

chronous or incomplete movement of the occluder can be seen in the absence of prosthetic dysfunction in certain cases, for example, irregular heart rhythm (atrial fibrillation, multiple extrasystole, or ventricular pacing). In the immediate/early post-CPB period, abnormal movement of the prosthesis occluder could be present and disappear just a few minutes after reestablishing normal circulation and LV function.

The identification of abnormal movement of the prosthesis occluder in the early post-CPB period in the operating room (OR) warrants immediate surgical reassessment and correction. This may sometimes simply consist of rotating the prosthesis within the sewing ring or resecting some "excess" subvalvular tissue (Figs. 17.11 and 17.12). This may prevent a late second look, which represents a high-risk early reoperation.

Reduced excursion of the mobile components could be due to the presence of foreign bodies such as thrombus or vegetation, interfering excess subvalvular apparatus, abnormal tissue growth (pannus), or intrinsic prosthetic valve failure. Sometimes, the cause of dysfunction may not be readily obvious as with thrombus at the prosthetic hinge points. The only clue to prosthetic dysfunction may simply be abnormal disc motion or increased transvalvular gradient. It is also important to remember that these abnormalities may be present intermittently necessitating prolonged careful 2D imaging.

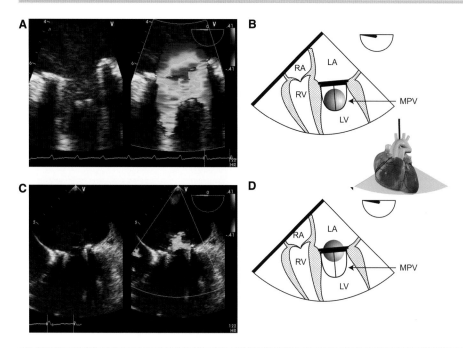

Figure 17.10 Starr-Edwards ball-in-cage prosthesis. Color compare mid-esophageal four-chamber views show a normal Starr-Edwards ball-in-cage prosthesis in diastole (**A,B**) and in systole (**C,D**) in the mitral position. *Abbreviations*: LA, left atrium; LV, left ventricle; PMV, prosthetic mitral valve; RA, right atrium; RV, right ventricle.

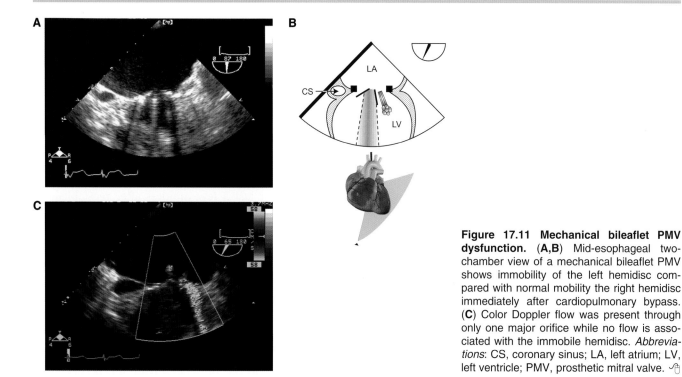

Figure 17.11 Mechanical bileaflet PMV dysfunction. (**A,B**) Mid-esophageal two-chamber view of a mechanical bileaflet PMV shows immobility of the left hemidisc compared with normal mobility the right hemidisc immediately after cardiopulmonary bypass. (**C**) Color Doppler flow was present through only one major orifice while no flow is associated with the immobile hemidisc. *Abbreviations*: CS, coronary sinus; LA, left atrium; LV, left ventricle; PMV, prosthetic mitral valve.

Thrombus (Figs. 17.13 and 17.14) and vegetation (Fig. 17.15) generally appear as echo-dense irregular masses attached to a leaflet, the disc, or to the sewing ring of the prosthesis. Their mobility and size are variable. These masses could be highly mobile and attached to the wall by a pedicle or fixed with a large base. Size could vary between a few millimeters to many centimeters in diameter. Masses could interfere with prosthetic function by causing obstruction, regurgitation, or a combination of both (Fig. 17.15).

Thrombus and vegetation can be very difficult to differentiate echocardiographically from one another. Certain clues within the clinical context may help to sort them out. The coexistence of spontaneous echo

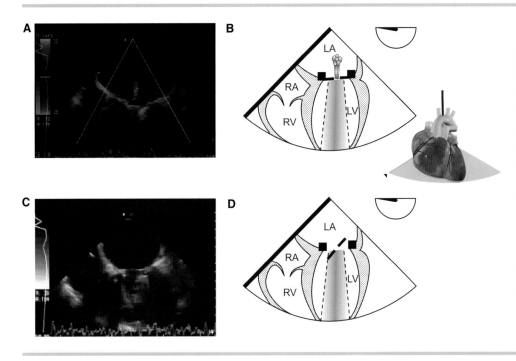

Figure 17.12 Mechanical tilting disk PMV dysfunction. Severe pulmonary hypertension was noted during weaning from CPB in a patient undergoing MV replacement with a tilting disk prosthesis. (**A,B**) The PMV was fixed in a closed position and only blood flowing through the central disk orifice could be seen both in systole and diastole. (**C,D**) CPB was reinstituted immediately and after rotation of the PMV normal motion was seen. *Abbreviations*: CPB, cardiopulmonary bypass; LA, left atrium; LV, left ventricle; MV, mitral valve; PMV, prosthetic mitral valve; RA, right atrium; RV, right ventricle. *Source*: Courtesy of Dr. Jocelyne Maucotel.

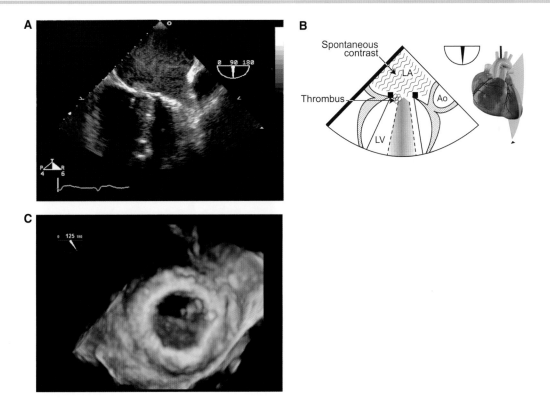

Figure 17.13 Thrombosed mechanical bileaflet PMV. (**A,B**) Mid-esophageal two-chamber view shows a thrombus protruding through one of the hemidiscs of a mechanical bileaflet PMV during diastole. Spontaneous echo contrast due to stasis is noted in the LA. (**C**) Full volume 3D transesophageal view of a thrombosed mechanical bileaflet PMV seen from the LA. *Abbreviations*: Ao, aorta; LA, left atrium; LV, left ventricle; PMV, prosthetic mitral valve.

contrast, atrial fibrillation, a significantly dilated LA with subtherapeutic anticoagulation are more commonly associated with thrombus. Conversely, fever, weight loss, positive blood cultures, and/or the iden-

tification of an abscess or a fistula make the diagnosis of vegetations more likely.

Abscesses are typically found at the level of the sewing ring, appearing as an echo-lucent area of

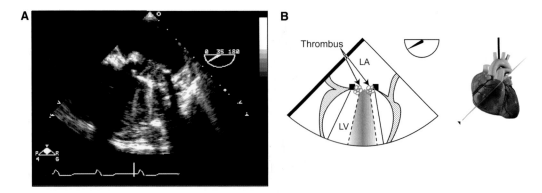

Figure 17.14   Thrombosed mechanical bileaflet PMV. (A,B) Mid-esophageal 35° view shows extensive thrombosis of a mechanical bileaflet PMV, with decreased mobility of the hemidiscs. This patient was deemed a poor candidate for reoperation because of concomitant severe LV dysfunction. The administration of an intravenous thrombolytic agent resulted in the disappearance of the thrombus and the patient recovered uneventfully. *Abbreviations*: LA, left atrium; LV, left ventricle; PMV, prosthetic mitral valve.

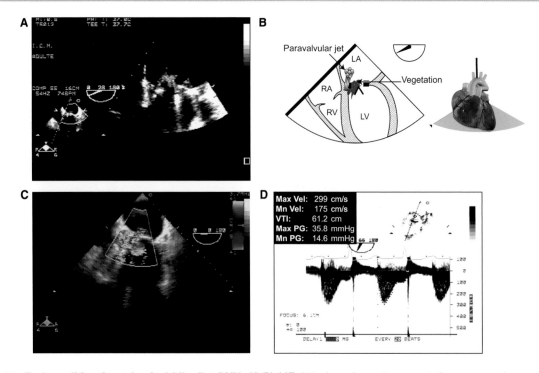

Figure 17.15   Endocarditis of mechanical bileaflet PMV. (A,B) ME 28° view shows two vegetations, a very large medial and a smaller lateral one, protruding through the orifices of a mechanical bileaflet PMV during both diastole and systole. **(C)** In the color Doppler ME four-chamber view, an associated color jet directed from the LV to the LA during systole is consistent with a ruptured abscess and perivalvular fistula secondary to an infectious process. **(D)** Continuous wave Doppler across the PMV demonstrates an increased transprosthetic PG due to the large obstructive vegetation. *Abbreviations*: LA, left atrium; LV, left ventricle; Max, maximum; ME, mid-esophageal; Mn, mean; PG, pressure gradient; PMV, prosthetic mitral valve; RA, right atrium; RV, right ventricle; Vel, velocity; VTI, velocity-time integral.

variable dimension. To-and-fro flow within the abscess (Fig. 17.15) or periprosthetic regurgitation with annular dehiscence (Fig. 17.16) can be visualized. Spontaneous rupture of abscess may lead to perivalvular fistulae between various cardiac chambers. During all phases of the cardiac cycle, a normal prosthetic valve should move en bloc with the base of the ventricle to

which it is sutured. Rocking represents abnormally exaggerated or independent motion of part of the sewing ring due to its dehiscence. Although rupture of a suture due to degenerescence could be the cause, endocarditis and abscess should be ruled out.

The leaflets of a normal bioprosthesis are thin and pliable. Thickening and calcification of the leaflets

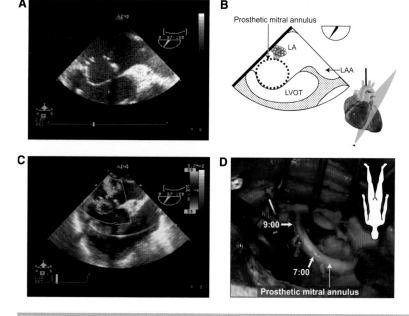

Figure 17.16 Dehiscence of a MAR. (A,B) Mid-esophageal view at 57° is shown from a 55-year-old man undergoing reoperation for dehiscence of a MAR. **(C)** Severe para-annular mitral regurgitation is present on color Doppler imaging of the same view. **(D)** The intraoperative findings confirmed the 7–9 o'clock dehiscence (arrows). *Abbreviations*: LA, left atrium; LAA, left atrial appendage; LVOT, left ventricular outflow tract; MAR, mitral annular ring. *Source*: Photo D courtesy of Dr. Michel Pellerin.

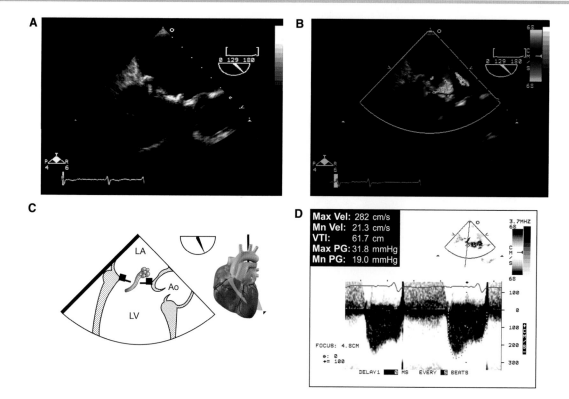

Figure 17.17 Degenerative bioprosthetic MV. (A–C) Mid-esophageal long-axis views of a dysfunctional MV bioprosthesis with thickened and calcified leaflets results in reduced mobility and an eccentric MR jet. **(D)** The continuous wave Doppler demonstrates a very high mean diastolic PG of 19 mmHg through the dysfunctional MV bioprosthesis. *Abbreviations*: Ao, aorta; LA, left atrium; LV, left ventricle; Max, maximum; Mn, mean; MR, mitral regurgitation; MV, mitral valve; PG, pressure gradient; VTI, velocity-time integral; Vel, velocity.

or the annulus can be demonstrated by 2D imaging. These degenerative changes decrease the mobility of the leaflets or may lead to fracture and tears of the cusps, with resulting stenosis and/or regurgitation detectable by color-flow imaging and CW Doppler (Fig. 17.17). Degenerative changes can also be seen in the cloth-covered model of the Starr–Edwards prosthesis (Figs. 17.18–17.20).

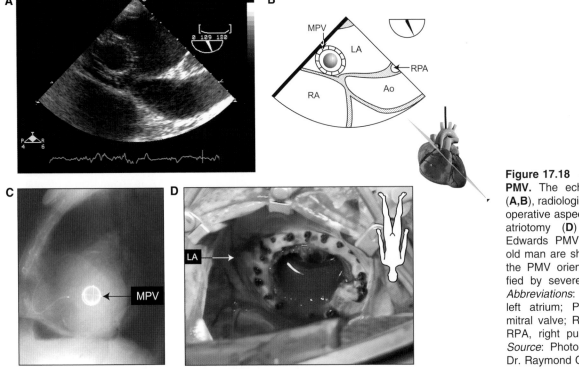

Figure 17.18 Starr–Edwards PMV. The echocardiographic (**A,B**), radiologic (**C**), and intraoperative aspect through a left atriotomy (**D**) of a Starr–Edwards PMV in a 59-year-old man are shown. Note that the PMV orientation is modified by severe LA dilatation. *Abbreviations*: Ao, aorta; LA, left atrium; PMV, prosthetic mitral valve; RA, right atrium; RPA, right pulmonary artery. *Source*: Photo D courtesy of Dr. Raymond Cartier.

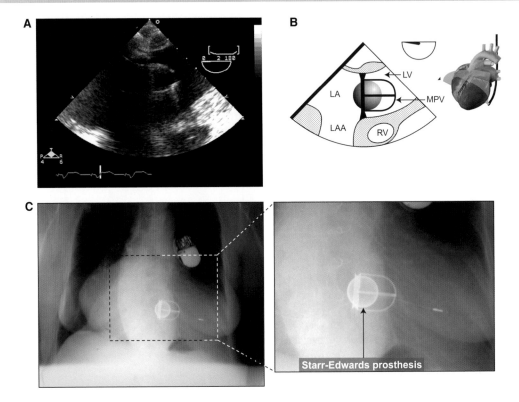

Figure 17.19 Starr–Edwards PMV. A 59-year-old man with a Starr–Edwards mechanical PMV is shown. (**A,B**) The transgastric 0° view is altered secondary to the atrial dilatation. (**C**) Note the similar position of the prosthesis on the chest X-ray. *Abbreviations*: LA, left atrium; LAA, left atrial appendage; LV, left ventricle; PMV, prosthetic mitral valve; RV, right ventricle.

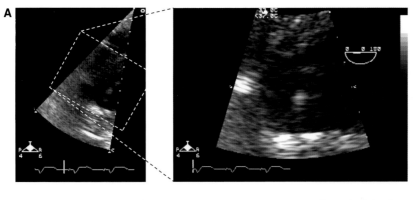

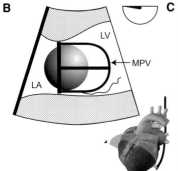

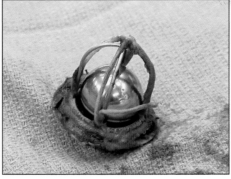

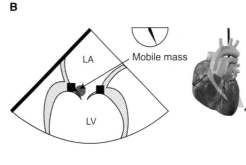

Figure 17.20 Starr–Edwards PMV dysfunction. (A,B) A 59-year-old man with a Starr–Edwards mechanical PMV shows mobile material in the transgastric view. **(C)** The sheath over the prosthesis struts, which was a feature of the cloth-covered model 6310, is broken. *Abbreviations*: LA, left atrium; LV, left ventricle; MV, mitral valve; PMV, prosthetic mitral valve. *Source*: Photo C courtesy of Dr. Raymond Cartier.

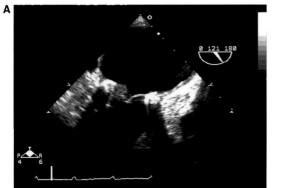

Figure 17.21 Mass on bioprosthetic MV. (A,B) Mid-esophageal long-axis view shows a mobile mass attached to the posterior aspect of the sewing ring of a MV bioprosthesis. This mass could represent a thrombus or vegetation. *Abbreviations*: LA, left atrium; LV, left ventricle; MV, mitral valve.

The presence of thrombus on a bioprosthetic valve is much less common than with mechanical valves but can sometimes be seen (Fig. 17.21). Valve degeneration or endocarditis may cause ring dehiscence and rocking with periprosthetic regurgitation. Endocarditis can also cause leaflet destruction and perforation with significant regurgitation.

Transvalvular Prosthetic Regurgitation

During TEE imaging, one must resist the urge to turn on the color flow imaging mode too early without

having properly performed a thorough 2D examination of all parts of the prosthesis. Similarly, during color flow imaging, the operator should not hesitate to turn off the color when a flow abnormality is found, to understand its underlying anatomical basis.

Thrombus, vegetation, abnormal tissue growth (pannus), interfering residual subvalvular apparatus, and intrinsic prosthetic valve failure (Fig. 17.22) could all be responsible for dysfunctional prosthetic regurgitation. This type of regurgitation will usually be transvalvular or intraprosthetic, meaning that the regurgitation originates from within the prosthetic

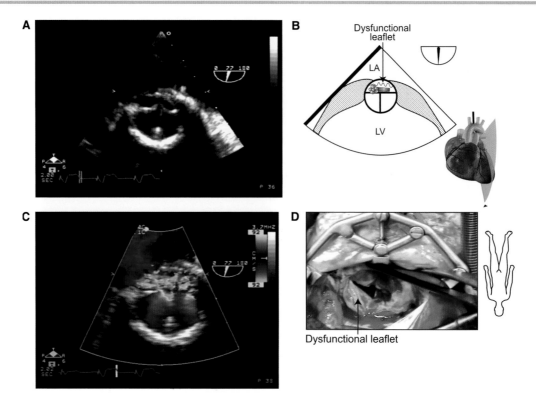

Figure 17.22 **Dysfunctional bioprosthetic MV. (A,B)** Mid-esophageal two-chamber view and **(C)** color flow imaging with severe mitral regurgitation due to a torn leaflet. **(D)** Corresponding intra-operative view. *Abbreviations*: LA, left atrium; LV, left ventricle; MV, mitral valve. Source: Photo D courtesy of Dr. Raymond Cartier.

sewing ring, due to incomplete closure of one of the mobile components (Figs. 17.17 and 17.22). Intraprosthetic dysfunctional regurgitation is uncommon in the immediate postoperative period. When present with a mechanical prosthesis, it is generally associated with abnormal disc closure due to interfering residual subvalvular tissue or apparatus. This can often be immediately corrected by rotating the valve within the sewing ring. Early postoperative bioprosthetic valve regurgitation could arise from suture misplacement or improper sizing. In rare cases, an intrinsic bioprosthetic manufacturing problem could be responsible.

As mentioned previously, normal prosthetic valves may present a mild degree of intraprosthetic functional regurgitation characteristic of their valve design. On the other hand, pathological intraprosthetic regurgitation will generally be ≥2/4, or moderate to severe, and could result from any of the abnormalities discussed earlier. It originates within the prosthetic ring but could sometimes be difficult to differentiate from periprosthetic regurgitation. Complete 2D and color Doppler imaging examination from one side of the sewing ring to the other in orthogonal planes will generally allow the localization of the origin of the jet and its cause. Indeed, careful observation of the location of the origin of the jet, the vena contracta, and the proximal flow convergence in reference to the prosthetic ring will help to identify the type of regurgitation (i.e., intraprosthetic vs.

periprosthetic). The severity of regurgitation is graded as for native valves (8).

Periprosthetic Regurgitation

Periprosthetic regurgitation is a common cause of reoperation for prosthetic valve dysfunction. It is a dysfunctional regurgitant jet occurring outside the prosthetic sewing ring as a result of a degenerative process or endocarditis. Occasionally, significant perivalvular regurgitation can be found at surgical closure in the OR.

One of the major indications and advantages of perioperative TEE is the identification of the presence, severity, and location of periprosthetic regurgitation to guide surgical intervention before CPB, or to reduce the morbidity associated with this condition by allowing immediate diagnosis and correction after CPB, thus avoiding unnecessary reoperation.

The severity of perivalvular regurgitation is highly variable, ranging from a tiny suture leak to severe regurgitation associated with partial dehiscence. The identification and quantification of periprosthetic regurgitation requires a careful and systematic TEE evaluation. As mentioned above for intraprosthetic regurgitant jets, periprosthetic regurgitant jets should be sought with a thorough 2D and color-flow imaging examinations not only limited to a tomographical view through the middle of the prosthesis, but starting from the outside of one flank to the opposite aspect of the sewing ring. This should be done in at least two orthogonal views, but other angles better adapted to the examination of suspicious findings can be used. Moreover, this inspection at the plane of the valve should be complemented by a similar sweep above and below the prosthesis level to improve the detection of perivalvular regurgitant jets or rocking of the sewing ring.

Localization of regurgitation can be reported in reference to neighboring anatomical landmarks, such as the atrial septum, the AoV, or the left atrial appendage (LAA). Others prefer to report jets following the polar coordinate system of a time-clock in reference to the surgeon's view (Figs. 17.23–17.27): at 0°, the left side of the display with the LA up or the side near the atrial septum corresponds to 12:00 on the clock; at 90°, the left side of the screen with the LA up corresponds to 03:00; and at 150°, the left side of the screen (opposite the AoV) corresponds to 05:00 and the AoV to 11:00; the LAA corresponds to 7:00–9:00. For example, a periprosthetic leak extending between 0°, atrial septal side (i.e., left side of the imaging screen with LA up), and 60°, opposite the LAA, at the left side of the screen corresponds to a regurgitation between 12:00 and 02:00 on the surgical field.

In transgastric views at 0°, the TEE probe could be angled to achieve a short-axis ("en-face") view (Fig. 17.28) of the MV prosthesis. The site and extent of regurgitation can also be evaluated from this level by flexing the probe and slightly advancing or withdrawing the shaft.

The severity of MR is graded as for native valves and based on the integrated evaluation of the regurgitant jet color Doppler surface area, the pulmonary venous systolic flow component on PW Doppler and the proximal flow convergence area (8). Several caveats must however be kept in mind: periprosthetic regurgitant jets often hug the LA wall (Coanda effect) and the jet area generally appears smaller than with central regurgitation. The quantification of periprosthetic MR by the proximal isovelocity surface area (PISA) method can also be used but has not been as well validated as for native valves. Finally, the severity of immediate post-CPB MR could be underestimated with color-flow imaging (see section "TEE Evaluation after MV Repair," p. 449).

Gradient Evaluation

An abnormal increase in transprosthetic gradient (Figs. 17.15 and 17.17) can be secondary to incomplete opening of the mobile components, most often due to thrombus, pannus, or calcific degeneration, but can also result from the increased flow due to significant regurgitation. The measurement of DT or PHT can prove very useful in distinguishing incomplete opening from high flow. The DT and PHT will be prolonged with increased gradients due to thrombosis or degeneration, whereas they will be within normal limits or reduced with severe regurgitation. The transvalvular diastolic gradient should be measured in the immediate

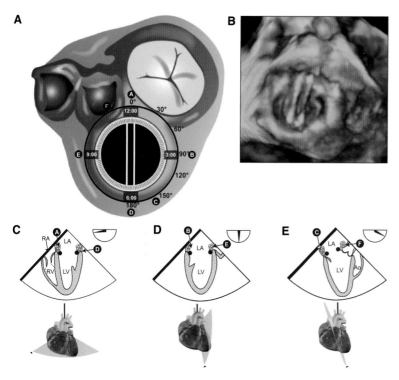

Figure 17.23 Localization of the paravalvular leaks of the MV prosthesis. (**A**) Schematic of surgeon's view of the MV prosthesis during systole is compared with a 3D transesophageal echocardiographic image (**B**) during diastole. (**C–E**) Three different 2D mid-esophageal views can be used to localize the paravalvular leaks. Note that the angle may vary ±15°. *Abbreviations*: LA, left atrium; LV, left ventricle; MV, mitral valve; RA, right atrium; RV, right ventricle.

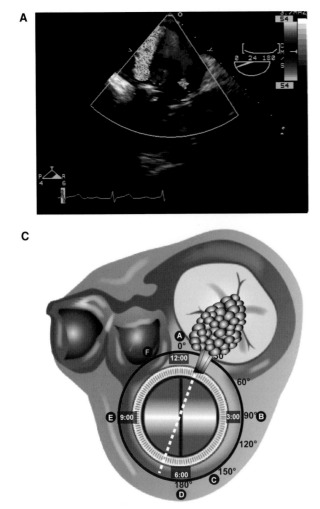

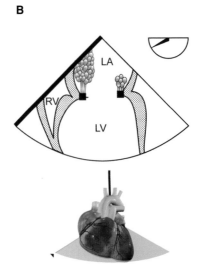

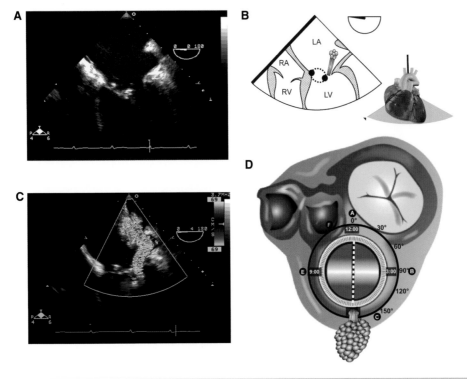

Figure 17.24 Periprosthetic MV regurgitation. (A,B) Color Doppler mid-esophageal view shows periprosthetic regurgitation passing outside the sewing ring as well as transvalvular prosthetic functional converging regurgitant jets in a mechanical bileaflet PMV. **(C)** Periprosthetic leak shown here corresponds to 01:00 in the surgeon's view. *Abbreviations*: LA, left atrium; LV, left ventricle; MV, mitral valve; PMV, prosthetic mitral valve; RV, right ventricle.

Figure 17.25 Periprosthetic MV regurgitation. (A,B) Mid-esophageal four-chamber view shows annular dehiscence; the annular ring has moved in an apical direction away from the atrioventricular groove. **(C)** Color Doppler of this view shows the mitral regurgitant jet lateral to the annular ring. **(D)** The location of periprosthetic regurgitation jet corresponds to 6:00 in the surgeon's view. *Abbreviations*: LA, left atrium; LV, left ventricle; MV, mitral valve; RA, right atrium; RV, right ventricle.

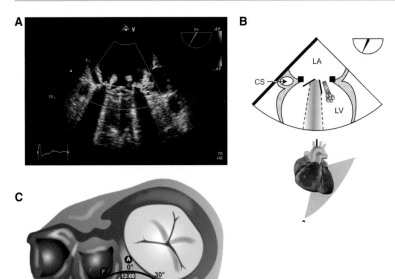

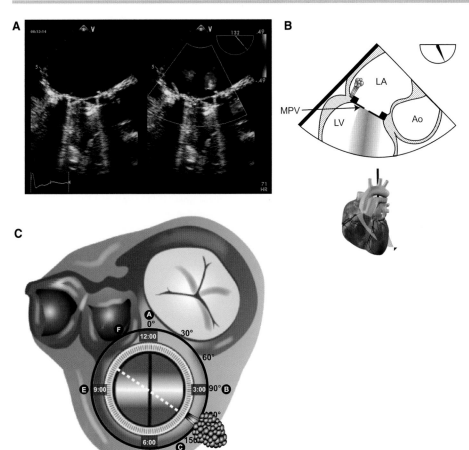

Figure 17.26 Periprosthetic MV regurgitation. (A,B) Color Doppler mid-esophageal two-chamber view shows two jets of periprosthetic regurgitation passing outside the sewing ring as well as transvalvular prosthetic functional converging regurgitant jets in this mechanical bileaflet PMV. **(C)** Periprosthetic leak shown here corresponds to 2:00 and 8:00 in the surgeon's view. *Abbreviations*: CS, coronary sinus; LA, left atrium; LV, left ventricle; MV, mitral valve; PMV, prosthetic mitral valve.

Figure 17.27 Periprosthetic MV regurgitation. (A,B) Color Doppler mid-esophageal long-axis view shows a small periprosthetic regurgitant jet passing outside the sewing ring in this mechanical bileaflet PMV. **(C)** This corresponds to 4:00 in the surgeon's view. *Abbreviations*: Ao, aorta; LA, left atrium; LV, left ventricle; MV, mitral valve; PMV, prosthetic mitral valve.

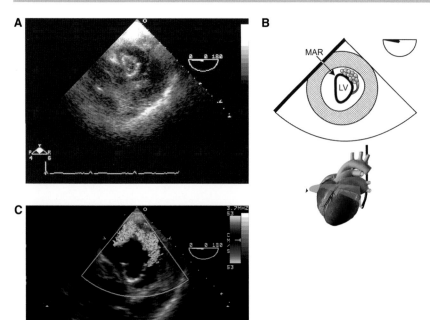

Figure 17.28 Periprosthetic MV regurgitation. (**A–C**) Transgastric basal short-axis views show dehiscence of a MAR with severe posterior periannular mitral regurgitation by color Doppler (**C**). The regurgitant jet appears clearly outside, lateral to, the MAR. *Abbreviations*: LV, left ventricle; MAR, mitral annuloplasty ring; MV, mitral valve.

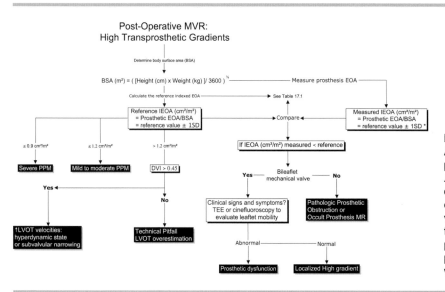

Figure 17.29 Transprosthetic gradient. Algorithm for the interpretation of high transprosthetic gradient after MVR is presented. *Abbreviations*: BSA, body surface area; DVI, dimensionless velocity index; EOA, effective orifice area; IEOA, indexed EOA; LVOT, left ventricular outflow tract; MR, mitral regurgitation; MVR, mitral valve replacement; PPM, patient-prosthesis mismatch; TEE, transesophageal echocardiography. *Source*: Adapted with permission from Ref. 16.

post-CPB period to serve as baseline hemodynamics for future comparison and detection of prosthetic dysfunction. An approach to the evaluation of increased transprosthetic gradient is shown in Figure 17.29 (9).

Patient-Prosthesis Mismatch

Patient-prosthesis mismatch (PPM) and its impact on morbidity and mortality for the AoV have been exten-

sively studied. For patients with MV replacement, however, the concept of PPM remains controversial and its consequences on morbidity and mortality are unclear. Initially described in the late 1970s by Rahimtoola and Murphy (10), interest in MV replacement, PPM, and its clinical impact has increased over the past few years. Many authors have tried to standardize the definition of PPM, but conflicts remain whether to use in vivo hemodynamic calculation of

Table 17.1 Normal Reference Values of Effective Orifice Areas for Mitral Prostheses

Prosthetic valve size (mm)	25	27	29	31	33
Stented bioprostheses					
Medtronic Mosaic	1.5 ± 0.4	1.7 ± 0.5	1.9 ± 0.5	1.9 ± 0.5	
Hancock II	1.5 ± 0.4	1.8 ± 0.5	1.9 ± 0.5	2.6 ± 0.5	2.6 ± 0.7
Carpentier–Edwards Perimount[a]	1.6 ± 0.4	1.8 ± 0.4	2.1 ± 0.5		
Mechanical prostheses					
St. Jude Medical Toronto SPV	1.5 ± 0.3	1.7 ± 0.4	1.8 ± 0.4	2.0 ± 0.5	2.0 ± 0.5
On-X®	2.2 ± 0.9	2.2 ± 0.9	2.2 ± 0.9	2.2 ± 0.9	2.2 ± 0.9

[a]These results are based on a limited number of patients and thus should be interpreted with caution.
[b]The strut and leaflets of the On-X® valve are identical for all sizes (25–33 mm).
Source: With permission from Ref.16.

an indexed effective orifice area rather than in vitro geometric orifice area provided by the manufacturer (11). Regardless of the absolute numerical value, PPM that mimics mitral stenosis leads, in the long run, to poorer clinical outcome. Indeed, it leads to pulmonary hypertension, recurrence of heart failure, impairment of atrioventricular remodeling, and predisposes to unwanted arrhythmias compromising cardiac output (12). Referring to criteria and values used in recent published articles, it is reasonable to assume that an IEOA (indexed effective orifice area, adjusted for body weight surface area) inferior to 1.2 cm^2/m^2 will confer higher pressure gradients through a fully functional prosthetic valve causing a mismatch between EOA and transmitral flow. The concept of MV PPM initially ignored and overlooked has an incidence higher than anticipated earlier that can reach up to 71% as stated in Li et al. (13). However, PPM seems to be lower in patients where mechanical prostheses have been implanted instead of bioprostheses and the majority of those had IEOA >1.5 cm^2/m^2 (14).

Echographic measurements utilized to determine the IEOA include PHT and the continuity equation methods. The PHT method seems to be less accurate as it tends to overestimate the EOA because it is influenced by the chronotropic and diastolic states and conditions of the heart (10).

Unfortunately, options to avoid PPM remain limited. When technically feasible, repairing and preserving the native valve should be the preferred course of action. For cases in which the valve cannot be repaired, careful selection of the prosthetic valve must be addressed prior to surgery. Selection of the highest projected IEOA prosthetic valve for a given annulus size should always be favored since occurrence of PPM could translate into higher postoperative and long-term mortality and morbidity in these patients (15) (Table 17.1).

SURGICAL INDICATIONS OF MV REPAIR AND REPLACEMENT

The American College of Cardiology (ACC) and the American Heart Association (AHA) established, in 1998 and updated in 2006, Guidelines for the Management of Patients with Valvular Heart Disease (2). The indications for MV repair and replacement are shown in Tables 17.2 and 17.3. The level of evidence is discussed in Chapter 16. Recent guidelines described

Table 17.2 Indications for Surgery in Mitral Stenosis

Class I	1.	MV surgery (repair if possible) is indicated in patients with symptomatic (NYHA functional class III–IV) moderate or severe MS[a] when (*i*) percutaneous mitral balloon valvotomy is unavailable, (*ii*) percutaneous mitral balloon valvotomy is contraindicated because of left atrial thrombus despite anticoagulation, or because concomitant moderate to severe MR is present, or (*iii*) the valve morphology is not favorable for percutaneous mitral balloon valvotomy in a patient with acceptable operative risk. (Level of Evidence: B)
	2.	Symptomatic patients with moderate to severe MS[a], who also have moderate to severe MR, should receive MV replacement, unless valve repair is possible at the time of surgery. (Level of Evidence: C)
Class IIa		MV replacement is reasonable for patients with severe MS[a], and severe pulmonary hypertension (pulmonary artery systolic pressure greater than 60) with NYHA functional class I to II symptoms who are not considered candidates for percutaneous mitral balloon valvotomy or surgical MV repair. (Level of Evidence: C)
Class IIb		MV repair may be considered for asymptomatic patients with moderate or severe MS[a] who have had recurrent embolic events while receiving adequate anticoagulation and who have valve morphology favorable for repair. (Level of Evidence: C)
Class III	1.	MV repair for MS is not indicated for patients with mild MS. (Level of Evidence: C)
	2.	Closed commissurotomy should not be performed in patients undergoing MV repair; open commissurotomy is the preferred approach. (Level of Evidence: C)

[a]See Table 16.5 for severity criteria.
Abbreviations: MR, mitral regurgitation; MV, mitral valve; MS, mitral stenosis; NYHA, New York Heart Association.
Source: Adapted from Ref. 2.

by the American Society of Echocardiography's Guidelines and Standards Committee and the Task Force on Prosthetic Valves (17) may be used to assess MV prosthetic stenosis (Table 17.4) and regurgitation (Tables 17.5 and 17.6).

Table 17.3 Indications for Mitral Valve Operation

Class I	1. MV surgery is recommended for the symptomatic patient with acute severe MR.[a] (Level of Evidence: B)
	2. MV surgery is beneficial for patients with chronic severe MR[a] and NYHA functional class II, III, or IV symptoms in the absence of severe LV dysfunction (severe LV dysfunction is defined as ejection fraction less than 0.30) and/or end-systolic dimension greater than 55 mm. (Level of Evidence: B)
	3. MV surgery is beneficial for asymptomatic patients with chronic severe MR[a] and mild to moderate LV dysfunction, ejection fraction 0.30 to 0.60, and/or end-systolic dimension greater than or equal to 40 mm. (Level of Evidence: B)
	4. MV repair is recommended over MV replacement in the majority of patients with severe chronic MR[a] who require surgery, and patients should be referred to surgical centers experienced in MV repair. (Level of Evidence: C)
Class IIa	1. MV repair is reasonable in experienced surgical centers for asymptomatic patients with chronic severe MR[a] with preserved LV function (ejection fraction greater than 0.60 and end-systolic dimension less than 40 mm) in whom the likelihood of successful repair without residual MR is greater than 90%. (Level of Evidence: B)
	2. MV surgery is reasonable for asymptomatic patients with chronic severe MR,[a] preserved LV function, and new onset of atrial fibrillation. (Level of Evidence: C)
	3. MV surgery is reasonable for asymptomatic patients with chronic severe MR,[a] preserved LV function, and pulmonary hypertension (pulmonary artery systolic pressure greater than 50 mmHg at rest or greater than 60 mmHg with exercise). (Level of Evidence: C)
	4. MV surgery is reasonable for patients with chronic severe MR[a] due to a primary abnormality of the mitral apparatus and NYHA functional class III to IV symptoms and severe LV dysfunction (ejection fraction less than 0.30 and/or end-systolic dimension greater than 55 mm) in whom MV repair is highly likely. (Level of Evidence: C)
Class IIb	MV repair may be considered for patients with chronic severe secondary MR[a] due to severe LV dysfunction (ejection fraction less than 0.30) who have persistent NYHA functional class III to IV symptoms despite optimal therapy for heart failure, including biventricular pacing. (Level of Evidence: C)
Class III	1. MV surgery is not indicated for asymptomatic patients with MR and preserved LV function (ejection fraction greater than 0.60 and end-systolic dimension less than 40 mm) in whom significant doubt about the feasibility of repair exists. (Level of Evidence: C)
	2. Isolated MV surgery is not indicated for patients with mild or moderate MR. (Level of Evidence: C)

[a]See Table 16.3 for severity criteria.
Abbreviations: LV, left ventricular; MR, mitral regurgitation; MV, mitral valve; NYHA, New York Heart Association.
Source: Adapted from Ref. 2.

Table 17.4 Doppler Parameters of Prosthetic Mitral Valve Function

	Normal[a]	Possible stenosis[b]	Suggests significant stenosis[a,b]
Peak velocity (m/s)[c,d]	<1.9	1.9–2.5	≥2.5
Mean gradient (mmHg)[c,d]	≤5	6–10	>10
VTI_{PMV}/VTI_{LVOT}[c,d]	<2.2	2.2–2.5	>2.5
EOA (cm^2)	≥2.0	1–2	<1
PHT (ms)	<130	130–200	>200

[a]Best specificity for normality or abnormality is seen if the majority of the parameters listed are normal or abnormal, respectively.
[b]Values of the parameters should prompt a closer evaluation of valve function and/or other considerations such as increased flow, increased heart rate, or PPM.
[c]Slightly higher cutoff values than shown may be seen in some bioprosthetic valves.
[d]These parameters are also abnormal in the presence of significant prosthetic MR.
Abbreviations: EOA, effective orifice area; LVOT, left ventricular outflow tract; PHT, pressure half-time; PMV, prosthetic mitral valve; VTI, velocity-time integral; PPM, patient-prosthesis mismatch.
Source: From Ref. 17.

Table 17.5 Transthoracic Echocardiographic Findings Suggestive of Significant Prosthetic MR in Mechanical Valves with Normal Pressure Half-Time

Finding	Sensitivity	Specificity	Comments
Peak mitral velocity $\geq$ 1.9 m/s[a]	90%	89%	Also consider high flow, PPM
VTI$_{PMV}$/VTI$_{LVOT}$ $\geq$ 2.5[a]	89%	91%	Measurement errors increase in atrial fibrillation due to difficulty in matching cardiac cycles; also consider PPM
Mean gradient $\geq$ 5 mmHg[a]	90%	70%	At physiological heart rates; also consider high flow, PPM
Maximal TR jet velocity > 3 m/s[a]	80%	71%	Consider residual postoperative pulmonary hypertension or other causes
LV stroke volume derived by 2D or 3D imaging is >30% higher than systemic stroke volume by Doppler	Moderate sensitivity	Specific	Validation lacking; significant MR is suspected when LV function is normal or hyperdynamic and VTI$_{LVO}$ is <16 cm
Systolic flow convergence seen in the left ventricle toward the prosthesis	Low sensitivity	Specific	Validation lacking; technically challenging to detect readily

[a]When both peak velocity and VTI ratio are elevated with a normal pressure half-time, specificity is close to 100% (data from Ref. 18).

Abbreviations: LV, left ventricular; LVOT, left ventricular outflow tract; MR, mitral regurgitation; PMV, prosthetic mitral valve; PPM, patient-prosthesis mismatch; TR, tricuspid regurgitation; VTI, velocity-time integral.

Source: From Ref. 17.

Table 17.6 Echocardiographic and Doppler Criteria for Severity of Prosthetic MR Using Findings from TTE and TEE

Parameter	Mild	Moderate	Severe
Structural parameters			
LV size	Normal[a]	Normal or dilated	Usually dilated[b]
Prosthetic valve[c]	Usually normal	Abnormal[d]	Abnormal[d]
Doppler parameters			
Color flow jet area[c,e]	Small, central jet (usually <4 cm^2 or <20% of LA area)	Variable	Large central jet (usually >8 cm^2 or >40% of LA area) or variable size wall impinging jet swirling in left atrium
Flow convergence[f]	None or minimal	Intermediate	Large
Jet density: CW Doppler[c]	Incomplete or faint	Dense	Dense
Jet contour: CW Doppler[c]	Parabolic	Usually parabolic	Early peaking, triangular
Pulmonary venous flow[c]	Systolic dominance[g]	Systolic blunting[g]	Systolic flow reversal[h]
Quantitative parameters[i]			
VC width (cm)[c]	<0.3	0.3–0.59	$\geq$0.6
R vol (mL/beat)	<30	30–59	$\geq$60
RF (%)	<30	30–49	$\geq$50
EROA (cm^2)	<0.20	0.20–0.49	$\geq$0.50

[a]LV size applied only to chronic lesions.

[b]In the absence of other etiologies of LV enlargement and acute MR.

[c]Parameter may be best evaluated or obtained with TEE, particularly in mechanical valves.

[d]Abnormal mechanical valves, for example, immobile occluder (valvular regurgitation), dehiscence or rocking (paravalvular regurgitation); abnormal biological valves, for example, leaflet thickening or prolapse (valvular), dehiscence or rocking (paravalvular regurgitation).

[e]At a Nyquist limit of 50 to 60 cm/s.

[f]Minimal and large flow convergence defined as a flow convergence radius <0.4 and >0.9 cm for central jets, respectively, with a baseline shift at a Nyquist limit of 40 cm/s; cutoffs for eccentric jets may be higher.

[g]Unless other reasons for systolic blunting (e.g., atrial fibrillation, elevated LA pressure).

[h]Pulmonary venous systolic flow reversal is specific but not sensitive for severe MR.

[i]These quantitative parameters are less well validated than in native MR.

Abbreviations: CW, continuous wave; EROA, effective regurgitant orifice area; LA, left atrial; LV, left ventricular; MR, mitral regurgitation; RF, regurgitant fraction; R vol, regurgitant volume; TEE, transesophageal echocardiography; TTE, transthoracic echocardiography; VC, vena contracta.

Source: From Ref. 17.

TEE EVALUATION AFTER MV REPAIR

After surgical repair, the MV often resembles a uni-leaflet valve with a large mobile and functional anterior leaflet and a fixed posterior leaflet (Fig. 17.30). The TEE evaluation of the MV after repair focuses on detecting residual MR that is generally within the annular ring and is usually eccentric. The causes include imperfect coaptation of the mitral leaflets, restricted leaflet motion, or residual prolapse. Color flow Doppler could underestimate the severity of immediate post-CPB MR if global and regional LV function and the patient's hemodynamics are not taken into consideration (19). When LV function or blood pressure are significantly reduced [i.e., left ventricular ejection fraction (LVEF) < 40% or systolic arterial pressure (SAP) $\leq$ 100 mmHg], stimulation with vasopressors such as phenylephrine should be considered to reevaluate the severity of MR with higher loading conditions (see Chapter 16).

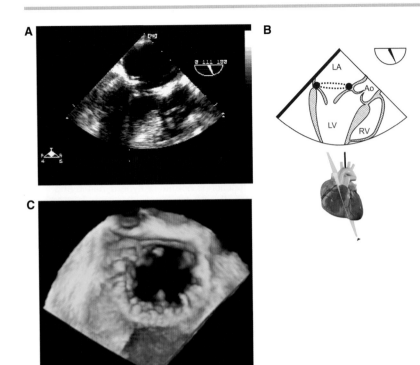

Figure 17.30   Mitral annuloplasty ring. (A,B) Mid-esophageal long-axis view shows adequate function of the MV immediately after annuloplasty. The MAR is viewed transversely by the 2D tomographic plane and thus appears as two small echodensities at the base of the MV leaflets on the atrial side. This is sometimes mistaken for annular calcifications. **(C)** 3D transesophageal view of a MAR seen from the LA orientation. *Abbreviations*: Ao, aorta; LA, left atrium; LV, left ventricle; MAR, mitral annuloplasty ring; MV, mitral valve; RV, right ventricle.

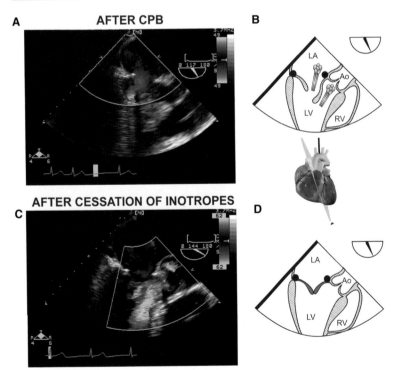

Figure 17.31   Systolic anterior motion. Mid-esophageal long-axis views immediately after coming off CPB for mitral valve repair shows SAM (**A,B**) which improves after cessation of inotropes (**C,D**). *Abbreviations*: Ao, aorta; CPB, cardiopulmonary bypass; LA, left atrium; LV, left ventricle; RV, right ventricle; SAM, systolic anterior motion.

Significant extra- or periannular leaks are uncommon after MV repair, but a search for their presence and evaluation of their severity should systematically be performed as with MV replacement. In the long term, annular dehiscence with periannular leak is an infrequent condition and often results from degenerative disease or endocarditis.

Systolic anterior motion (SAM) of the anterior mitral leaflet (20,21) may arise after MV repair as a result of changes in the LV geometry and in the relationship among the LV, the mitral leaflets, and the annulus. This is particularly prone to happen when LV function is hyperdynamic or under inotropic stimulation (Figs. 17.31 and 17.32) leading to variable

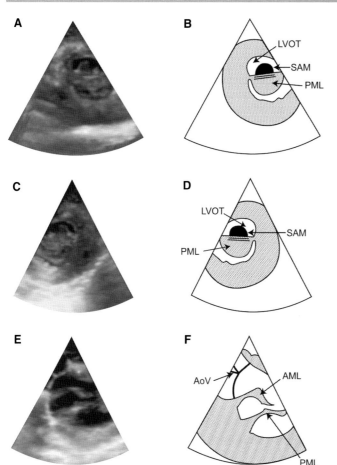

Figure 17.32 Systolic anterior motion. A 71-year-old man undergoing MV repair developed SAM of the MV during weaning from cardiopulmonary bypass. Epiaortic 3D (**A–D**) and 2D views (**E,F**) were obtained demonstrating partial obstruction of the LVOT. The long anterior mitral leaflet is seen displaced in the LVOT during systole. *Abbreviations*: AoV, aortic valve; LVOT, left ventricular outflow tract; MV, mitral valve; PML, posterior mitral leaflet; SAM, systolic anterior motion. *Source*: With permission from Ref. 32.

degrees of subaortic dynamic obstruction and a late-peaking pressure gradient. Color Doppler imaging demonstrates the presence of flow acceleration and color aliasing in the LVOT; properly aligned CW Doppler from the deep transgastric view estimates the severity of the dynamic gradient. Significant LVOT obstruction is remedied by volume loading, down-titrating vasopressor and inotropic agents, or β-blockers but sometimes requires reintervention. Left unrecognized, SAM and LVOT dynamic obstruction can complicate postoperative management.

Mitral valve repair often causes a mild obstruction to diastolic flow and consequently a small gradient of 2 to 4 mmHg between the LA and the LV, which can be higher with tachycardia. The transmitral gradient is measured with CW Doppler through the MV during diastole. A regurgitant systolic signal noted during this evaluation should trigger the search for previously unsuspected MR.

The TEE evaluation of MV repair for mitral stenosis (usually mitral commissurotomy) mostly involves evaluation of valvular and subvalvular anatomy as well as measurement of the mean diastolic MV gradient and the search for regurgitation.

Routine TEE is also useful after MV repair or replacement for evaluation of de-airing, exclusion of foreign material in the cardiac cavity (see Fig. 15.24), evaluation of LV and right ventricular (RV) function, and exclusion of de novo valvular or aortic disease and pleural effusions. The role of TEE in mitral valvular surgery is summarized in Table 17.7.

MV REPAIR TECHNIQUES

Mitral valve reconstruction is the procedure of choice for correcting MR. The issue of degenerative valve MR has been addressed by the pioneering work of Prof Alain F Carpentier, a world leader in the development and teaching of modern techniques of valve repair (23). Standardization of these techniques and favorable long-term results have resulted in an exponential expansion of the indications for surgery of MR. The purpose of this section is to review and describe the contemporary surgical techniques used to correct severe MR.

The initial steps of the operation are important to establish the basis for precise reconstructive surgical techniques.

Table 17.7 Summary of the Role of TEE in Patients Undergoing Mitral Valve Surgery

	Importance
Before the procedure	
• See Table 13.1 for the role of TEE in cardiac surgery	Anticipation of difficult valve repair with possible modification of the surgical approach, removal of thrombus
• Evaluate left atrial dimension, presence of unsuspected thrombus in LA and LAA	
• Confirm the mechanism of mitral dysfunction (importance of loading condition)	Confirmation of reparability or replacement
• Evaluation of the severity of pulmonary hypertension and tricuspid regurgitation	Tricuspid annuloplasty may be considered with modification of the surgical approach
During CPB	
• See Table 13.1	
After CPB	
• See Table 13.1	
• Evaluate result of repair or replacement	Early detection and correction of prosthetic dysfunction or suboptimal repair
• Measure the gradient	The mean gradient should be less than 5 mmHg. Higher gradient could indicate prosthetic dysfunction
• Rule out SAM and LVOT obstruction	SAM will modify the medical approach and could lead to surgical re-intervention
In the intensive care unit	
• See Table 13.1	

Abbreviations: CPB, cardiopulmonary bypass; LA, left atrium; LAA, left atrial appendage; LVOT, left ventricular outflow tract; SAM, systolic anterior motion; TEE, transesophageal echocardiography.

Cannulation and Extracorporeal Circulation

After induction of general anesthesia, invasive cardiovascular monitoring, and multiplane TEE probe insertion, the MV repair is classically performed through a median sternotomy. Mini-invasive approaches through the sternum or the right chest are becoming more popular as is robotic surgery (24).

The pericardium is opened longitudinally to the right of the midline using electrocautery. Special attention is given to the careful midline division of the thymus gland at the superior part of the anterior mediastinum. Traction sutures are applied to the right and left superior pericardium to elevate and induce a right lateral rotation of the heart. These maneuvers will later facilitate the arterial and venous cannulations and the exposure of the MV through the interatrial groove. Alternative exposures of the MV include various transseptal approaches. Systemic anticoagulation is achieved with intravenous heparin (3 mg/kg). Purse-string sutures are completed on the ascending aorta (Ao), and double venous cannulation of the superior and inferior venae cava is preferred to avoid cerebral congestion due to superior venae cava distortion by the left atrial retractor. A combined anterograde cardioplegia cannula and vent is inserted and secured in the ascending Ao. The final step is the introduction of the retrograde cardioplegia catheter in the coronary sinus through a stab incision in the right atrium (RA) guided into position by TEE.

Activated clotting time (ACT) is monitored after heparin injection (a level of >400 seconds will permit the establishment of CPB at 2.2 L/m²). Mechanical ventilation is then stopped and the Ao is cross-clamped followed by antegrade cold blood (4:1) cardioplegia infusion in the aortic root. Continuous retrograde cold blood cardioplegia is infused during the repair at a perfusion pressure <40 mmHg to prevent myocardial edema. The LA is opened and retractor blades are positioned with pump aspirators used to remove LA blood during surgery.

Valve Analysis

Functional analysis of the MV is then performed. This is of critical importance in valve reconstruction and should correlate with the perioperative TEE examination. There are three possible mechanisms responsible for MR: type 1, normal leaflet motion; type 2, increased leaflet motion; and type 3, restricted motion (see Fig. 16.17). Despite the fact that there are numerous possible valve lesions, they can always be categorized into these three functional groups.

Surgical valve analysis is systematically performed with specifically designed hooks. The P1 scallop of the valve is taken as the reference point and delicately stretched with the left-hand hook. The right-hand hook will alternatively evaluate the posterior leaflet P2 and P3 scallops for prolapse or restriction, which is defined as a coaptation plane above or below the plane of the native annulus of the MV, respectively. Then, attention is given to the anterior leaflet A1, A2, and A3 segments and finally to both anterolateral and posteromedian commissures defined by their fan-shaped chords (Fig. 17.33).

Once the surgeon has determined the mechanism of MR, specific techniques of repair will be performed to correct the pathological valve.

Annuloplasty

The annuloplasty ring has four functions: (*i*) to restore normal annular geometry, (*ii*) to prevent further annular dilation, (*iii*) to decrease tension of sutures on mitral leaflets and annulus, and (*iv*) to increase MV

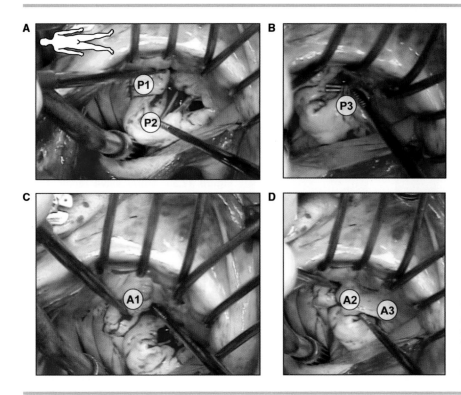

Figure 17.33 Intraoperative MV examination. (**A–D**) Intraoperative examination of the MV through a left atriotomy in a 71-year-old man with prolapse of P2 scallops due to chordal rupture. *Abbreviation*: MV, mitral valve.

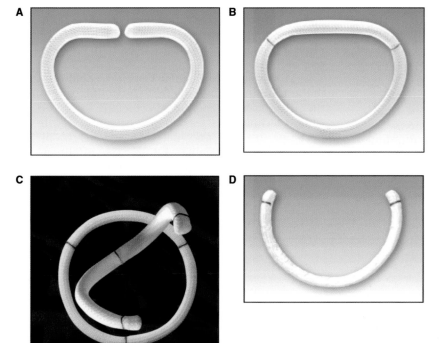

Figure 17.34 Annuloplasty rings. Various models of mitral annuloplasty rings. (**A**) Edwards Lifesciences Carpentier–Edwards Classic annuloplasty ring. (**B**) Edwards Lifesciences Carpentier–Edwards Physio ring. (**C**) Medtronic Duran AnCore flexible annuloplasty ring. (**D**) Edwards Lifesciences Cosgrove–Edwards ring. *Source*: Courtesy of the manufacturers.

coaptation surface. There are complete and incomplete annuloplasty rings (Fig. 17.34). All rings are associated with an excellent clinical outcome. In ischemic MR, experimental and clinical studies support the use of complete remodeling annuloplasties to provide circumferential support. In degenerative etiologies, posterior bands have been associated with good results, the anterior part of the mitral annulus being naturally fixed by the left and right fibrous trigone and the aortic annulus. The ring size is selected with specifically designed templates that measure the intercommissural distance or the intertrigonal distance and the surface

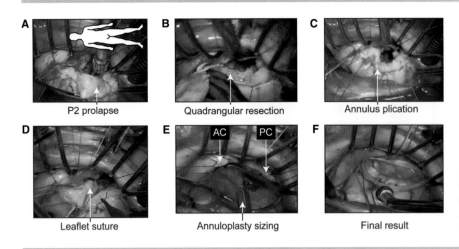

Figure 17.35 Mitral valve repair. (A–F) Operative steps for quadrangular resection are shown (see text for details). *Abbreviations*: AC, anterolateral commissure; PC, posteromedial commissure.

area of the anterior leaflet depending on the model of ring selected.

In degenerative MR, avoidance of an annuloplasty ring has been related to an increased recurrence rate of MR. However, in the case of an active acute bacterial endocarditis, an autologous pericardial posterior band can be used to avoid the presence of foreign material in the ring annuloplasty (25).

POSTERIOR LEAFLET PROLAPSE

The posterior MV leaflet is frequently involved in degenerative MR. Approximately 60% of cases of MV prolapse are located on the middle scallop of the posterior leaflet (26).

Quadrangular Resection

The classic technique is to perform a quadrangular resection (Fig. 17.35) of the prolapsed segment. After resection of the diseased scallop, the native annulus is plicated with several figures of eight polyester braided 2-0 sutures. Finally, the leaflet remnants are

reapproximated with simple everting mattress sutures or double running 5-0 propylene monofilament sutures (Cardionyl, Peters, Paris, France). The valve is then tested with intraventricular saline injection. The plane of coaptation should be symmetric without residual prolapse.

Sliding Plasty of the Posterior Leaflet

In some circumstances, the diseased portion is large and requires extensive resection accounting for >50% of the posterior leaflet. This should be recognized rapidly because it can be associated with an increased risk of SAM.

A simple quadrangular resection could decrease the aorto-mitral angle, thereby propelling in systole, the anterior leaflet of the MV toward the LVOT. A sliding technique is used progressively to plicate the posterior annulus and decrease the height of the posterior leaflet remnants (27) (see Chapter 11, Fig. 11.12). The posterior leaflet should be <2 cm after resection as excessive height is also linked with SAM (Fig. 17.36).

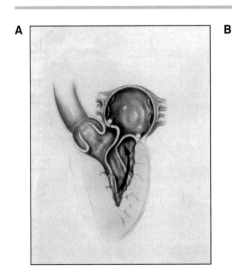

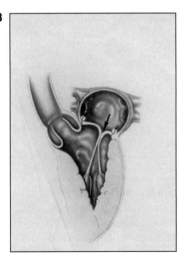

Figure 17.36 Sliding technique. (A) An inadequate repair will result in flow closing the posterior leaflet, which pushes the anterior leaflet toward the LVOT. **(B)** After the sliding leaflet technique, the height of the posterior leaflet is reduced and the anterior leaflet closes away from the LVOT. *Abbreviation*: LVOT, left ventricular outflow tract. *Source*: With permission from Ref. 27.

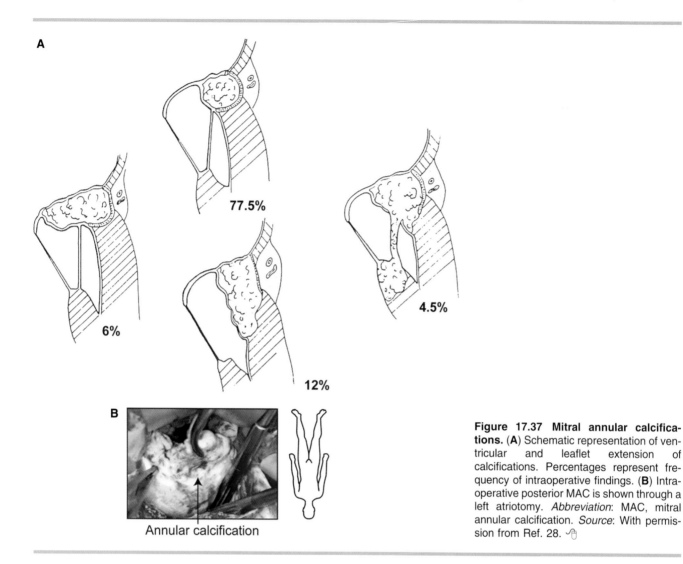

Figure 17.37 Mitral annular calcifications. (A) Schematic representation of ventricular and leaflet extension of calcifications. Percentages represent frequency of intraoperative findings. **(B)** Intraoperative posterior MAC is shown through a left atriotomy. *Abbreviation*: MAC, mitral annular calcification. *Source*: With permission from Ref. 28.

This technique involves detachment of the leaflet remnants from the MV annulus followed by a variable number of plication sutures (2-0 Ticron) to reapproximate the leaflets without tension. The leaflets are then reattached to the native annulus with a 4-0 Cardionyl running suture and sutured together with 5-0 Cardionyl sutures. The valve is then tested with saline injection, and an appropriate annuloplasty ring is selected. These technical points will maintain the normal aorto-mitral angle (Fig. 17.36).

Commissural Prolapse

Commissural prolapse and perforations are frequently associated with bacterial endocarditis. The treatment of a pure prolapse is simple resection and suture. In some cases, a plication of the commissural area without resection is possible. For extensive commissural prolapse and chord rupture, chordal transfer can be used.

Extensive Calcification of the Mitral Annulus

Extensive calcification of the mitral annulus, particularly the posterior portion, is occasionally encountered in degenerative MR. In >50% of cases, the calcifications involve >50% of the annulus (Fig. 17.37) (28). The etiology of this condition is related to increased tension forces at the native posterior annulus, induced by the increased surface area of the prolapsed leaflet. These repeated microtrauma generate fibrin deposition and progressive annular calcification.

In addition to degenerative MR, aging and hypertension have been linked to mitral annulus calcification. For the echocardiographer and the surgeon this condition should be differentiated from rheumatic valve calcification, which involves only the MV leaflets and subvalvular apparatus. The clinical problem related to extensive annular calcifications is the difficulty in plicating the underlying native annulus when a posterior leaflet resection is necessary.

If a MV repair is contemplated, a total decalcification of the mitral annulus is required (28). After standard resection of the prolapsed posterior leaflet, the posterior leaflet remnants are detached from the mitral annulus to the commissural level if there is complete posterior calcification. A sharp dissection plane is defined using a #15 blade scalpel and the resection of the calcified area is performed en bloc to avoid

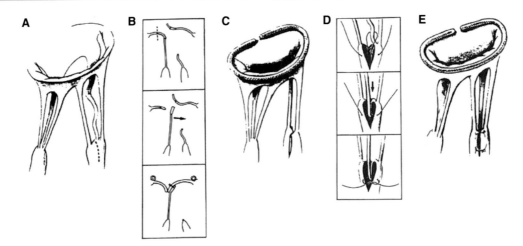

Figure 17.38   Mitral valve repair. Repair of anterior leaflet prolapse due to chordal rupture, by transposition of mural leaflet chordae (**A–C**) or by shortening plasty of the chordate (**D,E**). *Source*: With permission from Ref. 26.

fragmentation. After completion of this step the LA is disconnected from the LV, and the atrioventricular (AV) groove fat often becomes visible. The AV junction is then reconstructed using the LA as a cuff to cover the LV muscle. Alternatively, if the tissues are fragile, an autologous pericardial patch is used to reconstruct the AV junction (29). After reconstruction of the AV junction, the steps of a sliding plasty are completed with appropriate annuloplasty ring selection.

ANTERIOR LEAFLET PROLAPSE

Anterior leaflet prolapse is encountered in approximately 20% of all cases of degenerative MR. It can be associated with posterior leaflet prolapse. The lesion is suspected when the regurgitant jet is directed toward the posterior aspect of the LA. Repair of anterior lesions necessitates a mastery of surgical techniques.

Chordal Transfer

When ruptured chords are responsible for anterior leaflet prolapse, chordal transfer is the treatment of choice (30). The advantage of this approach is the constant length of the transferred scallop. The anterior leaflet segment is located and 2-0 Ticron traction sutures are placed on each side of the prolapsed area. A corresponding segment of the posterior leaflet is selected and two simple 4-0 Cardionyl sutures are applied directly on the lateral borders of the leaflet segment to be transferred. The posterior leaflet is excised and transferred to the corresponding area of the anterior leaflet (Fig. 17.38). The 4-0 Cardionyl sutures are inserted on the edge of the anterior

leaflet and tied to approximate the transferred portion. The posterior leaflet cleft is then repaired as in posterior resections. In a similar approach for limited prolapse, healthy anterior secondary chords can be transferred to the free margin of the anterior leaflet (26).

Artificial Gore-Tex® Chords

Synthetic chords can be used for diffuse anterior leaflet prolapse. This technique is now widely utilized with excellent long-term results. The anterior leaflet is assessed during valve analysis. A double armed 4-0 Gore-Tex® suture is passed through the papillary muscle and tied with Dacron pledgets. The two ends are then passed through the leaflet edge, at the site of ruptured or elongated chords from the LV side to the LA side, and then again passed through the leaflet and tied, using stay sutures on the posterior and anterior leaflet edges to assess proper length of the neo chordae (Fig. 17.39). Multiple chords can be placed on both papillary muscles, to correct the leaflet pathology completely.

Papillary Muscle Shortening

This technique has been associated with an increased rate of late recurrence due to chordal erosion. A trench (half the length to be shortened) is made in the papillary muscle and a 4-0 Cardionyl suture is passed around the selected chordae to be shortened. The chord is then buried in the papillary muscle and, finally, the trench is closed with figure of eight stitches (Fig. 17.38) (30). An alternative technique to shorten numerous chords is to perform a wedge resection of

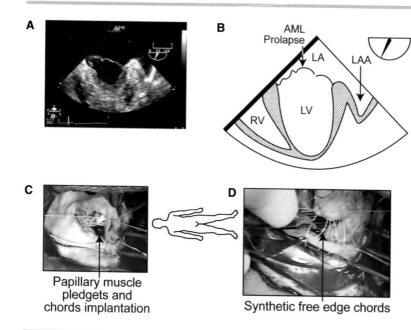

Figure 17.39 Mitral valve repair. (**A,B**) Mid-esophageal view at 68° of a patient shows AML prolapse. (**C,D**) Synthetic chords attached to the leaflet free edge are then implanted on the papillary muscle, preventing prolapse of the leaflet. *Abbreviations*: AML, anterior mitral leaflet; LA, left atrium; LAA, left atrial appendage; LV, left ventricle; RV, right ventricle.

the papillary muscle and to suture the parts close together with 4-0 Cardionyl simple sutures.

Alferi Operation (Edge-to-Edge Repair)

A central vertical pledgetted 2-0 Ticron suture can, occasionally, be applied as a bail out procedure for anterior or bileaflet prolapse. This should never be used as a primary procedure and only added when no other option can be used. This technique has been associated with early recurrence of MR.

Anterior Leaflet Resection

Anterior leaflet resection has been abandoned as the primary treatment for prolapse. Extensive leaflet resection will decrease the surface area of coaptation and may lead to early failure of the procedure. An exception is the occasional rupture of a primary chord attached to the free margin of the anterior leaflet without any other valve lesion. A small wedge resection of the involved segment can then be performed if it represents <10% of the anterior surface of the anterior leaflet.

EARLY COMPLICATIONS

There are few early complications of MV repair (see section "TEE Evaluation after MV Repair").

Systolic Anterior Motion

After MV repair for prolapse, SAM is a complication that must be specifically looked for while in the OR (see Chapter 11, section "Conditions Simulating Hypertrophic Cardiomyopathy"). The incidence of LVOT obstruction after MV repair varies from 2% to 14% (31) and is more frequent with myxomatous changes involving both leaflets. The underlying mechanisms include anterior displacement of the coaptation point, a longer and redundant posterior leaflet (with or without a more acute mitroaortic angle), causing the MV apparatus to be displaced toward the LVOT and be dragged by the outflow, provoking typical SAM and subsequent subvalvular obstruction. Preoperatively, a longer posterior leaflet relative to the anterior (anterior/posterior length ratio ≤1.3) and a shorter distance (≤2.5 cm) between the coaptation point and the septum are predictors of SAM development post repair (see Fig. 11.11) (32). For some patients the problem can be alleviated by increasing LV filling or by reducing inotropic support. However, other patients require MV replacement or subsequent repair.

Surgical risk factors are well known and include extensive posterior leaflet resection, a small LV, and excess posterior valve tissue. Perioperative conditions have also been identified, such as a hyperdynamic LV, hypovolemia, and tachycardia. Prevention remains the best approach to SAM. A sliding plasty of the posterior leaflet is the most important single technique to consider (Fig. 17.36). Perioperative management includes optimal TEE monitoring, judicious preload adjustment, and avoidance of excessive inotropic agents.

Success of the Repair

Mitral valve reconstructive surgery for degenerative lesions is based on the critical knowledge of mitral anatomy. Long-term clinical evolution has been extensively reported. The freedom rate from reoperation at 20 years is low (30).

CONCLUSION

Mitral valve reconstruction is now the procedure of choice for severe MR. Improvements in myocardial protection have allowed longer ischemic time to enable the repair of very complicated lesions. The better understanding of severe MR natural history, the standardization of surgical techniques, the excellent long-term postoperative clinical outcomes, together with the accurate identification of surgical candidates and the dedication to preserve the native MV, have resulted in an expansion of surgical indications to the asymptomatic patient before the onset of irreversible LV dysfunction.

REFERENCES

1. Braunwald E. Heart Disease: A Textbook of Cardiovascular Medicine. 5th ed. Philadelphia: Saunders, 1997.
2. Bonow RO, Carabello BA, Kanu C, et al. ACC/AHA 2006 guidelines for the management of patients with valvular heart disease: a report of the American College of Cardiology/American Heart Association Task Force on Practice Guidelines (writing committee to revise the 1998 Guidelines for the Management of Patients with Valvular Heart Disease): developed in collaboration with the Society of Cardiovascular Anesthesiologists: endorsed by the Society for Cardiovascular Angiography and Interventions and the Society of Thoracic Surgeons. Circulation 2006; 114:e84–e231.
3. Weyman AE. Principles and Practice of Echocardiography. 2nd ed. Philadelphia: Lea & Febiger, 1994.
4. Hammermeister K, Sethi GK, Henderson WG, et al. Outcomes 15 years after valve replacement with a mechanical versus a bioprosthetic valve: final report of the Veterans Affairs randomized trial. J Am Coll Cardiol 2000; 36: 1152–1158.
5. Solowiejczyk DE, Yamada I, Cape EG, et al. Simultaneous Doppler and catheter transvalvular pressure gradients across St Jude bileaflet mitral valve prosthesis: in vivo study in a chronic animal model with pediatric valve sizes. J Am Soc Echocardiogr 1998; 11:1145–1154.
6. Dumesnil JG, Honos GN, Lemieux M, et al. Validation and applications of indexed aortic prosthetic valve areas calculated by Doppler echocardiography. J Am Coll Cardiol 1990; 16:637–643.
7. Shanewise JS, Cheung AT, Aronson S, et al. ASE/SCA guidelines for performing a comprehensive intraoperative multiplane transesophageal echocardiography examination: recommendations of the American Society of Echocardiography Council for Intraoperative Echocardiography and the Society of Cardiovascular Anesthesiologists Task Force for Certification in Perioperative Transesophageal Echocardiography. Anesth Analg 1999; 89:870–884.
8. Zoghbi WA, Enriquez-Sarano M, Foster E, et al. Recommendations for evaluation of the severity of native valvular regurgitation with two-dimensional and Doppler echocardiography. J Am Soc Echocardiogr 2003; 16:777–802.
9. Fernandes V, Olmos L, Nagueh SF, et al. Peak early diastolic velocity rather than pressure half-time is the best index of mechanical prosthetic mitral valve function. Am J Cardiol 2002; 89:704–710.
10. Rahimtoola SH, Murphy E. Valve prosthesis—patient mismatch. A long-term sequela. Br Heart J 1981; 45:331–335.
11. Pibarot P, Dumesnil JG. Prosthesis-patient mismatch in the mitral position: old concept, new evidences. J Thorac Cardiovasc Surg 2007; 133:1405–1408.
12. Magne J, Mathieu P, Dumesnil JG, et al. Impact of prosthesis-patient mismatch on survival after mitral valve replacement. Circulation 2007; 115:1417–1425.
13. Li M, Dumesnil JG, Mathieu P, et al. Impact of valve prosthesis-patient mismatch on pulmonary arterial pressure after mitral valve replacement. J Am Coll Cardiol 2005; 45:1034–1040.
14. Lam BK, Chan V, Hendry P, et al. The impact of patient-prosthesis mismatch on late outcomes after mitral valve replacement. J Thorac Cardiovasc Surg 2007; 133:1464–1473.
15. Pibarot P, Dumesnil JG. Prosthesis-patient mismatch: definition, clinical impact, and prevention. Heart 2006; 92:1022–1029.
16. Pibarot P, Dumesnil JG. Prosthetic heart valves: selection of the optimal prosthesis and long-term management. Circulation 2009; 119:1034–1048.
17. Zoghbi WA, Chambers JB, Dumesnil JG, et al. Recommendations for evaluation of prosthetic valves with echocardiography and Doppler ultrasound: a report from the American Society of Echocardiography's Guidelines and Standards Committee and the Task Force on Prosthetic Valves, developed in conjunction with the American College of Cardiology Cardiovascular Imaging Committee, Cardiac Imaging Committee of the American Heart Association, the European Association of Echocardiography, a registered branch of the European Society of Cardiology, the Japanese Society of Echocardiography and the Canadian Society of Echocardiography, endorsed by the American College of Cardiology Foundation, American Heart Association, European Association of Echocardiography, a registered branch of the European Society of Cardiology, the Japanese Society of Echocardiography, and Canadian Society of Echocardiography. J Am Soc Echocardiogr 2009; 22:975–1014.
18. Olmos L, Salazar G, Barbetseas J, et al. Usefulness of transthoracic echocardiography in detecting significant prosthetic mitral valve regurgitation. Am J Cardiol 1999; 83:199–205.
19. Gisbert A, Souliere V, Denault AY, et al. Dynamic quantitative echocardiographic evaluation of mitral regurgitation in the operating department. J Am Soc Echocardiogr 2006; 19:140–146.
20. Kronzon I, Cohen ML, Winer HE, et al. Left ventricular outflow obstruction: a complication of mitral valvuloplasty. J Am Coll Cardiol 1984; 4:825–828.
21. Freeman WK, Schaff HV, Khandheria BK, et al. Intraoperative evaluation of mitral valve regurgitation and repair by transesophageal echocardiography: incidence and significance of systolic anterior motion. J Am Coll Cardiol 1992; 20:599–609.
22. Denault AY, Couture P, Pellerin M. Images in anesthesia: 3D systolic anterior motion of the mitral valve. Can J Anaesth 2004; 51:481.
23. Carpentier AF, Lessana A, Relland JY, et al. The "physio-ring": an advanced concept in mitral valve annuloplasty. Ann Thorac Surg 1995; 60:1177–1185.
24. Loulmet DF, Carpentier A, Cho PW, et al. Less invasive techniques for mitral valve surgery. J Thorac Cardiovasc Surg 1998; 115:772–779.
25. Dreyfus G, Serraf A, Jebara VA, et al. Valve repair in acute endocarditis. Ann Thorac Surg 1990; 49:706–711.
26. Carpentier A. Cardiac valve surgery—the "French correction". J Thorac Cardiovasc Surg 1983; 86:323–337.
27. Jebara VA, Mihaileanu S, Acar C, et al. Left ventricular outflow tract obstruction after mitral valve repair. Results of the sliding leaflet technique. Circulation 1993; 88:II30–II34.
28. Carpentier AF, Pellerin M, Fuzellier JF, et al. Extensive calcification of the mitral valve anulus: pathology and surgical management. J Thorac Cardiovasc Surg 1996; 111:718–729.

29. Feindel CM, Tufail Z, David TE, et al. Mitral valve surgery in patients with extensive calcification of the mitral annulus. J Thorac Cardiovasc Surg 2003; 126:777–782.
30. Braunberger E, Deloche A, Berrebi A, et al. Very long-term results (more than 20 years) of valve repair with Carpentier's techniques in nonrheumatic mitral valve insufficiency. Circulation 2001; 104:I8–I11.
31. Lee KS, Stewart WJ, Lever HM, et al. Mechanism of outflow tract obstruction causing failed mitral valve repair. Anterior displacement of leaflet coaptation. Circulation 1993; 88:II24–II29.
32. Maslow AD, Regan MM, Haering JM, et al. Echocardiographic predictors of left ventricular outflow tract obstruction and systolic anterior motion of the mitral valve after mitral valve reconstruction for myxomatous valve disease. J Am Coll Cardiol 1999; 34:2096–2104.

18

Pulmonic and Tricuspid Valves

François Marcotte and Denis Bouchard
Université de Montréal, Montreal, Quebec, Canada

Mark Hynes
University of Ottawa, Ottawa, Ontario, Canada

INTRODUCTION

Transesophageal echocardiography (TEE) is only occasionally requested for the primary evaluation of tricuspid valve (TV) and pulmonic valve (PV) disease. This is, in part, because isolated TV and PV diseases are relatively uncommon in comparison with left-sided valvular heart disease (1). Furthermore, compared with the mitral valve (MV) and aortic valve (AoV), these structures are more anterior and located in the TEE far field, making their assessment perhaps more difficult. Nevertheless, as transthoracic echocardiography (TTE) does not always allow the optimal evaluation of the TV and PV, particularly during cardiac surgery, TEE may yield very useful information complementary to TTE. A TEE examination, oblivious to the presence of right-sided valve disease in the operating room (OR), can lead to serious short- and long-term consequences for the patient. Right-heart failure secondary to right-sided valvulopathies can be extremely difficult to treat medically and may ultimately lead to a reduced event-free survival (2,3).

NORMAL TRICUSPID AND PULMONIC VALVE ANATOMY

Situated in the crescentic, pyramid-shaped right ventricle (RV) that supports the low-pressure pulmonary circulation, the TV is in the RV inlet or sinus, while the PV is anterior and superior to the TV in the RV outlet, or conus (Fig. 18.1). Unlike the AoV and MV, the TV and PV are anatomically discontiguous, separated by myocardium.

The TV is situated anterior, inferior, and to the right of the MV. Traditionally, the TV is described as having three leaflets: the septal, the anterior, and the posterior (or inferior) (Fig. 18.2). However, autopsy evidence suggests that there can be significant variability in this arrangement. A review of fifty "normal" morphological right-sided atrioventricular valves showed that 30% had only two leaflets, while 8% had four leaflets (4). There was even greater variability in the papillary muscles supporting the valve. A

medial group of chords arising from the posterior limb of the trabecula septomarginalis was the most consistent finding. Other frequent arrangements were an anterior papillary muscle arising from the apical limb of trabecula septomarginalis supporting highly variable portions of the anterior and inferior leaflets, direct chordal supports from the septum to the septal leaflet, and an inferior papillary muscle supporting the lateral edge of the septal leaflet.

The TV has a large orifice, usually >7 cm^2 and, like its left-sided counterpart, requires the coordination of multiple structures for proper function as described in Table 18.1 (5,6). Abnormalities affecting each of these components may in turn cause TV regurgitation and/or stenosis. The normal tricuspid annular circumference is 12 to 14 cm. Guidelines on the measurement of the tricuspid annulus have been published (7). The tricuspid annulus is defined as normal (2.0–2.8 cm), mildly abnormal (2.9–3.3 cm), moderately abnormal (3.4–3.8 cm), and severely abnormal (>3.9 cm) (see Fig. 5.9). Normal tricuspid leaflet thickness is <3 mm.

The PV is situated anterior and to the left of the AoV. It has two posterior cusps (right and left) and one anterior cusp, in mirror image to the AoV cusps (Fig. 18.3). Proper PV function requires normal cusp anatomy and support from the pulmonary artery and right ventricular outflow tract (RVOT).

From the recommended 22 views for performing a comprehensive TEE examination (see Fig. 4.3), 7 views are particularly useful for the evaluation of the right-sided structures (8) but up to 14 views can be used to evaluate RV anatomy and function (Fig. 18.4) (9). Basic TEE assessment of the right-sided valves begins with the mid-esophageal views that are typically used for valvular anatomy and atrial assessment. The mid-esophageal four-chamber view at $0°$ reveals the TV anterior and septal leaflets (Fig. 18.5). In this view, during early diastole, the tricuspid annulus measures approximately 2.9 ± 0.5 cm or $1.6 + 0.3$ cm/m^2 body surface area (BSA) (10) (see Chapter 5).

The assessment of tricuspid flow is often hindered by its perpendicular direction to the ultrasound beam as well as occasional shadowing by the left-sided valves

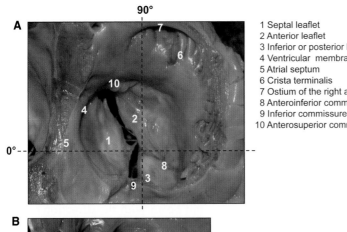

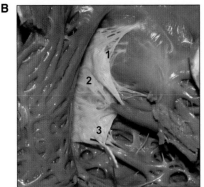

1 Septal leaflet
2 Anterior leaflet
3 Inferior or posterior leaflet
4 Ventricular membranous septum
5 Atrial septum
6 Crista terminalis
7 Ostium of the right atrial appendage
8 Anteroinferior commissure
9 Inferior commissure
10 Anterosuperior commissure

Figure 18.1 Normal TV anatomy. (A) The TV is seen from the right atrium with 0° and 90° echocardiographic planes indicated. **(B)** The TV is seen from the right ventricle. *Abbreviation*: TV, tricuspid valve. *Source*: Photos courtesy of Drs. Nicolas Dürrleman and Michel Pellerin.

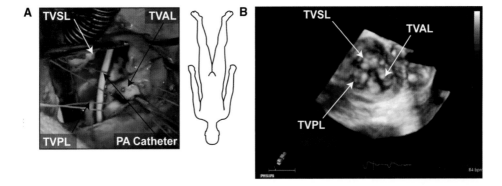

Figure 18.2 Normal TV. Intraoperative view **(A)** compared with a 3D transesophageal short-axis view **(B)** of a normal TV shown from the right atrium. *Abbreviations*: PA, pulmonary artery; TV, tricuspid valve; TVAL, tricuspid valve anterior leaflet; TVPL, tricuspid valve posterior leaflet; TVSL, tricuspid valve septal leaflet. *Source*: Photo A courtesy of Drs. Nicolas Dürrleman and Michel Pellerin, Photo B courtesy of Philips Healthcare.

and the septum. In the upper esophageal view at 0°, by withdrawing the probe cephalad, the PV is seen anteriorly and to the left of the ascending aorta (Ao), while the pulmonary artery courses posteriorly. The RVOT diameter usually measures 2.7 + 0.4 cm or 1.5 + 2 cm/m² BSA (10). Guidelines for the measurement of the

RVOT have been published (7). The RVOT is measured below the PV (RVOT1) and perpendicular to the non-coronary cusp in a mid-esophageal right ventricular inflow-outflow view (see Fig. 5.14). The RVOT1 is defined as normal (2.5–2.9 cm), mildly abnormal (3.0–3.2 cm), moderately abnormal (3.3–3.5 cm), and

Table 18.1 Components of Normal Tricuspid Valve Function

Structure	Pathological process
Right atrium	Right atrial dilatation
	atrial septal defect
	anomalous pulmonary venous return
	right ventricular diastolic dysfunction
	Tumor protrusion through the annulus
Tricuspid annulus	Annular enlargement
Tricuspid leaflets and chordae tendineae	Myxomatous degeneration
	Destruction by endocarditis
	Rheumatic heart disease
	Ebstein's anomaly
	Carcinoid tumor
	Anorectic drugs, ergot-derived drugs
	Radiation-induced scar
	Valve dysplasia
	Connective tissue disease
	Interference or damage by catheter or pacemaker wire
	Trauma from endomyocardial biopsy
	Unguarded tricuspid valve orifice
Atrioventricular septum	Septal defect producing septal leaflet clef
	Septal aneurysm
Papillary muscles	Destruction by endocarditis
	Rupture from right ventricular infarction
	Damage from trauma
Right ventricle	Pressure overload
	pulmonary hypertension
	pulmonic valve stenosis
	Volume overload
	atrial septal defect
	pulmonic valve regurgitation
	Regional dysfunction
	dysplasia
	infarction
	trauma
	radiation injury
	Dilated cardiomyopathy
	Restrictive cardiomyopathy

severely abnormal (>3.6 cm). The RVOT2 is defined as normal (1.7–2.3 cm), mildly abnormal (2.4–2.7 cm), moderately abnormal (2.8–3.1 cm), and severely abnormal (>3.2 cm) (see Fig. 5.14).

As the probe is further withdrawn, shadowing from air in the tracheobronchial tree frequently precludes visualization of the pulmonary artery, especially the left branch.

As the imaging plane is rotated to 30° to 70° and the probe is turned toward the right, the equivalent of the transthoracic parasternal short-axis view or RV inflow-outflow view becomes visible (Fig. 18.6). Below the atrial septum and the AoV, the TV anterior and septal leaflets are seen, with tricuspid regurgitation (TR) shown by color Doppler imaging.

Further rotation of the imaging plane to 90° in the mid- and upper esophageal views reveals the RV infundibulum, the PV, and the main pulmonary artery in a sagittal view of the heart (Fig. 18.7). Easy alignment of the ultrasound beam with the direction of the pulmonary artery flow makes this view particularly suited to spectral Doppler interrogation of the PV.

At 120°, rightward rotation of the probe shaft yields the equivalent of a transthoracic parasternal long-axis RV inflow view that demonstrates the TV anterior and posterior leaflets and may be useful to disclose a posteriorly directed TR jet by color Doppler imaging (Fig. 18.8).

The examination proceeds toward the transgastric views to demonstrate ventricular function and subvalvular atrioventricular apparatus anatomy. Advancing the probe from the mid-esophageal position first leads to the transitional (or gastroesophageal) view at 0° at the level of the coronary sinus, displays the TV posterior and septal leaflets, and is a useful view in the assessment of TR (Fig. 18.9). Further down, the transgastric view at 0° reveals the LV and RV side by side. This view may require some tilting of the probe in certain patients with unusual cardiac orientation (Fig. 18.10). The three leaflets of the TV can be seen "en face" when the RV is markedly dilated. More importantly, the RV contractility and the ventricular septal curvature can be assessed in this view.

Rotation of the imaging plane to 60° to 90°, with rightward rotation of the shaft past the plane of the ventricular septum, reveals a right sagittal view with the RV infundibulum and the subvalvular tricuspid

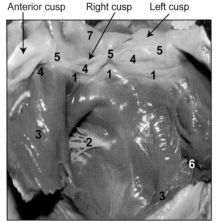

1 Pulmonic annulus
2 Septal leaflet of tricuspid valve
3 Right ventricle walls
4 Pulmonic cusps
5 Pulmonic commissures
6 Interventricular septum
7 Pulmonic artery

Figure 18.3 PV anatomy. The PV is seen from a right ventriculotomy in this anatomical specimen. *Abbreviation*: PV, pulmonic valve. *Source*: Courtesy of Dr. Nicolas Dürrleman.

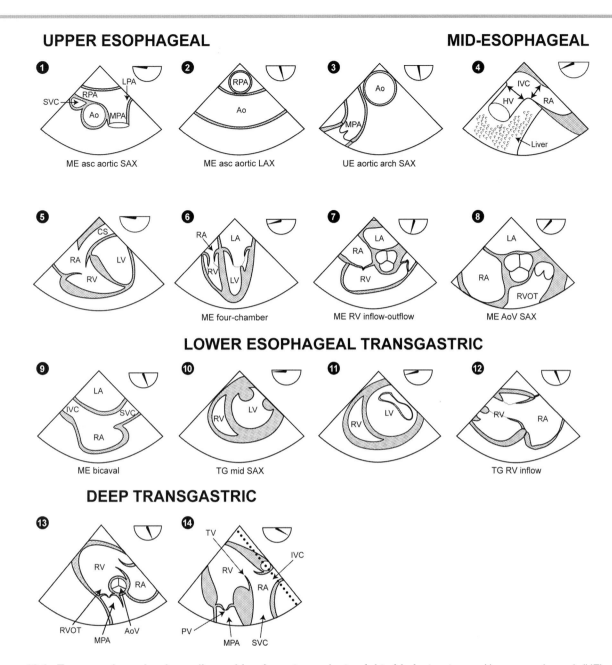

Figure 18.4 Transesophageal echocardiographic views to evaluate right-sided structures. Upper esophageal (UE), mid-esophageal (ME), low esophageal (LE), transgastric (TG), and deep TG views are useful in the evaluation of right ventricular (RV) function. *Abbreviations*: Asc, ascending; Ao, aorta; AoV, aortic valve; CS, coronary sinus; HV, hepatic vein; IVC, inferior vena cava; LA, left atrium; LAX, long-axis; LPA, left pulmonary artery; LV, left ventricle; MPA, main pulmonary artery; PV, pulmonic valve; RA, right atrium; RPA, right pulmonary artery; RV, right ventricle; RVOT, right ventricular outflow tract; SAX, short-axis; SVC, superior vena cava; TV, tricuspid valve. *Source*: Adapted with permission from Ref. 9.

apparatus (Fig. 18.11). The RVOT and the pulmonary trunk may be also visualized in the far field. Easy alignment of the ultrasound beam with the direction of the flow in this view is ideal for Doppler interrogation of the PV sub- and supravalvular velocities to diagnose stenosis.

A deeper transgastric view at 120° allows further visualization of the TV anterior and posterior leaflets and the subvalvular apparatus (Fig. 18.12).

ANATOMICAL MANIFESTATIONS OF VALVULAR LESIONS

Tricuspid Regurgitation

With the development of color Doppler imaging, TR is a frequent finding seen, to some degree, in almost all individuals. Hemodynamically and echocardiographically significant TR, however, is usually associated with right-sided cardiac chamber enlargement unless

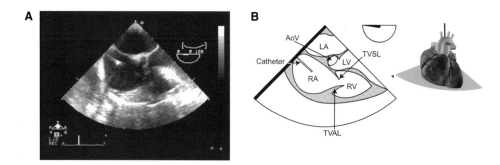

Figure 18.5   ME four-chamber view of the TV. (A,B) This rotated ME four-chamber view shows the TVAL and TVSL in a 74-year-old man before coronary revascularization. A pulmonary artery catheter is seen in the RA. *Abbreviations*: AoV, aortic valve; LA, left atrium; LV, left ventricle; ME, mid-esophageal; RA, right atrium; RV, right ventricle; TV, tricuspid valve; TVAL, TV anterior leaflet; TVSL, TV septal leaflet.

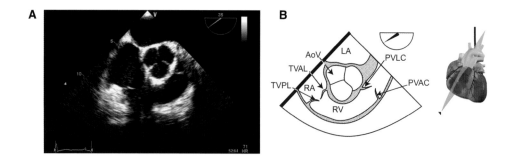

Figure 18.6   ME right ventricular inflow/outflow view. (A,B) This ME view shows both the tricuspid and pulmonic valves. *Abbreviations*: AoV, aortic valve; LA, left atrium; ME, mid-esophageal; PVAC, pulmonic valve anterior cusp; PVLC, pulmonic valve left cusp; RA, right atrium; RV, right ventricle; TVAL, tricuspid valve anterior leaflet; TVPL, tricuspid valve posterior leaflet.

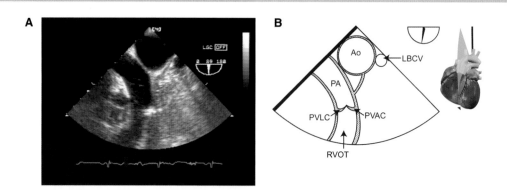

Figure 18.7   Upper esophageal view of the PV. (A,B) This sagittal view shows the RVOT and PV with good alignment for Doppler evaluation. *Abbreviations*: Ao, aorta; LBCV, left brachiocephalic vein; PA, pulmonary artery; PV, pulmonic valve; PVAC, pulmonic valve anterior cusp; PVLC, pulmonic valve left cusp; RVOT, right ventricular outflow tract.

A

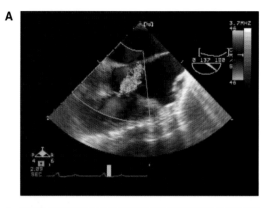

B

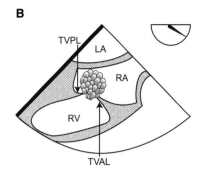

C

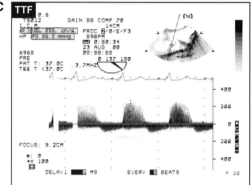

Vel: 259 cm/s
PG: 28.3 mmHg

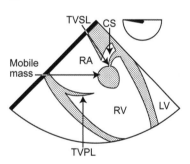

Figure 18.8 ME tricuspid valve view. (A,B) Color Doppler mid-esophageal 120° view with rightward rotation, demonstrates the TVAL and TVPL with TR, in a 77-year-old woman scheduled for TV annuloplasty. **(C)** The peak systolic PG of the TR signal is 28.3 mmHg measured by continuous wave Doppler of TTF. *Abbreviations*: LA, left atrium; ME, mid-esophageal; PG, pressure gradient; RA, right atrium; RV, right ventricle; TTF, transtricuspid flow; TR, tricuspid regurgitation; TV; tricuspid valve; TVAL, TV anterior leaflet; TVPL, TV posterior leaflet; Vel, velocity.

A

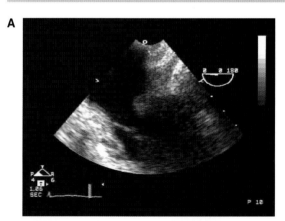

B

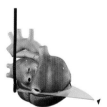

C

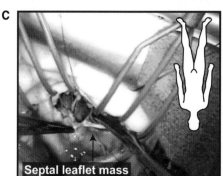

Septal leaflet mass

Figure 18.9 TV mass. (A,B) Low esophageal view in a 65-year-old woman undergoing surgery for a TV mass located near the TVSL close to the CS. **(C)** Intraoperative findings seen through a right atriotomy. The mass was diagnosed on pathology as a fibroelastoma. *Abbreviations*: CS, coronary sinus; LV, left ventricle; RA, right atrium; RV, right ventricle; TV, tricuspid valve; TVPL, TV posterior leaflet; TVSL, TV septal leaflet. *Source*: Photo C courtesy of Dr. Pierre Pagé.

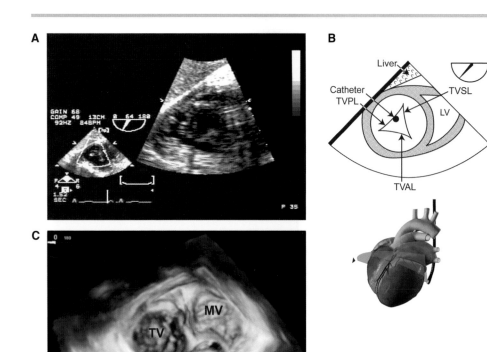

Figure 18.10 TG view of the TV. Modified TG basal view (**A,B**) of the right ventricle shows all three leaflets of the TV in a 50-year-old man compared with a 3D transesophageal echocardiographic view (**C**) of the base of the heart showing the TV in a similar orientation. *Abbreviations*: AoV, aortic valve; LV, left ventricle; MV, mitral valve; TG, transgastric; TV, tricuspid valve; TVAL, TV anterior leaflet; TVPL, TV posterior leaflet; TVSL, TV septal leaflet.

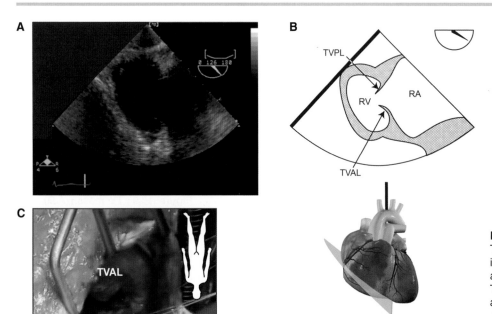

Figure 18.11 TG view of the TV. This TG RV inflow view (**A,B**) at 120° in a 70-year-old woman before TV annuloplasty shows the TVPL and TVAL. (**C**) Intraoperative findings are seen through a right atriotomy. *Abbreviations*: RA, right atrium; RV, right ventricle; TG, transgastric; TV, tricuspid valve; TVAL, TV anterior leaflet; TVPL, TV posterior leaflet. *Source*: Photo C courtesy of Dr. Denis Bouchard.

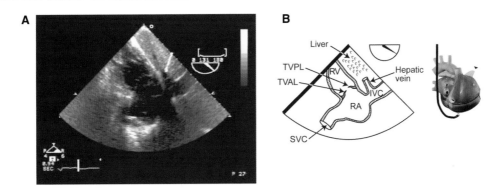

Figure 18.12 Deep TG long-axis view of the RV. (A,B) This view is obtained to complete the evaluation of RV function in this 63-year-old woman scheduled for coronary revascularization. The TVPL and TVAL are visualized. *Abbreviations*: IVC, inferior vena cava; RA, right atrium; RV, right ventricle; SVC, superior vena cava; TG, transgastric; TVAL, tricuspid valve anterior leaflet; TVPL, tricuspid valve posterior leaflet.

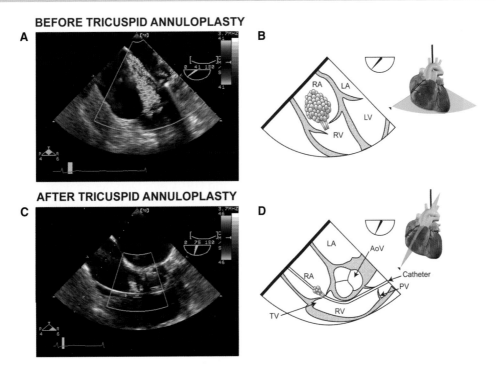

Figure 18.13 TV annuloplasty. (A,B) Color Doppler ME four-chamber view shows TR in a 70-year-old woman before TV annuloplasty. **(C,D)** Color Doppler ME right ventricular inflow/outflow view after TV repair reveals only mild residual TR around the pulmonary artery catheter. *Abbreviations*: AoV, aortic valve; LA, left atrium; LV, left ventricle; ME, mid-esophageal; PV, pulmonic valve; RA, right atrium; RV, right ventricle; TR, tricuspid regurgitation; TV, tricuspid valve.

it is of acute onset (Fig. 18.13). Most commonly, TR is of functional origin and less commonly from structural tricuspid disease (11). Functional TR implies normal valve leaflets and usually results from RV pressure overload from pulmonary hypertension or from RV dysfunction.

Functional TR results mostly from dilatation of the mural annulus, which supports the anterior and posterior leaflets, while there is little change in the septal annular dimensions (12,13). The mechanism of functional TR may also involve incomplete coaptation of the tricuspid leaflets as a result of the apical

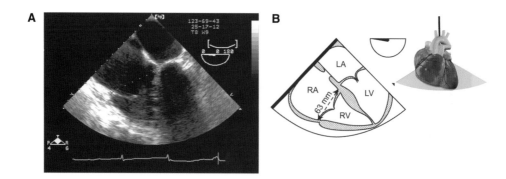

Figure 18.14   Dilated TV annulus. (A,B) Mid-esophageal four-chamber view in a 70-year-old woman scheduled for TV annuloplasty with a TV annulus diameter of 63 mm. *Abbreviations*: LA, left atrium; LV, left ventricle; RA, right atrium; RV, right ventricle; TV, tricuspid valve.

displacement of the tricuspid papillary muscles secondary to RV dilatation and dysfunction. This is best appreciated in the mid-esophageal four-chamber view (Fig. 18.14) (14). Significant TR is usually associated with dilatation of the tricuspid annulus diameter >2.7 cm/m² BSA (15). A diameter exceeding 30 mm is generally deemed enough to consider TV annuloplasty for significant TR in the setting of concomitant cardiac surgery. A tricuspid annular dilatation >50 mm is associated with a lower likelihood of RV function recovery following repair (Fig. 18.14) (16). Common causes of pulmonary hypertension leading to functional TR include left ventricular (LV) failure and MV disease, both easily identified by TEE. Other causes are thromboembolic pulmonary vascular disease, autoimmune pulmonary vascular disease, and primary pulmonary hypertension (14,17).

When TR is secondary to structural disease, this may implicate one of many mechanisms such as leaflet disease (e.g., endocarditis, rheumatic valvulitis, prolapse, and dysplasia), papillary muscle dysfunction or rupture (e.g., due to endocarditis, trauma, or infarction), or interference with proper tricuspid leaflet motion (e.g., by a pacemaker wire or an RV catheter) (Figs. 18.15–18.18) (18). The most common causes of TV disease are listed in Table 18.1 (6,11).

Color Doppler imaging has become the principal method to grade regurgitation severity by echocardiography, but few studies have looked at the assessment of right-sided valve regurgitation by TEE. A transthoracic TR jet color flow area >9 cm² is deemed significant, while a jet area <4 cm² is viewed as mild (19). Color Doppler imaging depicts the displacement of red blood cells in the right atrium (RA) caused

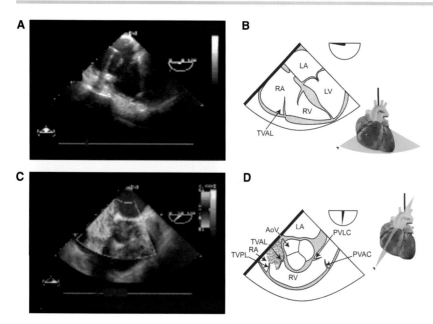

Figure 18.15   Flail TV. (A,B) ME four-chamber view shows a flail TVAL due to a ruptured anterior papillary muscle. **(C,D)** Color Doppler in the ME right ventricular inflow/outflow tract view shows severe tricuspid regurgitation. *Abbreviations*: LA, left atrium; LV, left ventricle; ME, mid-esophageal; PVAC, pulmonic valve anterior cusp; PVLC, pulmonic valve left cusp; RA, right atrium; RV, right ventricle; TV, tricuspid valve; TVAL, TV anterior leaflet; TVPL, TV posterior leaflet.

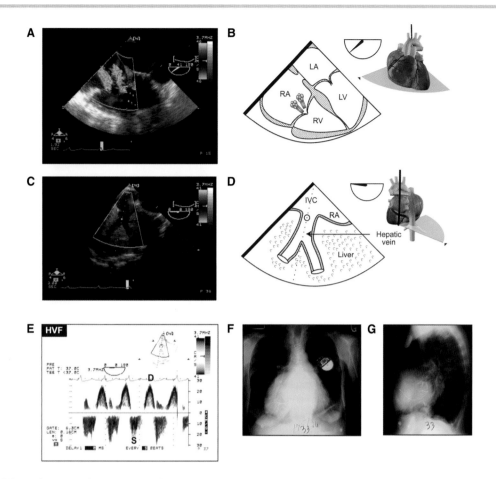

Figure 18.16 Tricuspid regurgitation. (A,B) Color Doppler mid-esophageal four-chamber view shows severe TR in a 77-year-old woman before tricuspid annuloplasty. **(C,D)** Transgastric IVC long-axis view indicates dilated hepatic veins. **(E)** Pulsed wave Doppler of HVF shows systolic flow reversal. **(F,G)** Chest radiography confirms the abnormal right heart border consistent with dilated right-sided structures. *Abbreviations*: D, peak diastolic HVF velocity; HVF, hepatic venous flow; IVC, inferior vena cava; LA, left atrium; LV, left ventricle; RA, right atrium; RV, right ventricle; S, peak systolic HVF velocity; TR, tricuspid regurgitation.

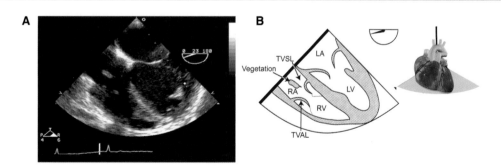

Figure 18.17 TV endocarditis. (A,B) Mid-esophageal four-chamber view of a patient with endocarditis shows a mobile echogenic mass between the TVSL and the TVAL consistent with a vegetation. *Abbreviations*: LA, left atrium; LV, left ventricle; RA, right atrium; RV, right ventricle; TV, tricuspid valve; TVAL, TV anterior leaflet; TVSL, TV septal leaflet.

by the TR jet, typically as a mosaic, predominantly red-orange jet directed posteriorly toward the probe. Although the magnitude of hemodynamic entrainment of red blood cells is assumed to represent regurgitant volume, the severity of TR may not exactly correspond to the regurgitant color jet area, though it is generally proportional (Figs. 18.15 and 18.16). Some factors, such as jet eccentricity and shadowing from left-sided structures, may limit the ability of regurgitant jet color flow area to grade TR.

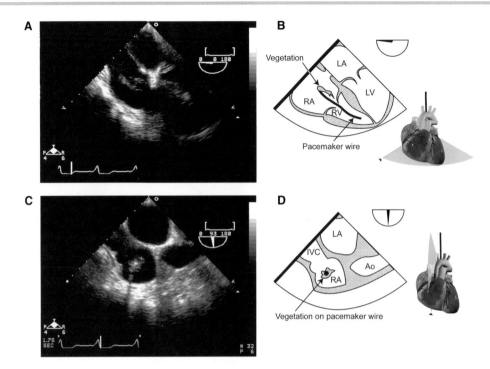

Figure 18.18   TV endocarditis. Echogenic material attached to a pacemaker wire is seen in mid-esophageal four-chamber (**A,B**) and 90° views (**C,D**). *Abbreviations*: Ao, aorta; IVC, inferior vena cava; LA, left atrium; LV, left ventricle; RA, right atrium; RV, right ventricle; TV, tricuspid valve.

Regurgitation severity can be best correlated with the width of the color regurgitant jet, as a surrogate of the vena contracta, and to the presence of a large zone of proximal flow convergence. Tribouilloy et al. (20) reported that a vena contracta >6.5 mm was a better predictor of severe TR than regurgitant jet color flow area. Hepatic vein systolic flow reversal due to severe TR is easily demonstrated by TTE and by TEE using the lower esophageal view at 0° or the transgastric view at 90° (Fig. 18.16) (19). Continuous wave (CW) Doppler is used to grade TR by weighing the amplitude of red blood cell displacement and right ventricular systolic pressure (RVSP), thus providing information on whether TR etiology is based on normal or high pulmonary artery pressures. The American Society of Echocardiography's (ASE) published guidelines on the evaluation of TR are summarized in Tables 18.2 and 18.3 (21).

Tricuspid Stenosis

Tricuspid stenosis (TS) is the least common valvular lesion. It is rarely an isolated lesion associated with rheumatic mitral stenosis (MS), carcinoid syndrome with TR, congenital heart disease, infected pacer wires, or extrinsic compression by masses.

Anatomic assessment by two-dimensional (2D) imaging demonstrates leaflet thickening, calcification, restricted mobility with diastolic doming, and right atrial (RA) enlargement. The leaflets may be completely frozen as occurs in carcinoid syndrome.

Color Doppler imaging shows a narrow turbulent diastolic inflow with associated TR. The CW Doppler signal, properly aligned, is preferably recorded during end-expiratory apnea in a spontaneous breathing patient. The heart rate (HR) should be <100 beats/min and averaged over several cardiac cycles if the patient has an irregular rhythm. The characteristic feature of TS is an increased peak transvalvular tricuspid inflow velocity of >1.0 m/s. Findings indicative of significant hemodynamic TS are based on specific findings using CW Doppler (Table 18.4) and supportive findings of moderate RA enlargement and dilated inferior vena cava (IVC) (24).

The tricuspid valve area (TVA) can be estimated using the pressure half-time (PHT) or continuity equation method, although both have limitations. The PHT method is similar to its use in MS but uses a constant of 190 ms, thus TVA = 190/PHT. The TVA obtained using this method may be less accurate than in MS. The continuity equation can be used provided an accurate measurement of the tricuspid inflow volume is obtained and compared with either RV or LV outflow.

ENDOCARDITIS

Vegetations

Endocarditis of right-sided valves has become a common problem with the advent of IV access used in various forms of therapy, especially with individuals who use contaminated needles for IV drug abuse. The

Table 18.2 Echocardiographic and Doppler Parameters Used in the Evaluation of Tricuspid Regurgitation Severity: Utility, Advantages, and Limitations

Parameter	Utility/Advantages	Limitations
RV/RA/IVC size	Enlargement sensitive for chronic significant TR Normal size virtually excludes significant chronic TR	Enlargement seen in other conditions May be normal in acute significant TR
TV leaflet alterations	Flail valve specific for significant significant TR	Other abnormalities do not imply TR
Paradoxical septal motion (volume overload pattern)	Simple sign of severe TR	Not specific for TR
Jet area—color flow	Simple, quick screen for TR	Subject to technical and hemodynamic factors Underestimates severity in eccentric jets
Vena contracta width	Simple, quantitative Separates mild from severe TR	Intermediate values require further confirmation
PISA method	Quantitative	Validated in only a few studies
Flow quantitation—PWD	Quantitative	Not validated for determining TR regurgitant fraction
Jet profile—CWD	Simple, readily available	Qualitative, complementary data
Peak tricuspid E velocity	Simple, usually increased in severe TR	Depends on RA pressure and RV relaxation, TV area, and atrial fibrillation; complementary data only
Hepatic vein flow	Simple Systolic flow reversal is sensitive for severe TR	Influenced by RA pressure, atrial fibrillation

Abbreviations: CWD, continuous wave Doppler; E, peak early diastolic TMF velocity; IVC, inferior vena cava; PISA, proximal isovelocity surface area; PWD, pulsed wave Doppler; RA, right atrium; RV, right ventricle; TMF, transmitral flow; TV, tricuspid valve; TR, tricuspid regurgitation.
Source: Adapted from Ref. 21.

Table 18.3 Echocardiographic and Doppler Parameters Used in Grading Tricuspid Regurgitation Severity

Parameter	Mild	Moderate	Severe
Tricuspid valve	Usually normal	Normal or abnormal	Abnormal/Flail leaflet/Poor coaptation
RV/RA/IVC size	Normal[a]	Normal or dilated	Usually dilated[b]
Jet area-central jets (cm^2)[c]	<5	5–10	>10
VC width (cm)[d]	Not defined	Not defined, but <0.7	>0.7
PISA radius (cm)[e]	<0.5	0.6–0.9	>0.9
Jet density and contour—CWD	Soft and parabolic	Dense, variable contour	Dense, triangular with early peaking
Hepatic vein flow[f]	Systolic dominance	Systolic blunting	Systolic reversal

[a]Unless there are other reasons for RA or RV dilation. Normal 2D measurements from the apical four-chamber view: RV mediolateral end-diastolic dimension <4.3 cm, RV end-diastolic area <35.5 cm^2, maximal RA mediolateral and superoinferior dimensions <4.6 cm and 4.9 cm, respectively, maximal RA volume <33 mL/m^2 (22,23).
[b]Exception: acute tricuspid regurgitation.
[c]At a Nyquist limit of 50 to 60 cm/s. Not valid in eccentric jets. Jet area is not recommended as the sole parameter of tricuspid regurgitation severity due to its dependence on hemodynamic and technical factors.
[d]At a Nyquist limit of 50 to 60 cm/s.
[e] Baseline shift with Nyquist limit of 28 cm/s.
[f]Other conditions may cause systolic blunting (e.g., atrial fibrillation, elevated RA pressure).
Abbreviations: CWD, continuous wave Doppler; IVC, inferior vena cava; PISA, proximal isovelocity surface area; RA, right atrium; RV, right ventricle; VC, vena contracta.
Source: Adapted from Ref. 21.

Table 18.4 Tricuspid Stenosis Severity

Specific findings	
Mean pressure gradient	≥5 mmHg
Inflow time-velocity integral	>60 cm
Pressure half-time	≥190 ms
Valve area by continuity equations[a]	≤1 cm^2
Supportive findings	
Enlarged right atrium ≥ moderate	
Dilated inferior vena cava	

[a]Stroke volume derived from left or right ventricular outflow. In the presence of more than mild tricuspid regurgitation, the derived valve area will be underestimated. Nevertheless, a value ≤1 cm^2 implies a significant hemodynamic burden imposed by the combined lesion.
Source: Adapted from Ref. 24.

agents most often involved in right-sided endocarditis come from the skin flora, in particular staphylococci. Structural heart disease is not a prerequisite but is often present. Vegetations classically appear as chaotically mobile echo-dense masses attached on the low-pressure aspect of a valve leaflet (Figs. 18.17 and 18.18). Thus, TV vegetations are typically found on the atrial aspect of the valve, while PV vegetations are seen on the ventricular aspect of the valve. Most investigators found that the sensitivity of TTE and TEE for right-sided endocarditis and TR were similar. Transesophageal echocardiography provides a superior characterization of vegetation size and extent as well as a greater specificity for endocarditis (25,26).

The mechanisms of TR, caused by endocarditis, include leaflet destruction or perforation, abnormal coaptation from chordal, or papillary muscle rupture (11). A vegetation size >10 mm is associated with an increased likelihood of pulmonary emboli (27).

Infection of indwelling central venous catheters and permanent pacemakers also occasionally predispose to right-sided endocarditis, which occurs in the face of valvular microtrauma, followed by bacteremia (28). The identification of vegetations on foreign material can be challenging with TTE as catheters often produce reverberations (29,30). Transesophageal echocardiography offers the advantage of a higher resolution to differentiate vegetation attachment to indwelling catheters or wires versus attachment to valves (30). Vegetations on pacemaker wires typically appear as sleeve-like with satellite vegetations on the TV associated in more than two-third of cases of pacemaker wire infections (Fig. 18.18) (29–32).

Transesophageal echocardiography also offers the ability to visualize a greater catheter length, including the superior vena cava, using the sagittal 90° to 120° bicaval view. Importantly, the site of pacemaker or defibrillator infection may be in the pulse generator pocket, remote from the imaging capabilities of TEE and sometimes even missed by clinical examination (32). Thus, a negative TEE does not preclude the diagnosis of cardiac device infection. In cases with a high level of suspicion, evaluation of the pacemaker generator pocket with a computed tomography (CT) scan can complement the TEE, especially in febrile patients soon after device implantation (<12 weeks) (32). Almost all patients with proven or strongly suspected endocarditis on permanent pacemaker or defibrillator wires must have these surgically removed (28,30,32,33). The imaging specialist in the OR is in a fortunate position to confirm the diagnosis and rule out the presence of TV and right-heart injury following the pacemaker lead extraction.

Abscess

An abscess is an encapsulated collection of necrotic and infected debris. The most common site of a cardiac abscess is the aortic root in association with an AoV infection (34,35). Left, and especially right, atrioventricular groove abscesses are uncommon, insidious, and associated with fistulous tracts and false aneurysms. They are more common in drug addiction–related endocarditis (35). A cardiac abscess appears typically as an oval or circular lesion containing different echo-densities, reflecting solid, fluid, and gaseous necrotic contents. Transesophageal echocardiography has been shown to be superior to TTE in disclosing perivalvular abscesses (see Fig. 14.35) (35). One should bear in mind that the right coronary artery is surrounded by adipose tissue in the right atrioventricular groove and may appear as a small echo-free space. This should not be mistaken for an abscess or tumor. Adipose tissue appears more homogeneous, echo-dense, and speckled, while a tricuspid abscess is usually associated with significant tricuspid leaflet infection with an RV to RA flow seen within an

annular perforation by color Doppler imaging. The presence of a pulmonary root abscess is usually associated with a prosthetic valve or conduit and is extremely rare. The diagnosis is generally difficult to establish by TEE because of the anterior location of the pulmonary artery trunk in the far field from the esophagus. Often, CT or magnetic resonance imaging is required to confirm the diagnosis.

RHEUMATIC VALVE DISEASE

Over the last 30 years, cases of rheumatic fever have been on the decline as a result of aggressive antibiotic treatment of streptococcal infections; however, rheumatic disease is still prevalent in regions of poor socioeconomic status. Rheumatic tricuspid valvulitis seldom accounts for tricuspid involvement in rheumatic disease in Western countries (36). Most commonly, functional TR occurs due to RV pressure overload and tricuspid annular dilatation as a result of pulmonary hypertension from rheumatic MS. Severe TR is substantially reduced following surgical mitral valvuloplasty or replacement (37).

When rheumatic tricuspid valvulitis occurs, the most common result is leaflet retraction and thickening with chordal fusion and shortening causing TR (Fig. 18.19). Sometimes the subvalvular involvement is the only major finding, and the leaflets are only mildly scarred (Fig. 18.20). Less frequently, rheumatic valvulitis leads to commissural fusion in the closed position with diffuse fibrosis, causing TS (11). The frequency of TS differs between reports, ranging between 5% and 38% of patients with rheumatic heart disease (5).

The 2D diagnosis of TS rests on echocardiographic visualization of tricuspid leaflet thickening and restricted motion. Doppler echocardiography provides insight into TS severity with the typical flattening of the tricuspid E-wave slope and prolongation of the tricuspid deceleration slope. Mild-to-moderate TS produces mean gradients of 3 to 9 mmHg, while severe TS is generally present with mean gradients >10 mmHg. The natural history of mild-to-moderate TS is generally benign and does not appear to benefit from surgery (38).

Other Inflammatory Valvulopathies

Another form of characteristically right-sided inflammatory valve disease is carcinoid heart disease. Carcinoid valvulitis is most commonly seen with small bowel carcinoid complicated by liver metastases, which produce high levels of circulating serotonin and systemic symptoms (e.g., flushing, bronchospasm, and diarrhea). However, occasionally, patients with primary ovarian carcinoid, in whom drainage from the ovarian veins bypasses the portal circulation, or patients with metastatic disease in lymph nodes in whom drainage via the thoracic duct may bypass the portal circulation present with carcinoid heart disease (39,40). Serotonin stimulates plaque development on the TV and PV, leading to leaflet thickening and

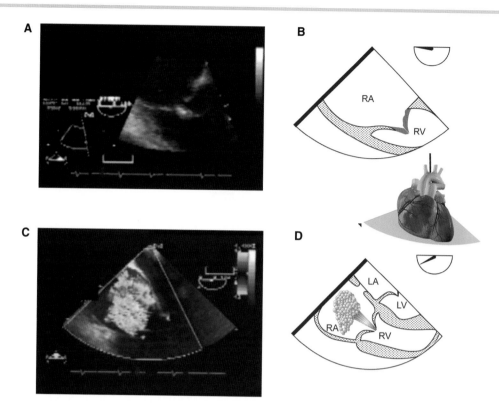

Figure 18.19 Rheumatic TV. Zoomed mid-esophageal four-chamber view (**A,B**) of the TV shows restricted motion from chordal shortening and fusion with severe tricuspid regurgitation (**C,D**). *Abbreviations*: LA, left atrium; LV, left ventricle; RA, right atrium; RV, right ventricle; TV, tricuspid valve.

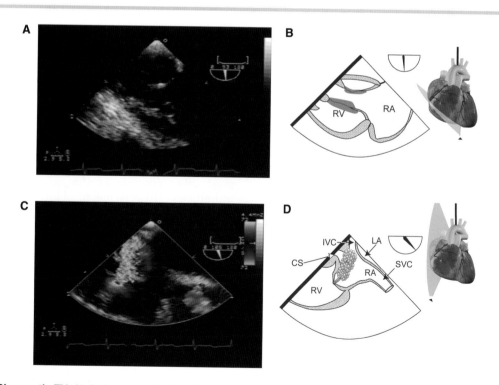

Figure 18.20 Rheumatic TV. (A,B) Transgastric RV inflow view at 90° shows shortened chordae to the TV anterior leaflet. **(C,D)** Mid-esophageal 120° view with rightward rotation demonstrates multiple tricuspid regurgitation jets. *Abbreviations*: CS, coronary sinus; IVC, inferior vena cava; LA, left atrium; RA, right atrium; RV, right ventricle; SVC, superior vena cava; TV, tricuspid valve.

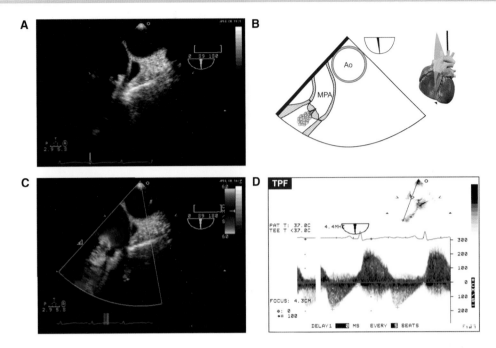

Figure 18.21   Carcinoid heart disease. (A–C) Upper esophageal aortic arch short-axis view in a patient with carcinoid heart disease shows retracted leaflets of the pulmonic valve in an open position with secondary pulmonic regurgitation. **(D)** Continuous wave Doppler of TPF confirms pulmonic regurgitation and stenosis with a diastolic pressure gradient of 14.3 mmHg. *Abbreviations*: Ao, aorta; MPA, main pulmonary artery; TPF, transpulmonic flow.

rigidity (Figs. 18.21 and 18.22) (11). The most common echocardiographic lesion, found in 97% of patients, with carcinoid heart disease is TR (41). It was moderate or severe in 90% of patients. In those patients in whom the PV could be examined with Doppler echocardiography, 81% had some degree of pulmonic regurgitation (PR), while 53% had some degree of pulmonic stenosis (PS). Cardiac metastases were identified in 4% of patients. Unless an intracardiac right-to-left shunt is present, it is unusual for the left heart to be involved in carcinoid disease as serotonin, and its metabolites are inactivated in the lung. Left-side lesions are only seen in 7% of patients (41). The short-term prognosis of carcinoid disease was formerly poor, but as a result of disease control by chemotherapy and with medium-term survival increasingly achieved, patients with significant right-heart failure symptoms are occasionally referred for valve surgery.

Connolly et al. (42) reported a nonrandomized series of 26 patients operated on for carcinoid valve disease. All had severe TR and significant mixed PV disease with (*i*) severe right-heart failure symptoms, (*ii*) controlled systemic disease, and (*iii*) no concurrent severe medical problems. All patients underwent TV replacement; most had pulmonic valvectomy; and in five, removal of endomyocardial metastases was carried out. The perioperative mortality was 35%, with a substantial number of deaths occurring as a result of right-heart failure or uncontrolled postoperative bleeding. Survival of surgically treated patients was 40% at two years compared with 8% for medically

treated patients. Furthermore, when PV disease was present, data from the same institution supports the use of PV replacement over simple valvectomy in reducing RV dilatation (43). However, it is possible that carcinoid disease may accelerate bioprosthetic tissue valve degeneration in the tricuspid and pulmonary positions (43).

MYXOID DEGENERATION

Degenerative myxoid, or myxomatous, valvular disease typically affects the MV, and TV involvement most often consists of functional TR secondary to pulmonary hypertension. However, myxomatous tricuspid degeneration is rarely seen and is usually encountered in the setting of concomitant MV disease. Inheritable disorders of connective tissue, such as Marfan's disease, may be a common link. Less is known about the 3D geometry of the TV than that of the saddle-shaped MV. Three-dimensional TTE in children has shown that the tricuspid annulus changes shape significantly throughout the cardiac cycle and that the greatest change in diameter is in a medial/lateral direction. There was also a larger degree of bending between the anterior (outflow) plane and the posterior plane of the annulus than seen in the MV (44). The typical appearance of tricuspid leaflet prolapse is mid-systolic coaptation posterior to the annular plane. Chordal rupture is usually easily identified and causes significant leaflet malcoaptation with the leaflet tip

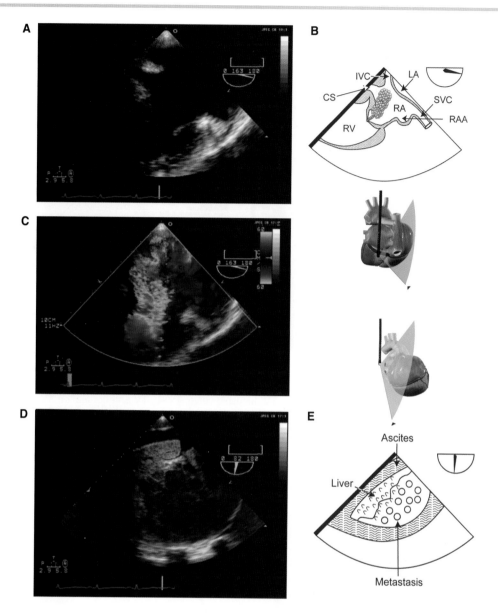

Figure 18.22 Carcinoid heart disease of TV. (A–C) Mid-esophageal views with rightward rotation shows severe tricuspid regurgitation with a huge regurgitant orifice due to thickened TV leaflets retracted in the open position. **(D,E)** Transgastric view at 82° of the liver in the same patient shows liver metastasis from the large carcinoid tumor. *Abbreviations*: CS, coronary sinus; IVC, inferior vena cava; LA, left atrium; RA, right atrium; RAA, right atrial appendage; SVC, superior vena cava; TV, tricuspid valve.

typically pointing toward the RA in association with severe eccentric TR directed opposite the diseased leaflet (Fig. 18.23).

PULMONIC VALVE DISEASE

Assessment, by TEE, of the PV remains challenging because of its anterior location relative to the esophagus in the far field (Figs. 18.24 and 18.25). In most cases, other than endocarditis or inflammatory disease, PV disease is congenital in origin. The normal PV is a semilunar valve with three cusps termed as the anterior, left posterior, and right posterior.

Pulmonic stenosis is almost always congenital and is valvular rather than sub- or supravalvular. In congenital PS, the valve can be unicuspid (usually acommissural), bicuspid (Figs. 18.26 and 18.27), or tricuspid with partial fusion of the commissures. Unicuspid valves are the most common finding in isolated PS (45). Bicuspid valves are usually found in patients with valvular PS and Tetralogy of Fallot (Fig. 18.28) (46). A PV with three cusps and extremely thickened and dysplastic leaflets is found only in 15% of cases of isolated PS (47) but is often found in Noonan's syndrome, which is characterized by short stature, abnormal facies (often with hypertelorism),

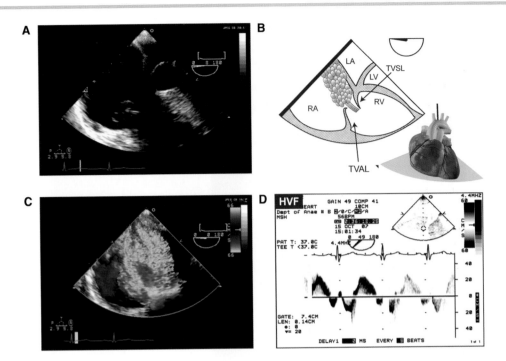

Figure 18.23 Flail anterior TV leaflet. Modified mid-esophageal four-chamber views (**A,B**) show a flail TVAL and torn chordae resulting in severe tricuspid regurgitation (**C**) with associated HVF systolic reversal (**D**). *Abbreviations*: HVF, hepatic venous flow; LA, left atrium; LV, left ventricle; RA, right atrium; RV, right ventricle; TV, tricuspid valve; TVAL, TV anterior leaflet; TVSL, TV septal leaflet. ⌐ᕁ

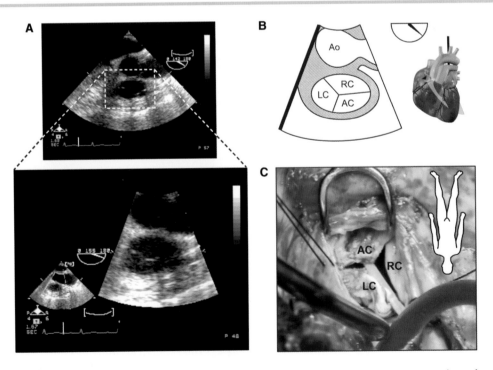

Figure 18.24 Normal PV. (**A,B**) Modified mid-esophageal long-axis view at 142° shows a transverse view of a normal PV. (**C**) Corresponding intraoperative view is shown. *Abbreviations*: AC, anterior cusp; Ao, aorta; LC, left cusp; PV, pulmonic valve; RC, right cusp. ⌐ᕁ

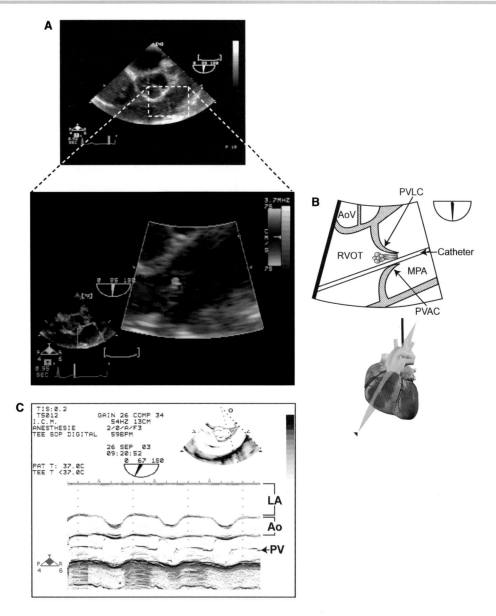

Figure 18.25 **Normal PV.** Mid-esophageal right ventricular inflow/outflow views at 85° (**A,B**) and M-mode (**C**) show the normal PV in a 23-year-old man undergoing mitral valve replacement. A small jet of PV regurgitation is present around the pulmonary artery catheter. *Abbreviations*: Ao, aorta; AoV, aortic valve; LA, left atrium; MPA, main pulmonary artery; PV, pulmonic valve; PVAC, PV anterior cusp; PVLC, PV left cusp; RVOT, right ventricular outflow tract.

webbed neck, and chest deformities (48). Quadricuspid valves are more common in the pulmonic position than the aortic but are usually functionally normal. Acquired PS is uncommon occurring in the presence of rheumatic, carcinoid disease, or compression from extra-cardiac masses.

Historically, PS is quantified using peak-to-peak gradients from catheterization data (49), although now peak gradients are often measured by CW Doppler echocardiography: mild PS defined as a peak gradient <36 mmHg, moderate PS as peak gradient 36 to 64 mmHg, and severe or critical PS as a peak gradient >64 mmHg (50).

A recent study has suggested that mean Doppler gradients agree better with invasively measured peak-to-peak gradients and should be used for clinical decision-making, although this has yet to be widely accepted (51). Measurement of the PV area is difficult and not typically used for clinical decision-making. Most individuals with severe PV stenosis are treated in childhood by either percutaneous valvuloplasty or surgical valvotomy. Variable degrees of residual regurgitation may ensue, producing RV dilatation when moderate or severe. The natural history of mild-to-moderate PV stenosis is benign and intervention is seldom required (52).

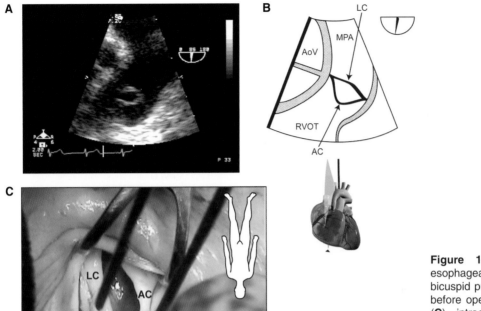

Figure 18.26 Pulmonic stenosis. Mid-esophageal view at 85° (**A,B**) shows a stenotic bicuspid pulmonic valve in a 29-year-old man before open commissurotomy confirmed with (**C**) intraoperative findings. *Abbreviations*: AoV, aortic valve; AC, anterior cusp; LC, left cusp; MPA, main pulmonary artery; RVOT, right ventricular outflow tract.

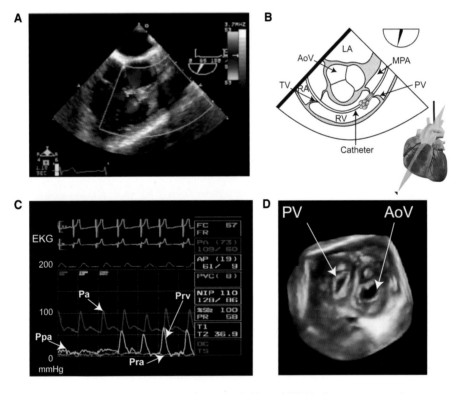

Figure 18.27   PV stenosis. A 29-year-old man presents with a stenotic bicuspid PV before open commissurotomy. (**A,B**) Color Doppler mid-esophageal right ventricular inflow/outflow view shows pulmonic regurgitation. (**C**) Hemodynamics measure the gradient between the Ppa and the Prv from a PAC. The Prv was obtained through the paceport lumen of the PAC. (**D**) Intraoperative epicardial 3D echocardiogram of PV stenosis viewed from the pulmonary artery. *Abbreviations*: AoV, aortic valve; EKG, electrocardiogram; LA, left atrium; MPA, main pulmonary artery; Pa, arterial pressure; PAC, pulmonary artery catheter; Ppa, pulmonary artery pressure; Pra, right atrial pressure; Prv, right ventricular pressure; PV, pulmonic valve; RA, right atrium; RV, right ventricle; TV, tricuspid valve. *Source*: Photo D courtesy of Philips Healthcare.

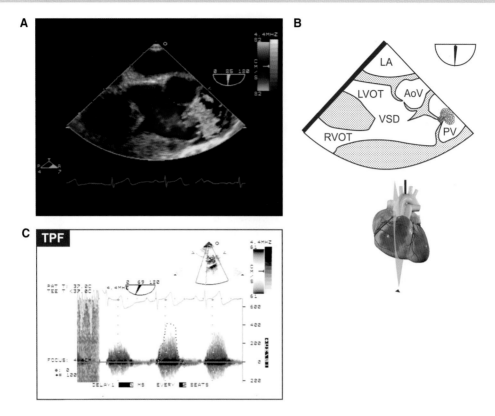

Figure 18.28 Tetralogy of Fallot. Pulmonic stenosis is present in a patient with unrepaired TOF. (**A,B**) Color Doppler mid-esophageal long-axis view shows thickened PV cusps doming in systole and infundibular narrowing, consistent with PS. Also present are a large VSD and an overriding aorta. The color Doppler shows aliased flow of PS at the PV level with free flow across the VSD and increased velocity across the RVOT. (**C**) Continuous wave Doppler of the TPF reveals a peak gradient of 70 mmHg with a mean gradient of 31 mmHg. *Abbreviations*: Ao, aorta; AoV, aortic valve; LA, left atrium; LVOT, left ventricular outflow tract; PS, pulmonic stenosis; PV, pulmonic valve; RVOT, right ventricular outflow tract; TOF, Tetralogy of Fallot; TPF, transpulmonic flow; VSD, ventricular septal defect.

Poststenotic dilatation of the pulmonary artery trunk is common in PS and can sometimes be severe enough to cause pulmonary artery aneurysms (Fig. 18.29). It is often out of proportion to the degree of PS. The left pulmonary artery is more often involved than the right, which is believed to be secondary to the fact that the high-velocity jet of PS is preferentially directed to the left main pulmonary artery because of the acute angle of the takeoff of the right main pulmonary artery (53).

Associated echocardiographic findings in PS include RV hypertrophy (>5-mm thickness). With progressive worsening, PS, RV, and RA dilatation also occurs. The RVSP should be estimated from the tricuspid regurgitant jet. In the presence of valvular PS, the pulmonary artery systolic pressure is determined by the RVSP minus the PV pressure gradient (see Fig. 5.27).

Pulmonic valve regurgitation can occur as a result of valvular abnormalities or annular dilatation, the latter being due either to increased flow through the valve (e.g., by an intracardiac systemic-to-pulmonary shunt) or secondary to significant chronic pulmonary hypertension (Fig. 18.26). Valvular abnormalities are almost always acquired as congenital significant PR is very rare. Although endocarditis, carcinoid, and rheumatic disease can all cause significant PR, the most common etiology is valve dysfunction after correction of a previous stenosis (48). Almost all patients in a recent series of patients with severe PR had a previous tetralogy repair with valvotomy (54) (Fig. 18.30) or endocarditis (Fig. 18.31).

The use of short-axis and sagittal views is helpful to visualize native or prosthetic PVs. Demonstration of PV stenosis and regurgitation by color and spectral Doppler is more easily done from above through the upper esophageal window in the sagittal view at 90° to 100° (Fig. 18.7) where pulmonary flow is nearly parallel to the ultrasound beam. PR appears as a blue, anteriorly directed color jet from the posteriorly situated pulmonary artery to the RV. Most jets are monochromic unless pulmonary hypertension is present and may only occur in early diastole. Because they are low velocity, laminar, and of short duration, they may sometimes be missed. Severe PV regurgitation leads to RV volume overload with dilatation and paradoxical septal motion and may ultimately cause RV systolic dysfunction (see Chapter 10). This may, in

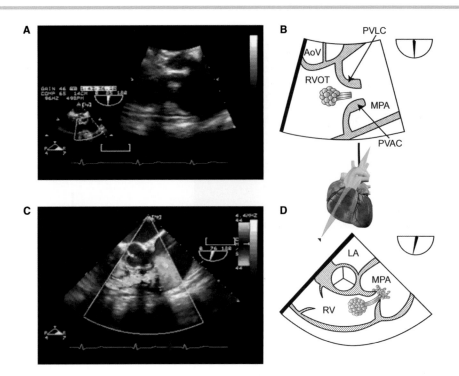

Figure 18.29 Pulmonary artery post-stenotic aneurysm. (A,B) Zoom of mid-esophageal right ventricular inflow/outflow view shows thickened PV cusps with systolic doming. **(C,D)** Color Doppler imaging shows a dilated MPA with mild pulmonic regurgitation. The gradient across the PV was measured at 19 mmHg by continuous wave Doppler (not shown). *Abbreviations*: AoV, aortic valve; LA, left atrium; MPA, main pulmonary artery; PV, pulmonic valve; PVAC, PV anterior cusp; PVLC, PV left cusp; RV, right ventricle; RVOT, right ventricular outflow tract.

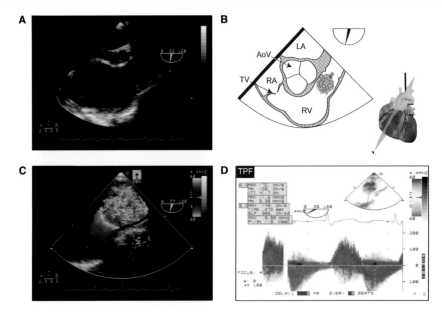

Figure 18.30 Severe PR. Severe pulmonic regurgitation (PR) is present in a patient with prior TOF repair. **(A,B)** Mid-esophageal right ventricular inflow/outflow tract view shows almost complete absence of the PV. **(C)** Color Doppler imaging demonstrates the low-velocity wide-open severe PR is associated with a high stroke volume across the PV and secondary aliased flow during systole. **(D)** By continuous wave Doppler of the TPF, a 5 mmHg mean systolic gradient is measured across the PV. *Abbreviations*: AoV, aortic valve; LA, left atrium; PR, pulmonic regurgitation; PV, pulmonic valve; RA, right atrium; RV, right ventricle; TOF, Tetralogy of Fallot; TPF, transpulmonic flow; TV, tricuspid valve.

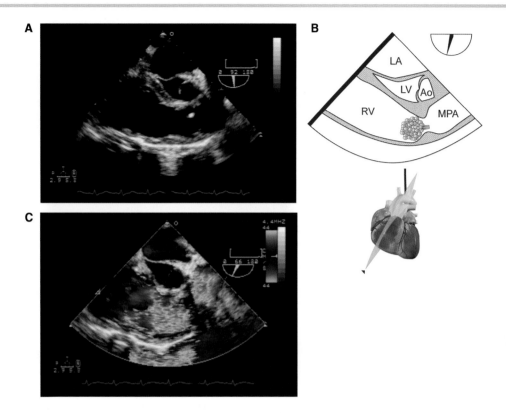

Figure 18.31 PV endocarditis. (A–C) Mid-esophageal right ventricular inflow/outflow views show a flail left posterior cusp of the PV with resulting severe pulmonic regurgitation on color Doppler imaging. *Abbreviations*: Ao, aorta; LA, left atrium; LV, left ventricle; MPA, main pulmonary artery; PV, pulmonic valve; RV, right ventricle.

Table 18.5 Echocardiographic and Doppler Parameters Used in the Evaluation of Pulmonic Regurgitation Severity: Utility, Advantages, and Limitations

Parameter	Utility/Advantages	Disadvantages
RV size	RV enlargement sensitive for chronic significant PR. Normal size virtually excludes significant PR	Enlargement seen in other conditions
Paradoxical septal motion (volume overload pattern)	Simple sign of severe PR	Not specific for PR
Jet length—color flow	Simple	Poor correlation with severity of PR
Vena contracta width	Simple quantitative method that works well for other valves	More difficult to perform; requires good images of pulmonic valve; lacks published validation
Jet deceleration rate—CWD	Simple	Steep deceleration not specific for severe PR
Flow quantitation—PWD	Quantitates regurgitant flow and fraction	Subject to significant errors due to difficulties of measurement of pulmonic annulus and a dynamic RVOT; not well validated

Abbreviations: CWD, continuous wave Doppler; PWD, pulsed wave Doppler; RV, right ventricle; PR, pulmonary regurgitation; RVOT, right ventricular outflow tract.
Source: Adapted from Ref. 21.

turn, lead to symptoms like dyspnea and atrial or ventricular arrhythmias (55). The ASE published guidelines (21) for the evaluation of PV regurgitation as summarized in Tables 18.5 and 18.6. Aside from these parameters, a recent study has shown that in patients with previously corrected congenital heart disease (most of whom had previous Tetralogy repairs or pulmonic valvotomies for PS), both a PHT of 100 ms and a diastolic "no flow" time of 80 ms (the time between cessation of regurgitant flow and onset of systolic ejection) correlated well with severe PR on pulmonary angiography (54).

Table 18.6 Echocardiographic and Doppler Parameters Used in Grading Pulmonic Regurgitation Severity

Parameter	Mild	Moderate	Severe
Pulmonic valve	Normal	Normal or abnormal	Abnormal
RV size	Normal[a]	Normal or dilated	Dilated[b]
Jet size by color Doppler[c]	Thin (usually <10 mm in length) with a narrow origin	Intermediate	Usually large, with a wide origin; may be brief in duration
Jet density and deceleration rate—CWD[d]	Soft; slow deceleration	Dense; variable deceleration	Dense; steep deceleration; early termination of diastolic flow
Pulmonary systolic flow compared to systemic flow—PWD[e]	Slightly increased	Intermediate	Greatly increased

[a]Unless there are other reasons for RV enlargement. Normal 2D measurements from the apical four-chamber view; RV mediolateral end-diastolic dimension <4.3 cm, RV end-diastolic area <35.5 cm² (23).
[b]Exception: acute PR.
[c]At a Nyquist limit of 50 to 60 cm/s.
[d]Steep deceleration is not specific for severe PR.
[e]Cutoff values for regurgitant volume and fraction are not well validated.
Abbreviations: CWD, continuous wave Doppler; PR, pulmonary regurgitation; PWD, pulsed wave Doppler; RA, right atrium; RF, regurgitant fraction; RV, right ventricle.
Source: Adapted from Ref. 21.

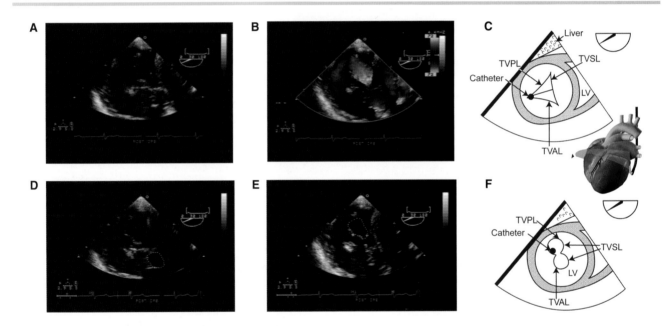

Figure 18.32 Alfieri stitch. (A–C) Transgastric short-axis view of the TV after a complex repair with bicuspidization (anterior/posterior commissure has been closed) and an Alfieri stitch joining the anterior/posterior leaflets to the TVSL. **(B)** Color Doppler imaging of this view shows flow through the two orifices. Flow directed through the posterior orifice is red, while flow directed anteriorly through the anterior orifice is blue. **(D–F)** Planimetry of the anterior and posterior orifices is shown. *Abbreviations*: LV, left ventricle; TV, tricuspid valve; TVAL, TV anterior leaflet; TVPL, TV posterior leaflet; TVSL, TV septal leaflet. 🖰

TV REPAIR—INDICATIONS AND METHODS OF REPAIR

The principal indication for TV repair is isolated moderate-to-severe TR, generally in the face of left-sided heart disease (33). For pure TV disease, surgery is generally performed for significant TR associated with right-sided heart failure. Surgical repair of the TV, using an annuloplasty ring or a suture annuloplasty (DeVega technique), is the technique of choice

as it retains the valve leaflets and provides adequate coaptation by reducing the diameter of the TV annulus (12). Alfieri has described applying his central "stitch" that he pioneered in MV repairs to the TV to create a "clover leaf" valve opening (Fig. 18.32) (56). Bicuspidization of the TV can also be done in complex cases (57). Tricuspid valve replacement is performed when severe valve destruction has occurred or when previous TV repair has failed to relieve significant TR. Residual moderate-to-severe TR on the postoperative

TEE should probably be addressed by replacement of the valve or re-repair if the patient is stable enough.

Predictors of adverse survival following TV surgery include severe TR as assessed echocardiographically, poor preoperative New York Heart Association functional class, LV systolic dysfunction, need for coronary revascularization, and need for TV replacement (3). Transesophageal echocardiography plays an important role in evaluating the success of surgical repair and was found to influence the surgical plan in 10% of cases in a large single-center study of 401 patients. The presence of residual TR (10–15%) disclosed by intraoperative TEE has a controversial ability in predicting long-term mortality following valve surgery but predicts at least a reduced event-free survival (2,3). More recent work has also shown that the amount of distortion of the TV apparatus were independent predictors of residual TR after annuloplasty in patients with TR undergoing left-sided heart surgery (58). The amount of tethering of the TV leaflets measured by the tethering distance from the annular plane to the point of coaptation and by the area subtended by the annular plane and the leaflets (the "tethering area") was measured. A tethering distance of >0.76 cm and a tethering area of >1.63 cm^2 were better predictors of postoperative moderate or severe TR than the degree of preoperative TR.

Suture Annuloplasty, Complications, Failed Repair

The TV suture annuloplasty by the DeVega technique is done with a 2.0 propylene suture button stressed with Teflon. A first suture line is started at the anteroseptal commissure and proceeds clockwise to a point just beyond the posteroseptal commissure (Fig. 18.33) (59).

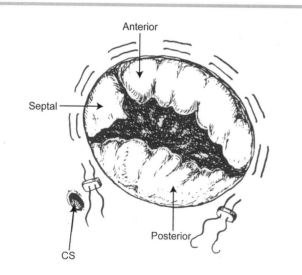

Figure 18.33 Tricuspid annuloplasty. DeVega's tricuspid annuloplasty technique, with a double purse-string suture is shown. *Abbreviation*: CS, coronary sinus. Source: Adapted with permission from Ref. 59.

A second suture line is similarly run 2 to 3 mm above the first one. The sutures are then tied with Teflon over a 27 valve sizer in the annulus to prevent valvular stenosis (60). Significant residual TR following repair usually becomes clinically evident with symptoms of fatigue and signs of right-sided heart failure on long-term follow-up. Perioperative TEE may be useful in detecting residual problems following cardiac surgery. Indeed, RV dimensions and systolic function remain important predictors of long-term success as the annuloplasty repair alone may not correct incomplete tricuspid leaflet closure in the setting of chronic RV remodeling. Dehiscence of a DeVega suture annuloplasty may appear on TEE as a horizontal linear echodensity running across the TV plane.

Annuloplasty Rings

Tricuspid annuloplasty rings appear on tomographic echo planes as two echo-dense annular structures located at the base of opposite leaflets on the atrial side of the valve, with variable acoustic shadowing (Figs. 18.34 and 18.35). Tricuspid leaflet mobility is expected to be somewhat reduced, but stenosis is rare as the annular dimensions remain large. Tricuspid regurgitation, or vegetation, is usually easily demonstrated at 30° to 90° in the mid-esophageal, the transitional gastroesophageal, and the sagittal transgastric views (Fig. 18.36).

VALVE REPLACEMENT

The American College of Cardiology and the American Heart Association established Guidelines for the Management of Patients with Valvular Heart Disease in 2006 (33). The recommendations for tricuspid surgery are summarized in Table 18.7. The level of evidence for each indication was discussed in Chapter 15. Recent guidelines described by the American Society of Echocardiography's Guidelines and Standards Committee and the Task Force on Prosthetic Valves may be used to assess TV or PV prosthetic stenosis (Tables 18.8 and 18.9) and regurgitation (Tables 18.10 and 18.11) (61).

The surgical decision to replace the TV is usually made preoperatively on the basis of extensive leaflet disease. Such is the case in Ebstein's anomaly, mixed or predominantly stenotic degenerated calcified leaflets, or extensive destruction by endocarditis. However, TV replacement does carry a higher operative mortality compared with repair, partly because it is often performed in light of previous cardiac surgery. In a series spanning 20 years, mortality approached 22% with about the same percentage of patients also requiring permanent pacing. This underscores the close relationship of the tricuspid annulus to the conduction system (62).

Replacement of the PV is increasingly performed, especially in patients with previous repair of Tetralogy of Fallot who present with RV volume overload from severe PV regurgitation (55). It is also done with implantation of a heterologous aortic or

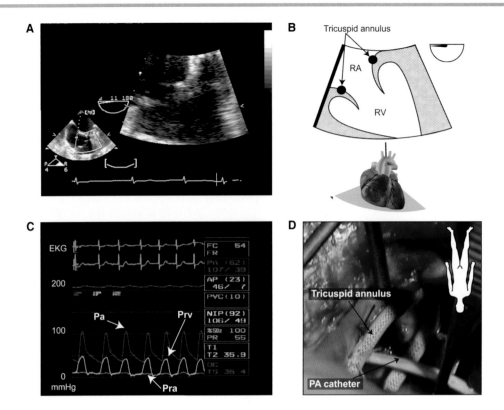

Figure 18.34 TV annuloplasty. (A,B) Zoomed mid-esophageal right ventricular view shows a TV annuloplasty ring. **(C)** After the procedure no significant stenosis is present as demonstrated by the absence of a diastolic gradient across the TV. This is confirmed on the simultaneous Pra and Prv tracings obtained through the paceport lumen of the PAC. **(D)** Corresponding intraoperative findings. *Abbreviations*: EKG, electrocardiogram; Pa, arterial pressure; PAC, pulmonary artery catheter; Pra, right atrial pressure; Prv, right ventricular pressure; RA, right atrium; RV, right ventricle; TV, tricuspid valve. *Source*: Photo D courtesy of Dr. Denis Bouchard.

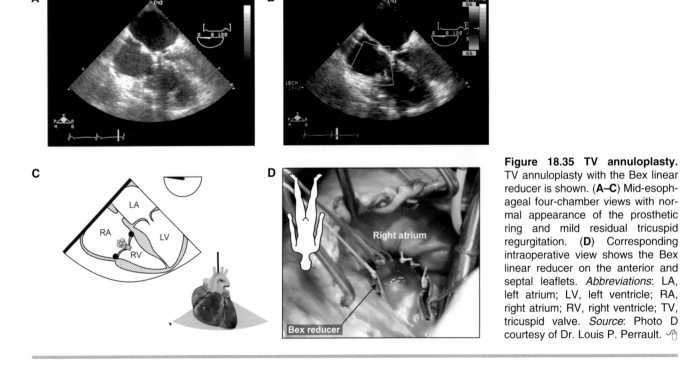

Figure 18.35 TV annuloplasty. TV annuloplasty with the Bex linear reducer is shown. **(A–C)** Mid-esophageal four-chamber views with normal appearance of the prosthetic ring and mild residual tricuspid regurgitation. **(D)** Corresponding intraoperative view shows the Bex linear reducer on the anterior and septal leaflets. *Abbreviations*: LA, left atrium; LV, left ventricle; RA, right atrium; RV, right ventricle; TV, tricuspid valve. *Source*: Photo D courtesy of Dr. Louis P. Perrault.

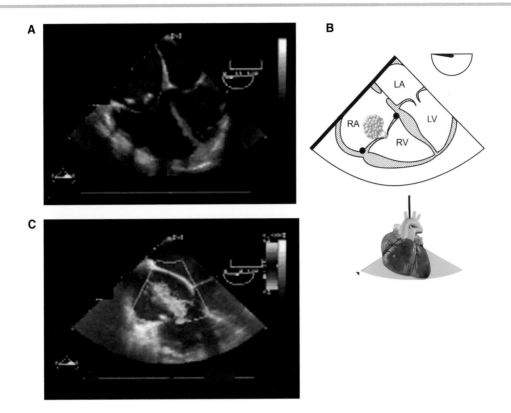

Figure 18.36 Dehisced TV annuloplasty. (A–C) Mid-esophageal four-chamber views in a patient with a previous TV annuloplasty shows the band has dehisced resulting in significant tricuspid regurgitation. *Abbreviations*: LA, left atrium; LV, left ventricle; RA, right atrium; RV, right ventricle; TV, tricuspid valve.

Table 18.7 Indications for Tricuspid Valve Replacement or Repair in Tricuspid Regurgitation

Class I	Tricuspid valve repair is beneficial for severe TR[a] in patients with MV disease requiring MV surgery. (Level of Evidence: B)
Class IIa	1. Tricuspid valve replacement or annuloplasty is reasonable for severe primary TR[a] when symptomatic. (Level of Evidence: C)
	2. Tricuspid valve replacement is reasonable for severe TR secondary to diseased/abnormal tricuspid valve leaflets not amenable to annuloplasty or repair. (Level of Evidence: C)
Class IIb	Tricuspid annuloplasty may be considered for less than severe TR[a] in patients undergoing MV surgery when there is pulmonary hypertension or tricuspid annular dilatation. (Level of Evidence: C)
Class III	1. Tricuspid valve replacement or annuloplasty is not indicated in asymptomatic patients with TR whose pulmonary artery systolic pressure is less than 60 mmHg in the presence of a normal MV. (Level of Evidence: C)
	2. Tricuspid valve replacement or annuloplasty is not indicated in patients with mild primary TR[a]. (Level of Evidence: C)

[a] See Table 18.3.
Abbreviations: MV, mitral valve; NYHA, New York Heart Association; TR, tricuspid regurgitation.
Source: Adapted from Ref. 33.

pulmonary homograft in pulmonary position as part of the Ross procedure, a treatment for congenital aortic stenosis in childhood and adolescence. In this procedure, AoV replacement is done by transplanting the native PV and root to the aortic position, thus avoiding the need for long-term anticoagulation while allowing the potential for the neoaortic valve to grow in children. Stenosis of the prosthetic heterologous aortic or pulmonic homograft in pulmonary position is a late complication (Fig. 18.37), sometimes difficult to diagnose by TTE alone.

Tricuspid Valvectomy

In the setting of significant endocarditis, total valvectomy is sometimes necessary and is, surprisingly, hemodynamically well tolerated initially. Once the infection is brought under control, a second-stage procedure with tricuspid prosthetic valve implantation is performed to prevent wide-open TR progression to severe right-heart failure. This technique has a definite place in the treatment of TV or PV endocarditis in IV drug abusers (63).

Table 18.8 Doppler Parameters of Prosthetic Tricuspid Valve Function

	Consider valve stenosis[a]
Peak velocity[b]	>1.7 m/s
Mean gradient[b]	≥6 mmHg
Pressure half-time	≥230 ms
EOA and VTI_{PRTV}/VTI_{LVO}	No data yet available for tricuspid prostheses

[a]Because of respiratory variation, average ≥5 cycles.
[b]May be increased also with valvular regurgitation.
Abbreviations: EOA, effective orifice area; LVO, left ventricular outflow; PRTV, prosthetic tricuspid valve; VTI, velocity-time integral.
Source: From Ref. 61.

Table 18.9 Findings Suspicious for Prosthetic Pulmonary Valve Stenosis

Cusp or leaflet thickening or immobility
Narrowing of forward color map
Peak velocity through the prosthesis >3 m/s or >2 m/s through a homograft[a]
Increase in peak velocity on serial studies[b]
Impaired RV function or elevated RV systolic pressure

[a]Suspicious but not diagnostic of stenosis.
[b]More reliable parameter.
Abbreviation: RV, right ventricle.
Source: From Ref. 61.

Table 18.10 Echocardiographic and Doppler Parameters Used in Grading Severity of Prosthetic Tricuspid Valve Regurgitation

Parameter	Mild	Moderate	Severe
Valve structure	Usually normal	Abnormal or valve dehiscence	Abnormal or valve dehiscence
Jet area by color Doppler, central jets only (cm^2)	<5	5–10	>10
VC width (cm)[a]	Not defined	Not defined, but <0.7	>0.7
Jet density and contour by CW Doppler	Incomplete or faint, parabolic	Dense, variable contour	Dense with early peaking
Doppler systolic hepatic flow	Normal or blunted	Blunted	Holosystolic reversal
Right atrium, right ventricle, IVC	Normal[b]	Dilated	Markedly dilated

[a]For a valvular TR jet, extrapolated from native TR; unknown cutoffs for paravalvular TR.
[b]If no other reason for dilatation.
Abbreviations: CW, continuous wave; IVC, inferior vena cava; TR, tricuspid regurgitation; VC, vena contracta.
Source: Adapted from Refs. 21 and 61.

Table 18.11 Evaluation of Severity of Prosthetic Pulmonary Valve Regurgitation

Parameter	Mild	Moderate	Severe
Valve structure	Usually normal	Abnormal or valve dehiscence	Abnormal or valve dehiscence
RV size	Normal[a]	Normal or dilated	Dilated[b]
Jet size by color Doppler (central jets)[c]	Thin with a narrow origin; jet width 25% of pulmonary annulus	Intermediate; jet width 26–50% of pulmonary annulus	Usually large, with a wide origin; jet width >50% of pulmonary annulus; may be brief in duration
Jet density by CW Doppler	Incomplete or faint	Dense	Dense
Jet deceleration rate by CW Doppler	Slow deceleration	Variable deceleration	Steep deceleration[d], early termination of diastolic flow
Pulmonary systolic flow vs. systemic flow by PW Doppler[e]	Slightly increased	Intermediate	Greatly increased
Diastolic flow reversal in the pulmonary artery	None	Present	Present

[a] Unless other cause of RV dilatation exists, including residual postsurgical dilatation.
[b] Unless there are other reasons for RV enlargement. Acute PR is an exception. RV volume overload is usually accompanied with typical paradoxical septal motion.
[c] At a Nyquist limit of 50 to 60 cm/s; parameter applies to central jets and not eccentric jets.
[d] Steep deceleration is not specific for severe PR.
[e] Cutoff values for regurgitant volume and fraction are not well validated.
Abbreviations: CW, continuous wave; PR, pulmonic regurgitation; RV, right ventricular.
Source: Adapted from Refs. 21 and 61.

Types of Valve Prosthesis

Bioprosthesis have been the most commonly implanted valves in the tricuspid and pulmonic position, usually in the setting of refractory right-sided endocarditis. The need for chronic anticoagulation is avoided in subjects at high risk of bleeding or deemed unreliable to benefit overall from such therapy. Unfortunately, bioprosthetic valve failure occurs in approximately 50% of patients at 10 years

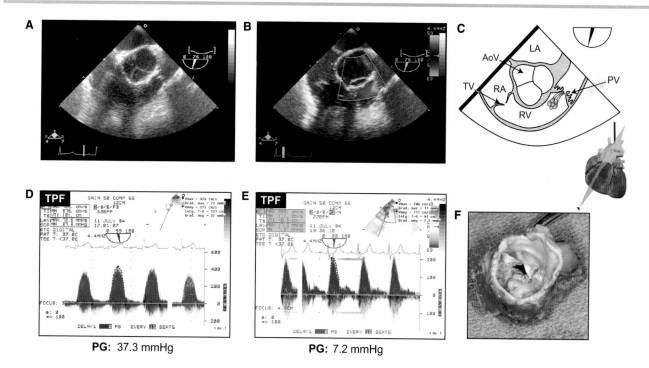

PG: 37.3 mmHg   **PG: 7.2 mmHg**

Figure 18.37   PV stenosis. A patient presents for reoperation for a stenotic pulmonary homograft after a Ross procedure for congenital aortic stenosis. (**A–C**) Mid-esophageal RV inflow/outflow views show the thickened and restricted PV cusps. (**D**) Continuous wave TPF Doppler identifies an elevated peak pressure gradient of 37.3 mmHg. (**E**) After reoperation, the latter gradient decreased to 7.2 mmHg. (**F**) Excised stenotic prosthetic pulmonary homograft is shown. *Abbreviations*: AoV, aortic valve; LA, left atrium; RA, right atrium; RV, right ventricle; PG, pressure gradient; PV, pulmonic valve; TPF, transpulmonic flow; TV, tricuspid valve. *Source*: Courtesy of Drs. André Saint-Pierre, André Martineau, and Jean Perron from Hôpital Laval, Quebec, Canada.

postimplantation and may require reoperation (64). Mechanical valve replacement offers greater durability but requires chronic anticoagulation (65). This may not be any more a significant issue in patients with rheumatic or degenerative disease where MV involvement and atrial fibrillation are commonly associated with TV pathology and warrant anticoagulation by themselves. However, mechanical prosthesis in tricuspid position prevents the implantation of endoventricular pacemaker leads in this group of patients in which atrioventricular block is common.

In view of the specific RV geometry, it was believed that the lower profile and the lesser procoagulant tendency of bioprosthesis in the setting of a low-pressure system would reduce thrombotic complications compared with mechanical valves. The poor performance of tilting-disk valves in the 1980s appeared to support this point, but more recent data on the good long-term performance of the low-profile bileaflet mechanical valves may outweigh the risk of long-term tissue valve failure in patients likely to be reliable in taking anticoagulant therapy (66). A new approach has been the implantation of a mitral homograft in tricuspid position with adjustment of papillary muscle tension obtained by two ventriculotomy apertures through which each papillary muscle is inserted (67).

Transesophageal echocardiography assessment of TV prosthesis begins, as for native valves, in the mid-esophageal four-chamber view (Fig. 18.38). The presence of coexisting mitral and aortic prostheses requires the use of further views, in particular sagittal views, so that the acoustic shadowing from the left-sided prosthesis located more superoposteriorly than their right-sided counterparts are circumvented. The atrial aspect of the tricuspid prosthesis can be shown with relative ease at 30° to 120° in the mid-esophageal and in the transitional gastroesophageal views. The transgastric views at 60° to 120° can also be used to inspect the diaphragmatic aspect of the TV. The normal tricuspid bioprosthesis has thin leaflets (2–4 mm) attached to three struts that protrude into the RV. Their appearance and movement resemble those of native leaflets (Fig. 18.38). Mechanical bileaflet valve hemidiscs have a more linear aspect and produce characteristic linear acoustic reverberations pivoting within the annulus (Fig. 18.39). In the open position, the two hemidiscs appear as two parallel lines, while in the closed position they assume a wide-open V shape against the prosthetic annulus.

Mechanical TV thrombosis should be ruled out when full range excursion of both hemidiscs cannot be demonstrated (68). Even by TEE, thrombus within the prosthesis associated with decreased mobility of the occluder is sometimes difficult to establish. A search for perivalvular regurgitation should be done

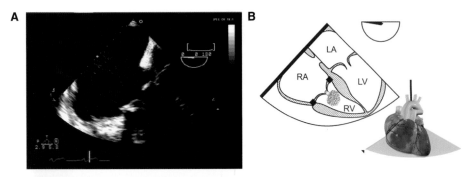

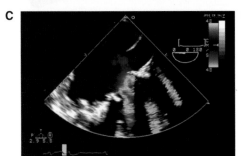

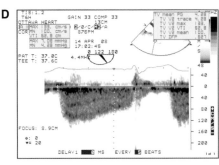

Figure 18.38 Bioprosthetic TV.
(**A–C**) Mid-esophageal RV views of a normal bioprosthetic valve in the tricuspid position with normal color Doppler imaging (**C**) and continuous wave Doppler tracing (**D**). *Abbreviations*: LA, left atrium; LV, left ventricle; RA, right atrium; RV, right ventricle; TV, tricuspid valve.

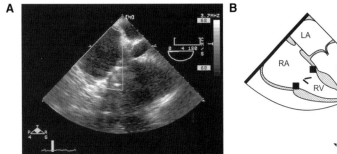

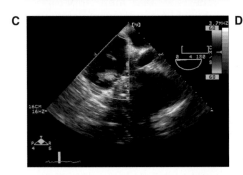

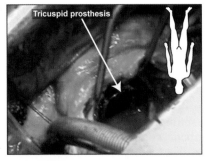

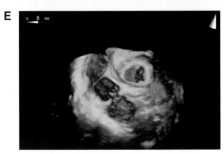

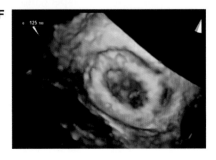

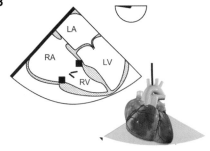

Figure 18.39 Mechanical tricuspid prosthesis. A 41-year-old man is reoperated on for tricuspid bileaflet prosthetic valve dysfunction. (**A–C**) Mid-esophageal four-chamber view shows a dilated RA and RV and mild tricuspid regurgitation. The lateral wall of the RV is obscured by acoustic shadowing from the tricuspid prosthesis. (**D**) Intraoperatively, one of the hemidiscs is found fixed in open position. (**E**) Full volume and (**F**) zoomed 3D transesophageal view of a thrombosed mechanical bileaflet valve as seen from the RA in another patient with L-transposition of the great vessels. *Abbreviations*: LA, left atrium; LV, left ventricle; RA, right atrium; RV, right ventricle. *Source*: Photo D Courtesy of Dr. Nancy Poirier.

Table 18.12 Summary of the Role of TEE in Patients Undergoing Tricuspid Valve Surgery

	Importance
Before the procedure	
• See Table 13.1 for the role of TEE in cardiac surgery	
• Evaluate right atrial dimension	Anticipation of difficult valve repair with possible modification of the surgical approach
• Evaluation of the severity of pulmonary hypertension and tricuspid regurgitation	Anticipate difficult separation from CPB
During CPB	
• See Table 13.1	
After CPB	
• See Table 13.1	
• Evaluate result of repair or replacement	Early detection and correction of prosthetic dysfunction or suboptimal repair
• Detect abnormal motion of PA catheter	The PA catheter could be accidentally entrapped during closure of the RA
In the intensive care unit	
• See Table 13.1	

Abbreviations: CPB, cardiopulmonary bypass; PA, pulmonary artery; RA, right atrium; TEE, transesophageal echocardiography.

by the color Doppler imaging in multiple planes to describe the sector, site, and width of the leak.

As for its native counterpart, the assessment of the PV prosthesis suffers from the distance between the TEE in the esophagus and the anterior position of the PV. In the absence of shadowing from the AoV, the PV can be seen in the mid-esophageal short-axis view at 30° to 80° and sometimes in the sagittal transgastric view. In these situations, the use of epicardial echocardiography can circumvent limitations (see Chapter 6).

THREE-DIMENSIONAL TECHNOLOGY

The TV is a complex structure. Unlike the AoV and MV, it is not possible to visualize all TV leaflets simultaneously in one cross-sectional view by standard 2D echocardiography, either transthoracic or transesophageal, due to the position of TV in the far field. Earlier experience with 3D TEE shows more accurate and reproducible anatomical and functional assessment of the TV (69), although not as good as the MV. As for the MV, the TV imaging with 3D TEE may have surgical implication by allowing the surgeon to make a more informed decision as to whether to repair the TV. Publications on the PV are mostly case reports (70). As 3D TEE becomes popular, there will be more literature to improve our understanding of the anatomy and function of the PV.

CONCLUSION

Despite limitations, TEE is a useful tool in the evaluation and of the TV and PV, and the quantification prosthetic dysfunction (Table 18.12). Its intraoperative use complements, or replaces, hemodynamic data from the pulmonary artery catheter and is likely to become an essential part of the postoperative evaluation of TV and PV surgery.

REFERENCES

1. Chaliki HP, Click RL, Abel MD. Comparison of intraoperative transesophageal echocardiographic examinations with the operative findings: prospective review of 1918 cases. J Am Soc Echocardiogr 1999; 12:237–240.
2. King RM, Schaff HV, Danielson GK, et al. Surgery for tricuspid regurgitation late after mitral valve replacement. Circulation 1984; 70:I193–I197.
3. Bajzer CT, Stewart WJ, Cosgrove DM, et al. Tricuspid valve surgery and intraoperative echocardiography: factors affecting survival, clinical outcome, and echocardiographic success. J Am Coll Cardiol 1998; 32:1023–1031.
4. Sutton JP III, Ho SY, Vogel M et al. Is the morphologically right atrioventricular valve tricuspid? J Heart Valve Dis 1995; 4:571–575.
5. Roguin A, Rinkevich D, Milo S, et al. Long-term follow-up of patients with severe rheumatic tricuspid stenosis. Am Heart J 1998; 136:103–108.
6. Ammash NM, Warnes CA, Connolly HM, et al. Mimics of Ebstein's anomaly. Am Heart J 1997; 134:508–513.
7. Lang RM, Bierig M, Devereux RB, et al. Recommendations for chamber quantification: a report from the American Society of Echocardiography's Guidelines and Standards Committee and the Chamber Quantification Writing Group, developed in conjunction with the European Association of Echocardiography, a branch of the European Society of Cardiology. J Am Soc Echocardiogr 2005; 18: 1440–1463.
8. Shanewise JS, Cheung AT, Aronson S, et al. ASE/SCA guidelines for performing a comprehensive intraoperative multiplane transesophageal echocardiography examination: recommendations of the American Society of Echocardiography Council for Intraoperative Echocardiography and the Society of Cardiovascular Anesthesiologists Task Force for Certification in Perioperative Transesophageal Echocardiography. Anesth Analg 1999; 89:870–884.
9. Haddad F, Couture P, Tousignant C, et al. The right ventricle in cardiac surgery, a perioperative perspective: I. Anatomy, physiology, and assessment. Anesth Analg 2009; 108:407–421.
10. Cohen GI, White M, Sochowski RA, et al. Reference values for normal adult transesophageal echocardiographic measurements. J Am Soc Echocardiogr 1995; 8:221–230.
11. Hauck AJ, Freeman DP, Ackermann DM, et al. Surgical pathology of the tricuspid valve: a study of 363 cases spanning 25 years. Mayo Clin Proc 1988; 63:851–863.

12. Yiwu L, Yingchun C, Jianqun Z, et al. Exact quantitative selective annuloplasty of the tricuspid valve. J Thorac Cardiovasc Surg 2001; 122:611–614.

13. Frater R. Tricuspid insufficiency. J Thorac Cardiovasc Surg 2001; 122:427–429.

14. Sagie A, Schwammenthal E, Padial LR, et al. Determinants of functional tricuspid regurgitation in incomplete tricuspid valve closure: Doppler color flow study of 109 patients. J Am Coll Cardiol 1994; 24:446–453.

15. Ubago JL, Figueroa A, Ochoteco A, et al. Analysis of the amount of tricuspid valve annular dilatation required to produce functional tricuspid regurgitation. Am J Cardiol 1983; 52:155–158.

16. Sugimoto T, Okada M, Ozaki N, et al. Influence of functional tricuspid regurgitation on right ventricular function. Ann Thorac Surg 1998; 66:2044–2050.

17. Enriquez-Sarano M, Rossi A, Seward JB, et al. Determinants of pulmonary hypertension in left ventricular dysfunction. J Am Coll Cardiol 1997; 29:153–159.

18. van Son JA, Danielson GK, Schaff HV, et al. Traumatic tricuspid valve insufficiency. Experience in thirteen patients. J Thorac Cardiovasc Surg 1994; 108:893–898.

19. Shapira Y, Porter A, Wurzel M, et al. Evaluation of tricuspid regurgitation severity: echocardiographic and clinical correlation. J Am Soc Echocardiogr 1998; 11:652–659.

20. Tribouilloy CM, Enriquez-Sarano M, Bailey KR, et al. Quantification of tricuspid regurgitation by measuring the width of the vena contracta with Doppler color flow imaging: a clinical study. J Am Coll Cardiol 2000; 36:472–478.

21. Zoghbi WA, Enriquez-Sarano M, Foster E, et al. Recommendations for evaluation of the severity of native valvular regurgitation with two-dimensional and Doppler echocardiography. J Am Soc Echocardiogr 2003; 16:777–802.

22. Wang Y, Gutman JM, Heilbron D, et al. Atrial volume in a normal adult population by two-dimensional echocardiography. Chest 1984; 86:595–601.

23. Weyman AE. Principles and Practice of Echocardiography. 2nd ed. Philadelphia: Lea & Febiger, 1994.

24. Baumgartner H, Hung J, Bermejo J, et al. Echocardiographic assessment of valve stenosis: EAE/ASE recommendations for clinical practice. J Am Soc Echocardiogr 2009; 22:1–23.

25. Herrera CJ, Mehlman DJ, Hartz RS, et al. Comparison of transesophageal and transthoracic echocardiography for diagnosis of right-sided cardiac lesions. Am J Cardiol 1992; 70:964–966.

26. San Roman JA, Vilacosta I, Zamorano JL, et al. Transesophageal echocardiography in right-sided endocarditis. J Am Coll Cardiol 1993; 21:1226–1230.

27. Robbins MJ, Frater RW, Soeiro R, et al. Influence of vegetation size on clinical outcome of right-sided infective endocarditis. Am J Med 1986; 80:165–171.

28. Rowley KM, Clubb KS, Smith GJ, et al. Right-sided infective endocarditis as a consequence of flow-directed pulmonary-artery catheterization. A clinicopathological study of 55 autopsied patients. N Engl J Med 1984; 311:1152–1156.

29. Vilacosta I, Sarria C, San Roman JA, et al. Usefulness of transesophageal echocardiography for diagnosis of infected transvenous permanent pacemakers. Circulation 1994; 89:2684–2687.

30. Klug D, Lacroix D, Savoye C, et al. Systemic infection related to endocarditis on pacemaker leads: clinical presentation and management. Circulation 1997; 95:2098–2107.

31. Tighe DA, Tejada LA, Kirchhoffer JB, et al. Pacemaker lead infection: detection by multiplane transesophageal echocardiography. Am Heart J 1996; 131:616–618.

32. Victor F, De Place C, Camus C, et al. Pacemaker lead infection: echocardiographic features, management, and outcome. Heart 1999; 81:82–87.

33. Bonow RO, Carabello BA, Kanu C, et al. ACC/AHA 2006 guidelines for the management of patients with valvular heart disease: a report of the American College of Cardiology/American Heart Association Task Force on Practice Guidelines (writing committee to revise the 1998 Guidelines for the Management of Patients With Valvular Heart Disease): developed in collaboration with the Society of Cardiovascular Anesthesiologists: endorsed by the Society for Cardiovascular Angiography and Interventions and the Society of Thoracic Surgeons. Circulation 2006; 114: e84–e231.

34. Arnett EN, Roberts WC. Valve ring abscess in active infective endocarditis. Frequency, location, and clues to clinical diagnosis from the study of 95 necropsy patients. Circulation 1976; 54:140–145.

35. Baumgartner FJ, Omari BO, Robertson JM, et al. Annular abscesses in surgical endocarditis: anatomic, clinical, and operative features. Ann Thorac Surg 2000; 70:442–447.

36. Eichelberger JP, Meltzer RS. Right-sided valvular pathology and rheumatic fever. Curr Opin Cardiol 1994; 9:181–185.

37. Sagie A, Schwammenthal E, Newell JB, et al. Significant tricuspid regurgitation is a marker for adverse outcome in patients undergoing percutaneous balloon mitral valvuloplasty. J Am Coll Cardiol 1994; 24:696–702.

38. Jamieson WR, Cartier PC, Allard M, et al. Surgical management of valvular heart disease 2004. Can J Cardiol 2004; 20(suppl E):7E–120E.

39. Chaowalit N, Connolly HM, Schaff HV, et al. Carcinoid heart disease associated with primary ovarian carcinoid tumor. Am J Cardiol 2004; 93:1314–1315.

40. Bernheim AM, Connolly HM, Pellikka PA. Carcinoid heart disease in patients without hepatic metastases. Am J Cardiol 2007; 99:292–294.

41. Pellikka PA, Tajik AJ, Khandheria BK, et al. Carcinoid heart disease. Clinical and echocardiographic spectrum in 74 patients. Circulation 1993; 87:1188–1196.

42. Connolly HM, Nishimura RA, Smith HC, et al. Outcome of cardiac surgery for carcinoid heart disease. J Am Coll Cardiol 1995; 25:410–416.

43. Connolly HM, Schaff HV, Mullany CJ, et al. Carcinoid heart disease: impact of pulmonary valve replacement in right ventricular function and remodeling. Circulation 2002; 106:I51–I56.

44. Nii M, Roman KS, Macgowan CK, et al. Insight into normal mitral and tricuspid annular dynamics in pediatrics: a real-time three-dimensional echocardiographic study. J Am Soc Echocardiogr 2005; 18:805–814.

45. Valdes-Cruz LM, Cayre RO. Echocardiographic Diagnosis of Congenital Heart Disease an Embryologic and Anatomic Approach. Philadelphia: Lippincott-Raven Publishers, 1999.

46. Altrichter PM, Olson LJ, Edwards WD, et al. Surgical pathology of the pulmonary valve: a study of 116 cases spanning 15 years. Mayo Clin Proc 1989; 64:1352–1360.

47. Franch RH. Recognition and management of valvular pulmonic stenosis. Heart Dis Stroke 1994; 3:365–370.

48. Mulhern KM, Skorton DJ. Echocardiographic evaluation of isolated pulmonary valve disease in adolescents and adults. Echocardiography 1993; 10:533–543.

49. Hayes CJ, Gersony WM, Driscoll DJ, et al. Second natural history study of congenital heart defects. Results of treatment of patients with pulmonary valvar stenosis. Circulation 1993; 87:I28–I37.

50. Therrien J, Gatzoulis M, Graham T, et al. Canadian Cardiovascular Society Consensus Conference 2001 update: Recommendations for the Management of Adults with Congenital Heart Disease—Part II. Can J Cardiol 2001; 17:1029–1050.

51. Silvilairat S, Cabalka AK, Cetta F, et al. Echocardiographic assessment of isolated pulmonary valve stenosis: which

outpatient Doppler gradient has the most clinical validity? J Am Soc Echocardiogr 2005; 18:1137–1142.

52. Nishimura RA, Pieroni DR, Bierman FZ, et al. Second natural history study of congenital heart defects. Pulmonary stenosis: echocardiography. Circulation 1993; 87:I73–I79.

53. Fernandes V, Kaluza GL, Zymek PT, et al. Successful balloon valvuloplasty in an adult patient with severe pulmonic stenosis and aneurysmal poststenotic dilatation. Catheter Cardiovasc Interv 2002; 55:376–380.

54. Yang H, Pu M, Chambers CE, et al. Quantitative assessment of pulmonary insufficiency by Doppler echocardiography in patients with adult congenital heart disease. J Am Soc Echocardiogr 2008; 21:157–164.

55. Gatzoulis MA, Balaji S, Webber SA, et al. Risk factors for arrhythmia and sudden cardiac death late after repair of tetralogy of Fallot: a multicentre study. Lancet 2000; 356: 975–981.

56. De Bonis M, Lapenna E, La Canna G, et al. A novel technique for correction of severe tricuspid valve regurgitation due to complex lesions. Eur J Cardiothorac Surg 2004; 25:760–765.

57. Ghanta RK, Chen R, Narayanasamy N, et al. Suture bicuspidization of the tricuspid valve versus ring annuloplasty for repair of functional tricuspid regurgitation: midterm results of 237 consecutive patients. J Thorac Cardiovasc Surg 2007; 133:117–126.

58. Fukuda S, Song JM, Gillinov AM, et al. Tricuspid valve tethering predicts residual tricuspid regurgitation after tricuspid annuloplasty. Circulation 2005; 111:975–979.

59. Rabago G, Fraile J, Martinell J, et al. Technique and results of tricuspid annuloplasty. J Card Surg 1986; 1:247–253.

60. Abe T, Tukamoto M, Yanagiya M, et al. De Vega's annuloplasty for acquired tricuspid disease: early and late results in 110 patients. Ann Thorac Surg 1989; 48:670–676.

61. Zoghbi WA, Chambers JB, Dumesnil JG, et al. Recommendations for evaluation of prosthetic valves with echocardiography and doppler ultrasound: a report From the American Society of Echocardiography's Guidelines and Standards Committee and the Task Force on Prosthetic Valves, developed in conjunction with the American College of Cardiology Cardiovascular Imaging Committee, Cardiac Imaging Committee of the American Heart Association, the European Association of Echocardiography, a registered branch of the European Society of Cardiology, the Japanese Society of Echocardiography and the Canadian Society of Echocardiography, endorsed by the American College of Cardiology Foundation, American Heart Association, European Association of Echocardiography, a registered branch of the European Society of Cardiology, the Japanese Society of Echocardiography, and Canadian Society of Echocardiography. J Am Soc Echocardiogr 2009; 22:975–1014.

62. Do QB, Pellerin M, Carrier M, et al. Clinical outcome after isolated tricuspid valve replacement: 20-year experience. Can J Cardiol 2000; 16:489–493.

63. Arbulu A, Holmes RJ, Asfaw I. Tricuspid valvulectomy without replacement. Twenty years' experience. J Thorac Cardiovasc Surg 1991; 102:917–922.

64. Glower DD, White WD, Smith LR, et al. In-hospital and long-term outcome after porcine tricuspid valve replacement. J Thorac Cardiovasc Surg 1995; 109:877–883.

65. Scully HE, Armstrong CS. Tricuspid valve replacement. Fifteen years of experience with mechanical prostheses and bioprostheses. J Thorac Cardiovasc Surg 1995; 109: 1035–1041.

66. Singh AK, Feng WC, Sanofsky SJ. Long-term results of St. Jude Medical valve in the tricuspid position. Ann Thorac Surg 1992; 54:538–540.

67. Hvass U, Baron F, Fourchy D, et al. Mitral homografts for total tricuspid valve replacement: comparison of two techniques. J Thorac Cardiovasc Surg 2001; 121:592–594.

68. Shapira Y, Sagie A, Jortner R, et al. Thrombosis of bileaflet tricuspid valve prosthesis: clinical spectrum and the role of nonsurgical treatment. Am Heart J 1999; 137:721–725.

69. Anwar AM, Soliman OI, Nemes A, et al. Value of assessment of tricuspid annulus: real-time three-dimensional echocardiography and magnetic resonance imaging. Int J Cardiovasc Imaging 2007; 23:701–705.

70. Citro R, Salustri A, Gregorio G. Images in cardiovascular medicine. Three-dimensional reconstruction of pulmonary valve endocarditis. Ital Heart J 2001; 2:938–939.

19

Transcatheter Aortic Valve Implantation

Yoan Lamarche and Arsène-J. Basmadjian
Montreal Heart Institute, Université de Montréal, Montreal, Quebec, Canada

Anson Cheung
St-Paul's Hospital, University of British Columbia, Vancouver, British Columbia, Canada

Massimiliano Meineri
Toronto General Hospital, University of Toronto, Toronto, Ontario, Canada

Jean Buithieu
McGill University Health Center, McGill University, Montreal, Quebec, Canada

INTRODUCTION

Aortic stenosis (AS) is the most common valvular pathology requiring intervention in adults. Some patients are denied surgery because of prohibitive risk of perioperative mortality and morbidity with conventional open aortic valve replacement. In 2002, Cribier described an endovascular transcatheter approach to aortic valve replacement (AVR) (1) for the high-risk surgical patient. In recent years different groups developed retrograde (2,3) and antegrade transapical (4–7) approaches to transcatheter aortic valve implantation (TAVI). Transesophageal echocardiography (TEE) has been a critical tool in the development and application of this new technology for candidate evaluation, for periprocedural monitoring and guidance, to rule out complications and for follow-up (8–10).

DEVICES

Transcatheter valvular prostheses are currently classified into two types with a different implantation procedure (Fig. 19.1). The self-expanding aortic valve (AoV) prosthesis intended for retrograde delivery across the AoV was originally developed by Core-Valve, Inc. The prosthesis originally consisted of a trileaflet bioprosthetic pericardial valve mounted and sutured in a self-expanding nitinol stent. The prosthetic AoV has three levels. The lower level of the prosthesis has high radial force to expand and exclude the native calcified leaflets from the orifice. The lower portion is the first to be deployed, anchoring the prosthetic nitinol stent proximally at the level of the aortic annulus. The middle level of the prosthesis carries the pericardial valve and is constrained to avoid occluding the coronary ostia. The upper portion of the valve is flared to anchor the prosthesis distally to the ascending aorta (Ao) and provide longitudinal stability. The first generation device required a 25F delivery sheath and extracorporeal circulatory support with a percutaneous femoro-femoral bypass as a safety measure to promote a hemodynamic standstill of the heart for positioning and deployment of the AoV prosthesis. With further development, the third generation Medtronic CoreValve porcine pericardial valve device (Medtronic, Minneapolis, Minnesota, U.S.) uses a 21/18F delivery sheath (Fig. 19.2) with a reduced profile while the extracorporeal circulatory support is no longer required for CoreValve implantation. As the proximal and middle portion of the AoV prosthesis are uncovered by retraction of the delivery sheath, the functioning of the AoV prosthesis can be ascertained, while the distal portion is still attached to the delivery catheter. This enables further pullback of the device if necessary for fine tuning of the position. If the position of the device is satisfactory, the upper portion self-expanding aortic nitinol prosthesis is completely uncovered and the device is released while the delivery catheter is removed. If not, complete bailing out of the device is still possible by withdrawing the whole prosthesis within the delivery sheath.

The other type of transcatheter prosthetic AoV, the Transcatheter Heart Valve™ (THV) (Edwards Lifesciences, Irvine, California, U.S.), is a stainless steel stent with pericardial leaflets and a fabric sealing cuff (Fig. 19.3). For implantation, it is crimped on a deflated aortic balloon for insertion and careful positioning before being deployed all at once by balloon inflation under rapid right ventricular pacing to reduce transvalvular aortic flow. It has been designed

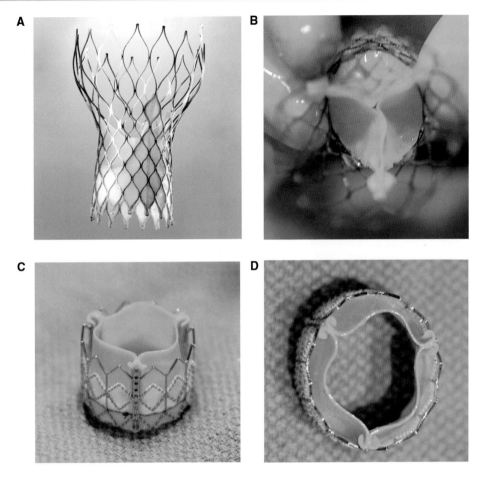

Figure 19.1 Percutaneous prosthesis. Transcatheter aortic valve prosthesis clinically available. (**A,B**) Medtronic CoreValve®. (**C,D**) Edwards SAPIEN Transcatheter Heart Valve™. *Source*: with permission from Medtronic CoreValve and Edwards Lifesciences.

for transfemoral insertion with the RetroFlex 3 delivery system or for transapical placement with the Ascendra delivery system. Both Edwards SAPIEN THV and CoreValve have been used clinically in patients with AS deemed to have excessive risk for standard open-heart procedures (2,3,11). The Medtronic Melody® transcatheter valve used with the Ensemble® Transcatheter Delivery System was developed for deployment in the pulmonic position and its successful implantation has been described (12,13). The system consists of a bovine jugular valve vein sewn inside a platinum iridium stent and is deployed by balloon inflation. There are many other transcatheter AoV, which are in different phases of preclinical and early clinical testing. As technology improves, eligibility criteria listed below may evolve and change and should be updated.

TECHNICAL ASPECTS

The main steps for TAVI are evaluation of access sites, evaluation of the AoV size and prosthesis model required, establishment of peripheral access and monitoring lines, correct positioning of the prosthesis, and deployment (Fig. 19.4). Different approaches to deliver prostheses exist. The antegrade transseptal approach was the first reported by Cribier (1) and is now rarely used. Retrograde delivery can be accomplished through a femoral artery (3) or axillary artery approach. The antegrade transapical approach (5,7) is currently employed for patients with limited peripheral access due to small size, tortuosity or disease of femoral and iliac arteries, or severe atheromatous disease of the aortic arch (Fig. 19.5). Implantation of a self-expandable or a balloon-expandable prosthesis in a degenerated bioprosthesis has been reported in the aortic and mitral position (14,15).

Potential complications in TAVI are suboptimal device positioning, device displacement or embolization, paraprosthetic leak, atrioventricular conduction disturbances, and atrial, ventricular, or aortic perforation causing pericardial tamponade. Paraprosthetic leaks have been corrected by balloon redilation or in situ deployment of a second valvular prosthesis (3). Tamponade can be drained percutaneously or surgically. Embolization of calcium, clot, intimal debris,

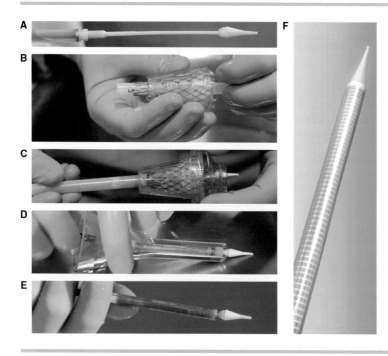

Figure 19.2   Medtronic CoreValve transcatheter aortic valve implantation system. (**A**) For implantation, after having soaked it in iced water, the Medtronic CoreValve is loaded onto a delivery catheter. (**B**) The outflow portion of the prosthesis is squeezed with the help of a reducing outflow cone, then a nontapered tube is inserted in the inflow end until the distal frame tabs are separated. (**C**) The tabs can then be attached to the catheter deployment end. (**D,E**) The covering sheath is advanced over the the prosthesis with the help of a reducing inflow cone until it reaches the distal end of the delivery catheter. (**F**) Appearance of the Medtronic CoreValve system for insertion and implantation.

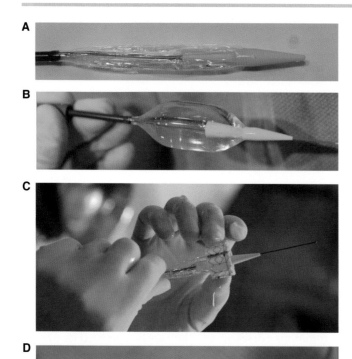

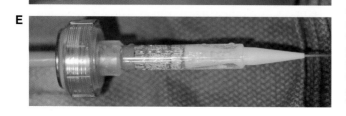

Figure 19.3   Edwards SAPIEN THV for transcatheter aortic valve implantation. (**A**) For implantation the Edwards SAPIEN THV is loaded onto a delivery balloon. (**B**) The balloon is first calibrated for specific inflation volume and diameter. (**C**) The prosthesis is then positioned over the deflated balloon. (**D**) Using a specialized device, the prosthesis is crimped over the deflated balloon, using a specialized device until it reaches the required minimum profile. During implantation, the system shows the typical appearance: the small space between the cone and the prosthesis may help identifying the end of the prosthesis for precise positioning before balloon deployment. (**E**) For insertion through the introducer sheath and the aorta, a protective sheath is covering the prosthesis. *Abbreviation*: THV, Transcatheter Heart Valve.

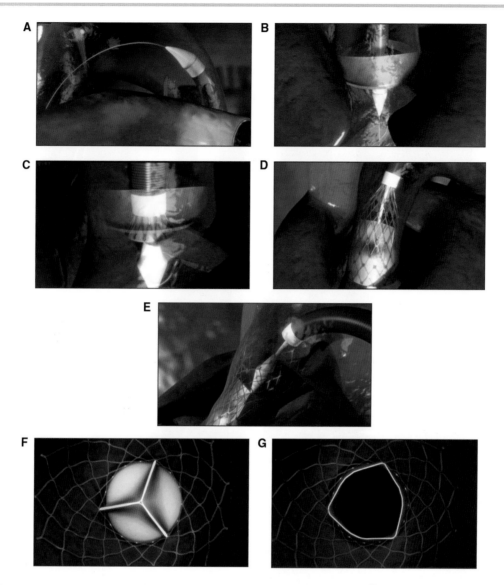

Figure 19.4 Transcatheter aortic valve implantation with the Medtronic CoreValve® system. (**A**) Positioning of the delivery catheter system in the ascending aorta. (**B**) Insertion through the native aortic valve. (**C,D**) Pull back of the covering sheath for deployment of the prosthesis. (**E**) Removal of the deployment system. (**F,G**) The prosthesis is shown in the closed (**F**) and open (**G**) positions. *Source*: Courtesy of Medtronic CoreValve.

and of the prosthesis itself have also been reported (3). Monitoring using TEE is the principal modality to detect and confirm diagnosis promptly and guide treatment of complications of TAVI.

CARDIOPULMONARY MANAGEMENT IN TAVI

There are several methods of cardiopulmonary support used to allow precise deployment of prostheses. Among these techniques, peripheral cardiopulmonary bypass (CPB) and partial left heart bypass have been used by several groups (2,7), but are no longer required. Rapid ventricular pacing (140–220 bpm) (see later in the chapter) can also be performed during

the short period of valvular deployment particularly for the Edwards SAPIEN THV prosthesis. Rapid pacing is associated with minimal transvalvular aortic flow and allows precise positioning of the valve during deployment (3). Finally, some have reported valvular deployment during normal beating heart without CPB support or alteration of normal hemodynamics (4,16).

ANESTHESIA AND MONITORING

The first case of TAVI described was performed under local anesthesia and minimal sedation (1); however, general anesthesia, with or without endotracheal intubation, is used in most centers (17,18). Most patients

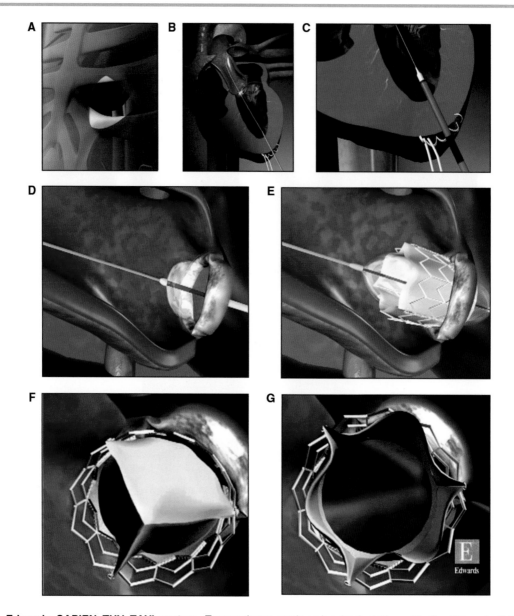

Figure 19.5 Edwards SAPIEN THV TAVI system. Transcatheter aortic valve implantation with the Edwards SAPIEN THV by transapical approach. (**A**) A small thoracotomy is performed near the left ventricular apex. (**B**) The apex is punctured and a guidewire is inserted. (**C**) The delivery catheter system is advanced in the left ventricle over the guidewire. (**D**) Predilatation with balloon valvuloplasty is first performed. (**E**) The transcatheter prosthesis is positioned through the native aortic valve and deployed. (**F,G**) The Edwards SAPIEN THV prosthesis is shown in the closed (**F**) and open (**G**) positions. *Abbreviations*: TAVI, transcatheter aortic valve implantation; THV, Transcatheter Heart Valve. *Source*: Courtesy of Edwards Lifesciences.

requiring TAVI have a frail status and are at risk of hemodynamic instability. Central venous and pulmonary arterial pressure measurements, as well as arterial pressure monitoring, are useful in the procedural and postprocedural period. Transesophageal echocardiographic monitoring is used in patients with general anesthesia and endotracheal intubation. Other imaging modalities include fluoroscopy and contrast angiography, and these are crucial for device positioning and deployment. Multidetector computed tomography (CT) and magnetic resonance imaging (MRI)

may prove to be useful for preprocedural evaluation and follow-up.

USE OF TEE AND SPECIAL CONSIDERATIONS FOR TAVI

Transesophageal echocardiography is used before, during, and after the TAVI procedure, as well as for follow-up in cases with a specific finding on TTE. The most commonly used views for TEE in TAVI are the same as those used for evaluating the native AoV (see Chapter 14), particularly the mid-esophageal long-axis (LAX) (120–150°) and short-axis (SAX) (30–50°) views. Frequent repositioning of the TEE probe is required to allow an unobstructed fluoroscopic evaluation.

PRE-PROCEDURAL USE OF TEE

Valvular Function

The morphology and function of AoV is studied in detail. Anatomy and calcifications are reported. A bicuspid AoV should be noted because it makes the expansion of the prosthesis less stable and increases the risk of subsequent embolization. The maximal and mean gradients are measured from transgastric views with angles appropriate for Doppler interrogation. The valvular area is calculated (see Chapter 14). The severity and mechanism of aortic regurgitation is also evaluated using published guidelines (19).

Precise measurement of the left ventricular outflow tract (LVOT) and annular diameters are critical in candidate selection and to aid in choosing the proper device size (Fig. 19.6). The aortic "annulus" should be properly measured at the hinge point of the aortic leaflets (Fig. 19.7). Two sizes are currently offered by CoreValve. The 26-mm inflow device is suitable for annulus size ranges from 20 to 23 mm, and the 29-mm inflow device is suitable for annulus size ranges from 23 to 27 mm. The risk for paravalvular regurgitation increases for aortic annuli greater than 25 mm in diameter. Edwards SAPIEN THV prostheses are also available in two sizes, 23 mm and 26 mm. The 23 mm valve is suitable for aortic annular sizes of 18 to 22 mm, and the 26 mm valve for annular sizes of 21 to 25 mm (3). The main rule is to oversize the prosthesis slightly in relation with the native aortic annulus to minimize paravalvular leak without significantly increasing the risk of perforation. Of note, TEE will generally yield measurements of the aortic annulus 1.0 to 1.5 mm greater than those achieved with transthoracic echocardiography (TTE) (9). Currently, a patient with an aortic annulus of 18 mm or less and greater than 27 mm is considered unsuitable for a percutaneous AoV replacement.

As the aortic-mitral continuity can be distorted by the placement of AoV prostheses, the anatomy and function of the mitral valve (MV) are studied extensively. The mechanism and severity of mitral regurgitation (MR) are evaluated, and the subvalvular apparatus is examined. The calcifications on aortic and MV leaflets and annuli can be used as landmarks for optimization of positioning using fluoroscopy (9). Post-implantation MR from MV tears has been described with transapical antegrade implantation. A transient increase in the degree of MR has also been observed in a small proportion of patients (8,9).

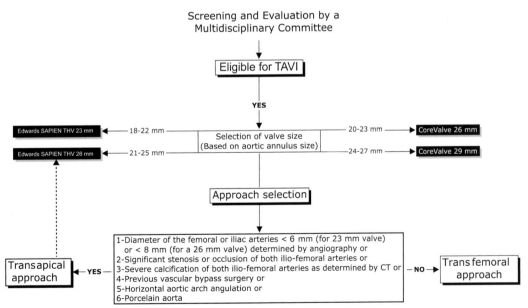

Figure 19.6 Algorithm for the use of TAVR. Schematic representation of patients' evaluation, enrollment, and approach for TAVI selection is presented. *Abbreviations*: CT, computed tomography; TAVI, transcatheter aortic valve implantation; THV, Transcatheter Heart Valve. *Source*: Adapted with permission from Ref. 20.

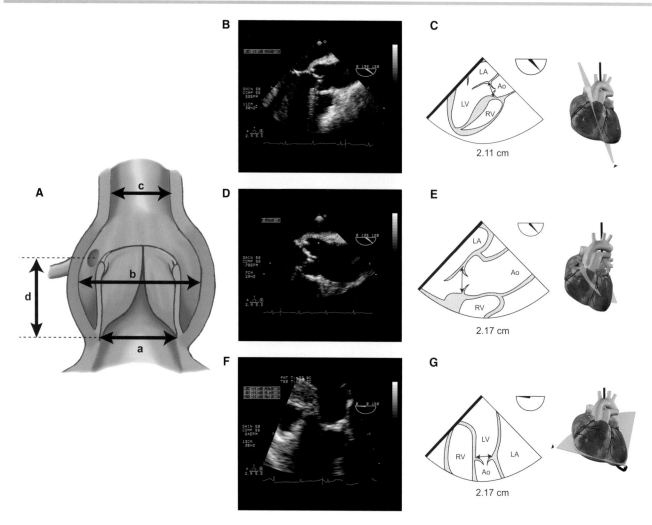

Figure 19.7 Measurements of the aortic annulus. Accurate aortic annulus diameter is a key measurement. (**A**) The AoV annulus (arrow a) should be measured between the hinge points of the AoV cusps. Other useful measurements are also performed: aortic root width at the level of the sinuses of Valsalva (arrow b), ascending aorta (arrow c), and distance from the coronary ostia to the native leaflet (arrow d). Multiple measurements are used from the ME LAX view (**B,C**), the ME AoV LAX view (**D,E**) and the deep transgastric LAX view (**F,G**). Shadowing from heavy cusp calcification as well as a mitral prosthesis can make accurate identification of the AoV annulus extremely difficult. The deep transgastric LAX view is useful in this situation. *Abbreviations*: Ao, aorta; AoV, aortic valve; LA, left atrium; LAX, long-axis; LV, left ventricle; ME, mid-esophageal; RV, right ventricle. *Source*: Diagram A, with permission, copyright of Gian-Marco Busato.

Ventricular Structure and Function

Left ventricular (LV) size is measured, LV mass is calculated (see Chapter 5), and LV regional wall motion (see Chapter 9) and diastolic function (see Chapter 10) are evaluated. The presence of aortic subvalvular stenosis is assessed. Right ventricular size and function are also evaluated.

Aorta

The ascending and descending Ao are evaluated pre-operatively. Advanced atherosclerotic disease with mobile plaque, dissection, intramural hematoma, or

aneurysmal dilatation should be communicated to the interventional team. Severely calcified or atherosclerotic lesions can limit peripheral access or represent a contraindication to retrograde transfemoral approach because of the risk of embolization and dissection. For the self-expanding CoreValve, since the prosthesis is anchored in the ascending Ao, the dimensions of that vessel segment are critical. The diameter of the ascending Ao must be inferior or equal to 43 mm at 3 cm above the aortic annulus. Larger aortic dimensions would lead to an unstable position and risk of dislodgement. The sinotubular junction diameter and tubular ascending aortic anatomy are also evaluated (Fig. 19.7). The distance from the plane of the aortic

Anatomy	Non-Invasive		Angiography				Selection Criteria		
	Echo	CT / MRI	LV gram	Ao gram	Coronary Argiogram	Ao & Runoffs	Preferred	Borderline	Not Acceptable
Atrial or Ventricular Thrombus	X						Not Present		Present
Mitral Regurgitation	X						≤ Grade 1	Grade 2	> Grade 2
LV Ejection Fraction	X		X				> 50%	30% to 50%	< 20% (w/o cardiac support)
LV Hypertrophy (wall thickness)	X						Normal to Mild (0.6 to 1.3 cm)	Moderate (1.4 to 1.6cm)	Severe (≥ 1.7cm)
Sub-Aortic Stenosis	X	X					Not Present		Present
Annulus (width)	X	X					20 to 23mm → 26mm device 24 to 27mm → 29mm device		< 20mm or > 27mm
Ao Root (width)		X	X	X			≥ 27mm → 26mm device ≥ 28mm → 29mm device		< 27mm
Coronary Ostia (from native leaflet)					X		≥ 14mm	13mm w/mod. Ca° 10 to 13mm w/o Ca°	< 27mm w/ severe Ca° < 13mm w/ mod. Ca° < 10mm w/o Ca°
Coronary Disease					X		None	Mid or Distal Stenosis < 70%	Proximal Stenosis ≥ 70%
Annulus-to-Aorta (angle) †		X	X	X			< 45°	45° to 70°	> 70°
Ascend Aorta (width)	X	X	X	X			≥ 40mm → 26mm device ≥ 43mm → 29mm device		> 43mm
Ao Arch Angulation		X		X		X	Large-Radius Turn		High Angulation or Sharp Bend
Aorta & Run-Off Vessels (Disease) ‡		X				X	None	Mild	Moderate to Severe
Iliac & Femoral Vessels (diameter)		X				X	≥ 7mm	Non-Diabetic Non-Dialyzed ≥ 6mm	< 6mm

† *Within the first 7cm of the ascending aorta versus a perpendicular line across the aortic valve.*
‡ *Evaluate for evidence and degree of calcification, obstruction, tortuosity, and ulceration.*

Figure 19.8 Medtronic CoreValve patient selection matrix. A specific patient selection matrix for the CoreValve is presented. *Abbreviations*: Ao, aorta; Ascend, ascending; Ca, calcium; CT, computed tomography; Echo, echocardiogram; LV, left ventricular; LV gram, left ventriculogram; MRI, magnetic resonance imaging; w/o, without. *Source*: With permission of Medtronic CoreValve.

annulus to the coronary ostia is evaluated. A short distance inferior to 10 mm increases the risk of occlusion by the excluded native leaflets during valvuloplasty and prosthesis deployment. The presence of moderate or severe valvular calcifications requires a larger 13 or 14 mm distance between the base of the native leaflets and the coronary ostia. The pre-implantation anatomical evaluation used for the CoreValve™ TAVI is summarized in Figure 19.8.

USE OF TEE DURING IMPLANTATION

During implantation, the adequate positioning of a venous cannula in the right atrium (RA) for peripheral CPB or through the interatrial septum for left heart bypass when necessary is guided by TEE. In addition, TEE will help to position the guidewires across the stenotic AoV (Fig. 19.9). The guidewire will be used to advance and position the prosthesis. The position of the guidewire must be verified constantly during the procedure to make sure that it did not move accidentally.

A balloon of appropriate size is selected for predilatation. It will be positioned in the AoV using TEE and fluoroscopic guidance. If CPB is used, it is initiated at that moment, and adequate venous drainage and absence of complications such as aortic dissection or pericardial effusion are documented.

During valvuloplasty or prosthesis deployment, the heart is adequately emptied if CPB is used or put under rapid ventricular pacing to minimize forward flow likely to move the balloon and/or the prosthesis from its accurate position. The efficacy of

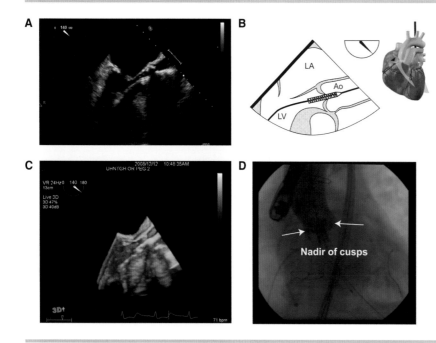

Figure 19.9 Approach to TAVI positioning. Anatomic landmarks for positioning must take into account forward displacement with TAVI deployment. The mid-esophageal AoV long-axis view (**A,B**), 3D echocardiography (**C**) and fluoroscopy (**D**) are used to guide positioning across the stenotic AoV. *Abbreviations*: Ao, aorta; AoV, aortic valve; LA, left atrium; LV, left ventricle; TAVI, transcatheter aortic valve implantation. ⁀

the ventricular pacing is confirmed by a decrease of the systolic pressure below 50 mmHg: pulse pressure must be minimal, ensuring a weak LV ejection and decreased output through the AoV (Fig. 19.10). To confirm this, a pulsed Doppler, in the ascending Ao, can be used to demonstrate the decrease in ejection volume during rapid ventricular pacing. During aortic valvuloplasty, proper positioning of the balloon through the valve is made first by fluoroscopy and then confirmed by echocardiography. The inflation of the balloon can be directly visualized by echocardiography (Fig. 19.10). LV function, degree of aortic regurgitation, and absence of coronary obstruction are assessed immediately after balloon deflation.

Positioning of the prosthesis is then guided with fluoroscopy and contrast injection before deployment. Transesophageal echocardiography will be particularly useful in assisting for correct positioning when minimal calcifications are present (9). For the Medtronic CoreValve TAVI, the proximal limit of the prosthesis should be positioned at 8 mm within the LVOT (from the aortic annulus). For the Edwards SAPIEN THV, the theoretical predicted final position of the prosthesis will be located at the point of inflection of the aortic cusps with the Ao (Fig. 19.11). Several indices exist to guide the deployment of the prosthesis but none are perfect. With fluoroscopy, the deployment site is defined by the nadir of the aortic cusp on aortography of the root. Calcifications are often misleading because of their variable position on the valve. The proximal one-half to two-thirds of the Edwards SAPIEN THV prosthesis should be located at this point before deployment for the femo-

ral approach and at half for the transapical approach (Fig. 19.11). It should be confirmed that the Edwards SAPIEN THV prosthesis completely covers the native aortic cusps before implantation (Fig. 19.12). With echocardiography, the major difficulty is to clearly delineate the proximal and the distal ends of the crimped prosthesis and to differentiate them from the cone and the balloon on which it is assembled and to visualize, with precision, the point of deployment when the valvular apparatus is heavily calcified. The aortic end is located by the notch that the prosthesis makes on the balloon. The ventricular part is often difficult to visualize but the prosthesis length can be useful to estimate it. Efforts must be made to visualize the prosthesis as a whole (Fig. 19.13). The prosthesis has a tendency to move, 2 to 4 mm in aortic direction, at time of the deployment. The optimal position of the Edwards SAPIEN THV prosthesis before deployment is approximately located at the same distance under the most ventricular portion of the native aortic cusp. This corresponds, in practice, to the position of the ventricular end at the inflection point of the anterior mitral valve leaflet (Fig. 19.12). It is important to remember that the balloon-deployed Edwards SAPIEN THV AoV final positioning must be decided before balloon inflation, as there will be no time to change the position of the prosthesis during or after deployment. In contrast, as the CoreValve prosthesis is gradually uncovered and deployed, there is still a possibility to reposition the prosthesis until the distal upper portion is definitively released. For this reason, it is not uncommon that the operator asks the echocardiographer to pull back slightly the

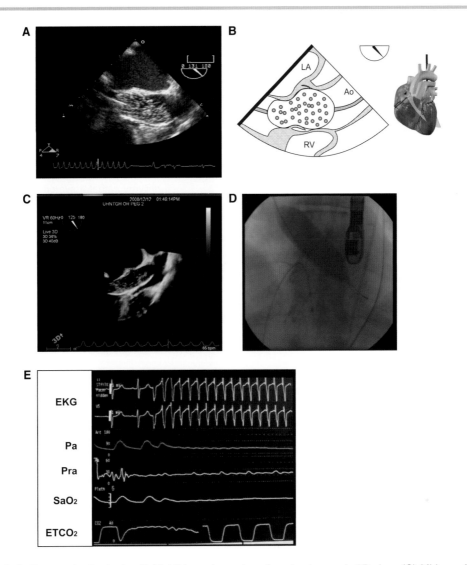

Figure 19.10 Aortic balloon valvuloplasty. (A,B) Mid-esophageal aortic valve long-axis 2D view. **(C)** Mid-esophageal aortic valve long-axis 3D view. **(D)** Fluoroscopy PA view. **(E)** ECG and hemodynamic pressure tracing during concomitant rapid ventricular pacing to reduce the ejection volume and minimize aortic balloon displacement during inflation. Note the secondary systemic aortic pressure decrease. *Abbreviations*: Ao, aorta, EKG, electrocardiogram; $ETCO_2$, end-tidal carbon dioxide; LA, left atrium; Pa, arterial pressure; Pra, right atrial pressure; RV, right ventricle; SaO_2, oxygen saturation; TAVI, transcatheter aortic valve implantation.

TEE probe to allow an unobstructed fluoroscopic view during deployment of the valve. The ideal positioning varies depending on the prosthesis type. It is usually 2 to 5 mm below the nadir of the aortic cusps insertion point for the ventricular end of the Edwards SAPIEN THV prosthesis during balloon inflation (Figs. 19.14 and 19.15) and 5 to 10 mm for the proximal (ventricular) portion of the CoreValve prothesis (Fig. 19.16).

USE OF TEE AFTER PROSTHETIC VALVE DEPLOYMENT

The aortic prosthesis is examined in LAX and SAX views for correct positioning and full deployment. The

function of the valve leaflets is examined and proper opening and closing, with absence of intraprosthetic or paraprosthetic leak (PPL) is documented (Figs. 19.16 and 19.17). Before complete withdrawal of the guidewire, the echocardiographer must identify and quantify PPL. Careful examination in the SAX view is particularly useful, as the prosthetic metallic material and the bulky native AoV calcifications may cause acoustic shadows hiding the regurgitant jets. A PPL of some degree is present in the majority of cases and translates the difficulty of completely affixing the prosthesis to the aortic annulus because of the bulky remains of the native AoV and calcifications. Most frequently PPL is presented in the posterior aspect (toward the mitral

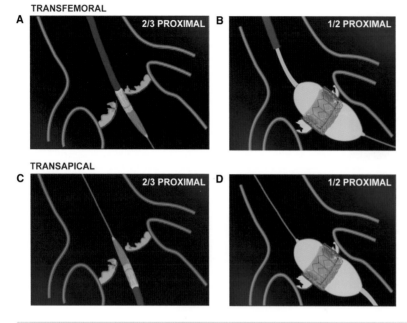

Figure 19.11 Step-by-step approach to TAVI. Correct positioning of the Edwards SAPIEN THV delivery catheter system for TAVI in both the transfemoral (**A,B**) and transapical (**C,D**) approaches are shown. (**A,C**) The catheter with the undeployed valve is positioned with one-half to two-thirds of the valve in the LVOT. (**B,D**) During valve deployment the valve moves forward slightly so the final prosthetic valve position is at the mid-point of the native aortic valve annulus. *Abbreviations*: LVOT, left ventricular outflow tract; TAVI, transcatheter aortic valve implantation; THV, Transcatheter Heart Valve. *Source*: Adapted with permission of Edwards Lifesciences.

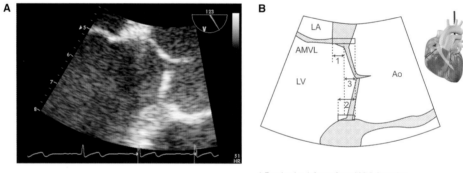

1 Proximal < 4-6 mm from AMVL insertion
2 Proximal < 2-4 mm below the most ventricular portion
3 Distal part should cover native Ao leaflets

Figure 19.12 Deployed Edwards SAPIEN THV prosthesis. The optimal final position of the deployed Edwards SAPIEN THV prosthesis on the ventricular and the aortic side is shown. *Abbreviations*: AMVL, anterior mitral valve leaflet; Ao, aorta; LA, left atrium; LV, left ventricle; TAVI, transcatheter aortic valve implantation; THV, Transcatheter Heart Valve.

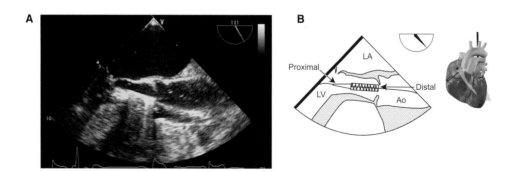

Figure 19.13 Balloon catheter positionning. (A,B) In the mid-esophageal AoV long-axis view the proximal and the distal edge of the AoV prosthesis on the balloon catheter have to be identified before implantation. In this example the prosthesis is completely below the aortic annulus, therefore too low. *Abbreviations*: Ao, aorta; AoV, aortic valve; LA, left atrium; LV, left ventricle; TAVI, transcatheter aortic valve implantation.

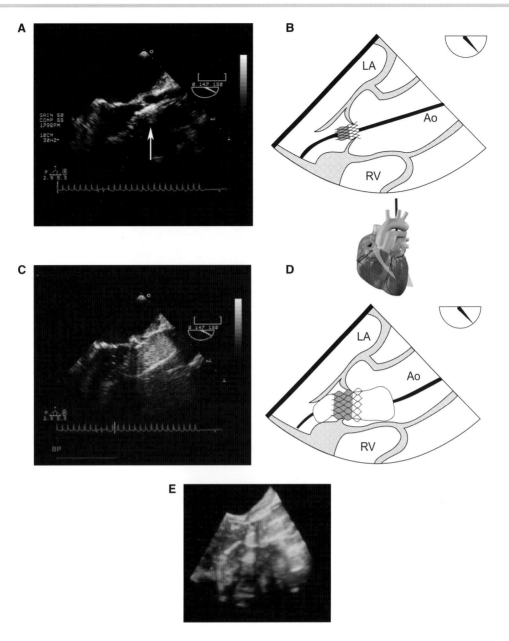

Figure 19.14 Deployment of an Edwards SAPIEN THV prosthesis. (A,B) Mid-esophageal long-axis views with correct positioning before deployment. Low positioning in the left ventricular outflow tract can cause prosthetic dysfunction or AV block. High positioning in the aorta (Ao) may result in obstruction of the coronary ostia or prosthesis dislodgement and embolization. **(C,D)** Immediate post-deployment imaging checking for complete expansion, cusp opening and appearance of the prosthesis: abnormal prosthetic movements or significant paraprosthetic leak may indicate early signs of prosthesis instability. **(E)** Real-time three-dimensional TEE view during deployment. *Abbreviations*: Ao, aorta; AV, atrio-ventricular; LA, left atrium; RV, right ventricle; TEE, transesophageal echocardiography; THV, Transcatheter Heart Valve.

valve) of the aortic annulus (Fig. 19.18). Small PPLs accounting for trace to mild AR are well tolerated and acceptable because they usually have no major clinical repercussions, remain stable, and sometimes regress over time particularly after intravenous heparin reversal with protamine (21). Moderate or severe PPL may

require more expansion of the prosthesis with repeat balloon inflation. However, this entails the potential risk of damaging the leaflets and inducing significant traumatic transvalvular regurgitation. Thus, the quantification of initial post-deployment aortic prosthetic regurgitation should be done meticulously and

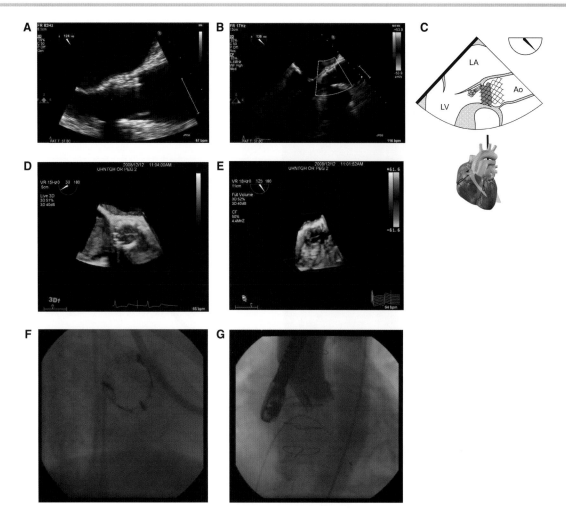

Figure 19.15   TAVI final result. The final result of TAVI shows a stable prosthesis with mild aortic paravalvular regurgitation (AR) in the mid-esophageal long-axis (**A–C**) and 3D short-axis (**D,E**) views. (**F,G**) Aortography confirms minimal prosthetic AR. *Abbreviations*: Ao, aorta; AR, aortic regurgitation; LA, left atrium; LV, left ventricle; TAVI, transcatheter aortic valve implantation. ᐁ

repeated serially over several minutes before deciding on repeat balloon inflation or observation. On the other hand, moderate to severe AR should be communicated immediately to the implanting team. Depending on the situation, reexpansion of the prosthesis using a balloon or in situ deployment of a second prosthesis within the first one in case of malposition of the initial prosthesis may be necessary (Fig. 19.19).

Intraprosthetic leaks must be evaluated after the withdrawal of the guidewire. A trace to mild central regurgitant jet is normal. Prosthesis function evaluation should be done according to usual standards. Special attention must be paid to the coronary circulation by evaluating global and regional LV function post prosthetic deployment. The proximal part of the left main coronary artery and the right coronary artery (RCA) could be examined using color and spectral

Doppler. A zone of turbulent flow or a maximal diastolic velocity higher than normal (>0.25 m/s in the RCA or >0.5 m/s in the left main coronary artery) may indicate a sign of a new stenosis secondary to embolization of material at the time of prosthesis implantation. Coronary embolization or obstruction should be suspected in the case of a new segmental motion abnormality in the LV (Fig. 19.20). Coronary angiography and percutaneous coronary intervention (PCI) with or without CPB for hemodynamic support may be warranted in such cases.

Finally, the aorta (Ao) and pericardium should be examined to rule out dissection or intramural hematoma. The absence of foreign objects or thrombus in the Ao is documented (Fig. 19.21), as well as absence of pericardial fluid (Fig. 19.22). The aortic-mitral continuity is examined and the degree of MR

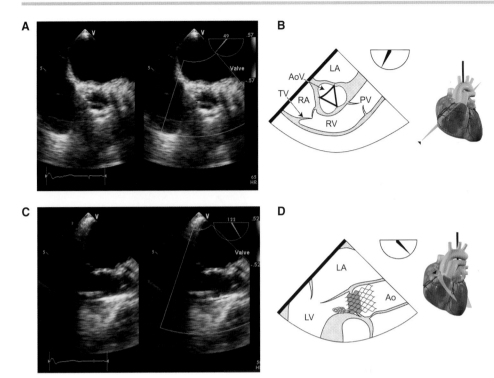

Figure 19.16 Normal Medtronic CoreValve. Color compare mid-esophageal AoV short-axis (**A,B**) and long-axis (**C,D**) views of the prosthesis confirm a good position with only trace anterior paravalvular aortic regurgitation. *Abbreviations*: Ao, aorta; AoV, aortic valve; LA, left atrium; LV, left ventricle; PV, pulmonic valve; RA, right atrium; RV, right ventricle; TV, tricuspid valve. *Source*: Courtesy of Dr. Robert R. Moss. ⌃

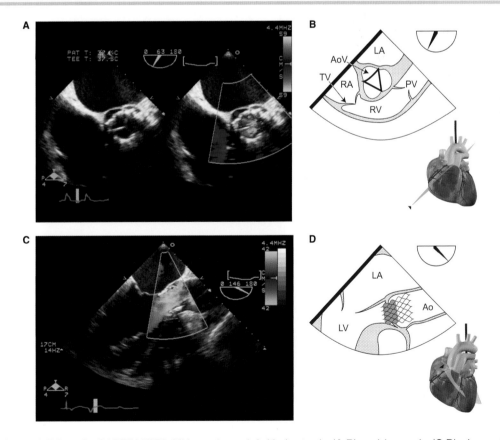

Figure 19.17 Normal Edwards SAPIEN THV. Mid-esophageal AoV short-axis (**A,B**) and long-axis (**C,D**) views of the prosthesis confirm a good position without significant aortic regurgitation. *Abbreviations*: Ao, aorta; AoV, aortic valve; LA, left atrium; LV, left ventricle; PV, pulmonic valve; RA, right atrium; RV, right ventricle; TV, tricuspid valve; THV, Transcatheter Heart Valve. *Source*: Courtesy of Dr. Robert R. Moss. ⌃

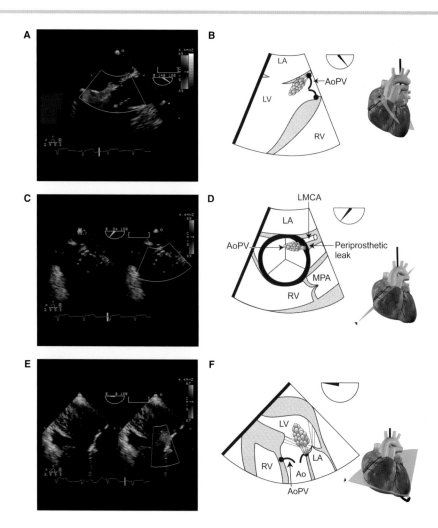

Figure 19.18 Paraprosthetic leaks. Paraprosthetic leak in a 77-year-old woman who underwent successful deployment of an Edwards SAPIEN THV 23 mm AoV is shown. (**A,B**) Color Doppler mid-esophageal (ME) AoV long-axis view with posterior paravalvular aortic regurgitation. The severity and localization of paravalvular leaks are also assessed in the color Doppler ME AoV short-axis (**C,D**) and in the deep transgastric long-axis (**E,F**) views. *Abbreviations*: Ao, aorta; AoPV, aortic valve prosthesis; AoV, aortic valve; ME, mid-esophageal; LA, left atrium; LMCA, left main coronary artery; LV, left ventricle; MPA, main pulmonary artery; RV, right ventricle; THV, Transcatheter Heart Valve.

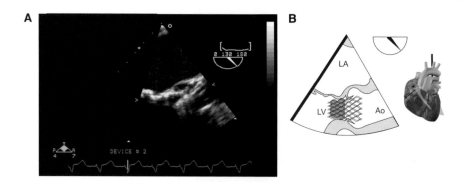

Figure 19.19 Prosthesis in a prosthesis. (**A,B**) Mid-esophageal aortic valve long-axis view following deployment of a second prosthesis within an initially malpositioned first one. Mild paraprosthetic leak is present. *Abbreviations*: Ao, aorta; LA, left atrium; LV, left ventricle. *Source*: Courtesy of Dr. Robert R. Moss.

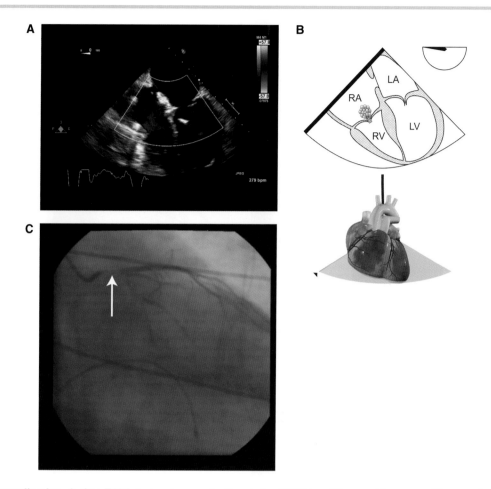

Figure 19.20 Complication during TAVI. Ischemic complication during TAVI in a 67-year-old woman with normal coronary arteries and left ventricular function. After balloon dilatation, she developed severe hypotension with significant QRS widening on the electrocardiogram. (**A,B**) Mid-esophageal four-chamber view shows severe left ventricular global hypokinesis. (**C**) Coronary angiography reveals acute left main occlusion. *Abbreviations*: LA, left atrium; LV, left ventricle; RA, right atrium; RV, right ventricle; TAVI, transcatheter aortic valve implantation.

assessed. The transprosthetic gradient is also evaluated. When the absence of complication is confirmed, TEE is used to guide weaning from CPB or left heart bypass when applicable.

USE OF TEE IN THE POST-PROCEDURAL PERIOD AND IN THE INTENSIVE CARE UNIT

In the event of hemodynamic instability after TAVI, TTE and TEE, when necessary, may help to identify complications. Tamponade, coronary ischemia with LV dysfunction, MR, aortic dissection, and device migration are among the considerations specific to TAVI that should be excluded. Assessment of fluid status, diastolic function, and right and left ventricular functions are evaluated as part of the postoperative echocardiographic examination of the unstable patient after TAVI.

In the stable patient, serial TTE (or TEE if indicated) is used in the days, weeks, and months following the procedure and can document aortic prosthetic valve function and area, transvalvular gradient, perivalvular leak, regression of LV hypertrophy, and changes in left ventricular ejection fraction (LVEF). Improvement in the degree of MR has been observed in some cases (9).

CONCLUSION

Transcatheter AoV implantation is a promising new technique with various approaches. During initial assessment, TEE provides important data helpful in the planning of the procedure (22) and in the identification of cardiac and aortic comorbidities. Data also suggests that periprocedural TEE may be helpful in optimizing the accurate positioning and subsequent deployment of the prosthesis (9). In addition, in the advent of hemodynamic instability or complications, TEE allows for rapid diagnostic clues important in their optimal management. TEE is therefore a highly useful tool for patient management in TAVI. The role of TEE in TAVI is summarized in Table 19.1.

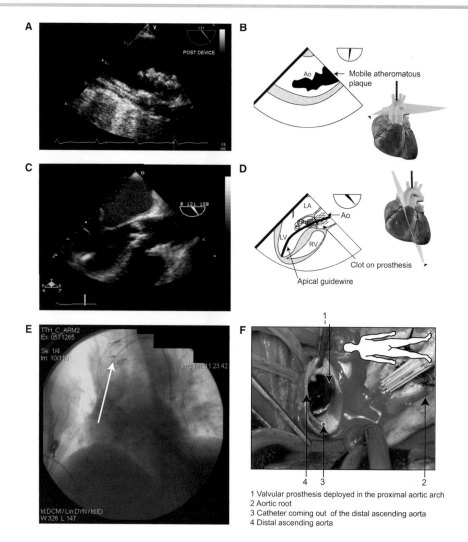

1 Valvular prosthesis deployed in the proximal aortic arch
2 Aortic root
3 Catheter coming out of the distal ascending aorta
4 Distal ascending aorta

Figure 19.21   Complications during TAVI. (A,B) Upper esophageal aortic arch long-axis view with embolized atherosclerotic material after deployment of a prosthesis in 76-year-old woman. Further imaging suggested that the atherosclerotic material originated from an iliac intimal flap stuck to the prosthesis during the transfemoral insertion of the crimped valve. **(C,D)** Mid-esophageal long-axis aortic valve view with thrombus near a deployed prosthesis. **(E,F)** Dislodged prosthesis with migration in the ascending Ao (arrow) visualized on fluoroscopy, requiring emergency conversion to an open AoV replacement. *Abbreviations*: Ao, aorta; LA, left atrium; LV, left ventricle; RV, right ventricle; TAVI, transcatheter aortic valve implantation. *Source*: A and C, courtesy of Dr. Robert R. Moss.

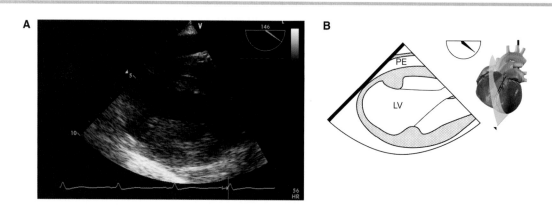

Figure 19.22   Pericardial complications in TAVI. (A,B) Transgastric long-axis view at 146° shows a new posterior PE after TAVI, worrisome for cardiac perforation or aortic dissection. *Abbreviations*: LV, left ventricle; PE, pericardial effusion; TAVI, transcatheter aortic valve implantation.

Table 19.1 Role of Transesophageal Echocardiography During TAVI

TAVI stage	Objectives
Baseline	1. Aortic valve assessment: calcification size and localization, leaflet mobility, AVA, aortic valve gradient, aortic regurgitation (grade and jet location) 2. Measurement of aortic root diameters (annulus and sinotubular junction) and left ventricular outflow tract dimension 3. Left ventricular function 4. Mitral valve function 5. Anatomic evaluation of thoracic aorta 6. Distance between valve and coronary ostia 7. Other cardiac structures: left atrial appendage
Balloon valvuloplasty	1. Effects of balloon valvuloplasty on aortic valve leaflet mobility, degree of aortic regurgitation 2. Left ventricular function 3. Anatomic evaluation of the aorta
Pre-TAVI deployment Post-TAVI deployment	Prosthetic valve position (with respect to aortic valve plane and the left ventricular outflow tract) 1. Prosthetic valve assessment—aortic valve annulus diameter, aortic valve area, aortic valve gradient (peak and mean), valve stability, leaflet mobility, regurgitation grade, and location (peri- vs. intra-prosthetic) 2. Morphology of aortic root and ascending aorta 3. Left ventricular outflow tract dimension and flows 4. Left ventricular function 5. Mitral valve function 6. Anatomic evaluation of thoracic aorta 7. Other cardiac structures: pericardium, interatrial septum, pleural space

Abbreviations: TAVI, transcatheter aortic valve implantation; AVA, aortic valve area.
Source: Adapted from Ref. 8.

ACKNOWLEDGMENTS

The authors would like to thank Dr John G. Webb and Dr Raoul Bonan for their help in the preparation of this chapter as well as Dr Robert R. Moss for images and echo clips.

REFERENCES

1. Cribier A, Eltchaninoff H, Bash A, et al. Percutaneous transcatheter implantation of an aortic valve prosthesis for calcific aortic stenosis: first human case description. Circulation 2002; 106:3006–3008.
2. Grube E, Laborde JC, Gerckens U, et al. Percutaneous implantation of the CoreValve self-expanding valve prosthesis in high-risk patients with aortic valve disease: the Siegburg first-in-man study. Circulation 2006; 114:1616–1624.
3. Webb JG, Chandavimol M, Thompson CR, et al. Percutaneous aortic valve implantation retrograde from the femoral artery. Circulation 2006; 113:842–850.
4. Ye J, Cheung A, Lichtenstein SV, et al. Transapical aortic valve implantation in humans. J Thorac Cardiovasc Surg 2006; 131:1194–1196.
5. Lichtenstein SV, Cheung A, Ye J, et al. Transapical transcatheter aortic valve implantation in humans: initial clinical experience. Circulation 2006; 114:591–596.
6. Webb JG, Lichtenstein S. Transcatheter percutaneous and transapical aortic valve replacement. Semin Thorac Cardiovasc Surg 2007; 19:304–310.
7. Walther T, Falk V, Kempfert J, et al. Transapical minimally invasive aortic valve implantation; the initial 50 patients. Eur J Cardiothorac Surg 2008; 33:983–988.
8. Berry C, Oukerraj L, Asgar A, et al. Role of transesophageal echocardiography in percutaneous aortic valve replacement with the CoreValve Revalving system. Echocardiography 2008; 25:840–848.
9. Moss R, Ivens E, Pasupati S, et al. Role of echocardiography in percutaneous aortic valve implantation. JACC Cardiovasc Imaging 2008; 1:15–24.
10. Chin D. Echocardiography for transcatheter aortic valve implantation. Eur J Echocardiogr 2009; 10:i21–i29.
11. Cribier A, Eltchaninoff H, Tron C, et al. Early experience with percutaneous transcatheter implantation of heart valve prosthesis for the treatment of end-stage inoperable patients with calcific aortic stenosis. J Am Coll Cardiol 2004; 43:698–703.
12. Khambadkone S, Nordmeyer J, Bonhoeffer P. Percutaneous implantation of the pulmonary and aortic valves: indications and limitations. J Cardiovasc Med (Hagerstown) 2007; 8:57–61.
13. Nordmeyer J, Coats L, Lurz P, et al. Percutaneous pulmonary valve-in-valve implantation: a successful treatment concept for early device failure. Eur Heart J 2008; 29:810–815.
14. Wenaweser P, Buellesfeld L, Gerckens U, et al. Percutaneous aortic valve replacement for severe aortic regurgitation in degenerated bioprosthesis: the first valve in valve procedure using the Corevalve Revalving system. Catheter Cardiovasc Interv 2007; 70:760–764.
15. Cheung A, Webb JG, Wong DR, et al. Transapical transcatheter mitral valve-in-valve implantation in a human. Ann Thorac Surg 2009; 87:e18–e20.

16. Grube E, Schuler G, Buellesfeld L, et al. Percutaneous aortic valve replacement for severe aortic stenosis in high-risk patients using the second- and current third-generation self-expanding CoreValve prosthesis: device success and 30-day clinical outcome. J Am Coll Cardiol 2007; 50:69–76.

17. Ree RM, Bowering JB, Schwarz SK. Case series: anesthesia for retrograde percutaneous aortic valve replacement—experience with the first 40 patients. Can J Anaesth 2008; 55:761–768.

18. Fassl J, Walther T, Groesdonk HV, et al. Anesthesia management for transapical transcatheter aortic valve implantation: a case series. J Cardiothorac Vasc Anesth 2009; 23:286–291.

19. Zoghbi WA, Enriquez-Sarano M, Foster E, et al. Recommendations for evaluation of the severity of native valvular regurgitation with two-dimensional and Doppler echocardiography. J Am Soc Echocardiogr 2003; 16: 777–802.

20. Rodés-Cabau J, Dumont E, De LaRochelliere R, et al. Feasibility and initial results of percutaneous aortic valve implantation including selection of the transfemoral or transapical approach in patients with severe aortic stenosis. Am J Cardiol 2008; 102:1240–1246.

21. Webb JG, Pasupati S, Humphries K, et al. Percutaneous transarterial aortic valve replacement in selected high-risk patients with aortic stenosis. Circulation 2007; 116:755–763.

22. Rodés-Cabau J, Webb JG, Cheung A, et al. Transcatheter aortic valve implantation for the treatment of severe symptomatic aortic stenosis in patients at very high or prohibitive surgical risk: acute and late outcomes of the Multicenter Canadian Experience. J Am Coll Cardiol 2010; 55:1080–1090.

20

Transesophageal Echocardiography for Minimally Invasive Cardiac Surgery

Jean-Sébastien Lebon
Université de Montréal, Montreal, Quebec, Canada

José Coddens and Hugo Vanermen
KUL University, Aalst, Belgium

INTRODUCTION

Cardiovascular surgery is, conventionally, performed through a median sternotomy enabling generous exposure to the operative field. This allows central cannulation for cardiopulmonary bypass (CPB) and performance of complex procedures under direct view. Concurrent advances in cardiopulmonary perfusion, intracardiac endoscopic visualization, instrumentation, and robotic telemanipulation have resulted in a dramatic shift toward efficient and safe cardiac procedures through minimal access.

The term minimally invasive, or minimal access, cardiac surgery refers to the size of the incision, the avoidance of sternotomy, and possible avoidance of CPB. Minimally invasive cardiac surgery is a nonspecific term that groups together different surgical procedures (Fig. 20.1).

Using this approach the surgeon must master levels of technical complexity starting with small incision, direct vision (level 1), then progressing toward more complex video-assisted procedures (level 2), video-directed and robot-assisted procedures (level 3), and, finally, to telemanipulation and robotic-assisted valve operations (level 4).

To be successful, the anesthesiologist must have detailed knowledge of each surgical procedure and the appropriate anesthesia technique, as well as being skilled in the use of transesophageal echocardiography (TEE). As the surgeon's visual field shrinks, the reliance on TEE to aid visualization increases. Transesophageal echocardiography is an indispensable tool in guiding venous and arterial catheter placement, monitoring cardiac function, and diagnosing complications and contraindications related to different procedures. The role of TEE in minimally invasive cardiac surgery is summarized in Table 20.1.

In this chapter, the emphasis will be placed on the use of perioperative TEE for diverse, minimally invasive, cardiac surgical procedures. For practical reasons, only the echographic considerations are presented for the different classes of well-established procedures (Table 20.2) available for cardiac surgery.

MITRAL VALVE PROCEDURE

The ultimate goal of a minimally invasive approach for mitral valve (MV) surgery is to offer a patient a valvular repair equivalent to that of an open approach while minimizing trauma. This different surgical attitude, developed in the 1990s following the undeniable success of abdominal surgery by endoscopy, aims to enable a patient to regain functional capacity rapidly and to diminish perioperative morbidity. However, scientifically proven clinical advantages as described in the literature are more modest. Esthetic advantages, better overall patient satisfaction, diminished systemic inflammation, as well as a reduction in reintervention morbidity and mortality have been proven (1–7). A few studies have reported a trend in reduced hospital stay, renal insufficiency, bleeding, atrial fibrillation incidence, and postoperative pain (2,3,8–10). As for all new techniques, a learning curve is inevitable and the results obtained by less experienced centers are truly interesting and cannot be ignored (6,11).

The principles of MV repair remain unchanged but a thoracoscopy approach modifies the classic technique (Fig. 20.2). The majority of minimally invasive mitral procedures are done on an arrested heart using PORT ACCESS technology (Fig. 20.3). This approach involves a small incision with soft tissue retraction at the fifth right intercostal space level (Fig. 20.4), exposure aided by thoracoscopic camera (Fig. 20.5), endovascular extracorporeal circulation, and aortic clamping.

The most significant change for the anesthesiologist is the use of CPB by an endovascular route (12,13). In this approach, venous return is maintained by one or two venous cannulae positioned in the right atrium (RA) by echocardiographic guidance from the femoral and right internal jugular veins. The oxygenized blood is returned to the patient by an arterial cannula inserted in the descending aorta (Ao) via the femoral artery. Aortic clamping is completed with the help of a balloon positioned by echocardiography in the ascending Ao or by an adapted clamp inserted through a thoracic port. After clamping, cardioplegia is administered by an antegrade route through the

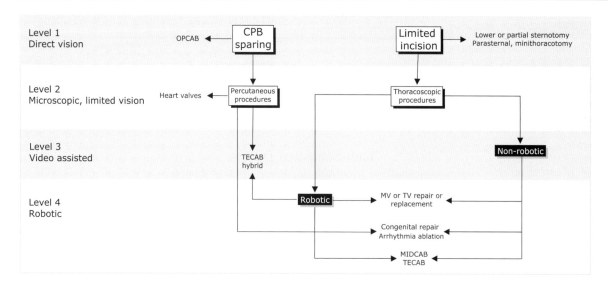

Figure 20.1 Minimally invasive cardiac surgery classification. This approach will involve increasingly complex and less invasive levels (1–4) to complete an array of various cardiac surgical procedures. *Abbreviations*: CPB, cardiopulmonary bypass; MIDCAB, minimally invasive direct coronary artery bypass; MV, mitral valve; OPCAB, off-pump coronary artery bypass; PAVR, percutaneous aortic valve replacement; PPVR, percutaneous pulmonary valve replacement; TECAB, total endoscopic coronary artery bypass; TV; tricuspid valve.

Table 20.1   Step-by-Step Approach to the Role of TEE in Minimally Invasive Cardiac Surgery

Before the procedure:

1. Careful insertion of the TEE probe under direct vision because of the use of double lumen endotracheal tube for single lung ventilation (Fig. 20.2).
2. Exclusion of any contraindication for minimally invasive cardiac surgery (Table 20.3 and Fig. 20.6).
3. Complete TEE exam (see Chapter 4) to evaluate biventricular systolic and diastolic function, coronary anatomy, complete valvular, aortic, pericardial and pleural evaluation.
4. Exclusion of a patent foramen ovale and a left pleural effusion.
5. Description of the mechanism of mitral regurgitation and the size of the left atrium and ventricle, determination of the risk factors for SAM, and exclusion of left atrial appendage thrombus.
6. Echocardiographic monitoring for the position of the guidewires (Fig. 20.7) retrograde sinus catheter (Fig. 20.8), the decompression cannula (Fig. 20.9), the superior and inferior vena cava venous cannula (Fig. 20.10), and the aortic endoclamp (Figs. 20.11 and 20.12).

During the procedure:

1. Monitoring of the adequate position of the various cannula (Figs. 20.14 and 20.15) and endovascular clamp (Figs. 20.17 and 20.18).
2. Monitoring of any complications related to the positioning of the various cannulae (Fig. 20.13).

After the procedure:

1. Confirmation of the adequacy of the surgical result.
2. Diagnosis of the causes of hemodynamic instability if present (Chapter 10). This includes new regional wall motion abnormalities (see Chapters 9 and 10), aortic dissection (Fig. 20.16), new valvular pathologies (Figs. 20.19 and 20.20), outflow tract obstructions, pericardial tamponade, pleural, peritoneal and retroperitoneal bleeding.

Abbreviations: SAM, systolic anterior motion; TEE, transesophageal echocardiography.

distal port of the intra-aortic balloon or by retrograde route via a coronary sinus catheter. These various components are necessary to ensure effective and secure CPB when direct access to the surgical site is limited and an unencumbered operating field is crucial. Additional anesthetic considerations include: positioning, single lung ventilation, cerebral perfusion monitoring, and the insertion of different catheters (Fig. 20.2).

Screening Exam

After induction of general anesthesia, a TEE probe is inserted, preferably aided by a laryngoscope to minimize

Table 20.2 Minimally Invasive Cardiac Surgery Procedures

1. Minimally invasive mitral valve surgery
   a. Direct-vision
   b. Video-assisted
   c. PORT ACCESS system
   d. Robot directed telemanipulation and computer enhanced
2. Minimally invasive aortic valve surgery
   a. Small thoracotomy
      i. J sternotomy
   b. Percutaneous aortic valve implantation
      i. Retrograde from femoral artery
      ii. Transapical transcatheter
3. Minimally invasive coronary artery surgery
   a. Off-pump coronary artery bypass (OPCAB)
   b. Minimally invasive direct coronary artery bypass (MIDCAB)
      i. Robotic enhanced MIDCAB
   c. Total endoscopic coronary artery revascularization (TECAB)
      i. TECAB—arrested heart
      ii. TECAB—beating heart
   d. Small thoracotomy
      i. Hemisternotomy
      ii. J sternotomy
4. Vascular stenting
   a. Aorta stent
   b. Carotid
5. Rhythm procedure
   a. A fib ablation
   b. Cardiac resynchronization

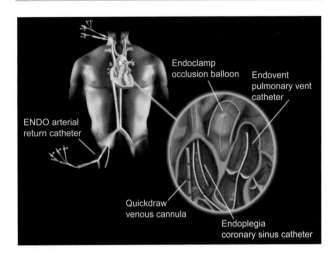

Figure 20.3 PORT ACCESS system. Components of various endovascular extracorporal circulation systems such as the EndoCPB and the InSite AVR systems. *Source*: With permission of Edwards Lifesciences. *http://www.edwards.com/products/portaccess/portaccess.htm.*

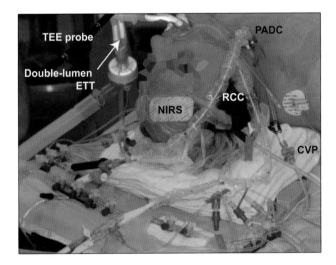

Figure 20.2 Minimally invasive cardiac surgery. Intraoperative photo shows the complex patient setup at the head of the bed. *Abbreviations*: CVP, central venous pressure catheter; ETT, endotracheal tube; PADC, pulmonary artery decompression catheter; NIRS, near-infrared spectroscopy monitoring; RCC, retrograde cardioplegia catheter; TEE, transesophageal echocardiography probe.

oral or esophageal trauma and avoid displacement of the double lumen endotracheal tube. The TEE exam is divided into two parts: a screening portion to rule out potential contraindications to PORT ACCESS surgery (Table 20.3) (14) followed by a complete exam. Absolute contraindications to PORT ACCESS surgery include (*i*) moderate to severe aortic regurgitation (AR), (*ii*) severe aortic disease, and (*iii*) right atrial and right ventricular inflow or outflow tract obstruction. These conditions must be ruled out before the installation of the central catheters to avoid exposing the patient to additional risks related to unnecessary procedures.

The presence of significant AR could inhibit the effective administration of the anterograde cardioplegia. Essentially, any AR severe enough to warrant surgical intervention would be a dissuasive argument for the use of an endovascular clamping. Furthermore, the thoracic Ao must be extensively evaluated to exclude any advanced atherosclerotic disease. The presence of mobile plaque, aneurysmal dilatation, dissection, intramural hematoma, or a penetrative ulceration constitutes relative contraindications to an endovascular approach. The ascending Ao must also be measured, as a diameter in excess of 40 mm is associated with incomplete endovascular aortic occlusion. Finally, the inflow anatomy of the right ventricle (RV) must be attentively examined to detect the presence of thrombus (Fig. 20.6) or vestigial embryonic development. The Eustachian and the Thebesian valves, the Chiari network, and a persistent left superior vena cava (SVC) with hypoplastic right SVC can make the positioning of venous cannulae and, especially, the coronary sinus catheter difficult. Finally, the complete absence of an inferior vena cava (IVC) is rare but excludes the PORT ACCESS approach since venous

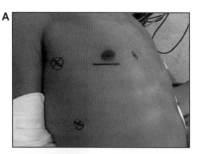

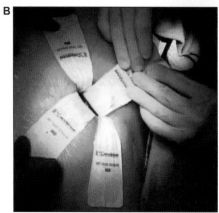

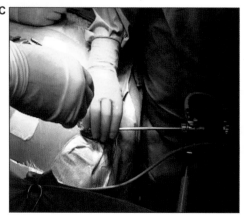

Figure 20.4 Minimally invasive cardiac surgery. Minimally invasive cardiac surgery with the PORT ACCESS MVR system. (**A**) Identification of the right thoracotomy incision site. (**B**) Application of the special soft tissue retractors. (**C**) Insertion of the thoracoscopic instruments for a nonrobotic thoracoscopic mitral valve repair. *Abbreviation*: MVR, mitral valve repair. *Source*: Courtesy of Dr. Michel Pellerin.

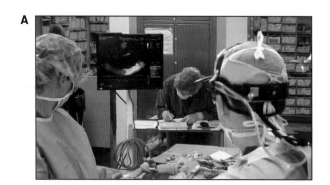

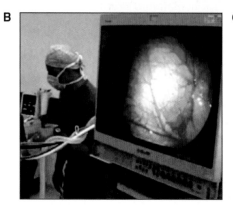

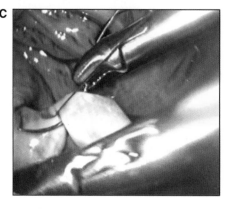

Figure 20.5 Monitoring during minimally invasive cardiac surgery. (**A**) Transesophageal echocardiography imaging is transmitted to other high resolution monitors in the OR for the benefit of the whole intervention team. (**B,C**) The thoracoscopic images displayed on high-resolution monitors enables a significantly magnified view of the surgical procedure. *Abbreviation*: OR, operating room. *Source*: Courtesy of Dr. Michel Pellerin.

Table 20.3 Contraindications for Minimally Invasive Surgery

1. Contraindications for TEE (see Chapter 8)
2. Moderate to severe aortic regurgitation (see Chapter 14)
3. Severe aortic disease: grade IV and V atheromatous disease, penetrating ulcers, dissection, hematomas, ascending aortic dilatation >40 mm (see Chapter 23)
4. Congenital or acquired right atrial and ventricular outflow tract obstruction (Fig. 20.6)
5. Absence of a superior or inferior vena cava

Abbreviation: TEE, transesophageal echocardiography.

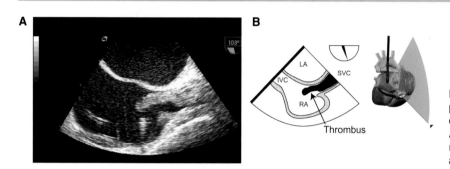

Figure 20.6 SVC thrombus. (A,B) Midesophageal bicaval view showing a SVC clot, a contraindication for the usage of the PORT ACCESS technique. *Abbreviations*: IVC, inferior vena cava; LA, left atrium; RA, right atrium; SVC, superior vena cava.

return from the azygos system prohibits the use of the IVC cannula.

Complete TEE

In a second order of things, an echocardiographic examination is completed in accordance to the Society of Cardiovascular Anesthesiologists (SCA)/American Heart Association (AHA) standards for perioperative monitoring of patients undergoing valvular surgery (15). Particular attention is given to RV and left ventricular (LV) systolic function, anatomy and function of the other valves, cardiac chamber dimensions, presence of ventricular hypertrophy, interatrial communication, thrombus in the left atrial appendage (LAA) and fluid in the pericardial, and pleural cavities.

The prevalence of atherosclerotic cardiac disease is high in patients with valvulopathy (16–18). This justifies preliminary coronary angiography for patients scheduled for MV repair. The presence of extensive coronary disease limits the use of the PORT ACCESS technique, considering the technical difficulty associated with complete revascularization. However, for certain single vessel disease, a hybrid approach can be suggested to the patient.

During the procedure, as coronary lesions are dynamic, it is important to look for the indirect signs of myocardial ischemia even without angiographic evidence of significant stenosis. A normal coronary angiogram does not invalidate the causal link between narrowing of the artery and the signs of ischemia observed during the perioperative period. In fact, myocardial ischemia should be suspected at the appearance of regional myocardial wall motion anomaly,

cavity dilatation, or de novo mitral regurgitation (MR). Myocardial ischemia is one of the most frequent causes of acute MR (16–18).

Furthermore, the anesthesiologist can directly monitor myocardial perfusion using TEE. The proximal part of the coronary arteries originating from their respective Valsalva sinus can be visualized in a short-axis (see Figs. 9.2 and 9.3) or long-axis (LAX) view of the aortic valve (AoV). In the presence of coronary artery disease, a zone of accelerated flow or turbulence can be detected (19–23). Moreover, a detailed exam of coronary circulation is important to detect any aberrant anatomy such as a circumflex artery passing close to the mitral annulus. Knowledge of this condition could prevent trauma to the circumflex artery during mitral annuloplasty.

Two-dimensional (2D) and color Doppler examination of the interatrial septum in search of a communication between atria must be done in all patients at the start of the surgery. The presence of a permeable foramen ovale in 10% to 35% of patients is significant (24,25). This finding should be relayed to the surgical team so that it can be closed at the beginning of the procedure. This avoids repeated flooding of the operating field and air embolism with air locked in the CPB endovascular circuit.

Recognizing a left pleural effusion before the surgery is fundamental because it interferes with adequate one lung ventilation and compromises oxygenation. Installation of a thoracic drain to empty the effusion is essential for safe unilateral ventilation.

A detailed exam of the MV is performed to guide the surgeon (see Chapter 16) (26,27). The anesthesiologist must evaluate the anatomy of the leaflets, the regurgitation mechanism and its importance, the presence of calcium, the annular dimensions, the left atrial (LA) and LV dimensions, the synchronism of wall contraction, as well as the absence of atrial or ventricular thrombus.

For patients scheduled for MV surgery, the preoperative risks of systolic anterior motion (SAM) of the MV anterior leaflet must be evaluated (see Chapter 11). Change made to the left ventricular outflow tract (LVOT) anatomy, when lowering the mitral annulus and the coaptation point with ring implantation, predisposes these patients to dynamic obstruction. Using mid-esophageal five-chamber or LAX views of the LV, three measurements are associated with a higher postoperative SAM risk (28–30). These are (*i*) a ratio of the length of the anterior leaflet/posterior leaflet <1.4, (*ii*) a distance between the coaptation point and the septum <2.5 cm, and (*iii*) an acute angle (≤130°) between the AoV and MV planes (see Fig. 11.11). This information should be communicated to the surgeon.

Finally, in view of a high association between MV and tricuspid valve (TV) pathologies, a careful evaluation of the tricuspid apparatus must be performed, especially when pulmonary hypertension is present. The increase in morbidity and mortality resulting from the presence of residual tricuspid regurgitation (TR) after the operation are well defined (31–33). However, the significance of diagnosing significant functional TR under anesthesia remains unclear. The difficulty stems from the underestimation of the importance of the TR jet in patients under general anesthesia and mechanical ventilation. Indirect criteria, other than jet quantification and hepatic venous flow, have been developed to offset this problem (see Chapter 18) (34,35). These criteria are based on TV anatomy and annular dilatation and also RV anatomy instead of the evaluation of the TR jet. They include (*i*) the eccentricity index of the RV (see Chapter 10), (*ii*) the subvalvular tenting area, and (*iii*) the tricuspid annulus diameter. They offer, in decreasing order, a sensitivity and a specificity superior to that of a qualitative evaluation of the regurgitating jet to diagnose the presence of significant functional TR. However, the use of these indices for patients under general anesthesia has not been validated.

Central Catheter Insertion

The insertion of various catheters at the jugular level, by an anesthesiologist, using the Seldinger method is

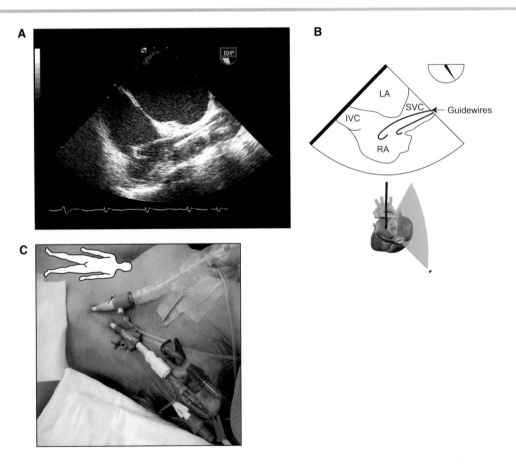

Figure 20.7 Guidewire position. (A,B) Mid-esophageal bicaval view at 104° shows two guidewires over which the decompression and retrograde cardioplegia catheters will be inserted. **(C)** Intraoperative view of the catheters at their insertion point in the neck. *Abbreviations*: IVC, inferior vena cava; LA, left atrium; RA, right atrium; SVC, superior vena cava.

guided by echocardiography or fluoroscopy to optimize their final position. In the operating room, confirmation by echocardiography is usually preferred for practical reasons; however a combined technique is always possible (36). The use of a cannula in the SVC, a coronary sinus catheter, and a pulmonary artery decompression catheter varies according to local practice. The rationale for use is guided by weighing individual risks and benefits for each patient.

SVC Venous Catheter

Optimal surgical conditions are achieved by reducing venous return to the heart and preventing flooding of the surgical field. Drainage of the right heart is primarily accomplished by a venous cannula positioned at the junction of the RA and the SVC supplemented by a cannula in the SVC. Installation of the SVC cannula is done in exactly the same manner as all other central catheters. However, due to its size, meticulous manipulation and a few rules exist to lessen the risk to the patient: (*i*) the guidewire must be visualized in the RA, in a bicaval view, before inserting this cannula (Fig. 20.7); (*ii*) insertion is greatly facilitated by a cutaneous incision adapted to the size of the cannula (21 French for men or women and 17 for small women, respectively) and a generous

dilation of the pathway; (*iii*) it is crucial to never use force. The cannula must glide easily without significant resistance as far as a full line indicating a distance to the skin of 10 cm. The utmost caution is essential; cases of perforation of the SVC and RA have been reported with disastrous results; (*iv*) the distal point of the cannula should be visualized at the junction of the SVC and the RA before skin fixation with a hemostatic stitch to ensure immobility and to facilitate postoperative hemostasis.

Coronary Sinus Catheter

The coronary sinus catheter is installed to enable the administration of retrograde cardioplegia. This is not an absolute indication as antegrade cardioplegia can be administered securely and effectively (3,6,7). However, in the presence of a permeable internal mammary artery graft or significant AR, administration of retrograde cardioplegia is necessary in certain patients to arrest the heart. Coronary sinus perforation is a risk inherent to catheter manipulation (Fig. 20.8) (37,38) (see Fig. 13.11) and the high rate of displacement during surgery accounts for its lack of popularity. The insertion of the coronary sinus catheter introducer is done using the Seldinger method at the right jugular level. A dirigible or preformed catheter is then advanced to the

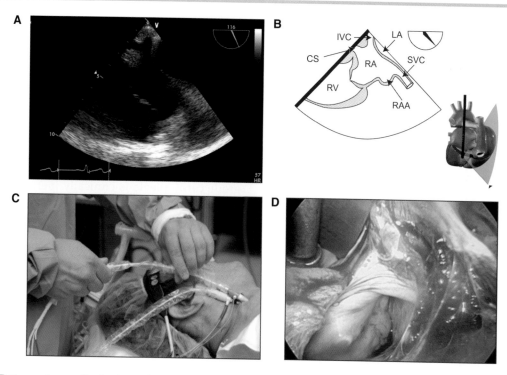

Figure 20.8 Retrograde cardioplegia catheter. Retrograde cardioplegia catheter insertion in the CS. (**A,B**) Modified lower midesophageal bicaval view at 110° where the IVC is at the top right, the TV on the left with the CS between them in the middle. (**C**) From a position at the head of the patient, the anesthesiologist tries to insert the retrograde cardioplegia catheter into the CS, clockwise from the IVC and counterclockwise from the TV. (**D**) Intraoperative thoracoscopic view of the retrograde cardioplegia catheter tenting (*arrow*) against the wall of the left atrium (LA). *Abbreviations*: CS, coronary sinus; IVC, inferior vena cava; LA, left atrium; ME, mid-esophageal; RA, right atrium; RAA, right atrial appendage; RV, right ventricle; SVC, superior vena cava; TV, tricuspid valve. *Source*: Courtesy of Dr. Michel Pellerin.

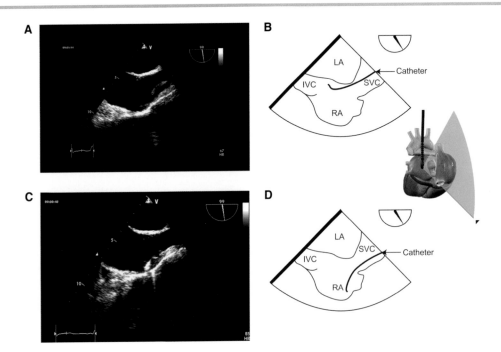

Figure 20.9 Retrograde cardioplegia catheter. Retrograde cardioplegia catheter insertion monitoring through the mid-esophageal bicaval view. **(A,B)** Ideal and **(C,D)** suboptimal starting position of the retrograde cardioplegia catheter. The latter should move along the interatrial septum. *Abbreviations*: IVC, inferior vena cava; LA, left atrium; RA, right atrium; SVC, superior vena cava.

RA and SVC junction. A bicaval view at 110 to 130° is the window of choice because it permits visualization of the entire catheter length (39). In this view, the coronary sinus is centrally located and bordered to the right by the IVC and to the left by the TV. The guidewire is handled at the exit of the SVC in such a way as to keep its concave face oriented toward the interatrial septum (Fig. 20.9). It is then advanced slowly in the direction of the sinus. At this moment, the catheter is mobilized using delicate movements toward the sinus ostium by turning clockwise from the IVC and counter clockwise from the TV (Fig. 20.10). Insertion into the sinus is confirmed by catheter visualization in a low esophageal view at 0°. Before inflating the balloon, sinus venography is done to verify position and to ensure that there is no extravasation of contrast fluid (Fig. 20.11). The catheter is then advanced as distally as possible to just before the great cardiac vein to increase its stability. The optimal position of the coronary sinus catheter reflects the conflict between stability and maximal cardioprotection. The many communications of the cardiac venous system forms a network ensuring a widespread distribution of cardioplegia irrespective of catheter depth (Fig. 20.11) (40).

The balloon is inflated under direct viewing and adequate positioning is corroborated by two functional tests. Firstly, a ventricularization of the pressure curve must be obtained (Fig. 20.11). Then, during injection of saline solution, bubbles should not escape from the coronary sinus ostium. If these two condi-

tions are not met, even if the echocardiographic position seems adequate, the catheter is not functionally well positioned and must be repositioned. The appearance of a pericardial effusion de novo during manipulations should be considered as a sign of cardiac perforation until proven otherwise. Finally, despite apparently adequate positioning at the start of the procedure, an insufficient perfusion pressure (≤20mmHg) (40) during cardioplegia administration, or failure to achieve asystole, are signs that the retrograde cardioplegia is clinically ineffective.

Pulmonary Artery Decompression Catheter

The pulmonary artery decompression catheter may be used to complete venous return as part of a strategy when using only one venous cannula in the RA. This catheter is inserted through an introducer in the right internal jugular vein, analogous to a pulmonary artery catheter. To ensure optimal decompression, the catheter tip must be placed exactly at the right and left pulmonary artery bifurcation, as verified by echocardiography or fluoroscopy.

Echocardiographic guidance begins with an RV inflow-outflow view at 60° to visualize the progression of the catheter through the TV and pulmonary valve (PV). An upper esophageal view at 0° enables final positioning while confirming that the catheter tip is at the junction of the right and left pulmonary artery (Fig. 20.12).

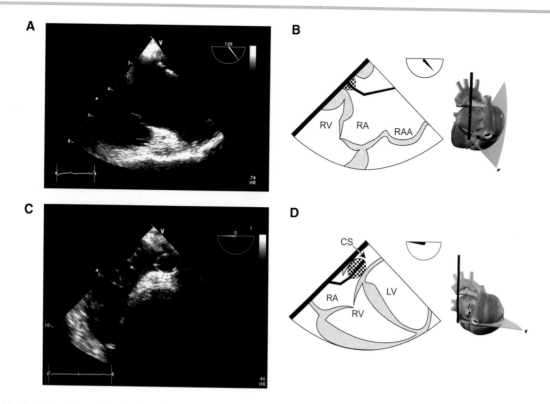

Figure 20.10 Retrograde cardioplegia catheter inadequate position. (A,B) Lower mid-esophageal bicaval view at 129°. **(C,D)** Lower-esophageal view from the four-chamber position at 0°. In both views, the retrograde cardioplegia catheter is not inserted deep enough in the CS. *Abbreviations*: CS, coronary sinus; LV, left ventricle; RA, right atrium; RAA, right atrial appendage; RV, right ventricle.

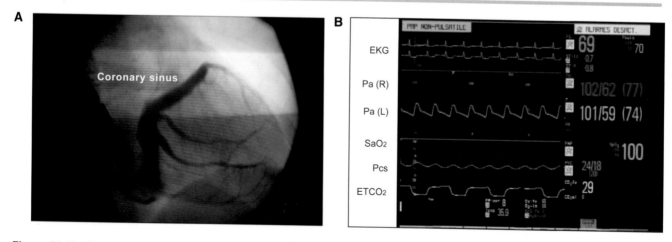

Figure 20.11 Retrograde cardioplegia catheter optimal position. (A) Coronary sinus venography. **(B)** Coronary sinus pressure (Pcs) hemodynamic tracing: note the ventricularized coronary sinus pressure at 24/18 mmHg. *Abbreviations*: EKG, electrocardiogram; ETCO₂, end-tidal CO₂; L, left; Pa, arterial pressure; Pra, radial artery pressure; R, right; SaO₂, oxygen saturation.

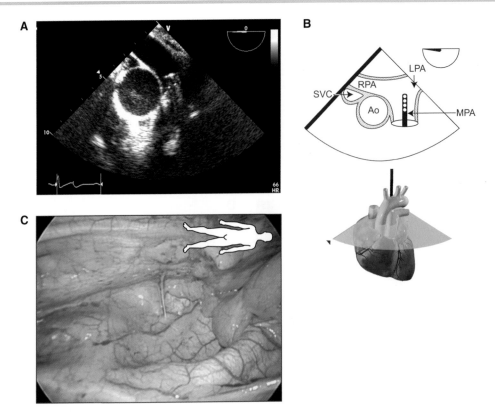

Figure 20.12 PA decompression catheter optimal position. (A,B) Mid-esophageal ascending Ao transverse view at 0°: the PA decompression catheter is ideally positioned at the bifurcation of the RPA and LPA. **(C)** Visual confirmation of the adequately decompressed heart. *Abbreviations*: Ao, aorta; LPA, left pulmonary artery; MPA, main pulmonary artery; PA, pulmonary artery; RPA, right pulmonary artery; SVC, superior vena cava. *Source*: Courtesy Dr. Michel Pellerin.

Central Catheter Positioning Guidance

After heparin administration, surgeons proceed to position the additional venous and arterial cannulae using a Seldinger technique with echocardiographic confirmation.

IVC Venous Cannula

A guidewire is first inserted into the femoral vein under direct vision and advanced until echocardiographic confirmation of its proper position in the SVC in a bicaval view. The cannula is then advanced over the guidewire until the junction of the RA and the SVC is reached (Fig. 20.13). This advanced position of the cannula in the atrium ensures adequate drainage after its distal displacement by the atrial retractor.

Femoral Arterial Cannula and the Aortic Balloon

A guidewire is introduced into the femoral artery using the same technique and its position in the descending aortic lumen is confirmed. An arterial cannula is inserted and the guidewire is removed. If an endoscopic aortic clamping strategy has been chosen, another guidewire is advanced through the hemostatic valve of the lateral port of the femoral arterial cannula. This new guidewire must first be

visualized in the descending aortic lumen, followed to the arch and then to the aortic root (Fig. 20.14). Before the balloon can be advanced, presence of the guidewire in the ascending aorta must be confirmed; in many cases the guidewire goes up the left internal carotid. In a mid-esophageal AoV LAX view, the intra-aortic balloon is slowly advanced until the sinotubular junction (STJ) is reached (Fig. 20.15). The guidewire is withdrawn and final proper positioning of the balloon will be done after the start of the endovascular CPB.

Endovascular CPB

Once the arterial and venous cannulae are in place and the anticoagulation allows it, CPB is started. To ensure the system's integrity, the following conditions must be met: a pulsatile flow in the arterial cannula, a sufficient assisted venous return to attain full flow, and a consistent pressure in the arterial line (Fig. 20.15). Despite well functioning of the CPB, a routine check of the descending Ao should be done to exclude aortic dissection. At the start of CPB by femoral technique, it is not unusual to see a pseudo-dissection in the descending aorta that reflects a separation of liquids only and not a loss of aortic wall integrity (Fig. 20.16).

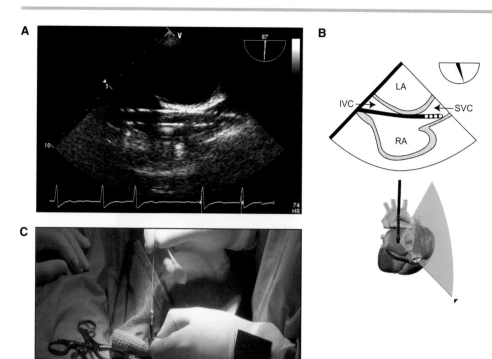

Figure 20.13 IVC venous drainage cannula optimal position. (**A,B**) Mid-esophageal bicaval view: the tip of the cannula should be ideally positioned at the junction of the right atrium (RA) and the superior vena cava (SVC). (**C**) Insertion of the cannula through the right femoral vein by the Seldinger technique. *Abbreviations*: IVC, inferior vena cava; LA, left atrium; RA, right atrium; SVC, superior vena cava. *Source*: Courtesy of Dr. Michel Pellerin.

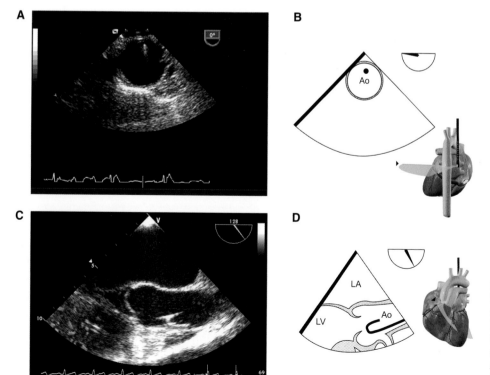

Figure 20.14 Aortic guidewire. Positioning of the guidewire for the aortic clamping endovascular balloon. Guidewire insertion is followed under TEE monitoring from the descending (**A,B**) to the ascending Ao (**C,D**). *Abbreviations*: Ao, aorta; LA, left atrium; LV, left ventricle.

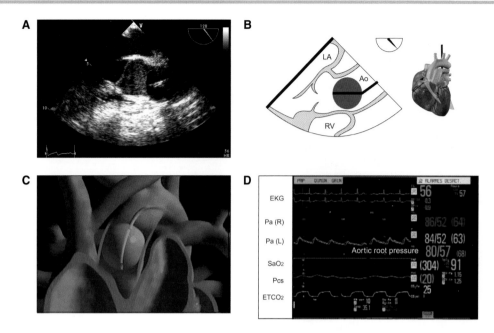

Figure 20.15 Endoclamp. Endovascular aortic clamping by balloon inflation of the EndoClamp aortic catheter. **(A–C)** Mid-esophageal AoV long-axis view and representation of the correct deployment of the EndoClamp catheter at the level of the sinotubular junction. **(D)** Hemodynamic monitoring during the procedure requires three Pa measurements: one from the right (R) radial artery (86/52 mmHg), one from the left (L) radial artery (84/52 mmHg), and the third directly from the EndoClamp catheter (80/57 mmHg) positioned in the aortic root. *Abbreviations*: Ao, aorta; AoV, aortic valve; EKG, electrocardiogram; ETCO$_2$, end-tidal CO$_2$; LA, left atrium; Pa, arterial pressure; Pcs, coronary sinus pressure; RV, right ventricle. *Source*: Diagram C with permission of Edwards Lifesciences.

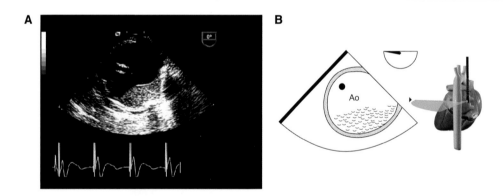

Figure 20.16 Pseudo-dissection. (A,B) Mid-esophageal descending Ao SAX view: upon initiation of peripheral extra-corporal circulation, separation of flows gives a pseudo-dissection appearance to the aorta. *Abbreviations*: Ao, aorta, SAX, short-axis.

Aortic Balloon Positioning

Under CPB, the pericardium is incised and the surgeon continues preparation of the surgical site. Aortic clamping can be done directly by a clamp introduced through a thoracic port or endovascularly. Endovascular clamping is achieved by the intra-aortic balloon previously introduced via the arterial femoral cannula. Team work is necessary for optimal positioning of the balloon. A good echocardiographic visualization of the AoV and the balloon in LAX must be

secured before endovascular clamping. The balloon must never be inflated if it is not visible. The balloon implantation zone is located between the STJ of the ascending aorta and the right brachiocephalic trunk. A position nearest to the STJ without obstructing the coronary ostia is deemed ideal (Fig. 20.17). During inflation, adenosine is given to obtain cardiac standstill.

In addition to direct balloon visualization, the optimal positioning is confirmed by an adequate flow of cardioplegia (Fig. 20.18) in the right coronary and left main coronary arteries after clamping. It is

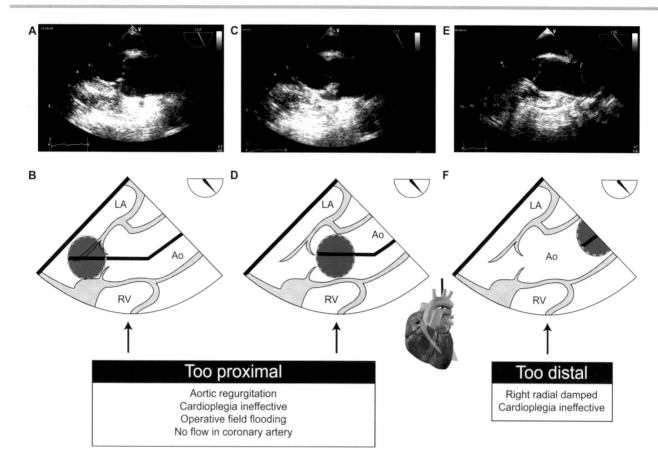

Too proximal

Aortic regurgitation
Cardioplegia ineffective
Operative field flooding
No flow in coronary artery

Too distal

Right radial damped
Cardioplegia ineffective

Figure 20.17 Endoclamp malposition. Proximal positions (**A–D**) compromises aortic valve motion and coronary perfusion, while distal positions (**E,F**) can impair cerebral perfusion. Transesophageal echocardiographic monitoring, right and left radial artery pressure monitoring and noninvasive continuous brain oximetry are routinely used to detect these potential complications. *Abbreviations*: Ao, aorta; LA, left atrium; RV, right ventricle.

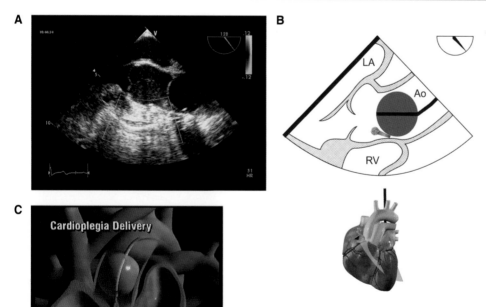

Figure 20.18 Antegrade cardioplegia delivery. (A,B) Mid-esophageal aortic valve long-axis view and representation of the deployed Endo-Clamp at the level of the sinotubular junction. (**C**). During antegrade cardioplegia administration, a small jet originating from the anterior aspect of the endoclamp can be seen. *Abbreviations*: Ao, aorta; LA, left atrium; RV, right ventricle. *Source*: With permission of Edwards Lifesciences.

important to visualize, by color Doppler, the flow of antegrade cardioplegia at the first injection as once the LA is opened, the echocardiographic window is reduced and visualization of the ascending Ao or the balloon becomes difficult. This characteristic becomes particularly important when the function of the intra-aortic balloon is suboptimal. When this situation occurs, flooding of the surgical field and direct palpation can help locate the balloon.

Hence, ensuring an exact and stable position of the intra-aortic balloon before atriotomy is critical because echographic monitoring of the balloon will become less reliable. Thereafter, the surgical team shall have to rely on indirect signs such as AR and cardioplegia response. The appearance of AR and flooding of the operating field can be signs of a balloon malpositioned proximally (Fig. 20.17). Once the

atrium is open, monitoring of the cardioplegia injection can only be done using aortic root pressure. During cardioplegia administration, this pressure should attain values close to that of the mean arterial pressure; proof that an adequate coronary perfusion pressure has developed in the aortic root (Fig. 20.15). If this is not the case, effective administration of antegrade cardioplegia cannot be ensured and the balloon positioning should be reevaluated immediately. In this situation, the balloon may have migrated proximally (causing AR and leakage of the cardioplegia solution into the LV) or distally (preventing its effective administration into the root).

To ensure that the endovascular clamp is proximal to the major vessels of the aortic arch, the best tool remains a reliable visualization of the balloon in the ascending Ao. However, when the surgery has

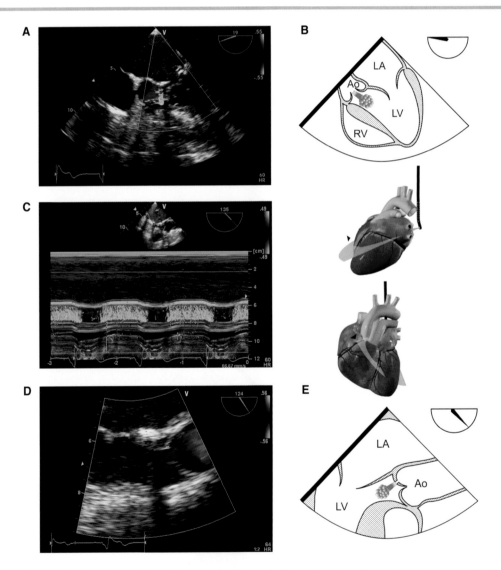

Figure 20.19   Aortic regurgitation after minimally invasive MV repair. Color Doppler mid-esophageal view at 19° (**A,B**) and M-mode of the ME AoV LAX view (**C**) show new-onset AR after MV repair in a 78-year-old woman. The left coronary cusp was inadvertently attached to the mitral ring. The surgeon went back on cardiopulmonary bypass and corrected the problem. The color Doppler ME AoV LAX view (**D,E**) shows the residual perforation from the anchoring stitch on the left coronary cusp of the AoV. *Abbreviations*: Ao, aorta; AoV, aortic valve; AR, aortic regurgitation; LA, left atrium; LAX, long-axis; LV, left ventricle; ME, mid-esophageal; MV, mitral valve; RV, right ventricle.

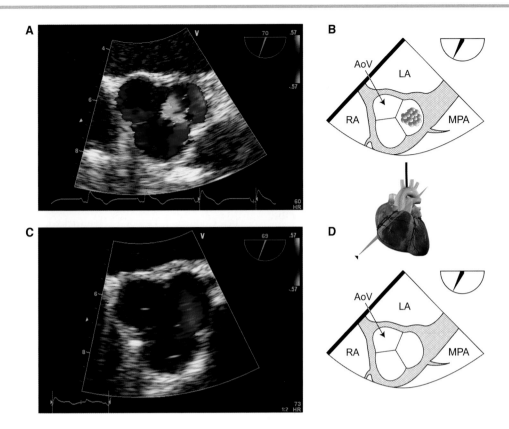

Figure 20.20   Aortic regurgitation after minimally invasive MV repair. Mid-esophageal AoV short-axis views of the same patient as in Figure 20.19. Compare before (**A,B**) and after (**C,D**) revision of the MV repair. *Abbreviations*: AoV, aortic valve; LA, left atrium; MPA, main pulmonary artery; MV, mitral valve; RA, right atrium.

started, it is better to rely on the right radial artery pressure curve in the absence of vascular abnormality (Fig. 20.15). Noninvasive brain oximetry can also be used to monitor for inadvertent displacement of the endovascular clamp in the innominate artery (41). Lastly, at the end of the cardioplegia injection, the root pressure must return to its initial value. If the pressure remains high, clamping could be nonocclusive or the pressure sensor could be oriented toward the wall, skewing the aortic root pressure estimation.

MV Repair Verification and Complication Monitoring

After aortic unclamping, the anesthesiologist must first evaluate the quantity of air present in the LA and LV. Continuous carbon dioxide insufflation in the chest during surgery promotes a more rapid resorption of the gas present in cardiac cavities. Sometimes a reperfusion period is needed before terminating CPB to allow dissipation of carbon dioxide from the cavities and coronaries. During this period, the surgical results should be evaluated. In MV repair, attention should focus on the coaptation surface of the anterior and posterior leaflets. Furthermore, a residual mitral leak, a significant transvalvular gradient and the presence of SAM should be sought out and communicated

to the surgeon. Following MV replacement, emphasis during TEE examination is placed in verifying prosthesis function, paravalvular leaks, and transvalvular gradient. In every case of MV repair by PORT ACCESS technique, the integrity of the AoV must be verified, as it could be compromised during the suture of anterior mitral ring by anchoring stitches (Figs. 20.19 and 20.20). Moreover, the LV and RV function and integrity of the aorta should be checked to exclude dissection.

REVASCULARIZATION AND ROBOTIC ASSISTED PROCEDURE

Minimally invasive revascularization procedures, with or without robotics, are performed on a beating heart. During this procedure the left lung is collapsed, both by selective ventilation and a pneumothorax. Intraoperative TEE is used to monitor right and left cardiac function and detect indirect signs of regional myocardial ischemia.

A decrease in RV contractility or an increase in TR associated with increases in pulmonary artery pressure measurements indicates increasing RV strain. Reducing the pressure produced by the pneumothorax may reduce the pulmonary artery pressure, with trocar pressures over 10 cmH$_2$O being associated with more complications. The use of nitroglycerin or milrinone may also reduce RV strain; however, right-sided dysfunction is a frequent cause of conversion to conventional CPB, especially in patients with associated right coronary artery disease.

Left ventricular dysfunction may also cause elevations in pulmonary artery pressures. Ischemia, a result of the underlying disease process, may lead to impaired relaxation or an increase in MR, both of which will elevate pulmonary artery pressure. Apical short-axis views are often of poor quality given the pneumothorax, therefore mid-esophageal four-chamber and two-chamber views may be necessary. MR during left internal mammary artery (LIMA) to the left anterior descending (LAD) grafting may be exacerbated by ischemia from vessel occlusion or from heart positioning. Shunts may be placed to minimize the effect of ischemia on myocardial function (42). Positioning of the heart is also restricted because of the intact sternum and does not usually cause hemodynamic changes. However, the use of a stabilizer may worsen MR (usually a result of the apex being pulled down from the base) (43).

CONCLUSION

In summary, minimally invasive cardiac surgery is a rapidly developing field where the role of the anesthesiologist has significantly increased. Detailed knowledge of the procedure, expertise in TEE, and communication skills are among the most important criteria for success in this challenging field.

REFERENCES

1. Glower DD, Landolfo KP, Clements F, et al. Mitral valve operation via Port Access versus median sternotomy. Eur J Cardiothorac Surg 1998; 14(suppl 1):S143–S147.
2. Grossi EA, Zakow PK, Ribakove G, et al. Comparison of post-operative pain, stress response, and quality of life in port access vs. standard sternotomy coronary bypass patients. Eur J Cardiothorac Surg 1999; 16(suppl 2):S39–S42.
3. Vanermen H, Farhat F, Wellens F, et al. Minimally invasive video-assisted mitral valve surgery: from Port-Access towards a totally endoscopic procedure. J Card Surg 2000; 15:51–60.
4. Schroeyers P, Wellens F, De Geest R, et al. Minimally invasive video-assisted mitral valve surgery: our lessons after a 4-year experience. Ann Thorac Surg 2001; 72:S1050–S1054.
5. Greco E, Barriuso C, Castro MA, et al. Port-Access cardiac surgery: from a learning process to the standard. Heart Surg Forum 2002; 5:145–149.
6. Casselman FP, Van Slycke S, Dom H, et al. Endoscopic mitral valve repair: feasible, reproducible, and durable. J Thorac Cardiovasc Surg 2003; 125:273–282.
7. Casselman FP, La Meir M, Jeanmart H, et al. Endoscopic mitral and tricuspid valve surgery after previous cardiac surgery. Circulation 2007; 116:I270–I275.
8. Chaney MA, Durazo-Arvizu RA, Fluder EM, et al. Port-access minimally invasive cardiac surgery increases surgical complexity, increases operating room time, and facilitates early postoperative hospital discharge. Anesthesiology 2000; 92:1637–1645.
9. McCreath BJ, Swaminathan M, Booth JV, et al. Mitral valve surgery and acute renal injury: port access versus median sternotomy. Ann Thorac Surg 2003; 75:812–819.
10. Richardson L, Richardson M, Hunter S. Is a port-access mitral valve repair superior to the sternotomy approach in accelerating postoperative recovery? Interact Cardiovasc Thorac Surg 2008; 7:678–683.
11. Mohr FW, Onnasch JF, Falk V, et al. The evolution of minimally invasive valve surgery—2 year experience. Eur J Cardiothorac Surg 1999; 15:233–238.
12. Toomasian JM, Peters WS, Siegel LC, et al. Extracorporeal circulation for port-access cardiac surgery. Perfusion 1997; 12:83–91.
13. Glower DD, Komtebedde J, Clements FM, et al. Direct aortic cannulation for port-access mitral or coronary artery bypass grafting. Ann Thorac Surg 1999; 68:1878–1880.
14. Coddens J, Deloof T, Hendrickx J, et al. Transesophageal echocardiography for port-access surgery. J Cardiothorac Vasc Anesth 1999; 13:614–622.
15. Bonow RO, Carabello BA, Kanu C, et al. ACC/AHA 2006 guidelines for the management of patients with valvular heart disease: a report of the American College of Cardiology/American Heart Association Task Force on Practice Guidelines (writing committee to revise the 1998 Guidelines for the Management of Patients with Valvular Heart Disease): developed in collaboration with the Society of Cardiovascular Anesthesiologists: endorsed by the Society for Cardiovascular Angiography and Interventions and the Society of Thoracic Surgeons. Circulation 2006; 114:e84–e231.
16. Trichon BH, Felker GM, Shaw LK, et al. Relation of frequency and severity of mitral regurgitation to survival among patients with left ventricular systolic dysfunction and heart failure. Am J Cardiol 2003; 91:538–543.
17. Grossi EA, Crooke GA, DiGiorgi PL, et al. Impact of moderate functional mitral insufficiency in patients undergoing surgical revascularization. Circulation 2006; 114:I573–I576.
18. Amigoni M, Meris A, Thune JJ, et al. Mitral regurgitation in myocardial infarction complicated by heart failure, left ventricular dysfunction, or both: prognostic significance and relation to ventricular size and function. Eur Heart J 2007; 28:326–333.
19. Vrublevsky AV, Boshchenko AA, Karpov RS. Simultaneous transesophageal Doppler assessment of coronary flow reserve in the left anterior descending artery and coronary sinus allows differentiation between proximal and nonproximal left anterior descending artery stenoses. Eur J Echocardiogr 2004; 5:25–33.
20. Florenciano-Sanchez R, de la Morena-Valenzuela G, Villegas-Garcia M, et al. Noninvasive assessment of coronary flow velocity reserve in left anterior descending artery adds diagnostic value to both clinical variables and dobutamine echocardiography: a study based on clinical practice. Eur J Echocardiogr 2005; 6:251–259.
21. Saraste M, Vesalainen RK, Ylitalo A, et al. Transthoracic Doppler echocardiography as a noninvasive tool to assess coronary artery stenoses—a comparison with quantitative coronary angiography. J Am Soc Echocardiogr 2005; 18:679–685.
22. Sobkowicz B, Hirnle T, Dobrzycki S, et al. Intraoperative echocardiographic assessment of the severe isolated ostial stenosis of left main coronary artery before and after surgical patch angioplasty. Eur J Echocardiogr 2005; 6:280–285.
23. Theunissen T, Coddens J, Foubert L, et al. Intraoperative severity assessment of coronary artery stenosis in patients at risk: the role of transesophageal echocardiography. Anesth Analg 2006; 102:366–368.
24. Hagen PT, Scholz DG, Edwards WD. Incidence and size of patent foramen ovale during the first 10 decades of life: an

autopsy study of 965 normal hearts. Mayo Clin Proc 1984; 59:17–20.

25. Fisher DC, Fisher EA, Budd JH, et al. The incidence of patent foramen ovale in 1,000 consecutive patients. A contrast transesophageal echocardiography study. Chest 1995; 107:1504–1509.

26. Omran AS, Woo A, David TE, et al. Intraoperative transesophageal echocardiography accurately predicts mitral valve anatomy and suitability for repair. J Am Soc Echocardiogr 2002; 15:950–957.

27. Agricola E, Oppizzi M, De Bonis M, et al. Multiplane transesophageal echocardiography performed according to the guidelines of the American Society of Echocardiography in patients with mitral valve prolapse, flail, and endocarditis: diagnostic accuracy in the identification of mitral regurgitant defects by correlation with surgical findings. J Am Soc Echocardiogr 2003; 16:61–66.

28. Lee KS, Stewart WJ, Lever HM, et al. Mechanism of outflow tract obstruction causing failed mitral valve repair. Anterior displacement of leaflet coaptation. Circulation 1993; 88:II24–II29.

29. Jebara VA, Mihaileanu S, Acar C, et al. Left ventricular outflow tract obstruction after mitral valve repair. Results of the sliding leaflet technique. Circulation 1993; 88:II30–II34.

30. Maslow AD, Regan MM, Haering JM, et al. Echocardiographic predictors of left ventricular outflow tract obstruction and systolic anterior motion of the mitral valve after mitral valve reconstruction for myxomatous valve disease. J Am Coll Cardiol 1999; 34:2096–2104.

31. Sagie A, Schwammenthal E, Newell JB, et al. Significant tricuspid regurgitation is a marker for adverse outcome in patients undergoing percutaneous balloon mitral valvuloplasty. J Am Coll Cardiol 1994; 24:696–702.

32. Boyaci A, Gokce V, Topaloglu S, et al. Outcome of significant functional tricuspid regurgitation late after mitral valve replacement for predominant rheumatic mitral stenosis. Angiology 2007; 58:336–342.

33. Chan V, Burwash IG, Lam BK, et al. Clinical and echocardiographic impact of functional tricuspid regurgitation repair at the time of mitral valve replacement. Ann Thorac Surg 2009; 88:1209–1215.

34. Fukuda S, Gillinov AM, Song JM, et al. Echocardiographic insights into atrial and ventricular mechanisms of functional tricuspid regurgitation. Am Heart J 2006; 152:1208–1214.

35. Kim HK, Kim YJ, Park JS, et al. Determinants of the severity of functional tricuspid regurgitation. Am J Cardiol 2006; 98:236–242.

36. Mierdl S, Meininger D, Byhahn C, et al. Transesophageal echocardiography or fluoroscopy during port-access surgery? Ann Acad Med Singapore 2002; 31:520–524.

37. Abramson DC, Giannoti AG. Perforation of the right ventricle with a coronary sinus catheter during preparation for minimally invasive cardiac surgery. Anesthesiology 1998; 89:519–521.

38. Deneu S, Coddens J, Deloof T. Catheter entrapment by atrial suture during minimally invasive port-access cardiac surgery. Can J Anaesth 1999; 46:983–986.

39. Akhtar S. Off-axis view using a multiplane transesophageal echocardiography probe facilitates cannulation of the coronary sinus. J Cardiothorac Vasc Anesth 1998; 12:374–375.

40. Clements F, Wright SJ, de Bruijn N. Coronary sinus catheterization made easy for Port-Access miimally invasive cardiac surgery. J Cardiothorac Vasc Anesth 1998; 12:96–101.

41. Denault AY, Deschamps A, Murkin JM. A proposed algorithm for the intraoperative use of cerebral near-infrared spectroscopy. Semin Cardiothorac Vasc Anesth 2007; 11:274–281.

42. Mishra M, Swaminathan M, Malhotra R, et al. Evaluation of right ventricular function during CABG: transesophageal echocardiographic assessment of hepatic venous flow versus conventional right ventricular performance indices. Echocardiography 1998; 15:51–58.

43. Lucchetti V, Capasso F, Caputo M, et al. Intracoronary shunt prevents left ventricular function impairment during beating heart coronary revascularization. Eur J Cardiothorac Surg 1999; 15:255–259.

21

TEE in Mechanical Circulatory Assistance

Yanick Beaulieu and Denis Bouchard
Université de Montréal, Montreal, Quebec, Canada

Annette Vegas
University of Toronto, Toronto, Ontario, Canada

INTRODUCTION

Over the last 20 years, considerable advances have been made in the field of mechanical circulatory support (1,2). The cardinal feature of the patient requiring implantation of a mechanical circulatory device is the presence of decompensated heart failure refractory to medical management (3,4). This population presents significant challenges to the medical team, specifically to the cardiac anesthesiologist in the perioperative setting (5). Several clinical features accompany the placement of a ventricular assist device (VAD) compared with other cardiovascular procedures, including the advanced degree of heart failure, the circulatory change induced by VAD therapy, complications specific to these devices, and the higher incidence of associated right ventricular (RV) failure and bleeding (6). Transesophageal echocardiography (TEE) has played an increasing role in the perioperative care of patients with severe heart failure and VAD placement, both as a diagnostic and a monitoring tool in the operating room (OR) and intensive care unit (ICU) (7). In this chapter, the essential role of TEE for VAD placement and monitoring will be reviewed.

DESCRIPTION OF ASSIST DEVICES AND ROLE OF TEE

General subsets of patients who may benefit from mechanical assist devices include (*i*) patients with severe hemodynamic instability who need a device *as a bridge to transplant*, (*ii*) patients in cardiogenic shock requiring a device *as a bridge to recovery*, and (*iii*) patients in whom a device is *destination therapy* (1,6,8–10). Approximately 5% of the patients undergoing open heart surgery develop postcardiotomy shock. Most of these patients will be weaned successfully from cardiopulmonary bypass (CPB) with aggressive medical treatment and an intra-aortic balloon pump (IABP) or counterpulsation system. However, 1% require temporary mechanical support until further recovery or a more prolonged type of assist device for subsequent transplantation (1).

Circulatory assist devices are available in different configurations tailored to specific clinical situations, from simple IABP to implantation of a total artificial heart. A number of these devices are Food and Drug Administration (FDA) approved, while the remainder are used extensively in Europe or are undergoing FDA evaluation (Table 21.1) (11). Selection of the specific type of mechanical assistance is based on a careful analysis of the factors underlying the cause of heart failure, the urgency of the situation, the patient's characteristics (body mass index, degree of organ dysfunction), the functional assistance needed [left ventricular (LV), RV, biventricular, implantable vs. paracorporeal], and the indication (bridge to transplant, bridge to recovery, or destination therapy).

Transesophageal echocardiography plays an important role in the perioperative management of these devices, especially those necessitating ventricular, atrial, and great vessel cannulation (7,12). In the updated perioperative TEE practice guidelines published in 2010 by the American Society of Anesthesiologists (ASA) and the Society of Cardiovascular Anesthesiologists (SCA) (8), the use of TEE for the monitoring of placement of VADs is strongly supported.

Intra-aortic Balloon Counterpulsation

The IABP is an intravascular, catheter-mounted, counterpulsation device with a balloon volume between 30 and 50 mL. It is usually inserted percutaneously (rarely surgically) via the femoral artery using the Seldinger technique. The intra-aortic balloon (IAB) is positioned in the descending thoracic aorta (Ao) (Figs. 21.1 and 21.2) and set to inflate at the dicrotic notch of the aortic arterial pressure waveform at the onset of isovolumic relaxation and deflate during the isovolumetric phase of LV contraction.

Table 21.1 Ventricular Assist Devices

	Pulsatile flow VADs				
Device manufacturer	Abiomed BVS5000 Abiomed Inc. (Danvers, Massachusetts, U.S.)	AB5OOO ventricle Abiomed Inc. (Danvers, Massachusetts, U.S.)	Thoratec VAS Thoratec Laboratories (Pleasanton, California, U.S.)	HeartMate Thoratec Corp. (Woburn, Massachusetts, U.S.)	Novacor WorldHeart Corp. (Ottawa, Canada)
FDA approval	1992	2003	1995	1994 (IP) 1998 (XVE)	1998
Body location		Extra/paracorporeal		Intracorporeal	
Ventricle support	Right, left, bilateral	Right, left, bilateral	Right, left, bilateral	Left	Left
Pump	Pneumatic	Pneumatic	Pneumatic	Electric	Electric
Valves	Polyurethane	Polyurethane	Mechanical	Porcine	Porcine
Anticoagulation	Heparin	Coumadin	Coumadin	Antiplatelet	Coumadin
Flows (L/min)	2.0–6.0	2.0–6.0	1.3–7.2	10	10
Advantages	Postcardiotomy shock bridge to survival, short-term support	Use existing cannulas Ambulatory	Small BSA Ambulatory	Low risk of thromboembolism Ambulatory BSA > 1.5 m^2	Durable Ambulatory
Disadvantages	Nonambulatory Systemic anticoagulation	Permanent anticoagulation	Permanent anticoagulation	Infection Only left VAD support	Permanent anticoagulation, high thrombotic stroke incidence despite anticoagulation, only left VAD support

	Continuous flow VADs		
Device manufacturer	HeartMate II Thoratec Corp. (Woburn, Massachusetts, U.S.)	Jarvik 2000 Jarvik Heart. Inc (New York, New York, U.S.)	DeBakey VAD MicroMed Technology (Houston, Texas, U.S.)
Ventricle support	Left	Left, bilateral	Left, bilateral
Flows (L/min)	6.0–10.0	2.5–6.0	5.0–10.0
Cannula	Left ventricle to ascending aorta	Left ventricle to descending aorta	Left ventricle apex to ascending aorta

Abbreviations: BSA, body surface area; FDA, Food and Drug Administration; L, liters; VAD, ventricular assist device.
Source: Adapted from Ref. 11.

The IABP creates a favorable shift in the myocardial oxygen supply/demand balance by decreasing myocardial O_2 consumption by approximately 15% to 20% while increasing systemic and diastolic coronary perfusion (Fig. 21.3) and cardiac output (CO) (Fig. 21.4).

Though of limited use, TEE is useful in confirming the correct position of the IABP in the descending thoracic Ao below the origin of the left subclavian artery, and to exclude an inappropriate location in the inferior vena cava (Fig. 21.5). Transesophageal echocardiography may help identify contraindications to IABP insertion, such as significant unsuspected aortic regurgitation (AR), complex atherosclerotic debris in the descending Ao at risk for embolization, and left ventricular outflow tract (LVOT) obstruction (Fig. 21.6). The correct operation of the balloon can be confirmed by visualization of its inflation and deflation (Fig. 21.2). In case of malfunction, the presence of aortic dissection or balloon perforation can be ascertained. Finally, TEE may be used postoperatively to reassess ventricular function before removing the IABP device.

Ventricular Assist Devices

Unlike the IABP, which provides only modest support to systemic perfusion, VADs are designed to unload the right ventricle (RV) and/or LV effectively while completely supporting the pulmonary and/or systemic circulation.

All VADs function in a similar way by draining blood from the patient through a device inflow (drainage) cannula into the mechanical pump that ejects the blood via an outflow (return) cannula back into the patient. In a left ventricular assist device (LVAD), blood flow is diverted from either the left atrium (LA) or the apex of the LV, passes through the LVAD, and is returned to the body by the ascending Ao (Figs. 21.7 and 21.8). In a right ventricular assist device (RVAD), blood is drained from the right atrium (RA) or RV and returned to the main pulmonary artery (MPA).

Three types of mechanical blood pumps, capable of replacing the function of one or both ventricles, are recognized based on their flow design: centrifugal, pulsatile, and axial (Table 21.1) (1,9). The respective

A

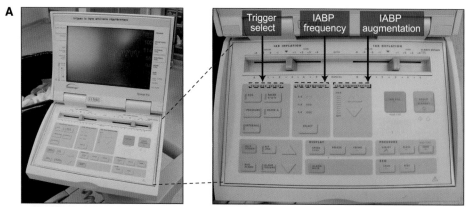

B

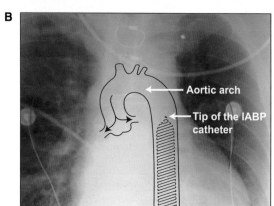

Aortic arch

Tip of the IABP catheter

Figure 21.1 IABP. (A) Adjustable controls on the IABP console are the trigger (most commonly the electrocardiogram), the inflation frequency (1:1, 1:2, and 1:3) and the degree of augmentation. **(B)** Correct intra-aortic balloon catheter position below the origin of the left subclavian artery is confirmed by chest X-ray or transesophageal echocardiography when inserted intraoperatively. *Abbreviation*: IABP, intra-aortic balloon pump.

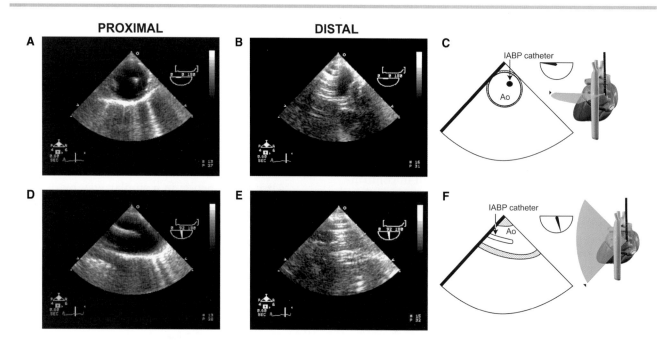

PROXIMAL

DISTAL

Figure 21.2 IABP. An intra-aortic balloon catheter is positioned in the Ao of a 75-year-old man before coronary revascularization. The descending Ao short-axis (**A–C**) and long-axis (**D–F**) views are shown. The tip of the catheter should ideally be located 5 to 10 cm below the origin of the left subclavian artery. Note that during inflation, air in the intra-aortic balloon catheter prevents visualization of the aortic wall. *Abbreviations*: Ao, aorta; IABP, intra-aortic balloon pump.

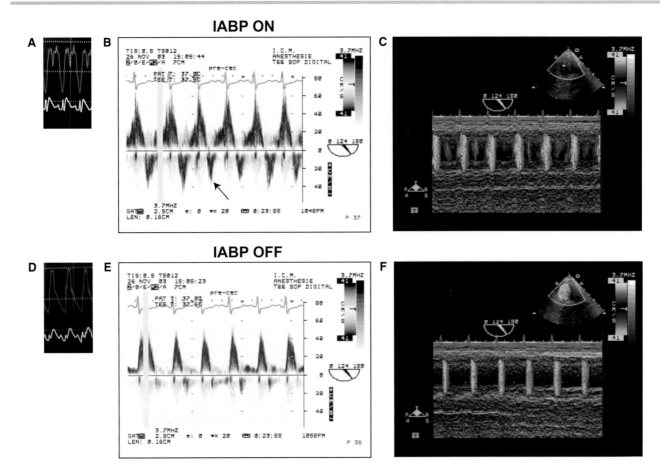

Figure 21.3 IABP. Compare the hemodynamic (**A,D**), pulsed wave Doppler profiles (**B,E**) and color M-mode tracings (**C,F**) in the ascending aorta when the IABP is on (**A–C**) and off (**D–F**). Diastolic velocities (arrow) almost disappear when the IABP is turned off. *Abbreviation*: IABP, intra-aortic balloon pump.

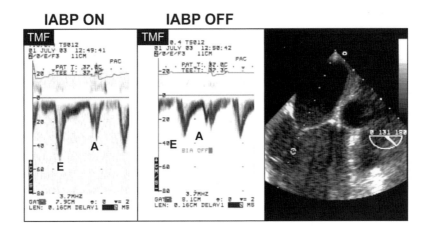

Figure 21.4 IABP. The pulsed wave Doppler TMF velocities obtained in the mid-esophageal aortic valve long-axis view are lower due to a reduction in stroke volume when the IABP is off compared to on. *Abbreviations*: A, peak late diastolic TMF velocity; E, peak early diastolic TMF velocity; IABP, intra-aortic balloon pump; TMF, transmitral flow.

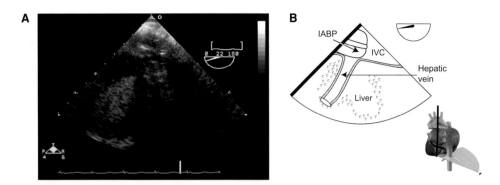

Figure 21.5   IABP catheter malposition. (A,B) Transgastric IVC long-axis view shows malposition of the intra-aortic balloon catheter in the IVC after emergency insertion in the operating room. *Abbreviations*: IABP, intra-aortic balloon pump; IVC, inferior vena cava.

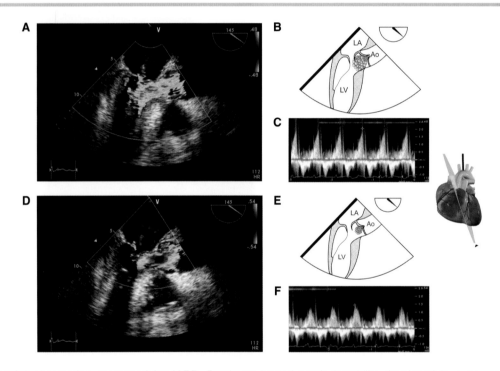

Figure 21.6   LVOT obstruction worsened by IABP. Persistent hemodynamic instability developed in a 64-year-old man after tamponade in whom an IABP was inserted. The color Doppler mid-esophageal long-axis views (**A,B**) show turbulent flow in the LVOT and a late peak systolic pressure gradient with continuous wave Doppler (**C**). When the IABP is turned off, the turbulent flow (**D,E**) and LVOT gradient (**F**) are reduced. *Abbreviations*: Ao, aorta; IABP, intra-aortic balloon pump; LA, left atrium; LV, left ventricle; LVOT, left ventricular outflow tract.

indications, contraindications, design features, and functional characteristics of these pumps will not be thoroughly discussed in this chapter, but the reader is referred to several reviews on the topic for further information (1,6,9).

Centrifugal Pumps

Centrifugal pumps are simple to use, relatively inexpensive, and readily available in most cardiovascular surgical centers. Standard CPB atrial and arterial cannulae are used and connected by polyvinyl chloride tubing to an extracorporeal centrifugal pump head. Internal cones, or an impeller, rotating at high speeds creates a vortex that drives blood through an inlet at the top of the pump, and blood exits via an outlet at the base. The adult model can rotate up to 5000 rpm to provide flow rates of up to 10 L/min. The device can provide short-term support to one or both ventricles, particularly in the setting of postcardiotomy shock.

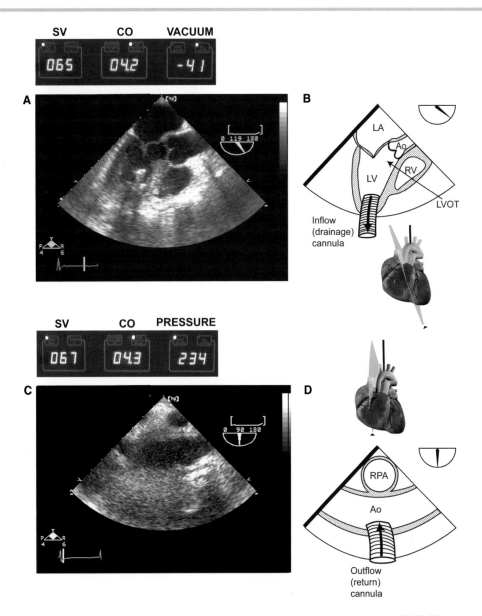

Figure 21.7 LVAD. A Thoratec LVAD is inserted in a 46-year-old woman in cardiogenic shock. **(A,B)** Blood is suctioned (vacuum pressure of −41 mmHg) from the LV into the LVAD through a device inflow (drainage) cannula inserted in the LV apex as shown in this ME LAX view. **(C,D)** ME ascending Ao LAX view shows the device outflow (return) cannula in the ascending Ao through which blood is injected into the patient at a pressure of 234 mmHg. *Abbreviations*: Ao, aorta; CO, cardiac output; LA, left atrium; LAX, long-axis; LV, left ventricle; LVAD, left ventricular assist device; LVOT, left ventricular outflow tract; ME, mid-esophageal; RPA, right pulmonary artery; RV, right ventricle; SV, stroke volume. 🖱

Cannulation may be performed centrally using the RA for venous drainage and the great vessels for arterial return, as discussed in Chapter 13. Besides its availability, this system has the advantage of enabling peripheral cannulation for full cardiopulmonary support. This can be performed either percutaneously or via open "cut-down" of the femoral artery and either the femoral or internal jugular vein (Fig. 21.9). This type of support is used as a bridge to recovery in postcardiotomy cardiogenic shock and can also be used as part of an extracorporeal membranous oxygenation (ECMO) circuit for cardiac or respiratory

decompensation (6). This device can also be used to supplement blood flow in the settings of liver transplant surgery to augment venous return or thoracic Ao surgery to decrease the incidence of renal and spinal cord ischemia.

TEE assessment. During implantation, TEE is useful to guide correct cannula position and optimize device function (12). On the venous side, with either the central or peripheral cannulation technique, the venous catheter tip is positioned in the RA. The arterial catheter is correctly placed in the ascending (central cannulation) or descending thoracic Ao

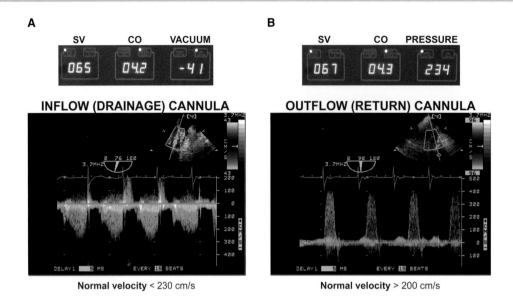

A

SV	CO	VACUUM
065	04.2	-41

INFLOW (DRAINAGE) CANNULA

Normal velocity < 230 cm/s

B

SV	CO	PRESSURE
067	043	234

OUTFLOW (RETURN) CANNULA

Normal velocity > 200 cm/s

Figure 21.8 Thoratec left ventricular assist device. Continuous wave Doppler tracing from the device inflow (drainage) and outflow (return) cannulae are interrogated from mid-esophageal views. The device inflow cannula in the LV apex should show normal laminar flow with a peak velocity <230 cm/s directed away from the probe. (**A**) In this example, the peak velocity is at the upper limit due to restricted cannula inflow secondary to left-sided ventricular septal shift from severe right ventricular dilatation. (**B**) Device outflow at the level of the ascending aorta is seen directed towards the transducer. The normal outflow velocity should be >200 cm/s. *Abbreviations*: CO, cardiac output; LV, left ventricular; SV, stroke volume.

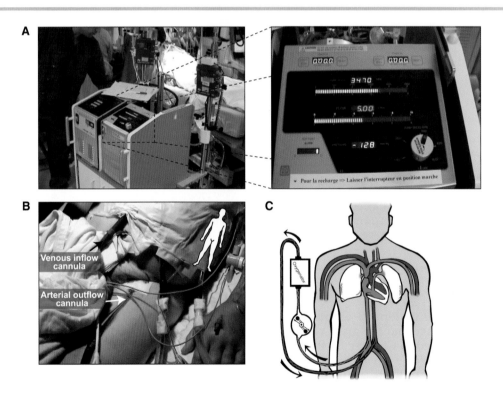

Figure 21.9 ECMO. (A,B) A centrifugal pump is used as veno-arterial ECMO in a 64-year-old man after a complicated heart transplant. The top number on the ECMO device indicates the number of revolutions per minute (RPM = 3470); the middle number, the cardiac output (5 L/min); and −128 mmHg correspond to the vacuum pressure. (**C**) Drainage to the ECMO inflow cannula is directly connected to the right atrium through the chest. The return via the ECMO outflow cannula is through the femoral artery. *Abbreviation*: ECMO; extracorporeal membrane oxygenator. *Source*: Courtesy of Dr. Y. Lamarche and illustration by A. Bérubé.

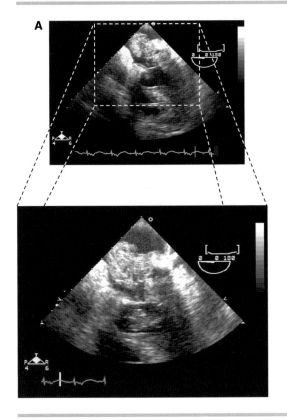

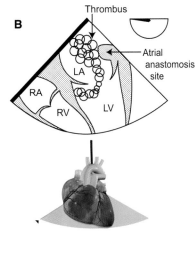

Figure 21.10 ECMO complication. A 64-year-old man is on a centrifugal pump for cardiogenic shock after heart transplantation. (**A,B**) The mid-esophageal four-chamber views show an unexpected LA and LV thrombus attached to the atrial anastomosis site on the third day. *Abbreviations*: ECMO, extracorporeal membrane oxygenator; LA, left atrium; LV, left ventricle; RA, right atrium; RV, right ventricle. ☞

(peripheral cannulation). At the onset of device operation, adequate venous drainage and optimal fluid balance benefit from the surveillance of the cardiac chamber size by TEE. Flow, at a given centrifugal pump speed, is preload and afterload dependent. With inadequate preload, the atrium will collapse about the inflow (drainage) cannula, causing cessation of blood inflow and hemodynamic instability.

The degree and timing of myocardial recovery can be periodically evaluated in the ICU by frequent assessment of LV and RV function by TEE or transthoracic echocardiography (TTE) (13). Progressive withdrawal of circulatory support can be initiated when signs of hemodynamic improvement are present. VADs should be removed as soon as hemodynamic competence and stability are restored, as morbidity significantly increases after 24 to 48 hours of support.

Weaning of LV centrifugal mechanical assistance can be monitored by the gradual pulse pressure restoration at reduced flow as LV function recovery is demonstrated by TEE. RV output may also be evaluated with thermodilution CO measurement. In our practice, by subtracting the assisted flow from this measurement, we can serially measure and follow the portion of CO originating from the recovering LV.

The weaning of a *biventricular* assist device is more difficult to assess: indeed, because venous mixing does not occur in the RV, CO determination by thermodilution is less accurate, while the relative contributions of RV and LV to forward flow cannot be precisely

determined (6). For those reasons, TEE may provide useful additional data in assessing right and left CO (14).

In addition to its role in assessing cardiac function, TEE can also be used to detect complications of centrifugal circulatory assistance in the postoperative period (15). Conditions causing hemodynamic instability can be diagnosed, such as the presence of intracardiac (or intracatheter) thrombus (Fig. 21.10), vegetations on the catheter tip, pericardial tamponade (Figs. 21.11 and 21.12), and the displacement or collapse of one of the cannulae.

Pulsatile Blood Pumps

Pulsatile VADs are more expensive and complex than centrifugal pump systems, both in their insertion and operation. However, their integrated sophisticated controls are largely self-regulating, and despite more operating modalities, they usually require minimal supervision beyond the first few days after device insertion. Different models of pulsatile VADs are available (Thoratec, Heartmate, Novacor, Abiomed) (Fig. 21.13) (2). Each has their own set of indications, contraindications, advantages, and disadvantages. Some are pneumatically driven, while others are electrically driven (Table 21.1). These types of mechanical assistance can offer complete circulatory support of RV and/or LV function. They are, in general, used in patients who need a high degree of circulatory support for an intermediate to long-term period as a

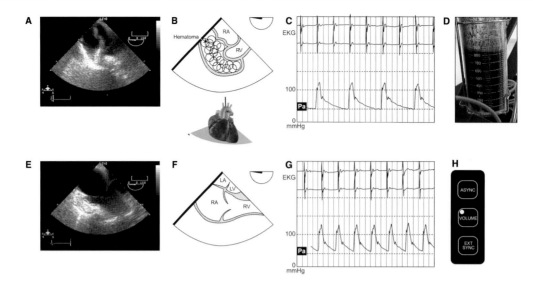

Figure 21.11 Tamponade. Tamponade and cardiogenic shock in a 46-year-old woman with a Thoratec LVAD. (**A,B**) Mid-esophageal four-chamber view rotated towards the right: compression of the RA. (**C**) Pa hemodynamic tracing: decreased rate of the pump, with insufficient LVAD output. (**D**) Therapeutic withdrawal of pericardial (600 mL) and pleural fluid (200 mL). (**E,F**) Disappearance of the RA compression with concomitant improvement of the LVAD output: (**G**) The LVAD pumping rate increases on the Pa tracing. (**H**) With the Thoratec LVAD in a volume-mode, the ejection is triggered when the pump chamber reaches the 90% fill level. The Pa is thus dissociated from the patient heart rate, which explains the reduced LVAD output with compromised filling due to tamponade. *Abbreviations*: ASYNC, asynchronous; EKG, electrocardiogram; EXT SYNC, external synchronization; LA, left atrium; LV, left ventricle; LVAD, left ventricular assist device; ME, mid-esophageal; Pa, arterial pressure; RA, right atrium; RV, right ventricle.

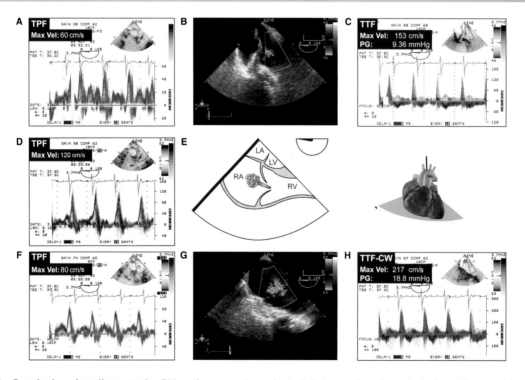

Figure 21.12 Surgical pericardiocentesis. RV performance is evaluated during pericardiocentesis in a 46-year-old woman with a Thoratec LVAD. (**A**) The maximum systolic TPF velocity by pulsed wave Doppler was 60 cm/s just before the pericardial drainage began. Modified mid-esophageal four-chamber views (**B,E**) show mild TR with a tricuspid systolic PG of 9.36 mmHg (**C**). With pericardiocentesis, the maximum TPF velocity increased to 120 cm/s (**D**) but then stabilized at 80 cm/s (**F**). This may have been due to unmasked RV dysfunction associated with increased TR (**G,H**). Of note, the cardiac output of the LVAD increased but the vasoactive support was unchanged. *Abbreviations*: CW, continuous wave; LA, left atrium; LV, left ventricle; LVAD, left ventricular assist device; Max, maximum; PG, pressure gradient; RA, right atrium; RV, right ventricle; TTF, transtricuspid flow; TPF, transpulmonary flow; TR, tricuspid regurgitation; Vel, velocity.

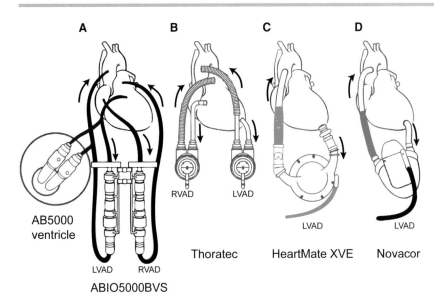

Figure 21.13 Pulsatile flow VADs. These devices provide augmented pulsatile peripheral flow. (**A**) The AB5000 and ABIO5000BVS VADs are extracorporeal devices that can support both ventricles using the same inflow (drainage) and outflow (return) cannulae for either the device. (**B**) The Thoratec VAD is an extracorporeal device that can support both ventricles. (**C**) The HeartMate XVE VAD and the (**D**) Novacor VAD are intracorporeal devices that support only the left ventricle. *Abbreviations*: LVAD, left ventricular assist device; RVAD, right ventricular assist device; VAD, ventricular assist device. *Source*: Adapted with permission from Ref. 11 and illustrations courtesy of Frances Yeung, University of Toronto.

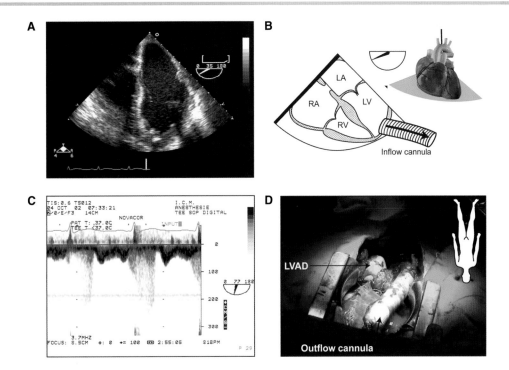

Figure 21.14   Novacor LVAD. Mid-esophageal four-chamber view (**A,B**) in a 37-year-old man with a Novacor LVAD system shows the device inflow (drainage) cannula in the LV apex. (**C**) Continuous wave Doppler velocities across the cannula. (**D**) Intraoperative view shows the device and device outflow (return) cannula in the aorta. *Abbreviations*: LA, left atrium; LV, left ventricle; LVAD, left ventricular assist device; RA, right atrium; RV, right ventricle. *Source*: Photo D courtesy of Dr. Michel Carrier.

bridge to recovery or cardiac transplantation or as destination therapy (6,9).

These devices have comparable cannulation setups, requiring a device inflow or drainage cannula, pump, and device outflow or return cannula. For support of the systemic circulation (Figs. 21.14 and 21.15), the inflow (drainage) cannula is usually inserted in the apex of the LV. In general, LA inflow (drainage) cannulation is technically easier to perform but may provide incomplete ventricular decompression. The device outflow (return) cannula goes from the LVAD to the ascending Ao. For support of the

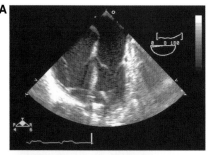

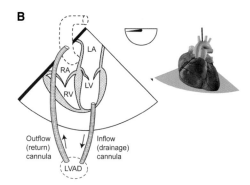

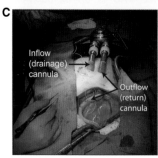

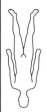

Figure 21.15 Thoratec LVAD. (A,B) The mid-esophageal four-chamber view shows an adequate position of the device inflow (drainage) cannula in a 21-year-old man with a Thoratec LVAD. Care must be taken to ensure that the cannula is at the LV apex not too close to the ventricular septal wall and directed toward the mitral valve. **(C)** Intraoperative view showing the Thoratec LVAD inflow (drainage) and outflow (return) cannulae. *Abbreviations*: LA, left atrium; LV, left ventricle; LVAD, left ventricular assist device; RA, right atrium; RV, right ventricle. *Source*: Photo C courtesy of Dr. Michel Carrier.

Table 21.2 Summary of the Role of TEE in Patients with Mechanical Circulatory Assistance

	Importance
Before insertion	
• Right and left ventricular function	Selection of device: right, left, or both
• Aortic valve competency	Regurgitation will have to be corrected
• Patent foramen ovale	Risk of hypoxia from right to left shunting
• Mitral and tricuspid valve evaluation	Usually improves with VAD
• Ventricular apex evaluation	An apical thrombus will complicate cannula insertion
• Aortic atheromatosis (epiaortic)	Grade 4 or 5 could complicate cannula insertion
During insertion	
• Assist the insertion	Inlet cannula well positioned in the LV and RV and outlet cannula in the ascending aorta or PA
• De-airing process	Air removed before activating the VAD
After insertion	
• Confirm ventricular decompression	VAD chamber is reduced in size
• Reevaluate aortic, mitral and tricuspid valve	Regurgitation could complicate VAD function
• Reconfirm the absence of PFO	Postoperative hypoxia
• Evaluate RV function (with LVAD)	Specific agents if RV dysfunction occurs
• Evaluate and measure drainage and return velocity	Normal drainage and return velocities should be <230 cm/s and >250 cm/s with no regurgitant signal
In the intensive care unit	
• Rule out specific complications if hemodynamically unstable	Tamponade, inlet or outlet valve incompetency, or obstruction, device malposition, RV failure (with LVAD), hypovolemia, shunting through a PFO, intracavitary thrombus
• Evaluation of RV and LV function during weaning	Estimation of ventricular recovery

Abbreviations: LV, left ventricle; LVAD, left ventricular assist device; PA, pulmonary artery; PFO, patent foramen ovale; RV, right ventricle; TEE, transesophageal echocardiography.

pulmonary circulation, the inflow (drainage) cannula is generally inserted in the RA or the apex of the RV, while the outflow (return) cannula goes from the RVAD to the pulmonary artery.

TEE assessment.   Again, TEE is useful for several aspects of the pre-, intra-, and postoperative management of patients undergoing pulsatile VAD implantation (Table 21.2) (7). It allows selection of the best type

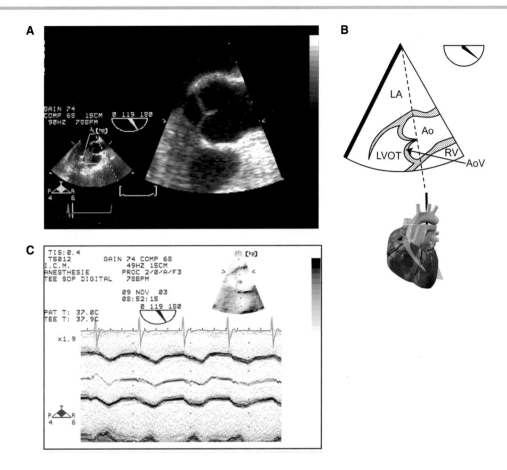

Figure 21.16 AoV evaluation in LVAD implantation. (A,B) Zoomed mid-esophageal AoV long-axis view in a 46-year-old woman with a Thoratec LVAD inserted for cardiogenic shock. The AoV is closed in systole. **(C)** The M-mode illustrates the continuous closure of the AoV throughout the cardiac cycle. No aortic regurgitation was present. *Abbreviations*: Ao, aorta; AoV, aortic valve; LA, left atrium; LVAD, left ventricular assist device; LVOT, left ventricular outflow tract; RV, right ventricle.

of support needed (left, right, or biventricular support), assists insertion and determination of optimal pump settings, expedites identification of VAD-related complications, and may help weaning attempts (often unsuccessful) from the device (16).

Before CPB In addition to a complete TEE examination, systematic evaluation of key anatomical structures is performed in the pre-CPB period:

1. The aortic valve (AoV) must be competent with minimal AR (Fig. 21.16). This is essential to avoid recirculation of blood from the outflow (return) aortic cannula back into the LV and ultimately back into the VAD via the inflow (drainage) cannula (6). This would greatly impair the efficacy of LVAD support. In the presence of moderate AR, the AoV must be repaired, replaced, or oversewn (17,18). This permanent closure of the AoV does not usually have hemodynamic consequences during full LVAD support, as the AoV normally remains closed (Fig. 21.16). However, it does have potential impacts in the advent of device failure or cardiac arrest and must be reversed for LVAD weaning in case of myocardial recovery.

2. The presence of intracardiac shunts such as *atrial septal defect* (ASD) or *patent foramen ovale* (PFO) must be methodically ruled out using two-dimensional (2D), color Doppler (see Figs. 26.6 and 30.4), and ultrasound contrast imaging (6). Because these patients often have an LA pressure exceeding RA pressure during the entire cardiac cycle, a PFO present in up to 20% to 30% of the general population (19) may not be readily obvious, even with IV injection of agitated saline ultrasound contrast (20). To elicit the presence of a potential right-to-left shunt, a maneuver equivalent to a Valsalva must be performed by inducing a sudden release of a sustained positive airway pressure previously achieved by inflating the lungs manually. This maneuver will transiently reverse the atrial transseptal gradient and may help uncover a PFO that would not have been seen otherwise. When a PFO or an ASD is

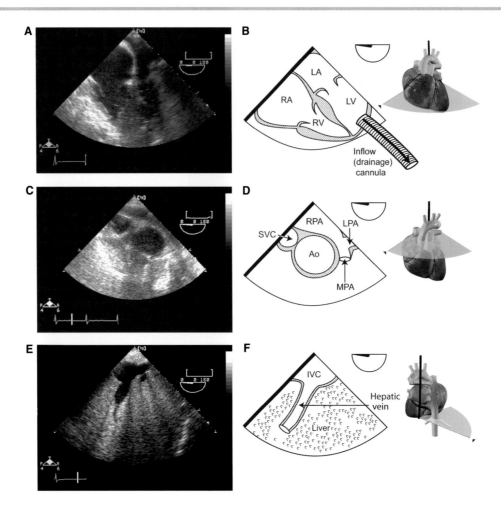

Figure 21.17   RV dysfunction with LVAD. (A,B) ME four-chamber view shows a dilated RA with compression of the LA and RV dysfunction in a 46-year-old woman with a Thoratec LVAD. This is associated with a dilated SVC shown in the ME ascending Ao short-axis view (**C,D**) and dilated IVC in the transgastric IVC long-axis view (**E,F**). *Abbreviations*: Ao, aorta; IVC, inferior vena cava; LA, left atrium; LPA, left pulmonary artery; LV, left ventricle; LVAD, left ventricular assist device; ME, mid-esophageal; MPA, main pulmonary artery; RA, right atrium; RPA, right pulmonary artery; RV, right ventricle; SVC, superior vena cava.

discovered, it must be repaired. Indeed, failure to recognize the presence of even a small right-to-left shunt, at baseline, can result in important arterial desaturation during LVAD support (21). This occurs from increased shunting due to the combination of frequently increased RA pressure and LA decompression by the LVAD.

3. A baseline dilated RV (Fig. 21.17) with poor RV function (RV fractional area change <20%) may further decompensate from improved RV preload after LVAD implantation and require insertion of an RVAD (22,23). The level of preoperative RV function also helps to predict the level of pharmacologic support required to support the RV to ensure adequate LVAD filling.

4. The degree of functional tricuspid regurgitation (TR) reflects RV dysfunction and influences RV function post LVAD implantation. Tricuspid valve (TV) repair should be considered in the presence of significant TR to improve functional TR and optimize RV function after LVAD insertion (18).

5. Insertion of an LVAD leads to reduced LV size, improved coaptation of the mitral valve (MV) leaflets, and, ultimately, decreased preexisting mitral regurgitation (MR) (24). Persistence of significant MR post-LVAD insertion may indicate inadequate LV decompression. The presence of significant MS restricts LVAD filling and requires surgical intervention with either a mitral commissurotomy or MV replacement (18).

6. The apices of both ventricles (and atrium) should be carefully inspected for thrombus. Ventricular cannulation with thrombi could induce catastrophic embolic events. Cautious removal of thrombus may be attempted by the surgeon to minimize embolic complications.

7. The ascending, transverse, and descending thoracic Ao are scrutinized for the presence of mobile atherosclerotic debris to facilitate the selection of a safe site for aortic cannulation (device outflow or return). Incomplete TEE visualization can be supplemented by epiaortic scanning.

During CPB   Surgical positioning of the device inflow (drainage) cannula in the atrium or the ventricle can be directly assisted by TEE. Effective decompression is best obtained when the inflow (drainage) cannula is positioned in the apex of the ventricle (Fig. 21.15). Moreover, to avoid cannula occlusion, it is crucial that the apical inflow (drainage) cannula be appropriately directed away from the interventricular septum (IVS) toward the MV for the LVAD (Fig. 21.15) and toward the TV for the RVAD (6). Device inflow (drainage) cannula position is examined in at least two views, the mid-esophageal long-axis (LAX) view (relation to IVS) and two-chamber view (anterior-posterior). The adequately aligned device inflow (drainage) cannula has laminar unidirectional flow with a peak velocity below 2.3 m/s (Fig. 21.8) (12).

The device outflow (return) cannula is typically anastomosed end to side of the right anterolateral aspect of the ascending Ao. It is best visualized by withdrawing the probe to image the ascending Ao in LAX and turning the probe slightly to the right. The RVAD outflow (return) cannula is anastomosed to the main PA and imaged in the mid-esophageal RV inflow-outflow view. Flow velocity in the LVAD outflow (return) cannula is measured by positioning the pulsed wave (PW) sample volume 1 cm proximal to the aortic anastomosis. The peak velocity is about 2.1 m/s in a normally functioning pulsatile LVAD.

Before initiating LVAD support, it is vital to check the adequacy of device and cardiac chamber de-airing by TEE. Various de-airing techniques have already been described in Chapter 13. The consequences of air emboli include migration in the coronary circulation with RV myocardial infarction and arrhythmias; migration in the systemic circulation with peripheral, visceral, or cerebral emboli; and migration in the venous circulation with pulmonary emboli. The occurrence of ischemic RV failure from air embolization could present a final insult to an already dysfunctional RV, requiring additional RVAD support.

Assessment of RV systolic function and loading conditions by TEE helps to identify the nature (inotropes, nitric oxide, peripheral and inhaled vasodilators, fluid) and adjust the level of the therapeutic support needed during weaning from CPB. Some patients (9–30%) may develop severe RV failure requiring RVAD insertion (25).

After CPB   Once fully weaned from CPB, the absence of significant AR and a PFO must absolutely be reascertained before leaving the OR. Reexamination of the LVAD inlet must also reconfirm the correct positioning of the cannula and adequate ventricular chamber decompression. Inadequate ventricular decompression may reflect insufficient device ejection or inflow (drainage) cannula obstruction. Finally, an independent measure of LVAD flow can be derived by the Doppler volumetric method (see Chapter 5) using the diameter of the outflow (return) aortic cannula and the velocity-time integral of the continuous wave (CW) Doppler signal in the cannula. There are inconsistent changes in the amount of TR after LVAD implantation, with occasional acute worsening (24).

Monitoring in the ICU   Complications may occur after LVAD implantation such as significant bleeding and hemodynamic instability. Maintenance of LVAD flow is a key indicator of the overall status. In the postoperative period, low LVAD flow is, in general, due to hypovolemia and/or RV dysfunction, easily assessed by TEE examination. RV failure has been reported in approximately 20% to 25% of patients supported by isolated LVADs (Fig. 21.17) (9).

The use of TEE is invaluable in assessing hemodynamic instability related to transient VAD dysfunction that may dramatically alter ventricular volumes (26). Not only can the inadequacy of VAD flow be confirmed but the etiology of the dysfunction may also be discovered by assessing the patency of both inflow (drainage) and outflow (return) cannulae, ruling out the presence of thrombi, air, collapse, or displacement of the cannulae. Spontaneous echocardiographic contrast in the LA or LV is also a sign of LVAD malfunction (27). The early diagnosis of cardiac tamponade warrants immediate pericardial drainage (Fig. 21.11). Severe hypoxemia in the ICU period may be due to pulmonary problems, but it is also prudent to rule out the presence of a new right-to-left shunting through a reopened PFO. The occurrence of cerebrovascular events during VAD support also warrants TEE examination to rule out the presence of intracavitary thrombus (Fig. 21.10).

Cases of successful weaning from LVAD support are infrequent (<5%) (6,9,28). As the patient's hemodynamic parameters improve and weaning from VAD is initiated, echocardiographic findings supportive of myocardial recovery include improved myocardial contractility, LVEF > 45% (29), left ventricular internal diameter in diastole (LVIDd) < 45 mm (30), and fractional area change > 40% (31). Experimental studies have shown that ventricular function and recovery could be monitored in the postoperative setting by obtaining pressure-area loops from transgastric two-chamber view using automated border detection and high-fidelity intraventricular pressure recording (32,33). Newer modalities such as tissue Doppler imaging have also been used to predict myocardial recovery during mechanical circulatory support (34).

Long-term monitoring   The cumulative probability of device failure increases from 6% at six months to 35% to 50% at two years (6,35). Device malfunction can be due to failure of the VAD components or changes in patient physiology (36).

Inflow valve regurgitation is the commonest cause of long-term LVAD malfunction. It is diagnosed by demonstrating turbulent color Doppler and inflow reversal with PW Doppler at the inflow (drainage) cannula during LVAD ejection. Additional TEE findings show a dilated LV, frequent AoV opening, and a reduced outflow (return) cannula velocity. Outflow valve regurgitation may also occur and can be demonstrated by the presence of retrograde Doppler flow in the outflow (return) cannula during LVAD diastole.

An obstructed inflow (drainage) cannula is suspected in the presence of turbulent flow in color Doppler images, intermittent diastolic flow, or peak

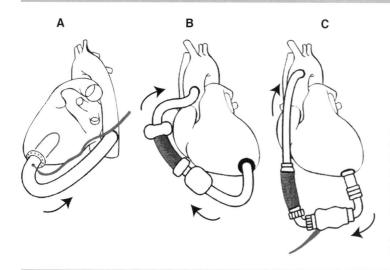

Figure 21.18 Continuous flow VADs. These are intracorporeal axial flow devices that provide augmented continuous peripheral flow. (**A**) The Jarvik 2000 uses a LV apical pump and descending aorta outflow (return) cannula. The DeBakey VAD (**B**) and the HeartMate 2 (**C**) devices use a LV apical inflow (drainage) cannula and an ascending aorta outflow (return) cannula. *Abbreviations*: LV, left ventricle; VAD, ventricular assist device. *Source*: Adapted with permission from Ref. 11 and illustrations courtesy of Frances Yeung, University of Toronto.

inflow velocity of >2.3 m/s (37). Outflow (return) cannula obstruction shows flow convergence and turbulent flow in color Doppler images as well as high peak velocity.

Continuous Flow Devices

Continuous flow (nonpulsatile) VAD devices provide continuous asynchronous flow independent of the native heart. Blood drains passively into the single-chamber pump that contains no valves. An axial or centrifugal pump rotates at a rapid rate continuously circulating blood forward. In the absence of any native heart ejection, the systemic flow is nonpulsatile.

The Jarvik 2000, DeBakey VAD, and HeartMate II (Fig. 21.18) are nonpulsatile intracorporeal valveless axial flow pump devices. These axial flow devices use a propeller screw-type design rotating at rapid rates to push blood continuously forward. The DeBakey VAD and HeartMate II provide only LVAD support with the intracorporeal axial pump using typical inflow (drainage) and outflow (return) cannulae. The impeller in the Jarvik 2000 device is implanted in the LV apex with the outflow (return) conduit in the descending Ao (left thoracotomy) or ascending Ao (sternotomy). All these nonpulsatile axial flow devices are currently used in Europe and are undergoing FDA approval trials as a bridge to transplant or destination therapy.

Transesophageal echocardiography. Initial TEE assessment in the pre-CPB period is similar for pulsatile LVADs as described previously (7). Specifically AR, PFO (Fig. 21.19), LV thrombus, and aortic atheroma must be ruled out and an assessment of RV function made. The LV apical cannula must also point toward the MV and away from the IVS. Dearing of the cannula and device occurs in a similar fashion to pulsatile LVADs. Air entrainment may occur through open suture lines as a result of the negative pressure suction created by the axial flow or the pump. Assessment of RV function and LV chamber size facilitates weaning from CPB.

Assessment of axial flow devices in the post-CPB period differs from pulsatile LVADs where the LV is significantly decompressed and the AoV rarely opens. Optimal function of an axial flow LVAD requires the IVS to remain in a neutral position. Typically, LVAD support results in increased RV preload and compliance with decreased RV afterload and contractility. The role of LV and RV interdependence is critical to understanding optimal RV and LVAD function. Complete decompression of the LV shifts the IVS to the left, creating a more spherical RV that compromises RV function (38). If there is insufficient decompression of the LV, the IVS remains to the right and also compromises RV function.

Spectral Doppler tracings from the outflow (return) cannula in the Ao of axial flow devices, such as the HeartMate II, shows a pulsatile pattern (peak velocity 1–2 m/s) synchronous to the patient's electrocardiogram superimposed on the continuous device flow. This pattern occurs even when the AoV remains closed during ventricular contraction.

Complications of nonpulsatile LVADs include bleeding, cannula obstruction, and rarely thrombus formation (39).

Percutaneous VADs

Percutaneous VADs are designed to provide temporary (5–14 days) partial or total circulatory support. These devices are inserted via the femoral artery and recirculate oxygenated blood from the left heart into the systemic circulation. Two types of devices are in use worldwide: the TandemHeart® (CardiacAssist, Inc., Pittsburgh, Pennsylvania, U.S.) and the Impella 2.5 LP System (Abiomed, Inc., Danvers, Massachusetts, U.S.) (40). Advantages of the Impella device include the use of a single arterial cannula, no transseptal puncture, and no extracorporeal pump. Both devices require systemic anticoagulation to prevent device clotting (Table 21.3).

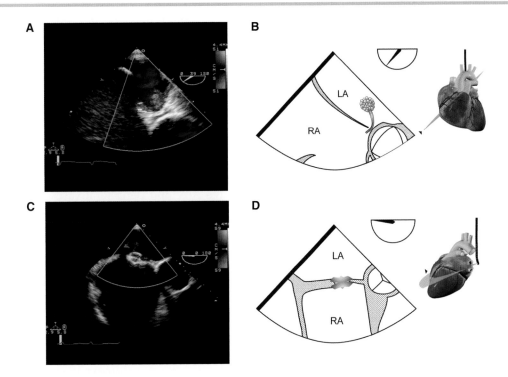

Figure 21.19   PFO with LVAD. (A,B) ME zoomed color Doppler right ventricular inflow/outflow tract view at 39° in a patient following implantation of a LVAD. Significant right-to-left shunt through a PFO is present. **(C,D)** Upper-esophageal color Doppler view after correction with trans-catheter Amplatzer device closure. *Abbreviations*: ME, mid-esophageal; PFO, patent foramen ovale; LA, left atrium; LVAD, left ventricular assist device; RA, right atrium.

Table 21.3   Percutaneous Ventricular Assist Devices

Device	TandemHeart®	Impella 2.5 system
Manufacturer	CardiacAssist, Inc., Pittsburgh, Pennsylvania, U.S.	Abiomed, Inc., Danvers, Massachusetts, U.S.
Approval	CE Mark, FDA 2003	CE Mark, Canada, FDA 2007
Cannula	Venous drainage, arterial outflow	Arterial only
Pump	Centrifugal, extracorporeal	Axial flow, intracorporeal
Circuit	Venous transseptal catheter in LA aspirates blood into pump and delivers into femoral artery	Retrograde aortic catheter in LV through aortic valve aspirates blood from LV below valve and delivers into ascending aorta above valve
Contraindications	RV failure (for left-sided devices), VSD, AR, Peripheral vascular disease	Mechanical aortic valve, calcific aortic stenosis, peripheral vascular disease
Anticoagulation	ACT > 300 s during insertion, Maintain ACT > 200	Maintain ACT > 160 ms
Hemodynamic effects	↑MAP, ↑CO, ↓afterload, ↓preload, ↑MVO$_2$	↑MAP, ↑CO, ↓PCWP
Complications	Cannula trauma (cardiac perforation), thromboembolism, hypothermia, bleeding, infection	Device malfunction, bleeding, infection, thrombus

Abbreviations: ACT, activated clotting time; AR, aortic regurgitation; CE, European Community; CO, cardiac output; FDA, Food and Drug Administration; LA, left atrium; MAP, mean arterial pressure; MVO$_2$, myocardial oxygen consumption; PCWP, pulmonary capillary wedge pressure; RV, right ventricle; VSD, ventricular septal defect.
Source: Adapted from Ref. 11.

The TandemHeart percutaneous LVAD is an LA to femoral artery bypass system consisting of three parts (Fig. 21.20A). A 21-F femoral venous cannula is inserted into the RA and directed transseptally into the LA under fluoroscopy or TEE guidance. This cannula is attached as inflow to an extracorporeal continuous flow centrifugal pump. Outflow (return) from the pump is a 15- to 17-F catheter inserted in the right femoral artery to the level of the aortic bifurcation. The device provides up to 5.0 L/min continuous flow. The TandemHeart is contraindicated in patients with RV failure, ventricular septal defect (VSD), AR,

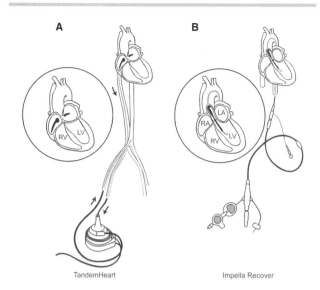

Figure 21.20 Percutaneous VADs. These devices are inserted via the femoral artery to provide partial or complete left ventricular support and continuous augmented peripheral flow. (**A**) The TandemHeart VAD is an extracorporeal centrifugal pump with device inflow (drainage) via a femoral vein cannula advanced across the interatrial septum into the LA. The device outflow (return) is through a cannula inserted via a femoral artery. (**B**) The Impella 2.5 VAD is a microaxial flow pump catheter inserted retrograde via the femoral artery up to the LV. Flow exits in the ascending aorta just above the aortic valve. *Abbreviations*: LA, left atrium; LV, left ventricle; RA, right atrium; RV, right ventricle; VAD, ventricular assist device. *Sources*: Adapted with from Ref. 11 and illustrations courtesy of Frances Yeung, University of Toronto.

from the LV and expels it into the ascending Ao using a microaxial flow blood pump (Fig. 21.20B). The 12-F catheter is inserted retrograde via a femoral artery and positioned across the AoV using fluoroscopy. The catheter is connected to an external console that monitors the pressure difference between the LV and Ao and permits adjustment of the motor speed to provide up to 2.5 to 5.0 L/min continuous flow. Oxygenated blood is aspirated from the LV into the tip of the catheter by the proximally located axial flow pump and expelled through the catheter side upstream from the pump into the Ao. Contraindications to the Impella 2.5 system are mechanical or heavily calcified native AoV and peripheral vascular disease (42).

It is likely that both devices provide more ventricular support than an IABP and can be implanted percutaneously in a prophylactic or emergent setting. The beneficial hemodynamic effects of these devices include increased CO and mean arterial pressure with decreased filling pressures (43,44). The devices are used prophylactically to support patients undergoing high-risk percutaneous coronary interventions or emergently in hemodynamically unstable patients as a bridge to recovery or stability pending implantable VAD or heart transplantation. Their role in the management of cardiogenic shock remains poorly defined (45).

Transesophageal echocardiography. Insertion of the TandemHeart can be guided using TEE (46). Adequate position of the needle tip, wire, and cannula for the transseptal placement of the device inflow (drainage) catheter is obtained from the mid-esophageal four-chamber view. The optimal position of the inflow cannula is entirely within the LA and directed toward the pulmonary veins. Adequate function is determined by color Doppler. The outflow (return) cannula is positioned in the lower descending abdominal Ao.

The correct position of the Impella catheter can be monitored by TEE (Fig. 21.21). The tip of the device is positioned in the LV at the anterior MV leaflet edge, 3 to 4 cm from the AoV annulus. Catheter tip

and peripheral vascular disease. At the time of explantation, a small residual ASD is formed, which usually closes over in a matter of weeks (41).

The Impella 2.5 or 5.0 system is a ventricular unloading catheter that aspirates oxygenated blood

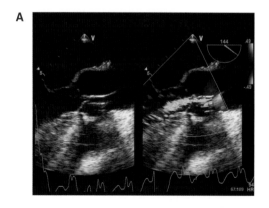
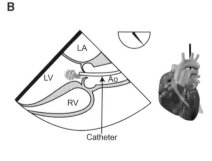

Figure 21.21 Impella 2.5 VAD. (**A,B**) Mid-esophageal long-axis view: the catheter is positioned across the AoV, causing intermittent aortic regurgitation. Visible color artefact within the catheter from the micro-axial endovascular impeller rotating device which aspirates blood from the LV below the AoV and pumps it into the ascending Ao above the AoV. *Abbreviations*: Ao, aorta; AoV, aortic valve; LA, left atrium; LV, left ventricle; RV, right ventricle; VAD, ventricular assist device. *Source*: Courtesy of Dr. Richard Cook.

occlusion by contact with the IVS or LV free wall should be excluded. The catheter outflow port is positioned in the ascending Ao 1.5 to 2 cm from the sinuses of Valsalva (47).

CONCLUSION

Transesophageal echocardiography appears to be an extremely valuable tool in the management of patients on mechanical circulatory assistance. It is an important component to the different aspects of assisted circulation, from the selection of the most appropriate form of ventricular assistance to the fine-tuning of pre-, intra-, and postoperative care. When TEE is combined with comprehensive hemodynamic assessment, it contributes to optimal management of this complex condition in patients with end-stage heart failure. As new modalities in TEE imaging evolve, further diagnostic applications and refinements of this technique in the management of mechanical circulatory support will likely emerge.

REFERENCES

1. Stevenson LW, Kormos RL. Mechanical cardiac support 2000: current applications and future trial design. J Thorac Cardiovasc Surg 2001; 121:418–424.
2. Ohuchi K, Takatani S. Currently available ventricular-assist devices: capabilities, limitations and future perspectives. Expert Rev Med Devices 2006; 3:195–205.
3. Mancini D, Burkhoff D. Mechanical device-based methods of managing and treating heart failure. Circulation 2005; 112:438–448.
4. Drakos SG, Charitos EI, Nanas SN, et al. Ventricular-assist devices for the treatment of chronic heart failure. Expert Rev Cardiovasc Ther 2007; 5:571–584.
5. Stone ME. Current status of mechanical circulatory assistance. Semin Cardiothorac Vasc Anesth 2007; 11:185–204.
6. Rose EA, Gelijns AC, Moskowitz AJ, et al. Long-term mechanical left ventricular assistance for end-stage heart failure. N Engl J Med 2001; 345:1435–1443.
7. Chumnanvej S, Wood MJ, Macgillivray TE, et al. Perioperative echocardiographic examination for ventricular assist device implantation. Anesth Analg 2007; 105:583–601.
8. Practice Guidelines for Perioperative Transesophageal Echocardiography: An Updated Report by the American Society of Anesthesiologists and the Society of Cardiovascular Anesthesiologists Task Force on Transesophageal Echocardiography. Anesthesiology 2010; 112:1–13.
9. Goldstein DJ, Oz MC, Rose EA. Implantable left ventricular assist devices. N Engl J Med 1998; 339:1522–1533.
10. Deng MC, Edwards LB, Hertz MI, et al. Mechanical circulatory support device database of the International Society for Heart and Lung Transplantation: third annual report—2005. J Heart Lung Transplant 2005; 24:1182–1187.
11. Vegas A. Assisting the failing heart. Anesthesiol Clin 2008; 26:539–564.
12. Scalia GM, McCarthy PM, Savage RM, et al. Clinical utility of echocardiography in the management of implantable ventricular assist devices. J Am Soc Echocardiogr 2000; 13:754–763.
13. Brack M, Olson JD, Pedersen WR, et al. Transesophageal echocardiography in patients with mechanical circulatory assistance. Ann Thorac Surg 1991; 52:1306–1309.
14. Barzilai B, Davila-Roman VG, Eaton MH, et al. Transesophageal echocardiography predicts successful withdrawal

15. of ventricular assist devices. J Thorac Cardiovasc Surg 1992; 104:1410–1416.
15. Pollock SG, Dent JM, Kaul S, et al. Diagnosis of ventricular assist device malfunction by transesophageal echocardiography. Am Heart J 1992; 124:793–794.
16. Simon P, Owen AN, Moritz A, et al. Transesophageal echocardiographic evaluation in mechanically assisted circulation. Eur J Cardiothorac Surg 1991; 5:492–497.
17. Bryant AS, Holman WL, Nanda NC, et al. Native aortic valve insufficiency in patients with left ventricular assist devices. Ann Thorac Surg 2006; 81:e6–e8.
18. Rao V, Slater JP, Edwards NM, et al. Surgical management of valvular disease in patients requiring left ventricular assist device support. Ann Thorac Surg 2001; 71:1448–1453.
19. Sukernik MR, Mets B, Bennett-Guerrero E. Patent foramen ovale and its significance in the perioperative period. Anesth Analg 2001; 93:1137–1146.
20. Liao KK, Miller L, Toher C, et al. Timing of transesophageal echocardiography in diagnosing patent foramen ovale in patients supported with left ventricular assist device. Ann Thorac Surg 2003; 75:1624–1626.
21. Baldwin RT, Duncan JM, Frazier OH, et al. Patent foramen ovale: a cause of hypoxemia in patients on left ventricular support. Ann Thorac Surg 1991; 52:865–867.
22. Fukamachi K, McCarthy PM, Smedira NG, et al. Preoperative risk factors for right ventricular failure after implantable left ventricular assist device insertion. Ann Thorac Surg 1999; 68:2181–2184.
23. Nakatani S, Thomas JD, Savage RM, et al. Prediction of right ventricular dysfunction after left ventricular assist device implantation. Circulation 1996; 94:II216–II221.
24. Holman WL, Bourge RC, Fan P, et al. Influence of left ventricular assist on valvular regurgitation. Circulation 1993; 88:II309–II318.
25. Ochiai Y, McCarthy PM, Smedira NG, et al. Predictors of severe right ventricular failure after implantable left ventricular assist device insertion: analysis of 245 patients. Circulation 2002; 106:I198–I202.
26. Farrar DJ. Ventricular interactions during mechanical circulatory support. Semin Thorac Cardiovasc Surg 1994; 6:163–168.
27. Peterson GE, Brickner ME, Reimold SC. Transesophageal echocardiography: clinical indications and applications. Circulation 2003; 107:2398–2402.
28. Leprince P, Combes A, Bonnet N, et al. Circulatory support for fulminant myocarditis: consideration for implantation, weaning and explantation. Eur J Cardiothorac Surg 2003; 24:399–403.
29. Hetzer R, Muller J, Weng Y, et al. Cardiac recovery in dilated cardiomyopathy by unloading with a left ventricular assist device. Ann Thorac Surg 1999; 68:742–749.
30. Leyvi G, Rhew E, Crooke G, et al. Transient right ventricular failure and transient weakness: a TEE diagnosis. J Cardiothorac Vasc Anesth 2005; 19:406–408.
31. Gorcsan J III, Severyn D, Murali S, et al. Non-invasive assessment of myocardial recovery on chronic left ventricular assist device: results associated with successful device removal. J Heart Lung Transplant 2003; 22: 1304–1313.
32. Gorcsan J III, Gasior TA, Mandarino WA, et al. Assessment of the immediate effects of cardiopulmonary bypass on left ventricular performance by on-line pressure-area relations. Circulation 1994; 89:180–190.
33. Mandarino WA, Winowich S, Gorcsan J III, et al. Right ventricular performance and left ventricular assist device filling. Ann Thorac Surg 1997; 63:1044–1049.
34. Vermes E, Houel R, Simon M, et al. Doppler tissue imaging to predict myocardial recovery during mechanical circulatory support. Ann Thorac Surg 2000; 70:2149–2151.

35. Long JW, Healy AH, Rasmusson BY, et al. Improving outcomes with long-term "destination" therapy using left ventricular assist devices. J Thorac Cardiovasc Surg 2008; 135:1353–1360.

36. Frazier OH, Rose EA, Oz MC, et al. Multicenter clinical evaluation of the HeartMate vented electric left ventricular assist system in patients awaiting heart transplantation. J Thorac Cardiovasc Surg 2001; 122:1186–1195.

37. Horton SC, Khodaverdian R, Chatelain P, et al. Left ventricular assist device malfunction: an approach to diagnosis by echocardiography. J Am Coll Cardiol 2005; 45:1435–1440.

38. Kawai A, Kormos RL, Mandarino WA, et al. Differential regional function of the right ventricle during the use of a left ventricular assist device. ASAIO J 1992; 38:M676–M678.

39. Catena E, Milazzo F, Montorsi E, et al. Left ventricular support by axial flow pump: the echocardiographic approach to device malfunction. J Am Soc Echocardiogr 2005; 18:1422.

40. Lee MS, Makkar RR. Percutaneous left ventricular support devices. Cardiol Clin 2006; 24:265–275, vii.

41. Fonger JD, Zhou Y, Matsuura H, et al. Enhanced preservation of acutely ischemic myocardium with transseptal left ventricular assist. Ann Thorac Surg 1994; 57:570–575.

42. Abiomed. Impella®—The System for Biventricular Cardiovascular Support. Electronic Citation, 2009. Available at: http://www.abiomed.com.

43. Thiele H, Lauer B, Hambrecht R, et al. Reversal of cardiogenic shock by percutaneous left atrial-to-femoral arterial bypass assistance. Circulation 2001; 104:2917–2922.

44. Valgimigli M, Steendijk P, Serruys PW, et al. Use of Impella Recover® LP 2.5 left ventricular assist device during high-risk percutaneous coronary interventions; clinical, haemodynamic and biochemical findings. EuroIntervention 2006; 2:91–100.

45. Burkhoff D, Cohen H, Brunckhorst C, et al. A randomized multicenter clinical study to evaluate the safety and efficacy of the TandemHeart percutaneous ventricular assist device versus conventional therapy with intraaortic balloon pumping for treatment of cardiogenic shock. Am Heart J 2006; 152:469–468.

46. Pretorius M, Hughes AK, Stahlman MB, et al. Placement of the TandemHeart percutaneous left ventricular assist device. Anesth Analg 2006; 103:1412–1413.

47. Catena E, Milazzo F, Pittella G, et al. Echocardiographic approach in a new left ventricular assist device: Impella Recover 100. J Am Soc Echocardiogr 2004; 17:470–473.

22

Heart Transplantation

Pierre Couture and Michel Carrier
Université de Montréal, Montreal, Quebec, Canada

François Haddad
Stanford University, Palo Alto, California, U.S.A.

INTRODUCTION

Orthotopic heart transplantation (OHT) is a valuable treatment option for selected patients with advanced heart failure refractory to surgical or medical management and poor short-term prognosis (1). Transesophageal echocardiography (TEE) is useful for monitoring patients undergoing heart transplantation. In this chapter, we will review the surgical technique and the role of TEE in the perioperative management of heart transplant patients.

DONORS AND RECIPIENTS

The availability of donor organs has led to a plateau of the annual number of heart transplants at 5000 cases worldwide (2). Broader donor eligibility criteria, to include older donors (>50-year-olds), marginal donors, and resuscitated hearts, have yet to have a substantial impact on the cardiac donor pool (2,3). Currently older donors (50–60 year olds) account for 12% of all donors (4). Marginal donor hearts may have coronary artery disease (CAD), mildly reduced left ventricular ejection fraction (LVEF), left ventricular (LV) hypertrophy, and successful resuscitation after asystole or exposure to high dose inotropes. A structurally normal young heart with LV dysfunction can recover normal function after hemodynamic and metabolic management. This form of donor heart resuscitation involves invasive monitoring to optimize fluid status; arginine vasopressin to maintain a normal systemic vascular resistance (SVR); and intravenous treatment of steroids, insulin, and thyroid hormone (3).

Donor ischemic time is defined as the time from aortic cross-clamp at harvest to cross-clamp release following implantation. Donor ischemic time has increased beyond the gold standard of four hours without a significant increase in mortality (5).

Immediately prior to transplantation recipients should have a pulmonary artery catheter (PAC) inserted to assess pulmonary artery (PA) pressures. Elevated PA pressures, whether fixed or reactive, are a risk factor for post-transplant right heart failure and may preclude

transplantation (6). General guidelines for unacceptable PA pressures and a relative contraindication to heart transplantation include (*i*) absolute systolic PA pressure >60mmHg, (*ii*) calculated pulmonary vascular resistance (PVR) >6 Wood units, (*iii*) transpulmonary gradient (TPG) = mean PA pressure − mean pulmonary capillary wedge pressure (PCWP) >16 to 20 mmHg (6). A vasodilator challenge using nitroprusside or inhaled nitric oxide may identify vasoreactive patients that may still be suitable transplant candidates (7).

SURGICAL CONSIDERATIONS

There are two surgical techniques of OHT currently used in clinical practice: the standard technique originally described by Lower and Shumway in 1966 (8,9) and the bicaval technique described by Dreyfus et al. (10) in 1991.

Standard Technique

A standard anesthetic preparation for routine cardiac surgery is performed including the use of a TEE probe for monitoring. The right internal jugular vein is left undisturbed for later use for endomyocardial biopsies. The Swan–Ganz catheter is initially inserted to measure real time RV and PA pressure but is pulled back during surgery. Both groins are prepared for emergency cannulation and initiation of cardiopulmonary bypass (CPB) if needed.

Through a median sternotomy following full systemic heparinization, standard cannulation of the ascending aorta (Ao) and both vena cava is performed. CBP is initiated when the donor heart arrives in the operating room (OR). Cross-clamping of the Ao is followed by removal of the recipient's failing heart leaving in place the posterior aspect of the left and right atria (LA, RA), and keeping as much as possible of the recipient's ascending Ao and PA tissue. Mild systemic hypothermia is easily reached and maintained throughout surgery (34°C).

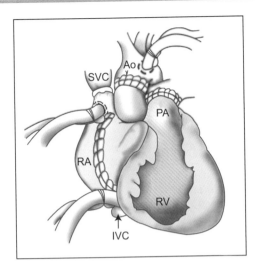

Figure 22.1 Classic biatrial technique of orthotopic heart transplantation. In this technique, the sites of anastomoses between the donor heart and recipient heart are at the level of the level of the atria. *Abbreviations*: Ao, aorta; IVC, inferior vena cava; PA, pulmonary artery; RA, right atrium; RV, right ventricle; SVC, superior vena cava.

While the cardiectomy is performed, the donor heart is inspected and prepared in a cold bath saline solution. The integrity of the atrial septum is ensured and corrected if, for instance, a foramen ovale is detected. The tricuspid and mitral valve (TV, MV) apparatus are also carefully inspected. Proper ligation of the superior vena cava (SVC) is secured, the right atrial wall is opened from the inferior vena cava (IVC) to the right atrial appendage (RAA) and the LA wall is trimmed and prepared. The ascending Ao and the PA are completely dissected and separated to facilitate proper exposure and suturing approach (Fig. 22.1).

The donor heart is brought into the thoracic cavity and the LA anastomosis is performed first with 3.0 polypropylene continuous sutures. To keep the heart as cold as possible during surgical implantation standard cold blood cardioplegia, at a rate of 100 to 200 mL/min, is administered retrograde through a coronary sinus catheter in addition to the application of ice slush onto the right ventricle (RV) (11). The RA anastomosis (Fig. 22.2) is completed with 3.0 polypropylene sutures, leaving a small gap for the coronary sinus catheter prior to completion of both the PA and aortic anastomoses. Donor and recipient pulmonary arteries are prepared, trimmed, and anastomosed with a continuous 4.0 polypropylene suture.

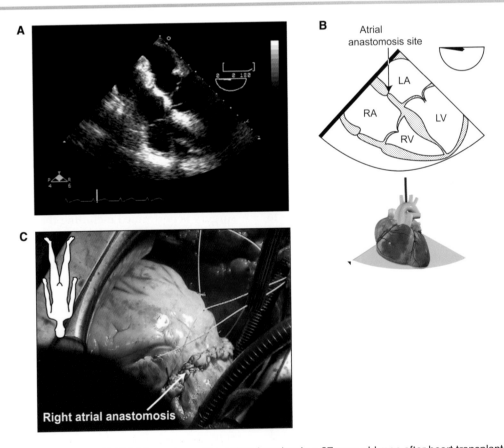

Figure 22.2 Atrial anastomosis. (A,B) Mid-esophageal four-chamber view in a 37-year-old man after heart transplantation shows the thickened atrial anastomotic ridge. **(C)** Intraoperative view of the right atrial anastomotic line. *Abbreviations*: LA, left atrium; LV, left ventricle; RA, right atrium; RV, right ventricle. *Source*: Courtesy of Dr. Denis Bouchard.

Next, snares on both vena cava are released, the coronary sinus catheter is removed, the operating table is put in the Trendelenburg position, and the ascending Ao clamp is released. With gentle massage of the heart, air is evacuated from the LV and the ascending Ao through the suture line via the puncture used to inject the antegrade cardioplegic solution at the donor site. The hole created in the left atrial appendage (LAA) to decompress the LV during the harvest of the donor heart is closed with a 3.0 polypropylene suture.

The patient is weaned from the CPB with a heart rate averaging 100 beats/min achieved by an isoproterenol infusion or atrial pacing and a good cardiac performance with systolic blood pressure (SBP) >90 to 100 mmHg. Atrial and aortic cannulae are removed while 500 mg of solumedrol is administered and protamine is injected intravenously. The Swan–Ganz catheter is refloated through the PA to monitor cardiac output (CO) and PA pressure. Two chest tubes are inserted in the mediastinum. Temporary pacing wires are sutured onto the RV. The sternum is then closed according to a standard technique.

Bicaval Technique

This alternative technique of cardiectomy and anastomoses is now more widely accepted as it minimizes the problems arising from oversized post-transplant atria, such as stasis, spontaneous echo contrast, and embolic complications (10). The right aspect of the LA is entered as for a routine MV surgical approach. The incision is extended superiorly under the SVC and inferiorly under the IVC (Fig. 22.3). During excision of the RA, generous portions of the SVC and IVC are left to facilitate donor and recipient anastomoses.

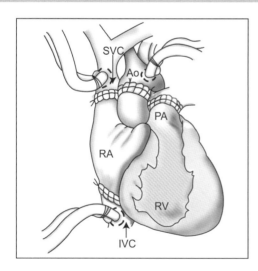

Figure 22.3 Bicaval technique of orthotopic heart transplantation. In this technique, the donor venae cavae are anastomosed to the recipient SVC and IVC. *Abbreviations*: Ao, aorta; IVC, inferior vena cava; PA, pulmonary artery; RA, right atrium; RV, right ventricle; SVC, superior vena cava.

The donor LA is anastomosed to the recipient LA as described in the standard method. The IVC and SVC are then anastomosed with 4.0 polypropylene suture. The rest of the procedure continues as described above for the standard approach to OHT.

TRANSESOPHAGEAL ECHOCARDIOGRAPHY IN THE PERIOPERATIVE PERIOD

In the updated perioperative TEE practice guidelines published in 2010 by the American Society of Anesthesiologists (ASA) and the Society of Cardiovascular Anesthesiologists (SCA) (12), the use of TEE during OHT is strongly supported. The role of TEE is less valuable during the pre-CPB period as the recipient's failing heart is completely removed. Rarely, thrombotic material in the native heart can be mobilized during manipulation and lead to pulmonary embolism (Fig. 22.4). During the CPB weaning process, TEE helps to define the etiology of hemodynamic instability, assesses the efficacy of de-airing procedures, and confirms the integrity of surgical anastomosis in the post-transplantation period.

Hemodynamic instability after heart transplantation may arise from a single or multiple causes such as primary graft failure, hyperacute rejection, RV dysfunction (Fig. 22.5), hypovolemia, vasodilatation, tamponade, right ventricular outflow tract (RVOT) obstruction (Fig. 22.6), or left ventricular outflow tract (LVOT) obstruction (Fig. 22.7).

Nonspecific graft failure is still the most common cause of death in the early postoperative period (13). Severe systolic dysfunction in the recipient may result from inadequate myocardial protection during the harvesting of the donor heart (role of cardioplegic solution, temperature, and duration of ischemia) and/or during transplantation. In rare instances, hyperacute rejection, rather than insufficient myocardial protection, may be responsible for the heart failure.

Right ventricular failure may occur in the recipient with preexisting and underestimated pulmonary hypertension (PH) (Fig. 22.5). Registry data from the International Society of Heart and Lung Transplantation show that, despite advances in perioperative management, RV dysfunction accounts for 50% of all cardiac complications and 19% of early death after heart transplantation (2,13,14) (Fig. 22.8). There is approximately a fourfold higher mortality among transplanted patients with fixed PH compared with patients without PH (13). PH, defined as a PVR >480 dyne s/cm^5 or 6 Wood units, is currently considered a contraindication to OHT. Patients with marked PH (PVR > 640 dyne s/cm^5 or 8 Wood units) should be considered for heart and lung transplantation and, more recently, long-term LV assistance followed by transplantation after significant improvement in PH. Patients with normal preoperative PVR have a significantly lower risk of postoperative RV failure following heart transplantation.

Organ preservation and CPB may have deleterious effects on ventricular function. Indeed CPB has

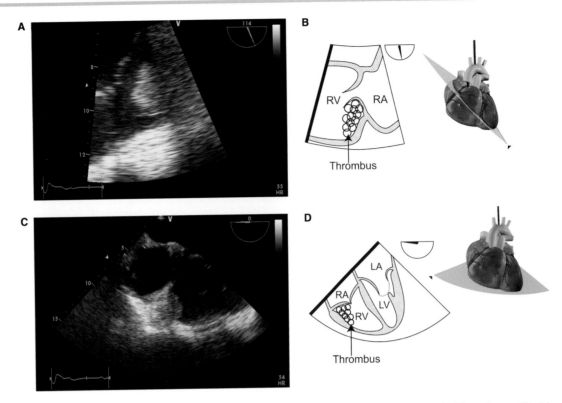

Figure 22.4   RV thrombus prior to OHT. Zoomed mid-esophageal right ventricular view at 114° (**A,B**) and a modified four-chamber view (**C,D**) show a laminated thrombus under the anterior leaflet of the tricuspid valve in a 49-year-old woman prior to OHT. *Abbreviations*: LA, left atrium; LV, left ventricle; OHT, orthotopic heart transplantation; RA, right atrium; RV, right ventricle.

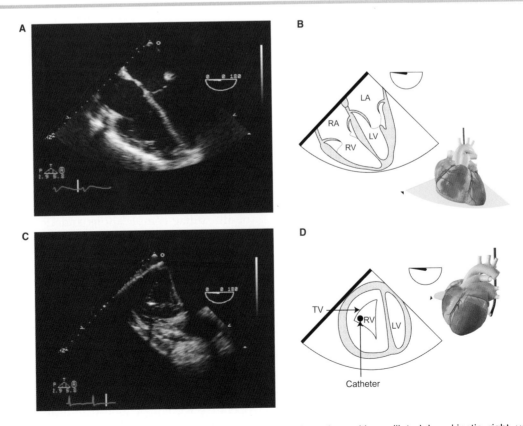

Figure 22.5   RV failure after OHT. (**A,B**) Mid-esophageal four-chamber view with a dilated hypokinetic right ventricle. (**C,D**) Transgastric view: note the D-shaped RV due to the flattened ventricular septum. *Abbreviations*: LA, left atrium; LV, left ventricle; OHT, orthotopic heart transplantation; RA, right atrium; RV, right ventricle.

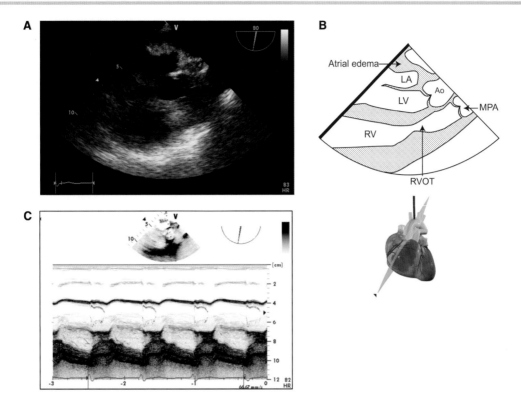

Figure 22.6 RVOT obstruction after OHT. (A,B) Mid-esophageal right ventricular inflow/outflow view shows dynamic RVOT obstruction. **(C)** Corresponding M-mode with systolic obliteration. *Abbreviations*: Ao, aorta; LA, left atrium; LV, left ventricle; MPA, main pulmonary artery; OHT, orthotopic heart transplantation; RV, right ventricle; RVOT, right ventricular outflow tract. ⌐🖱

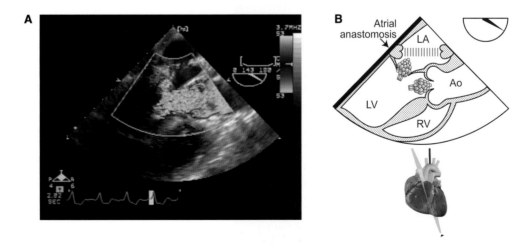

Figure 22.7 Atrial anastomosis after OHT. Left ventricular outflow tract (LVOT) obstruction due to the atrial anastomosis after OHT in a 47-year-old man. **(A,B)** Color Doppler mid-esophageal long-axis view showing flow acceleration in the LVOT upon weaning from cardiopulmonary bypass. Aliasing was also seen at the level of the mitral valve, most likely from the edematous atrial anastomosis, mimicking cor triatriatum sinister. *Abbreviations*: Ao, aorta; LA, left atrium; LV, left ventricle; OHT, orthotopic heart transplantation; RV, right ventricle. ⌐🖱

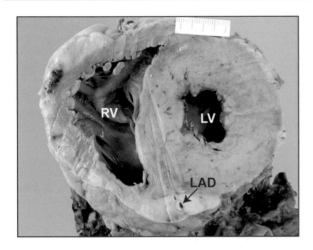

Figure 22.8 Acute rejection after heart transplantation. A 50-year-old man died from acute rejection after heart transplantation. The autopsy showed a hypertrophied LV and a dilated RV. *Abbreviations*: LAD, left anterior descending; LV, left ventricle; RV, right ventricle. *Source*: Courtesy of Dr. Tack Ki Leung.

been shown to cause an increase in PVR (13). Reviews have been published on the management of RV failure after heart transplantation and the role for inhaled nitric oxide (NO) treatment (13,15,16). These studies have demonstrated that inhaled nitric oxide may be useful in decreasing the risk of RV failure in high-risk patients.

Transesophageal echocardiography is also useful to evaluate surgical anastomosis in the post-transplantation period (Fig. 22.9). The main PA anastomosis appears as a suture ridge within the vessels. Stenosis should be ruled out by two-dimensional (2D) color Doppler imaging to detect turbulent flow and by continuous wave (CW) Doppler to measure the systolic gradient across the anastomosis. The PAC can also be used to document any gradient across the RV and the PA (Fig. 22.10) (17). The mid-esophageal long-axis (LAX) or two-chamber views show an elongated LA now composed of both donor and recipient atrial tissue (Fig. 22.11). The suture line within the LA and RA also appears predominantly as an echodense ridge (Fig. 22.9). Acquired cor triatriatum may develop secondary to infolding of the redundant tissue from excessive donor atrial tissue (Fig. 22.7). Anastamoses of both cavae are examined to rule out stenosis.

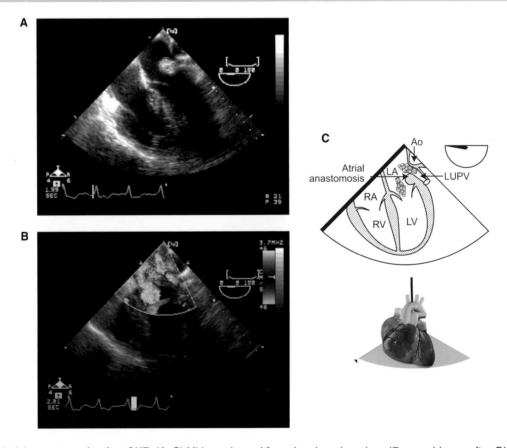

Figure 22.9 Atrial anastomosis after OHT. (A–C) Mid-esophageal four-chamber views in a 47-year-old man after OHT showing the edematous LA anastomotic site with flow acceleration in the LUPV. *Abbreviations*: Ao, aorta; LA, left atrium; LUPV, left upper pulmonary vein; LV, left ventricle; OHT, orthotopic heart transplantation; RA, right atrium; RV, right ventricle.

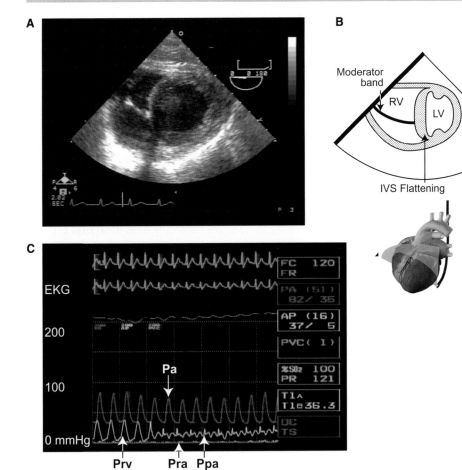

Figure 22.10 RV function after OHT. (**A,B**) The transgastric mid short-axis view in a 37-year-old man after OHT shows mild RV dilatation with a prominent moderator band and a flattened IVS. (**C**) A 10 mmHg systolic pressure gradient is present between the Prv and the Ppa. *Abbreviations*: EKG, electrocardiogram; IVS, interventricular septum; LV, left ventricle; OHT, orthotopic heart transplantation; Pa, arterial pressure; Ppa, pulmonary artery pressure; Pra, right atrial pressure; Prv, right ventricular pressure; RV, right ventricle. 🖱

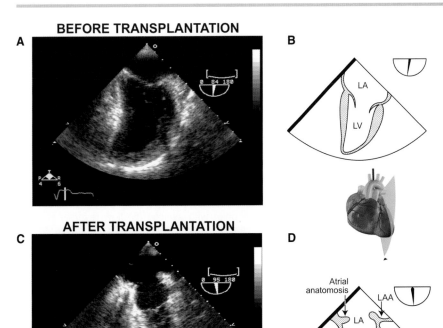

Figure 22.11 Atrial anastomosis after OHT. Mid-esophageal two-chamber views in a patient with end-stage hypertrophic cardiomyopathy (**A,B**) before and (**C,D**) after OHT are shown. Note the new LA suture anastomosis after the procedure and the LA elongation (increase in the anteroposterior size). *Abbreviations*: LA, left atrium; LAA, left atrial appendage; LV, left ventricle; OHT, orthotopic heart transplantation. 🖱

ECHOCARDIOGRAPHY IN THE POSTOPERATIVE PERIOD

The early postoperative changes following heart transplantation include RV remodeling, abnormal septal motion, increase in LV mass, presence of pericardial fluid, and abnormal LV and RV filling patterns (Fig. 22.12) (18).

Right Ventricular Remodeling, Tricuspid Regurgitation, and Abnormal Movement of the Ventricular Septum

The time course of the resolution of PH and RV remodeling after OHT has been described by Bhatia et al. (19). In 24 patients with moderate PH (mean PA pressure < 50 mmHg) after heart transplantation, the PH resolved rapidly, with the mean PA pressure approaching normal values at two weeks after surgery. In parallel, the PVR had returned to normal in 80% of patients by one year. Patients with the highest preoperative PVR had the greatest decrease after the transplantation (ranging from 10% to 84%). Right and left heart filling pressure also decreased to a nadir in the upper normal range at two weeks after surgery and remained unchanged over one year of follow-up.

The donor RV remodels in response to recipient perioperative PH. Initially enlarged, it dilates further during the first month and subsequently returns to its immediate perioperative dimensions at one year after surgery (Fig. 22.13) (19). The RV wall thickness does not increase significantly probably because the PVR declines to normal level. Thus, at one year, while resting hemodynamics are normal, the donor RV remains enlarged, probably as an adaptation to chronic volume overload.

Tricuspid regurgitation (TR) is common after heart transplantation due to the afterload mismatch and RV dilatation. The incidence of TR (grades 1–3) changes from 67% on day one after heart transplantation to 36% at one year. Nevertheless, TR is generally well tolerated and rarely of clinical significance (19). Finally, abnormal diastolic flattening of the ventricular septum was present in all patients immediately postoperatively (Fig. 22.10). This proportion decreased to 75% at one month and 42% at one year. This decline parallels the decrease in TR and RV dimensions. On the other hand, systolic paradoxical septal motion was uncommon, probably because the

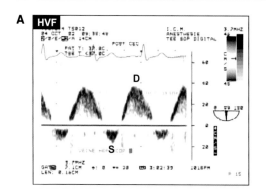

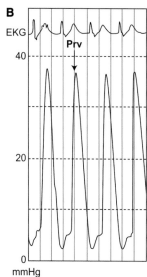

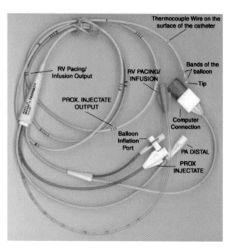

Figure 22.12   RV diastolic function after OHT. (**A**) Hepatic venous flow (HVF) pulsed wave Doppler with systolic (S) flow reversal in a 37-year-old man after OHT. (**B**) Right ventricular pressure (Prv) abnormal waveform with rapid increase in diastolic pressure consistent with abnormal right ventricular filling. (**C**) The tracing was obtained from the right ventricular pacing port of the pulmonary artery catheter. *Abbreviations*: D, peak diastolic HVF velocity; EKG, electrocardiogram; HVF, hepatic venous flow; OHT, orthotopic heart transplantation; PA, pulmonary artery; Prv, right ventricular pressure; PROX, proximal; RV, right ventricle; S, peak systolic HVF velocity.

TIME AFTER TRANSPLANTATION

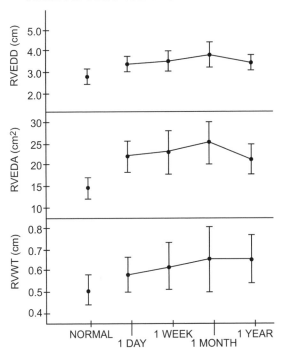

Figure 22.13 RV function after OHT. Serial RV echocardiographic measurements after OHT (±1 SD) are compared with control values (n = 10). Shown are right ventricular end-diastolic dimensions (RVEDD in cm^2), right ventricular end-diastolic area (RVEDA in cm^2) and right ventricular wall thickness (RVWT in cm). *Abbreviations*: OHT, orthotopic heart transplantation; RV, right ventricle. *Source*: Adapted with permission from Ref. 19.

mean PA pressure decreases significantly immediately after OHT (19).

Left Ventricular Mass and Mitral Valve Function

In the immediate postoperative period, both LV wall thickness and mass increase, most likely from perioperative myocardial ischemia and edema. Systemic hypertension and side effects from cyclosporine and corticosteroid administration can further contribute to LV mass augmentation seen at one year. Acute increase in myocardial thickness may also occur later with allograft rejection (Fig. 22.8) (20). Left ventricular contractility and contractile reserve both appear to be normal after heart transplantation (21).

Mild to moderate mitral regurgitation (MR) has been reported to occur with a frequency ranging from 55% to 87% without major clinical implications (19,22). It usually occurs in a donor heart without structural abnormality of the mitral apparatus or LV dysfunction. The MR may arise from biatrial enlargement that exerts tension on the posterior MV leaflet and causes incomplete closure of the valve and annuloventricular dis-

proportion (19). Moreover, the presence of both donor and recipient atria and sinus nodes results in asynchrony and inhomogenous atrial contraction, which may also play a role in the genesis of MR (19). Finally, MR can occur in association with LVOT obstruction.

Pericardial Effusion

Pericardial effusions are commonly observed in 85% of patients after heart transplantation (23). The loss of lymphatic drainage and the discrepancy in size between the new donor heart and the large remaining pericardial cavity are plausible explanations (20). Even though pericardial effusions are common, rarely do they precipitate hemodynamic instability, such as cardiac tamponade. While large but slowly accumulating pericardial effusions usually cause little hemodynamic impairment, a loculated hematoma developing at a critical location may conversely cause acute cardiac tamponade (see Chapter 12). Thus, the relationship between the size of the effusion and the clinical outcome is likely to show a poor correlation (20). Most effusions are nearly, or completely, resolved by 30 days after surgery (23).

Left Ventricular Diastolic Function

Diastolic function is also altered in the heart transplant recipient (in the absence of rejection) during the early postoperative period. Initial pulsed wave (PW) Doppler examination of the mitral inflow shows a profile comparable to previously defined restrictive parameters (see Chapter 10); this evolves into a nonrestrictive pattern over a six-week period, leading to progressive improvement in postoperative diastolic function parameters and decrease in left heart filling pressures (24). The presence of recurrent or persistent severe diastolic dysfunction with restrictive filling within six months after transplantation is associated with a reduced late-term actuarial survival, independent of graft rejection (25).

Evidence suggests that retaining normal LA size and shape by using the bicaval technique promotes ventricular filling dynamics that more closely approximates normal physiology (20). Ventricular filling is influenced by the mechanical activity of residual recipient atrial tissue over that of the donor heart. In addition, "parasystolic" contraction of residual recipient atrial tissue also modifies the pulmonary venous flow (PVF): recipient atrial contraction occurring in late systole results in an increase in the diastolic component (D-wave); if it happens in early systole the systolic component (S-wave) is decreased. End-diastolic atrial contraction will increase the velocity observed during atrial reversal (AR) (18).

Normal Echocardiographic Profile After Heart Transplantation

One year after OHT, echocardiograms of recipients doing clinically well are characterized by increased

LV wall thickness and mass. Left ventricular dimensions, volumes, and ejection fraction are within normal limits. Right ventricular wall thickness and cavity size are increased with preserved RV systolic function. The transplanted heart also shows an anteromedial translational motion during systole. The atria of the transplanted heart have unique echocardiographic features. The anastomotic suture line is easily identified on 2D imaging as the waist of these hourglass-shaped atria (Fig. 22.11). This waist creates a natural point of subdivision within the native and donor atria. The markedly enlarged atrial volume results primarily from an increased LAX dimension (Fig. 22.11), although maximal width or short axis dimension is also slightly larger than in controls (26). The increase in both donor and recipient atrial size is inversely correlated with survival (27).

Abnormal Echocardiographic Findings Following Heart Transplantation

The presence of the atrial suture line, increased atrial size with subcontractile portion of the recipient atrium, and asynchrony between the donor and recipient atria contraction promotes stasis and thrombosis. These factors may account for the high prevalence of atrial spontaneous echo contrast (55%) as assessed with TEE (28). Left atrial thrombi were observed in 38% by TEE and are often missed by transthoracic echocardiography (TTE). Thrombi were located in the donor LAA (10/18), on the posterior wall of the LA (6/18), on the donor component of the atrial septum (1/18), and on the left atrial suture (1/18) (28). Thrombi occurred only in patients displaying spontaneous echocardiographic contrast (Fig. 22.14). Episodes of arterial embolism were documented in 22% of patients with both spontaneous echocardiographic contrast and LA thrombus (6% of heart transplantation recipients) (28). The use of the modified bicaval OHT technique seems to decrease the incidence of this problem considerably (29).

Transesophageal echocardiography has also been found to be superior to TTE in demonstrating thickening of the atrial septum, bulging of the recipient and donor atrial septum, and shunt at the atrial level (28). It may identify uncommon patent foramen ovale after heart transplantation (30). Coronary fistula is another finding detected by TEE after heart transplantation. The incidence of this iatrogenic complication has been estimated between 5% and 15%, a 20-fold increase over the incidence of congenital

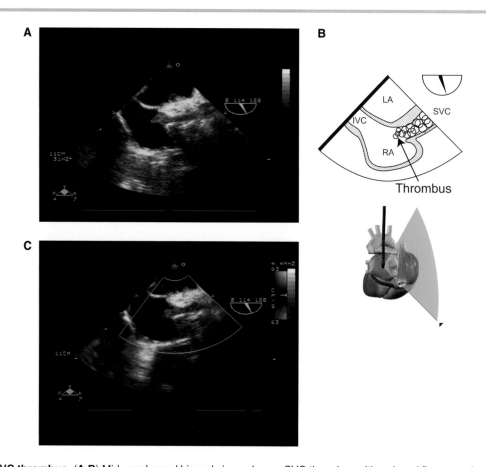

Figure 22.14   SVC thrombus. (A,B) Mid-esophageal bicaval views show a SVC thrombus with reduced flow on color Doppler (**C**) after heart transplantation. *Abbreviations*: IVC, inferior vena cava; LA, left atrium; RA, right atrium; SVC, superior vena cava.

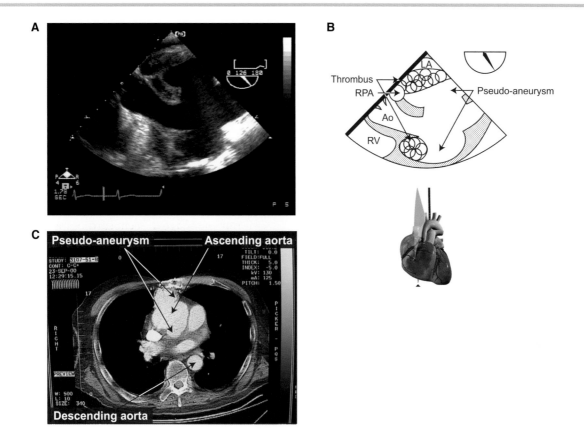

Figure 22.15 **Aortic pseudoaneurysm after OHT. (A,B)** Mid-esophageal ascending Ao long-axis view shows an aortic pseudoaneurysm in a 65-year-old man which developed nine months after OHT. The pseudoaneurysm was located at the anastomotic site of the native Ao. Blood flow in the pseudoaneurysm was present. **(C)** Chest CT scan with both posterior and anterior extension of the pseudoaneurysm close to the sternal border. *Abbreviations*: Ao, aorta; LA, left atrium; OHT, orthotopic heart transplantation; RPA, right pulmonary artery; RV, right ventricle.

coronary artery fistula (31). The increased incidence in this group is attributed to injury from multiple routine surveillance RV endomyocardial biopsy procedures for detection of cardiac rejection, which frequently involves the right coronary artery (RCA). The vast majority of these fistulas communicate directly with the RV, are usually diagnosed by routine coronary angiography, and are without hemodynamic significance (31). Finally, pseudoaneurysm can occur after cardiac transplantation at any site of major vessel anastomosis (Fig. 22.15).

Detection of Acute Allograft Rejection and Coronary Artery Disease

Acute allograft rejection is common, particularly in the first year after transplantation. It constitutes the most frequent cause of death during this period. Morphologic features suggestive of allograft rejection include an increase in myocardial mass due to inflammatory cell infiltration and myocardial edema (Fig. 22.8) (Table 22.1). However, with the addition of cyclosporine to the immunosuppressive medical regimen, cellular rejection is associated with less myocardial edema: the evaluation of ventricular systolic function

and myocardial mass has thus become less sensitive as a means of detecting early rejection. Doppler parameters of diastolic function have recently been used to detect acute rejection (Table 22.2).

Moderate to severe rejection has been associated with a fall of at least 15% in the mitral deceleration or the isovolemic relaxation time. However, wide interpatient variability in Doppler variables renders isolated measurement cut-offs less predictive. Each patient acting as her/his own control (from baseline) provides the basis for Doppler-based surveillance of allograft rejection. Currently, Doppler-derived parameters of diastolic function are used as an adjunct rather than a replacement for endomyocardial biopsy. Protocols now combine routine biopsies, with supplemental biopsy in the event of echocardiographic evidence of acutely restrictive physiology (20).

In patients who survive the first two years of transplantation, CAD constitutes an important cause of mortality. There is increasing interest in the ability of dobutamine stress echocardiography to predict adverse cardiac events in OHT recipients. A normal dobutamine stress echocardiography result is a very powerful determinant of a benign clinical course with a negative predictive value in excess of 90% to 95% (20).

Table 22.1 International Society of Heart and Lung Transplant (ISHLT) Standardized Cardiac Biopsy Grading[a]

1990	
Grade 0	No rejection
Grade 1, mild	
A – Focal	Focal perivascular and/or interstitial infiltrate without myocyte damage
B – Diffuse	Diffuse infiltrate without myocyte damage
Grade 2 moderate (focal)	One focus of infiltrate with associated myocyte damage
Grade 3, moderate	
A – Focal	Multifocal infiltrate with myocyte damage
B – Diffuse	Diffuse infiltrate with myocyte damage
Grade 4, severe	Diffuse, polymorphous infiltrate with extensive myocyte damage $\pm$ edema, $\pm$ hemorrhage $+$ vasculitis
2004	
Grade 0 R[b]	No rejection
Grade 1 R[b], mild	Interstitial and/or perivascular infiltrate with up to 1 focus of myocyte damage
Grade 2 R[b], moderate	Two or more foci of infiltrate with associated myocyte damage
Grade 3 R[b], severe	Diffuse infiltrate with multifocal myocyte damage $\pm$ edema, $\pm$ hemorrhage $\pm$ vasculitis

[a] The presence or absence of acute antibody-mediated rejection (AMR) may be recorded as AMR 0 or AMR 1, as required.
[b] Where "R" denotes revised grade to avoid confusion with 1990 scheme.
Source: With permission from Ref. 32.

Table 22.2 Detection of Heart Transplant Rejection by Echocardiographic Indices

Study	Design number	Criteria used for rejection[a]	Events	Index	Cut-off value	Se (%)	Sp (%)
Valantine et al. (33)	Retrospective n = 39	≥ 2	56	PHT	$\geq 15\%\downarrow$	82	79
				IVRT		82	79
Stork et al. (34)	Retrospective n = 21	$\geq 3a$	11	PHT	≥ 8 ms $\downarrow$	73	80
				IVRT	≥ 12 ms $\downarrow$	82	80
Ciliberto et al. (35)	Retrospective n = 130	≥ 1	95	PHT	≥ 20 ms $\downarrow$	44	98
				IVRT		28	98
Mouly-Bandini et al. (36)	Retrospective n = 23	≥ 1	84	PHT or IVRT	$\geq 20\%\downarrow$	31	93
Puleo et al. (37)	Retrospective n = 121	$\geq 3a$	16	E_m	ns	76	88
Stengel et al. (38)	Retrospective n = 41	$\geq 3a$	23	A_m	<0.087cm/s	82	53
Dandel et al. (39)	Retrospective n = 161	≥ 2	35	S_m	$>10\%\downarrow$	88	94
				E_m	$>10\%\downarrow$	92	92
Vivekananthan et al. (40)	Retrospective n = 40	$\geq 3a$	20	LVMPI	$\geq 20\%\downarrow$	90	90
Burgess et al. (41)	Retrospective n = 50	≥ 2	34	LVMPI	ns	–	–
Palka et al. (42)	Retrospective n = 44	$\geq 3a$		E_m	<0.12 m/s	69	59
Sun et al. (43)	Retrospective n = 264	$\geq 3a$	138	IVRT E/A PE	<90 ms >1.7	3 independent predictors of rejection	

[a]Criteria used to define significant rejection are based on the previous International Society of Heart and Lung Transplant (ISHLT) classification; Grade 3a or 2R rejection in the revised classification usually lead to an increase in immunosuppression (32).
Abbreviations: A, peak late diastolic TMF velocity; A_m, peak late diastolic MAV; E, peak early diastolic TMF velocity; E_m, peak early diastolic MAV; IVCT, isovolumic contraction time; IVRT, isovolumic contraction time; MAV, mitral annular velocity; MPI, myocardial performance index; n, number; na, not available; ns or –, nonsignificant; PE, pericardial effusion; PHT, pressure half-time; Se, sensitivity; S_m, peak systolic MAV; Sp, specificity; +, significant.

Table 22.3 Role of TEE in Cardiac Transplantation

Before the procedure in patient with ventricular assist device (see Table 21.3)

Perioperative period:
- Monitoring after cardiac surgery (see Table 13.1)
- Deairing of all four cardiac cavities
- Detection of stenotic anastomosis (pulmonary artery, pulmonary veins, inferior and superior vena cava)
- Detection of patent foramen ovale

Early and late postoperative period: evaluation of
- Left and right systolic and diastolic function
- Mitral and tricuspid valves
- Atrial anastomosis, thrombus, spontaneous echocardiographic contrast
- Presence of coronary fistula
- Aneurysm and pseudoaneurysm of the large vessels anastomoses

If hemodynamic instability: detection of
- Left and right ventricular acute systolic and diastolic dysfunction
- Left and right ventricular outflow tract dynamic obstruction
- Severe mitral or tricuspid regurgitation
- Hypovolemia and vasodilatation
- Cardiac tamponade from circumferential or loculated effusion
- Inferior vena cava stenosis

CONCLUSION

In summary, echocardiography may significantly contribute to the evaluation of patients at various stages of heart transplantation (Table 22.3). During the initial perioperative period, it provides timely assessment of cardiac anatomy and physiology and bestows the opportunity to detect specific problems. Later, detection of allograft rejection and accelerated CAD benefits from the addition of this noninvasive diagnostic tool.

REFERENCES

1. Hunt SA, Abraham WT, Chin MH et al. ACC/AHA 2005 Guideline Update for the Diagnosis and Management of Chronic Heart Failure in the Adult: a report of the American College of Cardiology/American Heart Association Task Force on Practice Guidelines (Writing Committee to Update the 2001 Guidelines for the Evaluation and Management of Heart Failure): developed in collaboration with the American College of Chest Physicians and the International Society for Heart and Lung Transplantation: endorsed by the Heart Rhythm Society. Circulation 2005; 112:e154–e235.

2. Taylor DO, Edwards LB, Boucek MM, et al. Registry of the International Society for Heart and Lung Transplantation: twenty-fourth official adult heart transplant report–2007. J Heart Lung Transplant 2007; 26:769–781.

3. Zaroff JG, Rosengard BR, Armstrong WF, et al. Consensus conference report: maximizing use of organs recovered from the cadaver donor: cardiac recommendations. March 28–29, 2001, Crystal City, Va. Circulation 2002; 106:836–841.

4. Renlund DG, Taylor DO, Kfoury AG, et al. New UNOS rules: historical background and implications for transplantation management. United Network for Organ Sharing. J Heart Lung Transplant 1999; 18:1065–1070.

5. Russo MJ, Chen JM, Sorabella RA, et al. The effect of ischemic time on survival after heart transplantation varies by donor age: an analysis of the United Network for Organ Sharing database. J Thorac Cardiovasc Surg 2007; 133:554–559.

6. Mehra MR, Kobashigawa J, Starling R, et al. Listing criteria for heart transplantation: International Society for Heart and Lung Transplantation guidelines for the care of cardiac transplant candidates-2006. J Heart Lung Transplant 2006; 25:1024–1042.

7. Butler J, Stankewicz MA, Wu J, et al. Pre-transplant reversible pulmonary hypertension predicts higher risk for mortality after cardiac transplantation. J Heart Lung Transplant 2005; 24:170–177.

8. Lower RR, Shumway NE. Studies on orthotopic homotransplantation of the canine heart. Surg Forum 1960; 11:18–19.

9. Shumway NE, Lower RR, Stofer RC. Transplantation of the heart. Adv Surg 1966; 2:265–284.

10. Dreyfus G, Jebara V, Mihaileanu S, et al. Total orthotopic heart transplantation: an alternative to the standard technique. Ann Thorac Surg 1991; 52:1181–1184.

11. Carrier M, Leung TK, Solymoss BC, et al. Clinical trial of retrograde warm blood reperfusion versus standard cold topical irrigation of transplanted hearts. Ann Thorac Surg 1996; 61:1310–1314.

12. Practice Guidelines for Perioperative Transesophageal Echocardiography: An Updated Report by the American Society of Anesthesiologists and the Society of Cardiovascular Anesthesiologists Task Force on Transesophageal Echocardiography. Anesthesiology 2010; 112:1–13.

13. Stobierska-Dzierzek B, Awad H, Michler RE. The evolving management of acute right-sided heart failure in cardiac transplant recipients. J Am Coll Cardiol 2001; 38:923–931.

14. Hosenpud JD, Bennett LE, Keck BM, et al. The Registry of the International Society for Heart and Lung Transplantation: seventeenth official report-2000. J Heart Lung Transplant 2000; 19:909–931.

15. Carrier M, Blaise G, Belisle S, et al. Nitric oxide inhalation in the treatment of primary graft failure following heart transplantation. J Heart Lung Transplant 1999; 18:664–667.

16. Haddad F, Couture P, Tousignant C, et al. The right ventricle in cardiac surgery, a perioperative perspective: II. Pathophysiology, clinical importance, and management. Anesth Analg 2009; 108:422–433.

17. Suriani RJ. Transesophageal echocardiography during organ transplantation. J Cardiothorac Vasc Anesth 1998; 12:686–694.

18. Durennes ME. Échocardiographie transoesophagienne chez le transplanté cardiaque. In: Cohen A, ed. Échocardiographie Transoesophagienne en Cardiologie et en Anesthésie. Édition Arnette, 1992:265–279.

19. Bhatia SJ, Kirshenbaum JM, Shemin RJ, et al. Time course of resolution of pulmonary hypertension and right ventricular remodeling after orthotopic cardiac transplantation. Circulation 1987; 76:819–826.

20. Burgess MI, Bhattacharyya A, Ray SG. Echocardiography after cardiac transplantation. J Am Soc Echocardiogr 2002; 15:917–925.

21. Borow KM, Neumann A, Arensman FW, et al. Left ventricular contractility and contractile reserve in humans after cardiac transplantation. Circulation 1985; 71:866–872.

22. Angermann CE, Spes CH, Tammen A, et al. Anatomic characteristics and valvular function of the transplanted heart: transthoracic versus transesophageal echocardiographic findings. J Heart Transplant 1990; 9:331–338.

23. Weitzman LB, Tinker WP, Kronzon I, et al. The incidence and natural history of pericardial effusion after cardiac surgery—an echocardiographic study. Circulation 1984; 69:506–511.

24. StGoar FG, Gibbons R, Schnittger I, et al. Left ventricular diastolic function. Doppler echocardiographic changes

soon after cardiac transplantation. Circulation 1990; 82:872–878.

25. Ross HJ, Gullestad L, Hunt SA, et al. Early Doppler echocardiographic dysfunction is associated with an increased mortality after orthotopic cardiac transplantation. Circulation 1996; 94:II289–II293.

26. Gorcsan J III, Snow FR, Paulsen W, et al. Echocardiographic profile of the transplanted human heart in clinically well recipients. J Heart Lung Transplant 1992; 11:80–89.

27. Gudmundsson GS, Smull DL, Pisani BA, et al. Increase in atrial size in long-term survivors of heart transplant. J Am Soc Echocardiogr 2003; 16:1043–1048.

28. Derumeaux G, Mouton-Schleifer D, Soyer R, et al. High incidence of left atrial thrombus detected by transoesophageal echocardiography in heart transplant recipients. Eur Heart J 1995; 16:120–125.

29. Riberi A, Ambrosi P, Habib G, et al. Systemic embolism: a serious complication after cardiac transplantation avoidable by bicaval technique. Eur J Cardiothorac Surg 2001; 19:307–311.

30. Ouseph R, Stoddard MF, Lederer ED. Patent foramen ovale presenting as refractory hypoxemia after heart transplantation. J Am Soc Echocardiogr 1997; 10:973–976.

31. Lowry RW, Young JB, Kleiman NS, et al. Transesophageal echocardiographic demonstration of right coronary artery-to-coronary sinus fistula in a heart transplant recipient. J Am Soc Echocardiogr 1993; 6:449–452.

32. Stewart S, Winters GL, Fishbein MC, et al. Revision of the 1990 working formulation for the standardization of nomenclature in the diagnosis of heart rejection. J Heart Lung Transplant 2005; 24:1710–1720.

33. Valantine HA, Yeoh TK, Gibbons R, et al. Sensitivity and specificity of diastolic indexes for rejection surveillance: temporal correlation with endomyocardial biopsy. J Heart Lung Transplant 1991; 10:757–765.

34. Stork T, Mockel M, Eichstadt H, et al. Noninvasive diagnosis of cardiac allograft rejection by means of pulsed Doppler and M-mode ultrasound. J Ultrasound Med 1991; 10:569–575.

35. Ciliberto GR, Mascarello M, Gronda E, et al. Acute rejection after heart transplantation: noninvasive echocardiographic evaluation. J Am Coll Cardiol 1994; 23:1156–1161.

36. Mouly-Bandini A, Vion-Dury J, Viout P, et al. Value of Doppler echocardiography in the detection of low-grade rejections after cardiac transplantation. Transpl Int 1996; 9:131–136.

37. Puleo JA, Aranda JM, Weston MW, et al. Noninvasive detection of allograft rejection in heart transplant recipients by use of Doppler tissue imaging. J Heart Lung Transplant 1998; 17:176–184.

38. Stengel SM, Allemann Y, Zimmerli M, et al. Doppler tissue imaging for assessing left ventricular diastolic dysfunction in heart transplant rejection. Heart 2001; 86:432–437.

39. Dandel M, Hummel M, Muller J, et al. Reliability of tissue Doppler wall motion monitoring after heart transplantation for replacement of invasive routine screenings by optimally timed cardiac biopsies and catheterizations. Circulation 2001; 104:I184–I191.

40. Vivekananthan K, Kalapura T, Mehra M, et al. Usefulness of the combined index of systolic and diastolic myocardial performance to identify cardiac allograft rejection. Am J Cardiol 2002; 90:517–520.

41. Burgess MI, Bright-Thomas RJ, Yonan N, et al. Can the index of myocardial performance be used to detect acute cellular rejection after heart transplantation? Am J Cardiol 2003; 92:308–311.

42. Palka P, Lange A, Galbraith A, et al. The role of left and right ventricular early diastolic Doppler tissue echocardiographic indices in the evaluation of acute rejection in orthotopic heart transplant. J Am Soc Echocardiogr 2005; 18:107–115.

43. Sun JP, Abdalla IA, Asher CR, et al. Non-invasive evaluation of orthotopic heart transplant rejection by echocardiography. J Heart Lung Transplant 2005; 24:160–165.

23

Aorta

Ivan Iglesias, Daniel Bainbridge, John M. Murkin, and Mackenzie Quantz
University of Western Ontario, London, Ontario, Canada

ANATOMICAL CONSIDERATIONS

The aortic wall is composed of three layers: the intima, the media, and the adventitia. The intima is a delicate endothelial layer. The media layer contains relatively little smooth muscle and collagen between mainly elastic fibers arranged in a spiral manner. The adventitia, the outer layer of the aortic wall, is predominantly comprised of elastic tissue, collagen, and the vasa vasorum. The elastic tissue is responsible for the distensibility (elastic recoil) of the aorta (Ao), while the collagen is the main determinant of the tensile strength. The vasa vasorum provides blood flow to the outer half of the aortic wall, including much of the media.

The Ao is divided anatomically into thoracic and abdominal components. The thoracic Ao is further subdivided into ascending, transverse (arch), and descending segments. The approximately 5-cm ascending Ao is divided into the proximal aortic root and a more distal tubular portion that joins the aortic arch. The aortic root extends from the aortic valve (AoV) to the sinotubular junction (STJ) and contains the sinuses of Valsalva, which bulge outward allowing full excursion of the AoV cusps during systole. This segment represents the widest portion of the Ao and measures approximately 3.3 cm (Fig. 23.1). The aortic annulus supports the AoV cusps and is crown shaped with three points extending to the STJ (see Chapter 14). The right and left main coronary arteries arise from the right and the left sinuses of Valsalva, respectively.

The ascending Ao sits just to the right of the midline and its proximal portion lies within the pericardial cavity. The aortic arch lies superior to the pulmonary artery bifurcation and to the right pulmonary artery. It courses slightly leftward in front of the trachea and then proceeds posteriorly. From the transverse Ao arise the arch vessels, that is, the right brachiocephalic, the left common carotid, and the left subclavian arteries (see Fig. 4.37). The aortic isthmus is the point at which the transverse Ao joins the descending Ao (Fig. 23.2). The Ao is relatively vulnerable to acceleration and deceleration injury at this point because it is anchored by the ligamentum arteriosum (see following text) (1).

TRANSESOPHAGEAL ECHOCARDIOGRAPHY AS A DIAGNOSTIC TOOL

Echocardiography is considered a good noninvasive tool for the assessment of aortic pathology. Compared with transthoracic echocardiography (TTE), transesophageal echocardiography (TEE) has a better resolution of the Ao due to the proximity of the esophagus to the thoracic Ao and the use of high-frequency transducers. TEE is considered accurate, time saving, and provides assessment of other involved structures such as valves. Moreover, contrary to computed tomography (CT) or magnetic resonance imaging (MRI) scanning, TEE can be easily brought to the patient's bedside and also be used intraoperatively. Using a multiplane probe, both short-axis (SAX) and long-axis (LAX) views of the ascending Ao are possible, with visualization up to 10 cm. The most cephalad portion of the ascending Ao and the proximal segment of the arch may not always be satisfactorily visualized due to interposition of the right mainstem bronchus and/or the trachea. The entire descending thoracic Ao can usually be scanned with comparable quality to CT scan imaging (2).

The normal aortic wall is usually <3-mm thick as measured with TEE. The overall diameter of the aortic root is 2.8 ± 0.3 cm at the level of the sinuses of Valsalva, 2.4 ± 0.4 cm at the STJ, and 2.6 ± 0.3 cm at the tubular portion of the ascending Ao (see Fig. 5.11), although, preferably, it should be indexed to body surface area (see Fig. 5.12) (3). The descending Ao diameter is 2.3 ± 0.5 by 1.6 ± 0.4 cm (see Fig. 5.13). The TEE examination of the thoracic Ao is shown in Figures 23.3 to 23.8.

TEE IMAGING OF THE THORACIC AORTA AND AORTIC ARCH VESSELS

See also Chapter 4.

Ascending Aorta

The TEE multiplane probe is positioned at the midesophageal (ME) level, at 30 to 40 cm from the incisors, at a 135° angle. From the ME AoV LAX

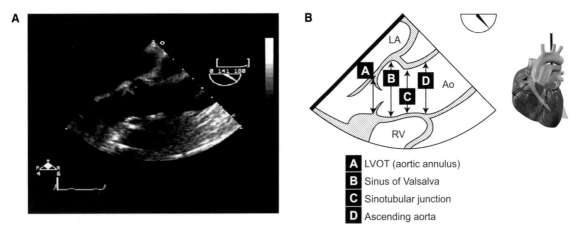

Figure 23.1 Aortic root measurements. (A,B) The sites of measurement for the LVOT, aortic annulus, sinus of Valsalva, sinotubular junction, and proximal ascending Ao are indicated in this mid-esophageal ascending Ao long-axis view. *Abbreviations*: Ao, aorta; LA, left atrium; LVOT, left ventricular outflow tract; RV, right ventricle.

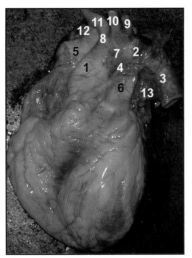

1 Ascending aorta
2 Transverse aorta
3 Descending aorta
4 Ligamentum arteriosum
5 Superior vena cava
6 Pulmonary artery trunk
7 Arch of aorta
8 Brachiocephalic artery
9 Left subclavian artery
10 Left common carotid artery
11 Right common carotid artery
12 Right subclavian artery
13 Left pulmonary vein

Figure 23.2 Large vessels. Anatomical description of the large intra-thoracic vessels and branches of the thoracic aortic arch. *Source*: Courtesy of Dr. Nicolas Dürrleman.

view, the aortic root and the initial 1 to 3 cm of the proximal ascending Ao are visible longitudinally (Fig. 23.4). The mid-portion of the ascending Ao will be visualized by withdrawing the probe and lowering the angle to approximately 100° (Fig. 23.6) until the distal ascending Ao is eventually obscured by the acoustic shadowing from the air in the right mainstem bronchus or trachea (5).

The TEE examination is unable to image, in any detail, the mid- and distal ascending Ao (42% of its length) and the proximal aortic arch (6). Sometimes, it is possible to visualize these structures in the far field of the deep transgastric LAX view, but the resulting images have a low resolution of detail (7). To circumvent this problem, Li et al. (8) described a saline-filled endotracheal balloon as a novel acoustic window to visualize the proximal aortic arch (Fig. 23.9). This approach allows for visualization of the aortic blind

spot (9,10) (Figs. 23.10 and 23.11). Furthermore, using a TEE probe, Mahajan et al. (11) proposed the use of a new proximal transgastric view to visualize the ascending Ao and aortic arch (Fig. 23.12).

The ME AoV SAX view, at a 45° angle, gives a transverse view of the AoV (Fig. 23.4). As the TEE probe is withdrawn, to an angle of 0° to 30°, the aortic root and proximal ascending Ao as well as the adjacent superior vena cava, main pulmonary artery (MPA), and its right and left branches are visualized (Fig. 23.5).

Descending Aorta

From the ME view at 0°, the multiplane TEE probe is rotated posteriorly a quarter turn toward the left to reveal the descending Ao SAX view (Fig. 23.7). The corresponding ME descending Ao LAX view is

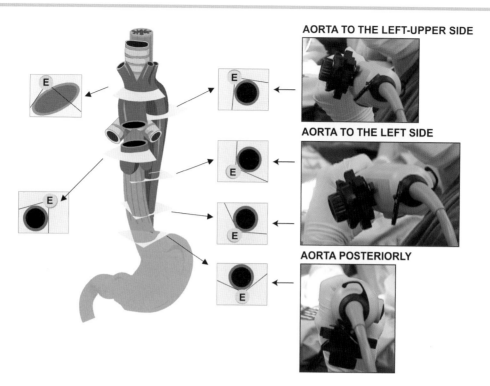

Figure 23.3 Echocardiographic examination of the aorta. Right-sided structures are represented on the left side of the image display. The descending Ao is initially anterior, left, and then becomes posterior in the distal portion. Consequently the anatomical orientation of the descending Ao varies according to the position of the transesophageal echocardiographic probe. *Abbreviations*: Ao, aorta; E, esophagus. *Source*: Adapted from Ref. 4.

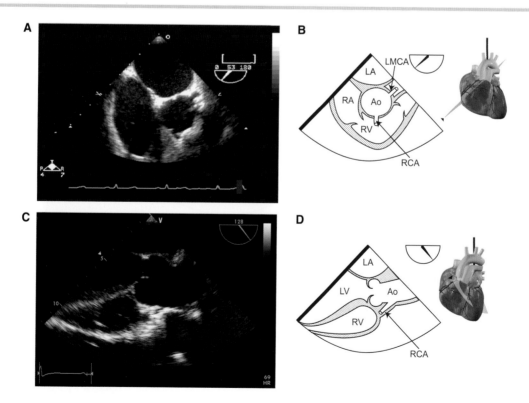

Figure 23.4 Coronary ostia. (A,B) Mid-esophageal short-axis view of the ascending Ao with both coronary ostia visualized above the aortic valve. **(C,D)** Mid-esophageal long-axis view of the ascending showing the RCA ostium. *Abbreviations*: Ao, aorta; AoV, aortic valve; LA, left atrium; LMCA, left main coronary artery; LV, left ventricle; RA, right atrium; RCA, right coronary artery; RV, right ventricle.

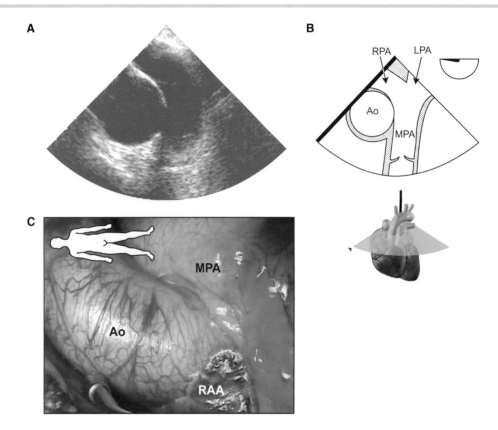

Figure 23.5   Ascending aorta. Mid-esophageal ascending Ao short-axis view (**A,B**) shows the MPA, RPA, and the origin of the LPA. (**C**) Corresponding intraoperative view of the ascending Ao. *Abbreviations*: Ao, aorta; LPA, left pulmonary artery; MPA, main pulmonary artery; RAA, right atrial appendage; RPA, right pulmonary artery. *Source*: Photo C courtesy of Dr. Michel Pellerin. ⌐⏃

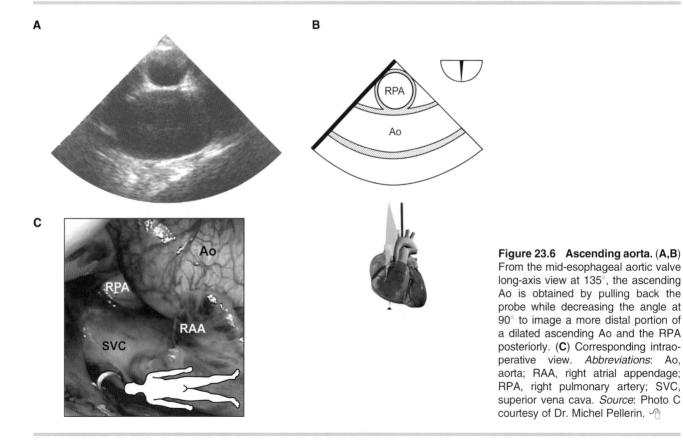

Figure 23.6   Ascending aorta. (A,B) From the mid-esophageal aortic valve long-axis view at 135°, the ascending Ao is obtained by pulling back the probe while decreasing the angle at 90° to image a more distal portion of a dilated ascending Ao and the RPA posteriorly. (**C**) Corresponding intraoperative view. *Abbreviations*: Ao, aorta; RAA, right atrial appendage; RPA, right pulmonary artery; SVC, superior vena cava. *Source*: Photo C courtesy of Dr. Michel Pellerin. ⌐⏃

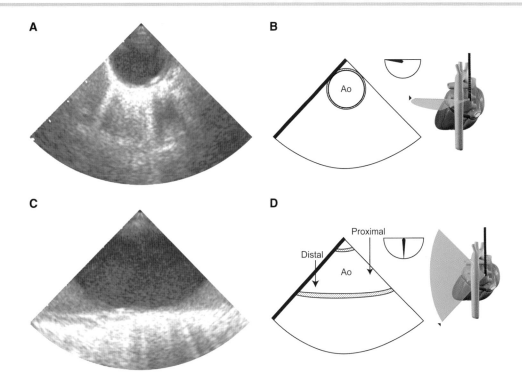

Figure 23.7 Descending aorta. (**A,B**) Mid esophageal short-axis view of the descending Ao, obtained from the four-chamber view at 0° with a counterclockwise leftward quarter turn of the TEE probe. (**C,D**) Corresponding long-axis view at 90°. *Abbreviation*: Ao, aorta.

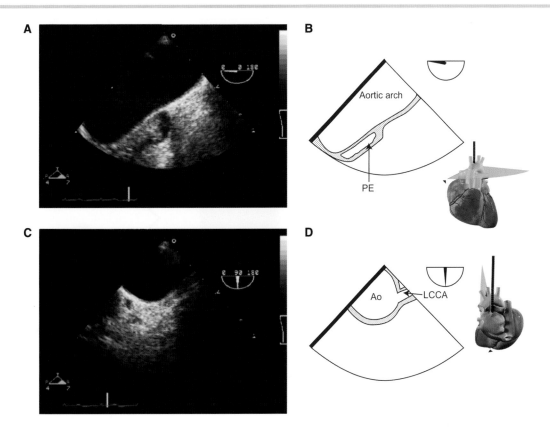

Figure 23.8 Transverse aorta. Upper esophageal aortic arch long-axis (**A,B**) and short-axis (**C,D**) views are shown. *Abbreviations*: Ao, aorta; LCCA, left common carotid artery; PE, pericardial effusion.

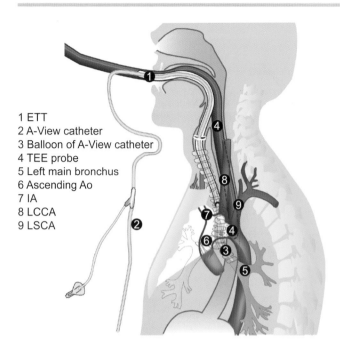

1 ETT
2 A-View catheter
3 Balloon of A-View catheter
4 TEE probe
5 Left main bronchus
6 Ascending Ao
7 IA
8 LCCA
9 LSCA

Figure 23.9   The A-View balloon catheter. Sagittal cross-section illustrates the anatomic interrelation of structures with an A-View balloon catheter, and TEE probe. *Abbreviations*: Ao, aorta; ETT, endotracheal tube; IA, innominate artery; LCCA, left common carotid artery; LSCA, left subclavian artery; TEE, transesophageal echocardiography. *Source*: Adapted with permission from Ref. 9.

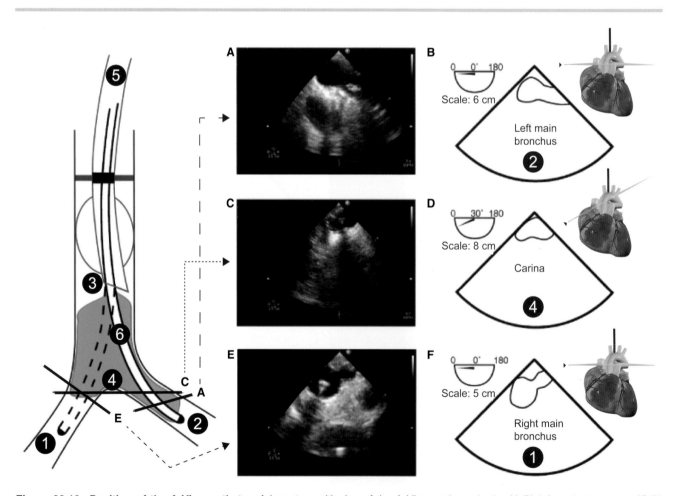

Figure 23.10   Position of the A-View catheter. Adequate positioning of the A-View catheter in the (**A,B**) left main bronchus, (**C,D**) carina and (**E,F**) right main bronchus is shown (1, right main bronchus; 2, left main bronchus; 3, trachea; 4, carina; 5, endotracheal tube; 6, A-View catheter). *Source*: Adapted with permission from Ref. 10.

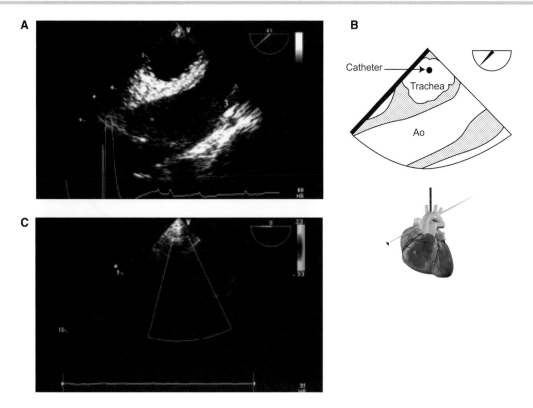

Figure 23.11 Blind spot "unblinded." Distal ascending and proximal transverse Ao blind spot "unblinded." Compare the upper esophageal views of the transverse Ao at 43° with (**A,B**) and without (**C**) the A-View catheter. *Abbreviation*: Ao, aorta. *Source*: Adapted courtesy of Cordatec (www.cordatec.be).

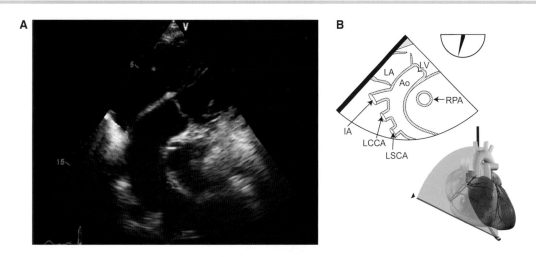

Figure 23.12 TG view of the aorta. (**A,B**) Deep TG view at 80° with right sided rotation shows the ascending and transverse Ao and the branch vessels. *Abbreviations*: Ao, aorta; IA, innominate artery; LA, left atrium; LCCA, left common carotid artery; LSCA, left subclavian artery; LV, left ventricle; TG, transgastric. *Source*: Adapted from Ref. 11.

readily obtained by rotating to a 90° angle. The probe is advanced into a deep gastric position to follow the descending Ao to the upper abdomen. Likewise, the proximal descending Ao is assessed by withdrawing the probe to the upper esophageal (UE) level, up to the junction with the distal transverse Ao at 20 to 25 cm from the incisors.

Aortic Arch

At the UE level, at a 0° angle reveals the distal aortic arch LAX view at the left of the display (Fig. 23.8) as the probe is rotated anteriorly toward the right. As the imaging plane is rotated to 90°, the mid-portion of the aortic arch SAX view is obtained. As the probe shaft is gradually rotated toward the right, the origins of the arch vessels are successively visualized (left subclavian, left common carotid, and right brachiocephalic arteries) (see Fig. 4.37). More rotation of the probe shaft toward the right will bring into view the distal ascending Ao and the adjacent MPA trunk.

EPIAORTIC SCANNING

Perioperative stroke following cardiac surgery is a cataclysmic complication that increases hospital length of stay twofold, mortality by a factor of 15, and carries a 47% rate of discharge to a facility for intermediate or long-term care (12,13).

Atherosclerotic disease of the ascending Ao is an independent risk factor for stroke and systemic embolization following cardiac surgery (14–16). A classification of aortic atherosclerosis is shown in Fig. 23.13. Conditions associated with atherosclerosis of the Ao include advanced age, presence of peripheral vascular disease (PVD), carotid stenosis, hypertension, a higher EuroSCORE, and disease of the descending thoracic Ao (14,17–19).

The "gold standard" for evaluating ascending aortic plaque is epiaortic ultrasound (EAU) and not TEE. Epiaortic ultrasound is performed using a 7- to 15-MHz probe directly applied to the Ao. This technique produces high-resolution images of the ascending Ao and proximal aortic arch. Imaging may be limited by the direct application of ultrasound gel within the surgical field, near-field artifacts, and the air-tissue interface. These may be minimized by the use of a linear array probe. The probe can also be immersed in a saline-filled sheath, using it as a standoff or intermediate acoustic medium (Figs. 23.14 and 23.15). The air-tissue interface may be eliminated by filling the upper mediastinum with warm saline and keeping the probe submerged. Epiaortic ultrasound requires a high-frequency probe, technical skills to perform and interpret the study, and an increase in the total operating time. Guidelines for EAU have been proposed (Figs. 23.16 and 23.17) (20). An experienced operator can evaluate the entire ascending Ao thoroughly in less than five minutes (20).

There appears little difference in the sensitivity of either two-dimensional (2D) or three-dimensional (3D) imaging to detect plaque within the Ao. We found that live 3D was superior to 2D imaging in identifying, localizing, and defining the true extent of plaque in the Ao (21) (Fig. 23.18).

AORTIC ATHEROSCLEROSIS

Aortic Atherosclerosis and Outcomes After Cardiac Surgery

Aortic atherosclerosis is present in 19% to 58% of patients undergoing cardiac procedures (14,15,19,22–25). Plaque is not uniformly distributed throughout the Ao. It is most prevalent in the anterior (48.4%) and posterior (31.4%) segments of the distal ascending Ao (Figs. 23.19 and 23.20) and less frequently involves

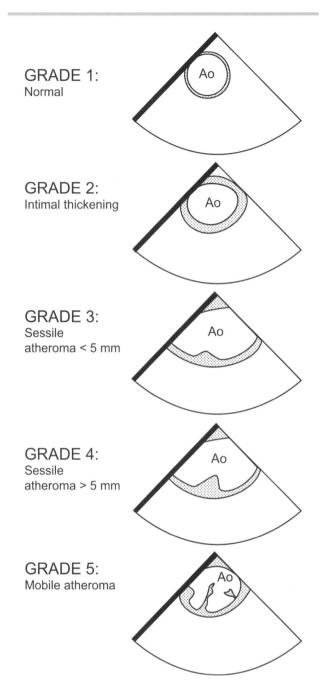

Figure 23.13 Classification of atheromatosis of the aorta. Grades of atheromatous disease of the Ao are represented. *Abbreviation*: Ao, aorta. *Source*: Adapted from Ref. 5.

the lateral wall of the proximal (7.6%) and middle (9.4%) ascending Ao (16). The frequent involvement of the distal segments of the ascending Ao has significant implications regarding the conduct of cardiac procedures as this is the usual site for the aortic cannula and cross clamp. The etiology of stroke, following cardiac surgery, is multifactorial. However, the relationship between aortic atherosclerosis and postoperative neurologic events is well established (12,14–16).

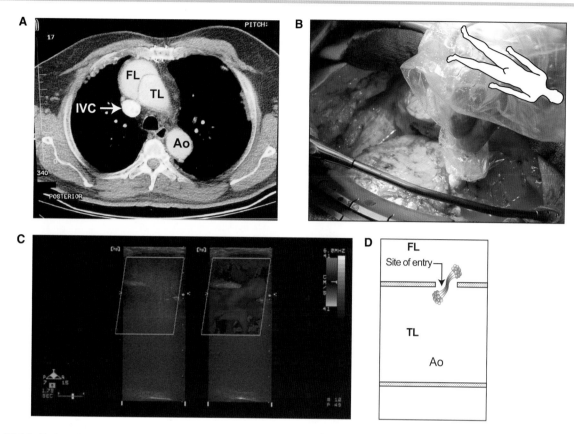

Figure 23.14 Epiaortic scanning. (**A**) A 69-year-old man after coronary artery revascularization is reoperated on for an aortic dissection diagnosed with a computed tomography scan. An epiaortic probe (**B**) is used to localize the site of the aortic rupture (**C,D**). *Abbreviations*: Ao, aorta; FL, false lumen; IVC, inferior vena cava; TL, true lumen. *Source*: Photo B courtesy of Dr. Raymond Cartier.

Patients with aortic atherosclerosis experience a higher incidence of stroke and neurologic dysfunction. There are no accepted criteria for what extent of increase in intimal thickness represents mild, moderate, or severe atherosclerotic disease. However, most investigators have considered intimal thicknesses of 3, 4, or 5 mm to represent severe disease. A number of grading systems have been described, and these are summarized in the guidelines for epiaortic ultrasound presented by the American Society of Echocardiography (20).

The likelihood of a neurologic event seems to correlate with the presence of more severe disease. In a number of studies, patients with no or minimal aortic disease experienced a stroke rate of 1.2% to 1.8% compared with a fourfold increase to a rate of 6.4% to 10.5% when severe disease was present (16,17,19). Neurologic dysfunction was also more prominent in those with atherosclerotic disease (26% vs. 8%) (17). Ulcerated lesions or mobile atheromas may pose an additional embolic risk and impart stroke rates of 23.5% (compared with 6.8% of patients with severe disease) (14).

The overall extent of atherosclerotic disease also influences neurologic outcome. Van der Linden et al. (16) identified an association between the incidence of perioperative stroke and the number of ascending Ao segments that had atherosclerotic plaque. Disease of a single aortic segment (out of a possible 12) was associated with an 8% stroke rate that increased to 33.3% when half of the Ao was involved. The specific location of aortic disease may also be a factor in neurologic outcome. For instance, disease of the middle-lateral and proximal-lateral segments were independent risk factors for stroke.

Aortic atherosclerosis, identified at the time of cardiac surgery, influences long-term outcomes. Freedom from stroke is less likely in patients with atherosclerotic Aos (88.7% vs. 95.7% at 5 years) (19). Disease in the distal left segment of the Ao carries a fivefold increase in stroke risk, with higher rates of stroke seen when disease involves the mid-left, distal posterior, and distal right segments (19). Similarly, six-year survival is negatively affected by aortic disease when the plaque measures ≥4 mm (72% vs. 85%) (22).

The presence of aortic atherosclerosis significantly increases the risk of plaque fracture and intimal flap formation after aortic cannulation and clamping as demonstrated by EAU (26). The potential for subsequent embolization of either plaque or thrombus is high and may account for many of the otherwise unexplained strokes that occur on the second or

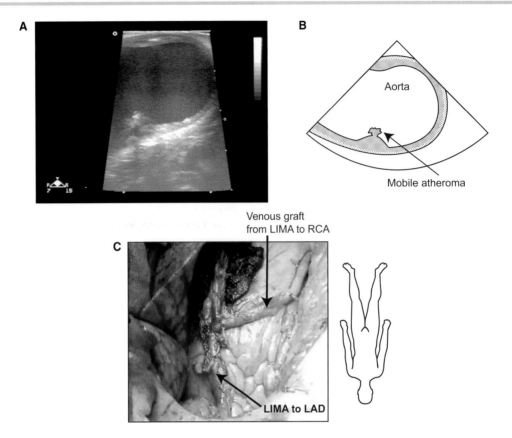

Figure 23.15   Epiaortic scanning. (A,B) Epiaortic images of the aortic arch reveal a mobile atheroma (Grade 5) in a 74-year-old woman before cardiopulmonary bypass. **(C)** To avoid aortic clamping during off-pump coronary artery bypass grafting, the saphenous vein graft to the RCA was anastomosed to the LIMA graft rather than on the aorta as is usually the case. *Abbreviations*: LAD, left anterior descending coronary artery; LIMA, left internal mammary artery; RCA, right coronary artery. *Source*: Photo C courtesy of Dr. Louis P. Perrault.

third postoperative day. Whether identification of such lesions warrants the administration of postoperative antithrombotic therapy to decrease the risk of stroke is unclear but is consistent with observations that aspirin decreases postoperative stroke (27).

Intraoperative Techniques for Assessment of Aortic Atheromatosis: TEE, Epiaortic Scan, Clinical Palpation

Identification of aortic atherosclerosis preoperatively is desirable and permits optimal planning of the operation. However, the preoperative chest X-ray (CXR) is an insensitive screen for aortic atherosclerosis. While noncontrast CT and MRI correlate well with TEE and have the advantage of being able to image the entire Ao, it is neither practical nor economically feasible to perform a preoperative study on every patient (28,29). Therefore, most patients will have the first evaluation of the Ao only following sternotomy.

Intraoperative evaluation includes digital palpation, EAU, and TEE. Since its description in 1989, EAU has been established as the most sensitive modality to image the ascending Ao (30). However, its routine use has not been widely adopted. Conversely, TEE is now readily available in most cardiac operating rooms (ORs).

A number of studies have examined the efficacy of different modalities of aortic evaluation to detect and quantify atherosclerotic disease. Digital palpation is unreliable in detecting aortic atherosclerosis, with a sensitivity of only 14% to 55% (18,23,24,30,31). Lesions that are comprised of soft plaque or located posteriorly are easily missed. The use of TEE has improved sensitivity (30–58%) (24,25,31) compared with digital palpation but still does not image the Ao as well as EAU. Ibrahim et al. (25) found that TEE identified 179 lesions in 60 patients, whereas EAU identified 362 lesions. Severe lesions (>4 mm or mobile atherosclerosis) were identified in only 5 instances with TEE compared with the 27 visualized with EAU. The techniques of TEE and EAU are complementary.

However, TEE cannot adequately visualize the distal ascending Ao because of interference from the airways (5), whereas EAU does not image the distal arch or descending Ao. TEE may also be advantageous for evaluating the proximal anterior ascending Ao when compared with EAU. A meta-analysis estimated that the sensitivity and specificity of TEE for detection of atherosclerosis is 21% and 99% compared with EAU (32). It has been reported that the epicardial

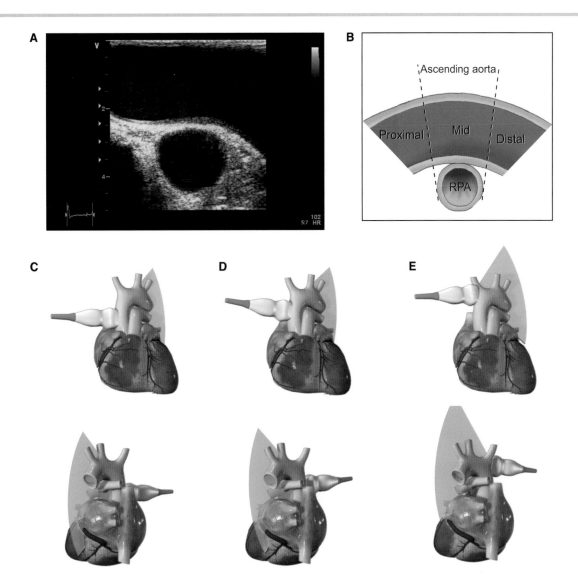

Figure 23.16 EAU long-axis view. (A,B) The EAU scanning is performed with a high resolution (>7MHz) ultrasound transducer inserted in a sterile sheath. The longitudinal ascending aorta is divided into proximal, mid and distal regions. **(C–E)** Anterior and posterior positions of the probe during EAU scanning are shown. *Abbreviations*: EAU, epiaortic ultrasound; RPA, right pulmonary artery. *Source*: Adapted from Ref. 20 and available at http://www.asefiles.org/EpiaorticDocument.pdf.

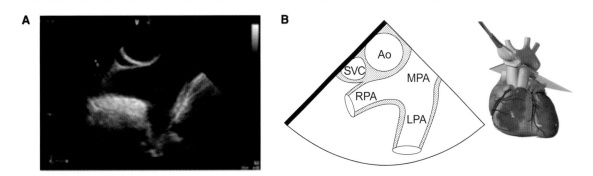

Figure 23.17 EAU short-axis view. (A,B) An EAU scan of the ascending aorta in short-axis view also shows the bifurcation of the MPA into the RPA and LPA. *Abbreviations*: Ao, aorta; EAU, epiaortic ultrasound; LPA, left pulmonary artery; MPA, main pulmonary artery; RPA, right pulmonary artery; SVC, superior vena cava. *Source*: Adapted from Ref. 20 and available at http://www.asefiles.org/EpiaorticDocument.pdf.

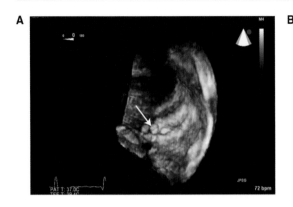

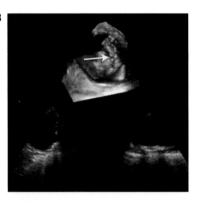

Figure 23.18 3D view of aortic atherosclerosis. Ulcerated plaques in the aorta are shown in these (**A**) 3D zoom and (**B**) 3D full volume (arrow) views.

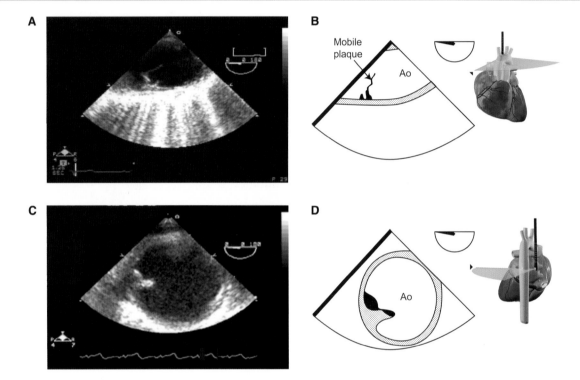

Figure 23.19   Aortic atherosclerosis. Mobile plaques (grade 5) in the distal transverse arch in upper esophageal aortic arch long-axis (**A,B**) and descending Ao short-axis views are shown (**C,D**). *Abbreviation*: Ao, aorta.

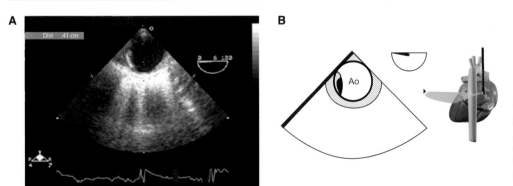

Figure 23.20   Aortic athero-sclerosis. (A,B) Descending Ao short-axis view shows a 4.1 mm thick plaque (grade 3) in the Ao before cardiopulmo-nary bypass. *Abbreviation*: Ao, aorta.

fat pad may obscure the proximal anterior area and reduce the accuracy of the examination with EAU (25). Epiaortic ultrasound has been applied selectively in some studies. If a selective approach to screening is used, patient selection should be based on the presence of risk factors that are associated with atherosclerotic disease (14–16) as opposed to findings on digital palpation. However, because of the inability to evaluate the ascending Ao independently and thoroughly, a combination of digital palpation, TEE, and EAU should be considered in all patients.

Related Echocardiographic Findings with Aortic Atherosclerosis

Further indication of the presence of atherosclerosis in the Ao may be inferred from the presence of cardiac valvular calcification. A significant association between the presence of AoV and mitral annular calcification and the presence and severity of ascending aortic atheroma has been demonstrated (33). Thus, AoV calcification may serve as a marker for atherosclerosis of the Ao. When preoperative TEE discloses AoV or mitral annular calcification and plaque in the ascending or descending Ao, some authors have recommended proceeding directly to EAU of the ascending Ao prior to cannulation and instrumentation (33,34).

Other indications for EAU include age (>60 years), calcified aortic knob on CXR or palpable calcifications in the ascending Ao, severe PVD, and previous history of transient ischemic attack or cerebrovascular accident.

AORTIC DILATATION AND ANEURYSMS

An aortic aneurysm is defined as a localized dilatation, or enlargement, of the Ao. As the Ao dilates, its wall tensile strength becomes progressively weakened and may lead to dissection and/or rupture (35). Aneurysms can result from a variety of congenital and acquired pathologies and involve any segment of the Ao. Aortic aneurysms are considered significant when their diameter exceeds two standard deviations above the normal diameter (35).

Thoracic aortic aneurysms are reported to occur with an incidence of 5.9/100,000 patients and are more commonly observed in the older age groups. Aortic aneurysms can be classified based on four characteristics: shape, location, etiology, and histology (Table 23.1). Ascending aortic aneurysms are located proximal to the origin of the brachiocephalic trunk (innominate artery); aortic arch aneurysms are located between the brachiocephalic trunk and the left subclavian artery; descending aortic aneurysms are located between the left subclavian artery and the diaphragm (Fig. 23.21). Aneurysms may have either a fusiform or saccular shape. Histologically, they may be classified into three categories: (*i*) true aneurysms, where all three normal layers (intima, media, and adventitia) are present in the aneurysm wall; (*ii*) dissecting aneurysms, where the normal aortic wall

Table 23.1 Classification of Aortic Aneurysms

Shape	Saccular
	Fusiform
Histology	True
	Dissecting
	False aneurysm
Location	Ascending
	Arch
	Descending
Etiology	Cystic medial degeneration/necrosis
	Atherosclerosis
	Congenital
	Inflammatory
	Other

See text for details.

layers are divided with the formation of a false lumen; and (*iii*) false aneurysms, due to aortic wall rupture that is contained only by the adventitia (35,37) (Table 23.1).

Aortic aneurysms involve the ascending Ao in approximately 50% of cases, the descending portion in 40%, and the arch in 10%. Descending aortic aneurysms are caused most often by atherosclerosis, while ascending and transverse aortic aneurysms are commonly due to cystic medial degeneration (Fig. 23.21) (2,38). Aortic aneurysms are frequently associated with hypertension, and their incidence is higher in the seventh decade of life.

TEE as a Diagnostic Tool for Thoracic Aortic Aneurysms

Characteristic findings on 2D echocardiography include dilatation of the Ao (Fig. 23.22), increased echogenicity of the aortic wall and presence of intraluminal spontaneous echo contrast reflecting decreased blood flow locally, and mural thrombus formation (Fig. 23.23). In the presence of a mural thrombus, differentiation of an aortic aneurysm from aortic dissection may become difficult (37,39,40).

Sinus of Valsalva Aneurysms

Aneurysms of the sinus of Valsalva are considered to be a congenital defect resulting from the discontinuity between the aortic media and the annulus fibrosus. The frequent association of sinus of Valsalva aneurysms with ventricular septal defects also supports a congenital etiology. These aneurysms arise from the right coronary sinus in 65% to 85% (Fig. 23.24), from the noncoronary sinus in 10% to 30%, but rarely (<5%) from the left coronary sinus (Fig. 23.25). Associated lesions include ventricular septal defects in 30% to 60% of cases, aortic regurgitation (AR) in 20% to 30%, and less commonly, bicuspid AoV, atrial septal defect (ASD), and pulmonic valve stenosis. Congenital aneurysms show a male-to-female ratio of 4:1 and a racial predominance of Asian patients.

Sinus of Valsalva aneurysms commonly cause symptoms from the compression of neighboring coronary arteries, obstruction of the right ventricular

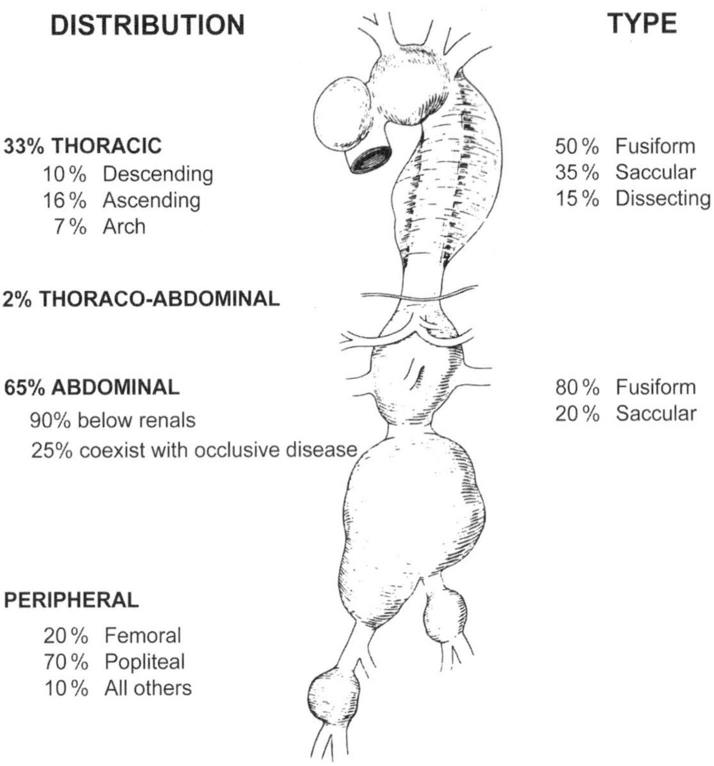

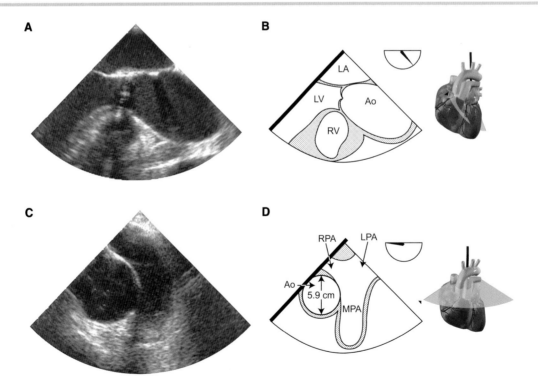

DISTRIBUTION
TYPE
33% THORACIC
10 % Descending
16 % Ascending
7 % Arch
50 % Fusiform
35 % Saccular
15 % Dissecting
2% THORACO-ABDOMINAL
65% ABDOMINAL
90% below renals
25% coexist with occlusive disease
80 % Fusiform
20 % Saccular
PERIPHERAL
20 % Femoral
70 % Popliteal
10 % All others

Figure 23.21 Aortic aneurysms. The frequency and distribution of aortic aneurysms are shown in this diagram. *Source*: With permission from Ref. 36.

A
B
LA
LV
Ao
RV
C
D
RPA
LPA
Ao
5.9 cm
MPA

Figure 23.22 Ascending aortic aneurysm. Mid-esophageal ascending Ao long-axis (**A,B**) and short-axis (**C,D**) views show an ascending aortic aneurysm with a 5.9 cm Ao diameter, that is almost twice the upper limit of normal. *Abbreviations*: Ao, aorta; LA, left atrium; LPA, left pulmonary artery; LV, left ventricle; MPA, main pulmonary artery; RPA, right pulmonary artery; RV, right ventricle.

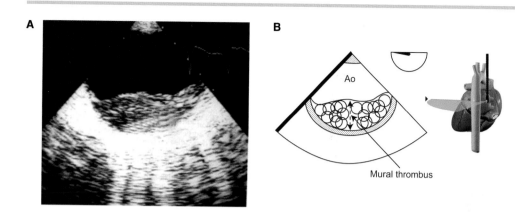

Figure 23.23 Aortic thrombus. Mid-esophageal descending aorta (Ao) short-axis view demonstrates ectasia of the Ao and mural thrombus formation. *Abbreviation*: Ao, aorta. *Source*: With permission from Ref. 37.

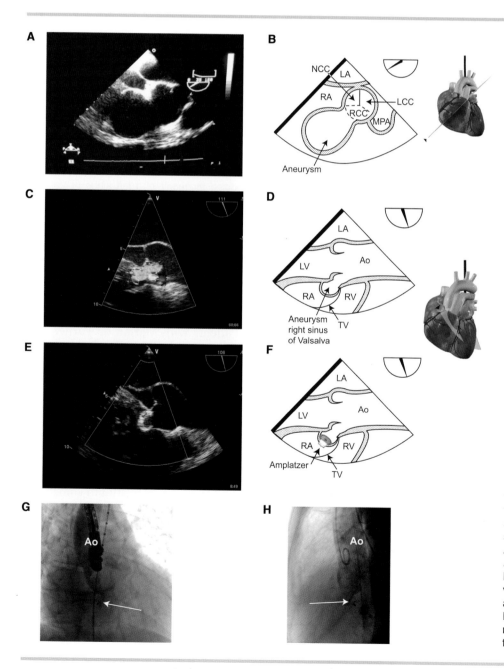

Figure 23.24 Aneurysm of the right sinus of Valsalva. (A,B) Mid-esophageal aortic valve short-axis view shows a large aneurysm of the right sinus of Valsalva. **(C,D)** Color Doppler mid-esophageal aortic valve long-axis view. **(E,F)** Same view after transcatheter device closure. **(G,H)** Corresponding fluoroscopic PA and lateral views of the Amplatzer device (arrow). *Abbreviations*: Ao, aorta; LA, left atrium; LCC, left coronary cusp; LV, left ventricle; MPA, main pulmonary artery; NCC, non-coronary cusp; RA, right atrium; RCC, right coronary cusp; RV, right ventricle; TV, tricuspid valve.

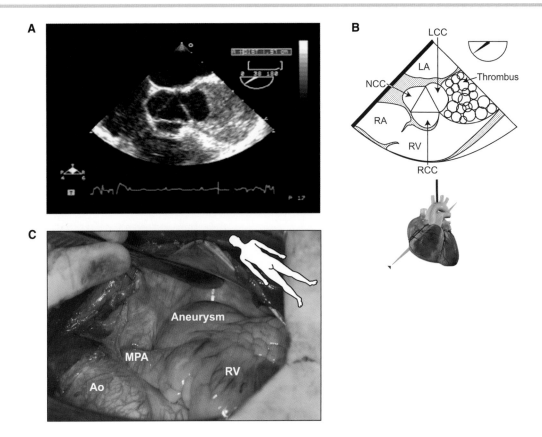

Figure 23.25 Aneurysm of the left sinus of Valsalva. A 64-year-old woman is scheduled for repair of a left sinus of Valsalva aneurysm. (**A,B**) Mid-esophageal aortic valve short-axis view showing a large, thrombus-filled, aneurysm originating from the left sinus of Valsalva. (**C**) Corresponding intraoperative view. *Abbreviations*: Ao, aorta; LA, left atrium; LCC, left coronary cusp; MPA, main pulmonary artery; NCC, noncoronary cusp; RA, right atrium; RCC, right coronary cusp; RV, right ventricle. *Source*: Photo C courtesy of Dr. Denis Bouchard.

outflow tract, or rupture into an adjacent chamber. The latter may be spontaneous, may occur after intense physical exercise or trauma, or result from complicated acute bacterial endocarditis. Aneurysms of the right coronary sinus tend to extend to the right atrium (RA) and right ventricle (RV), while those of the noncoronary sinus usually extend to the RA. Rarely, these aneurysms may rupture into the pericardium and cause a lethal tamponade.

On TEE imaging, these aneurysms present as a fingerlike "windsock" cavity extending from the affected sinus (Fig. 23.24). Potential involvement of the AoV and both coronary arteries, as well as extension or communication of the aneurysm with any of the heart chambers, must be ruled out using color flow Doppler (34,40,41).

AORTIC DISSECTION

Clinical Background

The incidence of aortic dissection in the general population is around five per million. However, several necropsy series have reported evidence of aortic dissection in approximately 0.2% of cases. Hypertension

is the most commonly reported risk factor. Males have a higher incidence than females, with ratios varying from 2:1 to 5:1. Patients with Marfan or Turner syndrome, as well as those with Ehlers–Danlos or coarctation, have an increased risk of aortic dissection. Patients with unicuspid or bicuspid AoVs are also at increased risk of aortic dissection. Interestingly, atherosclerosis is not considered an independent risk factor for aortic dissection but does increase the risk of free rupture following dissection (42).

Patients with acute aortic dissection typically describe sudden severe chest and/or back pain. At the onset, the pain is most severe, on occasion excruciating, with little or no change in the intensity but sometimes with migrating location, or in association with syncope. Sixty percent of patients will demonstrate a pulse deficit or asymmetry in arterial blood pressure in at least one limb due to the occlusion of one or more aortic branches caused by aortic dissection. Hypertension or hypotension may be present. Hypertension may be related to several factors including pain, anxiety, and preexisting elevated blood pressure. Hypotension may result from severe AR, dissection and occlusion of a coronary ostium, cardiac tamponade, or RV failure from right pulmonary artery compression. Patients may also

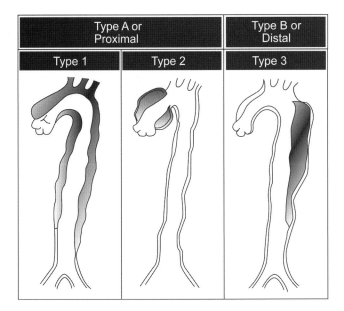

Figure 23.26 Classifications of aortic dissection. The Stanford type A or B and DeBakey types 1–3 classifications for aortic dissection are shown.

present with neurologic symptoms including stroke, Horner's syndrome, or paraplegia. These result from compromised perfusion or direct compression by expanding anatomical structures.

Classification of Aortic Dissection

Two classifications are currently used for aortic dissection and both are based on the anatomical location of the tear (Fig. 23.26). In the *Stanford* classification, any involvement of the ascending Ao is categorized as type A (Fig. 23.27) and all other tears are categorized as type B. The *DeBakey* system categorizes dissection, limited to the ascending Ao as type I; tears that propagate past this area are classified as type II; finally, tears limited to the descending Ao are labeled as type III with the IIIa designation denoting a tear limited to the supradiaphragmatic region and IIIb indicating extension below the diaphragm.

Imaging Modalities in Aortic Dissection

The diagnosis of aortic dissection has evolved as new diagnostic techniques have become available. In the past, conventional contrast angiography was the gold standard used to establish the diagnosis. However, this technique was invasive, required time and expertise in planar image acquisition and interpretation to demonstrate intimal flap. New techniques such as digital subtraction angiography, CT, and MRI scanning as well as TEE imaging have broadened the diagnostic armamentarium available to clinicians.

Many studies have examined the accuracy of these different diagnostic modalities. Erbel et al. (43) showed TEE to be 99% sensitive and 98% specific for the diagnosis of dissection. Adler et al. (33) reported a sensitivity (83%), specificity (100%), positive (100%),

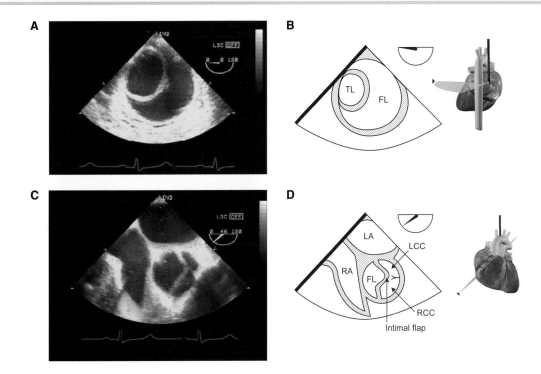

Figure 23.27 Aortic dissection Stanford type A. **(A,B)** Mid-esophageal descending aorta short-axis view. The TL has a smaller diameter and is more pulsatile compared with the FL. **(C,D)** Mid-esophageal AoV short-axis view: proximal extension of the intimal flap to the level of the sinuses of Valsalva above the AoV. *Abbreviations*: AoV, aorta valve; FL, false lumen; LA, left atrium; LCC, left coronary cusp; RA, right atrium; RCC, right coronary cusp; TL, true lumen.

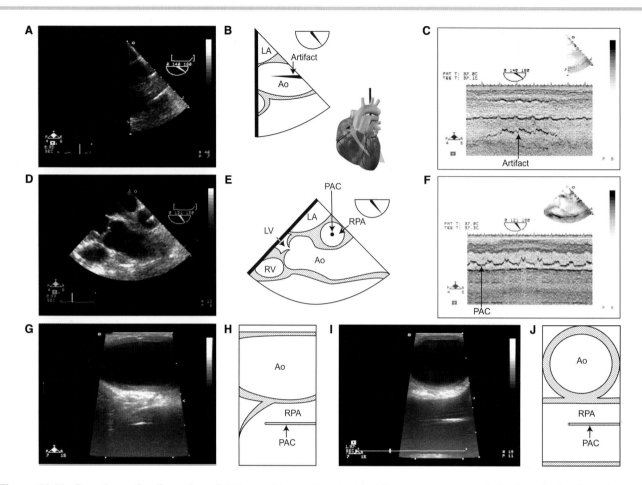

Figure 23.28 Pseudo-aortic dissection. A 57-year-old man is scheduled for coronary revascularization. Aortic dissection was suspected because of problematic insertion of the aortic cannula. (**A,B**) Mid-esophageal ascending Ao long-axis view with a mobile linear shadow suggestive of an intimal flap. (**C**) Corresponding M-mode of the suspected intimal flap (arrow) below the aortic wall. (**D,E**) Upper mid-esophageal ascending Ao long-axis view showing a PAC in the RPA. (**F**) On M-mode, the PAC motion (arrow) has an excursion quite similar to the suspected intimal flap. (**G–J**) Epiaortic scanning of the ascending Ao: the linear shadow is no longer visible in the aorta, while the PAC is still present in the RPA. Aortic dissection was ruled out, with a reverberation artefact in the aorta from the PAC in the RPA. *Abbreviations*: Ao, aorta; LA, left atrium; LV, left ventricle; PAC, pulmonary artery catheter; RPA, right pulmonary artery; RV, right ventricle.

and negative (86%) predictive values for CT scanning. Corresponding values for aortography were reported to be at 88%, 94%, 96%, and 84%. While Nienaber et al. (44) reported 100% sensitivity for both TEE and MRI, the specificity of TEE was lower (68%) than that of MRI (100%).

Nevertheless, TEE has the advantage of being more easily accessible at the bedside for hemodynamically unstable patients and may also be performed intraoperatively. This allows unstable patients to be monitored and treated in a safe environment. As mentioned previously, a complete evaluation of the entire ascending Ao with TEE may sometimes be impossible due to the trachea and/or the right mainstem bronchus interfering with the visualization of the mid- and distal ascending aortic segments. Dissections discretely limited to these blind areas could, therefore, be missed despite careful TEE examination (45). An erroneous diagnosis can also occur when there is increased aortic diameter (>5 cm), which is associated

with a higher incidence of linear artifacts (46). Other linear artifacts may also originate from pulmonary artery catheters (Fig. 23.28) and pericardial effusions (Fig. 23.29A). However, pericardial effusion can also complicate aortic dissection (Fig. 23.29C).

The diagnosis of aortic dissection is based on the identification of an intimal flap dividing the Ao into two separate channels, the true and the false lumen (Figs. 23.30–23.33). Determining which lumen is the false one may sometimes be difficult. Intuitively, blood should not flow freely through the false lumen if it is a blind pouch. On 2D imaging, the pulsatile lumen (showing a bigger diameter in systole) should represent the true lumen, while smoke-like or swirling spontaneous echo contrast suggests sluggish or absent flow in the false lumen. Color and pulsed wave (PW) Doppler imaging may also confirm decreased flow in the blind false lumen (Fig. 23.31). However, these criteria may also be misleading in certain settings: indeed if the false lumen has a large

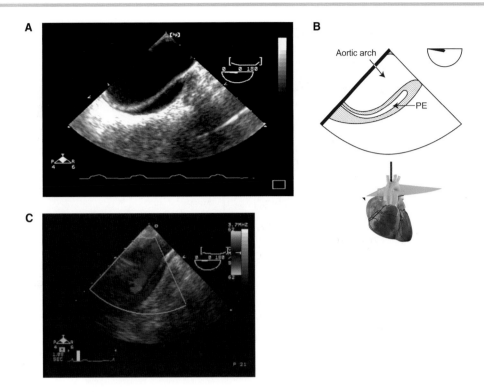

Figure 23.29 Pericardial effusion and aortic dissection. Similar upper esophageal aortic arch long-axis views of the transverse Ao in two patients are shown. (**A,B**) In a 25-year-old woman scheduled for aortic valve replacement, a PE along the distal aortic arch mimics an aortic dissection. (**C**) A 75-year-old woman presents with an acute aortic arch dissection complicated by a PE. *Abbreviations*: Ao, aorta; PE, pericardial effusion.

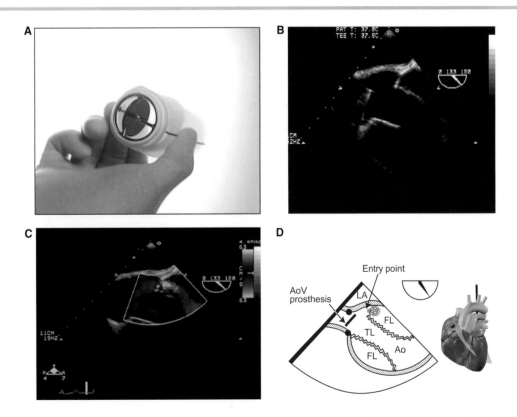

Figure 23.30 Aortic dissection. TL and FL in a patient with a previously placed ascending aortic conduit with a tilting-disk mechanical valve (**A**). (**B**) Mid-esophageal AoV long-axis view at 133° shows a FL next to the TL (**C,D**) color Doppler imaging at the entry point of the FL. *Abbreviations*: Ao, aorta; AoV, aortic valve; FL, false lumen; LA, left atrium; TL, true lumen.

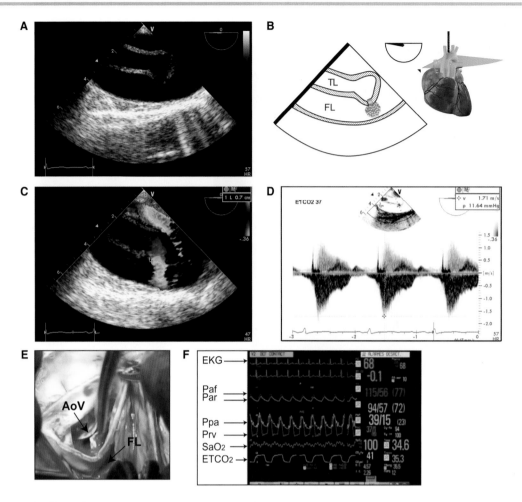

Figure 23.31   Aortic dissection. A 57-year-old man presents with an acute aortic dissection DeBakey type I. (**A–C**) Upper esophageal aortic arch long-axis views with a 7-mm opening between the TL and FL. (**D**) Continuous wave Doppler with an 11.6-mmHg PG across the communication. (**E**) Intraoperative view of the AoV and the FL. (**F**) Bedside hemodynamic tracings: note the 11 mmHg pressure difference between the femoral and the radial artery. *Abbreviations*: AoV, aortic valve; EKG, electrocardiogram; ETCO2, end-tidal carbon dioxide; FL, false lumen; Paf, femoral arterial pressure; Par, radial arterial pressure; PG, pressure gradient; Ppa, pulmonary artery pressure; Prv, right ventricular pressure; SaO2, oxygen saturation; TL, true lumen.

entry and exit site, free blood flow may be present in both false and true lumen. Epiaortic ultrasound can be helpful to localize the site of intimal rupture.

Associated Complications

In addition to identifying the location and extent of dissection, evidence of associated complications must also be sought. The mechanism of AR may result from both dilation of the aortic root and direct geometric disruption of the support by the false lumen. The extent and mechanism of AR should be evaluated and the potential for valve repair or the need for valve replacement (Fig. 23.33) assessed as described in Chapter 15. Free aortic rupture into the pericardial sac may be evident, but contained localized rupture should also be looked for actively. Although compression of the coronary arteries may be difficult to detect with TEE, attempts should be made to assess the patency of coronary ostia. Flow in the right and left main coronary arteries can be assessed by color and PW

Doppler interrogation. Finally, the presence of regional wall motion abnormalities may suggest impaired coronary perfusion.

Aortic Intramural Hematoma

Aortic intramural hematomas are presented as a possible early variant of aortic dissection (47) (Fig. 23.34). The aortic hematoma can be localized in the ascending Ao (type A) or in the descending Ao (type B). Hypertension and trauma are predisposing factors. The clinical presentation resembles that of aortic dissection, apart from less commonly associated AR, myocardial infarction, and extracardiac complications. On 2D imaging, intramural aortic hematomas appear as localized, often homogeneous, thickenings of the aortic wall (>7 mm) (Fig. 23.35), which are either crescent shaped (Fig. 23.36) or circumferential. The intramural accumulation of blood is evident in the absence of an intimal flap (48). Surgical therapy in type A lesions is associated with a reduction in mortality (49).

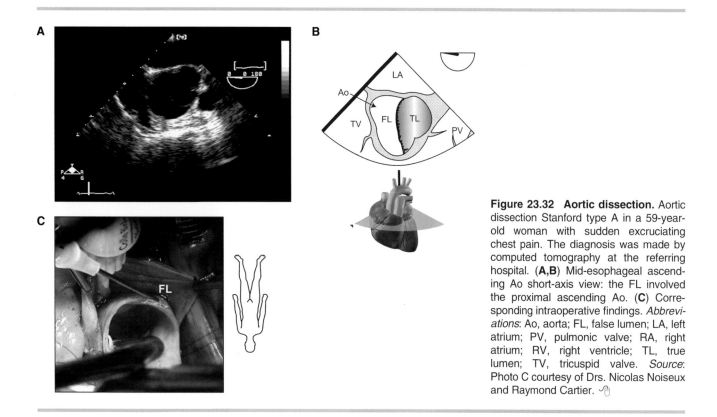

Figure 23.32 Aortic dissection. Aortic dissection Stanford type A in a 59-year-old woman with sudden excruciating chest pain. The diagnosis was made by computed tomography at the referring hospital. (**A,B**) Mid-esophageal ascending Ao short-axis view: the FL involved the proximal ascending Ao. (**C**) Corresponding intraoperative findings. *Abbreviations*: Ao, aorta; FL, false lumen; LA, left atrium; PV, pulmonic valve; RA, right atrium; RV, right ventricle; TL, true lumen; TV, tricuspid valve. *Source*: Photo C courtesy of Drs. Nicolas Noiseux and Raymond Cartier.

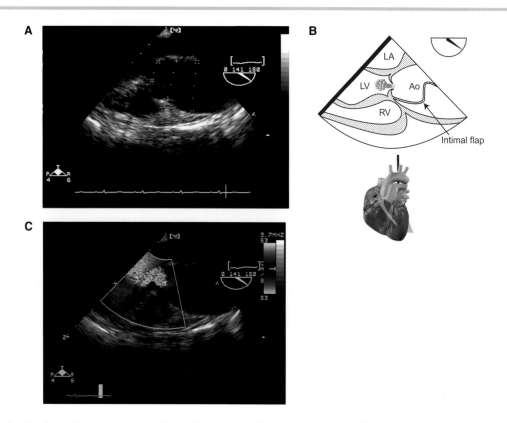

Figure 23.33 Aortic dissection. Aortic dissection with severe aortic regurgitation in a 59-year-old man. (**A,B**) Mid-esophageal aortic valve long-axis view with an intimal flap in a dilated ascending Ao at 41 mm. (**C**) Color flow imaging showing severe aortic regurgitation. *Abbreviations*: Ao, aorta; LA, left atrium; LV, left ventricle; RV, right ventricle.

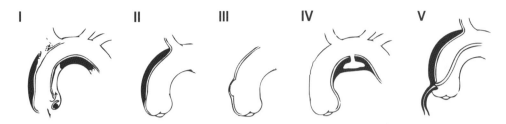

Figure 23.34   Classification of variants of aortic dissection. Type I is a classic dissection with lumen separation and a flap. Type II is an intramural hematoma. Type III is a localized intimal tear. Type IV is an atherosclerotic penetrating ulcer. Type V is iatrogenic or traumatic dissection. *Source*: Reprinted with permission from Ref. 47.

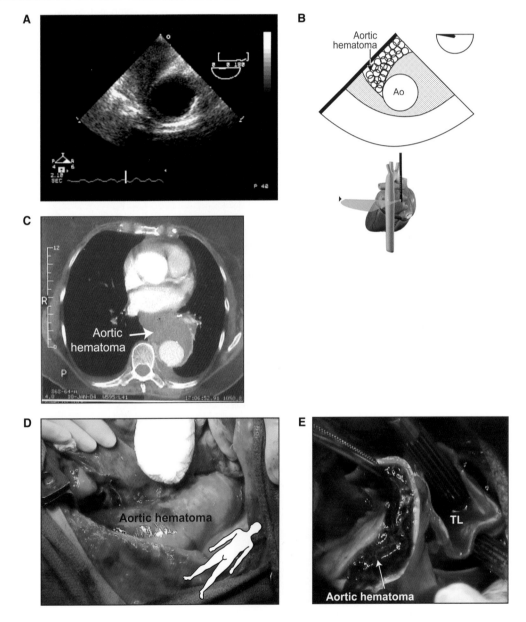

Figure 23.35   Aortic hematoma. Aortic hematoma in a 76-year-old patient. (**A,B**) Descending Ao short-axis view. (**C**) Computed tomography. (**D,E**) Intraoperative findings: the descending Ao is distended and edematous from the intramural hematoma, visible upon opening the Ao. *Abbreviations*: Ao, aorta; TL, true lumen. *Source*: Photos D and E courtesy of Dr. Philippe Demers.

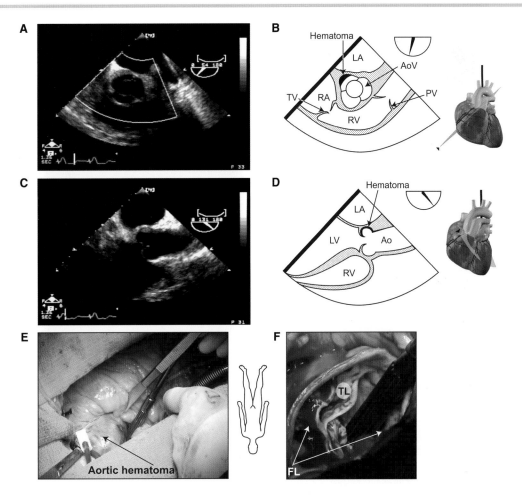

Figure 23.36 Aortic hematoma. Aortic hematoma localized to the aortic root in a 66-year-old man. **(A,B)** Mid-esophageal right ventricular inflow/outflow view: homogeneous thickening of the aortic root posterior aspect near the noncoronary cusp. **(C,D)** Mid-esophageal AoV long-axis views: the abnormality is restricted to the sinus of Valsalva, with no visible aortic regurgitation. **(E)** Intraoperative findings: the hematoma is seen on the surface of the proximal Ao with identification of the FL and TL after opening the Ao **(F)**. *Abbreviations*: Ao, aorta; AoV, aortic valve; FL, false lumen; LA, left atrium; LV, left ventricle; PV, pulmonic valve; RA, right atrium; RV, right ventricle; TL, true lumen; TV, tricuspid valve. *Source*: Photos E and F courtesy of Dr. Michel Pellerin.

TRAUMATIC RUPTURE OF AORTA

Traumatic rupture of the Ao is believed to account for up to 30% of motor vehicle accidental deaths. Mortality and morbidity are still significant in patients who survive to hospital admission (50). With sudden deceleration injuries, the lesion commonly occurs at the aortic isthmus where the ligamentum arteriosum and left subclavian artery firmly affix the Ao to the thoracic cage (Fig. 23.2).

Goarin et al. (51) published their experience in 28 patients diagnosed with traumatic disruption of the Ao: 19 showed thick stripes at the site of disruption, 15 presented an intimal flap, and 13 had fusiform aneurysms (>1.5 times normal) (Fig. 23.37). Vignon and Lang (52) examined 115 trauma patients and diagnosed 14 with aortic disruption (3 intimal and 11 subadventitial), yielding 91% sensitivity and 100% specificity compared with intraoperative pathology.

Medial flaps are caused by subadventitial tears and are thicker than intimal flaps as they contain both intimal and medial layers. In all cases, the medial flap runs perpendicular to the wall of the Ao unlike in dissections where it is most often parallel (Fig. 23.37). Medial flaps are mobile and influenced by the flow of blood within the Ao. Intimal tears appeared as thin flaps within the aortic lumen itself.

SURGICAL STRATEGY IN THE MANAGEMENT OF THE ATHEROSCLEROTIC ASCENDING AORTA

The detection of the atherosclerotic Ao by EAU and its impact on surgical outcomes is well established. Less clear, however, is the optimal technique for managing this finding. A number of strategies have been employed, ranging from EAU-guided placement of the cross clamp and aortic cannula to "no-touch" techniques and replacement of the atherosclerotic Ao (53–56). Minor alterations in surgical technique may improve patient outcomes. Several groups have used

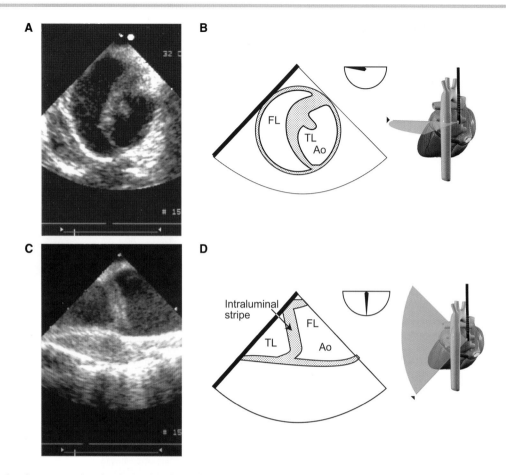

Figure 23.37 Aortic trauma. Intraluminal stripe due to intimal and medial laceration is seen in the descending Ao short-axis (**A,B**) and long-axis (**C,D**) views in a 32-year-old man with traumatic aortic injury. *Abbreviations*: Ao, aorta; FL, false lumen; TL, true lumen. *Source*: With permission from Ref. 51.

EAU to modify the placement of the aortic cannula, aortic cross clamp, and proximal anastomoses to avoid atherosclerotic plaque (53,57). They concluded that outcomes could be improved based on changes made with the ultrasound findings. Other studies, however, have reported significant stroke rates (8.7%) despite modification of techniques (16,58).

The use of a single cross clamp (i.e., proximal anastomoses constructed without the use of a side biting clamp) has been shown to reduce neurologic injury (3.2% vs. 9.6%, single clamp vs. double clamp) with a trend toward a lower stroke rate (59). The benefit is felt to be secondary to limited manipulation of the Ao. A number of "clampless" techniques have been described. These include the use of deep hypothermic circulatory arrest, fibrillatory arrest with venting, and resting heart techniques (53,55). In these situations, alternative proximal bypass graft anastomosis sites may be employed. Possibilities include the innominate and axillary arteries (60). When segments of disease-free Ao have been identified, proximal anastomotic devices (Guidant Heartstring) have been successfully used.

Off-pump coronary artery bypass surgery (OPCAB) has been advocated as being associated with a lower incidence of neurologic dysfunction. However,

a recent meta-analysis failed to support this (61). While neurologic outcomes may not differ in a general patient population, OPCAB may be beneficial in certain high-risk patient populations. Djaiani et al. (62) performed diffusion-weighted MRIs on patients with atherosclerotic Aos that were revascularized using either OPCAB or on-CPB methods. Patients in the OPCAB group did not demonstrate new ischemic brain lesions, whereas 61% of the on-CPB group did. Those having OPCAB surgery were also less confused during the first two postoperative days. Two propensity case-matched studies have examined only patients with atherosclerotic Aos. In both series, the OPCAB group demonstrated improved survival and lower rates of perioperative stroke compared with those who underwent CABG using conventional techniques (63,64).

Complete absence of aortic manipulation may provide the best outcomes in this high-risk patient population. A no-touch technique (Fig. 23.15) can be performed using arterial grafts constructed on a beating heart avoiding all instrumentation and manipulation of the Ao. Additional grafts are brought off the internal thoracic arteries in a "Y" configuration. Royse et al. (65) have reported that a no-touch technique improves late neurologic outcomes. Hangler et al. (54)

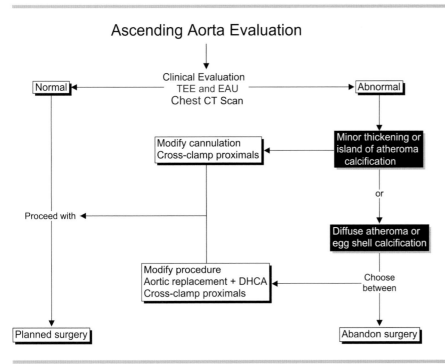

Figure 23.38 Aortic disease. Algorithm for the management of the ascending aorta during cardiac surgery is shown. *Abbreviations*: CT, computed tomography; DHCA, deep hypothermic cardiac arrest; EAU, epiaortic ultrasound; TEE, transesophageal echocardiography. *Source*: Adapted from Ref. 66.

employed a no-touch technique on a series of patients with severe aortic disease. Stroke rates in this group were not significantly different from those with less severely diseased Aos and less than predicted using the McSPI stroke risk model (2.9% actual vs. 4.4% predicted). In extreme cases or when valvular surgery is needed, replacement of the Ao has been employed with acceptable stroke rates (55).

The optimal treatment strategies for patients with aortic atherosclerosis have not been evaluated in the form of a randomized controlled trial. Until this time, surgeons will need to individualize their evaluation of the Ao as well as their approach to those patients who do have significant atherosclerotic burdens. An algorithm for the approach to the patient with ascending aortic atherosclerosis is shown in Figure 23.38.

REFERENCES

1. Kaplan JA. Cardiac Anesthesia. 4th ed. Philadelphia: W.B. Saunders Co, 1999.
2. Urban BA, Bluemke DA, Johnson KM, et al. Imaging of thoracic aortic disease. Cardiol Clin 1999; 17:659–82, viii.
3. Roman MJ, Devereux RB, Kramer-Fox R, et al. Two-dimensional echocardiographic aortic root dimensions in normal children and adults. Am J Cardiol 1989; 64:507–512.
4. Freeman WK, Seward JB, Khandheria BK, et al. Transesophageal Echocardiography. Boston: Little, Brown, 1994.
5. Katz ES, Tunick PA, Rusinek H, et al. Protruding aortic atheromas predict stroke in elderly patients undergoing cardiopulmonary bypass: experience with intraoperative transesophageal echocardiography. J Am Coll Cardiol 1992; 20:70–77.
6. Konstadt SN, Reich DL, Quintana C, et al. The ascending aorta: how much does transesophageal echocardiography see? Anesth Analg 1994; 78:240–244.
7. Darmon PL, Hillel Z, Mogtader A, et al. Cardiac output by transesophageal echocardiography using continuous-wave Doppler across the aortic valve. Anesthesiology 1994; 80:796–805.
8. Li YL, Wong DT, Wei W, et al. A novel acoustic window for trans-oesophageal echocardiography by using a saline-filled endotracheal balloon. Br J Anaesth 2006; 97:624–629.
9. van Zaane B, Nierich AP, Buhre WF, et al. Resolving the blind spot of transoesophageal echocardiography: a new diagnostic device for visualizing the ascending aorta in cardiac surgery. Br J Anaesth 2007; 98:434–441.
10. Nierich AP, van Zaane B, Buhre WF, et al. Visualization of the distal ascending aorta with A-Mode transesophageal echocardiography. J Cardiothorac Vasc Anesth 2008; 22: 766–773.
11. Mahajan A, Crowley R, Ho JK, et al. Imaging the ascending aorta and aortic arch using transesophageal echocardiography: the expanded aortic view. Echocardiography 2008; 25:408–413.
12. Roach GW, Kanchuger M, Mangano CM, et al. Adverse cerebral outcomes after coronary bypass surgery. Multicenter Study of Perioperative Ischemia Research Group and the Ischemia Research and Education Foundation Investigators. N Engl J Med 1996; 335:1857–1863.
13. John R, Choudhri AF, Weinberg AD, et al. Multicenter review of preoperative risk factors for stroke after coronary artery bypass grafting. Ann Thorac Surg 2000; 69:30–35.
14. Davila-Roman VG, Barzilai B, Wareing TH, et al. Atherosclerosis of the ascending aorta. Prevalence and role as an independent predictor of cerebrovascular events in cardiac patients. Stroke 1994; 25:2010–2016.
15. Hogue CW Jr., Murphy SF, Schechtman KB, et al. Risk factors for early or delayed stroke after cardiac surgery. Circulation 1999; 100:642–647.
16. Van der Linden J, Hadjinikolaou L, Bergman P, et al. Postoperative stroke in cardiac surgery is related to the location and extent of atherosclerotic disease in the ascending aorta. J Am Coll Cardiol 2001; 38:131–135.

17. Goto T, Baba T, Matsuyama K, et al. Aortic atherosclerosis and postoperative neurological dysfunction in elderly coronary surgical patients. Ann Thorac Surg 2003; 75:1912–1918.

18. Schachner T, Nagele G, Kacani A, et al. Factors associated with presence of ascending aortic atherosclerosis in CABG patients. Ann Thorac Surg 2004; 78:2028–2032.

19. Van der Linden J, Bergman P, Hadjinikolaou L. The topography of aortic atherosclerosis enhances its precision as a predictor of stroke. Ann Thorac Surg 2007; 83:2087–2092.

20. Glas KE, Swaminathan M, Reeves ST, et al. Guidelines for the performance of a comprehensive intraoperative epiaortic ultrasonographic examination: recommendations of the American Society of Echocardiography and the Society of Cardiovascular Anesthesiologists; endorsed by the Society of Thoracic Surgeons. Anesth Analg 2008; 106: 1376–1384.

21. Bainbridge D. 3-D imaging for aortic plaque assessment. Semin Cardiothorac Vasc Anesth 2005; 9:163–165.

22. Schachner T, Zimmer A, Nagele G, et al. The influence of ascending aortic atherosclerosis on the long-term survival after CABG. Eur J Cardiothorac Surg 2005; 28:558–562.

23. Bolotin G, Domany Y, de Perini L, et al. Use of intraoperative epiaortic ultrasonography to delineate aortic atheroma. Chest 2005; 127:60–65.

24. Suvarna S, Smith A, Stygall J, et al. An intraoperative assessment of the ascending aorta: a comparison of digital palpation, transesophageal echocardiography, and epiaortic ultrasonography. J Cardiothorac Vasc Anesth 2007; 21:805–809.

25. Ibrahim KS, Vitale N, Tromsdal A, et al. Enhanced intraoperative grading of ascending aorta atheroma by epiaortic ultrasound vs echocardiography. Int J Cardiol 2008; 128:218–223.

26. Ura M, Sakata R, Nakayama Y, et al. Ultrasonographic demonstration of manipulation-related aortic injuries after cardiac surgery. J Am Coll Cardiol 2000; 35:1303–1310.

27. Mangano DT. Aspirin and mortality from coronary bypass surgery. N Engl J Med 2002; 347:1309–1317.

28. Fayad ZA, Nahar T, Fallon JT, et al. In vivo magnetic resonance evaluation of atherosclerotic plaques in the human thoracic aorta: a comparison with transesophageal echocardiography. Circulation 2000; 101:2503–2509.

29. Lee R, Matsutani N, Polimenakos AC, et al. Preoperative noncontrast chest computed tomography identifies potential aortic emboli. Ann Thorac Surg 2007; 84:38–41.

30. Marshall WG Jr., Barzilai B, Kouchoukos NT, et al. Intraoperative ultrasonic imaging of the ascending aorta. Ann Thorac Surg 1989; 48:339–344.

31. Davila-Roman VG, Phillips KJ, Daily BB, et al. Intraoperative transesophageal echocardiography and epiaortic ultrasound for assessment of atherosclerosis of the thoracic aorta. J Am Coll Cardiol 1996; 28:942–947.

32. van Zaane B, Zuithoff NP, Reitsma JB, et al. Meta-analysis of the diagnostic accuracy of transesophageal echocardiography for assessment of atherosclerosis in the ascending aorta in patients undergoing cardiac surgery. Acta Anaesthesiol Scand 2008; 52:1179–1187.

33. Adler Y, Vaturi M, Wiser I, et al. Nonobstructive aortic valve calcium as a window to atherosclerosis of the aorta. Am J Cardiol 2000; 86:68–71.

34. Adler Y, Shohat-Zabarski R, Vaturi M, et al. Association between mitral annular calcium and aortic atheroma as detected by transesophageal echocardiographic study. Am J Cardiol 1998; 81:784–786.

35. Ring WS. Congenital Heart Surgery Nomenclature and Database Project: aortic aneurysm, sinus of Valsalva aneurysm, and aortic dissection. Ann Thorac Surg 2000; 69: S147–S163.

36. Jackson BB. Surgery of acquired vascular disorders. Springfield, Ill: Thomas, 1969.

37. Erbel R, Zamorano J. The aorta. Aortic aneurysm, trauma, and dissection. Crit Care Clin 1996; 12:733–766.

38. Coady MA, Rizzo JA, Goldstein LJ, et al. Natural history, pathogenesis, and etiology of thoracic aortic aneurysms and dissections. Cardiol Clin 1999; 17:615–635.

39. Feigenbaum H. Diseases of the aorta. In: Feigenbaum H, ed. Echocardiography. 5th ed. Philadelphia: Lea & Febiger, 1994:630–657.

40. King ME. Echocardiographic evaluation of the adult with unoperated congenital heart disease. In: Otto CM, ed. The Practice of Clinical Echocardiography. Philadelphia: W.B. Saunders, 1997:697–728.

41. Otto CM. Practice of Clinical Echocardiography. 1st ed. Philadelphia: W.B. Saunders Company, 1997.

42. Larson EW, Edwards WD. Risk factors for aortic dissection: a necropsy study of 161 cases. Am J Cardiol 1984; 53:849–855.

43. Erbel R, Engberding R, Daniel W, et al. Echocardiography in diagnosis of aortic dissection. Lancet 1989; 1:457–461.

44. Nienaber CA, Spielmann RP, von KY, et al. Diagnosis of thoracic aortic dissection. Magnetic resonance imaging versus transesophageal echocardiography. Circulation 1992; 85:434–447.

45. Bansal RC, Chandrasekaran K, Ayala K, et al. Frequency and explanation of false negative diagnosis of aortic dissection by aortography and transesophageal echocardiography. J Am Coll Cardiol 1995; 25:1393–1401.

46. Losi MA, Betocchi S, Briguori C, et al. Determinants of aortic artifacts during transesophageal echocardiography of the ascending aorta. Am Heart J 1999; 137:967–972.

47. Svensson LG, Labib SB, Eisenhauer AC, et al. Intimal tear without hematoma: an important variant of aortic dissection that can elude current imaging techniques. Circulation 1999; 99:1331–1336.

48. Vilacosta I, San Roman JA, Ferreiros J, et al. Natural history and serial morphology of aortic intramural hematoma: a novel variant of aortic dissection. Am Heart J 1997; 134: 495–507.

49. von Kodolitsch Y, Csosz SK, Koschyk DH, et al. Intramural hematoma of the aorta: predictors of progression to dissection and rupture. Circulation 2003; 107:1158–1163.

50. Schmidt CA, Jacobson JG. Thoracic aortic injury. A tenyear experience. Arch Surg 1984; 119:1244–1246.

51. Goarin JP, Catoire P, Jacquens Y, et al. Use of transesophageal echocardiography for diagnosis of traumatic aortic injury. Chest 1997; 112:71–80.

52. Vignon P, Lang RM. Use of Transesophageal Echocardiography for the assessment of traumatic aortic injuries. Echocardiography 1999; 16:207–219.

53. Duda AM, Letwin LB, Sutter FP, et al. Does routine use of aortic ultrasonography decrease the stroke rate in coronary artery bypass surgery? J Vasc Surg 1995; 21:98–107.

54. Hangler HB, Nagele G, Danzmayr M, et al. Modification of surgical technique for ascending aortic atherosclerosis: impact on stroke reduction in coronary artery bypass grafting. J Thorac Cardiovasc Surg 2003; 126:391–400.

55. Zingone B, Rauber E, Gatti G, et al. Diagnosis and management of severe atherosclerosis of the ascending aorta and aortic arch during cardiac surgery: focus on aortic replacement. Eur J Cardiothorac Surg 2007; 31: 990–997.

56. Rosenberger P, Shernan SK, Loffler M, et al. The influence of epiaortic ultrasonography on intraoperative surgical management in 6051 cardiac surgical patients. Ann Thorac Surg 2008; 85:548–553.

57. Trehan N, Mishra M, Dhole S, et al. Significantly reduced incidence of stroke during coronary artery bypass grafting using transesophageal echocardiography. Eur J Cardiothorac Surg 1997; 11:234–242.

58. Djaiani G, Ali M, Borger MA, et al. Epiaortic scanning modifies planned intraoperative surgical management but not cerebral embolic load during coronary artery bypass surgery. Anesth Analg 2008; 106:1611–1618.

59. Grega MA, Borowicz LM, Baumgartner WA. Impact of single clamp versus double clamp technique on neurologic outcome. Ann Thorac Surg 2003; 75:1387–1391.

60. Bonatti J, Coulson AS, Bakhshay SA, et al. The subclavian and axillary arteries as inflow vessels for coronary artery bypass grafts—combined experience from three cardiac surgery centers. Heart Surg Forum 2000; 3:307–311.

61. Bainbridge D, Cheng D, Martin J, et al. Does off-pump or minimally invasive coronary artery bypass reduce mortality, morbidity, and resource utilization when compared with percutaneous coronary intervention? A meta-analysis of randomized trials. J Thorac Cardiovasc Surg 2007; 133:623–631.

62. Djaiani G, Fedorko L, Cusimano RJ, et al. Off-pump coronary bypass surgery: risk of ischemic brain lesions in patients with atheromatous thoracic aorta. Can J Anaesth 2006; 53:795–801.

63. Sharony R, Grossi EA, Saunders PC, et al. Propensity case-matched analysis of off-pump coronary artery bypass grafting in patients with atheromatous aortic disease. J Thorac Cardiovasc Surg 2004; 127:406–413.

64. Mishra M, Malhotra R, Karlekar A, et al. Propensity case-matched analysis of off-pump versus on-pump coronary artery bypass grafting in patients with atheromatous aorta. Ann Thorac Surg 2006; 82:608–614.

65. Royse AG, Royse CF, Ajani AE, et al. Reduced neuropsychological dysfunction using epiaortic echocardiography and the exclusive Y graft. Ann Thorac Surg 2000; 69:1431–1438.

66. Bainbridge D, Murkin J, Calaritis C, et al. Aortic dissection in a patient with a previous ascending aortic dissection and repair: the role of new monitoring devices in the high-risk patient. Semin Cardiothorac Vasc Anesth 2004; 8:3–7.

24

Endograft Placement in Aortic Disease

Alain Deschamps and Eric Therasse
Université de Montréal, Montreal, Canada

Oren Steinmetz
McGill University and McGill University Health Centre, Montreal, Canada

George Nicolaou
London Health Sciences Centre, University of Western Ontario, London, Canada

INTRODUCTION

Endovascular aortic repair is a relatively new surgical alternative to the traditional open surgical techniques, as it has a lower mortality and morbidity (1). Despite the growing popularity of endovascular grafts or endografts, the optimal imaging modality for guidance, during an implantation procedure, is not well defined (2). At present, transesophageal echocardiography (TEE), in conjunction with intraoperative angiography, appears to be advantageous and adds incremental information to guide endograft placement safely in a descending thoracic aneurysm or in type-B aortic dissection (3,4). This chapter describes the approach to the treatment of aortic disease, chronic or traumatic, and the role of TEE in endovascular surgery.

OPEN VASCULAR AND ENDOVASCULAR SURGERY

The primary treatment goal for most thoracic aortic pathology, such as aortic aneurysms, posttraumatic tears, acute intramural hematomas, and acute aortic dissections, is to prevent aortic rupture. In some cases of acute aortic dissection the goal is to reverse malperfusion syndrome. Currently, two entirely different treatment strategies can be employed to manage lesions of the thoracic aorta (Ao). They include traditional open surgical repair and the newer closed endovascular repair (Table 24.1).

In open surgical repair, the dilated or diseased section of the Ao is replaced with a synthetic graft that is surgically sewn into unaffected sections of the Ao above and below the lesion (Fig. 24.1). The complexity and risk of surgery increases significantly when the lesion is located in the proximal Ao, involves a long section of the Ao, extends distally into the visceral Ao, or is performed emergently for an acute aortic syndrome. Branches of the Ao that arise within the aneurysmal or diseased section can be surgically reimplanted onto the graft, thereby maintaining perfusion

(see Chapter 23). Open aneurysm repair is applicable to all sections of the thoracic and abdominal Ao and is the gold standard with which newer treatments, such as endovascular repair, must be compared.

During endovascular repair a fabric graft, which is internally or externally supported by metallic stents, is deployed within the Ao. The endograft used to treat an aneurysm must extend from the proximal to the distal nonaneurysmal Ao, thus excluding the aneurysmal segment from the systemic circulation and arterial pressures. All instrumentation and steps of endograft delivery, together with deployment, are carried out from within the arterial lumen under fluoroscopic and TEE guidance. Arterial access to introduce the endograft is at a site remote from the lesion such as a femoral artery cutdown. This approach avoids large thoracic and/or abdominal incisions. Most procedures can be performed under local or regional anesthesia, unless TEE is required for endograft placement or for comorbidity concerns. Following endograft placement, patients will require follow-up imaging for the rest of their lives to ensure that the aneurysm or other lesion remains excluded by the endograft.

PATIENT SELECTION

Endovascular surgery is gaining popularity worldwide and is regarded as a "novel technique," even though the first endovascular endograft of an ascending thoracic aneurysm in humans was performed, in 1864, by Moore (6). With the progressive aging of the population and the associated increase in comorbidity, advantages of endovascular surgery include decreased stress response, less perioperative complications, shorter hospital stay, and quicker return to normal activities. One of the main disadvantages of endovascular aneurysmal repair is the requirement for a yearly computed tomography (CT) scan.

Recent technological advances are producing ever smaller, more maneuverable, catheter delivery systems, endografts with holes and side arms for

Table 24.1 Criteria for Endovascular Repair of Thoracic Aortic Disease

1. Thoracic aortic aneurysm
   Descending thoracic aneurysm >5.5 cm
   Aneurysm 4.5–5.5 cm with increase in size by 0.5 cm in the last six months or twice normal size
   Saccular aneurysm or penetrating ulcer
   Nonaneurysmal proximal and distal aortic neck measures between 22 and 40 mm (dependent on device availability)
   No extension of aneurysm into abdominal aorta (distal neck at least 2 cm above celiac artery)
   Devices available suitable for patient's anatomy
   Patent iliac or femoral arteries that allow introduction of a 22–25 F delivery system (device dependant)
   Life expectancy of at least six months
   Able to consent for appropriate trials and follow-up protocols

2. Type-B aortic dissection
   Acute dissection with intractable pain, uncontrollable hypertension, progression of dissection, or end-organ ischemia
   Chronic dissection with aneurismal dilatation of proximal descending aorta
   Chronic dissection with acute symptoms
   Early tear at least 1 cm from left subclavian artery (LSCA) orifice (potentially 2 cm if plan to cover LSCA)
   No entry site of dissection that is proximal to LSCA or involves the arch or the ascending portion of the aorta.
   Devices available suitable for patient's anatomy
   Patent iliac or femoral arteries that allow introduction of a 22–25 F delivery system (device dependant)
   Life expectancy of at least six months
   Able to consent for appropriate trials and follow-up protocols

Source: Adapted from Lee et al. (5).

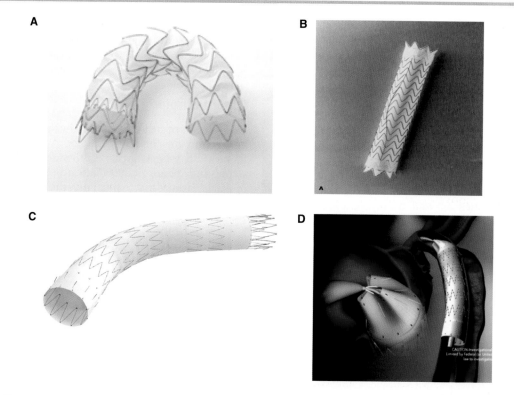

Figure 24.1 Types of endografts. Various endografts are shown including the (**A**) Valiant thoracic stent graft (Medtronic, Inc., Santa Rosa, California, USA), (**B**) Zenith TX2 (Cook, Inc., Bloomington, Indiana, USA) and (**C**) Gore (W. L. Gore & Associates, Flagstaff, Arizona, USA). (**D**) Example of the use of endograft during dissection. *Source*: Courtesy of Cook Medical, www.cookmedical.com.

branching of the renal arteries, self-expandable endografts, and devices within the endografts to monitor intra-aortic positioning. These advances facilitate installation in severely atherosclerotic patients and decrease the incidence of complications due to collateral artery occlusions.

The success of endovascular surgery in recent years has shifted the target population from patients deemed inoperable to patients with less severe comorbidities. Nevertheless, coronary artery disease (CAD) with silent ischemia, previous myocardial infarction, hypertension, chronic obstructive lung disease, chronic renal failure, and diabetes mellitus remain common in this patient population (7). Intraoperative TEE can be a useful tool to monitor patients with significant comorbid disease but also to help in the positioning and deployment of the endograft. While the use of TEE has the greatest benefits in the endovascular repair of the thoracic Ao, endovascular surgery for abdominal aortic disease can also benefit in cases where the risk for cardiac ischemia is very high.

Despite recent improvements, the operative mortality of conventional surgery for thoracic aortic pathology remains significant, especially for acute aortic syndromes involving the thoracic Ao (8–11). Given the less invasive and less traumatic nature of endovascular procedures, they have become an attractive alternative treatment option for many patients, particularly those who are elderly or considered at high risk due to multiple comorbidities. Since the successful implantation of an endograft for abdominal aortic aneurysm by Parodi et al. in 1991 (12), outcomes for endografts have been favorable in comparison with open surgery (13–18). These reports have made endovascular repairs a viable option in both the elective and emergent settings (19).

ROLE OF TEE DURING ENDOVASCULAR SURGERY

Patients undergoing major vascular surgery are at increased risk for perioperative cardiac complications (20,21). Early detection of the cardiac dysfunction and prompt treatment is crucial for a better outcome. The use of TEE as a hemodynamic monitor and a diagnostic tool provides the anesthesiologist with a detailed picture of both aortic pathology and cardiac function.

Unlike an angiogram, TEE has the unique advantages of portability and the ability to obtain high-resolution images of the normal and abnormal anatomy of the three layers of the aortic wall and lumen (see Chapter 23) (22). It is sufficiently sensitive to recognize simple aortic plaques as well more complex lesions protruding into the lumen (23) (see Chapter 23). TEE is also a highly sensitive and specific method of detecting injury to the thoracic Ao (24). Also, TEE provides additional critical information during endovascular thoracic aortic aneurysm repair, which impacts on early and late outcomes (25–28). In the operating room (OR), the initial TEE exam should rapidly confirm

the nature and extent of the aortic pathology and identify the proximal and distal landing zone sites.

Ventricular Function

Regional left ventricular (LV) dysfunction, due to newly appearing myocardial ischemia during endovascular surgery, can be evaluated using TEE. The presence of preexisting coronary atherosclerotic disease predisposes this patient population to ischemic events.

Although these events can occur at any time during the endovascular repair, they are more likely to occur during the deployment of the endograft. First, there can be a large increase in afterload if the heart is allowed to pump against the occlusion created by the deployment, or a significant decrease in blood pressure if the heart is stopped, through rapid pacing or with the administration of adenosine, to avoid the displacement of the deployed endograft. Either of these methods of deployment can result in decreased myocardial perfusion and ischemic events that can be evaluated using TEE.

A detailed description of TEE evaluation of LV function and ischemia is available in chapters 9 and 10. For the purpose of this chapter, mid-esophageal four-, two-chamber and long axis (LAX), as well as the transgastric views are sufficient to evaluate regional LV function (see Figs. 10.25–10.29).

Other Pathology

The degree of atherosclerosis in the ascending, transverse, and descending thoracic Ao can be evaluated using TEE (see Chapter 23). Studies have shown a strong independent association between the thickness of aortic atheroma (especially the ascending Ao and arch) and the risk factor of ischemic stroke (29,30). Evaluation of aortic arch atheroma with TEE is a recognized modality for the identification of patients at risk of stroke (31,32), and this evaluation should be performed for patients undergoing endovascular surgery (Fig. 24.2).

Aortic thrombus may easily form within the aortic aneurysm, and caution must be taken to exclude

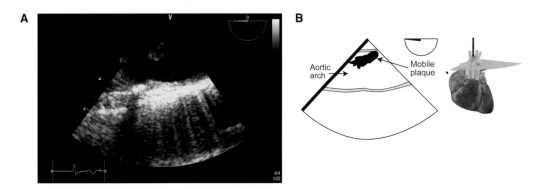

Figure 24.2 Aortic arch atheroma. (A,B) Upper esophageal aortic arch long-axis view shows a mobile atheroma (Grade V) in a 54-year-old patient scheduled for coronary artery bypass graft. Because of the unsuspected disease, the procedure was performed without clamping of the aorta and cardiopulmonary bypass.

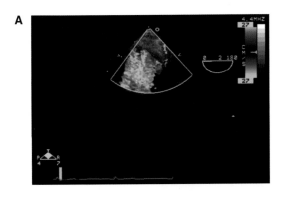

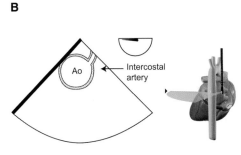

Figure 24.3 Intercostal artery. (A,B) Color Doppler descending Ao short-axis view shows flow in an intercostal artery. *Abbreviation*: Ao, aorta.

this thrombus from the landing zones. One of the advantages of utilizing the intraoperative TEE is its ability to visualize thrombus compared with the use of angiography (33). Cases where intraoperative angiography was unable to visualize mobile thrombus have been reported (34).

During the initial TEE exam, side branches (intercostals) may be identified in some patients and can provide information of the spinal cord blood supply (Fig. 24.3). Clinical reports estimate the risk of spinal cord ischemia to range from 3% to 12% in patients undergoing endovascular repair of thoracic or thoracoabdominal aneurysms (35). A complete description of the risk of paraplegia and organ ischemia is beyond the scope of this chapter.

Endograft Deployment

Endograft placement, under fluoroscopy, is usually straightforward for most aortic diseases because the lesion and endograft landing zones are easily assessable. Nevertheless, in cases where the aortic lesion is difficult to define or to localize, such as with the presence of small ulcers causing an intramural hematoma, or for the localization of the entry site of an aortic dissection, TEE imaging can be superior to fluoroscopy. For example, TEE can demonstrate that the normal Ao adjacent to the aneurysm is dilated and partially filled with mural thrombus making it a poor site for the endograft landing zone (Figs. 24.4 and 24.5).

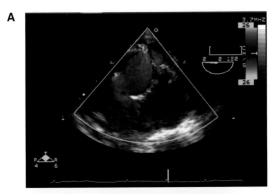

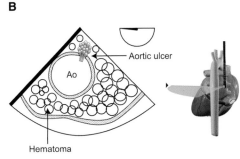

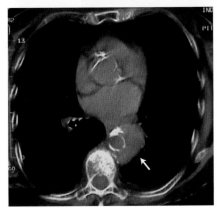

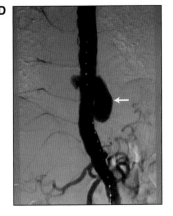

Figure 24.4 Aortic ulcer. An 84-year-old woman presents with a thoracic Ao pseudoaneurysm complicated by an aortic ulcer and hematoma seen in the descending Ao short-axis view (**A,B**), on computed tomographic scan (**C**) and angiography (**D**). *Abbreviation*: Ao, aorta.

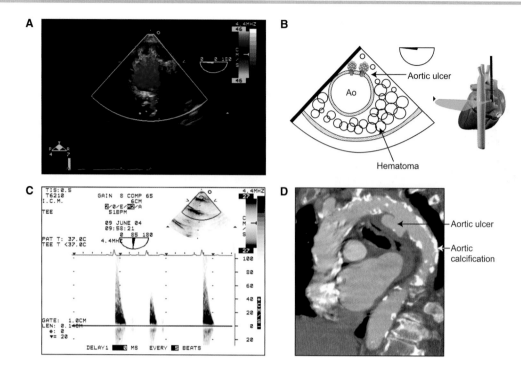

Figure 24.5 Endoleak type II. Evaluation of endograft landing zone for a proximal descending aortic ulcer. **(A,B)** Descending Ao short-axis view reveals on color flow imaging several abnormal flow jets exiting the lower descending Ao. **(C)** Pulsed wave Doppler of the jets yields a velocity >50 cm/s. **(D)** Computed tomography scan sagittal view showing the location of the nearby aortic ulcer and the extensive vascular calcifications. *Abbreviation*: Ao, aorta.

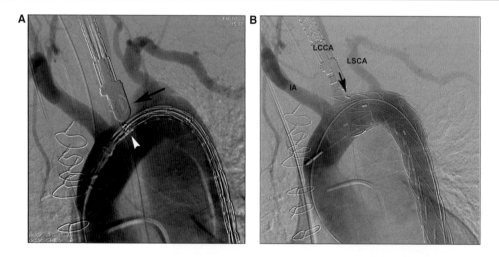

Figure 24.6 Fluoroscopy. (A) Left anterior oblique arteriography of the thoracic Ao before endograft deployment. The TEE probe (black arrow) was brought close to the proximal covered extremity of the endograft (white arrowhead) under fluoroscopic guidance to obtain a TEE image of the proximal landing zone site and as a fluoroscopic landmark during endograft deployment. **(B)** After deployment adequate positioning of the proximal covered part of the endograft (black arrow) is shown. The side branches and their relationship with the Ao can be assessed. *Abbreviations*: Ao, aorta; IA, innominate artery; LCCA, left common carotid artery; LSCA, left subclavian artery; TEE, transesophageal echocardiography. *Source*: Courtesy of Dr. E. Therasse.

The ability of TEE to localize the endograft extremities within the delivery system, when it is not deployed, is limited. The TEE probe may be used as a radiographic landmark, while the endograft is deployed under fluoroscopic guidance (Fig. 24.6). Once the endograft is released from the delivery system, it is visualized by fluoroscopy and its relationship with aortic side branches may be assessed.

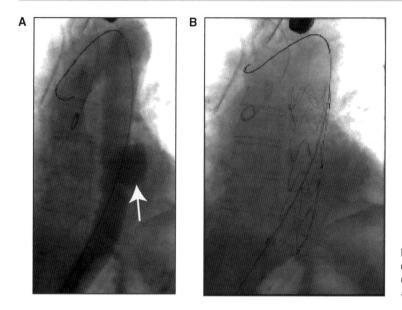

Figure 24.7 Aortic aneurysm. Angiography of a descending thoracic aortic aneurysm (arrow) before (**A**) and after (**B**) endograft implantation is shown. *Source*: Courtesy of Dr. Stéphane Coutu.

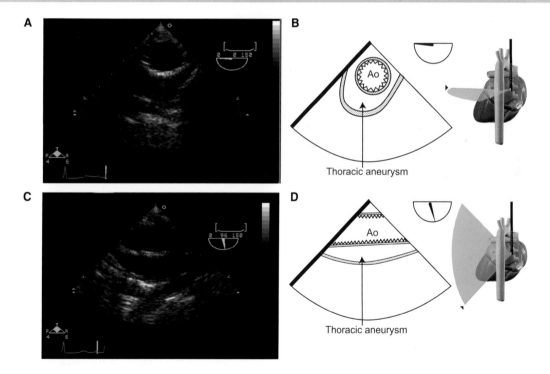

Figure 24.8 Aortic aneurysm after endograft implantation. Descending Ao short-axis (**A,B**) and long-axis (**C,D**) views. *Abbreviation*: Ao, aorta. *Source*: Courtesy of Dr. Stéphane Coutu.

Both intraoperative fluoroscopy (Fig. 24.7) and TEE (Fig. 24.8) can provide guidance for precise positioning of the device across an aortic lesion. However, when an aneurysm is located at the junction of the arch and descending Ao, intraoperative angiography may not be able to visualize it properly. While raising the patient's arms above his head may help to visualize this part of the Ao, a TEE probe positioned in the upper esophagus with the transducer angled between 50° and 70° may be helpful in providing a good image of this junction. Whenever possible, TEE should be the primary imaging modality used to minimize exposure to intravenous contrast associated with fluoroscopy.

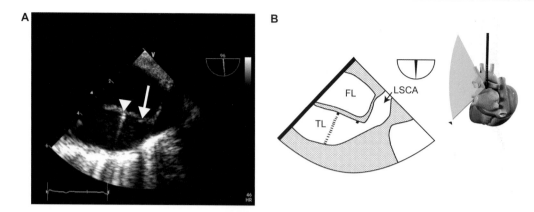

Figure 24.9 Endograft repair in aortic dissection. (A,B) Upper esophageal aortic arch long-axis view at 90° near the level of the LSCA shows an aortic dissection. The angiography catheter (arrowhead) and the stent-graft delivery catheter wire (small arrow) are located in the TL. *Abbreviations*: FL, false lumen; LSCA, left subclavian artery; TL, true lumen.

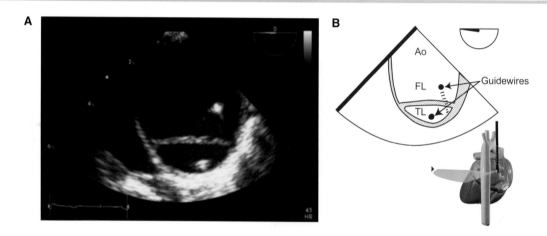

Figure 24.10 Guidewire position in aortic dissection. (A,B) Descending Ao short-axis view in a patient with an aortic dissection shows different guidewires in both the TL and in the FL. *Abbreviations*: Ao, aorta; FL, false lumen; TL, true lumen.

Guidewire and Delivery Device Insertion

Once the femoral artery is cannulated, TEE is used to confirm the proper location of the guidewire proximal to the aortic pathology both in the descending Ao short-axis (SAX) and LAX views. With aortic dissections, confirmation of the guidewire position in the true lumen of the Ao is much easier with TEE than with angiography as the course of the guidewire can be delineated throughout most of the descending thoracic Ao (Fig. 24.9). Unintentional insertion of the guidewire in the false lumen or into the pseudo-aneurysm has been documented (27,36) (Fig. 24.10).

Proximal Landing Zone

The proximal landing zone should be inspected for the presence of aortic plaque, mural thrombus, or calcification along the aortic wall with the purpose of avoiding endograft deployment in unfavorable aortic

segments. Once the endograft is deployed, it remains fixed in its position for the duration of its life and cannot be repositioned. Consequently, if the proximal landing zone is proximal to the left subclavian artery (LSCA), it is important to verify the patency of the left common carotid artery using either color Doppler with TTE (Fig. 24.11), surface ultrasonography (Fig. 24.12) (37), or near-infrared spectroscopy (38). As the aortic arch is a curvilinear structure, deployment of the endograft in this region forces it to recline on the inferior aortic arch. However, the proximal landing zone is usually at least 10 mm distal to the LSCA. In cases where there is less than 15 mm of normal Ao between the lesion and the LSCA, the covered part of the endograft may have to cross the origin of the LSCA to ensure adequate length of the proximal landing zone. A left carotid-subclavian artery bypass may be created beforehand, although many authors have reported coverage of the LSCA ostium without any sequelae (39).

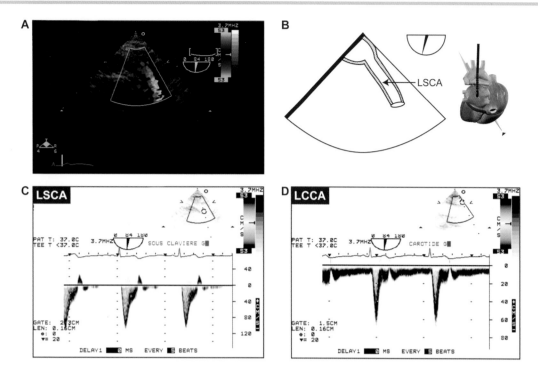

Figure 24.11 **Aortic arch vessel identification and monitoring.** (**A,B**) Color Doppler upper esophageal aortic arch short-axis view at 84° shows the LSCA. (**C**) Pulsed wave Doppler of LSCA: a peripheral artery has a typical triphasic appearance due to high vascular resistance of the downstream normal muscular vascular bed at rest. (**D**) Pulsed wave Doppler of LCCA: a diastolic flow component is usually present due to the low vascular resistance of the downstream normal cerebral vascular bed. *Abbreviations*: LCCA, left common carotid artery; LSCA, left subclavian artery.

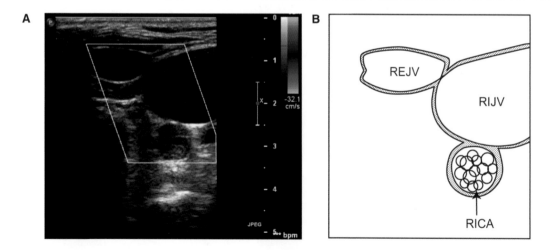

Figure 24.12 **Carotid occlusion.** (**A,B**) Surface ultrasound shows complete RICA occlusion in a patient with acute aortic dissection. Antegrade cardioplegia through the right innominate artery was aborted following this finding. *Abbreviations*: REJV, right external jugular vein; RICA, right internal carotid artery; RIJV, right internal jugular vein. *Source*: Courtesy of Dr. Stéphane Coutu.

Because aneurysms tend to elongate, producing vector forces that may eventually cause the endograft to migrate, it is advisable that the landing zones of the endograft be at least 2 cm long. For similar reasons, when multiple endografts are needed, they should generously overlap to prevent late disconnection (40).

Finally, after identification of the most favorable proximal landing zone in collaboration with the surgeon and/or radiologist, the aortic diameter is measured in both SAX and LAX to confirm the size of the endograft. Importantly, the size of the endograft selected should be 15% to 20% larger than the landing zone diameter. While the endograft size and the proximal landing zone site are usually selected preoperatively on the basis of CT scan and/or magnetic resonance imaging (MRI) studies, both TEE and fluoroscopy are used to confirm these.

Distal Landing Zone

While the proximal landing zone is the main determinant of the size and length of the required endograft, it is important not to underestimate the potential of a tortuous distal Ao resulting in misalignment and endoleak (28). In these cases, the use of more than one endograft should be considered. Another point to consider is the difference between the proximal and distal landing zone diameters. Should this difference be greater than 5 mm, the patient may require a special tapered endograft or may be considered for an open repair. The distal diameter should also be oversized by 15% to 20% in a manner similar to the proximal endograft diameter.

Length of Aortic Coverage

TEE is also used to confirm full coverage of the aneurysm or pseudo-aneurysm with the endograft ensuring the absence of endoleaks or retrograde

flow. Sometimes, more than one endograft may be required to cover the entire length of the aneurysm. In general, if the amount of coverage required is less than, or equal to, 12 cm, a single graft can be used. However, most of the times an aneurysmal segment is greater than 12 cm and two or more endografts will be required to achieve complete coverage of the aneurysm. In case multiple endografts are required, TEE should be focused on ensuring that sufficient overlap exists between endografts. Ballooning may be required at the landing zones and the sites of endograft overlap.

Thoracic aorta repairs require the use the shortest possible endograft to avoid the risk of occlusion of patent aortic branches and limit the likelihood of spinal cord ischemia. In these cases, proper endograft length and positioning is often more precise when TEE is used in association with fluoroscopy.

Aortic Dissections

The exit and reentry points of an aortic dissection cannot always be clearly visualized using fluoroscopy alone because of stagnant flow through sections of the false lumen extending proximally and distally. Transesophageal echocardiography is superior at locating the position and number of multiple exit and reentry tears (Fig. 24.13).

Indications for the treatment of distal aortic dissection include the obstruction of side branches

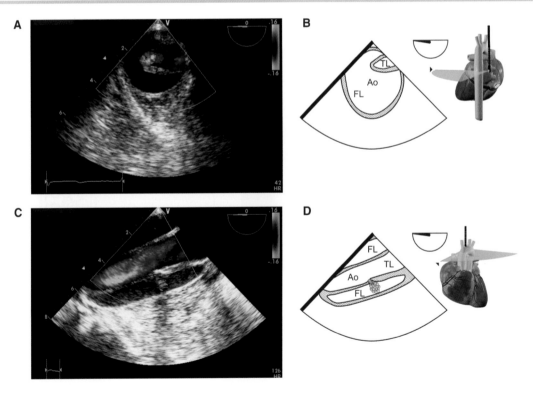

Figure 24.13   Aortic dissection. Color Doppler distal descending Ao short-axis (**A,B**) and aortic arch long-axis (**C,D**) views in a patient with aortic dissection easily identify the entry points between the TL and FL. *Abbreviations*: Ao, aorta; FL, false lumen; TL, true lumen.

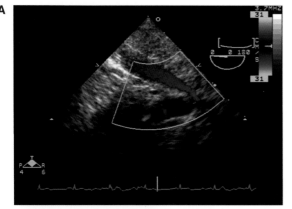

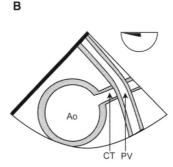

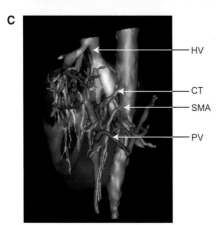

Figure 24.14 Celiac trunk and portal vein. (**A,B**) Color Doppler distal descending Ao short-axis view shows the origin of the celiac trunk and the PV. (**C**) 3D reconstruction of the large vessels of the abdomen as viewed from the left and behind demonstrate the relationship between the celiac trunk and the venous circulation. *Abbreviations*: Ao, aorta; CT, celiac trunk; HV, hepatic vein; PV, portal vein; SMA, superior mesenteric artery. *Source*: Courtesy of l'Institut de Recherche Contre les Cancers de l'Appareil Digestif, Strasbourg, France.

responsible for visceral ischemia. These obstructions are generally characterized as dynamic or static, and TEE can differentiate between the two. Dynamic vascular obstruction results when the intimal flap prolapses over the origin of the branch vessel, or collapses the true aortic lumen from above, and is related to blood flow dynamics between the true and false lumen. Static vascular obstruction results from the extension of the dissection flap directly into an aortic branch and is not related to blood flow distribution between the true and false lumen.

Aortic endograft insertion, used to redirect blood flow in the true lumen, may be useful to treat organ ischemia due to dynamic obstruction of the aortic branches but is unlikely to be effective in treating static vascular obstructions. Angiography is often inappropriate in the evaluation of significant obstructions, while TEE and color Doppler can be used to evaluate aortic side branch perfusion before and after endograft placement. Color Doppler imaging can demonstrate residual obstructions or adequate blood flow in aortic side branches (Fig. 24.14) such as renal arteries (Fig. 24.15) (41).

In the presence of residual obstruction, an additional aortic endograft or fenestration of the dissection flap or endograft of the aortic side branches may have to be considered. Percutaneous fenestration of the intimal flap may be required when endograft insertion

is either not indicated or is ineffective in reestablishing blood flow to the viscera or to the lower limb. TEE will be very useful to guide the needle across the intimal flap and to position the angioplasty balloon catheter through the fenestration (Figs. 24.16 and 24.17). Because of these considerations, combining TEE and fluoroscopy is thought to be superior to fluoroscopy alone in the treatment of aortic dissection (4).

Decreasing Aortic Blood Flow

Thoracic aortic lesions often arise close to the LSCA, and the success of the intervention frequently depends on exact positioning of the ends of the endograft. Inaccurate endograft positioning may compromise cerebral or visceral perfusion or predispose to post-deployment endoleaks. Precise positioning of the endograft in the thoracic Ao, which is critical when the landings zone are very short, may be hampered by the so-called "wind-sock effect" during endograft deployment. This effect is due to the blood flow entering the partially opened proximal portion of the endograft while the distal part is still closed, dragging the graft distally. To minimize this effect, different approaches are used to decrease blood flow during endograft deployment.

Nitrates or short-acting β-adrenergic blocking agents have often been used in the past. However,

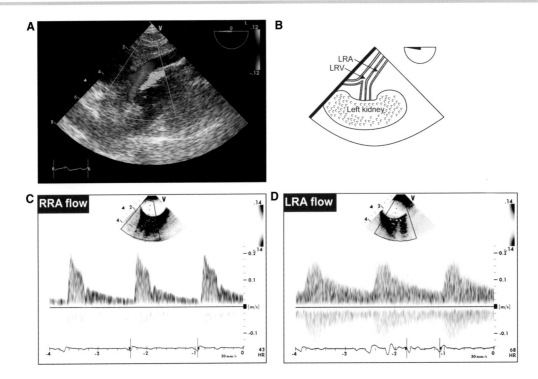

Figure 24.15 Renal artery Doppler monitoring. Renal artery Doppler monitoring during thoracic aortic endograft insertion to treat visceral ischemia associated with a type B aortic dissection. (**A,B**) Transgastric view at 0° of the left kidney with color Doppler of the LRV and LRA is shown. (**C,D**) Distal descending aorta short-axis view with pulsed wave Doppler interrogation of the RRA and LRA. There is a steep systolic rise associated with normal blood flow in the RRA, while the pulsus tardus in the LRA suggests residual partial obstruction. *Abbreviations*: LRA, left renal artery; LRV, left renal vein; RRA, right renal artery.

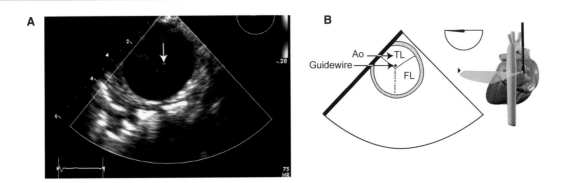

Figure 24.16 Guidewire fenestration. (**A,B**) Distal descending Ao short-axis view is shown during percutaneous fenestration of the intimal flap of an aortic dissection. The guidewire needle tip is in the smaller TL, orientated toward the FL to puncture the dissection flap. *Abbreviations*: Ao, aorta; FL, false lumen; TL, true lumen.

prolonged hypotension, especially when multiple endografts are deployed, may be hazardous for the patients, especially those with cerebrovascular disease or at risk of ischemic spine injury. Adenosine, an endogenous purine nucleoside, causes dose-dependent transient cardiac asystole and can be used to reduce blood flow just before endograft deployment

(42,43). However, it is short acting, and sometimes unpredictable, and the first strong heartbeats following cardiac asystole may drag the partially deployed device.

Rapid ventricular pacing, through a transvenous pacemaker, can be used to increase heart rate (HR) to 180 to 220 beats/minute resulting in an easily

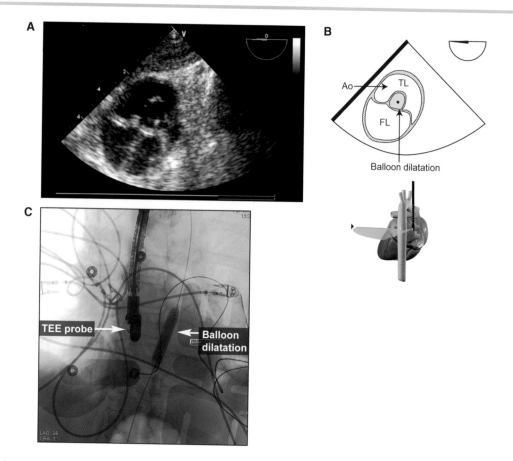

Figure 24.17 Guidewire fenestration. (A,B) Distal descending Ao short-axis view is shown during percutaneous fenestration of the intimal flap of an aortic dissection. The image shows the adequate positioning of the inflated balloon catheter across the dissection flap from the TL into the FL. **(C)** A postero-anterior fluoroscopic image shows the balloon catheter during inflation. *Abbreviations*: Ao, aorta; FL, false lumen; TEE, transesophageal echocardiography; TL, true lumen.

controlled decrease in blood flow that facilitates endograft deployment (43–45). This technique is the most convenient because it is predictable, starts and finishes on demand, and is readily reversible. Although rare, possible ventricular tachyarrhythmias, due to rapid ventricular pacing, require that radiolucent defibrillator pads be placed on the patient's thorax beforehand in case cardioversion is required.

COMPLICATIONS

Endoleaks

Endoleaks are defined as a persistence of blood flow outside the endograft (perigraft zone) after deployment. They result from a failure of the endograft to totally exclude blood flow to the aneurysm sac, causing continued pressurization of the aneurysm sac with risk of aortic rupture. Endoleak is one of the major complications following endograft insertion. The value of TEE color Doppler in the early detection of endoleaks, and in improving the immediate and late

procedural results, is well documented (46,47). The endoleaks classification is shown in Table 24.2 and Figure 24.18 (48).

Type I endoleak occurs at the attachment sites and can involve the proximal (type IA) and/or distal ends of the endograft (type IB). They are usually large and result from incomplete adhesion of the endograft to the aortic wall. To decrease their occurrence, balloon inflation after endograft deployment is normally performed at the proximal and distal ends to mould the endograft to the aortic wall. Type II endoleak, or branch leak, is due to retrograde blood flow into the aneurysm sac from one or more aortic collateral vessels. Type III endoleak, or graft defect, is a result of inadequate apposition of overlapping endograft joints or a tear of the graft fabric. Type IV endoleak is due to blood flow into the aneurysm sac due to the porosity of the graft fabric. Type I and III endoleaks are clearly associated with future aneurysm expansion and should, therefore, be corrected by balloon dilation or additional endograft insertion. Type IV endoleak generally does not require any further intervention (Fig. 24.19).

Table 24.2   Classification Scheme for Endoleaks[a]

I. Attachment Site Leaks[b]
   A. Proximal end of endograft
   B. Distal end of endograft
   C. Iliac occluder (plug)
II. Branch leaks[c] (without attachment site connection)
   A. Simple or to-and-fro (from only 1 patent branch)
   B. Complex or flow-through (with 2 or more patent branches)
III. Graft defect[b]
   A. Junctional leak or modular disconnect
   B. Fabric disruption (midgraft hole)
     Minor ($<$2 mm; e.g., suture holes)
     Major ($\geq$2 mm)
IV. Graft wall (fabric) porosity ($<$30 days after graft placement)

[a]Endoleaks also can be classified on basis of the time of first detection as: *perioperative*, within 24 hours of endovascular aortic aneurysm repair (EVAR); *early*, 1 to 90 days after EVAR; and *late*, after 90 days. In addition, they can be described as *primary*, from time of EVAR; *secondary*, appearing only after not being present at time of EVAR; and *delayed*, occurring after prior negative computed tomography (CT) scan results.
Endoleaks also can be described as *persistent*, *transient* or *sealed*, *recurrent*, *treated successfully*, or *treated unsuccessfully*.
Endoleaks and endotension may be associated with abdominal aortic aneurysm (AAA) enlargement, stability, or shrinkage.
[b]Some type I and type III leaks also may have patent branches opening from AAA sac and providing outflow for leak.
[c]From lumbar, inferior mesenteric, hypogastric, renal, or other arteries.
Source: Adapted from Veith et al. 48.

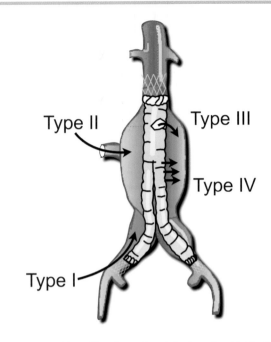

Figure 24.18   Classification of endoleaks. See Table 24.2.

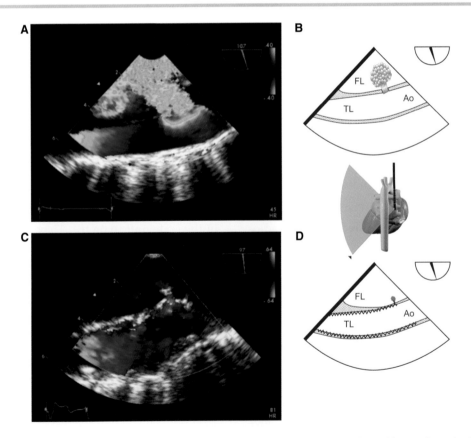

Figure 24.19   Type I endoleak. (A,B) Color Doppler descending Ao long-axis views in a patient with type B aortic dissection show the entry site between the TL and FL before repair. **(C,D)** After endograft insertion, residual flow at the proximal end of the device is still present (type I-A endoleak). *Abbreviations*: Ao, aorta; FL, false lumen; TL, true lumen.

TEE is the most sensitive tool for detecting endoleaks immediately after endograft deployment (49). Small endoleaks may be missed by angiography because the amount of dye within the leak is not detectable by fluoroscopy or because the imaging view is inadequate. The use of TEE is often superior to angiography in the detection and characterization of type I endoleaks, due to incomplete endograft apposition to the aortic wall. This is particularly useful in sections of the Ao that are highly curved such as the aortic arch. Endoleaks may also be better defined by TEE than by angiography because it is sometimes difficult to differentiate a transient type 4 endoleak from the more significant type 1 or 3 endoleaks immediately after endograft graft insertion (Fig. 24.19) (3,49). A pulsed wave (PW) Doppler velocity cutoff value of 50 cm/s has been advocated to enable differentiation of type IV endoleaks (slow blood flow) from type I or III endoleaks (high-velocity flows) (50) (Fig. 24.20).

Endoleaks that appear several weeks, months, or even years after the insertion of an endograft are called secondary endoleak. They are probably related to dislodgment of the endograft, to structural changes of the aortic wall, or to endoleaks that were simply not diagnosed at the time of insertion. Secondary endoleaks are the main cause of late treatment failure in the endovascular approach (51–53). Aneurysm expansion in the absence of visible endoleak has been reported with the hypothesis that endoleaks are not always visualized by current imaging methods, such as angiography or CT (54).

Side Branch Occlusion

Complete side branch occlusion following endograft insertion is a complication that is easy to identify by angiography. However, partial obstruction by the endograft membrane is difficult to demonstrate because the membrane is not radiopaque. Partial

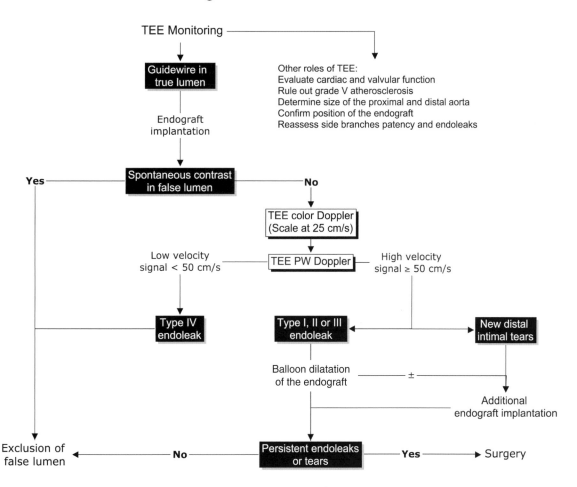

Figure 24.20 Endograft implantation for aortic dissection. The roles of TEE are to confirm the position of the guidewire in the true lumen, diagnose spontaneous echo contrast in the false lumen or persistent endoleaks and aortic wall tears. *Abbreviations*: PW, pulsed wave; TEE, transesophageal echocardiography. *Source*: Adapted from Ref. 50.

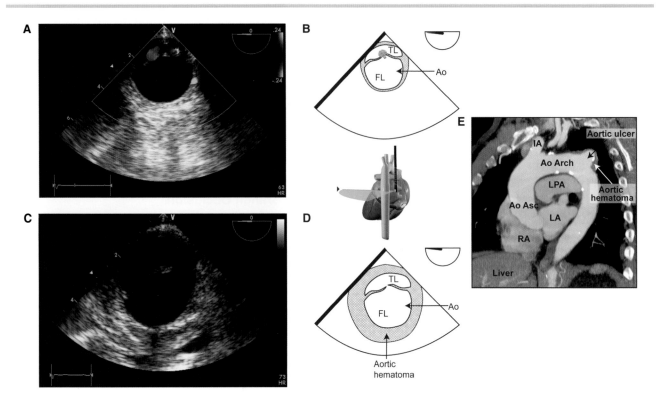

Figure 24.21   Complication of endograft procedure. A 62-year-old woman presents with a type B acute aortic dissection complicated by ischemic occlusion of the lower extremity. (**A,B**) Color Doppler descending Ao short-axis view shows the aortic dissection with the smaller TL. An endograft approach was selected. However, shortly following cannulation of the TL an acute aortic hematoma appeared (**C,D**) requiring urgent thoracotomy. *Abbreviations*: Ao, aorta; FL, false lumen; IA, innominate artery; LA, left atrium; LPA, left pulmonary artery; RA, right atrium; TL, true lumen.

obstruction may not be apparent during the intervention but may result in side branch vessel occlusion later on. Recognition of partial membranous obstruction during the intervention is important because this obstruction may be relieved by an endograft to the side branch ostium. The use of TEE may help identify these partial obstructions by demonstrating the membrane or the abnormal blood flow in the partially covered vessel.

Other Complications

During endograft implantation several complications, either immediate or delayed, can occur. The immediate complications include vascular access trauma, renal failure, bowel infarction, lower extremity embolism, paraplegia or paraparesis, and also lumen rupture that can manifest as spontaneous hematoma (Figs. 24.21 and 24.22) and the post-implantation syndrome. The latter consists of transient elevation of body temperature and C-reactive protein levels with back pain and mild leukocytosis. The role of TEE is paramount in the recognition of these immediate crit-

ical conditions that can mandate urgent surgical intervention. The other delayed complications can be related, or not, to the device. Those device-related complications include suture breakage, fabric erosion, endograft fracture, prolapse, migration, embolization, and infection. Bowel ischemia, expansion, and rupture of the treated aneurysm, and aortoesophageal or tracheal fistula have been described (55).

ENDOVASCULAR TREATMENT OF BLUNT TRAUMATIC THORACIC AORTIC INJURY

Blunt chest trauma is the most common cause of traumatic thoracic aortic injury (56). Four to 17% of patients with blunt chest trauma will have a thoracic aortic injury (57). The majority of aortic tears (80–90%) occur in the descending thoracic Ao at the aortic isthmus, just distal to the LSCA and proximal to the third intercostal artery (58). With sudden deceleration, the more mobile aortic arch swings forward, producing a combination of torsion, shearing, and bending stresses on the Ao at the isthmus, leading to disruption (58,59).

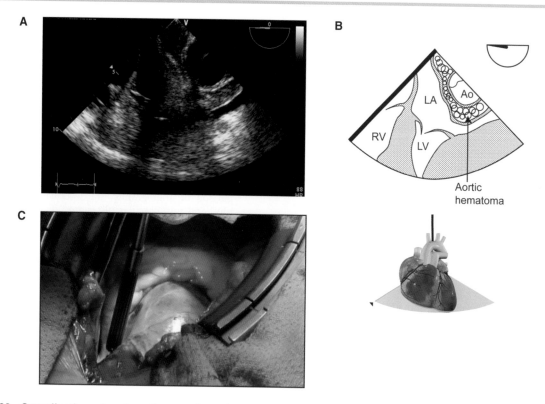

Figure 24.22 Complication of endograft procedure. (A,B) Mid-esophageal view shows an aortic hematoma compressing the LA causing an acute localized tamponade. **(C)** Intraoperative aspect the aortic dissection. *Abbreviations*: Ao, aorta; AoV, aortic valve; LA, left atrium; LV, left ventricle; RV, right ventricle.

Endovascular Endograft Repair

For nearly 50 years, open surgical repair of blunt traumatic thoracic aortic injury (BTTAI) has been the treatment of choice. This repair requires left thoracotomy, single lung ventilation, aortic-cross clamping with or without the adjunct use of partial or full cardiopulmonary bypass. The derived associated significant physiological stress leads to perioperative complications such as bleeding, myocardial infarction, stroke, respiratory failure, renal failure, bowel infarction, and paraplegia (59). The operative mortality rate from emergency open surgical repair of BTTAI is 15% to 30% and the incidence of paraplegia is 19% to 28.5%. Although distal perfusion techniques have reduced the rate of paraplegia, certain complications are associated with this technique partly because of the need for full systemic anticoagulation, which may adversely affect concomitant injuries involving the brain, liver, or lungs and result in fatal hemorrhagic outcome (59). Despite advances in critical care medicine, and refinement in surgical techniques, little change in perioperative mortality has occurred with open repair in patients with BTTAI. As a result endovascular repair of BTTAI has emerged as a less invasive treatment alternative (59).

Endovascular treatment of blunt thoracic aortic disruptions offers many practical benefits and technical advantages compared with conventional open repair. The deployment of an endograft in the descending Ao with a focal traumatic lesion allows immediate repair and avoidance of early mortality from aortic rupture.

Role of TEE in BTTAI

Aortography has long been considered the gold standard for the diagnosis of BTTAI (60). However, multiplane TEE and contrast-enhanced spiral CT of the chest have emerged as accurate alternative imaging modalities (61–63). Helical CT and TEE have a similar diagnostic accuracy in the identification of subadventitial injuries, located in the region of the aortic isthmus (64). The diagnostic accuracy of TEE for the identification of other aortic segments is unknown, and traumatic injuries to aortic branches are usually outside the scope of TEE. The TEE diagnosis of subadventitial BTTAI requires the presence of a disruption of the aortic wall with flow on both sides of the lesion that can be demonstrated by color Doppler imaging (63). The role of TEE in BTTAI is summarized in Table 24.3.

Table 24.3 Specific Steps for TEE Utilization in Endovascular Thoracic Aneurysm Repair

1. Before deployment of the endograft
   - Examine the entire ascending aorta, aortic arch, descending aorta.
   - Confirm the preoperative findings (CT scan or MRI).
   - Aortic pathology, plaques, dissection, aneurysm.
   - Aortic angulation and tortuosity.
   - Aortic thrombus and periaortic hematoma.
   - Aortic branch arteries.
   - Measurement of the landing zones (proximal and distal necks: aortic neck should be >15 mm) to confirm the proper size of the endograft. The size of the graft should be 15–20% larger than the aortic landing zone diameter. For example, a diameter of 40 mm will require an endograft of 46 mm.
   - Standard echocardiography exam and assess the systolic/diastolic functions.

2. During endograft deployment
   - Confirm the correct position of the guide wire.
   - Confirm the correct position of the device delivery system at the proximal landing zone immediately prior to deployment.
   - Confirm endograft deployment, expansion, and position.
   - If more than one endograft is used, advance the TEE probe to the distal end of the first endograft. The TEE probe can then be used as a landmark to position the next graft.

3. After deployment of the endograft
   - Document flow in the aorta with color flow Doppler.
   - Examine the graft for any endoleaks using color flow Doppler both in short and long axis.
   - Aliasing velocity for Doppler color flow may need to be reduced to 25 cm/s to detect low-flow endoleaks.
   - Results of ballooning at the site of a type I endoleak should be assessed with TEE and the presence of any residual leakage should be discussed with the vascular surgeon.
   - Efforts should be made to obtain the same aortic predeployment views.

Abbreviations: CT, computed tomography; MRI, magnetic resonance; TEE, transesophageal echocardiography.

CONCLUSION

Endovascular repair of aortic pathologies is a rapidly evolving field. Although fluoroscopy remains the main imaging device for the endovascular treatment of aortic pathologies, TEE is increasingly recognized as a valuable adjunct, especially in cases where low velocity flows are involved, or in cases of renal failure where the quantity of iodinated contrast media should be minimized. In patients with cardiac disease, TEE can be used to monitor cardiac function throughout the procedure. Limitations of TEE for the endovascular repair of aortic disease include the need for general anesthesia and inability to visualize the entire Ao. Despite these limitations the combination of fluoroscopy and TEE appears to be optimal for the proper placement, deployment, and identification of complications associated with endovascular devices.

REFERENCES

1. Dake MD, Miller DC, Semba CP, et al. Transluminal placement of endovascular stent-grafts for the treatment of descending thoracic aortic aneurysms. N Engl J Med 1994; 331:1729–1734.
2. Hagan PG, Nienaber CA, Isselbacher EM, et al. The International Registry of Acute Aortic Dissection (IRAD): new insights into an old disease. JAMA 2000; 283:897–903.
3. Fattori R, Caldarera I, Rapezzi C, et al. Primary endoleakage in endovascular treatment of the thoracic aorta: importance of intraoperative transesophageal echocardiography. J Thorac Cardiovasc Surg 2000; 120:490–495.
4. Koschyk DH, Nienaber CA, Knap M, et al. How to guide stent-graft implantation in type B aortic dissection? Comparison of angiography, transesophageal echocardiography, and intravascular ultrasound. Circulation 2005; 112: I260–I264.
5. Lee JT, White RA. Current status of thoracic aortic endograft repair. Surg Clin North Am 2004; 84:1295–1318, vi–vii.
6. Dale WA. The beginnings of vascular surgery. Surgery 1974; 76:849–866.
7. Baker B. Anaesthesia and endovascular surgery. Best Pract Res Clin Anaesthesiol 2002; 16:95–113.
8. Miller DC, Mitchell RS, Oyer PE, et al. Independent determinants of operative mortality for patients with aortic dissections. Circulation 1984; 70:I153–I164.
9. Crawford ES, Hess KR, Cohen ES, et al. Ruptured aneurysm of the descending thoracic and thoracoabdominal aorta. Analysis according to size and treatment. Ann Surg 1991; 213:417–425.
10. Fann JI, Smith JA, Miller DC et al. Surgical management of aortic dissection during a 30-year period. Circulation 1995; 92:II113–II121.
11. Brandt M, Hussel K, Walluscheck KP, et al. Early and long-term results of replacement of the descending aorta. Eur J Vasc Endovasc Surg 2005; 30:365–369.
12. Parodi JC, Palmaz JC, Barone HD. Transfemoral intraluminal graft implantation for abdominal aortic aneurysms. Ann Vasc Surg 1991; 5:491–499.
13. Duhaylongsod FG, Glower DD, Wolfe WG. Acute traumatic aortic aneurysm: the Duke experience from 1970 to 1990. J Vasc Surg 1992; 15:331–342.
14. Doss M, Balzer J, Martens S, et al. Surgical versus endovascular treatment of acute thoracic aortic rupture: a single-center experience. Ann Thorac Surg 2003; 76:1465–1469.
15. Nienaber CA, Ince H, Weber F, et al. Emergency stent-graft placement in thoracic aortic dissection and evolving rupture. J Card Surg 2003; 18:464–470.
16. Tse LW, MacKenzie KS, Montreuil B, et al. The proximal landing zone in endovascular repair of the thoracic aorta. Ann Vasc Surg 2004; 18:178–185.
17. Brandt M, Hussel K, Walluscheck KP, et al. Stent-graft repair versus open surgery for the descending aorta: a case-control study. J Endovasc Ther 2004; 11:535–538.
18. Rousseau H, Dambrin C, Marcheix B, et al. Acute traumatic aortic rupture: a comparison of surgical and stent-graft repair. J Thorac Cardiovasc Surg 2005; 129:1050–1055.
19. Iyer VS, MacKenzie KS, Tse LW, et al. Early outcomes after elective and emergent endovascular repair of the thoracic aorta. J Vasc Surg 2006; 43:677–683.
20. Mangano DT, Goldman L. Preoperative assessment of patients with known or suspected coronary disease. N Engl J Med 1995; 333:1750–1756.
21. Poldermans D, Boersma E, Bax JJ, et al. The effect of bisoprolol on perioperative mortality and myocardial infarction in high-risk patients undergoing vascular surgery. Dutch Echocardiographic Cardiac Risk Evaluation

Applying Stress Echocardiography Study Group. N Engl J Med 1999; 341:1789–1794.

22. Willens HJ, Kessler KM. Transesophageal echocardiography in the diagnosis of diseases of the thoracic aorta: part 1. Aortic dissection, aortic intramural hematoma, and penetrating atherosclerotic ulcer of the aorta. Chest 1999; 116:1772–1779.

23. Katz ES, Tunick PA, Rusinek H, et al. Protruding aortic atheromas predict stroke in elderly patients undergoing cardiopulmonary bypass: experience with intraoperative transesophageal echocardiography. J Am Coll Cardiol 1992; 20:70–77.

24. Smith DC, Bansal RC. Transesophageal echocardiography in the diagnosis of traumatic rupture of the aorta. N Engl J Med 1995; 333:457–458.

25. White GH, May J, Waugh RC, et al. Type I and Type II endoleaks: a more useful classification for reporting results of endoluminal AAA repair. J Endovasc Surg 1998; 5:189–191.

26. Fayad A. Images in Anesthesia. Transesophageal echocardiographic diagnosis of a failed balloon catheter during endovascular stenting of a descending thoracic aneurysm. Can J Anaesth 2007; 54:848–849.

27. Fayad A. A misplaced guide wire in the false lumen during endovascular repair of a type B aortic dissection. Can J Anaesth 2007; 54:947–948.

28. Fayad A. Echocardiography images of endovascular mal-aligned stent grafts. Can J Anaesth 2008; 55:306–307.

29. Amarenco P, Cohen A, Tzourio C, et al. Atherosclerotic disease of the aortic arch and the risk of ischemic stroke. N Engl J Med 1994; 331:1474–1479.

30. Davila-Roman VG, Murphy SF, Nickerson NJ, et al. Atherosclerosis of the ascending aorta is an independent predictor of long-term neurologic events and mortality. J Am Coll Cardiol 1999; 33:1308–1316.

31. Kazui S, Levi CR, Jones EF, et al. Lacunar stroke: transoesophageal echocardiographic factors influencing long-term prognosis. Cerebrovasc Dis 2001; 12:325–330.

32. Macleod MR, Amarenco P, Davis SM, et al. Atheroma of the aortic arch: an important and poorly recognised factor in the aetiology of stroke. Lancet Neurol 2004; 3:408–414.

33. Criado E, Wall P, Lucas P, et al. Transesophageal echo-guided endovascular exclusion of thoracic aortic mobile thrombi. J Vasc Surg 2004; 39:238–242.

34. Zhang WW, Abou-Zamzam AM, Hashisho M, et al. Staged endovascular stent grafts for concurrent mobile/ulcerated thrombi of thoracic and abdominal aorta causing recurrent spontaneous distal embolization. J Vasc Surg 2008; 47: 193–196.

35. Rossi PJ, Desai TR, Skelly CL, et al. Paravisceral aortic thrombus as a source of peripheral embolization—report of three cases and review of the literature. J Vasc Surg 2002; 36:839–843.

36. Dobson G, Petrasek P, Alvarez N. Images in Anesthesia: transesophageal echocardiography enhances endovascular stent placement in traumatic trans-section of the thoracic aorta. Can J Anaesth 2004; 51:931.

37. Orihashi K, Matsuura Y, Sueda T, et al. Flow velocity of central retinal artery and retrobulbar vessels during cardiovascular operations. J Thorac Cardiovasc Surg 1997; 114:1081–1087.

38. Denault AY, Deschamps A, Murkin JM. A proposed algorithm for the intraoperative use of cerebral near-infrared spectroscopy. Semin Cardiothorac Vasc Anesth 2007; 11:274–281.

39. Fattori R, Napoli G, Lovato L, et al. Indications for, timing of, and results of catheter-based treatment of traumatic injury to the aorta. AJR Am J Roentgenol 2002; 179:603–609.

40. Czermak BV, Waldenberger P, Perkmann R, et al. Placement of endovascular stent-grafts for emergency treatment of acute disease of the descending thoracic aorta. AJR Am J Roentgenol 2002; 179:337–345.

41. Royse CF, Bird H, Royse AG. Routine assessment of coeliac axis and renal artery flow is not feasible with transoesophageal echocardiography. Anaesthesia 2009; 64:103–104.

42. Kahn RA, Moskowitz DM, Marin ML, et al. Safety and efficacy of high-dose adenosine-induced asystole during endovascular AAA repair. J Endovasc Ther 2000; 7: 292–296.

43. Nienaber CA, Kische S, Rehders TC, et al. Rapid pacing for better placing: comparison of techniques for precise deployment of endografts in the thoracic aorta. J Endovasc Ther 2007; 14:506–512.

44. Pornratanarangsi S, Webster MW, Alison P, et al. Rapid ventricular pacing to lower blood pressure during endograft deployment in the thoracic aorta. Ann Thorac Surg 2006; 81:e21–e23.

45. Moon MC, Dowdall JF, Roselli EE. The use of right ventricular pacing to facilitate stent graft deployment in the distal aortic arch: a case report. J Vasc Surg 2008; 47:629–631.

46. Aadahl P, Saether OD, Aakhus S, et al. The importance of transesophageal echocardiography during surgery of the thoracic aorta. Eur J Vasc Endovasc Surg 1996; 12:401–406.

47. Moskowitz DM, Kahn RA, Konstadt SN, et al. Intraoperative transoesophageal echocardiography as an adjuvant to fluoroscopy during endovascular thoracic aortic repair. Eur J Vasc Endovasc Surg 1999; 17:22–27.

48. Veith FJ, Baum RA, Ohki T, et al. Nature and significance of endoleaks and endotension: summary of opinions expressed at an international conference. J Vasc Surg 2002; 35:1029–1035.

49. Swaminathan M, Lineberger CK, McCann RL, et al. The importance of intraoperative transesophageal echocardiography in endovascular repair of thoracic aortic aneurysms. Anesth Analg 2003; 97:1566–1572.

50. Rocchi G, Lofiego C, Biagini E, et al. Transesophageal echocardiography-guided algorithm for stent-graft implantation in aortic dissection. J Vasc Surg 2004; 40:880–885.

51. White GH, Yu W, May J, et al. Endoleak as a complication of endoluminal grafting of abdominal aortic aneurysms: classification, incidence, diagnosis, and management. J Endovasc Surg 1997; 4:152–168.

52. Golzarian J, Struyven J, Abada HT, et al. Endovascular aortic stent-grafts: transcatheter embolization of persistent perigraft leaks. Radiology 1997; 202:731–734.

53. Mitchell RS, Miller DC, Dake MD, et al. Thoracic aortic aneurysm repair with an endovascular stent graft: the "first generation". Ann Thorac Surg 1999; 67:1971–1974.

54. Alimi YS, Chakfe N, Rivoal E, et al. Rupture of an abdominal aortic aneurysm after endovascular graft placement and aneurysm size reduction. J Vasc Surg 1998; 28:178–183.

55. Gowda RM, Misra D, Tranbaugh RF, et al. Endovascular stent grafting of descending thoracic aortic aneurysms. Chest 2003; 124:714–719.

56. Marx JA, Hockberger RS, Walls RM, et al. Rosen's Emergency Medicine Concepts and Clinical Practice. 6th ed. St. Louis: Mosby, 2006.

57. Kaplan JA. Kaplan's Cardiac Anesthesia. 5th ed. Philadelphia, PA: Elsevier Saunders, 2006.

58. Schumacher H, Bockler D, von Tengg-Kobligk H, et al. Acute traumatic aortic tear: open versus stent-graft repair. Semin Vasc Surg 2006; 19:48–59.

59. Lin PH, Bush RL, Zhou W, et al. Endovascular treatment of traumatic thoracic aortic injury–should this be the new standard of treatment? J Vasc Surg 2006; 43(suppl A): 22A–29A.

60. Ben-Menachem Y. Assessment of blunt aortic-brachioce-phalic trauma: should angiography be supplanted by trans-esophageal echocardiography? J Trauma 1997; 42:969–972.

61. Patel NH, Stephens KE Jr., Mirvis SE, et al. Imaging of acute thoracic aortic injury due to blunt trauma: a review. Radiology 1998; 209:335–348.

62. Collier B, Hughes KM, Mishok K, et al. Is helical computed tomography effective for diagnosis of blunt aortic injury? Am J Emerg Med 2002; 20:558–561.

63. Cinnella G, Dambrosio M, Brienza N, et al. Transesopha-geal echocardiography for diagnosis of traumatic aortic injury: an appraisal of the evidence. J Trauma 2004; 57:1246–1255.

64. Vignon P, Boncoeur MP, Francois B, et al. Comparison of multiplane transesophageal echocardiography and con-trast-enhanced helical CT in the diagnosis of blunt trau-matic cardiovascular injuries. Anesthesiology 2001; 94: 615–622.

25

Intracavitary Contents

Maria Di Lorenzo, Robert Amyot, Réal Lebeau, and Claude Sauvé
Université de Montréal, Montreal, Canada

Marjan Jariani and R.J. Cusimano
University of Toronto, Toronto, Canada

INTRODUCTION

Transesophageal echocardiography (TEE) has become a powerful clinical tool that offers a wide range of diagnostic capabilities. It is, however, important to acknowledge its limitations. Although the improvement in image quality heightens the ability to detect cardiac masses, echocardiography still cannot define the histology of these masses.

Information about the size, location, origin, site of attachment, consistency, mobility of a mass, as well as associated heart disease can lead to a differential diagnosis that will suggest the most likely diagnosis. Using both clinical data and echocardiographic findings can then lead to the best therapeutic approach.

As discussed in Chapter 7, pitfalls are normal cardiac structures that can be misinterpreted as an abnormal mass or tumor. The majority of pathological cardiac masses, thrombus, tumor, or vegetations are reviewed in this chapter.

PRIMARY CARDIAC NEOPLASM

Tumors in the heart most often represent metastases from other primary neoplasms. Primary cardiac tumors are much less common with a prevalence of 0.02% reported in a large autopsy series (1). Benign tumors account for 75% of all primary cardiac tumors, three times more frequent than malignant tumors (Fig. 25.1). Myxoma, the most common benign tumor, has an incidence of approximately 0.5 per million population per year. On the other hand, sarcomas constitute the majority of malignant primary cardiac tumors. Tumors involving the heart may be intracavitary, intramural, or extracardiac, though most atrial tumors present as an intracavitary mass, whereas ventricular tumors are usually intramural.

Benign Cardiac Tumors

Myxomas

Myxomas represent nearly 50% of all histologically benign tumors of the heart. They occur most often in women at a mean age of 50. When present in a younger population, they are usually familial and part of a complex of multiple tumors that tend to recur. These tumors generally have a jellylike, globular appearance (Fig. 25.2). They are usually pedunculated, polypoid, and friable. Some may have a smooth surface and may be round. Echocardiographically they have a heterogeneous appearance with echo-free spaces present within the mass that correspond to areas of hemorrhage or necrosis and/or areas of calcification. At the time of diagnosis, myxomas have an average size of 4 to 8 cm but have been known to reach up to 15 cm.

Approximately 75% of cardiac myxomas classically involve the left atrium (LA), presenting as a mobile echogenic mass found in the body of the LA, usually attached to the interatrial septum by a stalk in the region of the fossa ovalis (Fig. 25.3). An additional 10% arise from other sites within the LA including the posterior wall, the anterior wall, or the left atrial appendage (LAA). Most remaining myxomas originate from the right atrium (RA); the right ventricle (RV) or left ventricle (LV) is implicated in approximately 5% of series. Some cases, arising from the mitral valve (MV) and the inferior vena cava (IVC), have also been reported. The diagnosis may be challenging when the stalk is short and difficult to visualize, and when the tumor is not very mobile or arises from an atypical location (1,2).

TEE is highly sensitive to detect LA tumors and is particularly useful in delineating the attachment or the tumor stalk that, as mentioned, narrows the differential diagnosis. Besides an accurate description of the size, shape, location, and attachment of the myxoma, TEE can also evaluate the degree of mitral inflow obstruction by the mass (Fig. 25.4). The mobility of the tumor and its variable excursion across the MV into the LV will depend both on the size of the mass and the length of the pedicle. Tumors with a long pedicle can be seen moving back and forth through the mitral orifice during the cardiac cycle.

Right atrial myxomas tend to be broader based than left-sided tumors and involve a larger area of the atrial wall or septum (Fig. 25.3). Ventricular myxomas may originate from the ventricular septum with either a pedunculated or a sessile appearance.

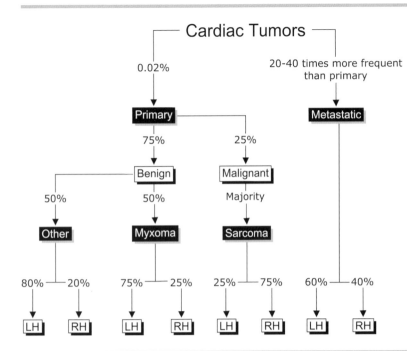

Figure 25.1 Cardiac tumors. A classification for cardiac tumors is presented. Abbreviations: LH, left heart; RH, right heart. *Source*: Adapted from Ref. 1.

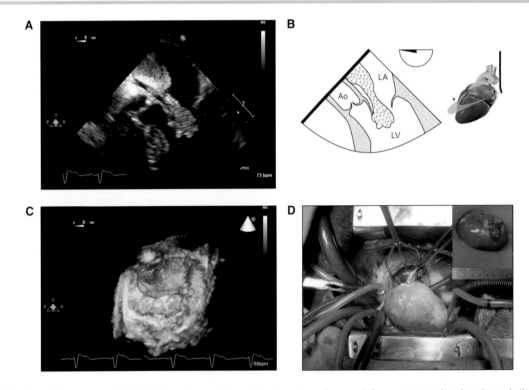

Figure 25.2 Left atrial myxoma. (A,B) Mid-esophageal four-chamber view shows a LA myxoma prolapsing through the mitral valve and partially obstructing flow. The mass is shown from the LA in the surgeon's orientation using 3D transesophageal echocardiography **(C)** confirmed with the intraoperative findings **(D)**. *Abbreviations*: Ao, aorta; LA, left atrium; LV, left ventricle.

Multiple tumors can be found in the same chamber or in different chambers. As multifocal myxomas have been reported in up to 5% of patients, a complete examination of all four cardiac chambers is mandatory. The most common pattern is biatrial (Fig. 25.3). Recurrence of tumors after surgical resection has been reported in 5% to 14% of cases, at the site of the original tumor, at multiple intracardiac sites, or

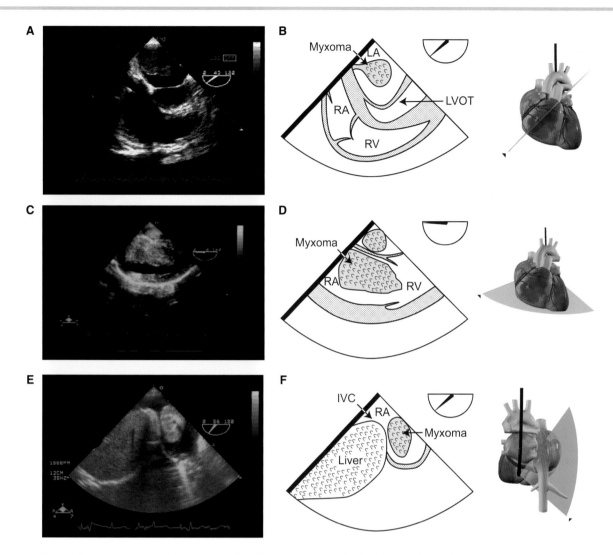

Figure 25.3 Atrial myxomas. (A,B) ME view at 42° shows a myxoma in the LA with the pedicle attached to the interatrial septum before surgical resection. **(C,D)** ME view displays a biatrial myxoma near the fossa ovalis. **(E,F)** Transgastric IVC long-axis view shows a right atrial myxoma at the junction of the IVC and RA. *Abbreviations*: IVC, inferior vena cava; LA, left atrium; LVOT, left ventricular outflow tract; ME, mid-esophageal; RA, right atrium; RV, right ventricle.

even at extracardiac sites (2–4). Serial follow-up echo-cardiographic studies are, therefore, recommended after surgical treatment. Left atrial myxoma arising from the interatrial septum is removed *en bloc* with a 5 mm margin of normal tissue. The fossa ovalis needs to be excised and is often repaired with a native pericardial patch (3).

Fibromas

Nearly all cardiac fibromas present as a solitary mass involving the ventricular myocardium, frequently in the septum, the apex, or the LV free wall. On two-dimensional (2D) echocardiography, they are recognized as a large mass well demarcated from the surrounding myocardium by multiple calcifications (Fig. 25.5) (5), which may be difficult to differentiate from a solitary rhabdomyoma. When located at the apex, they can mimic the apical form of hypertrophic cardiomyopathy.

Cardiac fibromas can occur in patients of all ages and in both sexes but they are more frequent in children, often diagnosed in the first year of life. It is the second most common primary cardiac tumor in the pediatric age group (2–4). Although it is a benign, low-grade connective tissue tumor, its slow continuous growth may interfere with LV filling and lead to obstruction. These tumors also encroach on, or invade, the conduction system resulting in the left and right bundle branches or generating various arrhythmias. Complete excision may be necessary when medical therapy does not control symptoms or arrhythmias (4).

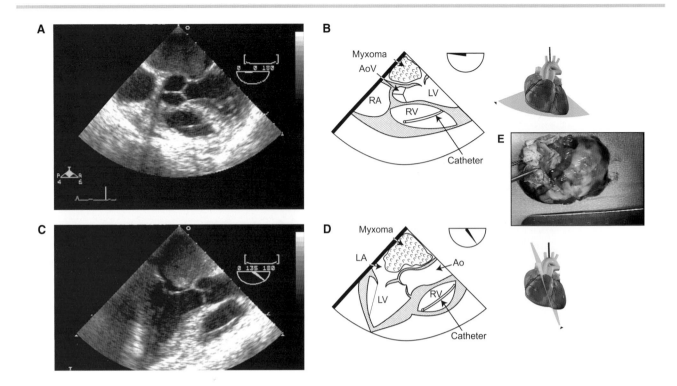

Figure 25.4   Left atrial myxoma. (A–D) Mid-esophageal views in a 61-year-old woman show a large myxoma occupying almost all the LA cavity compared with the intraoperative specimen (**E**). *Abbreviations*: Ao, aorta; AoV, aortic valve; LA, left atrium; LV, left ventricle; RA, right atrium; RV, right ventricle.

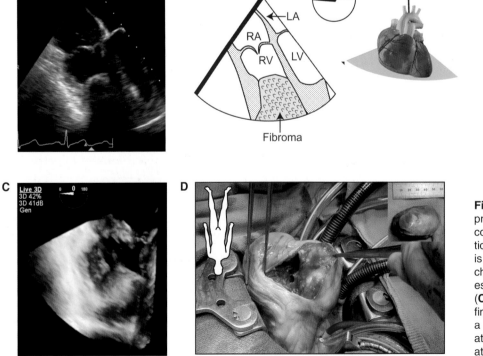

Figure 25.5 Fibroma. A patient presents with a tumor of the RV for complete resection and reconstruction with pericardial patch. The mass is seen in the mid-esophageal four-chamber view (**A,B**) and 3D trans-esophageal echocardiographic view (**C**) confirmed with the intraoperative findings (**D**). Pathology demonstrated a fibroma. *Abbreviations*: LA, left atrium; LV, left ventricle; RA, right atrium; RV, right ventricle.

Rhabdomyomas

Rhabdomyomas represent the most common benign cardiac tumors in infants and children. It is uncommon to find them at the atrial level as they tend to occur in the ventricles. No cases of rhabdomyomas attached to the cardiac valves have been reported. Most patients have multiple intramural or intracavitary tumors occurring with nearly equal frequency in the RV and LV, including the ventricular septum. Rhabdomyomas can present as a solitary intramural echo-dense mass in the ventricular septum or the LV free wall. A strong association between rhabdomyomas and tuberous sclerosis has been described (3,4). Most of these tumors regress spontaneously and thus surgery is required only if arrhythmias or obstruction to flow is not controlled by medical therapy.

Lipomas

Cardiac lipomas occur most often in the LV or the RA but can be seen throughout the heart including the pericardium and rarely attached to valves. These benign tumors occur at all ages and are seen with equal frequency in men and women. Cardiac lipomas can be subendocardial and have a sessile appearance. They can also present as a large subepicardial pedunculated mass. Approximately 25% of lipomas are completely intramyocardial. Compared with LV myxomas, lipomas are less mobile, generally more echo-dense and usually spare the fossa ovalis. The echocardiographic diagnosis of a lipoma remains difficult as it can mimic myxomas, fibromas, papillary fibroelastomas, and thrombi. Magnetic resonance imaging (MRI) may help confirm the fatty nature of the tumor (3,4).

Papillary Fibroelastomas and Lambl's Excrescences

Papillary fibroelastomas, or papillomas, are benign tumors that are clinically important because of their potential for systemic embolization. They represent a small fraction of all primary cardiac tumors but are the most common type of primary valve tumor. They can still be found anywhere in the heart (Fig. 25.5) and have been described in atypical locations such as the LAA (6). They can occur in any age group although they are most common in patients >60 years of age, usually affecting the aortic valve (AoV) (Fig. 25.6) (7). Fibroelastomas tend to arise in areas of endocardial damage such as the sites of valvular sclerosis, rheumatic heart disease, or cardiac surgery. When the atrioventricular valves are affected the tumor is usually attached on the atrial surface. When present on the semilunar valves, the tumor appears on either the ventricular or the arterial surface.

A typical papillary fibroelastoma appears on echocardiography as a small pedunculated, homogeneous, well-demarcated mobile mass attached by a small stalk (Fig. 25.7). Located at the mid portion or

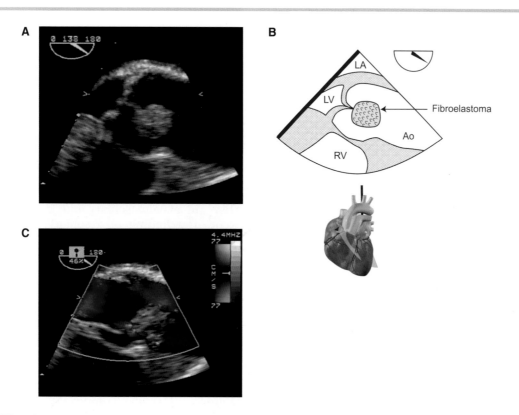

Figure 25.6 Fibroelastoma. (A,B) An asymptomatic 45-year-old woman presenting with a "pom-pom"–like mass attached to the AoV is shown in the mid-esophageal AoV long-axis view. **(C)** Color Doppler imaging shows no obstruction to flow through the AoV. Pathology demonstrated a fibroelastoma. *Abbreviations*: Ao, aorta; AoV, aortic valve; LA, left atrium; LV, left ventricle; LA, left atrium.

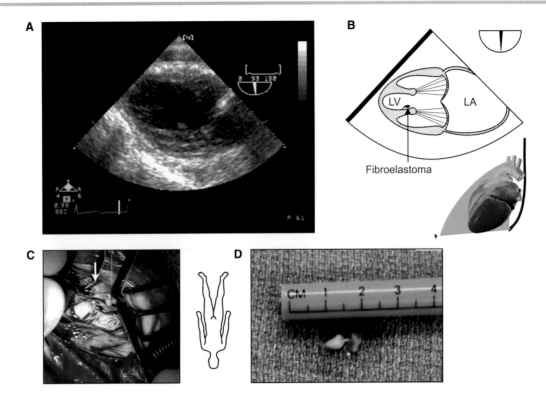

Figure 25.7   Fibroelastoma. Transgastric long-axis view (**A,B**) in a 65-year-old woman scheduled for mitral valve repair shows an incidental fibroelastoma attached to the anterior papillary muscle, confirmed with the intraoperative findings (**C**) and pathological specimen (**D**). *Abbreviations*: LA, left atrium; LV, left ventricle. *Source*: Photos C and D courtesy of Dr. Michel Pellerin.

body of the valve, the stalk usually has a broader base than a Lambl's excrescence.

As the resolution of echocardiography improves, so does the sensitivity of TEE in detecting intracardiac masses. Subtle structures can be seen and be confused with tumors or vegetations (Fig. 25.8).

Most important of these are Lambl's excrescences or valvular strands (Fig. 25.9), the prevalence of which increases with age. They consist of connective tissue with an elastin-like center, likely due to degenerative changes of the valves, but they have not been clearly associated with embolic events (8). They are more commonly seen attached to the free edge of the AoV cusps or on the ventricular surface of the cusps. They can also be found on the atrial surface of the MV. They can reach several millimeters in length but are usually very thin. Their independent random motion, particularly when they are long, mimics the appearance of filamentous vegetations and without the clinical context; the echocardiographic differentiation between the two may be difficult. The distinction between the Lambl's excrescence and a fibroelastoma can also be difficult.

Lambl's excrescences are also often detected on prosthetic valves in asymptomatic patients, in the absence of infection. Higher or harmonic frequencies and better temporal resolution make them increasingly common findings.

Surgical resection of a fibroelastoma is suggested if symptomatic emboli have occurred or if the lesion is highly mobile in an asymptomatic patient. Surgery is curative, safe, and well tolerated. Careful excision of the tumor to avoid fragmentation and embolization is usually followed by valve repair. It is the procedure of choice and has a high success rate.

Hemangiomas

Hemangiomas are benign proliferations of endothelial cells that form channels containing blood. These tumors can be intramural or intracavitary and can occur anywhere in the heart or pericardium, but are more common in the right-sided cardiac chambers. They are usually solitary but multiple tumors can occur. The finding of a solitary, sessile mass with echo-lucent areas associated with a pericardial effusion favors the diagnosis of a hemangioma rather than a myxoma or a rhabdomyoma (Fig. 25.10) (9). They are often an incidental lesion discovered on chest X-ray (CXR). Potential complications reported include chamber compression, ventricular outflow tract obstruction, pericardial effusion from tumor rupture, compression of the coronaries, and arrhythmias (10). Cardiac hemangiomas are usually cured by surgical resection. Insertion of a synthetic graft is often needed.

Malignant Cardiac Tumors

Thymomas

Thymomas are mainly tumors of the anterior mediastinum. They often present as an extracardiac mass

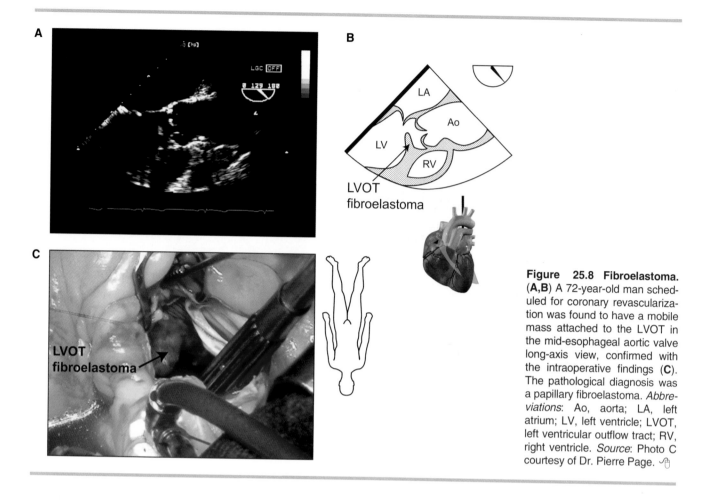

Figure 25.8 Fibroelastoma. **(A,B)** A 72-year-old man scheduled for coronary revascularization was found to have a mobile mass attached to the LVOT in the mid-esophageal aortic valve long-axis view, confirmed with the intraoperative findings (**C**). The pathological diagnosis was a papillary fibroelastoma. *Abbreviations*: Ao, aorta; LA, left atrium; LV, left ventricle; LVOT, left ventricular outflow tract; RV, right ventricle. *Source*: Photo C courtesy of Dr. Pierre Page. ⌐

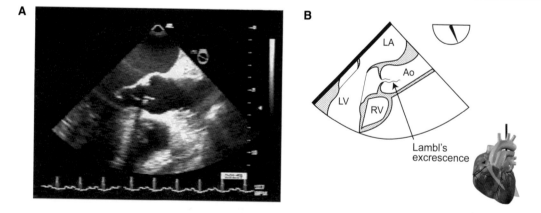

Figure 25.9 Lambl's excrescence. (A,B) Mid-esophageal long-axis view shows Lambl's excrescence on the aortic valve. *Abbreviations*: Ao, aorta; LA, left atrium; LV, left ventricle; RV, right ventricle. *Source*: Courtesy of Dr. François Béïque. ⌐

compressing a cardiac chamber. When no evidence of mediastinal involvement can be found, the pericardium can be deemed the primary site of origin (Fig. 25.11).

Lymphomas

Primary lymphomas of the heart, also known as lymphosarcomas, involve only the heart and the

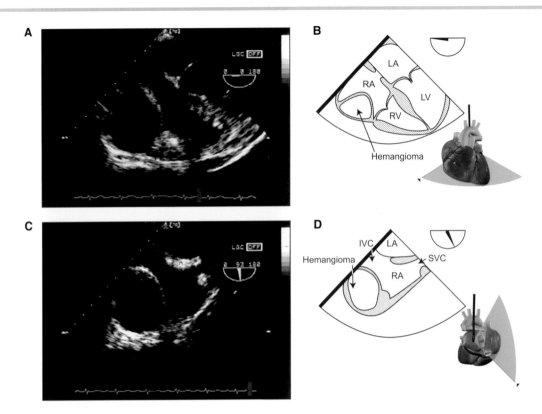

Figure 25.10 Cardiac hemangioma. Mid-esophageal four-chamber (**A,B**) and two-chamber (**C,D**) views show a large echolucent unilocular mass causing partial compression of the RA. A vague, curvilinear echodensity is seen within the mass, possibly representing trabeculum within the hemangioma. *Abbreviations*: IVC, inferior vena cava; LA, left atrium; LV, left ventricle; RA, right atrium; RV, right ventricle; SVC, superior vena cava. *Source*: Adapted with permission from Ref. 9.

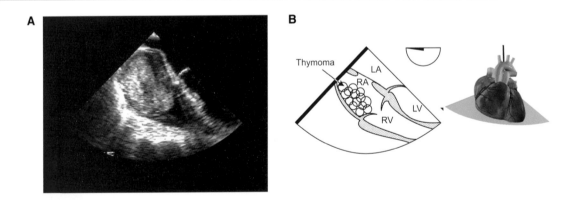

Figure 25.11 Thymoma. (A,B) Mid-esophageal four-chamber view in a 40-year-old man shows a recurrent thymoma in the RA. He presented a few months before with a large mediastinal mass and the diagnosis of a thymoma was made at the time. *Abbreviations*: LA, left atrium; LV, left ventricle; RA, right atrium; RV, right ventricle.

pericardium. They have been found in patients ranging from 14 months to 84 years of age but are extremely rare. An increased incidence of cardiac lymphomas has been noted in patients with acquired immunodeficiency syndrome (AIDS) and in trans-plant recipients under immunosuppressive therapy. Cardiac involvement in patient with non-Hodgkin's lymphoma and disseminated disease is more common than in primary cardiac lymphoma and occurs in up to 20% of cases.

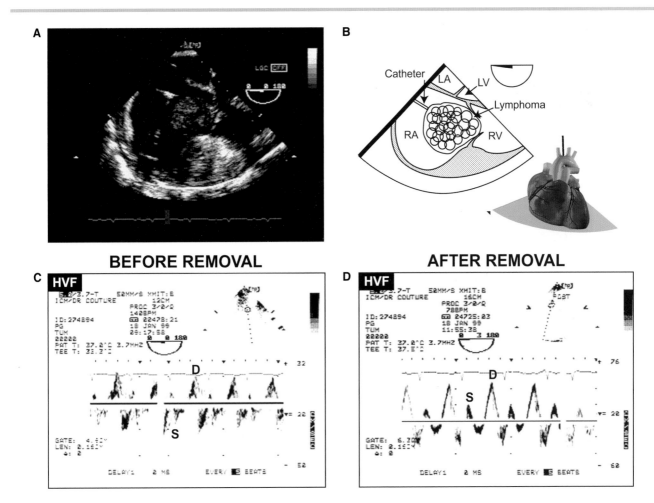

Figure 25.12 Lymphoma. (A,B) Mid-esophageal four-chamber view in a 62-year-old man shows a cardiac mass in the RA obstructing the tricuspid valve at the atrioventricular junction and infiltrating the lateral annulus. HVF pulsed wave Doppler demonstrates systolic flow reversal before removal (**C**) and improved systolic forward flow after removal of the mass (**D**). *Abbreviations*: D, peak diastolic HVF velocity; HVF, hepatic venous flow; LA, left atrium; LV, left ventricle; RA, right atrium; RV, right ventricle; S, peak systolic HVF velocity.

Lymphomas may involve various cardiac sites but right-sided involvement is more frequent followed by pericardium, RV, LA, and LV involvement. Myocardial infiltration can be diffuse or with multiple intracavitary nodules sometimes filling the LV apex resembling a thrombus. They can also mimic hypertrophic cardiomyopathy with thickening of the ventricular septum and lateral free wall (Fig. 25.12) (3,4,11). Treatment is usually not surgical. A combination of chemotherapy and radiotherapy is often used. Palliative surgery and tumor debulking can be done for relief of symptoms.

Angiosarcomas

Malignant cardiac tumors are predominantly sarcomas, most commonly angiosarcomas and rhabdomyosarcomas. Angiosarcoma occurs chiefly in men and 80% originate in the RA (Fig. 25.13). Some can be found within blood vessels (Fig. 25.14) giving rise to large mural masses that invade the pericardium, the

venae cavae, or the tricuspid valve (TV) (12). Extensive involvement of the pericardium resulting in constriction or hemopericardium is seen in 30% to 40% of cases (3,4).

Rhabdomyosarcomas

Rhabdomyosarcomas are the second most common primary sarcoma of the heart occurring in 25% of cases in patients <20 years of age. They can arise in any cardiac chamber and be multiple. Local pericardial and valvular invasion is frequent. They begin intramural but grow into adjacent cardiac chambers (3,4).

Primary Extraskeletal Osteosarcomas

Within the heart, primary extraskeletal osteosarcomas commonly arise from the LA, usually on the posterior wall close to the insertion of the pulmonary veins into the LA. These tumors can be mobile and prolapse into the mitral orifice at times. They can be

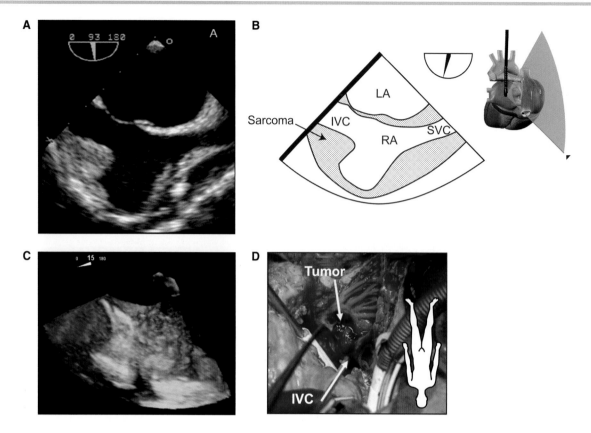

Figure 25.13 Right atrial sarcoma. A patient presents with a mass at the junction of the IVC and the RA. The tumor is visualized in the RA close to the IVC using 2D bicaval (**A,B**) and 3D TEE full volume (**C**) views confirmed by the intraoperative findings (**D**). Surgery consisted of resection of the tumor together with part of the IVC and RA under circulatory arrest. *Abbreviations*: IVC, inferior vena cava; LA, left atrium; RA, right atrium; SVC, superior vena cava.

differentiated from a myxoma by their site of attachment and their extension into the pulmonary veins. They often infiltrate the atrial wall. These tumors have also been described in the RA and RV. Metastatic osteosarcomas are more common. They can affect multiple sites within the heart. These tumors are often calcified, a useful feature for the diagnosis (3,4).

Mesotheliomas

Mesotheliomas represent the third most common malignant tumor of the heart and pericardium. They arise from the visceral or parietal pericardium and are more common in men than women. The majority of pericardial mesotheliomas diffusely cover the parietal and visceral pericardium encasing the heart. Solitary or localized tumors are extremely rare. Mesotheliomas invade adjacent structures, including the heart but only superficially. This may help differentiate between mesotheliomas and primary sarcomas as the latter can also invade the pericardium but almost always displays a large intramyocardial or intracavitary content (3,4). Primary cardiac mesothelioma is not associated with asbestosis exposure.

NONCARDIAC NEOPLASM INVADING THE HEART

Invasion of the heart by metastatic tumors occurs 20 to 40 times more frequently than primary cardiac tumors. Approximately 10% of patients with malignant neoplasm have cardiac metastases but only a small fraction of these patients have clinical evidence of such metastases. The most common neoplasms that produce cardiac metastases are lung tumors in men and breast cancer in women (Fig. 25.15). Lymphomas, leukemias, and melanomas are also often metastatic to the heart via hematogenous spread. Malignant tumors from every organ and tissue type have been reported to metastasize to the heart, with the exception of primary tumors of the central nervous system.

In most patients, clinical symptoms are the result of pericardial effusion, neoplastic thickening of the pericardium, or both. Wall thickening or protrusion of a tumor mass into a cardiac chamber may often produce obstruction. Lung tumors such as bronchogenic carcinomas can invade the heart through the pulmonary veins. Renal cell carcinomas, hepatomas, and uterine leiomyomas may all extend along the IVC into the RA (Fig. 25.16).

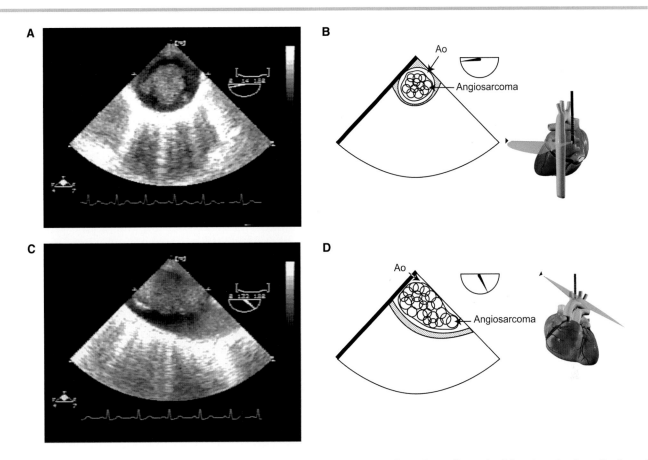

Figure 25.14 Aortic angiosarcoma. A 55-year-old woman was referred to the echocardiography laboratory for investigation of recurrent transient ischemic attacks. Mid-esophageal descending Ao short-axis (**A,B**) and upper esophageal aortic arch long-axis (**C,D**) views demonstrate a large aortic mass. Surgical removal was complicated with multiple emboli to the lower limbs. Biopsy revealed an angiosarcoma. *Abbreviation*: Ao, aorta.

CALCIFIED STRUCTURES

Calcified cardiac structures can be recognized by their bright, highly echogenic appearance associated with acoustic shadowing. Calcifications are not limited to the annular or submitral areas as they are frequently seen extending throughout the base of the heart to involve both the MV and AoV. Annular calcifications are usually immobile, and this immobility together with the location and their bright appearance are helpful in differentiating these masses from pathological tumors.

Calcification of the mitral apparatus is commonly associated with mitral regurgitation (MR) and sometimes with some degree of mitral inflow obstruction. Caseous calcification is a rare form of mitral annular calcification (13) (see Fig. 16.8) that appears as a large, round mass containing a central area of echolucencies. Misdiagnosis of this structure as myocardial abscess or tumor has led to cardiotomy in certain cases. Absence of systemic symptoms would favor the diagnosis of caseous calcification especially if located posteriorly and associated with dense calcification.

Extensive calcification of the mitral apparatus has been described in patients on chronic dialysis.

The calcification can extend to the papillary muscles and to the base of the mitral leaflets. They have also been described extending into the LA as unusual projecting nodules or excrescences (Fig. 25.17). Large calcific areas can also occur at the crux in the intervalvular fibrosa (14).

EXTRACARDIAC MASSES

Pericardial Cyst

Pericardial cysts are uncommon thoracic masses. They are usually detected on CXR in asymptomatic patients. The cysts are more commonly located at the right heart border and approximately 8% of them may project into the anterosuperior or the posterior mediastinum. Their dimensions range from 1 to 15 cm in diameter. They sometimes have a multilobular appearance and occasionally communicate with the pericardial cavity. Echocardiography reveals a spherical cystic echo-free space contiguous to the heart (see Fig. 12.24) and can, therefore, help rule out other tumors such as lipomas, lymphangiomas, leiomyomas, benign and malignant teratomas, mesotheliomas, thymomas, and sarcomas

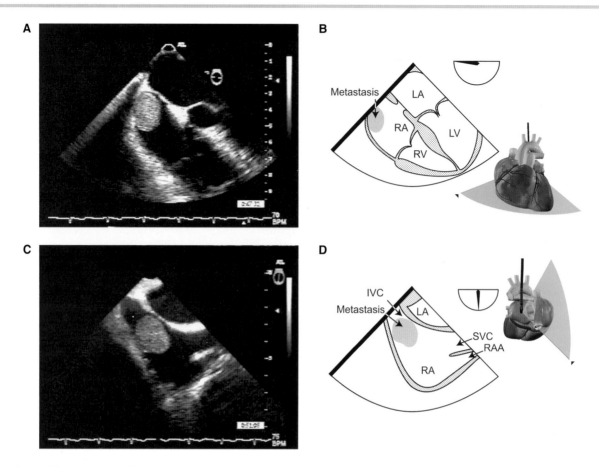

Figure 25.15   Breast cancer. Mid-esophageal four-chamber (**A,B**) and bicaval (**C,D**) views in a 60-year-old woman with a history of metastatic breast cancer, increasing dyspnea and right heart failure. A large mass was seen in the RA consistent with tumor metastasis. *Abbreviations*: IVC, inferior vena cava; LA, left atrium; LV, left ventricle; RA, right atrium; RAA, right atrial appendage; RV, right ventricle; SVC, superior vena cava. 🖰

(15). Aneurysms of saphenous venous bypass graft can also be similar in appearance (Fig. 25.18) (16).

Miscellaneous

Various extracardiac masses may compress the heart. A large thrombus, compressing the right or left cardiac chambers, is occasionally diagnosed in patients after cardiac surgery. As the usual clinical findings of cardiac tamponade may be absent and the localized cardiac compression may be missed by transthoracic echocardiography (TTE), TEE is required when the diagnosis is suspected in the hemodynamically unstable postoperative patient (see Chapter 12). Hiatal and diaphragmatic hernia, hepatic cyst, lung tumor, esophageal hematoma (Fig. 25.19), large goiter (Fig. 25.20), and aortic aneurysm have been also described as an extracardiac mass impinging on the heart.

INTUSSUSCEPTION OF THE LAA

Immediately following cardiac surgery, the finding of a new left atrial mass not present previously on the preoperative study has been reported as the result of an invagination of the LAA into the LA (Fig. 25.21). The long-term consequence of this phenomenon, if not corrected intraoperatively, remains unknown (17).

INTRACARDIAC THROMBI

Left Ventricular Thrombus

Left ventricular thrombi occur in conditions associated with stasis of blood and/or regional wall motion abnormalities such as severe LV systolic dysfunction, myocardial infarction, or LV aneurysm. Echocardiographically, it appears as a mass superimposed on and interrupting the normal endocardial contour of a myocardial wall with severely decreased contractility. These thrombi are most often located at the akinetic or dyskinetic apex of the LV (Fig. 25.22). The diagnosis is further supported by the presence of associated spontaneous echo contrast (SEC), an indicator of decreased blood flow velocity, described as dynamic smoke-like echoes with a characteristic swirling or layering pattern.

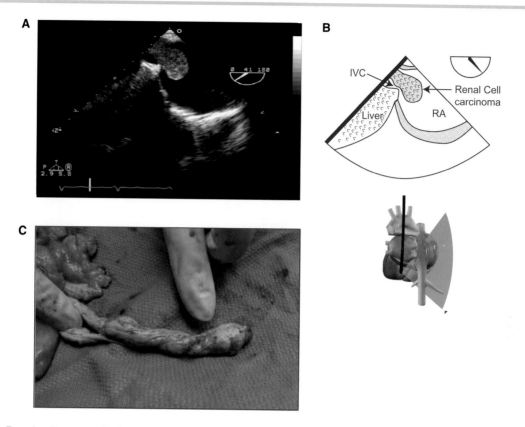

Figure 25.16   Renal cell cancer. An 80-year-old female presents with a history of palpitations and a left renal cell carcinoma extending into her IVC. (**A,B**) Lower esophageal view at 41° at the junction of the IVC and RA shows the mass partially obstructing the IVC. (**C**) Excised specimen showing the tumor portion in the IVC. *Abbreviations*: IVC, inferior vena cava; RA, right atrium.

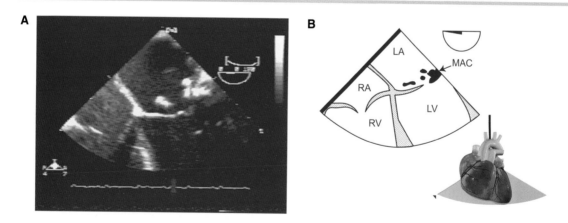

Figure 25.17   Mitral annular calcification. (**A,B**) Mid-esophageal four-chamber view demonstrates extensive calcification of the mitral valve annulus projecting into the LA in a patient on chronic hemodialysis. *Abbreviations*: LA, left atrium; LV, left ventricle; MAC, mitral annular calcification; RA, right atrium; RV, right ventricle.

Larger and more pedunculated thrombi are easier to identify than sessile thrombi. Thrombi that protrude into the LV cavity are freely mobile with an irregular shaggy border and are more likely to embolize. The differential diagnosis of LV thrombus includes benign and malignant tumors, transducer-related artifacts, as well as a variety of normal cardiac structures such as prominent papillary muscles (Fig. 25.23), apical hematomas after cardiopulmonary bypass from the decompression cannulas (Fig. 25.22E), trabeculations, and false tendons. Filling of the apex of a normal LV without regional wall abnormality can be

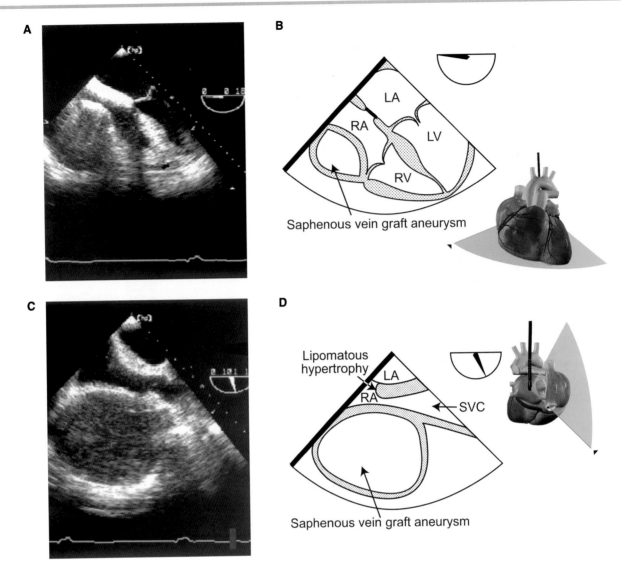

Figure 25.18 Saphenous vein graft aneurysm. Mid-esophageal four-chamber (**A,B**) and bicaval (**C,D**) views show a large circular mass compressing the RA in a patient with previous coronary artery bypass surgery. The saphenous vein graft appears filled with thrombus-like material. *Abbreviations*: LA, left atrium; LV, left ventricle; RA, right atrium; RV, right ventricle; SVC, superior vena cava. *Source*: Adapted from Ref. 16.

seen in patients with the hypereosinophilic syndrome, the apical form of hypertrophic cardiomyopathy or in patients with malignancies and hypercoagulable state. Primary lymphoma of the heart, or any metastatic malignancy, can also fill the apex of the LV.

Left Atrial Thrombus

Left atrial and LAA thrombi are associated with stasis of blood in the LA (Fig. 25.24). Predisposing factors in the formation of LA thrombi include LA and LAA enlargement, atrial fibrillation, MV disease (especially rheumatic MV stenosis), the presence of prosthetic mitral valve, and previous Maze procedure (see Fig. 29.36). As for LV thrombus, the presence of SEC

favors the diagnosis of a thrombus when a mass is found in the LA (Fig. 25.25A). Left atrial SEC is seen in >50% of patients with atrial fibrillation and in >80% of those with atrial fibrillation and LAA thrombi (18). Right atrial SEC is seen in only 14% of patients with atrial arrhythmias referred for TEE prior to cardioversion (19).

The texture of a large thrombus in the LAA, has an acoustic density different from the adjacent structures and the blood pool, may be helpful in distinguishing it from either pectinate muscles or the muscular walls of the LAA. The thrombus appears as a relatively well-circumscribed echo-dense mass with a defined border that has asynchronous motion with the underlying heart wall throughout the cardiac cycle (Fig. 25.24). Thrombus in the LAA can sometimes

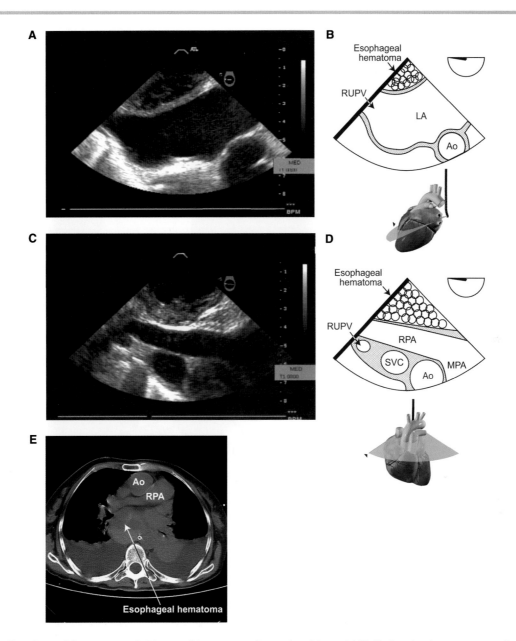

Figure 25.19 Esophageal hematoma. A 64-year-old woman anticoagulated for atrial fibrillation develops a retrocardiac isohomogeneous mass behind the LA. (**A,B**) ME view with a collection behind the LA (**C,D**). ME ascending Ao short-axis view shows its extension superiorly behind the RPA. (**E**) The computed tomography scan confirmed that the mass was a spontaneous esophageal hematoma. *Abbreviations*: Ao, aorta; LA, left atrium; ME, mid-esophageal; MPA, main pulmonary artery; RPA, right pulmonary artery; RUPV, right upper pulmonary vein; SVC, superior vena cava. *Source*: Photos A–C courtesy of Dr. Pierre Laramée.

appear as an ill-defined echogenic mass or sludge-like mass in the early stage of thrombus formation where the thrombus is in a more gelatinous form (Fig. 25.25C). When attached to the LA wall, it usually has a broad-based attachment and can be seen in several views. When uncertainty remains in regards to the presence of thrombus in the LAA, particularly in the evaluation of patients pre-cardioversion, contrast-enhanced harmonic imaging with a left cardiac chamber opacification agent (such as perflutren lipid microsphere) will reveal a filling defect in the presence of a clot.

Less commonly, the atrial thrombus may be attached to the mitral orifice, especially when rheumatic mitral stenosis (MS) is present or to the atrial anastomosis on the suture line after cardiac transplantation (see Fig. 22.9). Rarely, the thrombus may be free-floating, appearing as a LA ball thrombus (20).

The differential diagnosis of LA thrombus includes myxoma, fibroelastoma, other tumors, and artifacts (see Fig. 7.4). The clinical setting often aids in the diagnosis. The presence of SEC and the lack of

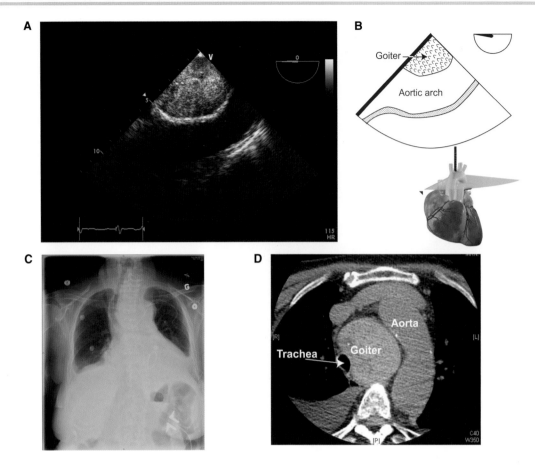

Figure 25.20   Goiter. (A,B) Upper esophageal aortic arch long-axis view in an 80-year-old woman shows a large mediastinal mass adjacent to the aortic arch. Corresponding chest X-ray **(C)** and computed tomography of the upper chest **(D)** confirm a goiter beside the aortic arch displacing the trachea to the right. 🖰

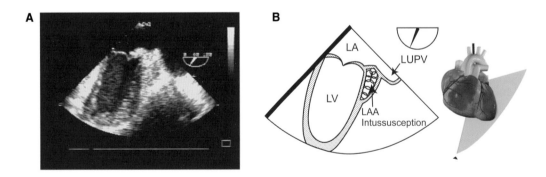

Figure 25.21   Intussusception of the LAA. (A,B) Mid-esophageal mitral commissural view in a patient shows an intussusception of the LAA after coronary revascularization. The preoperative examination was normal. *Abbreviations*: LA, left atrium; LAA, left atrial appendage; LUPV, left upper pulmonary vein; LV, left ventricle. 🖰

septal wall attachment favor the diagnosis of a thrombus rather than a tumor. Myxoma and LA thrombus can often have a similar appearance. A mass that spares the fossa ovalis is less likely to be a myxoma especially if MS or SEC is present. Thrombi are avascular masses and color Doppler flow within the mass rules out a thrombus but raise the possibility of a myxoma or a sarcoma.

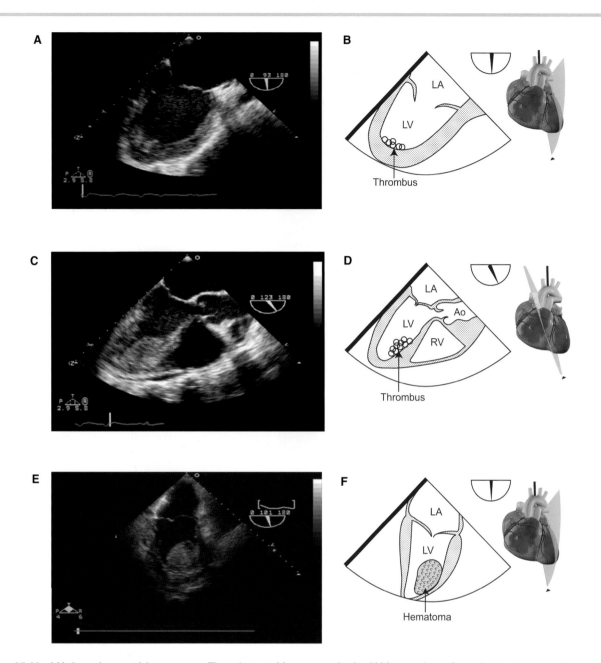

Figure 25.22 LV thrombus and hematoma. Thrombus and hematoma in the LV in a patient after a large anteroseptal myocardial infarction. (**A,B**) ME two-chamber view with thrombus seen at the LV apex. (**C,D**) ME long-axis view showing a concomitant hematoma of the anteroseptal wall. (**E,F**) ME two-chamber view in a different patient after cardiopulmonary bypass for aortic valve replacement: new apical mass /wall hematoma secondary to the decompression cannula positioned through the mitral valve toward the LV apex. *Abbreviations*: Ao, aorta; LA, left atrium; LV, left ventricle; ME, mid-esophageal.

Left Atrial Thrombus in Patients in Sinus Rhythm

Left atrial thrombus is usually detected in association with atrial arrhythmias and is uncommon in the presence of sinus rhythm. Thus, the yield of TEE in detecting LA thrombus in unselected patients in sinus rhythm is low. The incidence of LA thrombus and sinus rhythm was approximately 0.1% in a recent cohort of >20,000 TEE examinations (21). This low frequency is further supported by the rare occurrence of SEC in the LA in patients with sinus rhythm. Patients in whom LA thrombus is detected in sinus rhythm are characterized by the presence of significant LV dysfunction, MS, or previous episodes of paroxysmal atrial fibrillation. The latter is suspected when pulsed wave (PW) Doppler interrogation of the LAA orifice yields velocities <40 cm/s, suggestive of

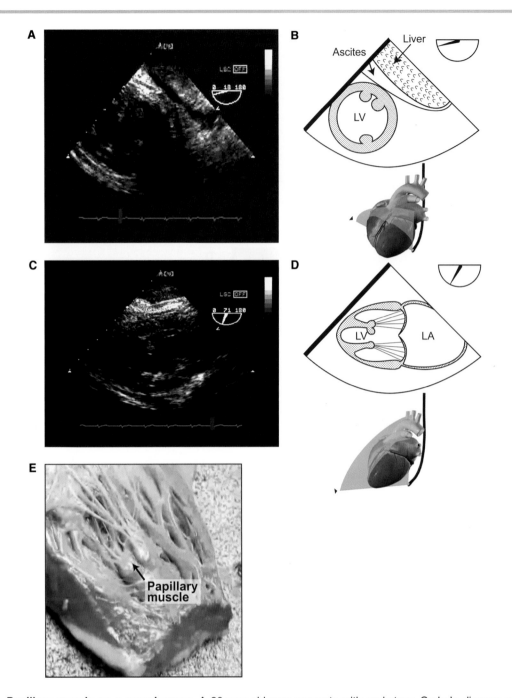

Figure 25.23 Papillary muscle as a pseudomass. A 36-year-old man presents with end-stage Crohn's disease complicated by respiratory insufficiency, renal failure and sepsis. (**A,B**) The transgastric mid short-axis and (**C,D**) 71° views show a mobile mass in the LV close to the posterior-medial papillary muscle. (**E**) The patient died from multiorgan failure and an autopsy confirmed a double-headed papillary muscle. *Abbreviations*: LA, left atrium; LV, left ventricle. *Source*: Photo E courtesy of Dr. Tak Ki Leung.

poor contractility and increased probability of thrombus formation. These features define a group of patients in sinus rhythm who are at higher risk for LA thrombus formation. Percutaneous closure of LAA are now being performed in patients with atrial fibrillation at risk of thrombus formation (22) (Fig. 25.24D).

Right Atrial Thrombus

Right atrial thrombi often originate from venous thromboemboli migrating through the right heart (Figs. 25.26–25.28). As large thrombi are often constituted from "casts" of large deep veins, they often get transiently entangled in the tricuspid valve apparatus

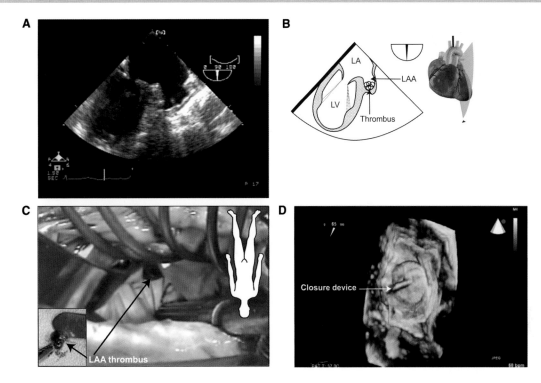

Figure 25.24 LAA thrombus. A 63-year-old woman is scheduled for mitral and tricuspid valve surgery. (**A,B**) A mid-esophageal two-chamber view was suggestive of thrombus in the LAA. (**C**) Upon opening the LA a small thrombus was seen and removed. (**D**) 3D view of an LAA percutaneous closure device in a different patient: before final release, the device is still seen attached to the catheter. *Abbreviations*: LA, left atrium; LAA, left atrial appendage; LV, left ventricle. *Source*: Figure D courtesy of Dr. Patrick Garceau.

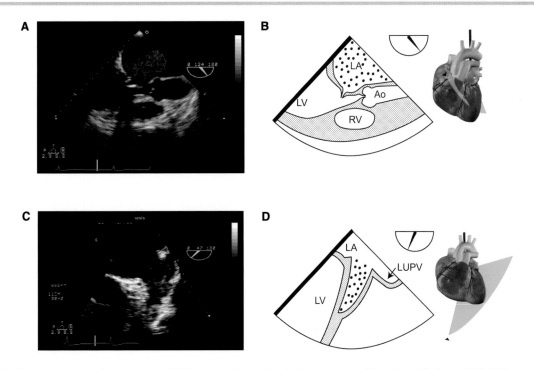

Figure 25.25 Spontaneous echo contrast. SEC in a patient with mitral stenosis and junctional rhythm. (**A,B**) Mid-esophageal AoV long-axis view showing significant SEC in a dilated left atrium (LA). (**C,D**) SEC in the left atrial appendage at 60°. *Abbreviations*: Ao, aorta; AoV, aortic valve; LA, left atrium; LV, left ventricle; ME, mid-esophageal; RA, right atrium; RV, right ventricle; SEC, spontaneous echo contrast.

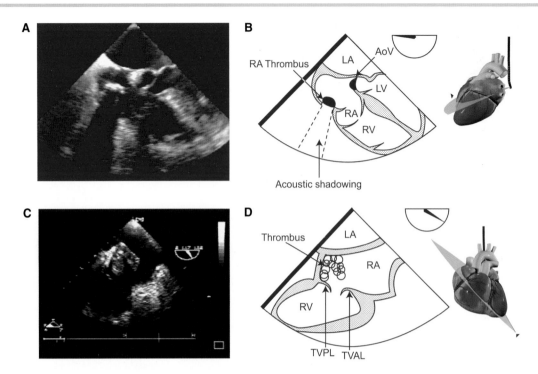

Figure 25.26 RA thrombus. (A,B) ME five-chamber view displays a calcified thrombus in the RA (proven at surgery) with secondary acoustic shadowing that extends from the thrombus surface to the far field. **(C,D)** Mid-esophageal right ventricular view at 117° with a "popcorn-like" thrombus in transit in a different patient two weeks after revascularization. *Abbreviations*: AoV, aortic valve; LA, left atrium; LV, left ventricle; ME, mid-esophageal; RA, right atrium; RV, right ventricle; TVAL, tricuspid valve anterior leaflet; TVPL, tricuspid valve posterior leaflet.

during their transit, giving a classical appearance of "popcorn." Patients present with acute cor pulmonale secondary to pulmonary embolus (see Figs. 30.4 and 30.5). The migrating nature of a thrombus in transit may be demonstrated by finding of additional clots in the SVC, RV, and right ventricular outflow tract (RVOT), as well as the main pulmonary trunk and the right and left pulmonary branches. A thrombus in transit can also be seen crossing a patent foramen ovale (see Fig. 30.4) and reaching the left-sided cardiac chambers and the systemic circulation as a paradoxical embolus.

Thrombus formation in situ in the RA also occurs in conditions associated with blood stasis or endocardial damage, such as in patients with RA dilatation, atrial arrhythmias, cardiomyopathies (see Fig. 22.4), or after right heart manipulation. Thrombi in situ may also form on foreign bodies present in the RA including central venous and Swan–Ganz pulmonary artery catheters, transvenous pacing electrodes (see Figs. 18.17 and 18.18), and ventriculoatrial shunts for hydrocephalus. This thrombus can be seen even after the removal of the catheter.

Right Ventricular Thrombi

Right ventricular thrombi are rarely diagnosed clinically. Besides conditions associated with decreased blood flow including RV infarction, RV failure and cor pulmonale, they have been also reported in patients with endomyocardial fibroelastosis, cardiomyopathy, and hypercoagulable states (Fig. 25.28). The differential diagnosis with other tumors is helped by the clinical context. Flow within the mass, evidenced by color Doppler, eliminates a thrombus and favors the diagnosis of a tumor. Thrombus in transit can also be seen within the RV or RVOT. This may be fully mobile or attached to the wall of the RV or RVOT.

Biventricular Thrombi

Biventricular thrombi are quite rare and have been described in dilated cardiomyopathy and severe biventricular systolic dysfunction as well as in patients with a hypercoagulable state (Fig. 25.28) (23).

MAN-MADE OBJECTS IN THE HEART

Intracardiac catheters are the most common objects seen in the heart and typically appear as a sharply defined linear intracardiac echo-density (see Chapter 13). Central venous catheters are a well-known nidus for infection and thrombosis. Careful examination should be performed to rule out the presence of superimposed thrombus, vegetation, and cardiac perforation. Echocardiography has become standard in the imaging of a venous catheter placed in the SVC or RA. TEE has been shown to be superior to TTE for

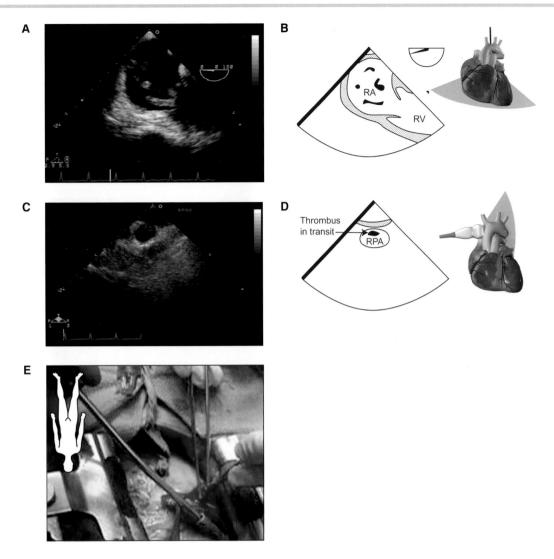

Figure 25.27 Thrombus in transit. (A,B) Mid-esophageal right ventricular view demonstrates a "popcorn-like" thrombus in transit through the RA in a patient two weeks after a prostatectomy. **(C,D)** A piece of the embolus is seen in the RPA using epiaortic scanning. **(E)** Removal of the thrombus at the time of surgery. *Abbreviations*: LA, left atrium; RA, right atrium; RPA, right pulmonary artery; RV, right ventricle.

diagnosis of right heart and SVC lesions (24). Other foreign bodies, including pacemaker wires, atrial septal occluding prosthesis, and embolized vena cava umbrella, can be easily recognized by the echogenic appearance characteristic of their design. They can also become a nidus for thrombus formation or vegetations that can persist even after removal of the foreign object.

VEGETATIONS

Echocardiographic detection of a mass suggestive of vegetation has become an important criterion in the clinical diagnosis of endocarditis. Complications of endocarditis such as periannular abscess, prosthetic valve dehiscence, leaflet perforation, and fistula are best seen by TEE and help confirm the diagnosis and

dictate important management decisions. Compared with TTE or monoplane transducers, multiplane TEE probes have improved diagnostic accuracy particularly with regard to prosthetic valves and abscess formation. The sensitivity of TEE imaging for the detection of vegetations approximates 100% on native valves and 86% to 94% for prosthetic valves, while its specificity ranges from 88% to 100%. False negative echocardiographic studies have been seen in the case of disappearance by embolization of the infected material, inadequate visualization due to acoustic shadowing, or with minute vegetation size falling below the resolution range of TEE. When both TTE and TEE studies are normal, the negative predictive value is 95% and, therefore, a single negative TEE study alone is insufficient to rule out infective endocarditis. Thus, TEE should be repeated within 7 to

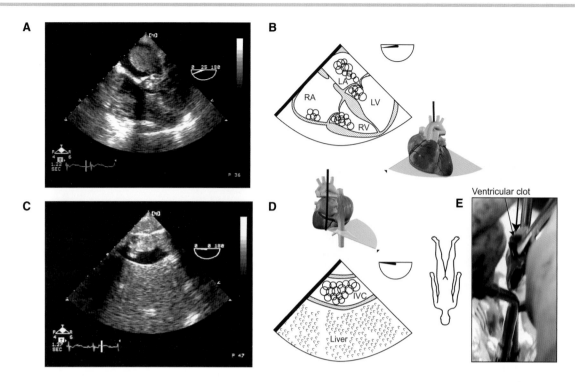

Figure 25.28 Intra-cardiac thrombus. A 73-year-old man reoperated for an aortic pseudoaneurysm develops an acute hyper-coagulable state after cardiac surgery. (**A,B**) Mid-esophageal four-chamber view showing clots in all the cardiac chambers. (**C,D**) Thrombus also present in the transgastric view of the IVC. (**E**) Intraoperative findings during reexploration. *Abbreviations*: IVC, inferior vena cava; LA, left atrium; LV, left ventricle; RA, right atrium; RV, right ventricle. ✍

10 days if the clinical findings strongly suggest the diagnosis of endocarditis (25).

Finding a mass on a valve is not necessarily specific of active infectious endocarditis. Noninfectious endocarditis also occurs in Libman–Sacks (lupus) and marantic (paraneoplastic) endocarditis. Endocarditis, secondary to granulomatous disease and scleroderma, has also been described. The non-infectious vegetations secondary to an inflammatory process tend to be sessile without independent motion, whereas marantic vegetations may appear identical to infectious vegetations (25).

Echocardiographic Appearance of Vegetations

The morphologic features of vegetations vary depending on the nature of the offending organism, the state of the involved valve, and the activity of the disease. Vegetations can appear as a discrete, sessile mass closely adherent to the valve, as pedunculated, friable clumps that prolapse freely, or as an elongated fibrous thickened strand (see Figs. 16.6 and 16.7). Fungal infections commonly give rise to larger vegetations that are less likely to cause significant leaflet destruction than bacterial vegetations. TV vegetations are generally larger than those located on the left heart.

In acute endocarditis, classic vegetation appears as a circumscribed, pedunculated echogenic mass arising from the leaflet tip with varying degrees of inde-

pendent motion. Active vegetations typically appear soft and friable, as opposed to chronic healed vegetations that are more echo-dense and fixed as they become fibrotic and calcified. Successful treatment of infectious endocarditis may not result in complete disappearance and resolution of the vegetation.

Vegetations can vary in size from a few millimeters, or less, to several centimeters and their appearance may dramatically change between studies because of growth, embolization, or valvular disruption. A complex appearance with cystic components may develop with certain vegetations, particularly those attached to foreign bodies. Vegetations typically occur at sites of endothelial damage due to impinging flow jets or on already structurally abnormal valves, their appearance is influenced by the underlying valvular disorder. In fact, the greater the degree of valvular deformity before infection, the more difficult the vegetation is to define. Extensive calcification may cause important shadowing and mask the presence of a small vegetation.

The MV is more frequently involved in infective endocarditis than any other valve (Fig. 25.29). The vegetations may involve either, or both, of its leaflets and are most often located on the atrial surface of the valve. Seeding of the chordae tendinae or the anterior mitral leaflet from an infected AoV can also occur. Mitral valve vegetations must be differentiated from a variety of other disorders affecting the valve including myxomatous degeneration that cause thickening of

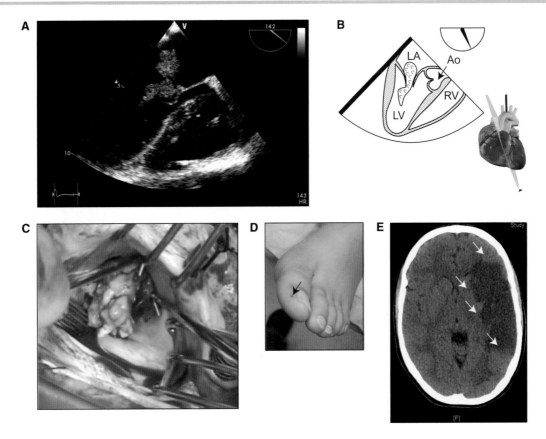

Figure 25.29 **Endocarditis.** Mid-esophageal long-axis view (**A,B**) in a 30-year-old woman with acute bacterial endocarditis of the mitral valve shows a large complex vegetation. (**C**) Corresponding intraoperative findings. (**D**) Peripheral embolic lesions in the big toe. (**E**) Large hemispheric temporal stroke on head computed tomography. *Abbreviations*: Ao, aorta; LA, left atrium; LV, left ventricle; RV, right ventricle. *Source*: Courtesy of Dr. Michel Pellerin.

both leaflets and increased echogenicity-simulating endocarditis. When there is associated leaflet prolapse or chordal rupture, the similarity may be even more striking. Primary leaflet tumor such as fibroelastoma or myxoma may also, at times, be impossible to differentiate from vegetations.

The AoV is a common site of involvement in bacterial endocarditis. Combined infection of both AoV and MV is also frequently observed. Predisposing factors in AoV endocarditis include rheumatic deformity of the valve cusps, bicuspid AoV, and degeneration and calcification of the aortic cusps frequently seen in the elderly. Aortic vegetation appears as a mass attached to the ventricular surface of the cusps, in the outflow tract during diastole, and prolapsing forward through the annulus during systole. Aortic vegetations characteristically involve the body or the free edges of the valve cusps. They are commonly focal and may involve one or two of the cusps. Endocarditis of the AoV can be complicated by the development of an abscess that appears initially as a periaortic asymmetric ill-defined thickening and swelling in which coalescing echo-free spaces gradually evolve into a newly formed cavity (see Fig. 14.35). Once a pseudoaneurysm has clearly formed, the presence of blood flow in and out of the cavity can be seen

with color Doppler imaging. The examination of AoV endocarditis should, therefore, warrant a careful evaluation of the periaortic area and the posterior mitral annulus (Fig. 25.30).

TV endocarditis is usually an acute, rather than a subacute, process. Staphylococcus aureus is the most common infecting organism, as predisposing factors include intravenous drug abuse, infected catheters, and virulent skin infection. In contrast to left-sided valves, infective endocarditis among intravenous drug users occurs on a structurally normal valve. Tricuspid vegetations generally appear as large echo-dense masses that disrupt the usual smooth contour of the TV (see Figs. 18.17 and 18.18). Vegetative growth may occur on the atrial surface, the leaflet margins, or the ventricular surface. Significant leaflet destruction and rupture of the chordae tendinea are common (25).

The pulmonic valve (PV) is the least commonly involved in infective endocarditis. It usually occurs in patients with congenital heart disease such as pulmonic stenosis (PS), patent ductus arteriosus, tetralogy of Fallot, or ventricular septal defect (VSD). As mentioned previously, vegetations develop on areas of endothelial damage by impinging flow jets. Thus, in patients with VSD, vegetations can appear at the site of the jet lesion on the endocardium of the RV.

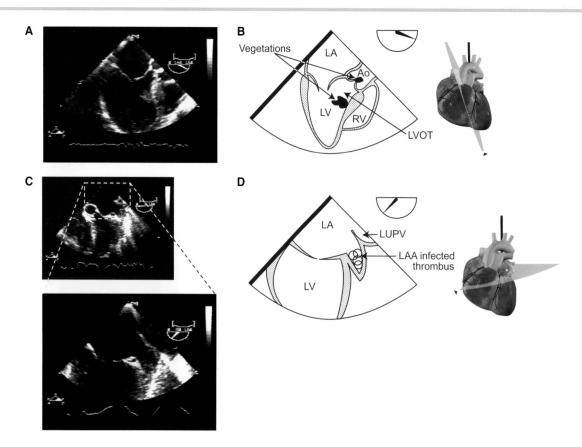

Figure 25.30 Endocarditis. Endocarditis in a 60-year-old woman with pneumococcal meningitis. (**A,B**) Mid-esophageal long-axis view with lesions on the AoV and the basal IVS where the jet of aortic regurgitation is directed. Note the multilobulated appearance suggestive of a vegetation. (**C,D**) Repeat TEE exam seven days later revealed a new multilobulated mass in the LAA. With persisting bacteremia and the absence of concomitant atrial fibrillation, this suggested uncontrolled infection and prompted surgical intervention where an infected thrombus was removed. *Abbreviations*: Ao, aorta; AoV, aortic valve; IVS, interventricular septum; LA, left atrium; LAA, left atrial appendage; LUPV, left upper pulmonary vein; LV, left ventricle; LVOT, left ventricular outflow tract; RV, right ventricle; TEE, transesophageal echocardiography.

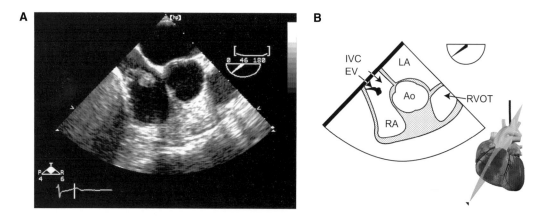

Figure 25.31 Vegetations on the Eustachian valve. (**A,B**) A 47-year-old woman is diagnosed with pacemaker endocarditis. Following removal of the infected pacing wire, echo-dense vegetations were seen at the tip of the EV in the mid-esophageal aortic valve short-axis view. *Abbreviations*: Ao, aorta, EV, Eustachian valve; IVC, inferior vena cava; LA, left atrium; RA, right atrium; RVOT, right ventricular outflow tract.

Table 25.1 Surgery for Native Valve Endocarditis

Class I	1.	Surgery of the native valve is indicated in patients with acute infective endocarditis who present with valve stenosis or regurgitation resulting in heart failure. (Level of evidence: B)
	2.	Surgery of the native valve is indicated in patients with acute infective endocarditis who present with AR or MR with hemodynamic evidence of elevated LV end-diastolic or left atrial pressures (e.g., premature closure of MV with AR, rapid decelerating MR signal by continuous-wave Doppler (v-wave cutoff sign), or moderate or severe pulmonary hypertension). (Level of evidence: B)
	3.	Surgery of the native valve is indicated in patients with infective endocarditis caused by fungal or other highly resistant organisms. (Level of evidence: B)
	4.	Surgery of the native valve is indicated in patients with infective endocarditis complicated by heart block, annular or aortic abscess, or destructive penetrating lesions (e.g., sinus of Valsalva to right atrium, right ventricle, or left atrium fistula; mitral leaflet perforation with aortic valve endocarditis; or infection in annulus fibrosa). (Level of evidence: B)
Class IIa		Surgery of the native valve is reasonable in patients with infective endocarditis who present with recurrent emboli and persistent vegetations despite appropriate antibiotic therapy. (Level of evidence: C)
Class IIb		Surgery of the native valve may be considered in patients with infective endocarditis who present with mobile vegetations in excess of 10 mm with or without emboli. (Level of evidence: C)

Abbreviations: AR, aortic regurgitation; LV, left ventricular; MR, mitral regurgitation; MV, mitral valve.
Source: Adapted from Ref. 26.

Vegetations on prosthetic valves are typically more difficult to detect than those involving native valves, as visualization of their components and specific design often requires specific angulations, complicated even more by acoustic shadowing from prosthetic material. The presence of both mitral and aortic prostheses is particularly challenging, as the aortic prosthesis obscures the MV in transthoracic imaging while the opposite occurs with transesophageal imaging. The advent of multiplane TEE transducers has been particularly helpful in enabling observation from multiple viewing positions and angles to detect the presence of vegetations.

Infection involving mechanical prosthetic valves usually begins in the perivalvular area at the annular insertion site and later extends along the struts where it may interfere with the motion of the occluder. Echocardiographically, the smooth contour of the ring may appear thickened, a finding sometimes difficult to differentiate from thrombus or pannus formation. When >40% of the sewing ring is involved by the infectious process, loosening of the sutures leads to dehiscence and rocking of the prosthesis. In bioprosthetic valves, in addition to similar involvement of the sewing ring, the infection may also deform and destroy the tissue cusps (3). Finally, any intracardiac structure or thrombus (Figs. 25.30 and 25.31) can become infected and the clinical evolution will be useful to make this diagnosis. Guidelines for surgery in endocarditis are summarized in Table 25.1 (26).

CONCLUSION

In summary, the diagnosis of abnormal intracavitary material is one of the most powerful applications of TEE in clinical practice and in the operating room (OR). Such abnormalities can appear in numerous medical conditions and in both cardiac and noncardiac surgeries. The impact of such observations can lead to important alteration in the medical and surgical management of these patients.

REFERENCES

1. Gopal AS, Stathopoulos JA, Arora N, et al. Differential diagnosis of intracavitary tumors obstructing the right ventricular outflow tract. J Am Soc Echocardiogr 2001; 14: 937–940.
2. Goldman JH, Foster E. Transesophageal echocardiographic (TEE) evaluation of intracardiac and pericardial masses. Cardiol Clin 2000; 18:849–860.
3. Weyman AE. Principles and Practice of Echocardiography. 2nd ed. Philadelphia: Lea & Febiger, 1994.
4. McAllister HA Jr., Hall RJ, Cooley DA. Tumors of the heart and pericardium. Curr Probl Cardiol 1999; 24:57–116.
5. Oh JK, Seward JB, Tajik AJ. The Echo Manual. 3rd ed. Philadelphia: Lippincott Williams & Wilkins, 2006.
6. Sidhu JS, Harries M, Senior R. Papillary fibroelastoma of the left atrial appendage. J Am Soc Echocardiogr 2001; 14:838–839.
7. Evans AJ, Butany J, Omran AS, et al. Incidental detection of an aortic valve papillary fibroelastoma by echocardiography in an asymptomatic patient presenting with hypertension. Can J Cardiol 1997; 13:905–908.
8. Roldan CA, Shively BK, Crawford MH. Valve excrescences: prevalence, evolution and risk for cardioembolism. J Am Coll Cardiol 1997; 30:1308–1314.
9. Landolphi DR, Belkin RN, Hjemdahl-Monsen CE, et al. Cardiac cavernous hemangioma mimicking pericardial cyst: atypical echocardiographic appearance of a rare cardiac tumor. J Am Soc Echocardiogr 1997; 10:579–581.
10. Chrissos DN, Agelopoulos NG, Garyfallos DJ, et al. Follow-Up of an unresectable hemangioma in the heart. Echocardiography 1998; 15:239–242.
11. Miller A, Mukhtar O, Aaluri SR, et al. Two- and three-dimensional TEE differentiation of lymphoma involving the atrial septum from lipomatous hypertrophy. Echocardiography 2001; 18:205–209.
12. Keller DI, Hunziker P, Buser P. Biopsy of right atrial angiosarcoma guided by transesophageal echocardiography. J Am Soc Echocardiogr 2002; 15:475–477.
13. Harpaz D, Auerbach I, Vered Z, et al. Caseous calcification of the mitral annulus: a neglected, unrecognized diagnosis. J Am Soc Echocardiogr 2001; 14:825–831.
14. Madu EC, D'Cruz IA, Wall B, et al. Transesophageal echocardiographic spectrum of calcific mitral abnormalities in patients with end-stage renal disease. Echocardiography 2000; 17:29–35.

15. Antonini-Canterin F, Piazza R, Ascione L, et al. Value of transesophageal echocardiography in the diagnosis of compressive, atypically located pericardial cysts. J Am Soc Echocardiogr 2002; 15:192–194.

16. Bansal RC. Echocardiographic diagnosis of an asymptomatic aneurysm of a saphenous vein graft. J Am Soc Echocardiogr 2002; 15:661–664.

17. Roberson DA, Arcilla RA, Sachsteder W, et al. Transesophageal echocardiography diagnosis of intussusception of the left atrial appendage. J Cardiovasc Ultrasound Allied Tech 1993; 10:619–622.

18. Otto CM, Pearlman AS. Textbook of Clinical Echocardiography. Philadelphia: W.B. Saunders, 1995.

19. Bashir M, Asher CR, Garcia MJ, et al. Right atrial spontaneous echo contrast and thrombi in atrial fibrillation: a transesophageal echocardiography study. J Am Soc Echocardiogr 2001; 14:122–127.

20. Feigenbaum H. Echocardiography. 5th ed. Baltimore: Williams & Williams, 1994.

21. Agmon Y, Khandheria BK, Gentile F, et al. Clinical and echocardiographic characteristics of patients with left atrial thrombus and sinus rhythm: experience in 20 643 consecutive transesophageal echocardiographic examinations. Circulation 2002; 105:27–31.

22. Holmes DR, Reddy VY, Turi ZG, et al. Percutaneous closure of the left atrial appendage versus warfarin therapy for prevention of stroke in patients with atrial fibrillation: a randomised non-inferiority trial. Lancet 2009; 374:534–542.

23. Wongpraparut N, Apiyasawat S, Jacobs LE, et al. Biventricular thrombi. Echocardiography 2001; 18:619–620.

24. Shapiro MA, Johnson M, Feinstein SB. A retrospective experience of right atrial and superior vena caval thrombi diagnosed by transesophageal echocardiography. J Am Soc Echocardiogr 2002; 15:76–79.

25. Ryan EW, Bolger AF. Transesophageal echocardiography (TEE) in the evaluation of infective endocarditis. Cardiol Clin 2000; 18:773–787.

26. Bonow RO, Carabello BA, Kanu C, et al. ACC/AHA 2006 guidelines for the management of patients with valvular heart disease: a report of the American College of Cardiology/American Heart Association Task Force on Practice Guidelines (writing committee to revise the 1998 Guidelines for the Management of Patients With Valvular Heart Disease): developed in collaboration with the Society of Cardiovascular Anesthesiologists: endorsed by the Society for Cardiovascular Angiography and Interventions and the Society of Thoracic Surgeons. Circulation 2006; 114:e84–e231.

26

Congenital Heart Disease

Jean-Marc Côté
Université Laval, Quebec City, Quebec, Canada

Jane Heggie and Annette Vegas
Toronto General Hospital, University of Toronto, Toronto, Ontario, Canada

INTRODUCTION

There are two basic categories of congenital heart disease in adults (1). The first includes defects that have been unrecognized in childhood but were diagnosed in the adult because of newly developed symptoms or as an incidental finding during an investigation for another reason. Coarctation of the aorta (Ao) and ostium secundum atrial septal defect (ASD) are examples of this category. It also includes patients with a previously diagnosed unrepaired congenital cardiac malformation such as a bicuspid aortic valve (AoV) that evolved to significant aortic stenosis (AS) in the adult. The second category involves patients surviving to adulthood with a previously diagnosed and repaired or palliated congenital heart defect, such as the patient with tetralogy of Fallot (TOF) or transposition of the great arteries. This chapter will review common congenital heart pathologies and their general echocardiographic findings.

ECHOCARDIOGRAPHY IN CONGENITAL HEART DISEASE

A simplified approach to understanding complex congenital heart disease is based on following blood flow into, through, and out of the heart. The comprehensive echocardiographic evaluation of the adult with a suspected or known congenital heart defect includes a detailed and systematic analysis of intracardiac and extracardiac structures. The segmental echocardiographic analysis of the heart requires identification of the various cardiac segments and components and involves four steps (Fig. 26.1). First, determine the cardiac and visceral sidedness (situs); second, the cardiac position and orientation; third, identify the atrial, ventricular, and arterial segments; and finally, define the atrial, the ventricular, and the arterial connections (Tables 26.1 and 26.2).

In practice, this begins by the evaluation of the venous connections (vena cava and pulmonary veins), atrial anatomy [right atrium (RA) and left atrium (LA)], atrioventricular (AV) valves, ventricles, outflow tracts, semilunar valves, and proximal portion of the

great arteries. The right and left sides of the heart can be examined in parallel or in sequence as long as the evaluation is complete. Over time, whether a ventricle is a morphological right ventricle (RV) or left ventricle (LV) can be difficult to distinguish as the ventricle will adapt to the loading conditions that it experiences.

UNREPAIRED CONGENITAL HEART DEFECTS

Septation Defects

Atrial Septal Defect

ASDs are common and can present at any age unrelated to the size of the defect or shunt (2). Many of the defects may evolve, unrecognized in childhood, and be diagnosed only in adulthood. Symptoms or signs that will usually prompt diagnosis in the adult are shortness of breath, exercise intolerance, right-heart failure, atrial arrhythmias, or a cardiac murmur (3). They can be managed either by surgical closure or, more recently in the case of secundum ASD, by percutaneous closure using one of the available devices (see Figure 29.1) (4).

A left-to-right shunt at the atrial level causes RV volume overload with RV and atrial dilatation in diastole (Fig. 26.2) and increased RV ejection volume in systole into a dilated pulmonary arterial bed. Hemodynamically significant ASDs rarely measure less than 10 mm in diameter. More quantitative assessment of the amount of shunting at the atrial level may be performed by measuring the Qp/Qs ratios from transgastric views at 60° to 90° [for the right ventricular outflow tract (RVOT) or the main pulmonary artery (PA)] and 90° to 120° [for the left ventricular outflow tract (LVOT) or Ao (see Fig. 5.37)]. In general, a left-to-right shunt is considered significant when the Qp/Qs ratio is 1.5 to 1.0 or causes dilatation of right-heart chambers (2).

The embryology of the interatrial septum is complex and includes the formation of a series of membranes and holes (foramen) (Fig. 26.3). There are four recognized types of ASDs based on location: ostium secundum (fossa ovalis), ostium primum,

Segmental Approach Congenital Heart Disease

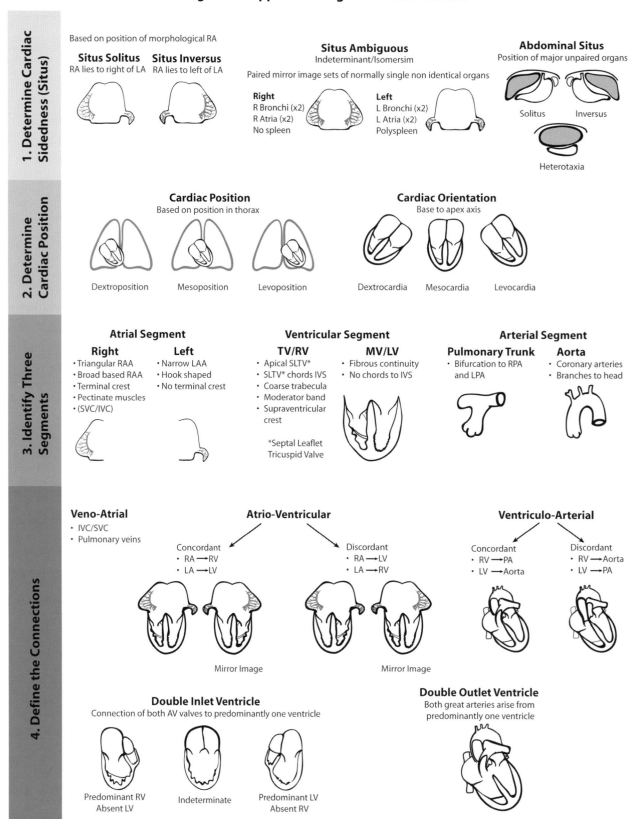

Figure 26.1   Segmental echocardiographic approach to congenital heart disease. *Abbreviations*: AV, atrioventricular; IVC, inferior vena cava; IVS, interventricular septum; L, left; LA, left atrium; LAA, left atrial appendage; LPA, left pulmonary artery; LV, left ventricle; MV, mitral valve; PA, pulmonary artery; R, right; RA, right atrium; RAA, right atrial appendage; RPA, right pulmonary artery; RV, right ventricle; SLTV, septal leaflet of tricuspid valve; SVC, superior vena cava; TV, tricuspid valve. *Source*: Courtesy of Dr. A. Vegas.

Table 26.1 Definitions of the Different Cardiac Segments and Components

Cardiac segments and connections	Definition
Visceroatrial situs	*Spatial positioning of abdominal organs and morphological right and left atria*
• Solitus (normal)	Morphologic RA, liver, and IVC to the right
	Morphologic LA, stomach, spleen, and descending aorta to the left
• Inversus	Opposite of solitus
• Ambiguous	Atrial situs undiagnosed with median liver
Atrioventricular connection	*Connection between the atria and the ventricles*
• Concordant	Morphologic RA connected to the morphologic RV and morphologic LA connected to the morphologic LV
• Discordant	Morphologic RA connected to the morphologic LV and morphologic LA connected to the morphologic RV
• Double inlet	Two atrioventricular valves are connected to the same ventricle
• Straddling	Subvalvular apparatus of one atrioventricular valve is connected to both sides of the interventricular septum
• Absent	Atresia of one atrioventricular valve
Ventriculoarterial connection	*Connection between the ventricles and the great arteries*
• Concordant	Morphologic RV connected to the pulmonary artery and the morphologic LV connected to the aorta
• Discordant	Morphologic RV connected to the aorta and morphologic LV connected to the pulmonary artery
• Double outlet	Aorta and pulmonary artery connected to the same ventricle, most commonly the RV
• Single outlet	Atresia of one great artery or fusion of the two (truncus arteriosus)

Abbreviations: IVC, inferior vena cava; LA, left atrium; LV, left ventricle; RA, right atrium; RV, right ventricle.

Table 26.2 Recommended TEE Views to Image Various Congenital Cardiac Malformations

Malformation	ME and UE views	TG view
Atrial septal defect	4 chamber (0°–20°) Aortic valve short axis (30°–60°) Bicaval (80°–110°)	
Ventricular septal defect	4 chamber (0°–20°) Aortic valve short axis (30°–60°) Aortic valve long axis (120°–160°)	Short axis (0°–30°) (Trabecular)
Patent ductus arteriosus	UE aortic short axis (90°) RV outflow (60°–90°)	
AV canal defect (AVSD, endocardial cushion defect)	4 chamber (0°–20°) Aortic valve long axis (120°–160°)	Basal short axis (0°–20°) Long axis (90°–110°)
Ebstein's anomaly	4 chamber (0°–20°) RV outflow (60°–90°)	Long axis of TV (60°–90°)
Pulmonary stenosis	UE RV outflow (60°–90°) Transgastric RV outflow (60°–90°)	
Tetralogy of Fallot	4 chamber (0°–20°) Aortic valve short axis (30°–60°) Aortic valve long axis (120°–160°) RV outflow (60°–90°)	
Cor triatriatum	4 chamber (0°–20°) 2 chamber (80°–100°)	
Mitral valve stenosis	4 chamber (0°–20°) 2 chamber (80°–100°) Long axis (120°–160°)	Basal short axis (0°–25°) Long axis (80°–100°)
Cleft mitral valve	4 chamber (0°–20°) 2 chamber (80°–100°)	Basal short axis (0°–20°)
Aortic valve stenosis	Aortic valve short axis (30°–60°) Aortic valve long axis (120°–160°) UE ascending aorta long axis (90°)	Long axis (90°–120°) Deep transgastric (apical) (0°–30°)
Subvalvular aortic stenosis	5 chamber (0°–20°)	Long axis (90°–120°)
Supravalvular aortic stenosis	Aortic valve long axis (120°–160°) UE ascending aorta long axis (90°)	Deep transgastric (apical) (0°–30°)
Coarctation of the aorta	UE aortic arch long axis (0°) UE aortic arch short axis (90°)	
Tetralogy of Fallot	4 chamber (0°–20°) Aortic valve short axis (30°–60°) Aortic valve long axis (120°–160°) RV outflow (60°–90°)	
Transposition of the great arteries	4 chamber (0°–20°) Bicaval (80°–110°) Aortic valve short axis (30°–60°) Aortic valve long axis (120°–160°)	Basal short axis (0°–20°) Mid short axis (0°–20°)

(Continued)

Table 26.2 Recommended TEE Views to Image Various Congenital Cardiac Malformations (*Continued*)

Malformation	ME and UE views	TG view
Complex single ventricle	4 chamber (0°–20°) Bicaval (80°–110°) Aortic valve short axis (30°–60°) Aortic valve long axis (120°–160°) RV outflow (60°–90°)	Basal short axis (0°–20°) Mid short axis (0°–20°)

Abbreviations: ME, mid-esophageal; RV, right ventricular; SD, septal defect; TEE, transesophageal echocardiography; TV, tricuspid valve; UE, upper esophageal.

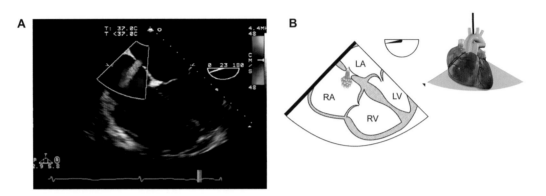

Figure 26.2 Right chamber dilatation in ASD. (**A,B**) Color Doppler mid-esophageal four-chamber view shows dilatation of the RV and RA compared with the left-sided chambers during diastole. Color Doppler shows left-to-right flow through the interatrial septum from an ASD. *Abbreviations*: ASD, atrial septal defect; LA, left atrium; LV, left ventricle; RA, right atrium; RV, right ventricle.

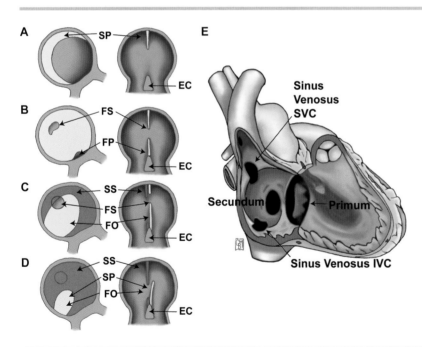

Figure 26.3 Embryology of the interatrial septum and ASD types. (**A**) Formation of the interatrial septum begins with the septum primum (SP) growing down from the dorsocranial wall of the atria towards the endocardial cushions (EC). (**B**) Above the EC a space remains called the foramen primum (FP). Perforations appear in the upper SP allowing partial resorption thus forming the foramen secundum (FS). (**C**) The septum secundum (SS) grows from the ventrocranial wall covering the FS and FP, but leaves an opening called the foramen ovale (FO) which is covered by the SP. (**D**) The upper SP disappears and the lower SP portion becomes the valve of the FO. (**E**) An ASD is a deficiency in the wall of the interatrial septum as shown. Comparative location of the types of ASD (coronary sinus ASD not shown). *Abbreviations*: ASD, atrial septal defect; IVC, inferior vena cava; SVC, superior vena cava. *Source*: Illustrations with permission, copyright of Gian-Marco Busato.

sinus venosus, and the seldom encountered unroofed coronary sinus.

Ostium secundum and patent foramen ovale. The ostium secundum (fossa ovalis) is the most common type of ASD (Figs. 26.4 and 26.5). It usually lies close to

the center of the interatrial septum occupying part, or all, of the fossa ovalis. It is caused by excessive resorption of the normal septum primum, leading to an absence of the LA portion of the atrial septum normally covering and closing the fossa ovalis (Fig. 26.3).

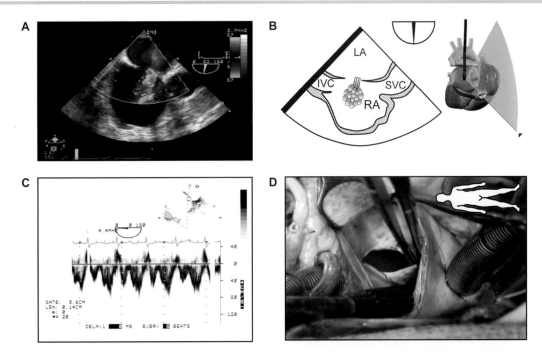

Figure 26.4 Ostium secundum ASD in a 50-year-old man undergoing coronary revascularization. (A,B) Color Doppler mid-esophageal bicaval view at 82° shows the left-to-right shunt from the LA to the RA. **(C)** Pulsed wave Doppler of an ASD demonstrates both systolic and diastolic flow. **(D)** Intraoperative aspect of the ASD from a right atriotomy. **(D)** Intraoperative aspect of an ASD is shown. *Abbreviations*: ASD, atrial septal defect; IVC, inferior vena cava; LA, left atrium; RA, right atrium; SVC, superior vena cava. *Source*: Photo D courtesy of Dr. Michel Carrier.

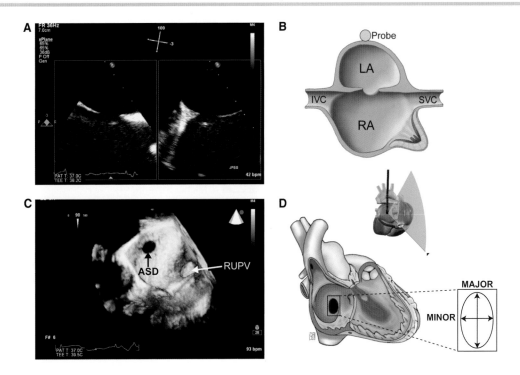

Figure 26.5 Ostium secundum ASD. (A,B) Mid-esophageal Xplane simultaneous bicaval view at 100° (left panel) and an orthogonal view at 0° (right panel), using a TEE 3D matrix probe. **(C)** 3D echocardiographic view of the ASD shown from the LA with the RUPV draining into the LA (arrow). **(D)** Measurement of the ASD size uses the minor axis obtained from ME right ventricular inflow/outflow or four-chamber views and the major axis obtained from a ME bicaval view. *Abbreviations*: ASD, atrial septal defect; IVC, inferior vena cava; LA, left atrium; LV, left ventricle; ME, mid-esophageal; RA, right atrium; RUPV, right upper pulmonary vein; SVC, superior vena cava. *Source*: Part D with permission, copyright of Gian-Marco Busato.

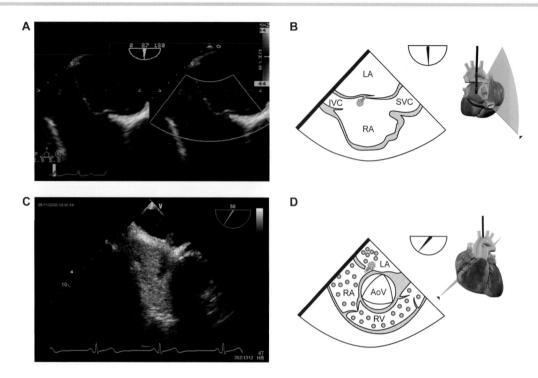

Figure 26.6 PFO. (A,B) Color Doppler ME bicaval view. **(C,D)** ME right ventricular inflow/outflow view with right-sided cardiac chambers opacification by intravenous injection of agitated normal saline. During the release phase of a Valsalva maneuver, microbubbles are seen crossing from the RA to the LA through the PFO. *Abbreviations*: AoV, aortic valve; IVC, inferior vena cava; ME, mid-esophageal; LA, left atrium; PFO, patent foramen ovale; RA, right atrium; RV, right ventricle; SVC, superior vena cava.

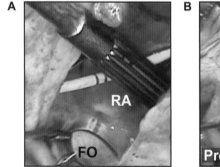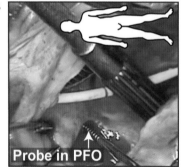

Figure 26.7 PFO. Intraoperative views through a right atriotomy of a PFO diagnosed and closed intraoperatively in a 67-year-old man undergoing tricuspid annuloplasty. **(A)** At baseline the fossa ovalis is visible at the lower part of the image. A suction device and a Swan-Ganz catheter are also visible in the RA. **(B)** Upon mild pressure on the fossa ovalis with a surgical probe, blood appears in the RA, coming from the left atrium through the PFO. *Abbreviations*: FO, fossa ovalis; PFO, patent foramen ovale; RA, right atrium. *Source*: Courtesy of Dr. Michel Pellerin.

This must be differentiated from a patent foramen ovale (PFO or "Trou de Botal") present in 20% of the adult population. A PFO has a normal amount of tissue as the septum primum is complete but does not fuse with the septum secundum to obliterate the foramen ovale (Fig. 26.3). A right-to-left shunt can be elicited with a Valsalva maneuver (Fig. 26.6). Patency of the foramen ovale can be demonstrated anatomically with a probe (Fig. 26.7). It usually has no consequences unless it is responsible for a cerebrovascular accident through paradoxical emboli (see Fig. 30.4). Some authors, however, suggest that it should be closed if found in a patient in whom a cardiac surgical procedure is performed (5). Closure is indicated if it does not significantly alter the surgical approach of the booked procedure. The presence of a PFO may alter the method of venous cannulation in the case of left-sided valve surgery or the need for cardioplegia in right-sided valve surgery. Cases in which the patient is at high risk of hypoxemia post bypass, such as left ventricular assist device insertion and heart transplant, closure of the PFO is warranted (see Fig. 21.20).

Secundum ASDs and PFOs can be demonstrated very easily with transesophageal echocardiography (TEE) using a combination of the mid-esophageal four-chamber (Fig. 26.2), AoV short-axis (SAX) (Fig. 26.6), and bicaval (Fig. 26.8) views (6). The location, anatomical size, and the amount of surrounding tissue in the rim of the defect (ridges) should be determined. The presence of a rim is necessary to secure an ASD

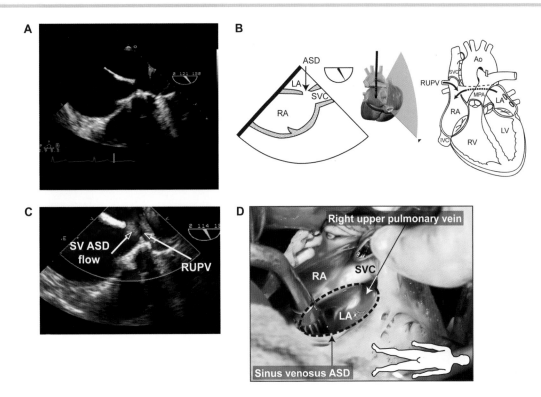

Figure 26.8 **Sinus venosus SVC type ASD. (A–C)** Mid-esophageal modified bicaval views at 121° with the defect located between the upper part of the atrial septum and the SVC. **(C)** Frequently associated anomalous right pulmonary venous connections to the SVC at its junction with the RA. **(D)** Intraoperative view of a sinus venosus ASD. The right pulmonary veins are here connected to the LA and can be seen through the ASD. *Abbreviations*: Ao, aorta; ASD, atrial septal defect; IVC, inferior vena cava; LA, left atrium; LV, left ventricle; MPA, main pulmonary artery; RA, right atrium; RUPV, right upper pulmonary vein; RV, right ventricle; SV, sinus venosus; SVC, superior vena cava. *Source*: Courtesy of Dr. Nancy Poirier.

percutaneous closure device. The shunt and its direction(s) can be visualized with color Doppler and will usually be from left to right because pressure in the LA is usually higher than in the RA (Fig. 26.4). The pulsed wave (PW) Doppler shows predominantly low velocity (<1 m/s) flow from mid-systole to mid-diastole (Fig. 26.4).

Sinus venosus ASDs. The sinus venosus ASD involves an interatrial communication at the superior and posterior aspect of the atrial septum adjacent to the superior vena cava (SVC) or inferior vena cava (IVC) (Fig. 26.3). It is often associated with a partial anomalous pulmonary venous connection of one or more of the right pulmonary veins to the junction of the SVC and the RA (Fig. 26.8). Less commonly, in the case of an IVC sinus venosus defect, there is a connection between the right lower pulmonary vein and the IVC (Fig. 26.9). The bicaval and ascending Ao SAX views in the mid-to-upper esophagus are helpful in assessing the SVC type of sinus venosus defect and the drainage of the anomalous right upper pulmonary vein into the SVC (Fig. 26.8).

Ostium primum ASD. The ostium primum (also called partial AV) septal defect is the consequence of an endocardial cushion defect with a resulting communication at the lower and posterior aspect of the interatrial septum at the level of the AV valves (Fig. 26.10). In this defect, there is a common AV junction with abnormalities of the AV valves. In the partial form, there are two separate AV valves and one common AV valve in the complete form. The left AV valve is trileaflet with a "cleft" in the anterior leaflet of the mitral valve (MV) and variable degrees of mitral regurgitation (MR). The presence of MR results in the patient becoming symptomatic at a younger age than those patients with other types of ASDs (Fig. 26.11). The distance from the left AV valve (mitral) annulus to the apex is much less than the distance from the apex to the aortic annulus, resulting in a "gooseneck" appearance to the LVOT. Adults may present for primary repair of the defect or for repair/replacement of the left AV valve or for LVOT obstruction (7).

The diagnostic hallmark using TEE is the absence of the atrial septum adjacent to the coplanar AV valves in the mid-esophageal four-chamber view (Fig. 26.10). A cleft anterior MV leaflet is best confirmed from the transgastric basal 0° "en face" transverse view of the MV (Fig. 26.12). The abnormal ventricular septal attachments of a cleft anterior mitral leaflet are seen in the mid-esophageal four-chamber and AoV long-axis (LAX) views of the MV and the

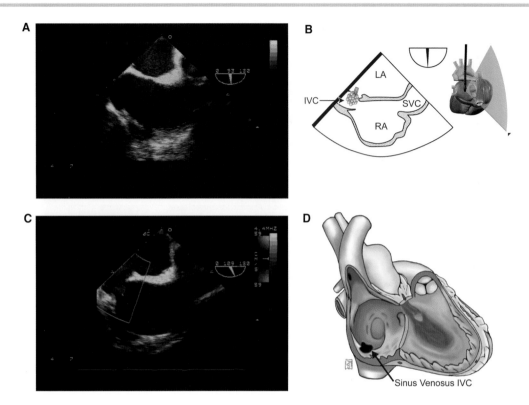

Figure 26.9 Sinus venosus ASD – inferior vena cava type. (A,B) Modified (lower) mid-esophageal bicaval view with the defect located between the lower part of the atrial septum and the IVC. **(C)** Color Doppler showing laminar left-to-right shunt flow from the LA into the RA. **(D)** Diagram illustrating the location of a sinus venosus ASD–IVC type. *Abbreviations*: ASD, atrial septal defect; IVC, inferior vena cava; LA, left atrium; RA, right atrium; SVC, superior vena cava. *Source*: Part D with permission, copyright of Gian-Marco Busato.

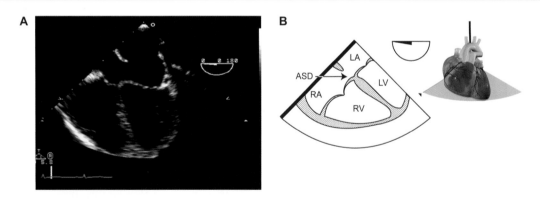

Figure 26.10 Ostium primum ASD. (A,B) Mid-esophageal four-chamber view shows, in addition to the ASD, the insertion of both atrioventricular valves at the same level of the superior aspect of the ventricular septum. *Abbreviations*: ASD, atrial septal defect; LA, left atrium; LV, left ventricle; RA, right atrium; RV, right ventricle.

LVOT. The gooseneck elongation of the LVOT as well as the presence of chordal attachments of the left AV valve to the ventricular septum can lead to LVOT obstruction (Fig. 26.12) (2).

Coronary sinus ASD. Finally, the coronary sinus defect is a rare but recognized type of ASD located around the orifice of an unroofed coronary sinus in association with a persistent left SVC that drains into the coronary sinus. Left-to-right shunt occurs as LA blood enters the RA via the unroofed coronary sinus (Fig. 26.13). This can be visualized in a mid-esophageal four-chamber view with mild probe retroflexion to see

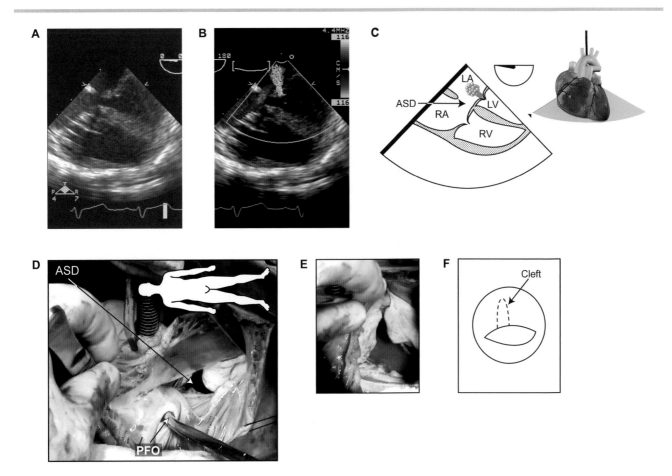

Figure 26.11 Cleft anterior MV leaflet in a 60-year-old man with an ostium primum ASD. (A–C) Color Doppler mid-esophageal four-chamber view shows the left-to-right shunt at the atrial level as well as left atrioventricular valve regurgitation through a cleft in the anterior MV leaflet. **(D–F)** Surgical views through a right atriotomy. *Abbreviations*: ASD, atrial septal defect; LA, left atrium; LV, left ventricle; MV, mitral valve; PFO, patent foramen ovale; RA, right atrium; RV, right ventricle. *Source*: Photos D and E courtesy of Dr. Nancy Poirier.

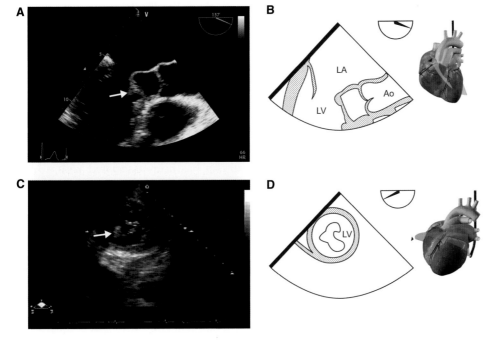

Figure 26.12 Cleft anterior MV leaflet. (A,B) Mid-esophageal aortic valve long-axis view showing the anterior mitral leaflet abnormal chordal attachment to the basal septum (arrow). This configuration can lead to left ventricular outflow tract obstruction. **(C,D)** Transgastric basal view, demonstrating the cleft in the anterior leaflet. *Abbreviations*: Ao, aorta; LA, left atrium; LV, left ventricle; MV, mitral valve. *Source*: Courtesy of Dr. A. Rochon.

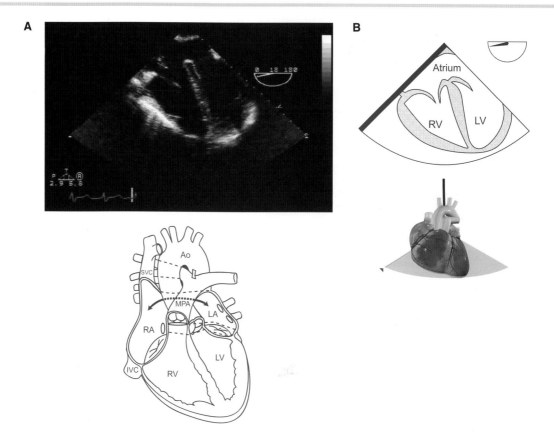

Figure 26.13 Unroofed coronary sinus ASD. (A,B) Low-esophageal four-chamber view shows an unroofed coronary sinus. *Abbreviation*: Ao, aorta; ASD, atrial septal defect; IVC, inferior vena cava; LA, left atrium; LV, left ventricle; MPA, main pulmonary artery; RA, right atrium; RV, right ventricle; SVC, superior vena cava.

the coronary sinus and persistent left SVC. Agitated saline injected into the left arm or left-sided neck vein will opacify the left SVC and coronary sinus before the right heart chambers (Fig. 26.14).

Ventricular Septal Defect

Ventricular septal defects (VSDs) are the commonest congenital cardiac anomalies identified in infancy and account for approximately 10% of adult congenital heart defects. A VSD with significant left-to-right shunt usually presents early in life with failure to thrive, pulmonary hypertension, and signs of heart failure. These shunts are diagnosed early and operated on before the development of irreversible obstructive pulmonary hypertension disease. Any VSDs persisting to adulthood are usually relatively small and restrictive, that is, with a systolic pressure gradient between the LV and RV unaccompanied by pulmonary hypertension.

Morphologically, the ventricular septum is a complex three-dimensional (3D) structure comprised of four distinct components: (*i*) membranous, (*ii*) inlet, (*iii*) muscular trabecular, and (*iv*) outlet or infundibular septum (see Fig. 4.16). The VSDs are classified according to their location as follows: (*i*) perimembranous, (*ii*) inlet, (*iii*) muscular, or (*iv*) outlet VSDs (Fig. 26.15) (2). The role of echocardiography for assessment of VSD is to identify the type and size, impact on ventricular function, and calculate the pulmonary (Qp) to systemic (Qs) shunt. The best TEE views to image the different types of VSDs are presented in Figure 26.15.

The most common defect, the perimembranous type (80%), is located near the tricuspid septal leaflet, just beneath the right and noncoronary aortic cusps in the LVOT (Fig. 26.15). The small membranous portion of the ventricular septum itself is divided into an AV portion above and an interventricular portion below the insertion of the septal tricuspid leaflet. The presence of a septal aneurysm has been associated with a high incidence of spontaneous defect closure (Fig. 26.16).

Inlet VSDs, also termed AV canal defects, are located in the posterior or inlet septum and lie in proximity to the AV valves. Echocardiographically, these defects are recognized by the fact that both AV valves insert at the same level instead of the normal offset inferior position of the tricuspid valve (TV) leaflets. These defects are usually large and do not close spontaneously, requiring surgical repair in the young. The TEE diagnosis is made using the mid-esophageal four-chamber, the AoV SAX and LAX

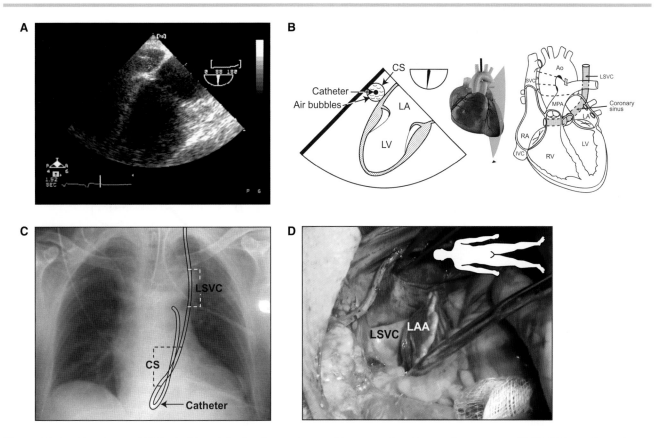

Figure 26.14 Persistent LSVC. Incidental finding in a 74-year-old man undergoing cardiac surgery. **(A,B)** Mid-esophageal two-chamber view: the diagnosis is evoked by a dilated CS in which a PAC and bubbles are visible. **(C)** Postoperative chest X-ray, showing the PAC inadvertent course through the LSVC and the CS, then normally in the RA, the RV, and the pulmonary artery. **(D)** Intraoperative view demonstrates the LSVC adjacent to the LAA. *Abbreviations*: Ao, aorta; CS, coronary sinus; IVC, inferior vena cava; LA, left atrium; LAA, left atrial appendage; LSVC, left superior vena cava; LV, left ventricle; MPA, main pulmonary artery; PA, pulmonary artery; PAC, pulmonary artery catheter; RA, right atrium; RV, right ventricle; SVC, superior vena cava. *Source*: Courtesy of Dr. Raymond Cartier.

views, and the deep transgastric LAX view of the ventricular septum.

Muscular (trabecular) VSD may persist to adult life but are usually very small, without significant shunt. The VSD can be seen with color Doppler anywhere along the trabecular (central or apical) part of the interventricular septum but may be quite difficult to see as they may be obscured by the multiple trabeculations of the RV (Fig. 26.17). These defects are rarely significant enough to require surgical closure. They can be seen using TEE in the mid-esophageal four-chamber view, LAX view, or deep transgastric LAX view.

Outlet VSDs are also referred to as supracristal, infundibular, conal, doubly committed, or subarterial ventricular defects (Fig. 26.18). They lie proximal to the right coronary cusp and pulmonic valve (PV) in the RV outflow portion lateral and inferior to the AoV. They are usually large and do not close spontaneously (Fig. 26.19). They are often associated with prolapse of the right aortic cusp due to decreased structural aortic valvular support or damage from a high-velocity impinging jet.

Surgical management for a VSD will be required if there is volume overload or if complications have developed, mainly bacterial endocarditis, or aortic cusp prolapse into the VSD with development of significant aortic regurgitation (AR). A large VSD has a small pressure gradient, and a smaller, restrictive defect displays a larger pressure difference between the LV and RV. The consequence of the VSD may also be reflected on the size of the right and the left cardiac chambers. In a significant VSD with Eisenmenger's physiology, RV dimensions and systolic function should be measured as well as the level of PA pressure (see Chapter 5).

Atrioventricular Septal Defect

Between the fourth and eighth week of gestation, fusion of the growing endocardial cushions with the muscular portion of the ventricular septum and the right and left ridges of the bulbus cordis results in the division of the single ventricle into two separate ventricles. The bulbus cordis is the caudal section of the heart tube and gives rise to the proximal portions of the Ao and PA. If the

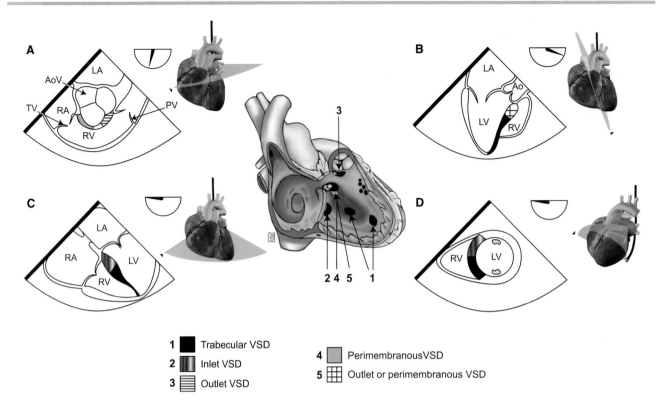

Figure 26.15   VSD classification. VSD location on various TEE views: (**A**) Mid-esophageal right ventricular inflow/outflow. (**B**) Mid-esophageal long-axis. (**C**) Mid-esophageal four-chamber. (**D**) Transgastric mid short-axis views. *Abbreviations*: Ao, aorta; AoV, aortic valve; LA, left atrium; LV, left ventricle; ME, mid-esophageal; PV, pulmonic valve; RA, right atrium; RV, right ventricle; TV, tricuspid valve; TEE, transesophageal echocardiographic; VSD, ventricular septal defect. *Source*: With permission, copyright of Gian-Marco Busato.

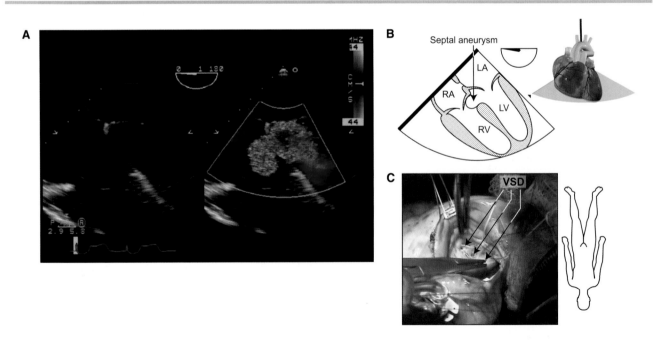

Figure 26.16   Perimembranous septal aneurysm and VSD in a 54-year-old man. (A,B) Color Doppler mid-esophageal four-chamber view: an aneurysmal membranous septum bulges toward the RV at the upper part of the interventricular septum. (**C**) Corresponding intraoperative view, showing three small perimembranous VSDs. *Abbreviations*: LA, left atrium; LV, left ventricle; RA, right atrium; RV, right ventricle; VSD, ventricular septal defect. *Source*: Photo C courtesy of Dr. Denis Bouchard.

A
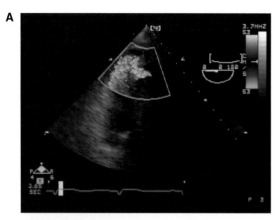

B
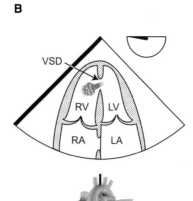

C
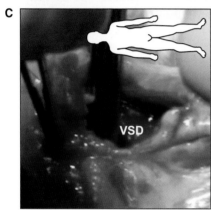

Figure 26.17 Trabecular or muscular VSD. (A,B) Color Doppler deep transgastric long-axis view with a trabecular muscular VSD and left-to-right shunt. **(C)** Corresponding intraoperative findings. *Abbreviations*: LA, left atrium; LV, left ventricle; RA, right atrium; RV, right ventricle; VSD, ventricular septal defect.

A
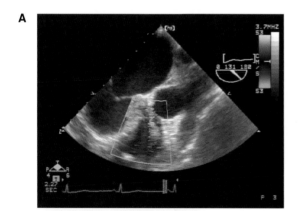

B
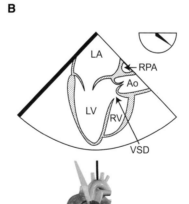

C
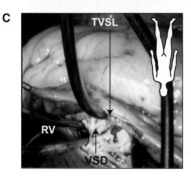

Figure 26.18 Outlet (or infundibular, subarterial membranous) VSD. (A,B) Color Doppler mid-esophageal long-axis view. **(C)** Corresponding intraoperative view from the opened pulmonary artery. *Abbreviations*: Ao, aorta; LA, left atrium; LV, left ventricle; RPA, right pulmonary artery; RV, right ventricle; TVSL, tricuspid valve septal leaflet; VSD, ventricular septal defect. *Source*: Photo courtesy of Dr. Nancy Poirier.

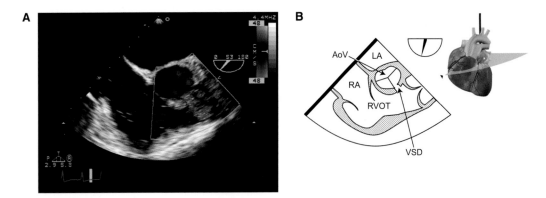

Figure 26.19   Outlet VSD. (A,B) Color Doppler mid-esophageal right ventricular inflow/outflow view shows an outlet VSD with flow from the LV to the RVOT. *Abbreviations*: AoV, aortic valve; LA, left atrium; LV, left ventricle; RA, right atrium; RVOT, right ventricular outflow tract; VSD, ventricular septal defect.

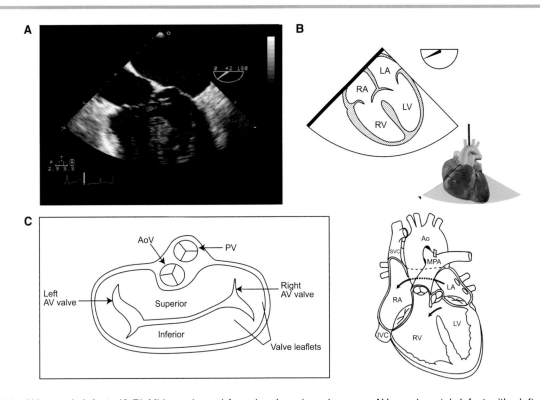

Figure 26.20   AV septal defect. (A,B) Mid-esophageal four-chamber view shows an AV canal septal defect with cleft valve leaflet dragged into the left ventricular outflow tract. **(C)** Diagram of the basal heart highlighting the common AV valve. *Abbreviations*: Ao, aorta; AoV, aortic valve; AV, atrioventricular; IVC, inferior vena cava; LA, left atrium; LV, left ventricle; MPA, main pulmonary artery; PV, pulmonic valve; RA, right atrium; RV, right ventricle; SVC, superior vena cava.

endocardial cushions fail to fuse, development of the AV valves, the lower portion of the atrial septum, and the upper portion of the ventricular septum will be deficient, leading to the AV septal defect. This condition is also referred to as AV canal defect, canal-type VSD, or endocardial cushion defect (Fig. 26.20).

The complete form of endocardial cushion defect will create a large primum ASD, a large inlet VSD, and a common AV valve (Fig. 26.20). The latter consists of five leaflets: the normal left posterior MV leaflet, the anterior and posterior tricuspid leaflets, and the remaining two, the anterosuperior and posteroinferior leaflets that straddle the atrial and ventricular septa and may be attached to the top of the ventricular septum by short chordae tendineae (Fig. 26.20). The diagnosis is sometimes made at an older age when the VSD is small or absent as in the partial form with only an interatrial communication, resulting in an ostium primum ASD and a cleft anterior mitral leaflet (Fig. 26.11). The TEE view that best displays this anomaly is the mid-esophageal four-chamber view (Fig. 26.20) that shows absence of atrial and ventricular septal tissue with abnormal flow using color Doppler. A cleft anterior MV may be more easily visualized in the transgastric basal view at the MV level (Fig. 26.12C). In a complete AV septal defect, a "bridging AV leaflet" may span the central defect with chordal insertion into both ventricles. At surgery, the bridging leaflet must be divided and resuspended to create separate AV orifices.

Patent Ductus Arteriosus

The ductus arteriosus serves, during fetal life, as a communication between the PA and the Ao and normally closes after birth. As it fibroses, it becomes the ligamentum arteriosum. The patient with a persistently patent ductus arteriosus (PDA) thus has a communication between the high-pressure Ao and the lower-pressure PA, leading to a left-to-right shunt beyond the RV level (Fig. 26.21). Therefore, the volume overload will result in dilatation of the pulmonary vessels, the left cardiac chambers, and the Ao but not the RA or RV. A significant PDA will present early in life with heart failure symptoms and pulmonary hypertension. On the other hand, a smaller PDA may

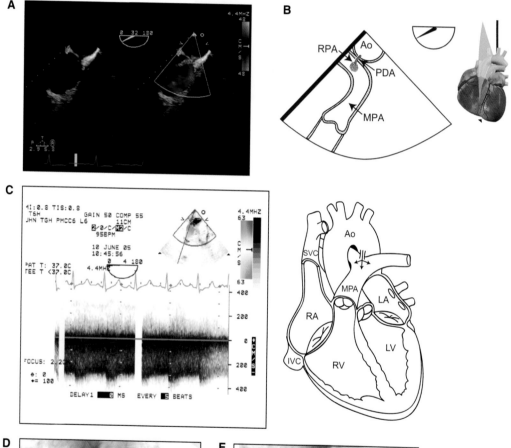

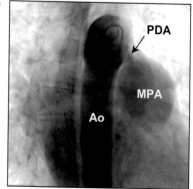

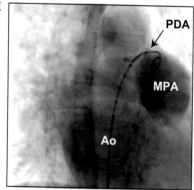

Figure 26.21 PDA. (A,B) Color Doppler upper-esophageal ascending Ao short-axis view with shunt flow from the Ao to the MPA. **(C)** Continuous wave Doppler revealing a 64-mmHg pressure gradient between the MPA and the Ao. **(D,E)** Fluoroscopic views demonstrating cannulation of the PDA with a catheter in the thoracic Ao. *Abbreviations*: Ao, aorta; IVC, inferior vena cava; LA, left atrium; LV, left ventricle; MPA, main pulmonary artery; PDA, patent ductus arteriosus; RA, right atrium; RPA, right pulmonary artery; RV, right ventricle; SVC, superior vena cava.

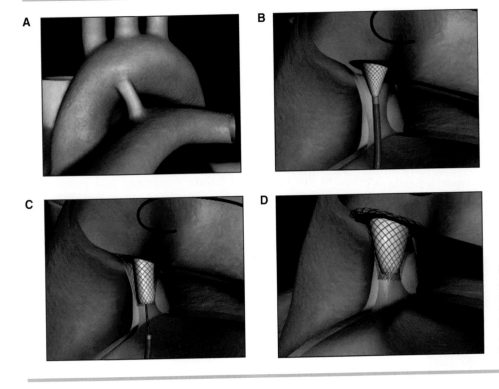

Figure 26.22 PDA catheter closure. Steps involved in PDA closure by a percutaneous catheter technique are shown. *Abbreviation*: PDA, patent ductus arteriosus. *Source*: Courtesy of AGA Medical Corporation.

remain unrecognized for years and be incidentally discovered during a work-up for other medical problems. A moderate shunt will cause decreased exercise tolerance and may predispose to the development of pulmonary hypertension and right-heart failure.

Closure of a PDA can be performed percutaneously by embolization with Gianturco coils or insertion of Rashkind double umbrella or Amplatzer closure device (Fig. 26.22) (see Chapter 29). The alternate approach is surgical, through an open left thoracotomy or by video-assisted thoracoscopic surgery.

Adequate TEE visualization is frequently difficult as the ductus arteriosus courses in front of the trachea and above the left main bronchus, draining most often to the superior aspect of the left side of the PA bifurcation. Withdrawal of the TEE probe from the mid-esophageal four-chamber view, to higher in the esophagus, reveals dilatation of the main, right, and left pulmonary arteries with presence of an abnormal turbulent shunt flow from the PDA. The PDA may be visualized in the upper esophageal aortic arch SAX and LAX views with rotation of the probe toward the right (see Fig. 5.29). The PDA should be assessed for the presence of an aneurysm, calcification, or atheroma. Continuous left-to-right flow with color and PW Doppler is seen from the transverse Ao to the main PA (Fig. 26.21). Both the LA and LV appear dilated in the mid-esophageal four-chamber view.

TV Anomaly

Ebstein's Anomaly of the TV

The classic findings in Ebstein's anomaly of the TV include a large sail-like anterior leaflet and apically displaced septal and posterior leaflets at a distance of greater than 8 mm/m^2 in adults (Fig. 26.23) (8,9). As a consequence of this displacement, the right heart is composed of three parts: the RA, the atrialized portion of the RV, and the functional RV that includes the trabecular and outlet RV. The displaced septal and posterior leaflets of the TV usually display impaired mobility because of short chordae, tethering, thickening, and fibrosis (Fig. 26.24). A variable degree of tricuspid regurgitation (TR) is present with the origin of the regurgitant jet at the coaptation level in the distal RV chamber. Tricuspid annular dilatation is the rule and can be severe. The severity of Ebstein's anomaly is described as the ratio between the functional RV and the combined area of both the RA and atrialized RV. Characteristic features include a dilated or aneurysmal RVOT, obstruction due to a redundant anterior TV leaflet, and altered geometry of the LV with regional (inferoseptal) dysfunction. The LV function may be difficult to evaluate by echocardiography because of the paradoxical motion of the interventricular septum and the crescentic shape of the LV due to bulging of the interventricular septum to the left. An ASD, or PFO, is a frequently associated finding (94%) and, less commonly, pulmonary atresia or stenosis, VSD, and partial AV canal (10).

The features of Ebstein's anomaly are best demonstrated with TEE in the mid-esophageal four-chamber view (Fig. 26.23): (*i*) degree of apical displacement of the origin of the TV septal leaflet from the AV junction, (*ii*) the location of leaflet coaptation within the RV cavity, (*iii*) the presence and severity of TR and/or stenosis, and (*iv*) the integrity of the TV leaflet

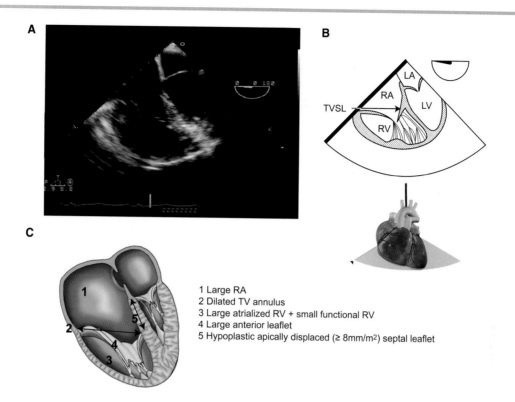

Figure 26.23 Ebstein's anomaly. (A,B) Mid-esophageal four-chamber view in a patient with Ebstein's anomaly shows a number of key findings as illustrated in the diagram (**C**). *Abbreviations*: LA, left atrium; LV, left ventricle; RA, right atrium; RV, right ventricle; TV, tricuspid valve; TVSL, tricuspid valve septal leaflet. *Source*: Part C with permission, copyright of Gian-Marco Busato.

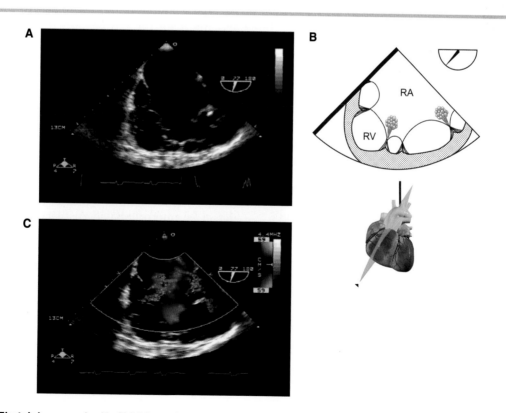

Figure 26.24 Ebstein's anomaly. (A–C) Mid-esophageal right ventricular inflow/outflow views show a tethered tricuspid valve anterior leaflet with multiple jets of tricuspid regurgitation originating below the annulus. *Abbreviations*: RA, right atrium; RV, right ventricle.

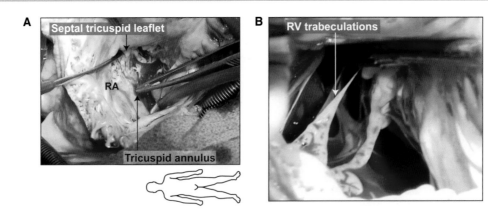

Figure 26.25 Ebstein's anomaly in a 63-year-old woman. Intraoperative views. (**A**) The origin of the tricuspid septal leaflet is displaced apically in relation to the position of the tricuspid annulus. (**B**) Prominent abnormal trabeculations from noncompaction of the RV. *Abbreviations*: RA, right atrium; RV, right ventricle. *Source*: Photos courtesy of Dr. Nancy Poirier.

and subvalvular apparatus to assess its suitability for repair versus replacement (Fig. 26.25). A large mobile anterior leaflet with a free leading edge is a factor that makes TV repair feasible. Leaflet tethering and presence of leaflet tissue in the RVOT makes a successful repair less likely (10). The transgastric RV inflow view at 60° to 90° can also add useful information about the presence and morphology of obstructive lesions within the infundibulum and the PV lesions (11).

In the immediate postoperative period following valve replacement and/or right-heart plication procedures, TEE examination is aimed at evaluating residual tricuspid stenosis or regurgitation and confirming the adequate function of the implanted prosthesis (9,10).

RVOT Anomaly

Pulmonic Stenosis (Subvalvular, Valvular, Supravalvular)

Valvular pulmonic stenosis (PS) is the most common form of RVOT obstruction; it is almost always congenital in origin and is found in approximately 10% of adults with congenital heart defects (see Figs. 18.26 and 18.27). Typically, the stenotic PV presents as a dome-shaped structure with thin, pliable tissue, and a narrow opening at the apex. In 10% to 15% of the cases, the valve is dysplastic with thickened and immobile cusps. When the peak systolic pressure gradient is moderate (50–79 mmHg) to severe (>80 mmHg) or the patient is symptomatic, percutaneous balloon valvuloplasty is recommended. Results are normally good except for dysplastic valves that often require a valvotomy. Assessment by echocardiography should include morphological examination of the PV, determination of annular size, severity of obstruction, sizing of the main PA and its branches, documentation of RV dilatation and/or hypertrophy, and other associated congenital lesions.

Subvalvular or infundibular stenosis is usually associated with other anomalies, especially VSD and TOF. A separate but similar entity is the double-chamber RV with mid-cavitary obstruction, often from a prominent moderator band, frequently associated with a VSD.

Supravalvular stenosis is rarely an isolated occurrence. It may be part of a TOF or William's syndrome, Noonan's syndrome, Allagyl's syndrome (arteriohepatic dysplasia), or congenital rubella syndrome.

The RVOT is best visualized using TEE with the mid-esophageal RV inflow/outflow view (see Fig. 18.6). Upper esophageal views of the RVOT, PV, and the main PA can be seen from "looking down" from the arch (see Fig. 18.7). This view as well as the transgastric views, usually at 90° to 120°, centered on the right heart may help to determine the gradient. Postoperatively, after reconstruction of the RVOT with a pericardial patch or repair with a conduit or a homograft, TEE should identify residual stenosis and flow across the PV.

Tetralogy of Fallot

TOF is one of the most common complex congenital cardiac malformations found in adults. The primary defect is anterocephalad displacement of the infundibular septum. The key anomaly is RVOT obstruction, which is usually infundibular but can also be valvular or supravalvular. The Ao overrides the septum and is doubly committed to both ventricles, although in TOF it is by definition at least 50% committed to the LV (Fig. 26.26). There is RV hypertrophy from systemic pressure in the RV due to the unrestrictive subaortic VSD. The severity of the disease depends largely on the degree of narrowing of the infundibulum, ranging from mild hypoplasia with good antegrade flow through the RVOT with mild cyanosis to complete atresia of the infundibulum with no antegrade flow to the pulmonary arteries. The patient is then dependent on pulmonary blood flow coming either from aortopulmonary collaterals or

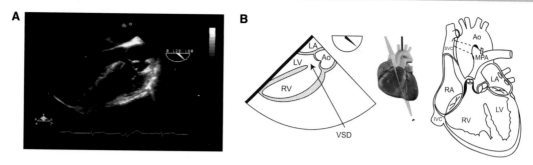

Figure 26.26 TOF. (A,B) Mid-esophageal long-axis view, demonstrates a VSD and the aortic root overriding the ventricular septum in a patient with an uncorrected TOF. *Abbreviations*: Ao, aorta; ASD, atrial septal defect; IVC, inferior vena cava; LA, left atrium; LV, left ventricle; MPA, main pulmonary artery; RA, right atrium; RV, right ventricle; SVC, superior vena cava; TOF, Tetralogy of Fallot; VSD, ventricular septal defect.

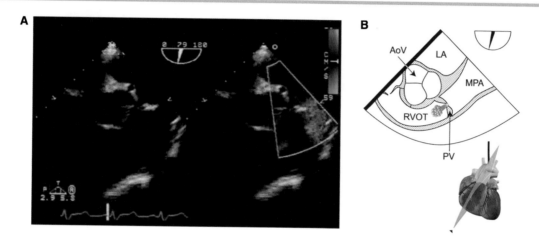

Figure 26.27 Pulmonic regurgitation in a patient with previously repaired TOF. (A,B) Color Doppler mid-esophageal right-ventricular inflow/outflow view with an abnormal PV and pulmonic regurgitation. *Abbreviations*: AoV, aortic valve; LA, left atrium; MPA, main pulmonary artery; PV, pulmonic valve; RVOT, right ventricular outflow tract; TOF, Tetralogy of Fallot.

from a PDA. Collaterals may originate anywhere in the arterial system but usually arise from the descending Ao and the transverse arch. Other associated features include additional muscular VSDs, anomalous coronary arteries, right aortic arch, PDA, aortic root dilation, and ASD. The major coronary artery anomalies include a prominent right conal artery or an anterior descending coronary originating from the right coronary artery.

The role of preoperative echocardiography in uncorrected TOF is mainly to evaluate the level and severity of the RVOT obstruction (Fig. 26.27), the VSD size, and rule out AR, which is sometimes associated with aortic root dilatation. Distal pulmonary arteries and coronary arteries are better evaluated with angiography. The large nonrestrictive VSD is best visualized in the mid-esophageal four-chamber view and AoV SAX and LAX views (Fig. 26.26). The appearance is similar to a truncus arteriosus and is differentiated by the identification of a separate origin of the PA (Fig. 26.28). Color Doppler evaluates the direction of

the ventricular shunt and the presence of other shunts, either at the atrial level or in the trabecular ventricular septum. The RVOT is best visualized with the upper and mid-esophageal RV outflow views (Fig. 26.27).

The immediate postoperative echocardiographic evaluation should attempt to detect residual RVOT obstruction and any leak across the VSD patch, demonstrating regurgitation of either the native PV, the valved conduit, or homograft. Evaluation of TR is important and can also be used to evaluate the RV systolic pressure. This should be completed by the evaluation of RV function, size and thickness, LV function, and AoV competence.

Left Atrial Anomaly

Cor Triatriatum

Cor triatriatum sinister is a rare congenital cardiac malformation involving the LA, resulting embryologically from failure of the common pulmonary vein to

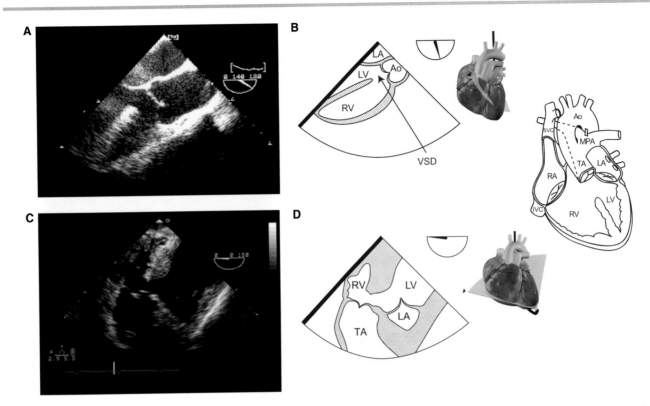

Figure 26.28   Truncus arteriosus. (A,B) Mid-esophageal long-axis view, bearing resemblance to Tetralogy of Fallot. However, the pulmonary artery has a separate origin in the latter. **(C,D)** Deep transgastric long-axis view of a patient with truncus arteriosus shows hypertrophy of the septum and the RV. *Abbreviations*: Ao, aorta; IVC, inferior vena cava; LA, left atrium; LV, left ventricle; MPA, main pulmonary artery; RA, right atrium; RV, right ventricle; SVC, superior vena cava; TOF, Tetralogy of Fallot; VSD, ventricular septal defect. *Source*: Photo A courtesy of Dr. François Béïque.

become incorporated into the LA. The incomplete absorption leaves a fibromuscular membrane dividing the left atrial chamber into a proximal compartment (the atrial accessory chamber) receiving the pulmonary veins and a distal compartment or true LA chamber, which most often contains the fossa ovalis and the left atrial appendage (LAA). The size of the communicating hole(s) between the proximal and the distal chambers determines the clinical picture (12). The degree of obstruction varies from being barely detectable to causing severe inflow obstruction and pulmonary venous congestion. There are many anatomic variations of that defect (Fig. 26.29). In severe forms, the diagnosis is usually made early in infancy and surgically corrected. Cyanosis may coexist if there is right-to-left shunt from the RA to the distal LA. Nonobstructive forms can be diagnosed as an incidental finding in adults during an echocardiographic study. Approximately 70% to 80% of cor triatriatums are associated with other congenital anomalies (13).

Because of its proximity with the LA and pulmonary veins, TEE is ideally suited for the characterization of cor triatriatum sinister. The fibromuscular membrane is classically seen coursing transversely in the LA in the mid-esophageal four- and two-chamber views (Fig. 26.30). The diagnosis requires documentation that the atrial accessory chamber does receive the

pulmonary veins while the LA proper chamber includes both the foramen ovale and the LAA. However, if the proximal chamber includes the ostium of the LAA or communicates with the ASD, the diagnosis of a supravalvular mitral ring should rather be considered. The connection of each pulmonary vein should be identified to rule out anomalous venous drainage in these patients. Other anomalous connections should also be identified such as an ASD connecting with the proximal atrial accessory chamber.

MV Anomalies

The normal MV has an anterior (aortic) and a posterior (mural) leaflet. The two commissures of these leaflets are subtended by the posteromedial and anterolateral papillary muscles and chordae tendineae. Congenital anomalies of the MV most frequently encountered include congenital mitral stenosis (MS) (including the parachute MV), an isolated cleft (see previous text), and double orifice.

Obstructions to LV inflow include congenital MS with two papillary muscles, parachute MV, supravalvular mitral ring, and cor triatriatum (see preceding text) (14).

Congenital MS can be classified according to which component of the MV apparatus is abnormal,

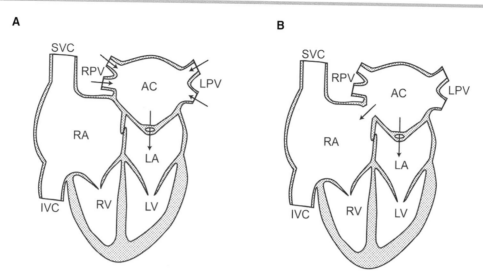

Figure 26.29   Cor triatriatum sinister variants. (A) Classic variant: the atrial AC receives the RPV and the LPV. The only outlet for pulmonary venous blood is the orifice of the fibromuscular transatrial membrane. (B) Cor triatriatum with anomalous connection between the atrial AC and the RA. The additional outlet decompresses the atrial AC and results in a left-to-right shunt at the atrial level. *Abbreviations*: AC, accessory chamber; IVC, inferior vena cava; LA, left atrium; LPV, left pulmonary veins; LV, left ventricle; RA, right atrium; RPV, right pulmonary veins; RA, right atrium; RV, right ventricle; SVC, superior vena cava. *Source*: Adapted with permission from Ref. 12.

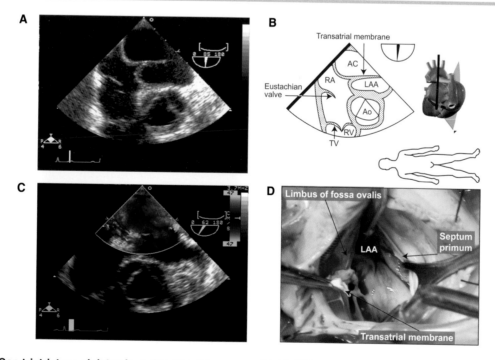

Figure 26.30   Cor triatriatum sinister in a 49-year-old woman. (A–C) Mid-esophageal views show a fibromuscular membrane coursing between the atrial septum and the junction of the LUPV and the LAA. The atrial AC receives the LUPV. (C) A left-to-right shunt through a patent foramen ovale is present. (D) Intraoperatively the fibromuscular membrane has a Swiss cheese appearance. *Abbreviations*: AC, accessory chamber; AoV, aortic valve; LAA, left atrial appendage; LUPV, left upper pulmonary vein; RA, right atrium; RV, right ventricle; TV, tricuspid valve. *Source*: Photo D courtesy of Dr. Nancy Poirier.

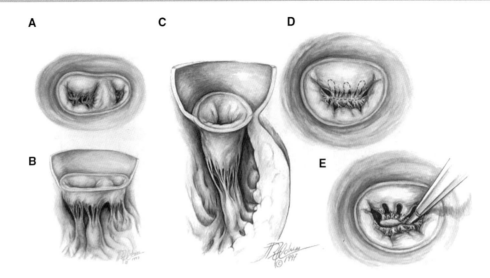

Figure 26.31 Congenital MV stenosis. (A,B) Double-orifice MV. Left atrial and cut-away atrioventricular views showing the more common variant where the smaller of the two orifices is in the right lateral position with a variable degree of stenosis. **(C–E)** Parachute MV. **(C)** Cut-away atrioventricular view with a single papillary muscle or fused papillary muscles usually arising from the posterior left ventricular wall. **(D)** Repair by leaflet fenestrations and papillary muscle incision (dotted line) to open the ventricular inlet. This technique is meant to maximize unrestricted blood flow into the left ventricle during diastole while preserving enough valvular tissue for effective coaptation during systole. **(E)** The fused papillary muscle is incised to facilitate valvular mobility. *Abbreviation*: MV, mitral valve. *Source*: Adapted with permission from Ref. 15.

including leaflets, annulus, chordae, or papillary muscles (Fig. 26.31) (15). Most cases, however, involve variable combinations of structural anomalies, including annulus hypoplasia, thickened rolled leaflet margins, commissural fusion, shortened and thickened chordae tendineae, fibrous obliteration of the interchordal spaces, abnormal chordal insertion, papillary muscle hypoplasia, and decreased interpapillary muscle distance or fusion. Echocardiographically, the MV leaflets appear thickened, dysplastic, and echo dense; they move poorly and dome during LV diastolic filling. The subvalvular mitral apparatus similarly presents an echo-dense, crowded appearance.

The parachute MV represents about half of the MS diagnosed in pediatric patients. It is characterized by insertion of all the chordae tendineae into a single papillary muscle group. The MV leaflets also appear dense, with restricted motion (Fig. 26.32). The chordae are generally shortened and thickened. The anatomy of the papillary muscles is highly variable. A single papillary muscle in the LV, the hallmark of this lesion, may be identified in the mid-esophageal four-chamber view, the transgastric SAX and LAX views. The parachute MV is often associated with other anomalies that constitute the Shone's syndrome: these include a supravalvular mitral ring, subaortic stenosis, and coarctation of the Ao. Nearly 70% of parachute MVs are associated with a supravalvular mitral ring, while 60% present a significant diastolic pressure gradient.

The supravalvular mitral ring rarely occurs as an isolated finding and most often occurs with the other component of the Shone's syndrome. A supravalvular ring is also found with 20% of congenital MS with two

anatomical papillary muscles. It originates from a collection of connective tissue arising from the atrial surface of the MV leaflets and consequently encroaches on the MV orifice. It may closely adhere to the anterior MV leaflet. The ring itself causes a significant obstruction in only 10% of cases. In the other cases, the ring does not add significant obstruction to the associated MV stenosis.

The MV is best evaluated with the mid-esophageal four- and two-chamber and LAX views using color Doppler, and spectral Doppler determination of mitral inflow diastolic pressure gradient. The transgastric views can also help evaluate the subvalvular apparatus.

AoV Anomalies

The bicuspid AoV is the most common congenital anomaly in adults. It occurs in approximately 2% to 3% of the general population. The lesions of bicuspid AoV, subvalvular and supra valvular stenosis are detailed in Chapter 14.

Coarctation of the Aorta

Coarctation of the Ao is narrowing of the Ao usually at the level of the ligamentum arteriosus. It is usually discrete but can be associated with diffuse hypoplasia of the aortic arch and isthmus. Coarctation is considered "simple" when it is discrete and without major intracardiac lesions. This is the form most commonly diagnosed de novo in teenagers and adults (Fig. 26.33). In contrast, "complex" aortic coarctation

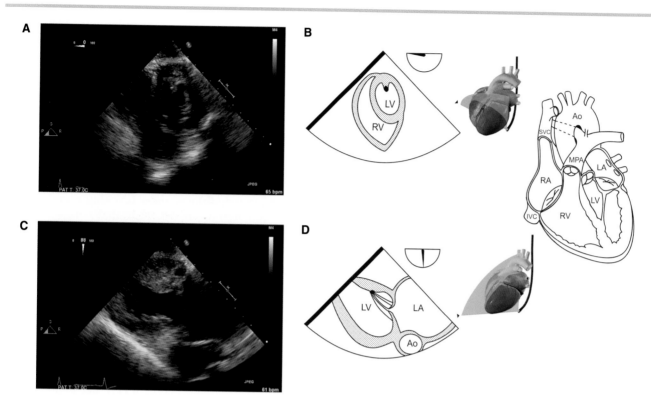

Figure 26.32 Parachute MV. Transgastric mid short-axis (**A,B**) and long-axis (**C,D**) views: note the presence of only a single papillary muscle. *Abbreviations*: Ao, aorta; IVC, inferior vena cava; LA, left atrium; LV, left ventricle; MPA, main pulmonary artery; MV, mitral valve; RA, right atrium; RV, right ventricle; SVC, superior vena cava.

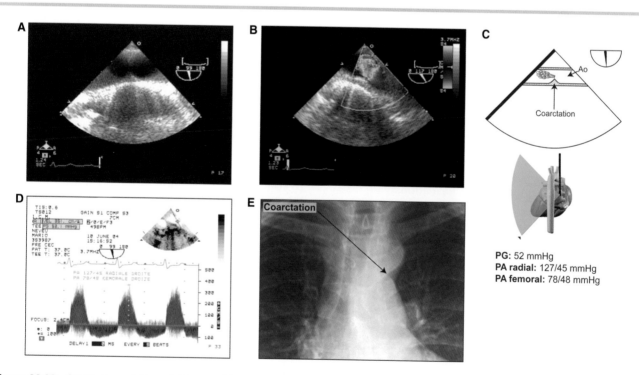

PG: 52 mmHg
PA radial: 127/45 mmHg
PA femoral: 78/48 mmHg

Figure 26.33 Aortic coarctation. A 48-year-old man with a bicuspid aortic valve scheduled for valve replacement also has an aortic coarctation. (**A–C**) Descending Ao long-axis views show the coarctation with color Doppler flow aliasing. (**D**) The continuous wave Doppler PG was 52 mmHg, close to the 49 mmHg PG obtained using the systolic radial to femoral Pa difference. (**E**) Chest X-ray with the classical "3" sign, due to the aortic indentation of coarctation. *Abbreviations*: Ao, aorta; Pa, arterial pressure; PG, pressure gradient.

is usually diagnosed in infancy and is associated with other important intracardiac anomalies, mainly VSD, subvalvular AS, and valvular AS.

The coarctation is hemodynamically significant in the presence of right arm hypertension and peak pull-back gradient of greater than 20 mmHg across the coarctation during catheterization. However, minimal or no-pressure gradient may be encountered in the presence of significant collateral circulation. Associated cardiovascular anomalies include bicuspid AoV in close to 85%, intracranial berry aneurysms of the circle of Willis in 3% to 5%, and anomalies of the brachiocephalic circulation such as anomalous origin of the right subclavian artery in 5%. Other anomalies include collaterals involving the internal mammary arteries anteriorly and the intercostal arteries posteriorly as well as VSD and aortic medial disease near the coarctation area and in the ascending Ao. In the absence of aneurysms in the area of the coarctation, these cases are dealt with in the interventional suite rather than the operating room.

The best echocardiographic window to visualize a coarctation is the transthoracic suprasternal notch view. It provides 2D imaging of the obstruction and allows acquisition of the Doppler-derived pressure gradient across the area of narrowing. Severe coarctation is suggested by high-velocity flow in systole with a gradient that persists in diastole. Abnormal flow will be found distally in the abdominal Ao. TEE evaluation can provide helpful information about the area of obstruction that is usually apparent just below the aortic arch beyond the origin of the left subclavian artery. In the upper esophageal SAX view, the coarctation will appear as narrowing of the cross-sectional area with a variable degree of hypoplasia proximally and dilatation distally. The aortic arch LAX view provides additional insight about the length and morphology of the coarctation (Fig. 26.33). However, in either view, Doppler determination of pressure gradient is frequently difficult due to inadequate alignment of the ultrasound beam with the blood flow. Hence, preoperative MRI or biplane aortography may be required to complete the evaluation in adults. Postsurgical evaluation includes determination of residual narrowing, recurrent obstruction, or aneurysmal formation.

PREVIOUSLY REPAIRED CONGENITAL HEART DEFECTS

Tetralogy of Fallot

Adults presenting with TOF can be separated into three groups (16): (*i*) adults who underwent a corrective procedure in infancy or childhood; (*ii*) adults with an unrepaired form of TOF, either the unusual patient with mild RVOT obstruction or an extreme form with aortopulmonary collaterals; and (*iii*) adults who underwent palliative surgery as a child without having undergone corrective surgery. The types of palliation includes Blalock–Taussig shunt or modification (subclavian artery to PA shunt), Waterston shunt (ascending Ao to right PA), Potts shunt (descending

Ao to left PA), central interposition tube graft, infundibulum resection (Brock), or pulmonary valvotomy, RV to PA conduit without VSD closure or partial closure of the VSD.

In TOF patients who underwent a complete repair in infancy and have survived to adulthood, evaluation must seek several conditions that may warrant reintervention. These include (*i*) residual VSD with a shunt greater than 1.5:1; (*ii*) residual PS with elevation of RV pressure to two-thirds or more of the systemic pressure (Fig. 26.34); (*iii*) severe pulmonary regurgitation associated with progressive RV enlargement (Fig. 26.35), TR, significant atrial, or ventricular arrhythmias and worsening exercise intolerance; (*iv*) significant AR associated with symptoms and LV enlargement and dysfunction; (*v*) aortic root enlargement; and (*vi*) large RVOT aneurysm (Fig. 26.36) (16–18). Patients with an RV to PA conduit as treatment for severe PS and TOF may require reoperation for conduit stenosis. These patients are also at risk for developing atrial and ventricular arrhythmias, and mapping with ablation may be part of the surgical procedure (17).

When TOF patients undergo reoperation, the preoperative TEE evaluation, in addition to evaluating the PV, is performed mainly to evaluate TV competence, RV and LV size and function, RVOT size and function. The presence of aortic root dilatation, AR, and residual VSD flow should also be assessed. The most useful TEE views include the mid-esophageal AoV SAX and LAX, mid-esophageal four-chamber, mid-esophageal RV inflow/outflow, upper esophageal aortic arch SAX as well as deep transgastric inflow outflow views of the RV. The immediate postoperative TEE evaluation will examine the result of the surgery and the need for further repair. The bioprosthetic PV is in proximity to the left main coronary artery. In addition to assessing the valve, both ventricles should be assessed for wall motion abnormalities in the post-cardiopulmonary bypass phase.

Transposition of the Great Arteries

D-TGA

In complete transposition of the great arteries (TGA), there is normal atrioventricular concordance but abnormal ventriculoarterial discordance (Fig. 26.37). Physiologically, the systemic venous deoxygenated blood is pumped by the RV back into the Ao and the systemic circulation, whereas the pulmonary venous oxygenated blood is ejected by the LV back into the pulmonary circuit. Delivery of oxygenated blood to the systemic circulation and peripheral tissues for survival is thus dependent on the mixing of blood between the two parallel circuits, either at the atrial, ventricular, or ductal level. Associated anomalies include ASD (mostly secundum), VSD (outlet type), pulmonary artery overriding, subaortic (RVOT) and subpulmonic (LVOT) obstruction, and tricuspid (systemic atrioventricular) valve abnormalities. Most patients present with cyanosis soon after birth. Nearly all patients seen in adolescence or adulthood will have

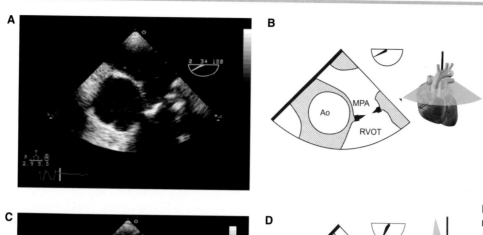

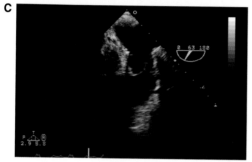

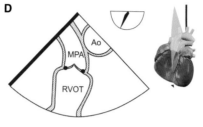

Figure 26.34 PS in a previously repaired TOF. (A,B) Mid-esophageal Ao short-axis view with a dysfunctional and stenotic calcified pulmonic prosthetic valve. **(C,D)** Same view after redo pulmonic valve replacement. Note the proximity of the coronary arteries. *Abbreviations*: Ao, aorta; AoV, aortic valve; MPA, main pulmonary artery; PS, pulmonic stenosis; RVOT, right ventricular outflow tract; TOF, Tetralogy of Fallot.

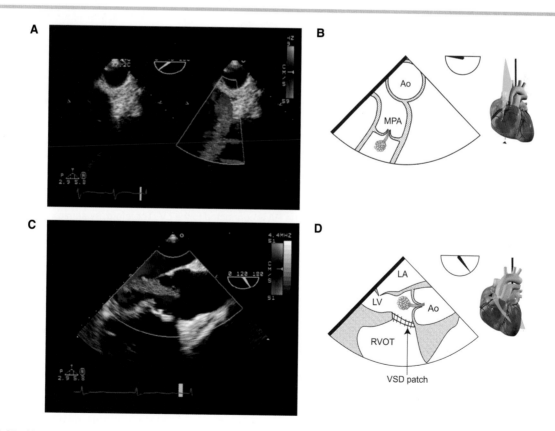

Figure 26.35 Valve regurgitation in previously repaired TOF. (A,B) Color Doppler upper esophageal aortic arch short-axis view with severe pulmonic regurgitation. **(C,D)** Color Doppler mid-esophageal AoV long-axis view with moderate aortic regurgitation. Note the VSD patch from previous repair. *Abbreviations*: AoV, aortic valve; LA, left atrium; LV, left ventricle; RVOT, right ventricular outflow tract; TOF, Tetralogy of Fallot; VSD, ventricular septal defect.

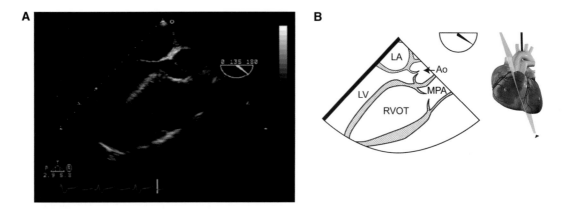

Figure 26.36   RVOT aneurysm in a patient with TOF. (A,B) Mid-esophageal long-axis view shows a RVOT aneurysm. *Abbreviations*: Ao, aorta; LA, left atrium; LV, left ventricle; MPA, main pulmonary artery; RVOT, right ventricular outflow tract; TOF, Tetralogy of Fallot.

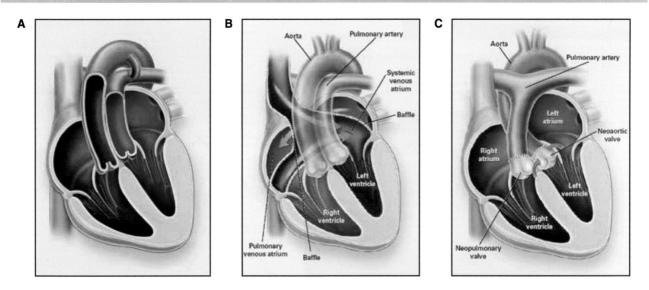

Figure 26.37   D-TGA. (A) The Ao is connected to the RV while the PA is connected to the LV. Therefore, systemic venous blood returns to the RA, from which it goes to the RV and then back to the systemic circulation through the Ao. Pulmonary venous blood returns to the LA, from which it goes to the LV and then to the PA. Survival is possible only if there is a communication between the two parallel circuits, such as a patent ductus arteriosus. **(B)** The "atrial switch" operation: a baffle is created in the atria, so that blood returning from the systemic venous circulation is diverted into the LV and then the PA (blue arrows), whereas blood returning from the pulmonary venous circulation is directed into the RV and then the Ao (red arrow). **(C)** The "arterial switch" operation: the PA and ascending Ao are transected above the semilunar valves and coronary arteries, are then switched (neoaortic and neopulmonary valves). *Abbreviations*: Ao, aorta; D-TGA, right (dextro) transposition of the great arteries; LA, left atrium; LV, left ventricle; PA, pulmonary artery; RA, right atrium; RV, right ventricle. *Source*: With permission from Ref. 20.

had surgery as unrepaired TGA is lethal with 90% mortality in the first year of life.

Two distinct surgical procedures have been advocated for the treatment of D-TGA. In the past, the most common form of repair was an atrial switch operation (Fig. 26.37), in which an intra-atrial baffle was made of a prosthetic patch (original Mustard procedure) (Fig. 26.38), supplemental pericardial tis-sue (modified Mustard procedure), or atrial tissue (Senning procedure). The baffle connects the venae cavae to the left atrium, the mitral valve, and the pulmonary circulation while it allows pulmonary venous blood to be redirected over the baffle to the right atrium and the systemic circulation. With this repair, the morphological RV has to support the increased pressures of the systemic circulation (19,20).

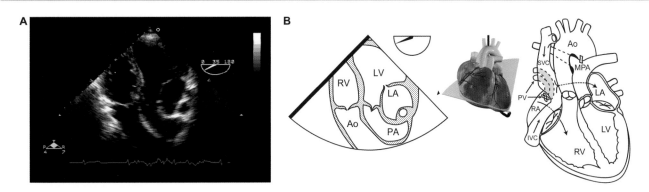

Figure 26.38 Mustard procedure for D-TGA. An intra-atrial baffle made of a prosthetic patch allows systemic venous return to be redirected, at the atrial level, to the subpulmonary morphologic LV while pulmonary venous blood is rerouted to the subaortic morphologic RV, thus achieving physiological correction. With this repair, the morphologic RV has to support the increased pressures of the systemic circulation. (**A,B**) The transgastric long-axis view shows the classic "double-barrel" parallel alignment of the great vessels and a portion of the atrial baffle. *Abbreviations*: Ao, aorta; D-TGA, right (dextro) transposition of the great arteries; IVC, inferior vena cava; LA, left atrium; LV, left ventricle; MPA, main pulmonary artery; PA, pulmonary artery; RA, right atrium; RV, right ventricle; SVC, superior vena cava.

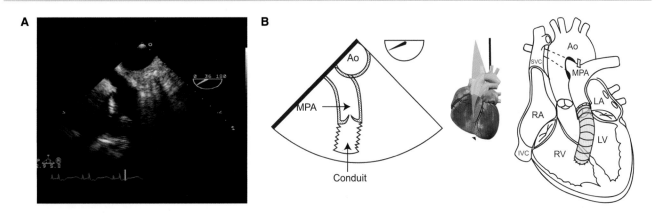

Figure 26.39 Rastelli procedure for D-TGA. In the Rastelli procedure, for patients with a VSD and pulmonic stenosis, the VSD is closed and blood is redirected at the ventricular level by tunneling the left ventricular outflow to the Ao whereas a valved conduit connects the RV to the MPA. (**A,B**) The upper esophageal aortic arch short-axis view shows the distal portion of the valved conduit as it connects with the PA. *Abbreviations*: Ao, aorta; D-TGA, right (dextro) transposition of the great arteries; IVC, inferior vena cava; LA, left atrium; LV, left ventricle; MPA, main pulmonary artery; PA, pulmonary artery; RA, right atrium; RV, right ventricle; SVC, superior vena cava; VSD, ventricular septal defect.

Starting in the late 1980s, the atrial switch operation has, progressively, been replaced by the arterial switch operation that consists of switching the great arteries and translocating the coronary arteries to the neoaorta (Fig. 26.37) (20). The theoretical advantage of this repair lies in the morphological LV being the systemic ventricle.

The Rastelli operation addressed patients with a VSD and PS (Fig. 26.39). Blood is redirected at the ventricular level by tunneling the LV outflow to the Ao and connecting the RV to the PA using a valved conduit. The morphological LV supports the systemic circulation. The RV to PA conduit lies retrosternal and may become compressed or obstructed over time. In addition, endocarditis is not an infrequent complication.

Long-term postoperative sequelae will vary according to the type of operation performed. Long-term recognized sequelae in patients who underwent an atrial switch operation include right (systemic) ventricular dysfunction, significant TR, symptomatic bradycardia, tachycardia, or sick sinus syndrome. Other potential late complications include obstruction of the SVC or IVC venous pathways, baffle leak resulting in significant left-to-right or right-to-left shunting, and progressive LV outflow subpulmonary obstruction (19,21). Some of those sequelae are best approached by percutaneous interventions: balloon angioplasty and stent insertion for baffle obstruction or occlusion devices for baffle leaks. Other sequelae such as AV valve regurgitation, subpulmonary obstruction, or ventricular dysfunction require surgery. The patient with a failing RV and severe TR may be considered for heart transplantation.

Late complications of the arterial switch procedure include significant RVOT obstruction, myocardial ischemia from coronary artery obstruction, and neoaortic valve regurgitation (22). Those complications need to be approached surgically. Rastelli patients may develop RV to PA conduit obstruction, subaortic obstruction across the left ventricular-Ao tunnel, VSD, and pulmonary branch stenosis.

L-TGA

Congenitally corrected transposition is characterized by AV discordance and ventriculoarterial discordance—essentially a "ventricular switch" (Figs. 26.1 and 26.40). Blood returning to the heart will pass through the cava into the RA, through the MV and the morphological LV, and then through the PV to the PA. The blood returning from the lungs passes from the pulmonary veins into the LA, through the TV and morphological RV, and across the AoV into the Ao.

The aortic root arises from the RV and is anterior and leftward of the PA trunk. The AV valves in transposition of the great arteries are coplanar (23). Normally, the PV and the AoV valve lie at orthogonal angles to each other, so one is seen in long axis while the other is seen in SAX. In TGA, both these valves lie in the same plane and, thus, are seen in SAX in the same view or LAX in the same view.

As these patients are "physiologically corrected," they may not present until later in life with progressive failure of the systemic morphological RV accompanied by dilatation and (left-sided) TR. Congenitally corrected transposition is commonly associated with perimembranous VSD, LVOT obstruction from valvular or subvalvular pulmonic stenosis, and with structural abnormalities of the left AV (tricuspid) valve, where the septal leaflet insertion is apically displaced (Ebstein-like anomaly). Conventional management has been to operate on the associated lesions and medical treatment of the failing systemic ventricle (23). Increasingly, these patients are referred for a "double switch procedure." The morphological LV is exposed to "training" of the systemic pressures by

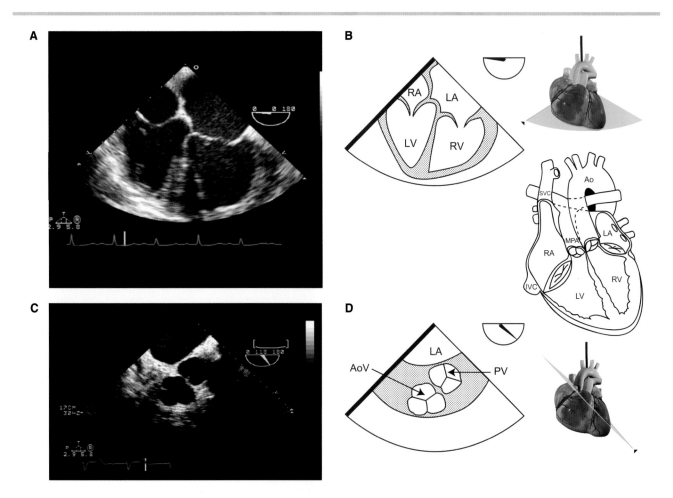

Figure 26.40 Congenitally corrected L-TGA. (A,B) Mid-esophageal four-chamber shows the higher insertion of the right atrioventricular valve consistent with a MV. **(C,D)** Mid-esophageal view at 118° shows the PV posterior to the AoV. *Abbreviations*: Ao, aorta; AoV, aortic valve; IVC, inferior vena cava; LA, left atrium; L-TGA, left transposition of the great arteries; LV, left ventricle; MV, mitral valve; MPA, main pulmonary artery; PV, pulmonic valve; RA, right atrium; RV, right ventricle; SVC, superior vena cava.

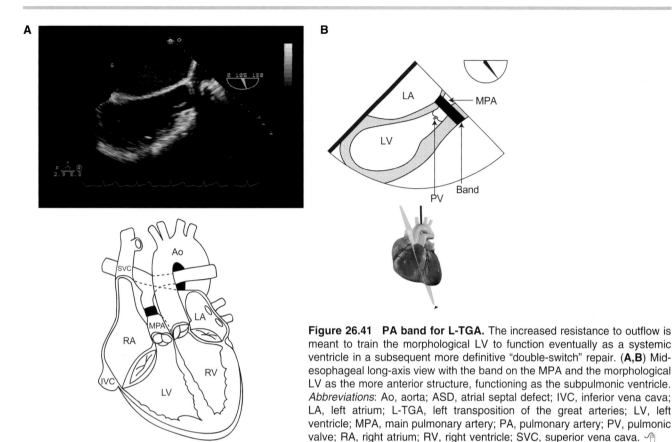

Figure 26.41   PA band for L-TGA. The increased resistance to outflow is meant to train the morphological LV to function eventually as a systemic ventricle in a subsequent more definitive "double-switch" repair. **(A,B)** Mid-esophageal long-axis view with the band on the MPA and the morphological LV as the more anterior structure, functioning as the subpulmonic ventricle. *Abbreviations*: Ao, aorta; ASD, atrial septal defect; IVC, inferior vena cava; LA, left atrium; L-TGA, left transposition of the great arteries; LV, left ventricle; MPA, main pulmonary artery; PA, pulmonary artery; PV, pulmonic valve; RA, right atrium; RV, right ventricle; SVC, superior vena cava.

means of PA banding (Fig. 26.41) in the absence of the morphological LV being exposed to increased resistance by means of an unrestricted VSD or pulmonary hypertension from pulmonary outflow tract obstruction. Once the morphological LV has been exposed to systemic or near systemic pressures and does not show signs of failure, the patient has a combined atrial and arterial switch procedure (24–26).

TEE will involve assessing the PA band as well as morphological LV function and the gradient pre and post deployment of the band. This can be done by the usual methods for the PA in the mid- and upper esophagus and the views usually used for assessment of RV function in the mid-esophageal and transgastric views (Fig. 26.41).

Complex Single Ventricle

Patients with a single ventricle have either a single anatomical ventricle comprised of a single pouch of indeterminate origin or, more commonly, a functional single ventricle with one well-formed ventricle accompanied by a second underdeveloped or rudimentary ventricle (Figs. 26.1 and 26.42). The atria can be solitus, inversus, or ambiguous (Table 26.1). The AV connection consists of a common valve or two separate valves, one patent and the other atretic. The well-developed ventricular chamber can be of the LV or RV

type. The ventriculoarterial connection can be concordant or discordant, or the great arteries can arise from the same ventricle and be either patent or stenotic. The most common types of single ventricle of LV morphology consist of tricuspid atresia, pulmonary atresia with intact ventricular septum, and double-inlet LV (Fig. 26.43). The most common single RV is the hypoplastic left-heart syndrome.

Adults with a single ventricle are separated into two groups: first, a group of patients who either never required surgery because of an acceptable well-balanced physiology or who have undergone one or several palliative (non-Fontan) surgical procedures (Fig. 26.44). The latter include the Glenn bidirectional cavopulmonary connection and a variety of other aortopulmonary shunts, such as the Blalock–Taussig subclavian to PA branch shunt (Fig. 26.44A), the Pott's shunt of the anterior wall of the descending Ao to the posterior wall of the left PA, and the Waterston shunt between the ascending Ao and the right PA. The Potts and Waterston shunt are rarely done now, but there are many adults that have residual shunts or physiological consequences of having had the shunt.

The other group includes patients who have undergone a repair where the systemic venous return is diverted to the PA circulation without passing through a subpulmonary ventricle, a principle that is now known as the Fontan procedure (Fig. 26.45).

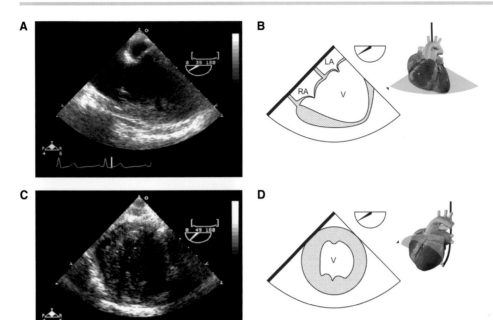

Figure 26.42 Single ventricle. Double inlet morphologic left ventricle in a 38-year-old woman who previously underwent a Blalock procedure. (**A,B**) Mid-esophageal view shows both atrioventricular valves (left and right) open into a single ventricle. (**C,D**) Transgastric view shows the thickened septal part of the ventricle. *Abbreviations*: LA, left atrium; RA, right atrium; V, ventricle. ⌐

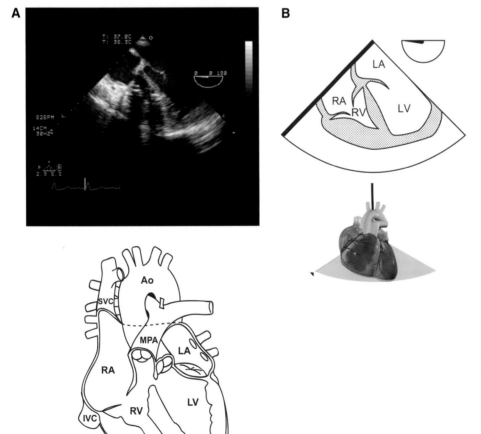

Figure 26.43 Tricuspid atresia. (**A,B**) Mid-esophageal four-chamber view in a patient demonstrates tricuspid atresia with a small rudimentary RV. *Abbreviations*: Ao, aorta; IVC, inferior vena cava; LA, left atrium; LV, left ventricle; MPA, main pulmonary artery; RA, right atrium; RV, right ventricle; SVC, superior vena cava. ⌐

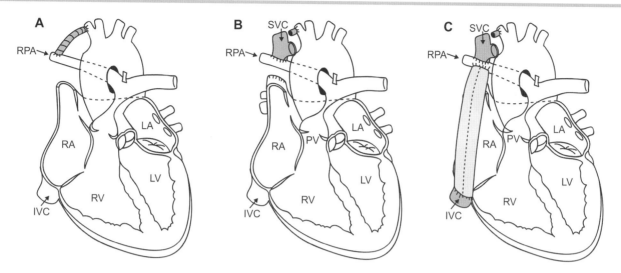

Figure 26.44 Palliative shunts in congenital heart disease. (A) Modified Blalock-Taussig shunt (from right subclavian artery to RPA) to supply venous blood to the pulmonary circuit in a single ventricle anomaly (tricuspid atresia). **(B)** Classic Glenn shunt (from SVC to RPA). **(C)** Fontan type procedure, where IVC blood has been routed to the RPA without passing through the subpulmonary ventricle, in this example using the extracardiac conduit technique. *Abbreviations*: IVC, inferior vena cava; LA, left atrium; LV, left ventricle; PA, pulmonary artery; PV, pulmonic valve; RA, right atrium; RPA, right pulmonary artery; RV, right ventricle; SVC, superior vena cava.

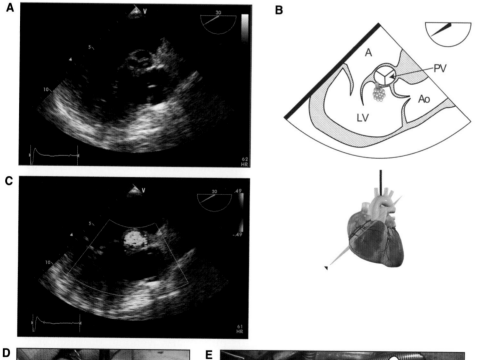

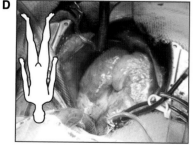

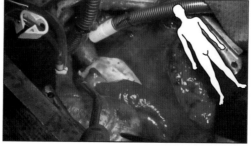

Figure 26.45 Fontan procedure. (A–C) Mid-esophageal views at 33° in a patient with D-TGA and situs inversus undergoing a Fontan procedure are shown. **(D,E)** Intraoperative views are shown. *Abbreviations*: A, atrium; Ao, aorta; D-TGA, right (dextro) transposition of the great arteries; LV, left ventricle; PV, pulmonic valve.

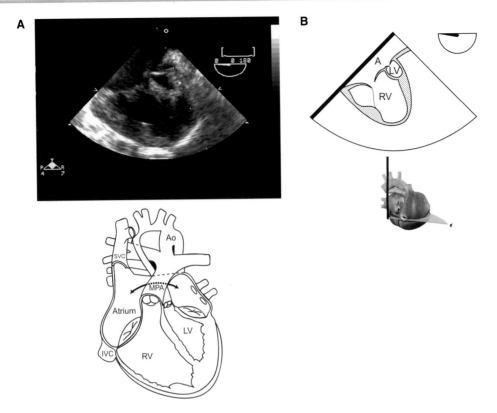

Figure 26.46   Hypoplastic LV. (A,B) Mid-esophageal view of a hypoplastic LV in a patient being evaluated for a third stage Fontan procedure. Note the small LV and the large RV and common atrium. *Abbreviations*: A, atrium; Ao, aorta; IVC, inferior vena cava; LA, left atrium; LV, left ventricle; MPA, main pulmonary artery; RA, right atrium; RV, right ventricle; SVC, superior vena cava.

There are many modifications of the original Fontan procedure (27). Although originally described as a treatment for tricuspid atresia, modifications to the original procedure are used for other forms of congenital heart disease with a single ventricle (Fig. 26.46) (28).

The non-Fontan adult with a single ventricle will require surgery in the presence of significant functional limitation, cyanosis (resting oxygen saturation <90%), dilated systemic ventricle from volume overload, and paradoxical embolism. Surgical options include performing a bidirectional Glenn, a bidirectional Glenn with additional pulmonary blood flow through a native PA with valvular stenosis or PA banding or the addition of a small aortopulmonary shunt, and Fontan procedure.

The Glenn shunt is a connection between a systemic vein, the SVC, and the right PA. As initially described, the classic Glenn shunt involved an end-to-side anastomosis of the SVC to the end of the right PA, which provides unidirectional pulmonary blood flow. The bidirectional Glenn involves the connection of the SVC end to side to the right PA, which is still connected to the main PA; hence, blood from the SVC can enter both the pulmonary arteries.

Numerous variants to the Fontan approach have been described. The most frequently encountered are the direct RA to PA connection, an RA to RV through a valved conduit, the total cavopulmonary connection (with SVC to PA and IVC to PA through an intra-atrial tunnel) (29), and the extracardiac conduit (SVC to PA and IVC to PA through an external conduit) (Fig. 26.45) (30).

Patients with a previous Fontan procedure may also require surgical reintervention (31,32) for the following indications: (*i*) residual ASD with right-to-left shunt and symptomatic cyanosis, (*ii*) significant AV valve regurgitation, (*iii*) obstruction in the Fontan conduit (see Fig. 13.17), (*iv*) development of venous collateral channels or pulmonary arteriovenous malformations, (*v*) development of sustained atrial flutter or fibrillation, (*vi*) protein-losing enteropathy, (*vii*) pulmonary venous obstruction, and (*viii*) heart block or sick sinus syndrome requiring a pacemaker. The Fontan "redo" procedures vary from the original Fontan procedure to more modern approaches with total cavopulmonary connection or extracardiac conduit.

The goal of a thorough perioperative TEE examination is mainly to evaluate ventricular function, AV competence or adequacy of the AV valve repair, semilunar valve function and competence, and pulmonary venous blood flow, and to exclude the presence of thrombus.

THREE-DIMENSIONAL ECHOCARDIOGRAPHY IN CONGENITAL HEART DISEASE

Congenital cardiology is probably the area that has gained the most from the development of 3D echocardiography. The emergence of new techniques in cardiac procedures, including minimally invasive surgeries and percutaneous catheter interventions, has increased the need for accurate assessment of cardiac structural defects size, morphology, and good understanding of the spatial relationship with adjacent structures. There is increasing literature showing that 3D TEE provides incremental information that can have an impact on therapeutic decision-making and prognosis in congenital heart disease, particularly in complex lesions.

In a study to determine the usefulness of 3D TEE in the assessment of secundum ASDs (Fig. 26.5) considered for device closure, Morgan et al. (33) compared the findings from 3D TEE with those from 2D TEE regarding dimensions, morphology, and suitability for device closure. They found that 3D TTE provides not only comparable data with 2D TEE but also useful additional dynamic and morphological information. Recent application of 3D TEE has shown great promise for imaging VSD with better display of the exact geometry, size, and location of the defect. Mercer-Rosa et al. (34) sought to answer the question of whether these additional morphological details

obtained with real-time 3D echocardiography imaging of muscular VSD have any significant impact on treatment options of individual patient. They concluded that 3D TEE can have significant impact on treatment strategies of individual patients and should be an important adjunct to the standard transthoracic echocardiographic and TEE imaging of these defect before any intervention.

Other more complex congenital heart disease will certainly benefit from this technology.

CONCLUSION

In summary, the role of TEE in congenital heart disease surgery, both in the pediatric and adult population, has been expanding (35,36). The preoperative characterization of the anomaly and its consequences and the evaluation of the postoperative results are important roles of TEE, as summarized in Table 26.3.

REFERENCES

1. Miller-Hance WC, Silverman NH. Transesophageal echocardiography (TEE) in congenital heart disease with focus on the adult. Cardiol Clin 2000; 18:861–892.
2. Webb G, Gatzoulis MA. Atrial septal defects in the adult: recent progress and overview. Circulation 2006; 114: 1645–1653.
3. Gatzoulis MA, Freeman MA, Siu SC, et al. Atrial arrhythmia after surgical closure of atrial septal defects in adults. N Engl J Med 1999; 340:839–846.
4. Chessa M, Carminati M, Butera G, et al. Early and late complications associated with transcatheter occlusion of secundum atrial septal defect. J Am Coll Cardiol 2002; 39:1061–1065.
5. Sukernik MR, Bennett-Guerrero E. The incidental finding of a patent foramen ovale during cardiac surgery: should it always be repaired? A core review. Anesth Analg 2007; 105:602–610.
6. Shanewise JS, Cheung AT, Aronson S, et al. ASE/SCA guidelines for performing a comprehensive intraoperative multiplane transesophageal echocardiography examination: recommendations of the American Society of Echocardiography Council for Intraoperative Echocardiography and the Society of Cardiovascular Anesthesiologists Task Force for Certification in Perioperative Transesophageal Echocardiography. Anesth Analg 1999; 89:870–884.
7. Gatzoulis MA, Hechter S, Webb GD, et al. Surgery for partial atrioventricular septal defect in the adult. Ann Thorac Surg 1999; 67:504–510.
8. Oechslin E, Buchholz S, Jenni R. Ebstein's anomaly in adults: Doppler-echocardiographic evaluation. Thorac Cardiovasc Surg 2000; 48:209–213.
9. Chen JM, Mosca RS, Altmann K, et al. Early and medium-term results for repair of Ebstein anomaly. J Thorac Cardiovasc Surg 2004; 127:990–998.
10. Dearani JA, Danielson GK. Surgical management of Ebstein's anomaly in the adult. Semin Thorac Cardiovasc Surg 2005; 17:148–154.
11. Boston US, Dearani JA, O'Leary PW, et al. Tricuspid valve repair for Ebstein's anomaly in young children: a 30-year experience. Ann Thorac Surg 2006; 81:690–695.
12. Moss AJ, Adams FH, Emmanouilides GC. Moss and Adams Heart Disease in Infants, Children, and Adolescents including the Fetus and Young Adult. 5th ed. Baltimore: Williams & Wilkins, 1995.

Table 26.3 Role of TEE in Congenital Heart Surgery

Before the procedure
- Systematic analysis of intra- and extracardiac structures (see Table 19.2)
- Evaluation of the anomalies and their impact on biventricular function
- Evaluation of all four cardiac valves
- Ruling out associated congenital anomalies
- Contrast examination and shunt calculation (see Chapter 5)

Perioperative period
- Monitoring during cardiac surgery (see Table 13.1)
- Ruling out stenotic or regurgitant anastomosis
- Detection of residual shunts
- De-airing of all (four) cardiac cavities
- Ruling out patent foramen ovale with color Doppler and contrast study

Early and late postoperative period
Systematic evaluation of:
- Left and right ventricular systolic and diastolic function
- Valvular (all four valves) integrity and function
- Vascular anastomosis, thrombus, spontaneous echocardiographic contrast
- Aneurysm and pseudoaneurysm of anastomosis

In the advent of hemodynamic instability: identification of
- Obstruction of the anastomosis
- Left and right ventricular systolic and diastolic function
- Left and right ventricular outflow tract dynamic or fixed obstruction
- Severe mitral or tricuspid regurgitation
- Hypovolemia
- Cardiac tamponade (circumferential or loculated)

Abbreviation: TEE, transesophageal echocardiography

13. Webb G, Gatzoulis M, Debauney P. Diagnosis and Management of Adult Congenital Heart Disease. London: Churchill Livingstone, 2003.

14. Banerjee A, Kohl T, Silverman NH. Echocardiographic evaluation of congenital mitral valve anomalies in children. Am J Cardiol 1995; 76:1284–1291.

15. Zias EA, Mavroudis C, Backer CL, et al. Surgical repair of the congenitally malformed mitral valve in infants and children. Ann Thorac Surg 1998; 66:1551–1559.

16. Therrien J, Warnes C, Daliento L, et al. Canadian Cardiovascular Society Consensus Conference 2001 update: recommendations for the management of adults with congenital heart disease part III. Can J Cardiol 2001; 17: 1135–1158.

17. Murphy JG, Gersh BJ, Mair DD, et al. Long-term outcome in patients undergoing surgical repair of tetralogy of Fallot. N Engl J Med 1993; 329:593–599.

18. Redington AN. Determinants and assessment of pulmonary regurgitation in tetralogy of Fallot: practice and pitfalls. Cardiol Clin 2006; 24:631–639, vii.

19. Gelatt M, Hamilton RM, McCrindle BW, et al. Arrhythmia and mortality after the Mustard procedure: a 30-year single-center experience. J Am Coll Cardiol 1997; 29:194–201.

20. Brickner ME, Hillis LD, Lange RA. Congenital heart disease in adults. Second of two parts. N Engl J Med 2000; 342:334–342.

21. Mee RB. Severe right ventricular failure after Mustard or Senning operation. Two-stage repair: pulmonary artery banding and switch. J Thorac Cardiovasc Surg 1986; 92: 385–390.

22. Haas F, Wottke M, Poppert H, et al. Long-term survival and functional follow-up in patients after the arterial switch operation. Ann Thorac Surg 1999; 68:1692–1697.

23. Sommer RJ, Hijazi ZM, Rhodes JF. Pathophysiology of congenital heart disease in the adult: part III: complex congenital heart disease. Circulation 2008; 117:1340–1350.

24. Devaney EJ, Charpie JR, Ohye RG, et al. Combined arterial switch and Senning operation for congenitally corrected transposition of the great arteries: patient selection and intermediate results. J Thorac Cardiovasc Surg 2003; 125:500–507.

25. Duncan BW, Mee RB, Mesia CI, et al. Results of the double switch operation for congenitally corrected transposition of the great arteries. Eur J Cardiothorac Surg 2003; 24:11–19.

26. Quinn DW, McGuirk SP, Metha C, et al. The morphologic left ventricle that requires training by means of pulmonary artery banding before the double-switch procedure for congenitally corrected transposition of the great arteries is at risk of late dysfunction. J Thorac Cardiovasc Surg 2008; 135:1137–1144.

27. Fontan F, Baudet E. Surgical repair of tricuspid atresia. Thorax 1971; 26:240–248.

28. Mott AR, Feltes TF, McKenzie ED, et al. Improved early results with the Fontan operation in adults with functional single ventricle. Ann Thorac Surg 2004; 77:1334–1340.

29. Kreutzer J, Keane JF, Lock JE, et al. Conversion of modified Fontan procedure to lateral atrial tunnel cavopulmonary anastomosis. J Thorac Cardiovasc Surg 1996; 111:1169–1176.

30. Mavroudis C, Backer CL, Deal BJ, et al. Total cavopulmonary conversion and maze procedure for patients with failure of the Fontan operation. J Thorac Cardiovasc Surg 2001; 122:863–871.

31. Driscoll DJ, Offord KP, Feldt RH, et al. Five- to fifteen-year follow-up after Fontan operation. Circulation 1992; 85:469–496.

32. Backer CL, Deal BJ, Mavroudis C, et al. Conversion of the failed Fontan circulation. Cardiol Young 2006; 16(suppl 1): 85–91.

33. Morgan GJ, Casey F, Craig B, et al. Assessing ASDs prior to device closure using 3D echocardiography. Just pretty pictures or a useful clinical tool? Eur J Echocardiogr 2008; 9:478–482.

34. Mercer-Rosa L, Seliem MA, Fedec A, et al. Illustration of the additional value of real-time 3-dimensional echocardiography to conventional transthoracic and transesophageal 2-dimensional echocardiography in imaging muscular ventricular septal defects: does this have any impact on individual patient treatment? J Am Soc Echocardiogr 2006; 19:1511–1519.

35. Therrien J, Dore A, Gersony W, et al. CCS Consensus Conference 2001 update: recommendations for the management of adults with congenital heart disease. Part I. Can J Cardiol 2001; 17:940–959.

36. Therrien J, Gatzoulis M, Graham T, et al. Canadian Cardiovascular Society Consensus Conference 2001 update: Recommendations for the Management of Adults with Congenital Heart Disease—Part II. Can J Cardiol 2001; 17:1029–1050.

27

TEE in Lung Transplantation and Thoracic Surgery

Jean Bussières
Université Laval, Quebec City, Quebec, Canada

Pasquale Ferraro
Université de Montréal, Montreal, Quebec, Canada

Peter Slinger
Toronto General Hospital, University of Toronto, Toronto, Ontario, Canada

INTRODUCTION

Transesophageal echocardiography (TEE) has, over the years, acquired an important role for patient monitoring in the operating room and the intensive care unit (ICU). Management of lung transplantation recipients requires extensive monitoring, as hemodynamic and ventilatory changes during and after surgery can be critical and precipitous. The American Society of Anesthesiologists (ASA) and Society of Cardiovascular Anesthesiologists (SCA) have published guidelines for the use of perioperative TEE (1) in thoracic surgery, which are summarized in Table 27.1.

Although not essential, TEE may also provide useful information when used in addition to other hemodynamic monitoring in selected high-risk patients undergoing thoracic surgery. In these patients, TEE allows the anesthesiologist to have a continuous real-time monitor of myocardial ischemic events, left and right heart function, cardiac preload during thoracic surgery. Some of this information, for example cardiac output and preload assessment, is difficult to obtain intraoperatively in the lateral position from other hemodynamic measures such as pulmonary artery or central venous pressure. Potential additional information provided by TEE that applies to thoracic surgery includes hemodynamic instability, pericardial effusions, cardiac involvement by tumor, air emboli, thoracic trauma, pleuropulmonary disease, and pulmonary thromboendarterectomy (PTE).

ROLE OF TEE IN LUNG TRANSPLANTATION

Lung transplant recipients generally fall into one of four major categories (by frequency of indication): First, chronic obstructive pulmonary disease (COPD) (e.g., emphysema); second, septic lung disease /bronchiectasis (e.g., cystic fibrosis); third, restrictive lung disease (e.g., idiopathic pulmonary fibrosis); and finally pulmonary vascular disease such as primary pulmonary hypertension (PPH). Although much less common,

there are a variety of other indications such as histiocytosis X, lymphangioleiomyomatosis, primary bronchoalveolar lung cancer (2).

Patients who become transplant candidates have severely limited pulmonary capacity as well as varying degrees of RV and LV dysfunction depending on the underlying disorder and coexisting medical conditions. Successful lung transplantation therefore requires careful perioperative patient management of which TEE has become a cornerstone. Depending on the patient's underlying disease and cardiopulmonary physiology, different surgical options exist: single-lung transplantation, bilateral sequential lung transplantation (Figs. 27.1 and 27.2), heart-lung transplantation, and living donor lobar transplantation. Indications and contraindications to lung transplantation are summarized in Table 27.2 (3).

TEE has, over the years, acquired an important role for patient monitoring in the operating room (OR) and the ICU. Management of lung transplantation recipients requires extensive monitoring, as hemodynamic and ventilatory changes during and after surgery can be critical and precipitous. The routine use of TEE during lung transplantation is considered a category II indication (1).

Before Lung Transplantation

The ability of TEE to assess the presence of pulmonary hypertension and RV dysfunction in transplant candidates on a waiting list has been shown by several authors (4–6). Interestingly, TEE also provided additional data that significantly altered surgical treatment in 25% of the 48 consecutive patients studied by Gorcsan et al. (4). At the time of the transplantation itself, the first role of TEE is to reassess the status of the RV function. Indeed, between the period of the initial transplant eligibility evaluation to the lung transplantation itself, worsening of the respiratory function and the development of pulmonary hypertension and RV failure is not uncommon. In patients with a mild degree of COPD, both RV and LV

Table 27.1   Indications for Transesophageal Echocardiography in Thoracic Surgery

- Hemodynamic instability (category 1)
- Assessment of pericardial effusion or tamponade (category 1)
- Cardiac and/or great vessel involvement by intrathoracic tumors (category 2)
- Pulmonary thromboendarterectomy (category 2)
- Air emboli (category 2)
- Lung transplantation (category 2)
- Thoracic trauma (category 2)
- Right ventricular function in pulmonary resection (category 3)

Category 1: Supported by the strongest evidence or expert opinion.
Category 2: Supported by weaker evidence or expert opinion.
Category 3: Little current scientific or expert support.
Source: From Ref. 1.

relaxation abnormalities are observed (7). As the disease progresses, these evolve toward an RV restrictive filling pattern that correlates with the severity of pulmonary hypertension. The diagnosis can be established using pulsed wave (PW) Doppler examination of the tricuspid inflow, hepatic venous flow (HVF), as well as tissue Doppler imaging of the tricuspid valve (TV) annulus (8) (see Fig. 10.46). Right ventricular systolic dysfunction has also been shown to be associated with an abnormal systolic (S) HVF wave (9). The use of a pulmonary artery catheter (PAC) for continuous pulmonary artery (PA) pressure measurement in conjunction with TEE is particularly useful in this setting. The need for pharmacological support,

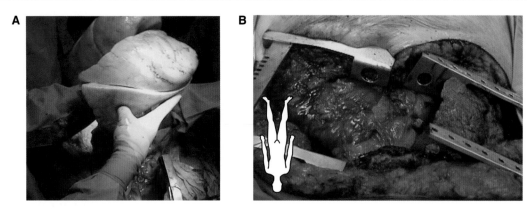

Figure 27.1   Lung transplantation. (**A**) Bilateral lung removal from the donor (**B**) prior to sequential single lung extraction from the recipient. ◌

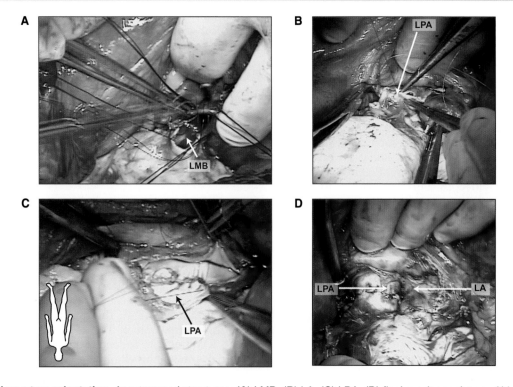

Figure 27.2   Lung transplantation. Anastomosed structures: (**A**) LMB, (**B**) LA, (**C**) LPA; (**D**) final result are shown. *Abbreviations*: LA, left atrium; LMB, left main bronchus; LPA, left pulmonary artery. ◌

Table 27.2 Indications and Contraindications for Lung Transplantation

Indications

Untreatable end-stage pulmonary parenchymal and/or vascular disease
Absence of other major medical illnesses
Substantial limitation of daily activities
Projected life expectancy: 2–3 yr predicted survival <50%
NYHA class III or IV functional level
Rehabilitation potential
Satisfactory psychosocial profile
Acceptable nutritional status
Disease-specific mortality exceeding transplant-specific mortality over 1–2 yr

Relative contraindications

Age >65 yr
Critical or unstable clinical conditions (e.g., shock, ECMO)
Severely limited functional status with poor rehabilitation potential
Severe obesity defined as a BMI >30 kg/m^2
Severe or symptomatic osteoporosis

Absolute contraindications

Untreatable advanced dysfunction of another major organ system (e.g., heart, liver, or kidney)
Active malignancy within the previous 2 yr
Noncurable chronic extrapulmonary infection
Chronic active viral hepatitis B, hepatitis C, or HIV
Significant chest wall or spinal deformity
Documented nonadherence or inability to comply with medical therapy
Untreatable psychiatric or psychologic condition
Absence of a reliable social support system
Substance addiction (e.g., alcohol, tobacco, or narcotics) that is either active or within the previous 6 mo

Abbreviations: BMI, body mass index; ECMO, extracorporal membrane oxygenation; HIV, human immunodeficiency virus; mo, months; NYHA, New York Heart Association; yr, years.
Source: From Ref. 3.

ventilatory management, and cardiopulmonary bypass (CPB) can thus be safely planned.

During Lung Transplantation

During the procedure, TEE can be used to evaluate LV and RV systolic and diastolic function, to rule out the presence of an unexpected patent foramen ovale (PFO) with a right-to-left shunt (10) (Fig. 27.3), to verify the integrity of the pulmonary vascular anastomoses (Fig. 27.4) and to exclude significant air embolus (1). The appearance of continuous air emboli observed by TEE at the end of a lung transplantation should prompt reexamination of the bronchial anastomosis integrity (11) (Fig. 27.5).

Although the need for CPB varies greatly, all lung transplantations are performed with CPB on standby. There are wide variations in the frequency of use of CPB during lung transplantation. In many centers, CPB is used in approximately 20% to 25% of lung transplantations. In approximately two-third of cases the use of CPB is anticipated at the start of the case due to high pulmonary artery pressures or RV failure. In the remaining one-third, the use of CPB is not initially predicted but is required because of hemodynamic instability or for technical reasons. The need for emergent CPB may occur before or after implantation of the first lung in bilateral procedures. Thus in all lung transplantations, anesthetic preparation is always made for emergent CPB (see Chapter 21). Although CPB may temporarily decrease postoperative gas exchange and increase intraoperative blood loss, there is no net increase in short- or long-term mortality attributable to CPB (12). In the absence of a formal indication for CPB such as the

A

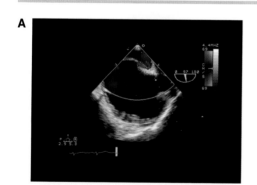

B

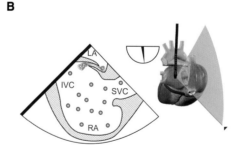

C

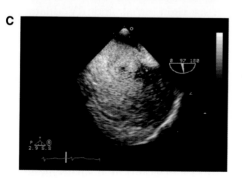

D

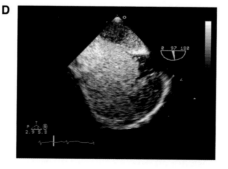

Figure 27.3 PFO in thoracic surgery. A patient with recurrent pulmonary emboli is undergoing a pulmonary thromboendarterectomy. (**A,B**) Color Doppler midesophageal bicaval view with a left-to-right flow suggestive of a previously undiagnosed PFO. (**C,D**) Right heart chamber contrast opacification with agitated saline intravenous injection during a Valsalva maneuver: (**C**) microbubbles initially fill the RA. (**D**) Upon sudden release of the Valsalva strain maneuver, microbubbles are seen crossing into the LA through the PFO. The latter was repaired during the surgery. *Abbreviations*: IVC, inferior vena cava; LA, left atrium; PFO, patent foramen ovale; RA, right atrium; SVC, superior vena cava.

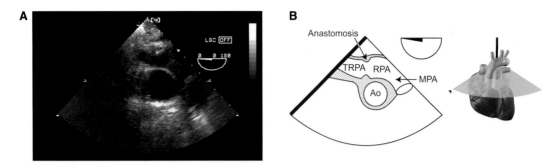

Figure 27.4   Pulmonary artery anastomosis. (A,B) Mid-esophageal ascending Ao short-axis view shows the anastomosis between the native RPA and the TRPA in a 45-year-old man after lung transplantation. *Abbreviations*: Ao, aorta; MPA, main pulmonary artery; RPA, right pulmonary artery; TRPA, transplanted right pulmonary artery.

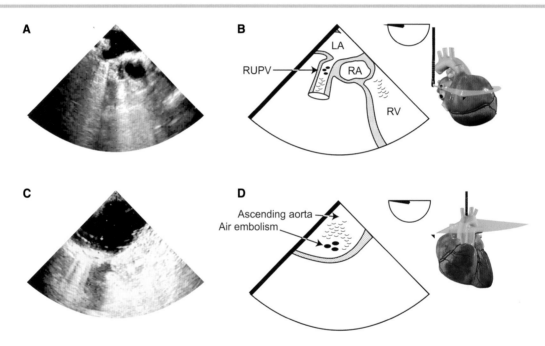

Figure 27.5   Air emboli in lung transplantation. (A,B) Mid-esophageal view with right-sided rotation showing air bubbles coming the RUPV at the completion of the vascular anastomosis. **(C,D)** Upper esophageal aortic arch long-axis view showing also air bubbles in the aorta. *Abbreviations*: LA, left atrium; RA, right atrium; RUPV, right upper pulmonary vein; RV, right ventricle.

presence of PPH or an Eisenmenger's syndrome, surgeons have yet to agree on whether CPB should be routinely used (13,14). The need for CPB is difficult to predict preoperatively as reported by de Hoyos et al. (15) and Triantafillou et al. (16). In these two studies, parameters such as preoperative PaO₂, mean pulmonary artery pressure (MPAP) and pulmonary vascular resistance (PVR) were not found to be reliable predictive indicators for the use of CPB. Intraoperatively however, the hemodynamic effects of PA clamping as evaluated by TEE are extremely useful in establishing the need for CPB: echocardiographic signs of low cardiac output (CO) or severe RV

dysfunction such as right atrial and RV dilatation with paradoxical septal motion (Fig. 27.6) and reduced systolic excursion of the tricuspid annulus (see Fig. 10.22) help determine precisely the need for circulatory support. Extracorporeal membrane oxygenation (ECMO) is used in some centers in place of CPB intraoperatively (17). ECMO or extracorporeal ventilation is also used increasingly for postoperative respiratory support in patients presenting severe primary graft dysfunction (PGD) (see Chapter 21).

A standard examination of all vascular anastomoses, including PW Doppler flow measurements, is performed in both the transverse and longitudinal

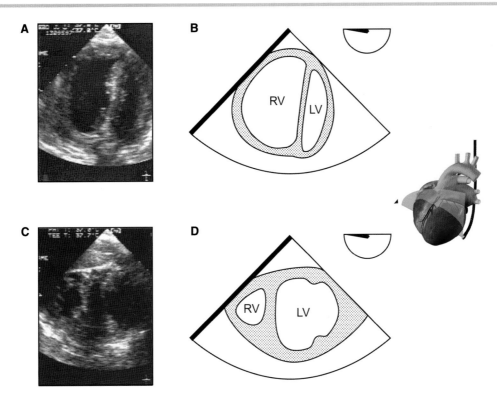

Figure 27.6   Transient RV dysfunction during bilateral lung transplantation. (A,B) Transgastric mid short-axis view with significant dilatation of the RV, flattened ventricular septum with paradoxical motion suggestive of RV failure, possibly secondary to clamping of the pulmonary artery or air embolization in the right coronary artery. **(C,D)** Improved RV dysfunction with administration of vasoactive support. *Abbreviations*: LV, left ventricle; RV, right ventricle.

planes. The examination should be repeated intraoperatively once the anastomoses have been completed. The presence of an arterial or pulmonary vein stenosis should be excluded by observing abnormal turbulence, by measuring the diameter of the donor and recipient vessels, and the corresponding pressure gradient (Figs. 27.7 and 27.8). The pulmonary veins and left atrium (LA) should be carefully examined for the presence of thrombus, and if there are any, their size, precise location, and associated flow abnormalities noted. The correction of such intraoperative findings is key in preventing life-threatening complications postoperatively (18).

Our approach in acquiring TEE two-dimentional Doppler data acquisition and hemodynamic evaluation of patients undergoing lung transplantation is summarized in Fig. 27.9.

After Lung Transplantation

TEE, whether used intraoperatively or postoperatively in the ICU, plays a valuable role in the assessment of arterial and venoatrial anastomotic complications following lung transplantation. As reported by Griffith et al. (19), all too often, even the most experienced transplant surgeons may underestimate these anastomotic problems. Generally, TEE will easily display the right pulmonary artery (RPA) anastomosis (Figs. 27.4

and 27.10) as well as those of the right upper pulmonary vein (RUPV) and right lower pulmonary vein (RLPV) to the LA (Figs. 27.7 and 27.8). However, on the left, due to the location of the left hilum, the left pulmonary artery (LPA) anastomosis can only be identified in 71% of the cases (20) while the left lower pulmonary vein (LLPV) is usually not adequately visualized beyond the ostium. A left upper pulmonary vein (LUPV) stenosis is shown in Fig. 27.8. Epicardial echocardiography is an option when the anastomosis cannot be visualized with TEE (21) or in patients who have contraindications to TEE such as those with esophageal disorders (e.g., scleroderma) (see Chapter 6).

Pulmonary venous obstruction or thrombosis is generally associated with early graft failure and a high mortality rate (22–24). The true incidence of these venous anastomotic complications is however difficult to establish and is probably underestimated. Early series, such as the one from the Pittsburgh group, described only two venous anastomotic complications from a series of 134 transplant patients. This low rate of 1.5% was, however, based on clinical grounds and not systematic use of TEE. Later, reports from Hausmann et al. (20) and Leibowitz et al. (25) quoted rates varying from 9% to 29% when TEE was routinely used in consecutive patients. In a recent prospective study by Schulman et al. (26), the incidence of venous anastomotic complications was recorded at 15%,

A

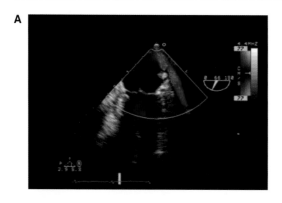

B

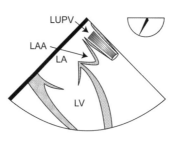

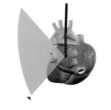

C

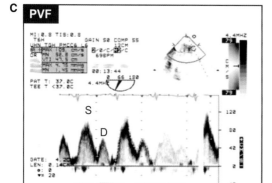

Figure 27.7 LUPV before lung transplantation. (A,B) Color Doppler mid-esophageal mitral commissural view at 66° of the LUPV. **(C)** Pulsed wave Doppler of the PVF showing normal laminar flow with systolic flow predominance. *Abbreviations*: D, peak diastolic PVF velocity; LA, left atrium; LAA, left atrial appendage; LUPV, left upper pulmonary vein; LV, left ventricle; PVF, pulmonary venous flow; S, peak systolic PVF velocity.

A

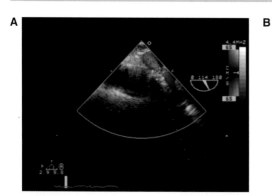

B

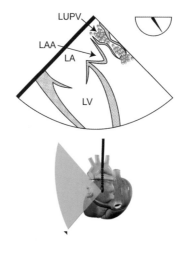

C

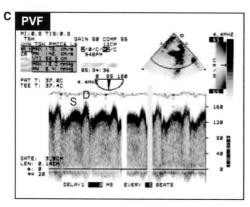

Figure 27.8 LUPV after lung transplantation. (A,B) Modified color Doppler mid-esophageal view at 114° with turbulence at the anastomosis of the LUPV. **(C)** Pulsed wave Doppler of the PVF showing elevated systolic (S) and diastolic (D) velocities with spectral broadening and abnormal diastolic flow predominance (S < D), consistent with increased pressure gradient across the anastomosis. No thrombus was present at the anastomosis. With satisfactory hemodynamics and gas exchange, the anastomosis was not revised and the patient had a satisfactory outcome. *Abbreviations*: D, peak diastolic PVF velocity; LA, left atrium; LAA, left atrial appendage; LUPV, left upper pulmonary vein; LV, left ventricle; PVF, pulmonary venous flow; S, peak systolic PVF velocity.

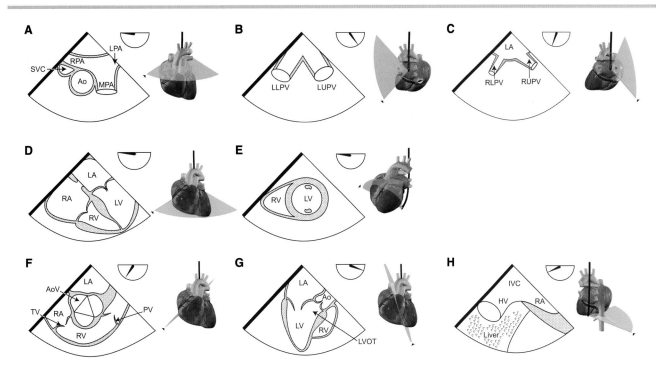

Figure 27.9 TEE evaluation of anatomy and function in lung transplantation. (A) ME ascending Ao short-axis view at 0° for the pulmonary arteries. **(B)** ME view at 120° with left rotation for the left-sided PVs. **(C)** ME view at 60° with right rotation for the right-sided PVs. PWD examination of the PVs is done for left ventricular diastolic function evaluation. **(D)** ME four-chamber and **(E)** transgastric mid short-axis views are used to evaluate systolic function of the RV and LV. **(F)** ME RV inflow/outflow and **(G)** ME long-axis views are obtained to exclude RVOT and LVOT obstruction. PWD of the mitral inflow and tissue Doppler of the mitral annulus in the ME long-axis view completes evaluation of LV diastolic function. Using views **(D)** or **(F)**, TV function is assessed with color Doppler while continuous wave Doppler enables estimation of the pulmonary artery pressure. **(H)** PWD of HVF assesses RV diastolic function. *Abbreviations*: Ao, aorta; HVF, hepatic venous flow; IVC, inferior vena cava; LA, left atrium; LLPV, left lower pulmonary vein; LPA, left pulmonary artery; LUPV, left upper pulmonary vein; LV, left ventricle; LVOT, left ventricular outflow tract; ME, mid-esophageal; MPA, main pulmonary artery; PVs, pulmonary veins; PWD, pulsed wave Doppler; RA, right atrium; RPA, right pulmonary artery; RLPV, right lower pulmonary vein; RV, right ventricle; RVOT, right ventricular outflow tract; RUPV, right upper pulmonary vein; SVC, superior vena cava; TV, tricuspid valve.

with 13 out of 87 consecutive transplant recipients diagnosed with a pulmonary vein thrombosis post-operatively. In 12 of the 13 cases, the thrombosis was localized in the upper lobe veins of the transplanted lung. The thrombi had a mean width of 0.9 ± 0.4 cm, with a mean pulmonary venous flow velocity of 127 ± 23 cm/s. The mortality in the presence of this complication was significant, with five of the 13 patients (38.5%) dying postoperatively. The incidence of the complication was similar regardless of the side of the transplant or the use of CPB. McIlroy et al. (27) reported pulmonary venous anastomosis thrombus in 3/81 (3.7%) cases, all detected by TEE intraoperatively at the left upper pulmonary venous anastomosis and all removed during surgery, with or without CPB. TEE was thought to be helpful by obviating the need for angiography.

Complications involving the PA anastomosis occur far less often. Indeed, from a surgical technical standpoint, this anastomosis is less difficult to accomplish while abnormalities are usually easily detected early intraoperatively. Clark et al. (28) reported five

cases of stenosis (2 RPAs and 3 LPA) from a series of 109 transplantations. Despite three surgical revisions of the PA anastomosis, all five patients ultimately died in the early postoperative period. Griffith et al. (19) also described fives cases of PA anastomotic complications, for a rate of 3.7%, in his review of 134 transplant recipients. Three of the five patients underwent reoperation and revision of the PA anastomosis. The author noted that excessive length of the donor PA and/or the recipient PA can create distortion or kinking of the anastomosis leading to reduced blood flow and thrombosis. This situation may arise particularly when an oversized lung is placed in a small chest during single lung transplantation. Careful tailoring of the vascular structures on the recipient and donor side as well as a meticulous surgical technique with the use of intraoperative TEE may account for the low incidence of vascular anastomotic complications.

In our experience with over 320 lung transplantations, over an 11-year period at the Centre Hospitalier de l'Université de Montreal, only one vascular anastomotic complication was observed postoperatively. In a

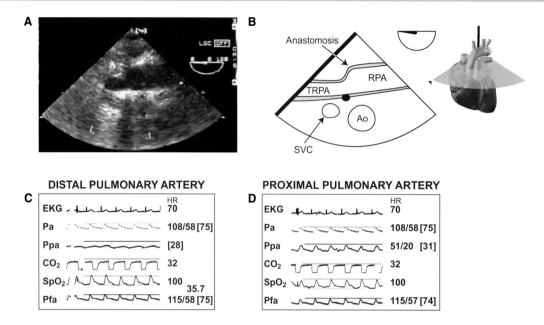

Figure 27.10 Pulmonary artery anastomosis. RPA anastomosis in a 65-year-old woman after right lung transplantation. (**A,B**) A mid-esophageal view at 0° shows a diameter reduction between the native and the TRPA. Its hemodynamic severity can be assessed by pulmonary artery catheter pullback from a distal (**C**) to a proximal position (**D**) revealing a mean pressure gradient of 3 mmHg (31 mmHg −28 mmHg). *Abbreviations*: Ao, aorta; CO_2, end-tidal carbon dioxide from capnography; EKG, electrocardiogram; HR, heart rate; Pa, arterial pressure (from radial artery); Pfa, arterial pressure from femoral artery; Ppa, pulmonary artery pressure; RPA, right pulmonary artery; SpO_2, saturation from pulse oximetry; SVC, superior vena cava; TRPA, transplanted right pulmonary artery.

cystic fibrosis patient who presented signs of a cerebral vascular accident in the postoperative period, a CT scan of the head showed multiple ischemic strokes. TEE confirmed the presence of large clots in the left atrium. Autopsy findings were consistent with fresh clots having formed along the anastomotic suture line in the left atrium. It is believed that the careful tailoring of the vascular structures on both the recipient and donor side as well as a meticulous surgical technique with the use of intraoperative TEE account for the rare occurrence of this complication.

After Lung Transplantation in the ICU

TEE also plays an essential role in the postoperative care of lung transplant recipients in the ICU. The early postoperative course of these patients is frequently characterized by hemodynamic, radiographic, and gas exchange abnormalities. Despite improved preservation techniques in recent years, severe PGD is still prevalent in 10% of patients following transplantation (Fig. 27.11).

This injury is usually associated with abundant frothy sputum from the endotracheal tube, a PaO_2/FiO_2 ratio <100, diffuse alveolar infiltrates on the side of the graft and hemodynamic instability. The differential diagnosis includes acute allograft rejection, cardiogenic pulmonary edema, noncardiogenic pulmonary edema other than ischemic reperfusion injury (IRI), sepsis, and vascular anastomotic complications. In this setting, TEE is useful in excluding

some of the etiologies listed earlier and in confirming the diagnosis of PGD suggested by the clinical history and the hemodynamic profile obtained from a PAC. Monitoring with TEE helps assess the response to therapy (Fig. 27.12) and determine the need for more invasive support such as ECMO.

During ECMO, based on the ASA-SCA guidelines (1), TEE is considered a category I indication (see Chapter 21). TEE can help evaluate ventricular recovery, assist in cannula positioning, and exclude the presence of intracardiac clot before initiating the weaning process (29) (see Table 21.3). The exact timing and the type of ECMO required can also be facilitated by TEE findings. Generally, when both RV and LV functions are preserved, the use of venovenous ECMO is sufficient but with RV or LV dysfunction venoarterial ECMO may be more appropriate. We reported a case in which continuous TEE in the ICU not only helped establish the indication for venoarterial ECMO in a transplant recipient with severe IRI, but also facilitated patient monitoring while on ECMO through a successful eventual weaning four days later (30). Other complications diagnosed with TEE following lung transplantation include LV (31) and RV dynamic outflow tract obstruction (32) precipitated by suboptimal preload, increased inotropy and RV hypertrophy (33) (Fig. 27.13), as well as thoracic tamponade (Figs. 27.14–27.16) (30). The role of TEE in lung transplantation is summarized on Table 27.3.

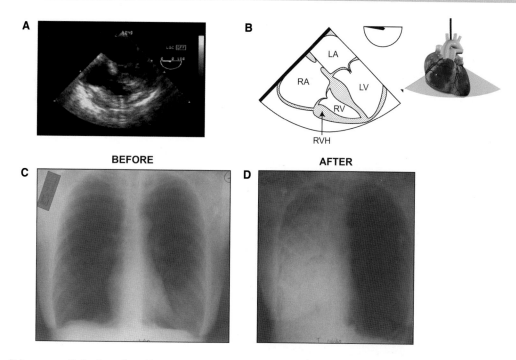

Figure 27.11 Primary graft dysfunction. Hemodynamic instability occurs after single lung transplantation in a 53-year-old woman with end-stage emphysema. (**A,B**) Mid-esophageal four-chamber view with RVH and abnormal tricuspid annular motion. She remained hemodynamically unstable despite administration of norepinephrine at 25 μg/min and displayed severe hypoxia from right-sided ischemic reperfusion injury and primary graft dysfunction, as evident on the chest X-ray (**C,D**). *Abbreviations*: LA, left atrium; LV, left ventricle; RA, right atrium; RV, right ventricle; RVH, right ventricular hypertrophy.

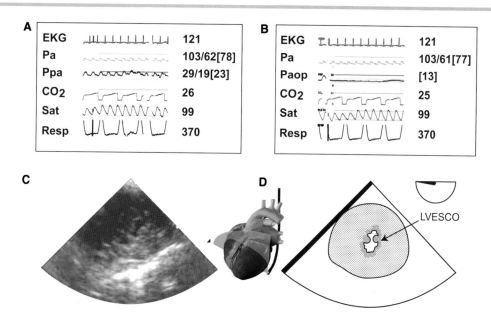

Figure 27.12 Fluid assessment. Preload evaluation during hemodynamic instability after single lung transplantation in a 53-year-old woman with end-stage emphysema. (**A,B**) Invasive hemodynamic monitoring shows a heart rate of 121 beats/min, a Pa of 103/62 mmHg, a Ppa of 29/19 mmHg with a Paop of 13 mmHg. The central venous pressure was 14 mmHg (not shown). The capnographic waveform (CO_2) is typical of a single lung transplant with the initial normal waveform from the transplanted lung followed by the ascending phase III typical of obstructive disease. Respiratory variation of the saturation signal from the pulse oximeter is seen. (**C,D**) Transgastric mid short-axis view: despite the above relatively normal filling pressures, the left ventricle appears suboptimally preloaded, with LVESCO. The patient's hemodynamic condition improved with intravenous fluid administration. *Abbreviations*: CO_2, carbon dioxide; EKG, electrocardiogram; LVESCO, left ventricular end-systolic cavity obliteration; Pa, arterial pressure; Paop, pulmonary artery occlusion (wedge) pressure; Ppa, pulmonary artery pressure; Resp, respiration; Sat, saturation.

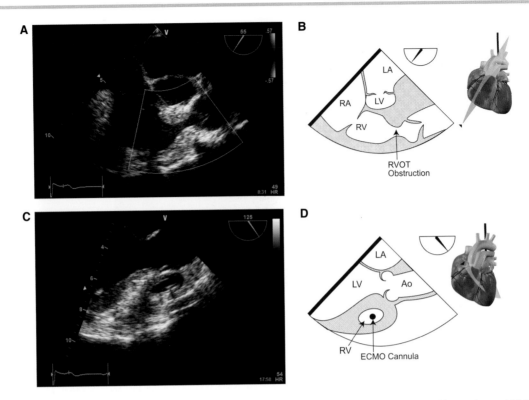

Figure 27.13 RVOT obstruction after single lung transplantation requiring ECMO. (A,B) The mid-esophageal RV inflow/outflow view shows significant edema causing RVOT obstruction just below the PV. **(C,D)** Mid-esophageal long-axis view also shows RVOT obstruction and the ECMO cannula in the RVOT. *Abbreviations*: ECMO, extra-corporeal membrane oxygenation; PV, pulmonic valve; RV, right ventricular; RVOT, right ventricular outflow tract. *Source*: Courtesy of Dr. Jens Lohser, Vancouver General Hospital.

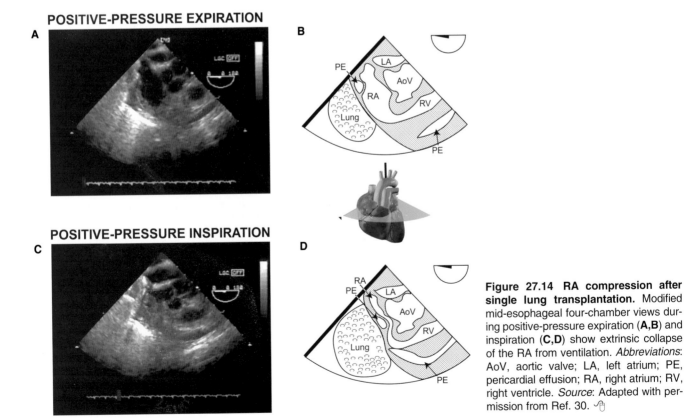

Figure 27.14 RA compression after single lung transplantation. Modified mid-esophageal four-chamber views during positive-pressure expiration **(A,B)** and inspiration **(C,D)** show extrinsic collapse of the RA from ventilation. *Abbreviations*: AoV, aortic valve; LA, left atrium; PE, pericardial effusion; RA, right atrium; RV, right ventricle. *Source*: Adapted with permission from Ref. 30.

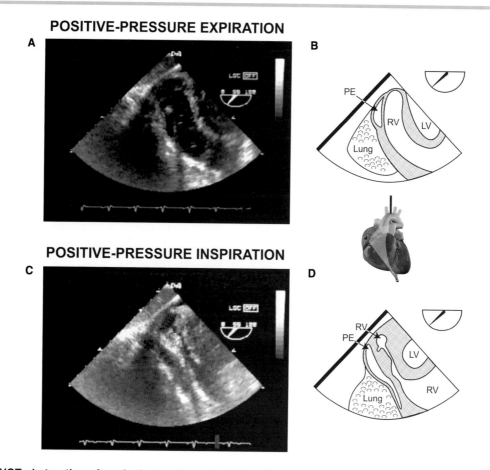

Figure 27.15 RVOT obstruction after single lung transplantation. Deep transgastric RVOT views at 55° during positive-pressure expiration (**A,B**) and inspiration (**C,D**) show extrinsic RVOT collapse from ventilation. *Abbreviations*: LV, left ventricle; PE, pericardial effusion; RV, right ventricle; RVOT, right ventricular outflow tract. *Source*: Adapted with permission from Ref. 30.

Table 27.3 Role of TEE in Lung Transplantation

Before the procedure
- Evaluation of left and right ventricular and valvular function
- Estimation of pulmonary artery pressure

Perioperative period
- If performed under CPB (see Table 21.3)
- De-airing of all four cardiac cavities
- Ruling out stenotic anastomosis (pulmonary artery, pulmonary veins)
- Ruling out patent foramen ovale

Early and Late postoperative period: evaluation of
- Left and right ventricular and valvular function
- Arterial and atrial anastomosis

If hemodynamic instability
- Ruling out left and right ventricular systolic and diastolic function
- Arterial or venous anastomotic obstruction
- Left and right ventricular outflow tract
- Hypovolemia and vasodilatation
- Air embolism
- Pericardial and thoracic tamponade
- If ECMO required (see Table 21.3)

Abbreviations: CPB, cardiopulmonary bypass; ECMO, extracorporeal membrane oxygenation; TEE, transesophageal echocardiography.

ROLE OF TEE IN NONCARDIAC THORACIC SURGERY

The clinical usefulness of TEE for pulmonary resection surgery is currently under investigation. Assessment of RV function is an appealing potential use for TEE, particularly in patients with limited cardiac reserve who undergo major pulmonary resections. Right ventricular ejection fraction catheters have been tried for this purpose but have not gained wide acceptance, probably due to the variability in the measurements. Because of its complex structure, RV function assessment with TEE has been commonly performed qualitatively. However, with the guidelines of chamber quantification (34), newer quantitative approach on the evaluation of RV function has been proposed (35).

Following the experience obtained with the use of TEE during lung transplantation (36), it is possible to measure flow velocities in the pulmonary veins in patients undergoing a pulmonary resection. It may be interesting to make clinical measurements of the blood flow through each lung independently (37). This has the potential to allow monitoring of physiologic

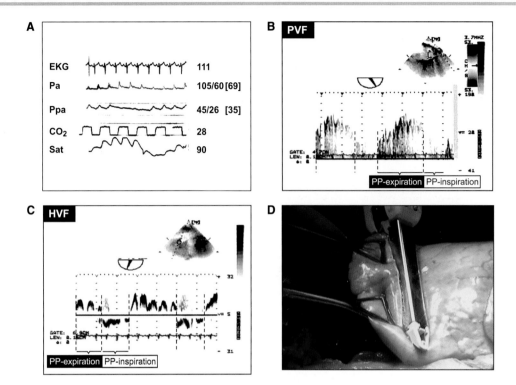

Figure 27.16 Thoracic tamponade after single lung transplantation. Hemodynamic instability occurs in a 65-year-old woman following single lung transplantation. (**A**) Fluctuation of the Pa or pulsus paradoxus coincident with the Sat signal, followed by the Ppa signal suggests tamponade physiology. Pulsed wave Doppler examination of the right upper PVF (**B**) and the HVF (**C**) demonstrates cyclic fluctuation with PP ventilation. The HVF flow reversal during PP inspiration is due to RA and RVOT compression (see Figs. 27.14 and 27.15). To avoid such complications as shown in (**D**), lung reduction can be performed. *Abbreviations*: CO_2, end-tidal CO_2; EKG, electrocardiogram; HVF, hepatic vein flow; Pa, arterial pressure; Ppa, pulmonary artery pressure; PP, positive-pressure; PVF, pulmonary venous flow; RA, right atrium; RVOT, right ventricular outflow tract; Sat, pulse oximetry saturation. *Source*: Adapted with permission from Ref. 30.

changes in blood flow redistribution during one lung ventilation (OLV) and to assess the effect of therapy of hypoxemia such positive end expiratory pressure (PEEP) administration. In 1996, an intraoperative TEE study evaluated the cardiovascular changes induced by pneumonectomy in eight patients without any cardiac involvement before surgery. The results suggested that the ligature of the RPA or LPA altered the geometry of the interventricular septum, mainly due to acute increase in RV afterload, and induced a transient LV diastolic dysfunction, associated with mild mitral regurgitation (MR). No alteration in LV systolic function was found. These events were transient and disappeared at the end of intervention, before chest closure (38).

TEE may also be useful in determining if there is unsuspected pericardial involvement (Fig. 27.17) or direct cardiac involvement from a tumor located in the pulmonary hilum (Fig. 27.18). It may be possible to estimate accurately the degree of atrial invasion (39). In addition, the extent of tumor invasion into the great vessels can be determined by TEE (Fig. 27.19) (40). Finally, a documented cause of hypoxemia associated with thoracic surgery is reversal of shunt flow through an undiagnosed PFO (Fig. 27.3) (41). When PEEP

(to 15 cm H_2O) was applied during controlled ventilation for nonthoracic surgery, 9% of patients developed a right to left intracardiac shunt (42). TEE should be capable of detecting these potential patients who might intraoperatively develop a right to left interatrial shunt during or after thoracic surgery (see Chapter 26)

ROLE OF TEE IN PTE

Pulmonary thromboendarterectomy (PTE) is a potentially curative procedure for chronic thromboembolic pulmonary hypertension (CTEPH). CTEPH is a progressive disorder that responds poorly to conservative therapy. PTE has become an effective treatment modality with a perioperative mortality of approximately 4% (43). The majority of patients with CTEPH present for medical evaluation late in the disease because many have not had an obvious episode of deep venous thrombosis or pulmonary embolus and the progression of the disease may be insidious. Patients present with severe dyspnea on exertion and signs of RV failure. Surgical candidates have hemodynamically significant pulmonary

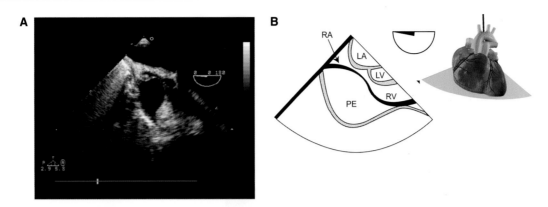

Figure 27.17 Pericardial effusion in metastatic breast cancer. The patient was scheduled for a video-thoracoscopic drainage of a left pleural effusion and experienced hemodynamic collapse after induction of general anesthesia. (**A,B**) Mid-esophageal right ventricular view revealed a previously undiagnosed large PE, with complete collapse of the RA during systole consistent with pericardial tamponade. The thoracoscopic procedure was modified to include the creation of a pericardial window. *Abbreviations*: LA, left atrium; LV, left ventricle; PE, pericardial effusion; RA, right atrium; RV, right ventricle. 🖰

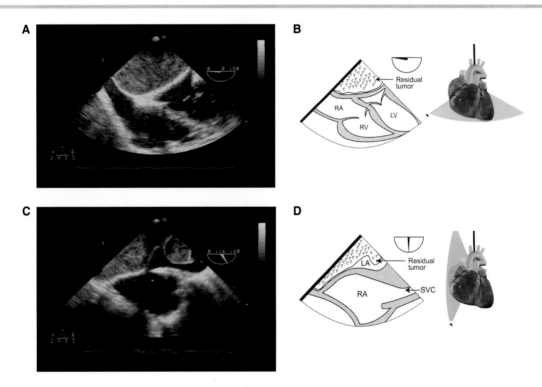

Figure 27.18 Posterior mediastinal neurogenic tumor invading the posterior pericardium. (**A,B**) Mid-esophageal four-chamber view with severe compression of the LA by the mass. (**C,D**) Bicaval view at 116° shows two distinct lobes in the tumor. *Abbreviations*: LA, left atrium; LV, left ventricle; RA, right atrium; RV, right ventricle; SVC, superior vena cava. 🖰

vascular obstruction (PVR >300 dynes sec/cm^5) with potentially accessible proximal areas of thromboembolus. Surgery is performed via a midline sternotomy with CPB with/without periods of deep hypothermic circulatory arrest (DHCA). These

patients are at risk of hemodynamic collapse due to RV failure from hypotension during induction of general anesthesia.

TEE is performed to rule out the presence of a PFO (Fig. 27.3). Significant hypoxemia could occur

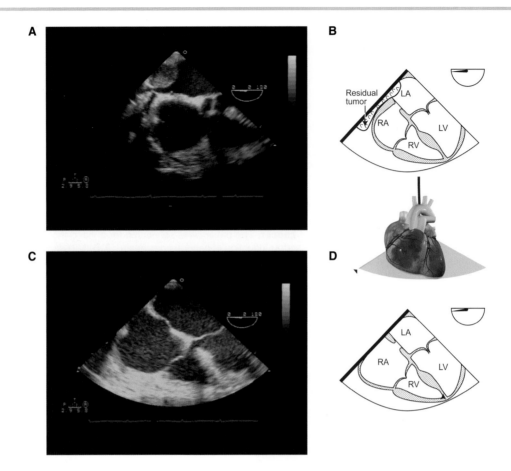

Figure 27.19   Residual posterior mediastinal neurogenic tumor after resection. Prior to chest closure in patient from Fig. 27.18, repeat TEE examination was performed. (**A,B**) Mid-esophageal four-chamber view revealed the presence of significant residual tumor in the LA. (**C,D**) Final results after further surgical excision. *Abbreviations*: LA, left atrium; LV, left ventricle; RA, right atrium; RV, right ventricle; TEE, transesophageal echocardiography.

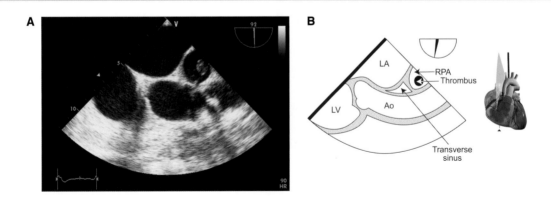

Figure 27.20   Chronic pulmonary embolism. (A,B) Mid-esophageal ascending Ao long-axis view in a 65-year-old woman with chronic pulmonary embolism shows the mobile clot adherent to the RPA wall. *Abbreviations*: Ao, aorta; LA, left atrium; LV, left ventricle; RPA, right pulmonary artery.

postoperatively from reversal of flow through the PFO with resulting right-to-left intra-atrial shunting (see Fig. 30.4), due to significant pulmonary hypertension from reperfusion injury of the lungs. Also TEE is performed to assess RV function and to examine for residual thrombus (Figs. 27.20–27.22).

Epicardial echocardiography can also be used for this purpose (see Fig. 6.18).

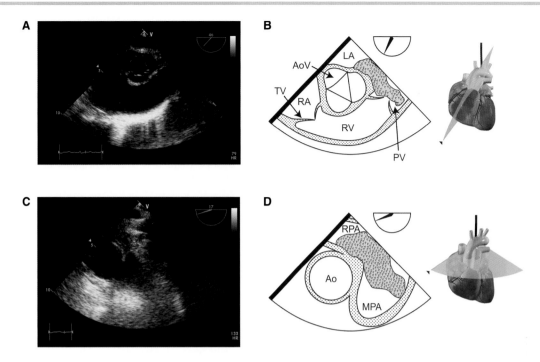

Figure 27.21   Acute pulmonary embolism. (A,B) Mid-esophageal RV inflow/outflow and **(C,D)** ascending aortic short-axis views show the MPA filled with thrombus. The patient underwent acute pulmonary thrombectomy under cardiopulmonary bypass. *Abbreviations*: Ao, aorta; AoV, aortic valve; LA, left atrium; LV, left ventricle; MPA, main pulmonary artery; PV, pulmonic valve; RA, right atrium; RPA, right pulmonary artery; RV, right ventricle; TV, tricuspid valve.

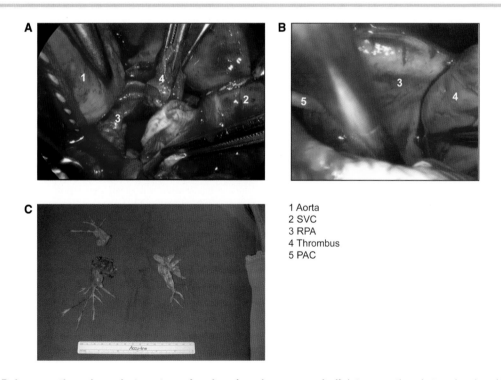

1 Aorta
2 SVC
3 RPA
4 Thrombus
5 PAC

Figure 27.22   Pulmonary thromboendarterectomy for chronic pulmonary emboli. Intraoperative photos showing: **(A)** the thrombus in situ. **(B)** Peeling of the thrombus away from the RPA. **(C)** Entire pathological specimen obtained at the end of the procedure. *Abbreviations*: PAC, pulmonary artery catheter; RPA, right pulmonary artery; SVC, superior vena cava. *Source*: Courtesy of Dr. Marc DePerrot, University of Toronto.

CONCLUSION

In summary, TEE is a promising diagnostic and monitoring modality in lung transplantation and thoracic surgery. It is likely to become a routine part of some of these life-saving procedures. Although not essential, TEE may also provide useful information when used in addition to other hemodynamic monitoring in selected high-risk patients undergoing thoracic surgery. The specific applications of TEE for hemodynamic instability, pericardial effusions, cardiac involvement by tumor, air emboli, thoracic trauma, pleuropulmonary disease and thromboatherectomy have proven to be extremely valuable.

REFERENCES

1. American Society of Anesthesiology. Practice guidelines for perioperative transesophageal echocardiography. A report by the American Society of Anesthesiologists and the Society of Cardiovascular Anesthesiologists Task Force on Transesophageal Echocardiography. Anesthesiology 1996; 84:986–1006.

2. Trulock EP, Christie JD, Edwards LB, et al. Registry of the International Society for Heart and Lung Transplantation: twenty-fourth official adult lung and heart-lung transplantation report-2007. J Heart Lung Transplant 2007; 26: 782–795.

3. Orens JB, Estenne M, Arcasoy S, et al. International guidelines for the selection of lung transplant candidates: 2006 update—a consensus report from the Pulmonary Scientific Council of the International Society for Heart and Lung Transplantation. J Heart Lung Transplant 2006; 25:745–755.

4. Gorcsan J III, Edwards TD, Ziady GM, et al. Transesophageal echocardiography to evaluate patients with severe pulmonary hypertension for lung transplantation. Ann Thorac Surg 1995; 59:717–722.

5. Schenk P, Globits S, Koller J, et al. Accuracy of echocardiographic right ventricular parameters in patients with different end-stage lung diseases prior to lung transplantation. J Heart Lung Transplant 2000; 19:145–154.

6. Bossone E, Paciocco G, Iarussi D, et al. The prognostic role of the ECG in primary pulmonary hypertension. Chest 2002; 121:513–518.

7. Ozer N, Tokgozoglu L, Coplu L, et al. Echocardiographic evaluation of left and right ventricular diastolic function in patients with chronic obstructive pulmonary disease. J Am Soc Echocardiogr 2001; 14:557–561.

8. Caso P, Galderisi M, Cicala S, et al. Association between myocardial right ventricular relaxation time and pulmonary arterial pressure in chronic obstructive lung disease: analysis by pulsed Doppler tissue imaging. J Am Soc Echocardiogr 2001; 14:970–977.

9. Mishra M, Swaminathan M, Malhotra R, et al. Evaluation of Right Ventricular Function During CABG: Transesophageal Echocardiographic Assessment of Hepatic Venous Flow Versus Conventional Right Ventricular Performance Indices. Echocardiography 1998; 15:51–58.

10. Sukernik MR, Mets B, Bennett-Guerrero E. Patent foramen ovale and its significance in the perioperative period. Anesth Analg 2001; 93:1137–1146.

11. Denault AY, Couture P, McKenty S, et al. Perioperative use of transesophageal echocardiography by anesthesiologists: impact in noncardiac surgery and in the intensive care unit. Can J Anaesth 2002; 49:287–293.

12. Gammie JS, Cheul LJ, Pham SM, et al. Cardiopulmonary bypass is associated with early allograft dysfunction but not death after double-lung transplantation. J Thorac Cardiovasc Surg 1998; 115:990–997.

13. McRae K. Con: lung transplantation should not be routinely performed with cardiopulmonary bypass. J Cardiothorac Vasc Anesth 2000; 14:746–750.

14. Marczin N, Royston D, Yacoub M. Pro: lung transplantation should be routinely performed with cardiopulmonary bypass. J Cardiothorac Vasc Anesth 2000; 14:739–745.

15. de Hoyos A, Demajo W, Snell G, et al. Preoperative prediction for the use of cardiopulmonary bypass in lung transplantation. J Thorac Cardiovasc Surg 1993; 106:787–795.

16. Triantafillou AN, Pasque MK, Huddleston CB, et al. Predictors, frequency, and indications for cardiopulmonary bypass during lung transplantation in adults. Ann Thorac Surg 1994; 57:1248–1251.

17. Bittner HB, Binner C, Lehmann S, et al. Replacing cardiopulmonary bypass with extracorporeal membrane oxygenation in lung transplantation operations. Eur J Cardiothorac Surg 2007; 31:462–467.

18. Michel-Cherqui M, Brusset A, Liu N, et al. Intraoperative transesophageal echocardiographic assessment of vascular anastomoses in lung transplantation. A report on 18 cases. Chest 1997; 111:1229–1235.

19. Griffith BP, Magee MJ, Gonzalez IF, et al. Anastomotic pitfalls in lung transplantation. J Thorac Cardiovasc Surg 1994; 107:743–753.

20. Hausmann D, Daniel WG, Mugge A, et al. Imaging of pulmonary artery and vein anastomoses by transesophageal echocardiography after lung transplantation. Circulation 1992; 86:II251–II258.

21. Catena E, Paino R, Fieschi S, et al. Lung transplantation and pulmonary vein thrombosis: a possible role of epicardial echocardiography. J Cardiothorac Vasc Anesth 2008; 22:167–168.

22. Sarsam MA, Yacoub M. Remodeling of the aortic valve anulus. J Thorac Cardiovasc Surg 1993; 105:435–438.

23. Shah AS, Smerling AJ, Quaegebeur JM, et al. Nitric oxide treatment for pulmonary hypertension after neonatal cardiac operation. Ann Thorac Surg 1995; 60:1791–1793.

24. Huang YC, Cheng YJ, Lin YH, et al. Graft failure caused by pulmonary venous obstruction diagnosed by intraoperative transesophageal echocardiography during lung transplantation. Anesth Analg 2000; 91:558–560.

25. Leibowitz DW, Smith CR, Michler RE, et al. Incidence of pulmonary vein complications after lung transplantation: a prospective transesophageal echocardiographic study. J Am Coll Cardiol 1994; 24:671–675.

26. Schulman LL, Anandarangam T, Leibowitz DW, et al. Four-year prospective study of pulmonary venous thrombosis after lung transplantation. J Am Soc Echocardiogr 2001; 14:806–812.

27. McIlroy DR, Sesto AC, Buckland MR. Pulmonary vein thrombosis, lung transplantation, and intraoperative transesophageal echocardiography. J Cardiothorac Vasc Anesth 2006; 20:712–715.

28. Clark SC, Levine AJ, Hasan A, et al. Vascular complications of lung transplantation. Ann Thorac Surg 1996; 61: 1079–1082.

29. Katz WE, Jafar MZ, Mankad S, et al. Transesophageal echocardiographic identification of a malpositioned extracorporeal membrane oxygenation cannula. J Heart Lung Transplant 1995; 14:790–792.

30. Denault AY, Ferraro P, Couture P, et al. Transesophageal echocardiography monitoring in the intensive care department: the management of hemodynamic instability secondary to thoracic tamponade after single lung transplantation. J Am Soc Echocardiogr 2003; 16:688–692.

31. Murtha W, Guenther C. Dynamic left ventricular outflow tract obstruction complicating bilateral lung transplantation. Anesth Analg 2002; 94:558–559.

32. Gorcsan J III, Reddy SC, Armitage JM, et al. Acquired right ventricular outflow tract obstruction after lung transplantation: diagnosis by transesophageal echocardiography. J Am Soc Echocardiogr 1993; 6:324–326.

33. Kirshbom PM, Tapson VF, Harrison JK, et al. Delayed right heart failure following lung transplantation. Chest 1996; 109:575–577.

34. Lang RM, Bierig M, Devereux RB, et al. Recommendations for chamber quantification: a report from the American Society of Echocardiography's Guidelines and Standards Committee and the Chamber Quantification Writing Group, developed in conjunction with the European Association of Echocardiography, a branch of the European Society of Cardiology. J Am Soc Echocardiogr 2005; 18:1440–1463.

35. Haddad F, Couture P, Tousignant C, et al. The right ventricle in cardiac surgery, a perioperative perspective: I. Anatomy, physiology, and assessment. Anesth Analg 2009; 108:407–421.

36. Serra E, Feltracco P, Barbieri S, et al. Transesophageal echocardiography during lung transplantation. Transplant Proc 2007; 39:1981–1982.

37. Boyd SY, Sako EY, Trinkle JK, et al. Calculation of lung flow differential after single-lung transplantation: a transesophageal echocardiographic study. Am J Cardiol 2001; 87:1170–1173.

38. Barletta G, Del Bene MR, Palminiello A, et al. Left-ventricular diastolic dysfunction during pneumonectomy—a transesophageal echocardiographic study. Thorac Cardiovasc Surg 1996; 44:92–96.

39. Torre W, Rabago G, Barba J, et al. Combined surgical approach for sarcoma lung metastasis with atrial involvement. Thorac Cardiovasc Surg 1999; 47:125–127.

40. Neustein SM, Cohen E, Reich D, et al. Transoesophageal echocardiography and the intraoperative diagnosis of left atrial invasion by carcinoid tumour. Can J Anaesth 1993; 40:664–666.

41. Dlabal PW, Stutts BS, Jenkins DW, et al. Cyanosis following right pneumonectomy: importance of patent foramen ovale. Chest 1982; 81:370–372.

42. Jaffe RA, Pinto FJ, Schnittger I, et al. Aspects of mechanical ventilation affecting interatrial shunt flow during general anesthesia. Anesth Analg 1992; 75:484–488.

43. Jamieson SW, Kapelanski DP, Sakakibara N, et al. Pulmonary endarterectomy: experience and lessons learned in 1,500 cases. Ann Thorac Surg 2003; 76:1457–1462.

28

Liver Transplantation

Michel-Antoine Perrault
Centre Hospitalier Universitaire de Sherbrooke, Sherbrooke, Quebec, Canada

Franck Vandenbroucke-Menu, François Plante, and Luc Massicotte
Université de Montréal, Montreal, Quebec, Canada

ORTHOTOPIC LIVER TRANSPLANTATION PROCEDURE

In the last 20 years, both pediatric and adult orthotopic liver transplantation (OLT) procedures have increased in the United States from approximately 2000 in 1988 to 6492 in 2007. Moreover, since 1999, nearly 5% of the transplanted livers each year have come from living donors (1). There are three distinct stages during OLT procedure: preanhepatic, anhepatic, and postanhepatic. Each stage is characterized by hemodynamic, metabolic, and hematological phenomena. Over the last decade, transesophageal echocardiography (TEE) has emerged as an invaluable tool to help the anesthesiologist adjust treatment for the complex hemodynamic fluctuations specific to OLT patients. After an overview of the surgical procedure, this chapter will present the role of perioperative TEE for OLT.

Preanhepatic Stage

The normal anatomy of the liver is shown in Figure 28.1 and Table 28.1. The preanhepatic stage begins with the skin incision and ends with the completion of the hepatic vascular dissection. Several problems may occur (Fig. 28.2).

1. *Hypotension*: Preload may decrease for many reasons. First, surgical bleeding may occur due to portal hypertension with intra-abdominal and parietal venous dilatation. Second, a preexisting coagulopathy may worsen due to blood replacement, lack of hepatic production of coagulation factors, platelet consumption or dilution, and ongoing hypothermia worsening blood loss. Lack of clearance of plasminogen activators, due to ongoing hepatic dysfunction, can accentuate fibrinolysis and aggravate the bleeding diathesis. Third, insensible fluid loss and formation of a third space due to a large wound will reduce the effective circulating volume. Finally, drainage of ascites, compression or torsion of major blood vessels, compartment syndrome (2,3), low systemic vascular resistance, preexisting right and left cardiac dysfunction worsened with arrhythmia from electrolyte disturbances,

and acid-base abnormalities can also contribute to hemodynamic instability.

2. *Hypothermia*: May develop from heat loss, administration of cold fluids, skin vasodilatation from anesthetic agents, and lack of heat production by the liver.
3. *Hypocalcemia*: Most commonly originates from citrate toxicity from the blood products. This can also contribute to the decrease in blood pressure.
4. *Hypoglycemia*: Results from decreased glucose production by the liver glycogenolysis.
5. *Metabolic acidosis*: Occurs secondary to impaired hepatic clearance of acidotic products.
6. *Reduced urine output*: Can be caused by hypotension, hypovolemia, fluid retention from stress hormones, and the hepatorenal syndrome.

During the last few years, improvements in surgical technique, the use of antifibrinolytic agents, and the development of new anesthetic strategies have contributed to a steady reduction in all these problems. For instance, some centers will use a postinduction phlebotomy to reduce splanchnic congestion (4), and TEE can monitor the efficacy of volume reduction. In those liver transplantation centers, the intraoperative transfusion rate has decreased to a median of zero for all blood products (5).

Anhepatic Stage

The anhepatic stage begins with the occlusion of all liver vessels. If a trial clamping test is hemodynamically well tolerated, the hepatic artery, portal vein, and both the suprahepatic and infrahepatic portions of the inferior vena cava (IVC) are clamped and divided (Figs. 28.3–28.8). During this phase, the problems described in the previous stage may worsen. Occlusion of the IVC and portal vein dramatically reduces venous return to the right heart, but it is usually well tolerated because of collateral vasculature and the hyperdynamic state of the cirrhotic patient. Vessel clamping also produces renal and intestinal congestion of the infracaval and portal vein drainage areas.

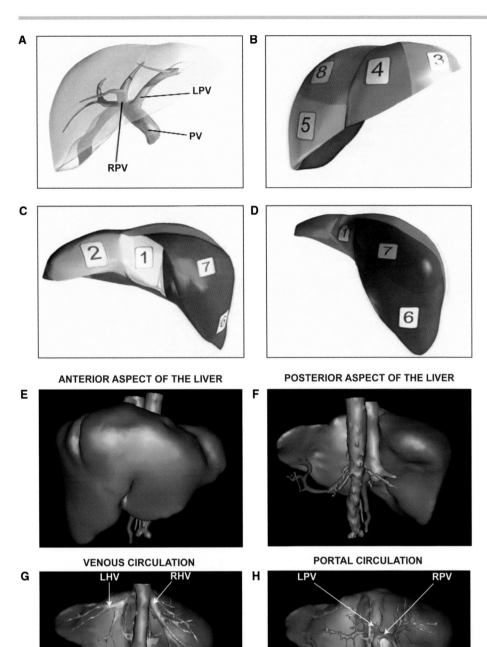

Figure 28.1 Normal liver anatomy. The Couinaud classification divides the liver into 8 independent segments each of which has its own vascular inflow, outflow, and biliary drainage. Anterior (**A,B**) and posterior (**C,D**) views are shown compared with a 3D anterior (**E**) and posterior (**F–H**) reconstruction of the hepatic circulation. *Abbreviations*: LHV, left hepatic vein; LPV, left portal vein; PV, portal vein; SMV, superior mesenteric vein; RHV, right hepatic vein; RPV, right portal vein; SV, splenic vein. *Source*: Courtesy of Sanofi Aventis and l'Institut de Recherche Contre les Cancers de l'Appareil Digestif, Strasbourg, France.

Table 28.1 Hepatic Anatomy

Couinaud	Traditional
Segment I	Caudate lobe
Segment II	Lateral segment left lobe (superior)
Segment III	Lateral segment left lobe (inferior)
Segment IV	Medial segment left lobe
Segment V	Anterior segment right lobe (inferior)
Segment VI	Posterior segment right lobe (inferior)
Segment VII	Posterior segment right lobe (superior)
Segment VIII	Anterior segment right lobe (superior)

The suprahepatic IVC anastomosis is performed first followed by the infrahepatic IVC and then the portal vein anastomoses. If a hyperkalemic preservation solution is used, the donor liver graft is flushed with colloid, crystalloid, or autologous blood through the incomplete portal vein anastomosis. The flushed fluid is recovered through the infrahepatic IVC anastomosis before the sutures are tied. Finally, the portal vein anastomosis is completed.

The graft is then reperfused. Consequently, cold, acidotic, hyperkalemic fluid, containing metabolically

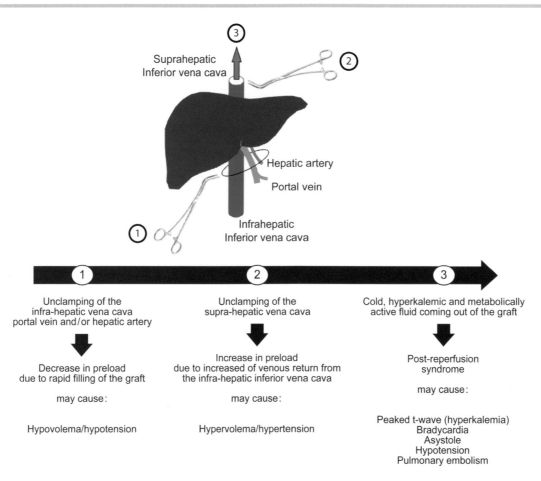

Figure 28.2 Hemodynamics during liver transplantation. Hemodynamic consequences during the reperfusion phase of a liver transplant procedure are presented in the sequence of occurrence.

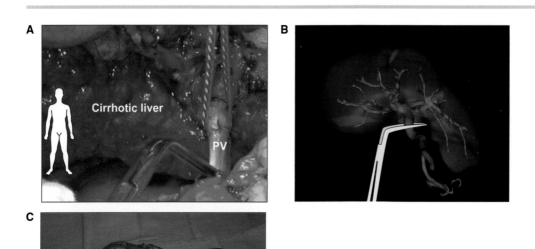

Figure 28.3 Portal vein identification and clamping during liver transplantation. (**A**) Intraoperative view. (**B**) Corresponding 3D reconstruction. (**C**) Pathological specimen of the excised cirrhotic liver. *Abbreviation*: PV, portal vein. *Source*: Part B courtesy of l'Institut de Recherche Contre les Cancers de l'Appareil Digestif, Strasbourg, France.

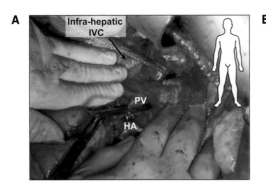
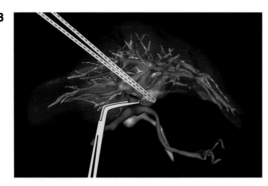

Figure 28.4 Hepatic vasculature during liver transplantation. (**A**) Intraoperative view. (**B**) Corresponding 3D reconstruction. *Abbreviations*: HA, hepatic artery; IVC, inferior vena cava; PV, portal vein. *Source*: Part B courtesy of l'Institut de Recherche Contre les Cancers de l'Appareil Digestif, Strasbourg, France.

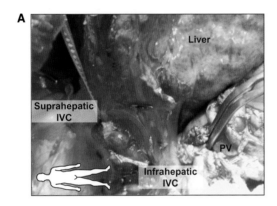
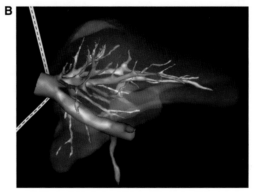

Figure 28.5 Identification of supra- and infra-hepatic IVC during liver transplantation. (**A**) Intraoperative view. A clamp is on the PV. (**B**) Corresponding 3D reconstruction. *Abbreviations*: IVC, inferior vena cava; PV, portal vein. *Source*: Part B courtesy of l'Institut de Recherche Contre les Cancers de l'Appareil Digestif, Strasbourg, France.

active byproducts, is released from the graft into the systemic circulation. Hypotension, peaked T-waves, and dysrhythmias (blocks, asystole) may ensue, causing the so-called postreperfusion syndrome (PRS). Its duration is usually short but may require aggressive resuscitation.

Alternative strategies can be used to avoid reduction of venous return: First, the "piggyback" technique, described first in 1989 by Tzakis (6), preserves the retrohepatic IVC with clamping of only the hepatic veins (Fig. 28.9). The reconstruction of the hepatic outflow is with an anastomosis between the donor IVC and the joined ostium of the recipient hepatic veins. This technique requires more time for dissection but may allow, based on some studies, better hemodynamic stability, lower blood transfusion, and shorter warm ischemic time (7,8). It also avoids dissection of the IVC from the retroperito-

neum. Alternatively, current trials have shown very good results with minimal blood transfusion requirements without performing vena cava preservation (4).

Second, a venovenous bypass circuit may be used. The IVC and the portal vein are cannulated with heparin-coated tubes through the saphenous vein. A vortex pump is used to return blood to the patient's circulation through the axillary vein (9). This circuit may offer more stable hemodynamics, especially during the clamping phase, and allow decompression of the splanchnic venous territory. The venovenous bypass cannula can also be inserted into the internal jugular vein with TEE guidance (10).

Third, a temporary portacaval shunt can be used with the piggyback technique to decompress the portal territory. Portal vein clamping induces major portal hypertension with splanchnic congestion and renal

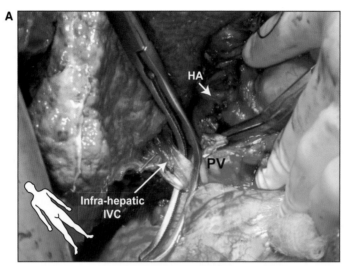

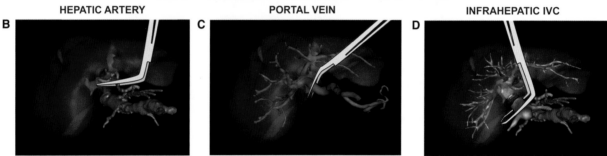

Figure 28.6 Clamping of the infrahepatic IVC and PV during orthotopic liver transplantation. (A) Intraoperative view. **(B–D)** Corresponding 3D reconstruction of clamping of the major hepatic vessels. *Abbreviations*: HA, hepatic artery; IVC, inferior vena cava; PV, portal vein. *Source*: Parts B to D courtesy of l'Institut de Recherche Contre les Cancers de l'Appareil Digestif, Strasbourg, France.

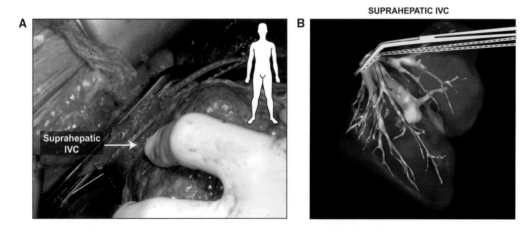

Figure 28.7 Clamping of the suprahepatic IVC during orthotopic liver transplantation. (A) Intraoperative view. **(B)** Corresponding 3D reconstruction. *Abbreviations*: IVC, inferior vena cava. *Source*: Part B courtesy of l'Institut de Recherche Contre les Cancers de l'Appareil Digestif, Strasbourg, France.

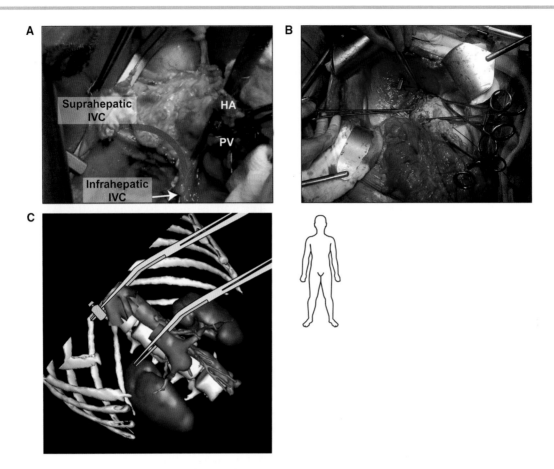

Figure 28.8 **Anhepatic phase of the orthotopic liver transplantation. (A,B)** Intraoperative view showing residual supra- and infra-hepatic IVC after removal of the liver and the retrohepatic portion of the IVC. (**C**) Corresponding 3D reconstruction. *Abbreviations*: HA, hepatic artery; IVC, inferior vena cava. *Source*: Part C courtesy of l'Institut de Recherche Contre les Cancers de l'Appareil Digestif, Strasbourg, France.

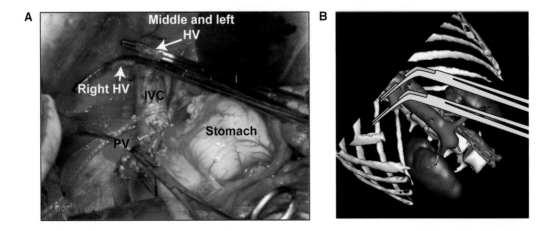

Figure 28.9 **Anhepatic phase of the liver transplantation by piggy-back technique. (A)** Intraoperative view shows the retrohepatic inferior vena cava left intact while the liver has been removed at the level of the hepatic veins. (**B**) Corresponding 3D reconstruction. *Abbreviations*: HV, hepatic vein; IVC, inferior vena cava; PV, portal vein. *Source*: Part B courtesy of l'Institut de Recherche Contre les Cancers de l'Appareil Digestif, Strasbourg, France.

dysfunction. In 1993, Tzakis et al. described a tempo-rary portacaval shunt (11). This shunt is particularly effective for patients with fulminant liver failure. These patients lack collaterals from portal hyperten-sion so they do not tolerate portal vein clamping very well. This led to severe splanchnic fluid retention (12). At the time of portal anastomosis, the shunt is taken down with a vascular stapler and the recipient and donor portal veins are anastomosed.

Postanhepatic Stage

The postanhepatic stage usually has less potential for complications than the previous stages. Once the reper-fusion phase has passed, the new liver gradually cor-rects the metabolic abnormalities. The hepatic artery reconstruction is performed, and the adequacy of this anastomosis is controlled by the surgeon with direct surface Doppler ultrasound. The resistance index nor-mal range is between 0.55 and 0.80 (Fig. 28.10) (13). Criteria for hepatic artery stenosis also include increased peak velocity greater than 2 m/s, focal color aliasing, and prolonged systolic acceleration time greater than 80 ms (*tardus*). In the presence of severe stenosis or occlusion, velocities may instead be significantly reduced (Fig. 28.11). Finally, the bile duct reconstruction is performed either with a duct-to-duct anastomosis or with a Roux-en-Y hepaticojejunostomy.

ROLE OF TEE

TEE may be useful in many instances as patients with liver failure are at risk of altered cardiopulmonary condition. Although TEE for OLT is considered a cate-gory III indication (14), this recommendation dates from 1996 and was recently reviewed (see Chapter 31). Some authors advocate the use of TEE as a routine monitor for OLT (15–17). In addition to the cardiac assessment, TEE can be used to evaluate the IVC, hepatic veins (Figs. 28.12 and 28.13) (18), portal vessels (Fig. 28.14), aorta (Ao) and major branches (Fig. 28.15), hepatic arteries (Figs. 28.16 and 28.17), lung and pleural region (Fig. 28.18) (19), and the abdominal cavity (Fig. 28.19) before, during, and after OLT.

Preoperatively

Hemodynamically, OLT is one of the most stressful surgeries for patients and a challenge for the anesthesi-ologist. Apart from the hemodynamic characteristics,

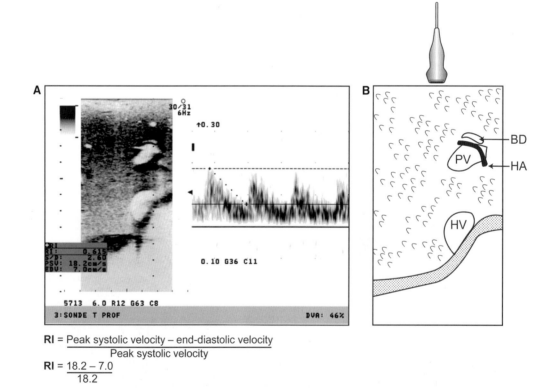

RI = Peak systolic velocity – end-diastolic velocity
         Peak systolic velocity

$$RI = \frac{18.2 - 7.0}{18.2}$$

RI = 0.62   (Normal value 0.55-0.80)

Figure 28.10   Resistance index of the HA. (A,B) Direct surface spectral Doppler interrogation of the HA is obtained intraoperatively by the liver transplant surgeon. The RI is calculated as the difference between the peak systolic and the end-diastolic velocities, divided by the peak systolic velocity. In the advent of HA anastomotic stenosis, the RI will be increased, while the systolic acceleration time (from end-diastole to the first systolic peak) will be prolonged (>80 ms). Surface spectral Doppler interrogation of the HA is obtained intraoperatively by the liver transplant surgeon. *Abbreviations*: BD, bile duct; HA, hepatic artery; HV, hepatic vein; PV, portal vein; RI, resistance index.

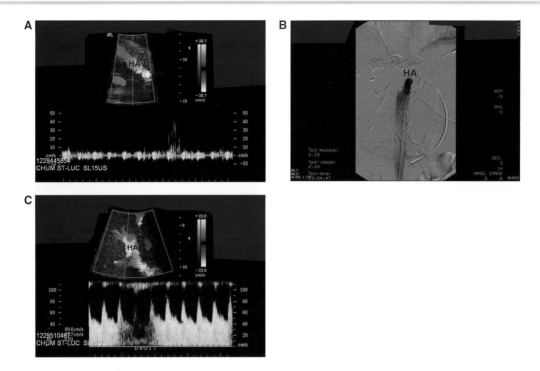

Figure 28.11 HA occlusion. (A) Significantly reduced velocities in the HA were noted on color and spectral Doppler after liver transplantation. **(B)** Angiography shows absent flow due to dissection of the HA. **(C)** Normal HA flow is re-established after reoperation. The velocity upstroke is rapid with a resistance index of 0.51. *Abbreviation*: HA, hepatic artery.

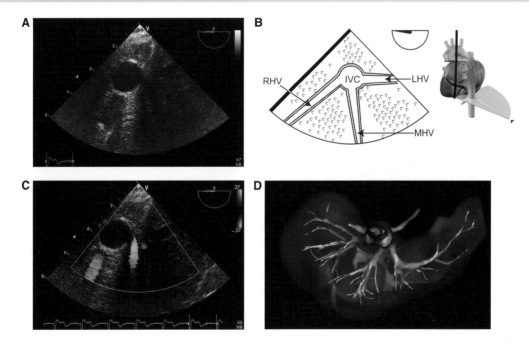

Figure 28.12 Hepatic veins. (A,B) Transgastric views with right-sided rotation showing the three branches of the hepatic veins. **(C)** Color Doppler with a 37 cm/s Nyquist limit. **(D)** Corresponding 3D reconstruction. *Abbreviations*: IVC, inferior vena cava; LHV, left hepatic vein; MHV, middle hepatic vein; RHV, right hepatic vein. *Sources*: Courtesy of Dr. Jean-Sébastien Bilodeau and l'Institut de Recherche Contre les Cancers de l'Appareil Digestif, Strasbourg, France.

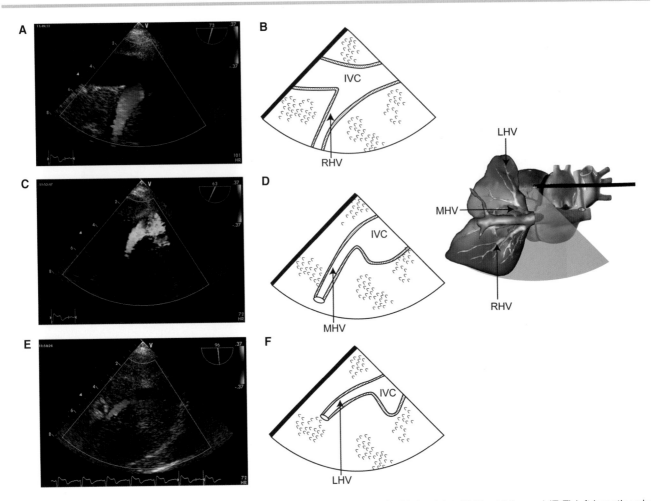

Figure 28.13 Hepatic veins. Transgastric views between 60° to 90° display: (**A,B**) the right, (**C,D**) middle, and (**E,F**) left hepatic veins in the majority of patients. *Abbreviations*: IVC, inferior vena cava; LHV, left hepatic vein; MHV, middle hepatic vein; RHV, right hepatic vein. ⌃🖱

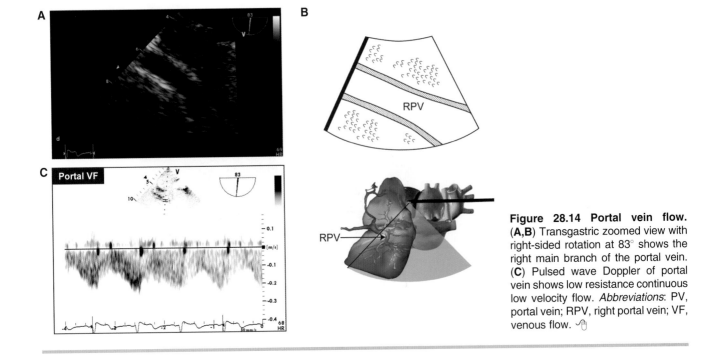

Figure 28.14 Portal vein flow. (**A,B**) Transgastric zoomed view with right-sided rotation at 83° shows the right main branch of the portal vein. (**C**) Pulsed wave Doppler of portal vein shows low resistance continuous low velocity flow. *Abbreviations*: PV, portal vein; RPV, right portal vein; VF, venous flow. ⌃🖱

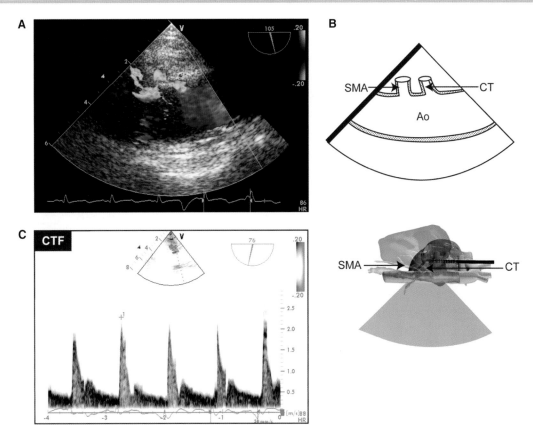

Figure 28.15 Abdominal aorta and visceral branches. (A,B) Color Doppler transgastric Ao long-axis view at 105° in which the CT and SMA are seen and can be interrogated using continuous wave Doppler (**C**). *Abbreviations*: Ao, aorta; CT, celiac trunk; CTF, celiac trunk flow; SMA, superior mesenteric artery.

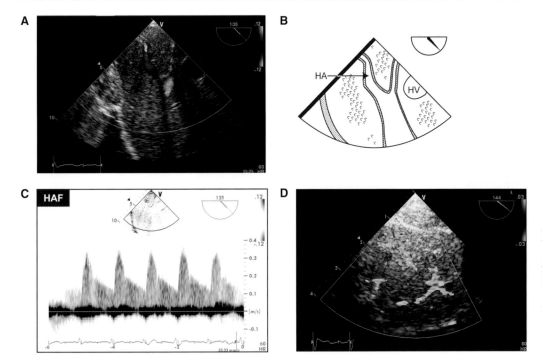

Figure 28.16 Hepatic artery. (**A,B**) Color Doppler transgastric view with right-side rotation at 135° shows the HA. (**C**) Continuous wave Doppler of normal HAF. (**D**) Vascular flow in the liver is shown. *Abbreviations*: HA, hepatic artery; HAF, hepatic artery flow; HV, hepatic vein.

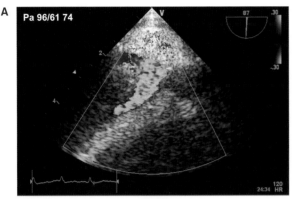

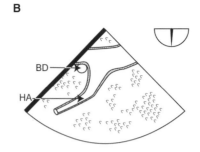

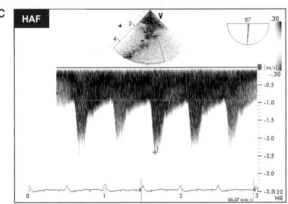

Figure 28.17 **Doppler imaging of the HA.** A 58-year-old woman is hemodynamically unstable following liver transplantation. (**A,B**) A color Doppler transgastric view at 87° shows turbulent flow in the HA. (**C**) Continuous wave Doppler interrogation of HAF reveals a peak systolic flow of 2.39 m/s with a normal resistance index of 62%. *Abbreviations*: BD, bile duct; HA, hepatic artery; HAF, hepatic artery flow, Pa, arterial pressure.

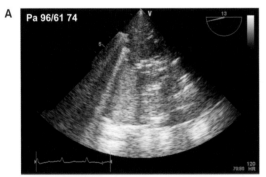

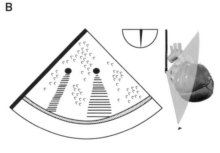

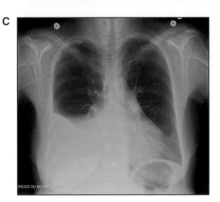

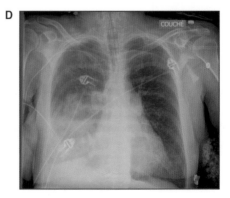

Figure 28.18 **Pulmonary examination using TEE.** A 58-year-old woman is hemodynamically unstable after liver transplantation. (**A,B**) TEE scanning of the chest reveals significant consolidation of the lung parenchyma. Chest radiographs (**C**) before intensive care unit admission and (**D**) during hemodynamic instability show a new right-sided lung infiltrate. *Abbreviation*: TEE, transesophageal echocardiography.

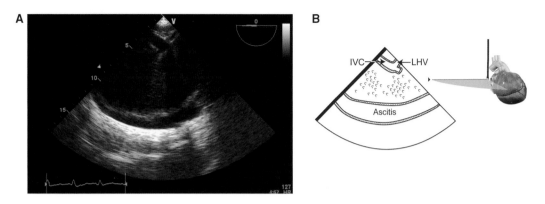

Figure 28.19 **Ascites. (A,B)** A transgastric IVC long-axis view reveals ascites in a hemodynamically unstable 58-year-old woman after liver transplantation. *Abbreviations*: IVC, inferior vena cava; LHV, left hepatic vein.

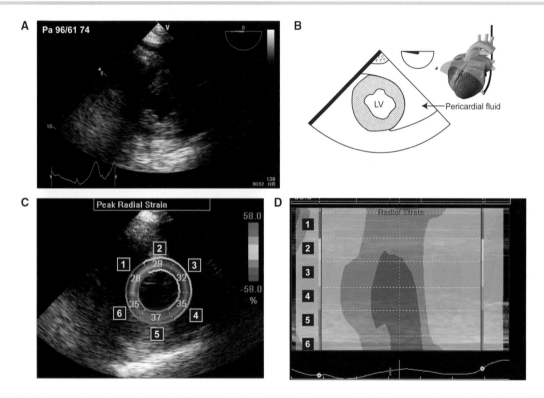

Figure 28.20 **Strain rate in a hemodynamically unstable 58-year-old woman after liver transplantation. (A,B)** Transgastric mid short-axis view with a posterior pericardial effusion. **(C,D)** 2D speckle tracking in the same view. The strain is lowest in the inferoseptal region where the patient was previously known to have a myocardial infarction. *Abbreviations*: LV, left ventricle; Pa, arterial pressure.

which will be discussed here, Carey et al. demonstrated that a third of patients presenting for OLT had at least a moderate degree of coronary artery disease as demonstrated on coronary angiography (20), which could manifest as abnormal segmental wall motion perioperatively (Fig. 28.20) (21–23). Consequently, preoperative assessment of the cardiac function is of prime importance to ensure the best outcome possible.

The patient with compensated end-stage liver failure usually presents with a hyperdynamic state characterized by high cardiac output, normal left ventricular ejection fraction (LVEF), low systemic vascular resistance, and elevated heart rate. More specifically, anomalies due to the hemodynamic consequences of hepatic failure on the systemic and pulmonary circulation include hepatopulmonary syndrome, plexogenic

Table 28.2 Associated Cardiac and Hepatic Disorders

Heart diseases affecting the liver
- Mild alterations of liver function tests in heart failure
- Cardiogenic IH and its variants
- CLF and congestive (cardiac) cirrhosis

Liver diseases affecting the heart
- Hepatopulmonary syndrome
- PPHTN in liver cirrhosis
- Pericardial effusion in cirrhosis
- Cirrhotic cardiomyopathy
- High-output failure caused by intrahepatic arteriovenous fistulas in the noncirrhotic liver

Cardiac and hepatic disorders with joint etiology

Infectious and parasitic, metabolic, immune and vasculitic, toxic

Abbreviations: CLF, congestive liver fibrosis; IH, ischemic hepatitis; PPHTN, portopulmonary hypertension.
Source: With permission from Ref. 23.

pulmonary hypertension, pericardial effusion, cardio-myopathy, and high-output heart failure caused by arteriovenous shunts (Table 28.2).

Hepatopulmonary Syndrome

Symptomatic hepatopulmonary syndrome (HPS) occurs in approximately 15% of patient with end-stage liver failure (24) and may be reversed by OLT. It is characterized by liver dysfunction, hypoxemia (PaO_2 <70 mmHg on room air), and intrapulmonary vascular dilatations. Liver dysfunction provokes an imbalance between vasoconstricting and vasodilating mediators as well as between hepatic factors control-ling endothelial cell growth. Consequently, pulmo-nary capillary vessels grow and dilate. During their passage through the dilated pulmonary capillaries,

red blood cells do not optimally pick up diffused oxygen in a patient breathing room air. Diffusion/perfusion mismatch causes hypoxemia (Fig. 28.21).

Contrast-enhanced echocardiography, with IV injection of agitated saline, is the current gold stan-dard for detection of pulmonary vascular dilatations (24). Bubbles are usually trapped in the pulmonary capillaries and are not seen in the left cardiac cham-bers. If an intracardiac shunt exists, such as an atrial septal defect, contrast bubbles will appear in the left atrium (LA) within three beats after their appearance in the right atrium (RA). In the case of HPS, contrast will be delayed but will still appear in the LA after four to six beats.

Portopulmonary Hypertension

Although not a common disease in liver failure, portopulmonary hypertension (PPHTN) can severely affect the outcome of OLT. The mechanisms are unknown. The severity appears to be related to the duration of portal hypertension, and, as in the case of HPS, substances not cleared by the liver (coming from the splanchnic blood) might cause vascular changes. On echocardiography, the diagnosis of PPHTN should be considered in the presence of signs of pul-monary hypertension such as dilated RA or ventricle, pulmonic regurgitation, or abnormal ventricular sep-tal curvature toward the left ventricle (LV).

Pericardial and Pleural Effusions

Pericardial and pleural effusions, due to fluid reten-tion, are frequently seen in decompensated liver dis-ease, and echocardiography is a useful tool to assess the presence of pericardial effusion in those patients. A baseline echocardiographic examination becomes useful as a pericardial effusion can happen

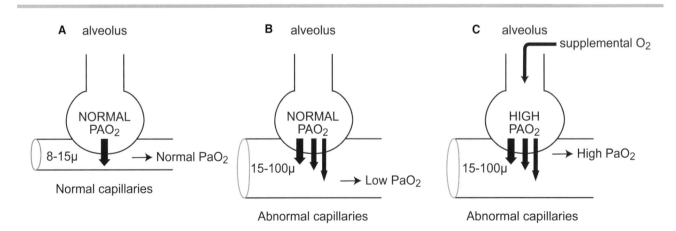

Figure 28.21 Hepatopulmonary syndrome. (A) Normal gas exchange with matched capillaries and alveolus. **(B)** In the hepato-pulmonary syndrome, capillaries become dilated and blood does not receive diffused oxygen in a patient breathing room air, causing hypoxemia. When the patient goes from a supine to a standing position, blood flow is increased at the lung base, exacerbating hypoxemia and causing orthodeoxia and platypnea. **(C)** Hypoxemia in severe diffusion-perfusion mismatch is improved by supplemental oxygen, as opposed to true right-to-left shunting. *Abbreviations*: A, alveolar; a, arterial; PaO_2, oxygen partial pressure.

iatrogenically intraoperatively and cause acute hemo-dynamic instability (Fig. 28.20) (16).

Cardiomyopathy

As previously mentioned, OLT presents one of the most important hemodynamic stressful procedures. Therefore, hypercontractility secondary to important preload variations, tachycardia, and circulation of vaso-active substances seen during the reperfusion syndrome can exacerbate conditions such as dynamic left ventricular outflow tract obstruction (25,26). Therefore, preoperative assessment of the LV function, before the procedure, is a mandatory part of the work-up.

Intraoperatively

After induction of anesthesia and before skin incision, a routine TEE examination provides essential information before the "storm." Baseline, under anesthesia, LV and right ventricular (RV) filling and global function are determined as well as regional wall motion abnormalities, valvular function, and the presence of an intracardiac shunt (foramen ovale) (Fig. 28.22). This last pathology has to be carefully assessed because of the possibility of RV failure following the anastomosis of the donor liver (27). As right-heart pressure can become superior to the left side, risk of paradoxical emboli arises (see Fig. 30.4). Postanhepatic RV failure

may account for some of the hemodynamic instability during OLT (28). Furthermore, as pulmonary hypertension may also be present in many of the OLT patients, rapid shifts in intravascular volume with transfusions and clamping of vessels may be poorly tolerated by the RV. As central venous pressure (CVP) is an incomplete and unreliable method for monitoring RV preload and function (29), TEE provides useful information on RV filling pressure, global function, and response to therapy.

As with CVP for the RV, the pulmonary capillary wedge pressure presents several shortcomings as an indicator of LV volumes (29). Measurement of end-diastolic volume and transmitral pulsed wave Doppler using TEE is a better reflection of LV preload alterations than CVP (30). During OLT, TEE has shown significant changes in end-systolic and end-diastolic volumes without changes in LVEF. This suggests that LV function was maintained and that volume fluctuations were the most likely cause of hypotension (22). Krenn et al. (23) confirmed this using TEE, during the three surgical phases of OLT, by measuring LV fractional area change (FAC) in 10 patients using a transgastric mid short-axis view. The LV FAC went from a baseline 51% ± 13% to 36% ± 10% in the anhepatic phase and back to 53% ± 15% during reperfusion. These changes were not clinically significant and can be explained by changes in loading conditions.

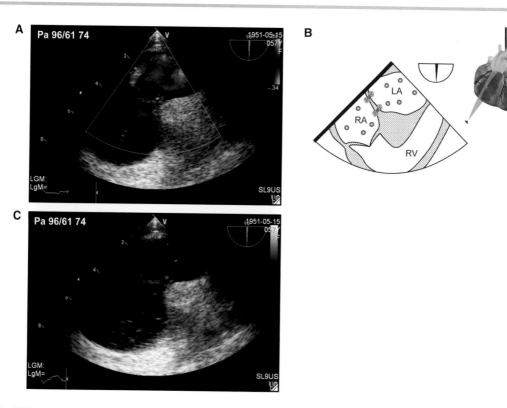

Figure 28.22 PFO in a severely hypoxic patient after liver transplantation. **(A,B)** Mid-esophageal right ventricular inflow/outflow view with color Doppler interrogation of the interatrial septum. **(C)** Right cardiac chamber opacification with agitated saline shows right-to-left shunting through a PFO. *Abbreviations*: LA, left atrium; Pa, arterial pressure; PFO, patent foramen ovale; RA, right atrium; RV, right ventricle.

OLT carries an important risk of thromboembolic phenomena. Although those patients seldom have normal coagulation profiles, they have often been found in a hypercoagulable state (15,31). Moreover, increasing use of antifibrinolytic agents in the last few years may have worsened this imbalance (32). Only TEE can rapidly diagnose the presence of an intracardiac thrombus and monitor subsequent treatment. Particular attention has to be paid during the reperfusion phase as embolic material from the graft can commonly appear in the right heart and aggravate an already very unstable condition (Fig. 28.23) (33). The mid-esophageal RV inflow-outflow view is useful to monitor in these situations.

Although global LV systolic function is maintained (34), some patients may present with diastolic dysfunction after reperfusion (Fig. 28.24). The LV filling pressures are higher after reperfusion, while the end-diastolic volume is not changed significantly. This change in LV compliance may be due to toxic effects

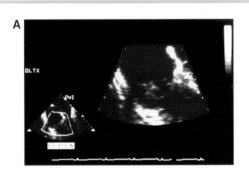
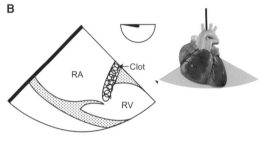

Figure 28.23   Thromboembolism during liver transplantation in a 44-year-old man. (A,B) Within five minutes after reperfusion of the transplanted liver, the mid-esophageal four-chamber view shows a large thrombus in the RA attached to the tricuspid valve. *Abbreviations*: RA, right atrium; RV, right ventricle. *Source*: Adapted with permission from Ref. 33.

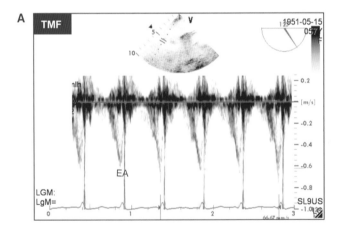
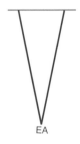

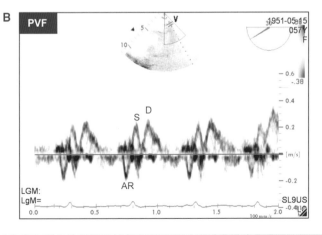
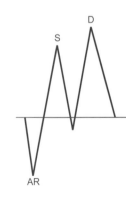

Figure 28.24 Diastolic dysfunction after liver transplantation in a hemodynamically unstable 58-year-old woman following liver transplantation. (A) Pulsed wave Doppler examination of the TMF: fusion of the *E* and *A* waves is secondary to tachycardia. **(B)** Pulsed wave Doppler examination of the PVF shows abnormal diastolic flow predominance with elevated AR velocity. This is consistent with moderate diastolic dysfunction. *Abbreviations*: A, peak late diastolic TMF velocity; AR, peak atrial reversal PVF velocity; D, peak diastolic PVF velocity; E, peak early diastolic TMF velocity; PVF, pulmonary venous flow; S, peak systolic PVF velocity; TMF, transmitral flow.

Table 28.3 Role of Transesophageal Echocardiography in Orthotopic Liver Transplantation

	Importance
Before the procedure	
• Left and right ventricular function	Loading condition and need for postoperative inotropic
• Aortic, mitral, tricuspid, and pulmonic valve competency	Detect unrecognized valvular disease
• PFO and PPHTN	Risk of hypoxia by right-to-left shunt if right ventricular dysfunction
• Detection of pleural effusion and ascites	Optimization of oxygenation and ventilation
During liver transplantation	
• Monitor the presence of embolic material	Embolism could cause hemodynamic instability
After liver transplantation	
• Reevaluate left and right ventricular function	Loading condition and need for postoperative inotropic support
• Reevaluate valvular function	LVOT and RVOT dynamic obstruction could complicate management
• Evaluate inferior vena cava anastomosis	Rule out new iatrogenic obstruction
• Evaluate hepatic artery RI	Rule out mechanical obstruction
• Rule out significant pleural effusion and ascites	Optimize chest tube drainage and ascites removal
In the intensive care unit	
• Rule out specific complications if hemodynamically unstable	Tamponade, ventricular dysfunction, valvular insufficiency, LVOT and RVOT dynamic obstruction hypovolemia, shunting through a PFO, persistent PPHTN, intracavitary thrombus

Abbreviations: LVOT, left ventricular outflow tract; PFO, patent foramen ovale; PPHTN, portopulmonary hypertension; RI, resistance index; RVOT, right ventricular outflow tract.

related to the graft fluid or cardiac edema secondary to massive volume infusion of blood products, crystalloids, and colloids.

The integrity of the suprahepatic IVC anastomosis can also be assessed using two-dimensional TEE (Fig. 28.12). The permeability of the hepatic artery and portal vein is best assessed using Doppler imaging (Figs. 28.14–28.17) (35–37).

In 1996, the clinical impact of 100 TEE examinations during OLT was reported by Suriani et al. (38). In their experience, unanticipated findings during the initial TEE examination, as well as the evaluation of intraoperative events, resulted in a major impact on patient management in 11% of patients. Despite the increased prevalence of esophageal varices in liver failure patients, only one OLT recipient suffered from upper gastrointestinal bleeding, with no significant clinical outcome. This suggests that the benefits of TEE in OLT outweigh the risks and that TEE may become important, if not essential, as a monitoring tool in patients undergoing this procedure. In the last few years, increasing publications on this subject support the observations of the Suriani study. A recent review could not find any reports of significantly adverse events due to the use of TEE in patients with end-stage liver disease undergoing OLT, even in the presence of documented esophageal varices (17). Training guidelines for the use of TEE in liver transplantation have been suggested (39).

CONCLUSION

In summary, TEE plays an important role in OLT, as it is performed in a population at high risk for perioperative hemodynamic instability. The role of TEE extends beyond the diagnosis of several potential etiologies for this condition but can help the liver transplantation team to recognize unanticipated surgical complications

and, therefore, improve patient outcome. The role of TEE in OLT is summarized in Table 28.3.

ACKNOWLEDGMENTS

The authors wish to thank Dr. André Roy, Dr. Réal Lapointe, and Dr. Marylène Plasse from the Unit of Hepatobiliary and Pancreatic Surgery, Liver Transplantation, Centre Hospitalier de l'Université de Montréal, Canada, for their contribution.

REFERENCES

1. The United Network for Organ Sharing. Electronic Citation, 2009. Available at: http://unos.org/.
2. Malbrain ML, Cheatham ML, Kirkpatrick A, et al. Results from the International Conference of Experts on Intra-abdominal Hypertension and Abdominal Compartment Syndrome. I. Definitions. Intensive Care Med 2006; 32: 1722–1732.
3. Cheatham ML, Malbrain ML, Kirkpatrick A, et al. Results from the International Conference of Experts on Intra-abdominal Hypertension and Abdominal Compartment Syndrome. II. Recommendations. Intensive Care Med 2007; 33:951–962.
4. Massicotte L, Lenis S, Thibeault L, et al. Effect of low central venous pressure and phlebotomy on blood product transfusion requirements during liver transplantations. Liver Transpl 2006; 12:117–123.
5. Massicotte L, Beaulieu D, Thibeault L, et al. Coagulation defects do not predict blood product requirements during liver transplantation. Transplantation 2008; 85:956–962.
6. Tzakis A, Todo S, Starzl TE. Orthotopic liver transplantation with preservation of the inferior vena cava. Ann Surg 1989; 210:649–652.
7. Moreno-Gonzalez E, Meneu-Diaz JG, Fundora Y, et al. Advantages of the piggy back technique on intraoperative transfusion, fluid consumption, and vasoactive drugs requirements in liver transplantation: a comparative study. Transplant Proc 2003; 35:1918–1919.

8. Nishida S, Nakamura N, Vaidya A, et al. Piggyback technique in adult orthotopic liver transplantation: an analysis of 1067 liver transplants at a single center. HPB (Oxford) 2006; 8:182–188.

9. Maddrey WC, Schiff ER, Sorrell MF. Transplantation of the Liver. 3rd ed. Philadelphia: Lippincott Williams & Wilkins, 2001.

10. Planinsic RM, Nicolau-Raducu R, Caldwell JC, et al. Transesophageal echocardiography-guided placement of internal jugular percutaneous venovenous bypass cannula in orthotopic liver transplantation. Anesth Analg 2003; 97:648–649.

11. Tzakis AG, Reyes J, Nour B, et al. Temporary end to side portacaval shunt in orthotopic hepatic transplantation in humans. Surg Gynecol Obstet 1993; 176:180–182.

12. Llado L, Figueras J. Techniques of orthotopic liver transplantation. HPB (Oxford) 2004; 6:69–75.

13. Dodd GD III, Memel DS, Zajko AB, et al. Hepatic artery stenosis and thrombosis in transplant recipients: Doppler diagnosis with resistive index and systolic acceleration time. Radiology 1994; 192:657–661.

14. Practice guidelines for perioperative transesophageal echocardiography. A report by the American Society of Anesthesiologists and the Society of Cardiovascular Anesthesiologists Task Force on Transesophageal Echocardiography. Anesthesiology 1996; 84:986–1006.

15. Planinsic RM, Nicolau-Raducu R, Eghtesad B, et al. Diagnosis and treatment of intracardiac thrombosis during orthotopic liver transplantation. Anesth Analg 2004; 99:353–356.

16. Sharma A, Pagel PS, Bhatia A. Intraoperative iatrogenic acute pericardial tamponade: use of rescue transesophageal echocardiography in a patient undergoing orthotopic liver transplantation. J Cardiothorac Vasc Anesth 2005; 19:364–366.

17. Burtenshaw AJ, Isaac JL. The role of trans-oesophageal echocardiography for perioperative cardiovascular monitoring during orthotopic liver transplantation. Liver Transpl 2006; 12:1577–1583.

18. Meierhenric R, Gauss A, Georgieff M, et al. Use of multiplane transoesophageal echocardiography in visualization of the main hepatic veins and acquisition of Doppler sonography curves. Comparison with the transabdominal approach. Br J Anaesth 2001; 87:711–717.

19. Lichtenstein D, Meziere G, Seitz J. The dynamic air bronchogram. A lung ultrasound sign of alveolar consolidation ruling out atelectasis. Chest 2009; 135:1421–1425.

20. Carey WD, Dumot JA, Pimentel RR, et al. The prevalence of coronary artery disease in liver transplant candidates over age 50. Transplantation 1995; 59:859–864.

21. Steltzer H, Blazek G, Gabriel A, et al. Two-dimensional transesophageal echocardiography in early diagnosis and treatment of hemodynamic disturbances during liver transplantation. Transplant Proc 1991; 23:1957–1958.

22. de la Morena G, Acosta F, Villegas M, et al. Transesophageal echocardiographic evaluation of left ventricular function during orthotopic liver transplantation. Transplant Proc 1993; 25:1832.

23. Krenn CG, Hoda R, Nikolic A, et al. Assessment of ventricular contractile function during orthotopic liver transplantation. Transpl Int 2004; 17:101–104.

24. Naschitz JE, Slobodin G, Lewis RJ, et al. Heart diseases affecting the liver and liver diseases affecting the heart. Am Heart J 2000; 140:111–120.

25. Cywinski JB, Argalious M, Marks TN, et al. Dynamic left ventricular outflow tract obstruction in an orthotopic liver transplant recipient. Liver Transpl 2005; 11:692–695.

26. Aniskevich S, Shine TS, Feinglass NG, et al. Dynamic left ventricular outflow tract obstruction during liver transplantation: the role of transesophageal echocardiography. J Cardiothorac Vasc Anesth 2007; 21:577–580.

27. Saada M, Liu N, Cherqui D, et al. Opening of a foramen ovale during liver transplantation. The value of transesophageal echocardiography. Ann Fr Anesth Reanim 1990; 9:412–414.

28. Ellis JE, Lichtor JL, Feinstein SB, et al. Right heart dysfunction, pulmonary embolism, and paradoxical embolization during liver transplantation. A transesophageal two-dimensional echocardiographic study. Anesth Analg 1989; 68:777–782.

29. Gelman S. Venous function and central venous pressure: a physiologic story. Anesthesiology 2008; 108:735–748.

30. Nishimura RA, Abel MD, Hatle LK, et al. Relation of pulmonary vein to mitral flow velocities by transesophageal Doppler echocardiography. Effect of different loading conditions. Circulation 1990; 81:1488–1497.

31. Pivalizza EG, Ekpenyong UU, Sheinbaum R, et al. Very early intraoperative cardiac thromboembolism during liver transplantation. J Cardiothorac Vasc Anesth 2006; 20: 232–235.

32. Ellenberger C, Mentha G, Giostra E, et al. Cardiovascular collapse due to massive pulmonary thromboembolism during orthotopic liver transplantation. J Clin Anesth 2006; 18:367–371.

33. Gologorsky E, De Wolf AM, Scott V, et al. Intracardiac thrombus formation and pulmonary thromboembolism immediately after graft reperfusion in 7 patients undergoing liver transplantation. Liver Transpl 2001; 7:783–789.

34. Kuo PC, Schroeder RA, Vagelos RH, et al. Volume-mediated pulmonary responses in liver transplant candidates. Clin Transplant 1996; 10:521–527.

35. Bjerke RJ, Mieles LA, Borsky BJ, et al. The use of transesophageal ultrasonography for the diagnosis of inferior vena caval outflow obstruction during liver transplantation. Transplantation 1992; 54:939–941.

36. De Wolf AM, Scott VL, Kang Y, et al. Hepatic venous outflow obstruction during hepatic resection diagnosed by transesophageal echocardiography. Anesthesiology 1994; 80:1398–1400.

37. Rumi MN, Schumann R, Freeman RB, et al. Acute transjugular intrahepatic portosystemic shunt migration into pulmonary artery during liver transplantation. Transplantation 1999; 67:1492–1494.

38. Suriani RJ, Cutrone A, Feierman D, et al. Intraoperative transesophageal echocardiography during liver transplantation. J Cardiothorac Vasc Anesth 1996; 10:699–707.

39. Wax DB, Torres A, Scher C, et al. Transesophageal echocardiography utilization in high-volume liver transplantation centers in the United States. J Cardiothorac Vasc Anesth 2008; 22:811–813.

29

TEE in the Hemodynamic and Electrophysiology Suite

Antoine G. Rochon, Reda Ibrahim and Annie Dore
Université de Montréal, Montreal, Quebec, Canada

André Saint-Pierre and Jean Champagne
Université Laval, Quebec City, Quebec, Canada

Viviane Nguyen and Jean Buithieu
McGill University, Montreal, Quebec, Canada

INTRODUCTION

Transesophageal echocardiography (TEE) is useful in many interventional and electrophysiological cardiac procedures (Table 29.1) as it provides access to real time information at all stages, thus improving efficiency and safety. Guidelines have been published, although the role of TEE in these settings is evolving (1,2). This chapter will first review the use of TEE during percutaneous closure of patent foramen ovale (PFO), atrial septal defects (ASDs), ventricular septal defects (VSDs), and paravalvular leaks (PVLs). The usefulness of TEE in atrial ablation procedures and its emerging role in cardiac resynchronization therapy will then be presented.

TEE GUIDANCE DURING PERCUTANEOUS CLOSURE PROCEDURES

The most frequent use of TEE guidance in the interventional setting is for percutaneous closure of PFO, ASDs, VSDs, PDAs, and PVLs using several types of occluding devices (Table 29.2 and Fig. 29.1). Amplatzer devices designed to percutaneously close congenital heart defects consist of self-expanding stents made of nitinol, a nontoxic metal alloy made of nickel and titanium with shape memory. The nitinol wires are bound together to form a closed frame that is collapsed within a delivery sheath for percutaneous insertion and reassumes its original shape at body temperature as it exits the sheath. The shape is designed to fit specific heart defects at its central waist while its two retention disks will help to secure the device on each side of the defect. The devices contain polyester fabric inserts to promote thrombosis that will eventually be covered by protein, cellular layers, and endothelium. Each device has a female microbolt at its end to which it is attached to a delivery cable with a microthreaded screw: the device can thus be retained as it is deployed and carefully positioned. Once the optimal position and stability has

been achieved, the device is finally released by unscrewing the delivery cable. Other percutaneous closure devices differ by their shape design (clamshell or double umbrellas, helix) and their delivery mechanism (bioptome, sutures, retrieval cord). Echocardiographic guidance, either by TEE or intracardiac echocardiography (ICE) is crucial to the safety and success of these procedures. It should be noted that when TEE is used, percutaneous closures should be done under general anesthesia with endotracheal intubation to avoid patient movement and ensure patient comfort. General anesthesia is not essential for ICE.

PFO Closure

The foramen ovale is an opening in the fossa ovalis originating from an overlap of the primum and secundum atrial septa (Fig. 29.2). During fetal life, right-sided pressures are higher, secondary to the pulmonary circulation resistance from the collapsed fetal lung. Oxygenated blood from the fetal vein thus crosses to the systemic circulation through the foramen ovale. At birth, inflation of the lungs with lowering of the pulmonary vascular resistance and increase of the left atrial pressure (LAP) functionally closes the foramen ovale by pushing the primum and secundum septa together. Over time, fibrous adhesions then usually seal the foramen ovale. However, in a significant number of individuals, fibrous adhesions fail to permanently close the foramen ovale, which therefore remains patent: left-to-right shunting at the atrial level usually ensues, with occasional right-to-left shunting when the right atrial pressure transiently exceeds the LAP, for example, during the Valsalva maneuver release phase. The prevalence of a PFO has been reported to be as high as 25.6% in the general population (see Chapter 26) (3,4).

Some PFOs are associated with an atrial septal aneurysm (ASA) caused by redundant tissue in the fossa ovalis, resulting in excessive interatrial septal

Table 29.1 Usefulness of Transesophagel Echocardiography During Interventional Cardiology Procedures

1. Pericardiocentesis
2. Trans-septal catheterization
3. Percutaneous balloon valvuloplasty
4. Percutaneous transcatheter closure of septal defects
5. Alcohol septal ablation in hypertrophic obstructive cardiomyopathy
6. Placement of percutaneous ventricular assist devices
7. Placement of atrial and ventricular occlusion devices
8. Placement of stented valve prosthesis
9. Echocardiographically guided right and left ventricular biopsies
10. Laser extraction of pacemaker and defibrillator leads
11. Congenital heart disease applications such as Fontan completion, coarctation repair
12. Electrophysiological procedures, such as pulmonary vein isolation for atrial fibrillation, sinoatrial node modification for inappropriate sinus tachycardia, and ablation of left ventricular tachycardia
13. Cardiac resynchronization therapy

Table 29.2 Available Devices for Percutaneous Closure

Company	Device name	Design	Indicated use	Defect diameter (mm)	Regulatory status
AGA Medical Corporation (Plymouth, Minnesota, U.S.)	AMPLATZER® Septal Occluder	Double flat disk made of nitinol wire mesh, polyester fabric inserts	Secundum ASD	4–40	United States CE mark
	AMPLATZER Multifenestrated Septal Occluder "Cribiform"	Double flat disk made of nitinol wire mesh, narrow waist polyester fabric inserts	Fenestrated Secundum ASD	18–40	United States CE mark
	AMPLATZER PFO Occluder	Double flat disk made of nitinol wire mesh, narrow waist polyester fabric inserts	PFO		Investigational
	AMPLATZER Muscular VSD Occluder	Two concentric disks, 7 mm long waist made of nitinol wire mesh polyester fabric inserts	Muscular VSD	4–18	United States CE mark
	AMPLATZER P.I. Muscular VSD Occluder	Two concentric disks, 10 mm long waist made of nitinol wire mesh polyester fabric inserts	Post-infarction muscular VSD	16–24	
	AMPLATZER Membranous VSD Occluder	Double flat disk made of nitinol wire mesh, asymmetrical rims polyester fabric inserts	Membranous VSD	4–18	
	AMPLATZER Duct Occluder I	Cylindrical plug with flared collar made of nitinol wire mesh polyester fabric inserts	PDA	4–14 (PA) 5–16 (Ao)	United States CE mark
	AMPLATZER Duct Occluder II	Cylindrical waist with 2 retention disks made of nitinol wire mesh polyester fabric inserts		3–6	CE mark
Cardia, Inc. (Eagan, Minnesota, U.S.)	Atriasept ASD	Dual articulating polyvinyl alcohol (PVA) umbrella sails 6-arm nitinol frame	ASD	8–32	CE mark
	Atriasept PFO	Dual articulating polyvinyl alcohol (PVA) umbrella sails 6-arm nitinol frame	PFO	17.5	CE mark
	Intrasept Fontan	Dual articulating polyvinyl alcohol (PVA) umbrella sails 6-arm nitinol frame	Fenestrated Fontan	75	CE mark

(Continued)

Table 29.2 (*Continued*)

Company	Device name	Design	Indicated use	Defect diameter (mm)	Regulatory status
Coherex Medical (Salt Lake City, Utah, U.S.)	FlatStent™ EF PFO Closure System	Planar nitinol structure (moose horns) Polyurethane substrate	PFO	6–13	CE mark
W.L. Gore & Associates, Inc. (Flagstaff, Arizona, U.S.)	GORE HELEX Spetal Occluder	Circular shape helix made of ePTFE membrane Nitinol circumferential single wire frame	Secundum ASD PFO	6–18	United States, CE mark CE mark
NMT Medical, Inc. (Boston, Massachusetts, U.S.)	CardioSEAL®	Two umbrella shaped disks MP35N framework knitted Dacron fabric	ASD VSD		CE mark United States
	STARFlex®	Two umbrella shaped disks MP35N framework surgical polyester mesh matrix	ASD VSD		CE mark United States
	BioSTAR®	Two umbrella-shaped disks Bioabsorbable purified acellular type-1 collagen matrix and a heparin coating	PFO		CE mark
Occlutech GmnH (Jena, Germany)	Figulla® PFO Occluder N Flexible Single Disk LA	Single layer LA retention disk, RA side hub nitinol meshwire Ultrathin polyethylene terephthalate patch	PFO	≤13.0	CE mark
	Figulla® PFO Occluder N Standard Double Disk	Double flat disk made of nitinol wire mesh, narrow waist	PFO	≤15.0	CE mark
	Figulla® ASD Occluder N	Double flat disk made of nitinol wire mesh	ASD	6–40	CE mark
Swissimplant AG (Solothum, Switzerland)	Solysafe® Septal Occluder	Two-folding patches Fixed to eight wires	ASD PFO	4–30	CE mark
St. Jude Medical (St. Paul, Minnesota, U.S.)	PREMERE™	Flexible low-profile nitinol left and right independent anchors Adjustable length tether connecting the two anchors	PFO	≤15 mm	CE mark
Nobles Medical Technology (Fountain Valley, California, U.S.)	NobleStitch	Percutaneous suture device	PFO		CE mark United States

Abbreviations: ASD, atrial septal defect; CE, European conformity; LA, left atrium; PFO, patent foramen ovale; RA, right atrium; VSD, ventricular septal defect.

movement with respiration. Isolated ASA are uncommon (2.2%) (3); however, up to 75% of patients presenting with an ASA also have a PFO (5). The TEE diagnosis of ASA is made by measuring the total excursion of the interatrial septum into the LA and RA. Excessive excursion is considered with 10 to 15 mm of interatrial septal movement (6).

As mentioned earlier, the membrane of the fossa ovalis usually closes the foramen ovale when LA pressure is higher than the RA pressure. In patients with a PFO, when RA pressure transiently exceed LA pressure during respiration, coughing or during a Valsalva maneuver, the fossa ovalis may open by the movement of the membrane, allowing right-to-left shunt (see Fig. 26.6). Both PFO and ASA have been associated with the occurrence of transient ischemic attacks (TIAs) and cryptogenic stroke (7). Paradoxical emboli are the most likely pathophysiologic mechanism (see Fig. 30.4). There is, however, no strong evidence correlating the risk of a first stroke in patients with either of these two anomalies. A PFO closure is usually performed in patients with

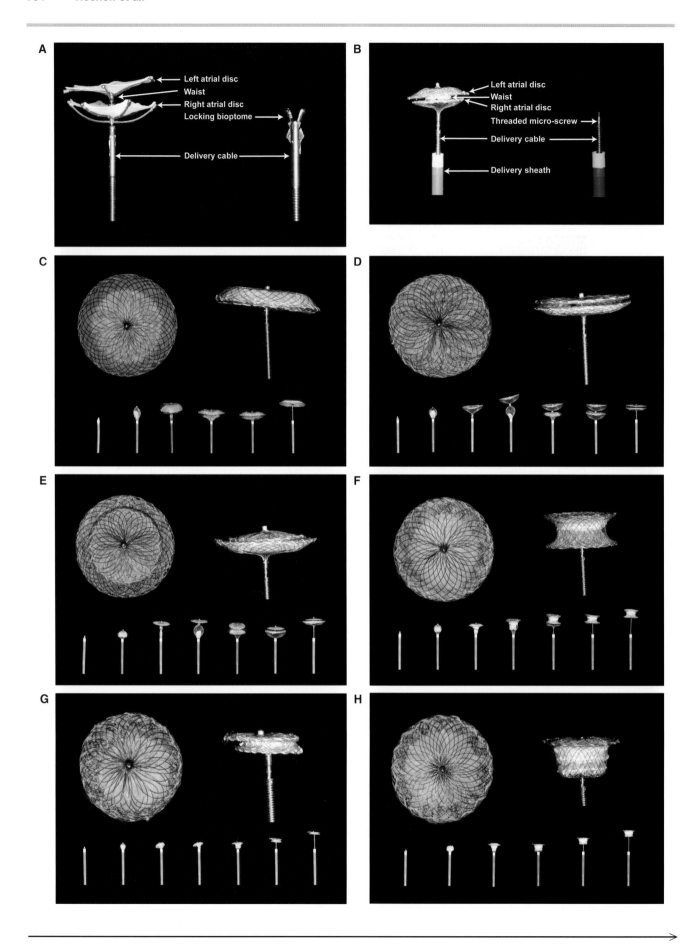

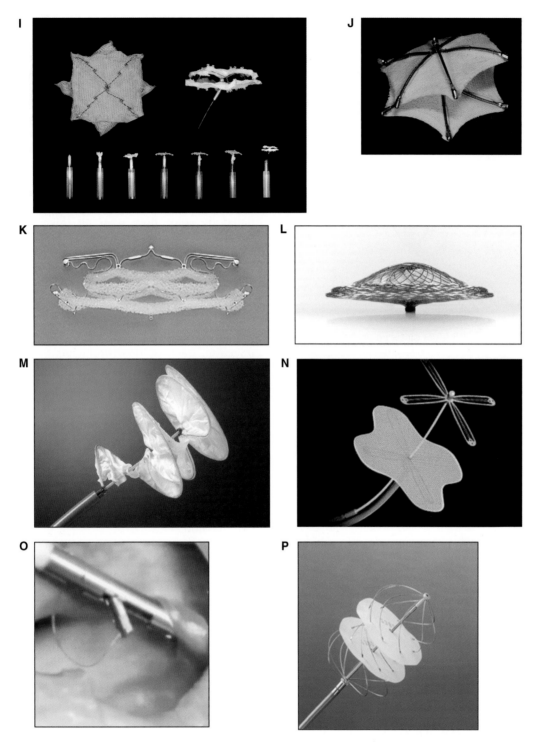

Figure 29.1 Percutaneous closure devices. (A) Components of a double-umbrella-type closure device system (Atriasept, Cardia Inc.). **(B)** Components of a double disk wire mesh-type closure device system (Amplatzer, AGA Medical Corporation). Various types of Amplatzer closure device (AGA Medical Corporation), with appearance through several stages of deployment: **(C)** Amplatzer septal occluder. **(D)** Amplatzer multi-fenestrated septal occluder "cribiform," with a smaller waist. **(E)** Amplatzer PFO occluder. **(F)** Amplatzer muscular VSD occluder, with a greater distance between the discs to accommodate the thicker ventricular septum. **(G)** Amplatzer membranous VSD occluder with a minimal rim on the left ventricular disc to sit beneath the aortic valve, a longer left ventricular apical rim and a short waist to keep the right ventricular disc away from the tricuspid leaflets. **(H)** Amplatzer Duct occluder, shaped like a plug with an aortic retention disc. **(I)** STARFlex Septal Occluder (Nitinol Medical Technologies). **(J)** Cardia Atriasept PFO Closure System (Cardia Inc.). **(K)** Coherex FlatStent™ EF PFO Closure System (Photo courtesy of Coherex Medical). **(L)** Occlutech Figulla® PFO Occluder (Photo courtesy of Occlutech International AB). **(M)** Gore Helex ASD Occluder (Photo courtesy of W.L. Gore & Associates, Inc.). **(N)** Premere™ PFO Closure System (Photo courtesy of St. Jude Medical). **(O)** NobleStitch percutaneous PFO suture device (Photo courtesy of Nobles Medical Technology). **(P)** Swissimplant Solysafe® Septal Occluder (Photo courtesy of Swissimplant AG). *Abbreviations*: ASD, atrial septal defect; PFO, patent foramen ovale; VSD, ventricular septal defect.

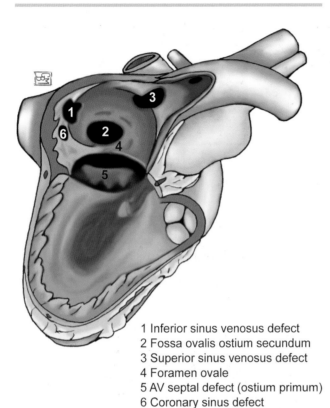

1 Inferior sinus venosus defect
2 Fossa ovalis ostium secundum
3 Superior sinus venosus defect
4 Foramen ovale
5 AV septal defect (ostium primum)
6 Coronary sinus defect

Figure 29.2 Types of atrial septal defects. Diagram shows various types of atrial septal defects viewed through the right atrium. *Abbreviation*: AV, atrioventricular. *Source*: with permission, copyright Gian-Marco Busato.

recurrent neurological symptoms despite medical therapy. Surgical closure of simple PFO is rarely needed as percutaneous closure represents an attractive and safe therapeutic option. Two randomized multicenter trials, comparing percutaneous PFO closure to medical therapy alone, are currently under way (CLOSURE and RESPECT) and will eventually clarify the indications for closure.

Depending on the size of the PFO, diagnosis is made using TEE, with color Doppler alone, with the use of agitated saline, or with agitated saline plus a Valsalva maneuver (see Fig. 26.6) (8). Preprocedure evaluation should focus on confirming the diagnosis and excluding additional pathology, especially an additional ASD or anomalous pulmonary vein connections. Estimation of right heart pressures is also correlated with direct hemodynamic invasive measurements. Echocardiographic guidance, either by TEE or ICE, is recommended for percutaneous closure. However, some centers use only fluoroscopic and angiographic guidance.

During the procedure, the interventional cardiologist will place a catheter through the PFO via the inferior vena cava (IVC) and the RA (Fig. 29.3A). A guidewire is then anchored within the left upper pulmonary vein (LUPV). There is usually no need for device sizing with an inflatable balloon. A delivery sheath is inserted (Fig. 29.3B) and the occluding device is loaded (screwed) on a delivery cable and its distal end positioned in the LA. The LA disk is deployed and abutted against the LA septal surface, after which the RA disk is deployed (Fig. 29.3C). The stability of the device anchoring is tested by pulling on it with the delivery cable (Fig. 29.3D). When the correct position is confirmed by TEE (Fig. 29.4A), the device is released from its delivery cable by unscrewing the latter (in the case of Amplatzer® device) or opening up the locking bioptome (for the BioSTAR® device).

Immediately after the procedure, the presence of any residual left-to-right shunting should be evaluated by color flow imaging (Fig. 29.5B). Agitated saline is injected and a Valsalva maneuver is performed to assess the degree of any residual right-to-left shunting (Fig. 29.5C). If right-to-left shunting is still present, TEE is usually repeated three to six months after the procedure when endothelialization of the device is completed. Complications may include device embolization, erosion in the cardiac structures, pericardial effusion, device thrombosis, infection, fracture, or dislodgement of the device (9) (Fig. 29.6).

ASD Closure

ASDs are a common congenital heart anomaly with an incidence of 1 in 1500 live births (10,11). Depending on the ASD location (Fig. 29.2), four anatomic types are described: ostium primum, ostium secundum, sinus venosus (inferior and superior), and coronary sinus (CS) (12). Ostium secundum ASDs are the most frequent (70%) and the only ones currently amenable to percutaneous closure.

The direction and importance of shunting of blood from one atrium to the other is relative to the size of the defect, as well as compliance and pressure gradients in the cardiac chambers. Defects <0.5 cm rarely have hemodynamic consequences. Larger ASDs may result in increased pulmonary blood flow, dilatation of right-sided chambers with occasional pressure overload, atrial tachyarrhythmias, exercise limitation, and late right heart failure (13). Any condition that increases left ventricular end-diastolic pressure (LVEDP) (ischemia, hypertension, hypertrophy) will increase left to right shunting and promote the development of symptoms.

Closure of an ASD is indicated in the presence of a hemodynamically significant ASD with or without symptoms. A hemodynamically significant ASD is defined in the presence of right ventricular dilatation or a significant shunt fraction (Qp:Qs >1.5) (14,15). Closure of an ASD may also be indicated in the presence of paradoxical emboli.

When an ASD is suspected in an adult, TEE is essential to confirm the location of the defect, its size, and its suitability for percutaneous closure (16,17). The size of the defect is measured by two-dimensional (2D) TEE in different views (Fig. 29.7). Color Doppler then confirms the presence of the ASD and rules out multiple ASDs or a fenestrated septum (Fig. 29.8) for

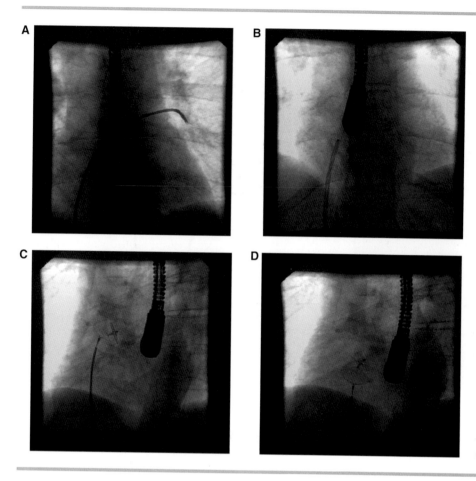

Figure 29.3 Angiographic views during percutaneous closure of a PFO. (A) A guidewire is passed through the PFO and anchored in the left superior pulmonary vein. **(B)** Once the occluding device is loaded inside a delivery catheter the distal end of the latter is positioned in the left atrium under TEE monitoring. **(C)** The left atrial disk is deployed in the left atrial cavity and then abutted against the left atrial septal surface. The right atrial disk must be deployed on the other side of the septum in the right atrial cavity. **(D)** Under TEE and fluoroscopy monitoring, pulling on the occluding device enables visualization of the atrial septum correctly sandwiched between the two disks as well as confirmation of the stability of the device against the rims of the atrial septal defect before final release. *Abbreviations*: PFO, patent foramen ovale; TEE, transesophageal echocardiography.

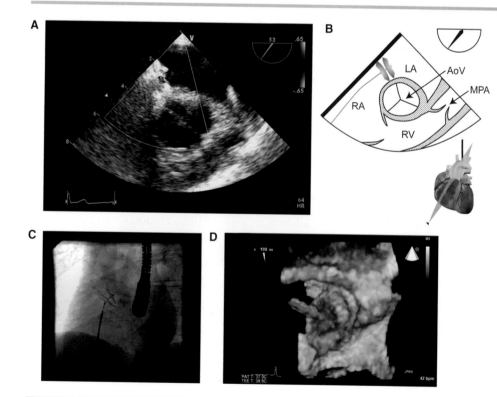

Figure 29.4 Verification of the Amplatzer PFO closure device position. (A,B) Mid-esophageal right ventricular inflow/outflow showing the correct position of a successfully deployed Amplatzer device discs on each side of the interatrial septum. **(C,D)** Corresponding fluoroscopic and 3D echocardiographic views. *Abbreviations*: AoV, aortic valve; MPA, main pulmonary artery; LA, left atrium; PFO, patent foramen ovale; RA, right atrium; RV, right ventricle.

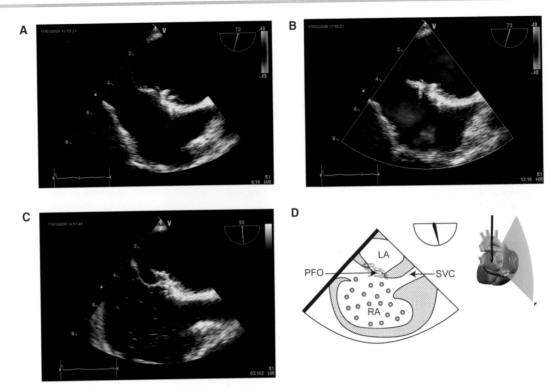

Figure 29.5 Assessment of residual shunt through the PFO after device implantation. (**A**) Mid-esophageal bicaval view after successfully deployed BioSTAR® device through a PFO. (**B**) Assessment of residual left-to-right shunt with color flow imaging. (**C,D**) Assessment of residual right-to-left shunt with agitated saline micro-bubble contrast injection. *Abbreviations*: LA, left atrium; PFO, patent foramen ovale; RA, right atrium; SVC, superior vena cava.

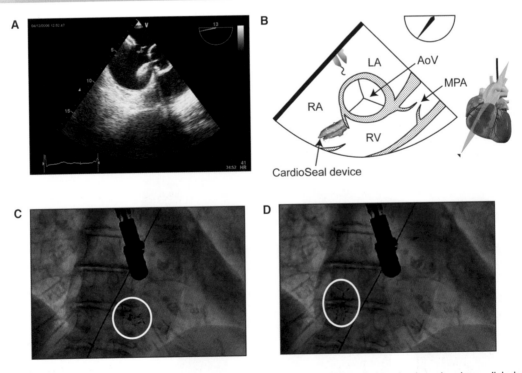

Figure 29.6 Dislodged percutaneous closure device. (**A,B**) Mid-esophageal aortic short-axis view showing a dislodged Amplatzer device randomly moving in the left atrium. (**C,D**) Fluoroscopic views with a dislodged CardioSeal device freely moving into a cardiac cavity. *Abbreviations*: AoV, aortic valve; LA, left atrium; MPA, main pulmonary artery; RA, right atrium; RV, right ventricle.

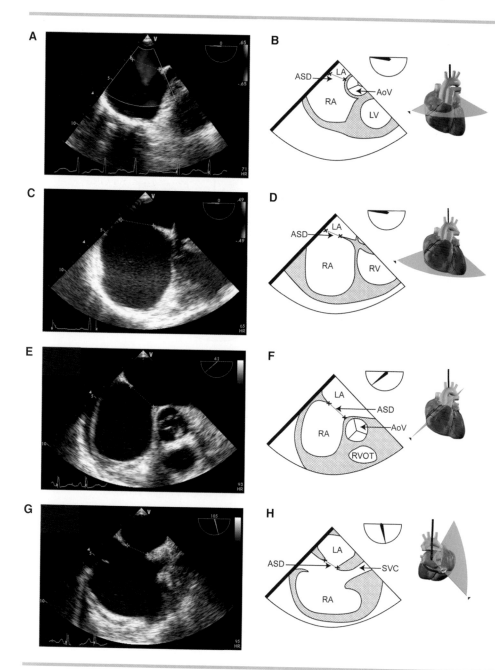

Figure 29.7 Measurement of the ASD. Various mid-esophageal views are used to assess the size of the ASD and its rims. (**A,B**) ME five-chamber view: the superior portion and minor axis of the ASD can be measured. (**C,D**) ME four-chamber view: superior rim and AoV rim. (**E,F**) ME AoV short-axis view: posterior rim and aortic rim. (**G,H**) ME bicaval view: IVC and SVC rims and the major axis of the ASD. See also Figure 26.5. *Abbreviations*: AoV, aortic valve; ASD, atrial septal defect; IVC, inferior vena cava; LA, left atrium; LV, left ventricle; ME, mid-esophageal; RA, right atrium; RV, right ventricle; RVOT, right ventricular outflow tract; SVC, superior vena cava.

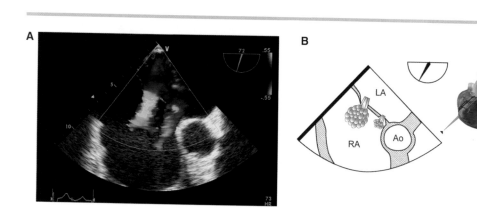

Figure 29.8 Multi-fenestrated ASD. (**A,B**) Color Doppler mid-esophageal right ventricular inflow/outflow view shows at least two defects in the interatrial septum with predominantly left-to-right flow. *Abbreviations*: Ao, aorta; ASD, atrial septal defect; LA, left atrium; RA, right atrium.

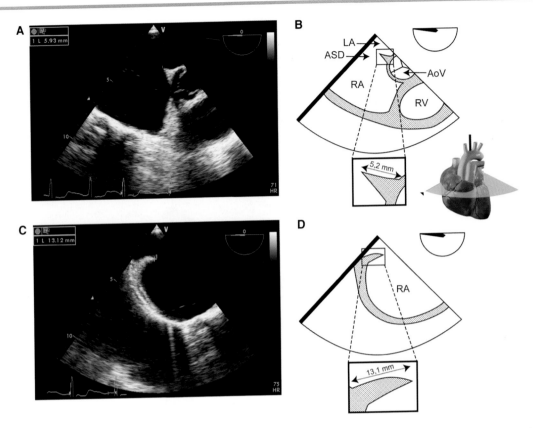

Figure 29.9 **Measurement of the rims of the ASD. (A,B)** Rotated mid-esophageal four-chamber view shows a secundum ASD with the medial portion of the surrounding rim of tissue required to anchor the device adjacent to the aorta. **(C,D)** Further rotation of the mid-esophageal four-chamber view brings the more lateral portion of the ASD for measurement of the rim of tissue needed to anchor the device. *Abbreviations*: AoV, aortic valve; ASD, atrial septal defect; LA, left atrium; RA, right atrium; RV, right ventricle.

Table 29.3 Eligibility Criteria for ASD Percutaneous Device Closure

- Ostium secundum ASD <40 mm measured by 2D TEE
- Rims > 5 mm (SVC, IVC, posterior, coronary sinus, and atrioventricular)
- The aortic rim can be absent
- Normal pulmonary venous drainage
- No other heart defect
- No intracavitary thrombi

Abbreviations: ASD, atrial septal defect; IVC, inferior vena cava; SVC, superior vena cava; TEE, transesophageal echocardiography.

which different devices may be used (Fig. 29.1). Adequacy of the various rims must also be evaluated before the procedure: the posterior, superior/superior vena cava (SVC), the right upper pulmonary vein, the inferior/IVC, the CS, and the atrioventricular rim posteriorly at the crux of the heart must all be >5 mm (Fig. 29.9). The aortic rim can be absent. The eligibility criteria for percutaneous closure are listed in Table 29.3.

If the patient has a suitable ASD, percutaneous closure can be offered (Fig. 29.10), and it can be done under TEE or ICE guidance. An appropriate sizing balloon is prepared and advanced over a guidewire previously positioned in the LUPV (Fig. 29.3). It is placed across the defect under both fluoroscopic and echocardiographic guidance. The sizing balloon is then inflated with diluted contrast until the left to right shunt ceases, as confirmed by color Doppler on TEE. The diameter of the balloon is measured by both TEE and fluoroscopy. There is usually a good correlation between these techniques (Fig. 29.11). After sizing, the balloon is deflated and pulled back, leaving the wire in the LUPV. A device 0 to 2 mm larger than the inflated balloon diameter is selected for closure. The selected delivery sheath is then advanced over the guidewire to the LUPV. The LA disk is deployed first under fluoroscopic and echocardiographic guidance by retracting the sheath over the cable (Figs. 29.1 and 29.12). During deployment, care must be taken not to interfere or occlude the LUPV or the left atrial appendage (LAA). With constant pulling, the delivery sheath is retracted off the wire, and the connecting waist and the RA disk are deployed in the ASD itself and in the RA, respectively. On TEE, the correctly deployed Amplatzer ASD closure device should have the two disks on each side of the septum—one in the LA and the other in the RA (Fig. 29.13). To help confirm this, while the interventional cardiologist

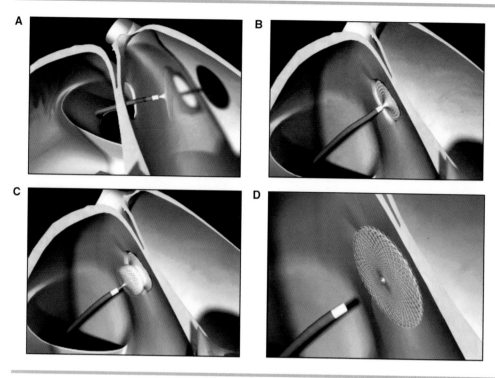

Figure 29.10 Percutaneous ASD device closure. Diagrams illustrating the sequence of events for percutaneous Amplatzer device closure of a secundum ASD are shown. (**A**) The catheter with the device is passed through the ASD from the RA to the LA. (**B**) The left atrial disk is deployed and pulled snugly against the LA side of the IAS. (**C**) The right atrial disk is deployed against the RA side of the IAS. (**D**) The device is definitively released in place by unscrewing the cable from it and retrieving both the cable and the delivery sheath. *Abbreviations*: ASD, atrial septal defect; IAS, interatrial septum; LA, left atrium; RA, right atrium. *Source*: Courtesy of AGA Medical.

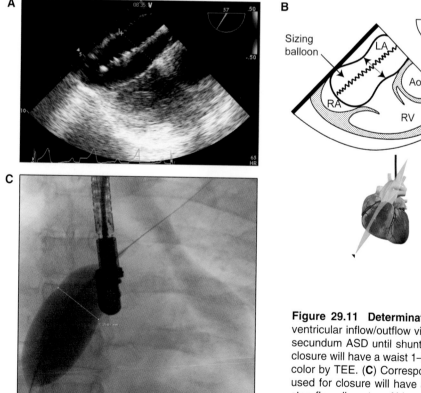

Figure 29.11 Determination of ASD size. (**A,B**) Mid-esophageal right ventricular inflow/outflow view showing a balloon catheter inflated across a secundum ASD until shunting disappears. The size of the device used for closure will have a waist 1–2 mm greater than the largest size measured on color by TEE. (**C**) Corresponding fluoroscopic view: The size of the device used for closure will have a waist 1–2 mm greater than the sizing balloon stop-flow diameter. *Abbreviations*: Ao, aorta; ASD, atrial septal defect; LA, left atrium; RA, right atrium; RV, right ventricle; TEE, transesophageal echocardiography.

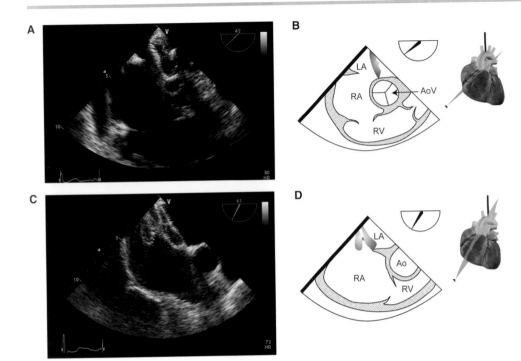

Figure 29.12 ASD Amplatzer closure device deployment. (A–D) Mid-esophageal right ventricular inflow/outflow views show the progressive deployment of an Amplatzer percutaneous device across a secundum ASD. Compare with figure 29.1C. *Abbreviations*: Ao, aorta; AoV, aortic valve; ASD, atrial septal defect; LA, left atrium; RA, right atrium; RV, right ventricle.

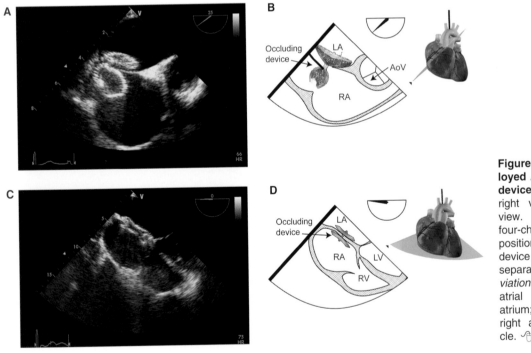

Figure 29.13 Correctly deployed ASD Amplatzer closure device. (A,B) Mid-esophageal right ventricular inflow/outflow view. **(C,D)** Mid-esophageal four-chamber view: adequate positioning of the ASD occluding device with the septum seen separating the two disks. *Abbreviations*: AoV, aortic valve; ASD, atrial septal defect; LA, left atrium; LV, left ventricle; RA, right atrium; RV, right ventricle.

pulls on the device with the cable to separate the two disks, the echocardiographer confirms the presence of the ASD rims between the two disks and also ascertains that with pulling, the LA disk does not slip out past the rim into the RA. Once satisfactory positioning and stability is confirmed by TEE, the device is released by unscrewing the cable from the Amplatzer device (Fig. 29.13).

Immediately after the device's release, the echocardiographer must again seek signs of device instability (Fig. 29.14) and evaluate the presence of residual shunt. Early after the occluder deployment, it is

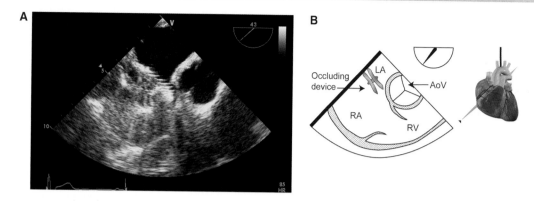

Figure 29.14   Dislodged ASD Amplatzer closure device. (A,B) Mid-esophageal right ventricular inflow/outflow view shows a mobile Amplatzer prosthesis suggestive of dislodgement at the aortic rim from the interatrial septum. *Abbreviations*: AoV, aortic valve; LA, left atrium; RA, right atrium; RV, right ventricle.

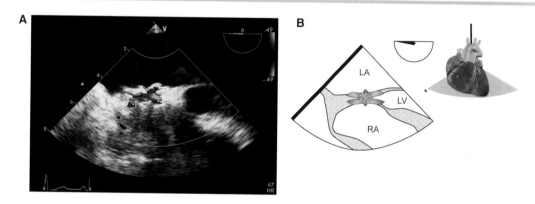

Figure 29.15   Residual shunt. (A,B) Color Doppler mid-esophageal right ventricular inflow/outflow view shows some residual flow around the device but little shunt through the interatrial septum. *Abbreviations*: LA, left atrium; LV, left ventricle; RA, right atrium.

normal to see a small residual intraprosthetic shunt through the device mesh (Fig. 29.15), which should resolve with complete endothelialization of the device after several weeks. Finally, evaluation of the pulmonary and systemic venous return for potential obstruction by the device, the degree of atrioventricular valve regurgitation, and the presence of a new pericardial effusion should be carried out. Complications may again include device embolization, erosion in the cardiac structures, pericardial effusion, device thrombosis, infection, fracture, or dislodgement of the device (Fig. 29.6).

VSD Closure

VSDs account for almost 20% of congenital cardiac anomalies (18). They can be classified in four different types according to their anatomic position: subarterial, perimembranous, inlet, and muscular (see Chapter 26) (Fig. 29.16) (19). Small VSDs present as systolic murmurs and are associated with a normal life

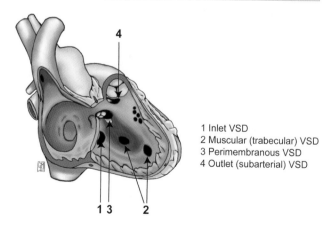

1 Inlet VSD
2 Muscular (trabecular) VSD
3 Perimembranous VSD
4 Outlet (subarterial) VSD

Figure 29.16   Types of VSD. Diagram shows various types of ventricular septal defects viewed from the right ventricle. *Abbreviation*: VSD, ventricular septal defects. *Source*: With permission, copyright Gian-Marco Busato.

expectancy. They can close spontaneously, most often during childhood. Moderate VSDs may cause left ventricular (LV) dilatation and symptoms of heart failure in infancy. They are unusual in the adult but may occur when a prolapsing aortic valve (AoV) cusp partially obstructs the defect. Large VSDs will be associated with the development of pulmonary hypertension and if not closed early in life will result in the Eisenmenger's syndrome. The VSDs reported after myocardial infarction (MI) and trauma have a poor prognosis. Without surgical or percutaneous VSD closure, their mortality exceeds 90%, and even with surgical intervention, reported early mortality ranges between 19% to 46% (20).

The following situations warrant VSD closure: a significant VSD with a Qp/Qs>2:1, pulmonary systolic pressure >50 mmHg or deteriorating ventricular function due to LV volume and right ventricular (RV) pressure overload, significant right ventricular outflow tract (RVOT) obstruction, a perimembranous or subarterial VSD with more than mild aortic regurgitation (AR) and recurrent endocarditis (14,15). Surgical closure has been advocated as the gold standard for VSD. Device closure may be performed in experienced centers in the setting of isolated trabecular muscular VSDs (Fig. 29.17) remote from the tricuspid valve and the aorta, perimembranous VSD, if the defect is far enough from the AoV, and in high-risk surgical patients (multiple previous cardiac surgical interventions, poorly accessible muscular VSDs, post myocardial infarction) (14,15).

The diagnosis is usually made by transthoracic echocardiography (TTE). Assessment will include LV size and function, right ventricular systolic pressure (RVSP), VSD location, LV to RV peak systolic gradient (the higher the gradient, the more restrictive is the VSD), AoV deformation and degree of AR. Unlike ASDs, a TEE is rarely needed to confirm the diagnosis before the procedure (Fig. 29.18).

During the procedure (21–23), TEE (Fig. 29.19) is preferred to ICE and general anesthesia is needed. The VSD is usually approached from the LV. A wire is placed across the defect into the right-sided chambers, snared and exteriorized via the right internal jugular or femoral vein (Fig. 29.20). Over this arterio-venous wire loop, the delivery catheter is inserted through the right venous introducer sheath and advanced in the RA and the RV until it reaches the vicinity of the ascending aorta (Ao). Under TEE guidance, the tip of the delivery catheter is then pushed inside the LV (Fig. 29.21A). The prosthesis is advanced into the LV, where the LV disk is carefully deployed to avoid impingement of the mitral valve (MV) (Fig. 29.21B). After TEE and fluoroscopic confirmation of adequate positioning (Fig. 29.21C), the RV disk is deployed (Fig. 29.21D). The device can then be released and its proper position confirmed with TEE (Fig. 29.22).

During VSD closure, complications, including right bundle branch block (RBBB), stroke, AR, ventricular arrhythmias, and device embolization, have been reported. The usefulness of echocardiography in identifying device- or procedure-related complications such as pericardial effusion cannot be understated. The major concern of device closure for perimembranous VSD is the 5% to 10% incidence of complete atrioventricular block that can occur early or late after closure.

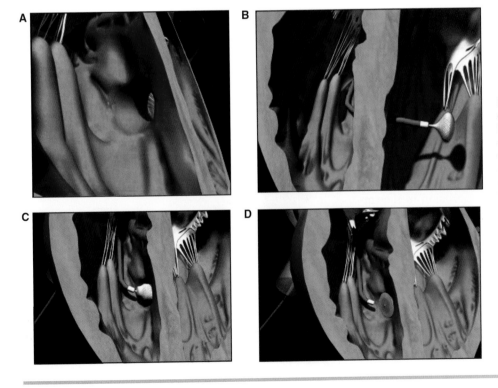

Figure 29.17 Percutaneous VSD device closure. Diagrams illustrating the sequence of events for percutaneous Amplatzer device closure of a muscular VSD are shown. (**A**) The catheter with the device is passed through the VSD from the RV to the LV. (**B**) The left ventricular disk is deployed and pulled snugly against the LV side of the IVS. (**C**) The right ventricular disk is deployed against the RV side of the IVS. (**D**) The introducer cable is detached from the device and removed with its delivery sheath. *Abbreviations*: IVS, interventricular septum; LV, left ventricle; RV, right ventricle; VSD, ventricular septal defects. *Source*: Courtesy of AGA Medical.

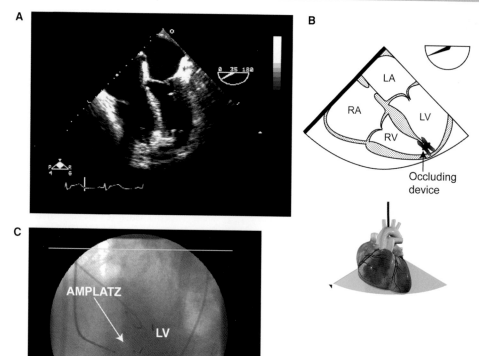

Figure 29.18   Percutaneous VSD device closure after myocardial infarction. (A,B) Mid-esophageal four-chamber view showing a successfully deployed Amplatzer prosthesis across an apical VSD secondary to an acute myocardial infarction chamber. **(C)** Corresponding fluoroscopic view. *Abbreviations*: LA, left atrium; LV, left ventricle; RA, right atrium; RV, right ventricle; VSD, ventricular septal defects.

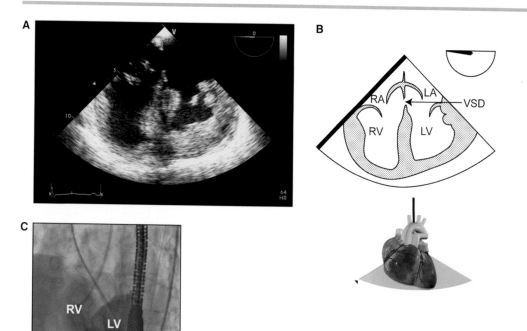

Figure 29.19   Perimembranous VSD. (A,B) Mid-esophageal four-chamber view with a perimembranous VSD. **(C)** Fluoroscopic visualization of flow through the VSD during left ventriculography. *Abbreviations*: LA, left atrium; LV, left ventricle; RA, right atrium; RV, right ventricle; VSD, ventricular septal defects.

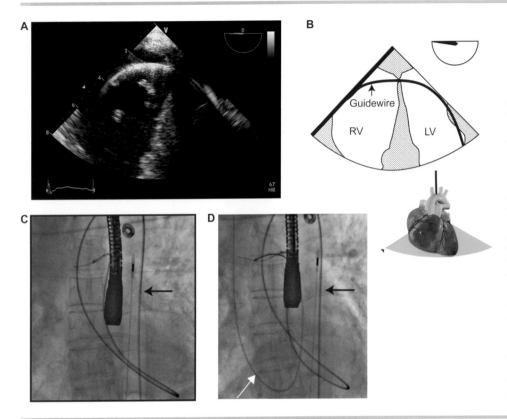

Figure 29.20 Arterio-venous wire loop positioning during VSD transcatheter closure. (**A,B**) Zoomed mid-esophageal four-chamber view showing a guidewire positioned across a perimembranous VSD. (**C,D**) Fluoroscopic views: the VSD is approached from the LV. (**C**) A wire is retrogradely passed in the VSD via the thoracic Ao (black arrow) and the LV. (**D**) To secure the position of the wire across the VSD, an additional wire inserted through the superior vena cava, right atrium and RV is used to snare the left-sided wire (white arrow). The ensemble will then be pulled back up and exteriorized through the right introducer sheath. *Abbreviations*: Ao, aorta; LV, left ventricle; RV, right ventricle; VSD, ventricular septal defects.

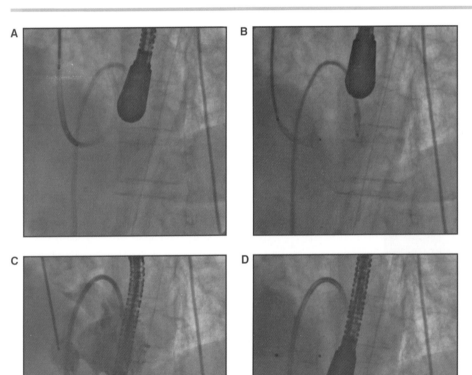

Figure 29.21 VSD transcatheter device closure. (**A**) Fluoroscopic view of the delivery catheter advanced through the SVC, the RA and the RV until it reaches the vicinity of the ascending aorta with the tip pushed inside the left ventricle through the VSD. (**B**) Under TEE guidance, the prosthesis is advanced into the left ventricle where the left ventricular disk is carefully deployed to avoid impingement of the mitral valve. (**C**) Adequate positioning of the left disk is confirmed by transesophageal echocardiography and fluroscopy. (**D**) The right ventricular disk is then deployed. *Abbreviations*: RA, right atrium; RV, right ventricle; SVC, superior vena cava; TEE, transesophageal echocardiography; VSD, ventricular septal defect.

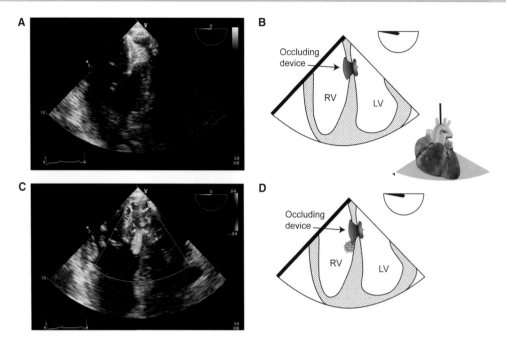

Figure 29.22   VSD occlude prosthesis. (A,B) Mid-esophageal four-chamber view after deployment of an occluding device shows mild residual left-to-right flow **(C,D)** across the VSD. *Abbreviations*: LV, left ventricle; RV, right ventricle; VSD, ventricular septal defect.

Patent Ductus Arteriosus

The ductus arteriosus is a remnant of the distal sixth aortic arch and connects the pulmonary artery at the junction of the main pulmonary artery (MPA) and the origin of the left pulmonary artery (LPA) to the proximal descending thoracic aorta just after the origin of the left subclavian artery. During fetal life, the ductus arteriosus is a normal structure that allows up to 90% of the RV output to bypass the pulmonary circulation through collapsed lungs and pump deoxygenated systemic blood via the descending thoracic aorta to the placenta for oxygenation. Normal closure of the ductus occurs within the first 12 hours after birth by smooth muscle contraction ultimately followed by cellular changes leading to the transformation into the ligamentum arteriosum. In 1/2000 live births, particularly in premature babies, this process of closure fails to complete and leads to variable left-to-right shunt depending on the pulmonary vascular resistance. Patent ductus arteriosus (PDA) is the persistence of a normal connection in fetal life between the proximal descending thoracic aorta and the proximal left pulmonary artery. Treatment with nonsteroidal anti-inflammatory medications (vg indomethacin) with or without fluid restriction may be tried with premature infants but not in term babies. If the ductus arteriosus fails to close, surgical or catheter-based correction is indicated. Preprocedure echocardiographic evaluation should confirm the presence of PDA with typical abnormal systolic left-to-right color flow jet into the MPA or proximal LPA, typically directed anteriorly, sometimes superiorly.

Differential diagnosis includes a small coronary to pulmonary artery fistula with a color flow jet directed posteriorly from the anterior wall of the MPA.

Small PDAs (diameter < 3 mm) can be closed with Gianturco embolization coils. Larger PDAs (diameter ≥ 3 mm) may be treated by transcatheter closure with an Amplatzer duct occluder (see Fig. 26.22).

Paravalvular Leak

One of the complications associated with valve replacement surgery is the development of a PVL from incomplete sewing of the prosthesis to the native tissue or dehiscence of the sutures. Clinically significant PVLs, not to be confused with the normal transvalvular prosthesis backflow, occur in 1% to 5% of patients with prosthetic valves. A PVL is more frequent with mitral than aortic prosthesis, and rarely in the tricuspid and pulmonic positions (24,25). The percutaneous closure techniques used for ASD and VSD can be applied to paravalvular defects in patients who are not candidates to reoperation. A variety of occluders have been used with relatively good results (26). Occluder devices have also been used to percutaneously correct other defects, such as ruptured sinus of Valsalva (see Fig. 23.24). During the procedure (Fig. 29.23), TEE is crucial as it locates the optimal trans-septal puncture site, guides the interventional cardiologist to introduce the guidewire through the defect allowing proper device delivery and deployment, monitors the immediate occurrence of complications (thrombi, interference with prosthesis), and evaluates the success of the procedure (27).

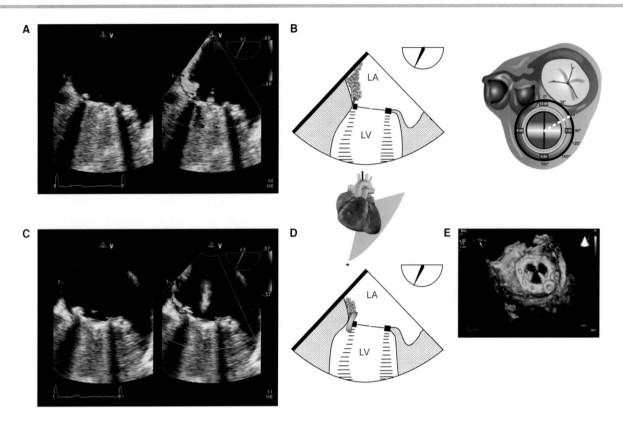

Figure 29.23 Paravalvular MR. Color compare mid-esophageal two-chamber views show a paravalvular leak at the posterior annulus (2 o'clock) resulting in moderate MR in a patient with a bileaflet mechanical mitral valve prosthesis before (**A,B**) and after (**C,D**) percutaneous closure. (**E**) Left atrial three-dimensional surgical view of Amplatz devices used for paravalvular leak closure in a different patient. *Abbreviations*: LA, left atrium; LV, left ventricle; MR, mitral regurgitation. *Source*: Figure E courtesy of Dr. Patrick Garceau.

CATHETER ABLATION PROCEDURES

Introduction

Cardiac tachyarrhythmias are expressed through electrical channels of facilitated conduction. In the electrophysiological suite (EPS), the cardiologist may insert intravascular catheters to identify the pathways responsible for a specific arrhythmia. Positioning an ablation catheter over the conductive part of the endocardium, which is responsible for the transmission of the faulty pathway, and delivering a radiofrequency current can interrupt the arrhythmia. Atrial fibrillation (AF), atrial flutter, atrioventricular node reentry, atrioventricular reentry and ventricular tachycardia are the arrhythmias that are amenable to this form of therapy (22). In the process of identification and management of these arrhythmias, echocardiography can be of interest when inserting various catheters to verify their correct position, to describe cardiac function before and after the procedure, and to identify the potential complications.

Procedure Overview

AF in the General Population

AF is one of the most frequent arrhythmias in the general population and is present in 9% of patients in

their eighth decade. The incidence increases with age, the presence of valvular heart disease, congestive heart failure (CHF), hypertension, and diabetes (23). Following cardiac surgery, AF is the most frequently occurring arrhythmia, present in 25% to 60% of patients by the second to third postoperative day (24). It is also reported in the structurally normal heart, affecting 2.7% of patients over 60 years of age (25). Chronic AF is difficult to treat medically, and many patients experience side effects of antiarrhythmic drugs without sustained relief (26). Surgical treatment for AF is possible with exposure of the LA and making cauterization lines to diminish to a critical point, the muscular mass subjected to the fibrillation wavelets. It is seldom made for its sole benefit, but as an adjuvant during another surgical procedure (27) or by a minimally invasive approach (28).

AF Catheter Ablation Technique

The interest of percutaneous AF ablation is a consequence of the discovery of a locus responsible for initiating the arrhythmia and the relative efficiency of that therapeutic compared with medical therapy alone. It has been demonstrated that a particular layer of muscular fibers (29) extending from the LA to the pulmonary veins is the most frequent site of origin of the impulses initiating as much as 95% of the documented AF occurring in patients (30). Other sites described are the SVC-RA junction or the ligament of Marshall. The therapeutic technique consists of the isolation of the pulmonary vein-LA junction by the creation of continuous lines of thermocoagulation lesions.

Before the procedure, the patient's mediastinal anatomy may be imaged with magnetic resonance (MRI) or with a computerized tomography (CT) scan to describe the precise pulmonary vein branching pattern and the number of venous connections to the LA (31). TEE is performed to rule out the presence of any LA thrombus (32).

The AF ablation procedure is often done under light sedation and ICE may be used to guide the manipulations. As an alternative to ICE, TEE under general anesthesia has also been used (33,34). The monitoring for the procedure is installed, including a three-dimensional (3D) mapping system, if required (35).

A complete echocardiographic examination (36) is performed to assess cardiac function and identification of any wall motion anomaly, valvular dysfunction, pericardial effusion, intracardiac shunt, or aortic root dilation. After the preliminary TEE examination, the catheters required for the procedure are introduced from a central vein to the right heart and through the interatrial septum to access the LA.

Trans-septal Left Heart Catheterization

The septum is imaged in different planes to identify the fossa ovalis, delineate its dimension, and identify the presence of an aneurysm, septal defect, or foramen that may be of concern for the trans-septal puncture (Fig. 29.24). The LA dimensions (37) are noted as well as its relationship with the surrounding structures for the secure septal catheterization using the Brockenbrough needle (38). Combined with fluoroscopic imaging, the needle is guided by TEE as it approaches the septum. The pressure made by the needle on the middle of the fossa ovalis creates a tenting of the thin membrane (Fig. 29.25). The general orientation of the needle is verified to ascertain that the increase of pressure on the needle, and, therefore, the small movement made by entering the LA will clear the aortic root, the pulmonary artery (PA), and the LA free wall. Once in the LA, the pressure on the catheter is relieved and the echo exam demonstrates that the interatrial septum has lost the tenting aspect to regain its usual form with the catheter in the LA (Fig. 29.26). A dilator and sheath catheter is then passed over the needle and its distal position is again ascertained to be at a safe distance from any

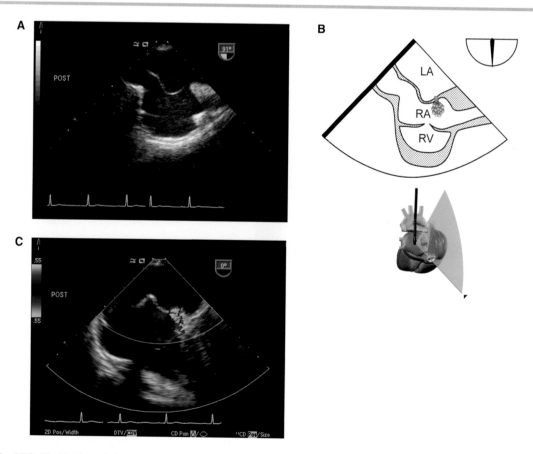

Figure 29.24   PFO. (A–C) Bicaval views show an apparently intact fossa ovalis but turbulent flow nearby on color Doppler is suggestive of a PFO. *Abbreviations*: LA, left atrium; PFO, patent foramen ovale; RA, right atrium; RV, right ventricle.

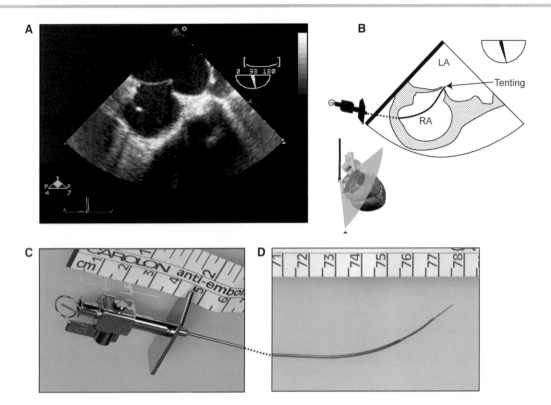

Figure 29.25   Brockenbrough needle. (A,B) Bicaval view guides the Brockenbrough needle as it tents against the right atrial side of the interatrial septal in preparation for a transseptal puncture. Details of the proximal (**C**) and distal (**D**) portions of the Brockenbrough needle are shown. *Abbreviations*: LA, left atrium; RA, right atrium.

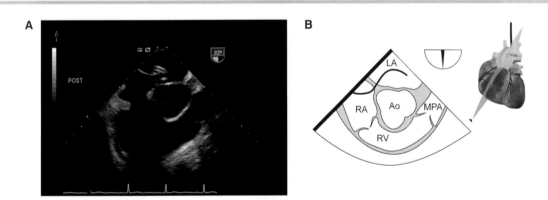

Figure 29.26   Transseptal puncture. (A,B) Mid-esophageal right ventricular inflow/outflow view following trans-septal puncture shows a non-tented interatrial septum and the catheter inserted into the LA. *Abbreviations*: Ao, aorta; LA, left atrium; MPA, main pulmonary artery; RA, right atrium; RV, right ventricle.

structure, including the LAA and pulmonary veins (39). Contrast media, radiopaque or agitated saline, is injected into the LA to verify the intracavitary position of the catheter, and a TEE exam is done to exclude the presence of any newly formed pericardial effusion (40). The patient is then heparinized, and the circular mapping catheter or the ablation catheter is passed through the sheath into the LA.

Difficulties occurring during the puncture may be caused by anatomic deformation such as scoliosis, severe atrial or aortic root dilatation (41,42), or atrial septal aneurysm. Coherent anatomic localization of the catheter by fluoroscopy and echocardiography must be obtained before the puncture. Most extracardiac perforation occurs in the posterior part of the atrium (38).

Anatomical Correlation

Anatomic variations of the pulmonary veins are frequently noted. The pulmonary vein ostium is defined as the point of inflection between the LA and the vein (43). Up to 19% of patients have a third ostium for a unique right pulmonary vein draining the middle lobe. The merging of two or three veins on the same side is described as a common ostium and occurs in 32% of patients for the right side and in up to 71% for the left side (Fig. 29.27) (43).

If the 3D mapping system is used, establishing cartography of the inside of the LA with the junction of the pulmonary vein and LAA is made by correlating the radiographic position of the ablation catheter with the echocardiographic image (Fig. 29.28). After a sufficient number of identification points have been

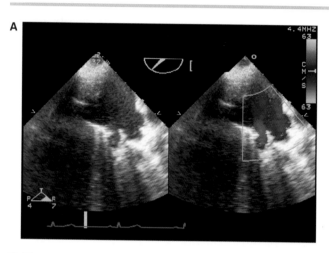

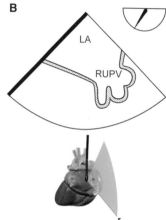

Figure 29.27 Right upper pulmonary vein. (A,B) Color Doppler mid-esophageal view at 30° rotated to the right side of the LA showing laminar flow in the RUPV. *Abbreviations*: LA, left atrium; RUPV, right upper pulmonary vein.

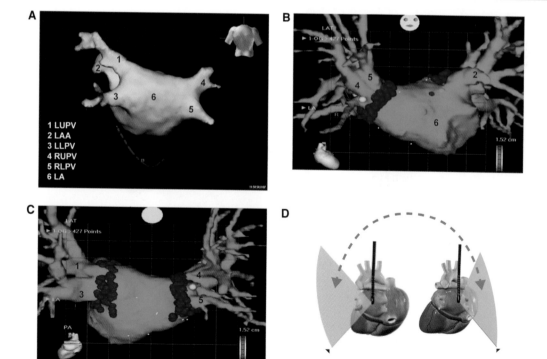

Figure 29.28 Three-dimensional (3D) mapping of LA. (A) 3D representation of the LA, LAA and pulmonary veins. **(B–C)** 3D mapping system used to establish the cartography of the LA during the electrophysiologic study. **(D)** 3D schematic representation of the rotation of the transesophageal echocardiographic probe used in order to monitor the ablation catheter. *Abbreviations*: LA, left atrium; LAA, left atrial appendage; LLPV, left lower pulmonary vein; LUPV, left upper pulmonary vein; RLPV, right lower pulmonary vein; RUPV, right upper pulmonary vein.

obtained, a numerical merging operation is made with the previously obtained MRI or CT image of the LA. This will facilitate the localization of the catheter during the ablation procedure with a minimum of radiation (44), reducing the risk of fluoroscopy (45).

The anatomic position of the catheter for those correlations is obtained by a TEE view made at the 90° plane and turning the probe clockwise back and forth (Fig. 29.29). By doing so, a partial sector of a sphere is imaged and the position of the catheter relative to the adjacent structures is identified. The catheter tip may, therefore, be imaged close to the atrial wall and structures amenable to radiofrequency cauterization. This apposition has been found to be of importance

for the efficiency of energy transmission to the myocardial wall. The displacement of the catheter from the target site, or its floating position, is noted throughout the procedure.

The relative position of the esophagus to the LA posterior wall is noted before the radiofrequency isolation of the pulmonary veins. The echocardiography probe can serve as a marker and its proximity noted, when lesions are made. The pulmonary veins isolation technique may be done by cauterization of different areas adjacent to the pulmonary vein ostia using the catheter tip to transmit the required energy to the apposed endocardium (Fig. 29.30). Other catheters, such as a circular or balloon mapping one, may be

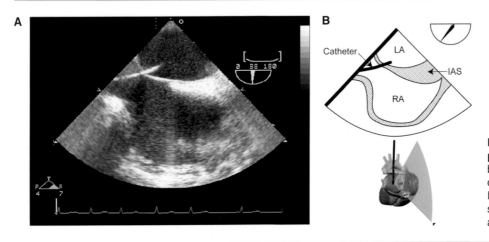

Figure 29.29 Ablation catheter positioning. (A,B) Mid-esophageal bicaval view shows the ablation catheter as it passes across the IAS. *Abbreviations*: IAS, interatrial septum; LA, left atrium; RA, right atrium.

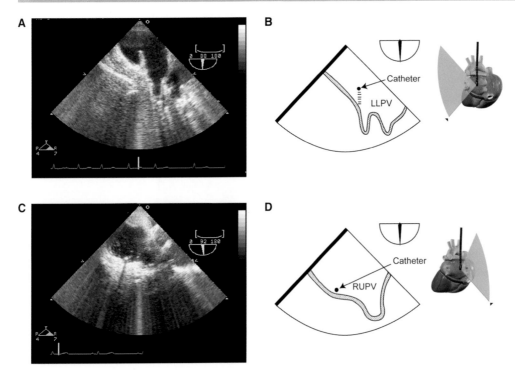

Figure 29.30 Ablation catheter position monitoring. (A,B) Mid-esophageal views at 90° rotated to the left side of the LA to show the LLPV and adequate catheter position at the orifice. **(C,D)** Turning the probe to the right side of the LA shows the RUPV with adequate catheter position close to the left atrial wall. *Abbreviations*: LA, left atrium; LLPV, left lower pulmonary vein; RUPV, right upper pulmonary vein.

inserted. A continuous flow of cold irrigating solution may divert the transmitted energy from the endocardium to diffuse in deeper layers and is visualized by the echocardiographic appearance of bubbles at the tip of the catheter. Different cauterization patterns may be used and may include all venous ostia. During the procedure, the catheter tip is visualized using the 3D localization antenna and a correlation is made with its echocardiographic position. The inadvertent migration of the ablation catheter into anatomical zones prone to perforation such as the LAA or its proximity to the circumflex artery or to the MV is carefully monitored (Figs. 29.31 and 29.32). Frequent atrial echocardiographic monitoring facilitates the observation of any new or evolving pericardial effusion as it becomes apparent.

When the cauterization pattern and the electric isolation of the pulmonary veins are satisfactory, a

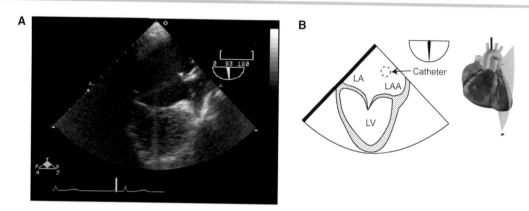

Figure 29.31   Ablation catheter malposition. (A,B) Mid-esophageal two-chamber view shows the inadvertent migration of the ablation catheter into the orifice of the LAA. Delivery of radiofrequency energy for fulguration in this position may result in cardiac perforation. *Abbreviations*: LA, left atrium; LAA, left atrial appendage; LV, left ventricle.

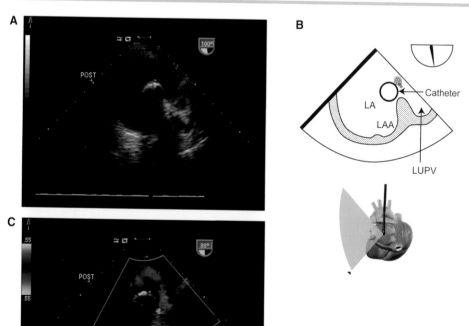

Figure 29.32 Ablation catheter malposition. (A–C) Color Doppler mid-esophageal two-chamber view shows the inadvertent migration of the ablation catheter into the orifice of the LAA. Cauterization in this location may cause cardiac perforation. *Abbreviations*: LA, left atrium; LAA, left atrial appendage; LUPV, left upper pulmonary vein.

final echocardiographic examination, similar to the one made at the end of a cardiac procedure, is made (see Chapter 13), including LAA fractional area change and velocity (46). Atrial stunning, indicated by the latter measurements and the presence of spontaneous echo contrast, is associated to the risk of a post-procedural thrombus formation (47). It also includes a visualization of all pulmonary vein ostia and the diameter at the connection with the atrium is noted, and their inflow velocities are recorded by pulsed wave (PW) Doppler.

Echocardiographic Issues

As described in the procedure, the echocardiographic exam serves as a baseline for the anatomical and physiologic description of the heart, more precisely for the pulmonary veins and atrium, and as a comparison after the procedure. By defining the position of the catheter and marking the correlation with the 3D imaging system, it reduces the radiographic exposure time and its consequences (44) (Table 29.4). The advantages of the procedure have been outlined in adults (48), in children, and in adolescents (44).

Catheter Ablation Procedure Complications

Echocardiography contributes to the early identification and follow-up of the procedure complications as described in a large series or occasional reports (49) (Table 29.5).

Table 29.4 Echocardiographic Sequence During Atrial Fibrillation Ablation Procedure

Preliminary examination
Oesophagus localization
Identification of thrombus
Pulmononary vein velocity and ostia diameters before, during, and after the procedure
Trans-septal puncture guidance
Identification of pericardial effusion
Position correlation with the ablation catheter
Thrombus and bubble monitoring
Identification of potential complication
Post-procedural examination

Table 29.5 Complications Associated with the Catheter Ablation Procedure of Cardiac Arrhythmias (41,50,51)

Pulmonary vein stenosis
Oesophageal perforation
Thrombus formation
Persistent atrial septal defect
Atrial dissection
Cardiac perforation (52)
Tamponade (53)
Mitral valve apparatus entrapment (54)
Vagal reflex (55)
Arrhythmia (38)
Cerebrovascular insult (56)
Phrenic nerve injury (57)
Gastroparesis (58)

The reported complications include those inherent to the trans-septal catheterization and to the radio frequency (RF) ablation procedure by itself.

Pulmonary Vein Stenosis

Pulmonary vein function is defined by its dynamic ability to serve as a conduit for the return of oxygenated blood to the LA. It is assessed at the pulmonary vein-atrial junction by measuring the modification of the pulmonary vein diameters and flows that are indicated by the mean and peak velocities and velocity-time integral (VTI) are calculated by PW Doppler.

Echocardiography, MRI, and CT scan have been evaluated for the measurement of the pulmonary vein diameter. The differences obtained were thought to be due to the plane of interrogation of the different compared modalities and to the fact that the cross-sectional area of the pulmonary vein at their atrial junction is not circular but elliptic (59). At that point, the pulmonary veins are funnel shaped and their connection to the atrial wall is at an oblique angle (60).

The degree of stenosis is defined by angiography as mild if the post-ablation diameter is reduced between 30% to 50% of the pre-ablation one, moderate between 50% to 70%, and severe if it is >70%. It has been reported that 1% to 20% of the patients have some reduction of their pulmonary vein diameters following the ablation procedure. A significant difference in velocities was found between normal and mild stenotic veins versus moderate and severely stenotic ones. In severe stenosis, the pulmonary vein diameter was ≤6 mm, PW Doppler peak and mean velocities were respectively >185 and >110 cm/s, and the VTI was >105 cm (Fig. 29.33) (61). In the early days of pulmonary vein isolation using only fluoroscopy, the reports indicated up to 42% of pulmonary vein stenosis, possibly due to unrecognized ostial catheter migration (62).

Microbubbles

Microbubble formation occurs when there is a high energy output at the endocardial surface and poor catheter contact (63). The risk of scar and clot formation at that point may thus be increased. The initial production of bubbles (type 1) is a signal that the RF output must be lowered before the appearance of the type 2 bubbles (Fig. 29.34). Those are characterized by their brisk appearance associated with a rise of impedance, signs that the endocardium has received an amount of RF energy sufficient for the surface to boil. This observation is to be correlated with the increased incidence of pulmonary vein stenosis and high RF output (64).

Esophageal Perforation

This syndrome has been described with the surgical (65) and the endocardial ablation procedure (66) (see Chapter 8). The clinical presentation is an intermittent neurological defect happening on the second to third week after the procedure (66). Usually the symptoms

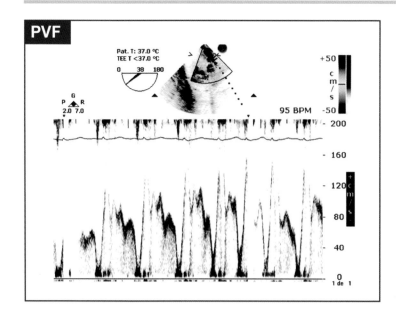

Figure 29.33 Pulmonary vein stenosis. Pulsed wave Doppler of PVF shows an elevated velocity suggestive of pulmonary vein stenosis. *Abbreviation*: PVF, pulmonary vein flow.

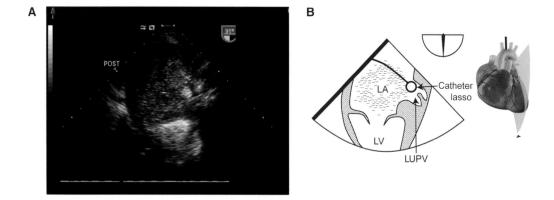

Figure 29.34 Micro-bubbles type II. (A,B) Mid-esophageal two-chamber view shows the presence of brisk micro-bubbles associated with a rise of impedence in the ablation catheter. This is suggestive of excessive high energy output at the endocardial surface, sufficient to induce boiling. The energy output should be reduced to prevent the risk of subsequent pulmonary vein stenosis. *Abbreviations*: LA, left atrium; LUPV, left upper pulmonary vein; LV, left ventricle.

that appear after a meal can be of different intensity and time duration. It is associated with a gaseous LA embolism secondary to an esophageal perforation. Death may occur during an esophageal endoscopic exam (65).

This complication has prompted an anatomic description of the relation of the posterior LA with the esophagus. The LA contact with the esophagus is identified on the mid to inferior atrial portion, and more frequently on the left or middle part of the LA than on its right side (67). The esophageal position has been observed to modify its anatomical relationship with the posterior part of the atrium during the ablation procedure, with lateral movements of a few centimeters (68). One can infer that a patient with a small atrium may be at higher risk of perforation (69). The position of the esophagus may be estimated by the intermittent radiographic projection of the echocardiographic probe adherent to the LA posterior wall. The latter view modality is useful to assess the proximity of the ablation catheter to the esophagus.

The recent interest for the circumferential atrial approach versus the pulmonary ostia isolation puts an emphasis on the importance of ablation catheter localization (70). The anatomical proximity of the esophagus to the LA (within a centimeter) (71) and the little amount of fat between both structures is thought to be responsible for the heat transmission during the ablation. Temperature monitoring is advised by passing an esophageal temperature probe after the TEE probe.

The most frequent location of an increase temperature is close to the LUPV, but it has been described at the back of all veins (72). If the ablation catheter is very close to the LA posterior wall and the TEE probe, the latter is momentarily withdrawn into the upper esophageal position. This will prevent any mucosal tension while applying the radiofrequency heat. The increase of esophageal temperature is better correlated with the presence of microbubbles than the radio-frequency power output (73).

Trans-septal Catheterization Complications

In a recent review of >5500 patients (74), a complication rate of 0.8% was observed for the trans-septal procedure. Cardiac, aortic root and RA perforation, tamponade (Fig. 29.35), arterial, and thromboembolism were reported. The trans-septal approach was also abandoned in 0.8% of the cases mainly because of the interatrial septal anatomy, or the occasional needle puncture of the RA or aortic root.

Thrombus Formation

Introduction of catheter into the left heart carries the risk of thrombus formation, which has been noted in 10.3% of procedures. Those thrombi are attached to the catheter or to the sheath and can frequently be withdrawn into the RA without left heart embolism. They are also associated with the presence of spontaneous echo contrast (75). The presence of a thrombus or vegetation at the localization of a previous RF ablation has also been reported (76) (Fig. 29.36).

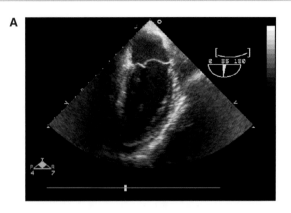

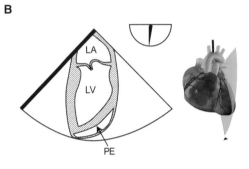

Figure 29.35 Pericardial effusion. (A,B) Mid-esophageal two-chamber view shows shows a small amount of pericardial fluid at the apex of the LV during transseptal perforation. *Abbreviations*: LA, left atrium; LV, left ventricle; PE, pericardial effusion.

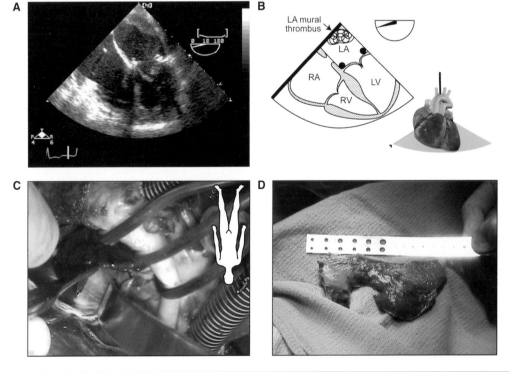

Figure 29.36 Left atrial mural thrombus after mitral valve repair and Maze procedure for chronic atrial fibrillation. (A,B) Mid-esophageal four-chamber view in a 78-year-old woman showing a large left atrial mural thrombus. **(C)** Intraoperative findings through a left atriotomy. **(D)** Excised specimen. *Abbreviations*: LA, left atrium; LV, left ventricle; RA, right atrium; RV, right ventricle. *Source*: Photos C and D courtesy of Dr. Michel Pellerin.

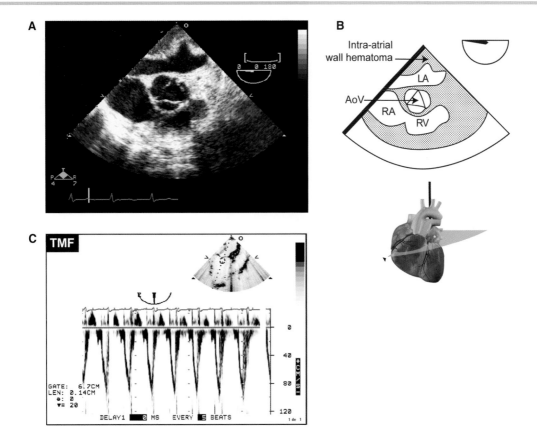

Figure 29.37   Intra-atrial wall hematoma during an ablation procedure. (**A,B**) Mid-esophageal AoV short-axis view at 0° shows significant thickening of the posterior wall of the LA consistent with an intra-atrial wall hematoma from dissection of the left atrial wall. (**C**) Pulsed wave Doppler of TMF shows normal flow without evidence of tamponade physiology. *Abbreviations*: AoV, aortic valve; LA, left atrium; RA, right atrium; RV, right ventricle; TMF, transmitral flow.

Persistent Atrial Septal Defect

The long-term persistence of an ASD has been documented (77). An interatrial shunt was noted only if two catheters were passed through the same introducer instead of by two different punctures. A pre-procedural increased pulmonary pressure was associated with an increase incidence of right to left shunt.

Atrial Dissection

An endocardial flap occurring after a catheter ablation has been described to occur at the junction of the LUPV with the LA (78). Dissection of the LA wall during the procedure is a rare event that may rapidly obstruct the blood passage to the LV (Fig. 29.37). If the LA has not been perforated in its full thickness, no extrapericardial effusion will be seen (79).

Tamponade

In a multicenter survey involving 8745 patients, cardiac tamponade was observed in 1.2% of cases (Fig. 29.38) (80).

Procedure Results

Although the rate of success is increasing, up to 32% of the patients must have a second ablation (81). A second procedure done for a recurrence has achieved a success rate of over 90% (82). Trans-septal catheterization has been reported to be more difficult in these patients, possibly due to the increased interatrial thickness induced by the first ablation procedure (83).

ROLE OF ECHOCARDIOGRAPHY IN CARDIAC RESYNCHRONIZATION THERAPY

Introduction

Cardiac resynchronization therapy (CRT) is an effective nonpharmacological strategy used in the management of chronic heart failure. Its benefits include the improvement of functional capacity and quality of life, as well as a reduction in the number of hospitalizations and a prolonged survival; these have been demonstrated in several large scale randomized clinical trials (84–90). This is likely due to a structural improvement in LV function, dimension and volume, combined with the reduction of MR through reverse

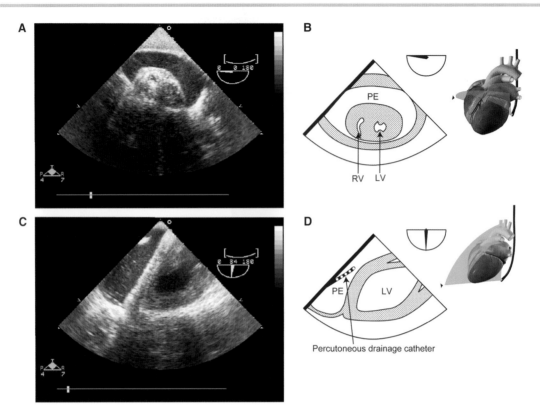

Figure 29.38   Pericardial tamponade. (A,B) Transgastric mid-papillary short-axis and **(C,D)** two-chamber views show a large PE surrounding the posterior aspect of the LV and RV. This was treated with a percutaneous drainage catheter. *Abbreviations*: LV, left ventricle; PE, pericardial effusion; RV, right ventricle.

remodeling (86,91–95). Echocardiography has often been used to help understand the different types and mechanisms of dyssynchrony and patient response to CRT.

The currently accepted patient selection criteria for CRT are based on clinical trial data and consists of severe heart failure, classified as functional class III and IV by the New York Heart Association (NYHA) despite adequate medical treatment, prolonged QRS duration >120 ms, left ventricular ejection fraction (LVEF) <35%, and left ventricular end-systolic dimension (LVESD) >55 mm (96). On the basis of these selection criteria, a relatively high proportion of patients still do not respond to this strategy (25–35%) (97). The etiology of nonresponse is multifactorial (e.g., lead placement, ischemic scar, AF, severity of heart failure, etc.); however, using QRS duration as the main screening tool for CRT is likely the main factor contributing to nonresponse, as it is a relatively crude and suboptimal estimate of true mechanical dyssynchrony.

Recently, the focus has been put on the use of echocardiography to identify patients with mechanical dyssynchrony who may derive benefits from CRT (97). Despite a theoretical advantage in using echocardiography in this setting, the reproducibility and reliability of the technique as a selection tool are

disputed (98). This section will review the applications of various echocardiographic modalities to identify mechanical dyssynchrony and, thus, possibly to improve patient selection, guide lead placement during implantation and its role in optimizing post-implantation CRT device settings.

Principle of Mechanical Dyssynchrony

Mechanical dyssynchrony can be defined as a timing of contraction differential between regions of the heart (99). Although frequently associated with a widened QRS of left bundle branch block (LBBB) morphology on surface electrocardiogram EKG, it can occur in a subset of patients with a narrow QRS as well. There are three types of dyssynchrony: atrioventricular (between atrium and ventricle), interventricular (between RV and LV), and intraventricular (between different regions within the LV) (Table 29.6).

Intraventricular dyssynchrony is thought to be the main factor contributing to LV contractile impairment. In LBBB, the interventricular septum typically contracts early, whereas the lateral and posterior LV walls contract much later, giving rise to a heterogeneous regional contraction pattern; the latter renders LV ejection inefficient, increases LV volume and wall stress, further perpetuating LV remodeling and

Table 29.6 Classification of Dyssynchrony

1-Intraventricular	Criteria for dyssynchrony
Diagnostic modalities:	
M-mode: using conventional or radial TDI	Septal to posterior wall motion delay >130 ms
Longitudinal TDI in the basal regions	
Offline: color coded TDI	Basal peak velocity delay >65 ms
Online: pulsed wave Doppler	QRS to early basal S_m delay >100 ms
Tissue synchronization imaging	Septal to posterior wall motion delay >65 ms
Radial TDI or strain	
TDI derived displacement	Septal to posterior wall motion delay in ejection phase >130 ms
Two-dimensional speckle strain	Septal to posterior wall motion delay in ejection phase >130 ms
2-Interventricular	
Diagnostic modalities:	
M-mode	Onset of Q wave to AVO
Pulsed wave (PW) Doppler	
LV PEP: QRS to LV to AVO	Interval >140 ms is considered abnormal
RV PEP: QRS to RV to PVO	
IVMD: LV PEP–RV PEP	Duration >40 ms is considered abnormal
Longitudinal TDI	Time from Q onset to peak St velocity of the RV free wall vs. the basal lateral wall S_m velocity of the LV
3-Atrioventricular (AV)	
Diagnostic modality:	
PW Doppler at the mitral annulus	
A wave	A wave absent if AV delay too short
A wave nontruncated during MVC	A wave termination <40 ms before MVC if AV delay too short
A wave and E wave	A wave merging with E wave if AV delay too long
	Diastolic mitral regurgitation if AV delay too long
4-Ventricular to ventricular (VV)	
Diagnostic modality	
PW Doppler	
LVOT PW Doppler VTI	No consensus on definition
	LV pacing 40 ms before RV with the highest LVOT VTI

Abbreviations: A, peak late diastolic TMF velocity; AVO, aortic valve opening; E, peak early diastolic TMF velocity; IVMD, interventricular mechanical delay; LV, left ventricular; LVOT, left ventricular outflow tract; MVC, mitral valve closure; PEP, pre-ejection period; PVO, pulmonic valve opening; RV, right ventricular; S_m, systolic mitral; St, systolic tricuspid; TDI, tissue Doppler imaging; TMF, transmitral flow; VTI, velocity time integral.
Source: Adapted from Ref. 97.

systolic dysfunction as well as increasing mitral regurgitation (MR) (Fig. 29.39). In cardiac surgery, the use of a single chamber pacemaker can also lead to reduced LV ejection (Figs. 29.40 and 29.41).

Echocardiographic Quantification of Mechanical Dyssynchrony

Absence of mechanical dyssynchrony is the main factor contributing to nonresponse to CRT (100). Echocardiographic strategies to identify mechanical dyssynchrony are evolving, and there is currently no single uniform approach to quantification. Several parameters using different echocardiographic techniques have been studied, either individually or in combination.

Interventricular dyssynchrony is the time difference between RV and LV ejection, and is described as interventricular mechanical delay (IVMD). It can be quantified using PW Doppler of the pulmonary and aortic outflow velocities (Fig. 29.42) or M-mode (see Fig. 10.16). Measuring the difference in timing between the onset of the Q wave (on EKG) to the onset of pulmonary and aortic flow velocities, one can calculate

the delay in the onset of ventricular contraction (Fig. 29.43). An abnormal IVMD has been described as >40 ms. Tissue Doppler imaging (TDI) can also be used to determine interventricular dyssynchrony by measuring the time from Q onset to peak systolic velocity (S_m) of the RV free wall versus the basal lateral wall of the LV (90). Despite its good reproducibility, interventricular dyssynchrony as represented by IVMD has been shown to be, at best, a nonspecific predictor of response to CRT with sensitivities and specificities as low as 66% and 55% for a cutoff of 44 ms (101,102).

Most studies have shown that response to CRT seems to be better predicted by intraventricular dyssynchrony indices. The latter has been more extensively studied and can be quantified using several different echocardiographic methods, including M-mode, TDI, longitudinal strain and strain rate, radial strain with speckle tracking, and 3D echocardiography. The septal-to-posterior wall motion delay (SPWMD) can be calculated by M-mode at the midventricular level in parasternal long or short axis views. A delay of >130 ms between peak systolic inward posterior wall motion compared with peak inward septal motion is considered significant intraventricular dyssynchrony with a sensitivity of 100%

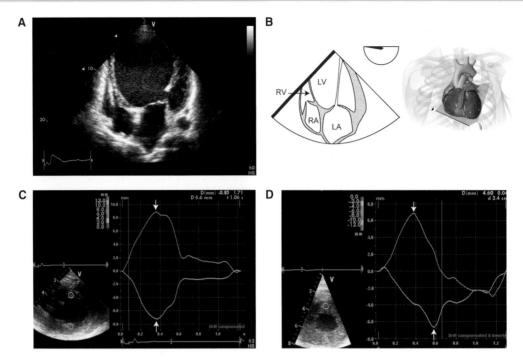

Figure 29.39 Dyssynchrony of the LV. (A,B) Apical four-chamber view demonstrating swinging pattern of contraction associated with LBBB on EKG. **(C)** Transgastric mid-papillary short-axis view of a 56-year-old man after coronary revascularization. Using tissue Doppler imaging to assess radial displacement, note the normal symmetrical and simultaneous displacement of the inferior and anterior walls in opposite direction. **(D)** When the pacemaker is turned on, there is now dyssynchrony with a significant delay in the anterior wall contraction. *Abbreviations*: EKG, electrocardiogram; LA, left atrium; LBBB, left bundle branch block; LV, left ventricle; RA, right atrium; RV, right ventricle. ⌐⊕

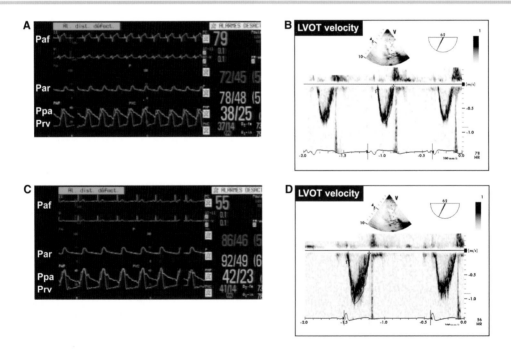

Figure 29.40 Pacemaker-induced dyssynchrony. Hemodynamic pressure tracings and pulsed wave Doppler interrogation of the LVOT in a patient after cardiac surgery with the ventricular pacemaker on **(A,B)** and off **(C,D)**. With the pacemaker turned off, although the heart rate dropped from 79 to 55 beats per minute, note the significant increase in stroke volume as the velocity time integral rose from 12.5 to 21.5 cm and the arterial blood pressure, from 78/48 to 92/49. The mechanism could be the result of an underlying filling abnormality or interventricular dyssynchrony. Indeed, in post-operative cardiac patients, the pacemaker wires are typically fixed on the right ventricle. *Abbreviations*: LVOT, left ventricular outflow tract; Paf, femoral arterial pressure; Par, radial arterial pressure; Ppa, pulmonary artery pressure; Prv, right ventricular pressure.

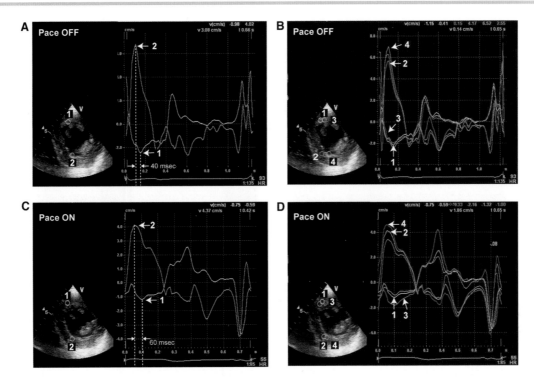

Figure 29.41 Pacemaker-induced intraventricular dyssynchrony by TDI analysis. Offline quantitative analysis of TDI through the transgastric mid-papillary short-axis view in a patient after cardiopulmonary bypass (the same as in Figure 29.40). (**A,B**) Pacemaker turned off: regional TDI velocities of the anterior wall (2 & 4) are higher than the inferior wall (1 & 3). (**C,D**) Pacemaker turned on: both anteroseptal and inferior TDI velocities are decreased. Note the different delay in peak systolic velocity between the two ventricular regions. *Abbreviation*: TDI, tissue Doppler imaging.

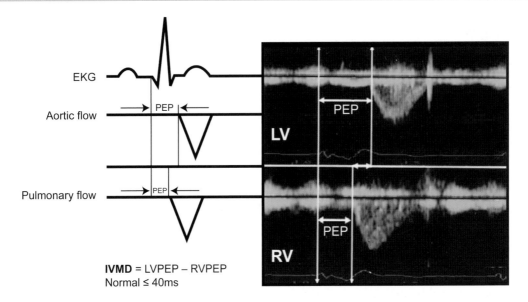

Figure 29.42 Interventricular mechanical delay measured by pulsed wave Doppler. The IVMD is the difference in onset of ventricular contraction between the LV and the RV. It can be obtained by calculating the difference between the left and the right pre-ejection period, measured from the onset of the QRS to the onset of ejection of each ventricle. *Abbreviations*: EKG, electrocardiogram; IVMD, interventricular mechanical delay; LV, left ventricle; PEP, pre-ejection period; RV, right ventricle.

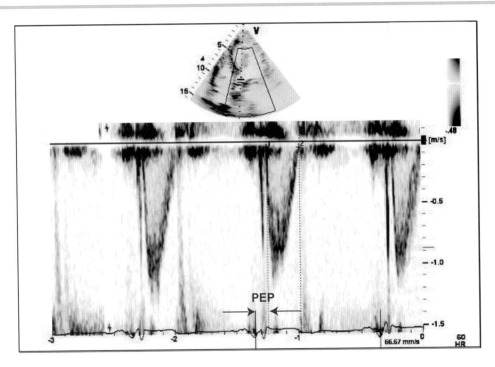

Figure 29.43   Identification of the pre-ejection and ejection period by pulsed wave Doppler. Transthoracic five-chamber view with pulsed wave Doppler sample in the LVOT. The AVO is identified at the onset of systolic forward flow. The AVC occurs at the end of the ejection, frequently accompanied by a vertical closing click. The LV PEP starts from the QRS to the beginning of the systolic forward flow. The proper identification of the systolic period between AVO and AVC in relation with the QRS is an important step to perform before assessing intraventricular dyssynchrony by longitudinal tissue Doppler imaging. *Abbreviations*: AVC, aortic valve closure; AVO, aortic valve opening; LV, left ventricular; LVOT, left ventricular outflow tract; PEP, pre-ejection period.

and a specificity of 63% in predicting reverse remodeling [15% decrease in left ventricular end-systolic volume (LVESV) index] (Fig. 29.44) (103,104). The main caveat of this technique is the presence of akinesis of either the septum or posterior wall that precludes the proper identification of peak inward motion. The reproducibility of this technique is, therefore, unsatisfactory on its own to identify intraventricular dyssynchrony and should, therefore, be used in conjunction with other parameters.

Tissue Doppler imaging has been used, almost exclusively, in the quantification of intraventricular dyssynchrony (Fig. 29.41). Using color-coded TDI, longitudinal LV shortening velocities in all three apical windows are identified by placing the regions of interest at the level of the basal and mid-inferoseptal, lateral, inferior, anterior, inferolateral, or anteroseptal walls. With offline quantitative analysis of stored myocardial velocity data, one can display longitudinal shortening velocities against time and calculate the time difference between peak systolic velocities in various regions to evaluate the maximum opposing wall delay. Care must be taken to properly identify first the LV ejection interval by determining the exact timing of aortic valve opening and closing: this will ensure that peak systolic myocardial velocities recorded do indeed belong to the systolic period. This is done using PW Doppler flow at the left

ventricular outflow tract (LVOT) in the five-chamber view to identify AoV opening and closure (Fig. 29.43). It can also be used for a composite index of inter- and intraventricular dyssynchrony, with a cutoff of 102 ms yielding an 88% accuracy (Fig. 29.45) (105).

The Yu index, or dyssynchrony index, another index of intraventricular dyssynchrony, is calculated as the standard deviation of the time-to-peak systolic velocities (Ts) at 12 LV sites (taken from mid and basal segments of opposing walls in all three standard apical views). A Yu dyssynchrony index of 33 ms has a sensitivity of 100% and a specificity of 78% in patients with QRS duration >150 ms in predicting reverse remodeling ($\geq$15% reduction in LV end-systolic volume) (106).

Caveats of doing offline quantitative analysis from color-coded TDI lie in the inability to identify the peak systolic velocity due to akinesis of a segment, multiple peaks, or signal noise. Moreover, the Yu index has been demonstrated, in the Prospect trial, to be technically too complex for good reproducibility (98). Parametric imaging with automated color coding, such as in tissue synchronization imaging (TSI), codes the different time to peak velocity data according to a given scale (with red representing the longest and green the shortest delays) and displays them superimposed on the 2D images, thus allowing a more visual evaluation of regional mechanical

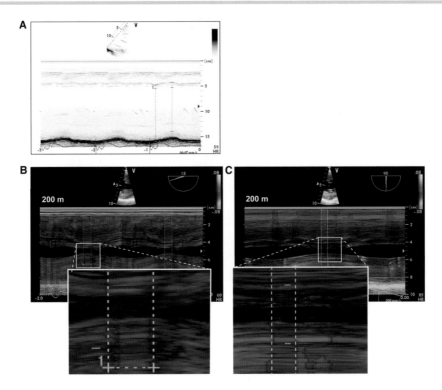

Figure 29.44 Intraventricular dyssynchrony by M-mode. (A) M-mode of the left ventricle through a transthoracic parasternal long-axis view. The septal-to-posterior wall motion delay is measured from the peak inward septal motion to the peak inward posterior wall motion. This is calculated to be superior to 130 ms, although determining the precise timing of each peak may be difficult particularly in the presence of severe hypokinesis. **(B,C)** Color M-mode of tissue Doppler imaging through a transgastric mid-papillary in an 80-year-old woman with a left bundle branch block (100 ms) present before (red inferior wall on top and red anterior wall below) **(B)** but absent after cardiac surgery (normal red inferior wall on top and blue anterior wall below) **(C)**. The change in myocardial velocity direction (and thus color) facilitates the precise determination of the timing of peak inward motion.

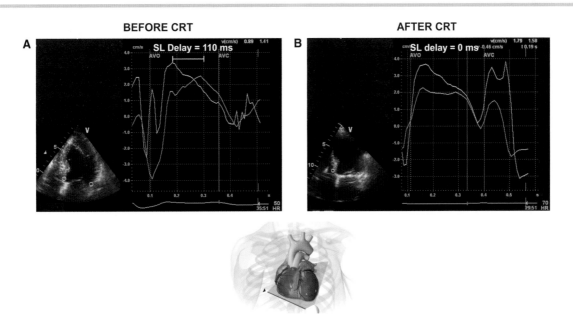

Figure 29.45 Intraventricular dyssynchrony assessed by tissue Doppler imaging in CRT. Quantitative analysis off stored tissue Doppler imaging in a patient before **(A)** and after **(B)** cardiac resynchronization therapy with biventricular pacing. The SL delay before CRT was 110 ms, consistent with significant intraventricular dyssynchrony (≥ 65 ms). Post CRT, the peak systolic velocities occurred almost simultaneously in the same two segments with a delay close to 0 ms, consistent with favorable response. *Abbreviations*: CRT, cardiac resynchronization therapy; MAV, mitral annular velocity; SL, septal to lateral; Sm, peak systolic MAV.

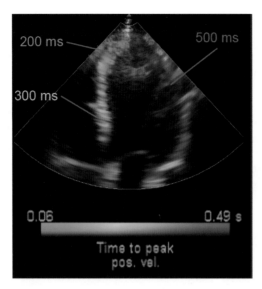
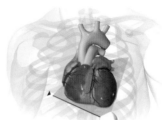

Green = 60 - 200 ms
Yellow = 201 - 350 ms
Red   = 350 - 500 ms

Figure 29.46 Intraventricular dyssynchrony assessed by parametric imaging. In parametric imaging with TSI, the time to peak velocity data is color-coded according to the scale at the bottom and superimposed on the two-dimensional image. This allows a more visual evaluation of regional mechanical delay, red representing the longest and green the shortest delays. *Abbreviation*: TSI, tissue synchronization imaging.

delay (Fig. 29.46). Gorcsan et al. (95) used TSI to derive a septal-to-posterior wall delay of 65 ms to predict improvement of stroke volume (SV) post CRT. Of note, current evidence suggests analyzing peak velocities within the ejection interval, because using post-systolic shortening velocities, that is, peaks that occur after AoV closure, significantly decreases specificity in predicting LV reverse remodeling (107). Currently used indices of intraventricular dyssynchrony, which have been studied together with corresponding response to CRT, have been the topic of an expert consensus statement (97).

Longitudinal strain and strain rate are indices of deformation rather than displacement; they are less subject to passive motion and have been used to assess dyssynchrony. So far the data has been mixed due to poor signal-to-noise ratio, which affects reproducibility. Moreover, there are not enough trials studying longitudinal strain and strain rate to come up with cut-off values that allow the prediction of the response to CRT. Radial strain is also an index of deformation used to assess radial deformation. By collecting data from the anteroseptal and infero-lateral wall in a parasternal short axis view, one can calculate the mechanical delay between those two segments.

More recently, speckle tracking has been used as it can be applied to routine gray-scale echocardio-graphic views. In one study, a time difference in peak anteroseptal to inferolateral wall radial strain >130 ms had a sensitivity and specificity of 89%

and 83%, respectively, in predicting LVEF increase in 50 patients (108). It is likely that combining both longitudinal and radial dyssynchrony patterns will best predict a patient's response to CRT (109).

Three-dimensional echocardiography could potentially be used as a tool to assess the dyssyn-chrony of all LV segments during the same cardiac cycle, as opposed to conventional 2D echo which requires three separate views to assess the whole LV. In one study, a 3D systolic velocity index was derived and was predictive of reverse remodeling (110). Unfortunately 3D imaging has the caveats of decreased spatial and temporal resolution with low frame rates; for this reason, it is not used uniformly in most institutions.

Echocardiography-Guided Lead Placement

Most CRT lead placements are done by implanting the LV lead adjacent to the lateral or posterolateral walls, as it is thought that in the majority of cases these are the segments showing the latest mechanical activa-tion. Several reports have indicated that using color-coded TDI to target LV lead location could result in better response rates, both hemodynamically and clin-ically (111,112). More studies are warranted to assess the reproducibility and practicality of this method, as the implantation procedure tended to be prolonged when more contrast agents were used in the echocar-diography-guided group.

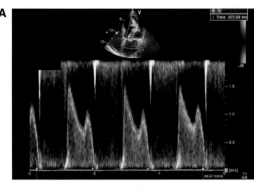 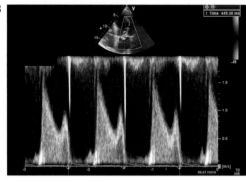

AV delay 200 ms   AV delay 120 ms

Figure 29.47   Optimization of the AV pacing interval with pulsed wave Doppler of TMF. This example was performed using the iterative method. At an AV delay of 200 ms, the DFT is 423 ms. With the AV delay set at 100 ms, the DFT was improved at 449 ms but the A wave contribution to filling was decreased by the beginning of mitral valve closure and left ventricular contraction. The AV pacing interval was thus set at 120 ms, the AV delay giving the longest DFT without A wave truncation. *Abbreviations*: A, peak late diastolic TMF velocity; AV, atrioventricular; DFT, diastolic filling time; TMF, transmitral flow.

Post-Implantation Device Optimization

Echocardiography can also be used in device optimization post implantation. Two intervals can be adjusted: the atrioventricular delay and the ventricular-to-ventricular (VV) delay.

Atrioventricular delay optimization can provide the most favorable preload to the LV. An atrioventricular delay that is too short will interrupt atrial contribution to diastolic filling by premature LV contraction, whereas an atrioventricular delay that is too long will result in diastolic MR. Although theoretically useful, routine atrioventricular delay optimization by echocardiography has not been demonstrated to be superior to standard out-of-the-box settings (atrioventricular delay 100–130 ms) in improving LV hemodynamics (113).

In our experience, the simplest approach has been to use the iterative method of atrioventricular delay optimization. A PW Doppler is placed slightly below the MV leaflet tips and different atrioventricular delays are tested sequentially while ensuring complete ventricular entrainment. The best atrioventricular delay is the shortest that provides the longest diastolic filling time (duration of E + A) but without A wave truncation by MV closure (which represents beginning of LV systole) (Fig. 29.47). Most of the time, the optimized atrioventricular delay will only marginally differ from the initial manufacturer's settings, thus calling into question the need of doing routine atrioventricular delay optimization on every patient with CRT. Important caveats to atrioventricular optimization are AF and presence of MV prosthesis precluding adequate E and A wave interrogation.

Ventricular-to-ventricular delay optimization has been shown to improve ejection fraction (EF) and decrease MR in a small number of patients with CRT (114–116). Currently, there is no consensus on the best method of VV delay optimization. A proposed approach suggests the testing of various VV intervals, starting with simultaneous RV and LV pacing (VV 0 ms), and increasing the intervals by 20 ms at a time with LV pacing preceding RV pacing, and vice versa, with the goal of obtaining the highest aortic VTI or best LV intraventricular synchrony by a few of the TDI color-coded methods.

Role of TEE in CRT

There are a few studies evaluating the effect of biventricular pacing with TEE in the perioperative period in cardiac surgery. Cannesson et al. have recently found that atriobiventricular pacing (RV and LV epicardial pacing) improves cardiac output when compared to atrioright ventricular pacing, and this increase was related to an improvement in left ventricular synchronicity. Although this observation has potential clinical applications, further studies are needed to explore the role of this strategy in the cardiac surgical patient (117). The data on the use of intraoperative TEE in CRT may also be useful for guiding CS lead placement. Small reports have shown that when conventional fluoroscopy has failed with special leads and cannulas, TEE improved the success rate of CS lead placement and decreased operative time (118,119).

CONCLUSION

Despite the theoretical advantages of using echocardiography to predict responders to CRT and optimizing the device post-implantation, there is still a lot of uncertainty with regard to the best echocardiographic approach. The Prospect trial, which tested real-life assessment of dyssynchrony in different centers worldwide, failed to show significant predictive value or reproducibility of a large number of echocardiographic parameters (98). Nevertheless, as with most operator-dependent techniques, there is a learning curve and many studies currently focus on finding simpler and more reproducible ways of evaluating dyssynchrony.

REFERENCES

1. Cheitlin MD, Armstrong WF, Aurigemma GP, et al. ACC/AHA/ASE 2003 guideline update for the clinical application of echocardiography: summary article: a report of the American College of Cardiology/American Heart Association Task Force on Practice Guidelines (ACC/AHA/ASE Committee to Update the 1997 Guidelines for the Clinical Application of Echocardiography). Circulation 2003; 108:1146–1162.
2. Silvestry FE, Kerber RE, Brook MM, et al. Echocardiography-guided interventions. J Am Soc Echocardiogr 2009; 22:213–231.
3. Meissner I, Whisnant JP, Khandheria BK, et al. Prevalence of potential risk factors for stroke assessed by transesophageal echocardiography and carotid ultrasonography: the SPARC Study. Mayo Clin Proc 1999; 74:862–869.
4. Hagen PT, Scholz DG, Edwards WD. Incidence and size of patent foramen ovale during the first 10 decades of life: an autopsy study of 965 normal hearts. Mayo Clin Proc 1984; 59:17–20.
5. Cabanes L, Mas JL, Cohen A, et al. Atrial septal aneurysm and patent foramen ovale as risk factors for cryptogenic stroke in patients less than 55 years of age. A study using transesophageal echocardiography. Stroke 1993; 24:1865–1873.
6. Pearson AC, Nagelhout D, Castello R, et al. Atrial septal aneurysm and stroke: a transesophageal echocardiographic study. J Am Coll Cardiol 1991; 18:1223–1229.
7. Overell JR, Bone I, Lees KR. Interatrial septal abnormalities and stroke: a meta-analysis of case-control studies. Neurology 2000; 55:1172–1179.
8. Pfleger S, Konstantin Haase K, Stark S, et al. Haemodynamic quantification of different provocation manoeuvres by simultaneous measurement of right and left atrial pressure: implications for the echocardiographic detection of persistent foramen ovale. Eur J Echocardiogr 2001; 2:88–93.
9. Braun MU, Fassbender D, Schoen SP, et al. Transcatheter closure of patent foramen ovale in patients with cerebral ischemia. J Am Coll Cardiol 2002; 39:2019–2025.
10. Dickinson DF, Arnold R, Wilkinson JL. Congenital heart disease among 160,480 liveborn children in Liverpool 1960 to 1969. Implications for surgical treatment. Br Heart J 1981; 46:55–62.
11. Samanek M, Slavik Z, Zborilova B, et al. Prevalence, treatment, and outcome of heart disease in live-born children: a prospective analysis of 91,823 live-born children. Pediatr Cardiol 1989; 10:205–211.
12. Hudson JK, Deshpande JK. Septal and endocardial cushion defects. In: Lake CL, Booker PD, eds. Pediatric Cardiac Anesthesia. Lippincott Williams & Wilkins: Philadelphia, 2005:329–343.
13. Brickner ME, Hillis LD, Lange RA. Congenital heart disease in adults. First of two parts. N Engl J Med 2000; 342:256–263.
14. Therrien J, Dore A, Gersonny A, et al. CCS Consensus Conference 2001 update: Recommendations for the Management of Adults with Congenital Heart Disease Part 1. Can J Cardiol 2001; 17:940–959.
15. Warnes CA, Williams RG, Bashore TM, et al. ACC/AHA 2008 Guidelines for the Management of Adults with Congenital Heart Disease: A Report of the American College of Cardiology/American Heart Association Task Force on Practice Guidelines (Writing Committee to Develop Guidelines on the Management of Adults with Congenital Heart Disease) Developed in Collaboration with the American Society of Echocardiography, Heart Rhythm Society, International Society for Adult Congenital Heart Disease, Society for Cardiovascular Angiography and Interventions, and Society of Thoracic Surgeons. J Am Coll Cardiol 2008; 52:e143–e263.
16. Konstantinides S, Geibel A, Olschewski M, et al. A comparison of surgical and medical therapy for atrial septal defect in adults. N Engl J Med 1995; 333:469–473.
17. Fischer G, Stieh J, Uebing A, et al. Experience with transcatheter closure of secundum atrial septal defects using the Amplatzer septal occluder: a single centre study in 236 consecutive patients. Heart 2003; 89:199–204.
18. Mcdaniel NL, Gutgesell HP. Ventricular septal defects. In: Allen HD, Gutgesell HP, Clark EB, et al., eds. Moss and Adams' Heart disease in infants, children and adolescents. Lippincott Williams & Wilkins: Philadelphia, 2001:636–651.
19. Jacobs JP, Burke RP, Quintessenza JA, et al. Congenital Heart Surgery Nomenclature and Database Project: ventricular septal defect. Ann Thorac Surg 2000; 69(4 suppl): S25–S35.
20. Holzer R, Balzer D, Amin Z, et al. Transcatheter closure of postinfarction ventricular septal defects using the new Amplatzer muscular VSD occluder: Results of a U.S. Registry. Catheter Cardiovasc Interv 2004; 61:196–201.
21. Holzer R, Balzer D, Cao QL, et al. Device closure of muscular ventricular septal defects using the Amplatzer muscular ventricular septal defect occluder: immediate and mid-term results of a U.S. registry. J Am Coll Cardiol 2004; 43:1257–1263.
22. Butera G, Carminati M, Chessa M, et al. Transcatheter closure of perimembranous ventricular septal defects: early and long-term results. J Am Coll Cardiol 2007; 50:1189–1195.
23. Masura J, Gao W, Gavora P, et al. Percutaneous closure of perimembranous ventricular septal defects with the eccentric Amplatzer device: multicenter follow-up study. Pediatric Cardiol 2005; 26:216–219.
24. Rallidis LS, Moyssakis IE, Ikonomidis I, et al. Natural history of early aortic paraprosthetic regurgitation: a five-year follow-up. Am Heart J 1999; 138:351–357.
25. Hassan A, Newman AM, Gong Y, et al. Use of valve surgery in Canada. Can J Cardiol 2004; 20:149–154.
26. Pate GE, Al Zubaidi A, Chandavimol M, et al. Percutaneous closure of prosthetic paravalvular leaks: case series and review. Catheter Cardiovasc Interv 2006; 68:528–533.
27. Cortès M, Garcia E, Garcia-Fernandez MA, et al. Usefulness of transesophageal echocardiography in percutaneous transcatheter repairs of paravalvular mitral regurgitation. Am J Cardiol 2008; 101:382–386.
28. Kottkamp H, Hindricks G, Autschbach R, et al. Specific linear left atrial lesions in atrial fibrillation: intraoperative radiofrequency ablation using minimally invasive surgical techniques. J Am Coll Cardiol 2002; 40:475–480.
29. Nathan H, Eliakim M. The junction between the left atrium and the pulmonary veins. An anatomic study of human hearts. Circulation 1966; 34:412–422.
30. Haissaguerre M, Jais P, Shah DC, et al. Spontaneous initiation of atrial fibrillation by ectopic beats originating in the pulmonary veins. N Engl J Med 1998; 339:659–666.

31. Wood MA, Wittkamp M, Henry D, et al. A comparison of pulmonary vein ostial anatomy by computerized tomography, echocardiography, and venography in patients with atrial fibrillation having radiofrequency catheter ablation. Am J Cardiol 2004; 93:49–53.

32. Calkins H, Brugada J, Packer DL, et al. HRS/EHRA/ECAS expert Consensus Statement on catheter and surgical ablation of atrial fibrillation: recommendations for personnel, policy, procedures and follow-up. A report of the Heart Rhythm Society (HRS) Task Force on catheter and surgical ablation of atrial fibrillation. Heart Rhythm 2007; 4:816–861.

33. Kinnaird TD, Uzun O, Munt BI, et al. Transesophageal echocardiography to guide pulmonary vein mapping and ablation for atrial fibrillation. J Am Soc Echocardiogr 2004; 17:769–774.

34. Champagne J, Echahidi N, Philippon F, et al. Usefulness of transesophageal echocardiography in the isolation of pulmonary veins in the treatment of atrial fibrillation. Pacing Clin Electrophysiol 2007; 30 Suppl 1:S116–S119.

35. Pappone C, Oreto G, Lamberti F, et al. Catheter ablation of paroxysmal atrial fibrillation using a 3D mapping system. Circulation 1999; 100:1203–1208.

36. Shanewise JS, Cheung AT, Aronson S, et al. ASE/SCA guidelines for performing a comprehensive intraoperative multiplane transesophageal echocardiography examination: recommendations of the American Society of Echocardiography Council for Intraoperative Echocardiography and the Society of Cardiovascular Anesthesiologists Task Force for Certification in Perioperative Transesophageal Echocardiography. Anesth Analg 1999; 89:870–884.

37. Lang RM, Bierig M, Devereux RB, et al. Recommendations for chamber quantification: a report from the American Society of Echocardiography's Guidelines and Standards Committee and the Chamber Quantification Writing Group, developed in conjunction with the European Association of Echocardiography, a branch of the European Society of Cardiology. J Am Soc Echocardiogr 2005; 18:1440–1463.

38. Tucker KJ, Curtis AB, Murphy J, et al. Transesophageal echocardiographic guidance of transseptal left heart catheterization during radiofrequency ablation of left-sided accessory pathways in humans. Pacing Clin Electrophysiol 1996; 19:272–281.

39. Weiner RI, Maranhao V. Development and application of transseptal left heart catheterization. Cathet Cardiovasc Diagn 1988; 15:112–120.

40. Bommer WJ, Shah PM, Allen H, et al. The safety of contrast echocardiography: report of the Committee on Contrast Echocardiography for the American Society of Echocardiography. J Am Coll Cardiol 1984; 3:6–13.

41. Hahn K, Gal R, Sarnoski J, et al. Transesophageal echocardiographically guided atrial transseptal catheterization in patients with normal-sized atria: incidence of complications. Clin Cardiol 1995; 18:217–220.

42. Hahn K, Bajwa T, Sarnoski J, et al. Transseptal Catheterization with Transesophageal Guidance in High Risk Patients. Echocardiography 1997; 14:475–480.

43. Jongbloed MR, Bax JJ, Zeppenfeld K, et al. Anatomical observations of the pulmonary veins with intracardiac echocardiography and hemodynamic consequences of narrowing of pulmonary vein ostial diameters after radiofrequency catheter ablation of atrial fibrillation. Am J Cardiol 2004; 93:1298–1302.

44. Kantoch MJ, Frost GF, Robertson MA. Use of transesophageal echocardiography in radiofrequency catheter ablation in children and adolescents. Can J Cardiol 1998; 14:519–523.

45. Calkins H, Niklason L, Sousa J, et al. Radiation exposure during radiofrequency catheter ablation of accessory atrioventricular connections. Circulation 1991; 84:2376–2382.

46. Pollick C, Taylor D. Assessment of left atrial appendage function by transesophageal echocardiography. Implications for the development of thrombus. Circulation 1991; 84:223–231.

47. Grimm RA, Stewart WJ, Arheart K, et al. Left atrial appendage "stunning" after electrical cardioversion of atrial flutter: an attenuated response compared with atrial fibrillation as the mechanism for lower susceptibility to thromboembolic events. J Am Coll Cardiol 1997; 29:582–589.

48. Saad EB, Marrouche NF, Natale A. Ablation of focal atrial fibrillation. Card Electrophysiol Rev 2002; 6:389–396.

49. Thakur RK, Klein GJ, Yee R, et al. Complications of radiofrequency catheter ablation: a review. Can J Cardiol 1994; 10:835–839.

50. Angkeow P, Calkins HG. Complications associated with radiofrequency catheter ablation of cardiac arrhythmias. Cardiol Rev 2001; 9:121–130.

51. O'Neill MD, Jais P, Hocini M, et al. Catheter ablation for atrial fibrillation. Circulation 2007; 116:1515–1523.

52. Kultursay H, Turkoglu C, Akin M, et al. Mitral balloon valvuloplasty with transesophageal echocardiography without using fluoroscopy. Cathet Cardiovasc Diagn 1992; 27:317–321.

53. Lundqvist C, Olsson SB, Varnauskas E. Transseptal left heart catheterization: a review of 278 studies. Clin Cardiol 1986; 9:21–26.

54. Wu RC, Brinker JA, Yuh DD, et al. Circular mapping catheter entrapment in the mitral valve apparatus: a previously unrecognized complication of focal atrial fibrillation ablation. J Cardiovasc Electrophysiol 2002; 13:819–821.

55. Pappone C, Santinelli V, Manguso F, et al. Pulmonary vein denervation enhances long-term benefit after circumferential ablation for paroxysmal atrial fibrillation. Circulation 2004; 109:327–334.

56. Kok LC, Mangrum JM, Haines DE, et al. Cerebrovascular complication associated with pulmonary vein ablation. J Cardiovasc Electrophysiol 2002; 13:764–767.

57. Sacher F, Monahan KH, Thomas SP, et al. Phrenic nerve injury after atrial fibrillation catheter ablation: characterization and outcome in a multicenter study. J Am Coll Cardiol 2006; 47:2498–2503.

58. Shah D, Dumonceau JM, Burri H, et al. Acute pyloric spasm and gastric hypomotility: an extracardiac adverse effect of percutaneous radiofrequency ablation for atrial fibrillation. J Am Coll Cardiol 2005; 46:327–330.

59. Wittkampf FH, Vonken EJ, Derksen R, et al. Pulmonary vein ostium geometry: analysis by magnetic resonance angiography. Circulation 2003; 107:21–23.

60. Verma A, Marrouche NF, Natale A. Pulmonary vein antrum isolation: intracardiac echocardiography-guided technique. J Cardiovasc Electrophysiol 2004; 15:1335–1340.

61. Schneider C, Ernst S, Malisius R, et al. Transesophageal echocardiography: a follow-up tool after catheter ablation of atrial fibrillation and interventional therapy of pulmonary vein stenosis and occlusion. J Interv Card Electrophysiol 2007; 18:195–205.

62. Chen SA, Hsieh MH, Tai CT, et al. Initiation of atrial fibrillation by ectopic beats originating from the pulmonary veins: electrophysiological characteristics, pharmacological responses, and effects of radiofrequency ablation. Circulation 1999; 100:1879–1886.

63. Kalman JM, Fitzpatrick AP, Olgin JE, et al. Biophysical characteristics of radiofrequency lesion formation in vivo: dynamics of catheter tip-tissue contact evaluated by intracardiac echocardiography. Am Heart J 1997; 133:8–18.

64. Haissaguerre M, Jais P, Shah DC, et al. Electrophysiological end point for catheter ablation of atrial fibrillation initiated from multiple pulmonary venous foci. Circulation 2000; 101:1409–1417.

65. Doll N, Borger MA, Fabricius A, et al. Esophageal perforation during left atrial radiofrequency ablation: Is the risk too high? J Thorac Cardiovasc Surg 2003; 125:836–842.

66. Pappone C, Oral H, Santinelli V, et al. Atrio-esophageal fistula as a complication of percutaneous transcatheter ablation of atrial fibrillation. Circulation 2004; 109:2724–2726.

67. Kottkamp H, Piorkowski C, Tanner H, et al. Topographic variability of the esophageal left atrial relation influencing ablation lines in patients with atrial fibrillation. J Cardiovasc Electrophysiol 2005; 16:146–150.

68. Han J, Good E, Morady F, et al. Images in cardiovascular medicine. Esophageal migration during left atrial catheter ablation for atrial fibrillation. Circulation 2004; 110:e528.

69. Good E, Oral H, Lemola K, et al. Movement of the esophagus during left atrial catheter ablation for atrial fibrillation. J Am Coll Cardiol 2005; 46:2107–2110.

70. Oral H, Scharf C, Chugh A, et al. Catheter ablation for paroxysmal atrial fibrillation: segmental pulmonary vein ostial ablation versus left atrial ablation. Circulation 2003; 108:2355–2360.

71. Lemola K, Sneider M, Desjardins B, et al. Computed tomographic analysis of the anatomy of the left atrium and the esophagus: implications for left atrial catheter ablation. Circulation 2004; 110:3655–3660.

72. Redfearn DP, Trim GM, Skanes AC, et al. Esophageal temperature monitoring during radiofrequency ablation of atrial fibrillation. J Cardiovasc Electrophysiol 2005; 16:589–593.

73. Cummings JE, Schweikert RA, Saliba WI, et al. Assessment of temperature, proximity, and course of the esophagus during radiofrequency ablation within the left atrium. Circulation 2005; 112:459–464.

74. De Ponti R, Cappato R, Curnis A, et al. Trans-septal catheterization in the electrophysiology laboratory: data from a multicenter survey spanning 12 years. J Am Coll Cardiol 2006; 47:1037–1042.

75. Ren JF, Marchlinski FE, Callans DJ. Left atrial thrombus associated with ablation for atrial fibrillation: identification with intracardiac echocardiography. J Am Coll Cardiol 2004; 43:1861–1867.

76. Kunze KP, Schluter M, Costard A, et al. Right atrial thrombus formation after transvenous catheter ablation of the atrioventricular node. J Am Coll Cardiol 1985; 6:1428–1430.

77. Hammerstingl C, Lickfett L, Jeong KM, et al. Persistence of iatrogenic atrial septal defect after pulmonary vein isolation—an underestimated risk? Am Heart J 2006; 152:362–365.

78. Ramakrishna G, Cote AV, Chandrasekaran K, et al. Endocardial flap of left atrial dissection following radiofrequency ablation. Pacing Clin Electrophysiol 2003; 26:1771–1773.

79. Echahidi N, Philippon F, O'hara G, et al. Life-threatening left atrial wall hematoma secondary to a pulmonary vein laceration: an unusual complication of catheter ablation for atrial fibrillation. J Cardiovasc Electrophysiol 2008; 19:556–558.

80. Cappato R, Calkins H, Chen SA, et al. Worldwide survey on the methods, efficacy, and safety of catheter ablation for human atrial fibrillation. Circulation 2005; 111:1100–1105.

81. Oral H, Pappone C, Chugh A, et al. Circumferential pulmonary-vein ablation for chronic atrial fibrillation. N Engl J Med 2006; 354:934–941.

82. Marrouche NF, Martin DO, Wazni O, et al. Phased-array intracardiac echocardiography monitoring during pulmonary vein isolation in patients with atrial fibrillation: impact on outcome and complications. Circulation 2003; 107:2710–2716.

83. Marcus GM, Ren X, Tseng ZH, et al. Repeat transseptal catheterization after ablation for atrial fibrillation. J Cardiovasc Electrophysiol 2007; 18:55–59.

84. Butter C, Auricchio A, Stellbrink C, et al. Effect of resynchronization therapy stimulation site on the systolic function of heart failure patients. Circulation 2001; 104:3026–3029.

85. Abraham WT, Hayes DL. Cardiac resynchronization therapy for heart failure. Circulation 2003; 108:2596–2603.

86. Young JB, Abraham WT, Smith AL, et al. Combined cardiac resynchronization and implantable cardioversion defibrillation in advanced chronic heart failure: the MIRACLE ICD Trial. JAMA 2003; 289:2685–2694.

87. Bradley DJ, Bradley EA, Baughman KL, et al. Cardiac resynchronization and death from progressive heart failure: a meta-analysis of randomized controlled trials. JAMA 2003; 289:730–740.

88. Bristow MR, Saxon LA, Boehmer J, et al. Cardiac-resynchronization therapy with or without an implantable defibrillator in advanced chronic heart failure. N Engl J Med 2004; 350:2140–2150.

89. Cleland JG, Daubert JC, Erdmann E, et al. The effect of cardiac resynchronization on morbidity and mortality in heart failure. N Engl J Med 2005; 352:1539–1549.

90. McSwain RL, Schwartz RA, Delurgio DB, et al. The impact of cardiac resynchronization therapy on ventricular tachycardia/fibrillation: an analysis from the combined Contak-CD and InSync-ICD studies. J Cardiovasc Electrophysiol 2005; 16:1168–1171.

91. Breithardt OA, Sinha AM, Schwammenthal E, et al. Acute effects of cardiac resynchronization therapy on functional mitral regurgitation in advanced systolic heart failure. J Am Coll Cardiol 2003; 41:765–770.

92. Lancellotti P, Melon P, Sakalihasan N, et al. Effect of cardiac resynchronization therapy on functional mitral regurgitation in heart failure. Am J Cardiol 2004; 94:1462–1465.

93. Porciani MC, Dondina C, Macioce R, et al. Echocardiographic examination of atrioventricular and interventricular delay optimization in cardiac resynchronization therapy. Am J Cardiol 2005; 95:1108–1110.

94. Turner MS, Bleasdale RA, Vinereanu D, et al. Electrical and mechanical components of dyssynchrony in heart failure patients with normal QRS duration and left bundle-branch block: impact of left and biventricular pacing. Circulation 2004; 109:2544–2549.

95. Gorcsan J, III, Kanzaki H, Bazaz R, et al. Usefulness of echocardiographic tissue synchronization imaging to predict acute response to cardiac resynchronization therapy. Am J Cardiol 2004; 93:1178–1181.

96. Hunt SA. ACC/AHA 2005 guideline update for the diagnosis and management of chronic heart failure in the adult: a report of the American College of Cardiology/American Heart Association Task Force on Practice Guidelines (Writing Committee to Update the 2001 Guidelines for the Evaluation and Management of Heart Failure). J Am Coll Cardiol 2005; 46:e1–e82.

97. Gorcsan J 3rd, Abraham T, Agler DA, et al. Echocardiography for cardiac resynchronization therapy: recommendations for performance and reporting—a report from the American Society of Echocardiography Dyssynchrony Writing Group endorsed by the Heart Rhythm Society. J Am Soc Echocardiogr 2008; 21:191–213.

98. Chung ES, Leon AR, Tavazzi L, et al. Results of the Predictors of Response to CRT (PROSPECT) trial. Circulation 2008; 117:2608–2616.

99. Grines CL, Bashore TM, Boudoulas H, et al. Functional abnormalities in isolated left bundle branch block. The effect of interventricular asynchrony. Circulation 1989; 79:845–853.

100. Bax JJ, Bleeker GB, Marwick TH, et al. Left ventricular dyssynchrony predicts response and prognosis after cardiac resynchronization therapy. J Am Coll Cardiol 2004; 44:1834–1840.

101. Bax JJ, Abraham T, Barold SS, et al. Cardiac resynchronization therapy: Part 2–issues during and after device implantation and unresolved questions. J Am Coll Cardiol 2005; 46:2168–2182.

102. Achilli A, Peraldo C, Sassara M, et al. Prediction of response to cardiac resynchronization therapy: the selection of candidates for CRT (SCART) study. Pacing Clin Electrophysiol 2006; 29(suppl 2):S11–S19.

103. Pitzalis MV, Iacoviello M, Romito R, et al. Cardiac resynchronization therapy tailored by echocardiographic evaluation of ventricular asynchrony. J Am Coll Cardiol 2002; 40:1615–1622.

104. Pitzalis MV, Iacoviello M, Romito R, et al. Ventricular asynchrony predicts a better outcome in patients with chronic heart failure receiving cardiac resynchronization therapy. J Am Coll Cardiol 2005; 45:65–69.

105. Penicka M, Bartunek J, de Bruyne B, et al. Improvement of left ventricular function after cardiac resynchronization therapy is predicted by tissue Doppler imaging echocardiography. Circulation 2004; 109:978–983.

106. Yu CM, Fung JW, Zhang Q, et al. Tissue Doppler imaging is superior to strain rate imaging and postsystolic shortening on the prediction of reverse remodeling in both ischemic and nonischemic heart failure after cardiac resynchronization therapy. Circulation 2004; 110:66–73.

107. Notabartolo D, Merlino JD, Smith AL, et al. Usefulness of the peak velocity difference by tissue Doppler imaging technique as an effective predictor of response to cardiac resynchronization therapy. Am J Cardiol 2004; 94:817–820.

108. Suffoletto MS, Dohi K, Cannesson M, et al. Novel speckle-tracking radial strain from routine black-and-white echocardiographic images to quantify dyssynchrony and predict response to cardiac resynchronization therapy. Circulation 2006; 113:960–968.

109. Gorcsan J III, Tanabe M, Bleeker GB, et al. Combined longitudinal and radial dyssynchrony predicts ventricular response after resynchronization therapy. J Am Coll Cardiol 2007; 50:1476–1483.

110. Kapetanakis S, Kearney MT, Siva A, et al. Real-time three-dimensional echocardiography: a novel technique to quantify global left ventricular mechanical dyssynchrony. Circulation 2005; 112:992–1000.

111. Ansalone G, Giannantoni P, Ricci R, et al. Doppler myocardial imaging to evaluate the effectiveness of pacing sites in patients receiving biventricular pacing. J Am Coll Cardiol 2002; 39:489–499.

112. Murphy RT, Sigurdsson G, Mulamalla S, et al. Tissue synchronization imaging and optimal left ventricular pacing site in cardiac resynchronization therapy. Am J Cardiol 2006; 97:1615–1621.

113. Kedia N, Ng K, Apperson-Hansen C, et al. Usefulness of atrioventricular delay optimization using Doppler assessment of mitral inflow in patients undergoing cardiac resynchronization therapy. Am J Cardiol 2006; 98:780–785.

114. Bordachar P, Garrigue S, Reuter S, et al. Hemodynamic assessment of right, left, and biventricular pacing by peak endocardial acceleration and echocardiography in patients with end-stage heart failure. Pacing Clin Electrophysiol 2000; 23:1726–1730.

115. Sogaard P, Egeblad H, Pedersen AK, et al. Sequential versus simultaneous biventricular resynchronization for severe heart failure: evaluation by tissue Doppler imaging. Circulation 2002; 106:2078–2084.

116. Bordachar P, Garrigue S, Lafitte S, et al. Interventricular and intra-left ventricular electromechanical delays in right ventricular paced patients with heart failure: implications for upgrading to biventricular stimulation. Heart 2003; 89:1401–1405.

117. Cannesson M, Farhat F, Scarlata M, et al. The impact of atrio-biventricular pacing on hemodynamics and left ventricular dyssynchrony compared with atrio-right ventricular pacing alone in the postoperative period after cardiac surgery. J Cardiothorac Vasc Anesth 2009; 23:306–311.

118. Artrip JH, Sukerman D, Dickstein ML, et al. Transesophageal echocardiography guided placement of a coronary sinus pacing lead. Ann Thorac Surg 2002; 74:1254–1256.

119. Bashir JG, Frank G, Tyers O, et al. Combined use of transesophageal ECHO and fluoroscopy for the placement of left ventricular pacing leads via the coronary sinus. Pacing Clin Electrophysiol 2003; 26:1951–1954.

30

TEE in the Intensive Care Unit and in Noncardiac Surgery

Martin Girard
Université de Montréal, Montreal, Quebec, Canada

Ashraf Fayad
University of Ottawa, Ottawa, Ontario, Canada

Antoine Vieillard-Baron
Hôpital Ambroise-Paré, Boulogne, France

INTRODUCTION

Since the introduction of intraoperative transesophageal echocardiography (TEE) during cardiac surgery in the 1980s, technological advances have dramatically influenced the way physicians use TEE. In the very early stages, the main application of TEE was assessment of global and regional left ventricular (LV) function. Now, the use of TEE has expanded beyond the cardiac operating room (OR), and its clinical usefulness is recognized in various noncardiac surgical procedures and in the intensive care unit (ICU).

While TEE can be used to diagnose a variety of pathologies, such as pulmonary embolism, infective endocarditis, and right-to-left shunts, it is first, and foremost, the most powerful hemodynamic monitoring tool available to physicians. Unexpected findings have consistently been reported with its use leading to changes in patients' management both in the noncardiac OR (1–6) and in the ICU (3,7–10). Another important feature of TEE is its portability that allows it to be performed at the bedside while other measures to stabilize the patient continue. As an example, the use of TEE during cardiopulmonary resuscitation (CPR) may lead to more specific and potentially life-saving therapy (11). Finally, with a complication rate of 3% and no procedure-related mortality, TEE should be considered a safe technique when performed in intubated patients (see Chapter 8) (10).

This chapter will focus on the use of TEE as a diagnostic and hemodynamic monitoring tool in the ICU and during noncardiac surgery.

TEE AS A DIAGNOSTIC TOOL

Thoracic Aorta Dissection

Aortic dissection is associated with a high mortality rate especially when diagnosis and treatment are unduly delayed. The test of choice in hemodynamically unstable patients when aortic dissection is suspected is TEE (12). By visualizing two distinct lumens, separated by an intimal flap, TEE can establish a diagnosis of dissection (Fig. 30.1). More importantly, TEE allows identification of the sites of intimal tear and can distinguish between communicating and noncommunicating dissections (12). In addition, TEE has the ability to identify related complications of dissection such as pleural and pericardial effusion (Fig. 30.2), aortic regurgitation (AR) (Fig. 30.1), and involvement of aortic side branches. In a meta-analysis comparing various imaging modalities to diagnose aortic dissection, TEE was found to have a sensitivity of 98% and a specificity of 95% (13). This topic is discussed in detail in Chapter 23.

Endocarditis

Although infective endocarditis is a relatively infrequent entity, it still has a reported in-hospital mortality of over 15% (14). Diagnosis of endocarditis is based on the modified Duke criteria that integrate clinical, microbiological, and echocardiographic data (see Chapter 25). According to the American Heart Association (AHA), when high clinical suspicion of endocarditis exists, TEE is the examination of choice (15). TEE is also the examination of choice in patients who are at high risk of endocarditis such as those with a prosthetic valve, previous endocarditis, congenital heart disease, new murmur, new heart failure, or stigmata of endocarditis (15). Despite technical advances in transthoracic echocardiography (TTE) imaging, TEE is still considered to be a superior modality to detect vegetations with high sensitivity (95%) and specificity (98%) (16).

Echocardiographic features of valve masses suggestive of endocarditis include (*i*) chaotic motion that is independent of other cardiac structures with fine vibrations; (*ii*) location along a high-velocity jet and/ or on the upstream side of the valve when it regurgitates; (*iii*) gray scale texture and reflectance in relation to the myocardium with calcification; (*iv*) amorphous

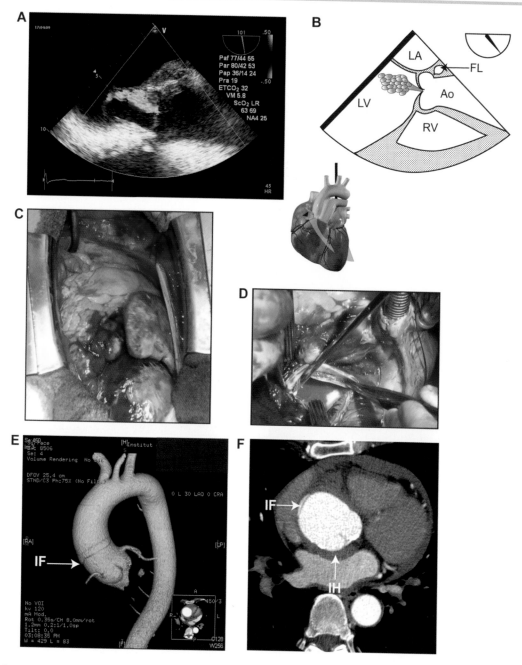

Figure 30.1 Acute aortic dissection in a 62-year-old man with known aortic regurgitation. The patient presented in the emergency room with acute chest pain irradiating to his back. He was initially hemodynamically stable. (**A,B**) Mid-esophageal aortic long-axis view showing moderate aortic regurgitation eccentrically directed toward the anterior mitral leaflet due to a prolapsed right coronary cusp. (**C,D**) Corresponding intraoperative findings before (**C**) and after (**D**) opening of the ascending Ao just above a visible IH. (**E,F**) Computed tomography showing the hematoma as well as an IF 2 cm above the origin of the right coronary artery. *Abbreviations*: Ao, aorta; ETCO$_2$, end-tidal carbon dioxide; IF, intimal flap; IH, intramural hematoma; FL, false lumen; L, left; LA, left atrium; LV, left ventricle; NA, noradrenaline; Paf, femoral arterial pressure; Pap, pulmonary artery pressure; Par, radial arterial pressure; Pra, right atrial pressure; R, right; RV, right ventricle; ScO$_2$, regional brain saturation; VM, minute ventilation. *Source*: Courtesy of Drs. Michel Carrier and Carl Chartrand-Lefebvre.

shape; and (*v*) associated abscess, fistula, new valve regurgitation or obstruction, prosthetic valve dehiscence, paravalvular leaks, valve perforation, or other endovascular prosthetic material superinfection (see Chapter 25) (Fig. 30.3).

Cardioembolic Stroke

Stroke is the second leading cause of death worldwide (17). It has been estimated that up to one-sixth of strokes are of cardioembolic origin (18). After a negative

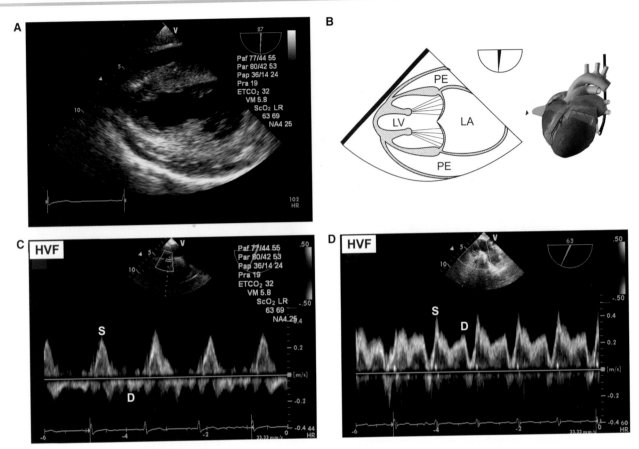

Figure 30.2   Pericardial tamponade in a patient with aortic dissection. The same patient as in Figure 30.1 became hemodynami-cally unstable after the induction of anesthesia, requiring vasoactive support with noradrenaline up to 6.7 µg/min. (**A,B**) Transgastric long-axis view at 87° with a PE present. (**C**) Pulsed wave Doppler of the HVF flow with absent diastolic forward flow, consistent with tamponade (see chap. 12). (**D**) Normalization of the HVF after pericardial drainage, with diastolic forward flow restored. *Abbreviations*: D, peak diastolic HVF velocity; ETCO₂, end-tidal carbon dioxide; HVF, hepatic venous flow; L, left; LA, left atrium; LV, left ventricle; NA, noradrenaline; Paf, femoral arterial pressure; Pap, pulmonary artery pressure; Par, radial arterial pressure; Pra, right atrial pressure; PE, pericardial effusion; R, right; ScO₂, regional brain saturation; S, peak systolic HVF velocity; VM, minute ventilation.

workup, consisting of electrocardiography (EKG), vas-cular ultrasound, computed tomography (CT), and/or magnetic resonance (MRI), and TTE, 30% of patients with acute ischemic stroke will see their treatment changed on the basis of new TEE findings (19). Potential sources of cardioembolic stroke can be classified into three broad categories: atrial fibrillation (i.e., left atrial or left atrial appendage clot), cardiovascular masses, and paradoxical emboli (Fig. 30.4).

Acute Pulmonary Embolism

In the United States, an estimated 300,000 people die each year from an acute pulmonary embolus (APE) (20). Untreated, APE has a mortality rate of 25% to 30%, while early diagnosis and treatment reduces mortality to 2%–8% (20). Unfortunately, a diagnosis of clinically significant APE is not made until autopsy in 20% of hospitalized patients (20). As death usually results from right ventricular (RV) failure secondary to the increased afterload, the European Society of

Cardiology has defined the term of massive APE for patients with RV failure and shock and the term of submassive APE in hemodynamically stable patients with RV dysfunction (21).

Diagnosis

Diagnosis of APE is a complex issue, and various diagnostic algorithms have been proposed (20). Because of its general availability and accuracy, CT angiography has played in recent years an increas-ingly important role in these algorithms (22). Impor-tantly, CT angiography has also been shown to be able to detect RV dysfunction that has prognostic and possible treatment implications. However, unstable patients and patients with contrast allergy or renal failure have relative contraindications to CT angiog-raphy (22). Furthermore, patients undergoing surgery or CPR simply cannot be moved to the radiology or nuclear medicine department. Consequently, echocar-diography has an important, albeit limited, role to play in the diagnosis of APE. An echocardiographic

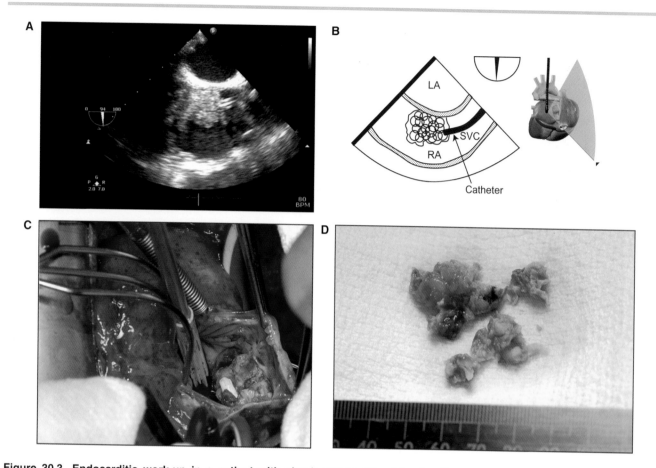

Figure 30.3 Endocarditis work-up in a patient with shock and positive blood cultures. (A,B) Mid-esophageal bicaval view showing a mass attached to a dialysis catheter in the RA, suspected as the nidus of infection. **(C,D)** Corresponding intraoperative findings and pathological specimen. *Abbreviation*: LA, left atrium; RA, right atrium; SVC, superior vena cava. *Source*: Courtesy of Drs. André Martineau and Éric Charbonneau.

diagnosis of APE can be made by either directly visualizing thrombus (Fig. 30.5) or, more frequently, by assessing the impact of APE on the RV. For safety reasons, we do not recommend that TEE be performed in patients who are not intubated.

Direct Visualization

Direct visualization of thrombi, in either the right heart cavities or the pulmonary vasculature, is sufficient evidence to diagnose APE (Fig. 30.5). Thrombus originating from lower extremity deep veins or central abdominal veins often represents an inner cast of the large vessels. As it travels through the RA, the long thrombus gets entangled in the tricuspid valve apparatus and presents the characteristic "popcorn" appearance of a thrombus-in-transit (see Fig. 25.26). Mostly seen in the right atrium (RA), right heart thrombi have been reported in approximately 4% of cases (range 0–8%) (23–25), while a higher incidence (~20%) is reported in massive APE (range 4–26%) (26,27).

With the exception of the middle segment of the left pulmonary artery (PA), TEE can detect thrombi in the central pulmonary vasculature up to the beginning of lobar arteries (28). However, only approximately 60% of patients with massive or submassive APE have thrombi in their central pulmonary vasculature (28). In those patients, TEE is accurate in diagnosing APE (sensitivity ~85%, specificity ~95%) but has low sensitivity for locating individual thrombi (26,28). This apparent discrepancy can be explained by the frequent, simultaneous, presence of multiple thrombi in the pulmonary vasculature. Use of TEE in pulmonary embolectomy to ensure complete removal of thrombi is a category 2 indication of the Society of Cardiovascular Anesthesiology (SCA) guidelines (29). However, more recent TEE guidelines would support the routine use of TEE in the high-risk patients (see Chapter 31). Because of the limited sensitivity of TEE for localizing all thrombi, it is doubtful that TEE can accomplish this role. However, TEE is extremely useful to locate extrapulmonary thrombi, which also need to be removed, and can potentially lead to a change in cannulation site prior to cardiopulmonary bypass (CPB) to prevent thrombi dislodgement and embolization (see Fig. 22.4) (26).

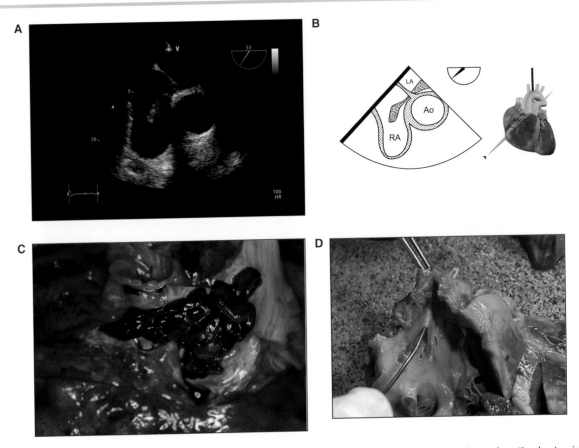

Figure 30.4 **Paradoxical embolism in a 48-year-old man with acute hypotension. (A,B)** Mid-esophageal aortic short-axis view at 55° showing a thrombus crossing a PFO. **(C)** Corresponding intraoperative findings of other thrombi in the pulmonary arteries. **(D)** Autopsy finding of a PFO from another patient who died of refractory hypoxia. *Abbreviations*: Ao, aorta; LA, left atrium; PFO, patent formamen ovale; RA, right atrium. *Source*: Courtesy of Drs. Michel Pellerin and Tack Ki Leung.

Indirect Signs—General Population

In most cases, actual thrombi will not be visualized and signs of acute pulmonary hypertension and secondary RV dysfunction will be helpful and strongly suggestive, but not pathognomonic, of APE. Only a few echocardiographic signs have been tested in more than one prospective cohort study. These include the right-to-left ventricular end-diastolic area (RVEDA/LVEDA) ratio (cutoff >1, sensitivity ~45%, specificity ~90%) and tricuspid regurgitation (TR) peak velocity (cutoff >2.7 cm/s, sensitivity ~60%, specificity ~90%) (30,31). Combining the RVEDA/LVEDA ratio and the TR peak velocity, and more complex indices do not significantly improve accuracy. However, the precision of the above heavily depends on the enrolled patients' comorbidities. A major decrease in specificity followed the inclusion of a significant number of patients with chronic cardiorespiratory diseases (32).

Other echocardiographic signs have been studied in single prospective cohort studies. These include the right-to-left ventricular end-diastolic diameter ratio (33), the presence of abnormal septal motion (33), different cutoffs of the TR peak velocity (33), and RV hypokinesis (31). Originally thought to be very specific for APE (32,34), the McConnell sign, a pattern of preserved contraction of the RV basal and apical segment with concomitant severe hypokinesis of the mid free wall, is also seen in the majority of patients with RV infarcts (35). Using two-dimensional strain imaging, regional RV dysfunction can also be observed in non-ischemic conditions such as fluid overload (Fig. 30.6) and in ischemic RV dysfunction (Fig. 30.7). Not as well known, the 60/60 sign, a combination of pulmonary flow acceleration time ≤60 ms and TR pressure gradient ≤60 mmHg (36), seems very specific but nevertheless insensitive (32). Finally, promising new indices include the assessment of tricuspid annular motion (37), the M-index (mitral E wave/RV myocardial performance index) (38), and the percentage difference in left and right pulmonary artery (LPA, RPA) time-velocity integral [(TVI$_{LPA}$–TVI$_{RPA}$)/mean TVI], a marker of flow asymmetry in the LPA/RPA (39).

Indirect Signs—Hemodynamically Unstable Patients

Echocardiographic indices of RV dysfunction are more sensitive as indirect signs of APE in patients with hemodynamic instability. Studies using a different

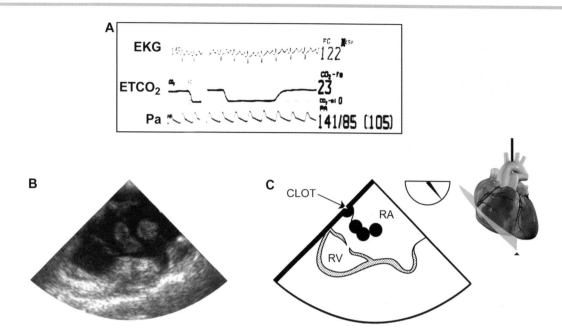

Figure 30.5 Acute pulmonary emboli. This 68-year-old woman presented with dyspnea and hypotension four weeks after a brain meningioma removal. **(A)** Hemodynamic data: heart rate of 122 beats/min, Pa of 141/85 mmHg on noradrenaline at 10 μg/min with ET CO_2 of 22 mmHg. Note the peaked P-waves on the EKG waveform suggesting right atrial dilatation. **(B,C)** Mid-esophageal modified bicaval view at 120° showing highly mobile clots floating in the RA. *Abbreviations*: EKG, electrocardiogram; $ETCO_2$, end-tidal carbon dioxide; Pa, arterial pressure; RA, right atrium; RV, right ventricle. *Source*: Photo B courtesy of Dr. Guy Cousineau.

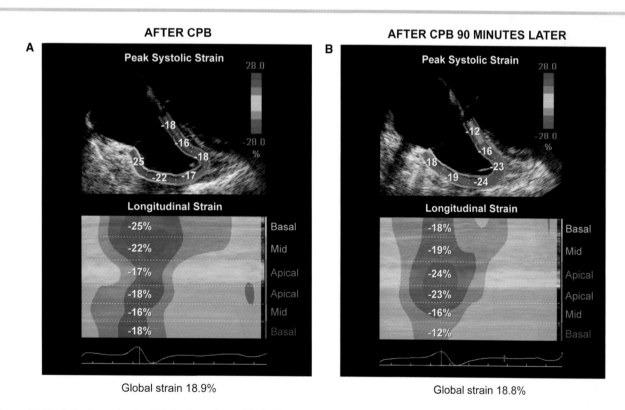

Figure 30.6 Apical sparing in RV dysfunction with fluid overload, assessed by 2D speckle tracking strain imaging. (A,B) Mid-esophageal four-chamber view of the RV in a patient with hemorrhagic shock. With massive fluid resuscitation, gradual reduction in the basal function of the RV was observed with compensatory increase in the apical strain. *Abbreviations*: CPB, cardiopulmonary bypass; RV, right ventricle.

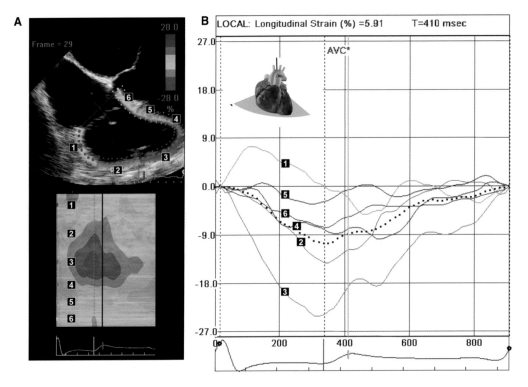

Figure 30.7   Apical sparing in RV dysfunction from RCA occlusion, assessed by 2D speckle tracking strain imaging. (A,B) Mid-esophageal right ventricular view with basal dysfunction in a patient after cardiac arrest and right coronary occlusion. Note the gradual reduction in the longitudinal strain values in basal segments (mostly 1) with preservation of the apical segments. *Abbreviations*: AVC, aortic valve closure; RCA, right coronary artery; RV, right ventricle.

composite index of echocardiographic signs of RV dysfunction demonstrated a sensitivity of approximately 98% for the diagnosis of APE in hemodynamically compromised patients compared with a sensitivity of approximately 50% in normotensive patients (40,41). Finally, TEE has also been shown to be useful for the diagnosis of APE during ongoing CPR in the wards, in the OR, and in the immediate postarrest period (42–44). Anticoagulation is the cornerstone of treatment for APE. The presence of right heart thrombi is a particular situation where thrombolysis is associated with a lower mortality and is rapidly efficacious (45). TEE may have a role in documenting the effect of thrombolysis on visible thrombi.

Assessment of Unexplained Hypoxemia

Hypoxia is a frequently encountered problem in the ICU. Few studies have reported echocardiographic findings in critically ill patients with unexplained hypoxemia. However, right-to-left shunting through a patent foramen ovale (PFO) or an atrial septal defect (ASD) has consistently been found to be the main mechanism responsible for the unexplained hypoxemia in these patients (2) (see Chapter 26).

Right-to-left shunting should be suspected in any ventilated patient with a PaO_2 <400 mmHg while receiving 100% FiO_2 and with no or minimal pulmonary infiltrate on chest X-ray (46). Right-to-left

shunting is not physiological and, with few exceptions (47), requires conditions of increased right-sided pressures such as the use of positive end-expiratory pressure (PEEP), RV infarction, APE, postpneumonectomy and post-CPB states. A PFO, or any right-to-left shunt, can be detected by injecting agitated saline as contrast medium in a peripheral vein (see Chapter 26). In the presence of severe hypoxemia, closure of the PFO or ASD with an occlusion device leads to an immediate improvement in SaO_2 (see Chapter 29). Because of the relatively frequent occurrence of postoperative shunting, prophylactic closure of a PFO has been advocated by some before pneumonectomy (48). Finally, while infrequent, intrapulmonary right-to-left shunting, responsible for severe hypoxemia, can occur in diseases such as hepatopulmonary syndrome and Osler–Weber–Rendu disease (46).

TEE AS A HEMODYNAMIC MONITORING TOOL

Advantages of TEE over the Pulmonary Artery Catheter

The pulmonary artery catheter (PAC) is a tool familiar to the majority of physicians, but in a large randomized controlled trial, its use has not been shown to result in improved outcome (49). As more than one mechanism is often present in hemodynamically unstable patients, their interplay makes PAC-based diagnosis difficult and often misleading (50). When used in PAC-equipped patients, TEE consistently identifies new causes of hemodynamic instability that leads to changes in the management (50,51). Accordingly, hemodynamic instability is a class I indication of the SCA TEE practice guidelines (29). As will be detailed below, TEE has the unique ability to assess, simultaneously, the major determinants of cardiac function and venous return. Finally, TEE, like the PAC, can measure SV, and its evolution should be followed to assess the impact of therapeutic interventions.

Assessment of Acute Hemodynamic Decompensation

Vascular Volume Assessment

A monitoring tool, with good sensitivity and specificity, to assess the fluid-responsiveness status of patients is highly desirable. Echocardiographic parameters of fluid responsiveness and other indices such as ΔP_{pleth} (respiratory variations of the plethysmographic pulse wave), ΔPP_{art} (respiratory variations of the pulse pressure measured using an arterial catheter), and esophageal Doppler-derived dynamic indices can be useful in the OR (52) and in the ICU (53) (see Table 10.1). Static volumetric indices such as LVEDA and Doppler indices are inaccurate markers of fluid responsiveness and should not be relied upon. Depending on the clinical setting, we recommend the use of one of the indices of cardiorespiratory interactions (see Table 10.1) or the use of indices obtained after passive leg raising (PLR) for the assessment of fluid responsiveness.

To circumvent the limitations of cardiorespiratory interactions, the PLR maneuver has been advocated as a way to generate, transiently, an increased preload and evaluate its effect on cardiac output (CO). Early results studying the effect of PLR on changes in aortic velocity-time integral ($\%VTI_{Ao}$) are very encouraging. A significant increase of aortic VTI following PLR has been shown to predict an increase in CO following IV fluid administration. Notably, these studies included spontaneously breathing patients (54,55) or patients with atrial fibrillation (55). The use of automated beds makes this technique relatively simple to perform (56). Preload (e.g., LVEDA) should be monitored to ensure that sufficient volume is recruited by PLR. Unfortunately, by its very nature, PLR-guided assessment of fluid responsiveness cannot be automated or be continuously available. Finally, it will not be possible to implement the PLR maneuver in a number of clinical settings, including most situations in the OR.

Left or Right Ventricular Dysfunction

LV systolic dysfunction. LV systolic dysfunction is thought to be the main factor causing hemodynamic instability in 15% to 27% of critically ill patients (7–10). In high-risk patients undergoing noncardiac surgery, 10% to 20% are found to have unexpected LV systolic dysfunction (1,4). Common causes of acute LV systolic dysfunction include myocardial infarction (MI), septic shock, stress cardiomyopathy, toxic ingestion, medication side effect, and myocarditis.

From a physiological point of view, contractility is the fundamental determinant of CO reflecting systolic function, even though no simple echocardiographic method allows it to be easily quantified. Although left ventricular ejection fraction (LVEF) is an imperfect surrogate for contractility, it is a marker of the adequacy of the ventricle's contractile state for its current loading conditions as significant changes in either preload or afterload can markedly affect it (see Chapter 10). For example, while not affecting contractility per se, increased afterload from sudden severe hypertension or aortic cross clamping will lead to a drop in LVEF. In such a case, measurement of contractility would be falsely reassuring, while the decreased LVEF will accurately reflect the drop in SV from the increased afterload. Conversely, as can be seen in septic shock, a normal LVEF in a severely vasoplegic patient may not indicate a normal systolic function. Restoration of a proper blood pressure and the ensuing increase in afterload may unmask underlying systolic dysfunction and a severely depressed LVEF (57). For similar reasons, LVEF should be used carefully in patients with significant mitral regurgitation (MR) as it provides a low-pressure outlet to the LV. This afterload-reducing effect will result in an increased LVEF, which will then reflect both the ejected and regurgitated fractions of the LV.

Another important physiological consideration in the evaluation of LV systolic function is the ventricle's low compliance that is responsible for its limited ability to acutely dilate under an increased load (58,59). LV dilation is a chronic compensatory mechanism that aims to maintain SV despite low contractility. Thus, an acute drop in LVEF is more likely to require inotropic support because of low SV compared with a chronically dilated LV with similar LVEF.

RV systolic dysfunction. Often neglected, RV failure is the main mechanism of shock in 3% to 18% of critically ill patients and is unexpectedly found in 4% to 6% of high-risk patients undergoing noncardiac surgery (1,4,7,8,10). Common causes of acute RV systolic dysfunction include fluid overload (Fig. 30.6), MI (Fig. 30.7), septic shock, acute respiratory distress syndrome (ARDS), and APE.

Acute RV failure with signs of increased afterload defines acute cor pulmonale. Regardless of the mechanism of RV failure, an important corollary of acute RV dilatation in the fixed pericardial space is direct LV compression with resulting impaired LV filling (see Chapter 10). In addition to the already decreased RV stroke volume, this will cause an even greater decrease in LV output and mean arterial pressure (MAP).

Decreased MAP from a failing RV is an ominous sign and may lead to RV ischemia. A relatively stable situation can rapidly deteriorate with RV ischemia as the resulting additional drop in MAP can further compromise blood supply to the RV and lead to a vicious cycle of autoaggravation (60,61).

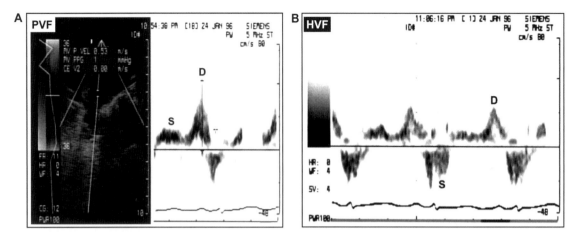

Figure 30.8   Diastolic dysfunction in a hemodynamically unstable patient with subarachnoid hemorrhage. (**A**) Pulsed wave Doppler of the PVF with abnormal diastolic flow predominance with prominent atrial reversal. (**B**) Pulsed wave Doppler of the HVF flow showing similar findings. *Abbreviations*: D, peak diastolic velocity; HVF, hepatic venous flow; PVF, pulmonary venous flow; S, peak systolic velocity. *Source*: Adapted with permission of McLaughin et al. from Ref. 67.

Left and right ventricular diastolic dysfunction. Affecting up to 35% of individuals above 60 years of age (62), chronic LV diastolic dysfunction is a frequent disease whose clinical importance has only recently been appreciated. For example, roughly half of patients with clinical heart failure have a normal ejection fraction, and these patients have a similar prognosis to patients with decreased LVEF (63). Up until recently, most echocardiographic markers of diastolic function were very dependent on loading conditions that made them impractical to study in critically ill patients. Less influenced by preload, a new generation of echocardiographic tools such as annular early diastolic velocity (E' or E_m) and mitral inflow propagation velocity (V_p) has created renewed interest in the study of diastolic dysfunction in the OR and the ICU. A detailed description of the echocardiographic assessment of diastolic function and of chronic left and right diastolic dysfunction is presented in Chapter 10.

Acute left diastolic dysfunction has been described in situations as varied as sepsis (64), cross clamping in vascular surgery (65), myocardial ischemia (66), subarachnoid hemorrhage (67) (Fig. 30.8), post-CPB (68), and RV dilatation (69), while acute right diastolic dysfunction has been described in APE (70), RV MI (71), ARDS, and post-CPB (72).

Suspected Tamponade

Depending on the studied population, cardiac tamponade is identified as the principal factor responsible for hemodynamic instability in 4% to 11% of critically ill patients (7,9,10). Frequent causes of pericardial effusion leading to tamponade include malignancy, cardiac surgery, acute pericarditis, and iatrogenic perforation during catheter-based procedures (73). Neither physical examination nor echocardiography allow for a definitive diagnosis, an approach that

combines the clinical context, findings on physical examination, and echocardiography is necessary (74).

Importantly, positive pressure ventilation makes analysis of respiratory variations in transvalvular flows challenging (see Chapter 12). However, in the presence of RV collapse (Fig. 30.9) or, in patients not subjected to positive pressure ventilation, of respiratory changes in transvalvular and central venous flow provides good supporting evidence for tamponade, while the absence of RA collapse is a strong argument against it (75). Finally, in cardiac surgery patients, atypical findings are the norm and tamponade should be considered in any hemodynamically unstable patient (Fig. 30.9). In more than half of the patients, tamponade will be secondary to compression of the LA and/or ventricle from a loculated posterior effusion (77).

Dynamic Outflow Tract Obstruction

Dynamic left ventricular outflow tract (LVOT) obstruction may show elevated wedge pressure and low cardiac index (CI) on PAC monitoring and masquerade as cardiogenic shock (78) (Fig. 30.10). Proper diagnosis is crucial since the treatment for the latter (i.e., diuretics, inotropes, intra-aortic balloon counterpulsation, and afterload-reducing agents) will likely exacerbate the hemodynamic instability due to dynamic LVOT obstruction (see Fig. 21.6), whereas administration of fluid, vasopressors, and even β-blockers should instead be the appropriate intervention (see Fig 11.13). In unselected ICU patients who underwent TEE for hemodynamic instability, dynamic LVOT obstruction was a rare finding and its incidence ranged from 1% to 3% (7,8). The occurrence of dynamic LVOT obstruction after aortic valve (AoV) replacement (see Fig 10.30) is not a benign finding and carries adverse prognostic value, with longer hospital stays and increased morbidity and mortality as discussed in Chapter 15 (79,80).

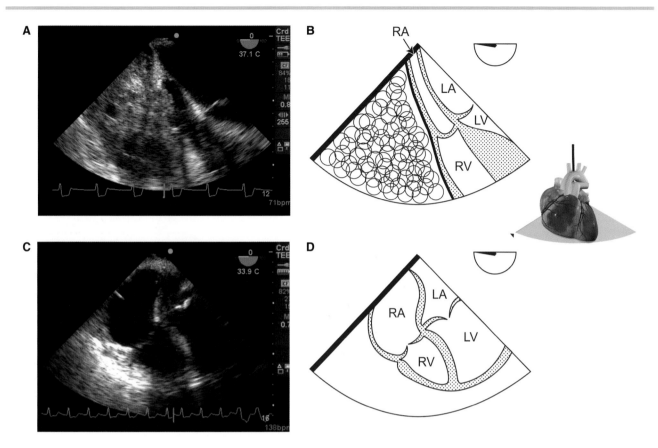

Figure 30.9 Cardiac tamponade in a 68-year-old woman hemodynamically unstable after cardiac surgery. (A,B) Mid-esophageal four-chamber view with a clot compressing the RA. **(C,D)** Control after clot evacuation. *Abbreviations*: LA, left atrium; LV, left ventricle; RA, right atrium; RV, right ventricle. *Source*: With permission of Durand et al. Ref. 76.

Acute Valvular Insufficiency

Acute severe regurgitation of the mitral valve (MV) and AoV has been reported as a cause of hemodynamic instability in 2% to 3% of critically ill patients (8,9). The acuteness of the valvular lesion is an important prerequisite to the development of hemodynamic instability as this prevents development of any meaningful physiological adaptation.

In the SHOCK trial registry, acute severe MR following MI was thought to be responsible for cardiogenic shock in 8% of cases (81). Other important etiologies of acute severe MR include degenerative MV disease and acute endocarditis. While less common than acute severe MR, acute severe AR is also an important cause of hemodynamic instability and is most frequently caused by acute aortic dissection, acute endocarditis, and thoracic trauma (82). Acute severe TR is an exceptionally rare cause of cardiovascular collapse but can occur following endocarditis or thoracic trauma. Finally, because of their chronic development, severe aortic stenosis and mitral stenosis rarely present with cardiovascular collapse without an intercurrent disease responsible for their decompensation. A complete description of valvular assessment is presented in chapters 14, 16, and 18.

Others

Because of the diversity involved, a complete list of the various causes of hemodynamic instability is impossible to compile. A few examples of less-frequent mechanisms that can lead to cardiovascular collapse include intracardiac obstruction [e.g., obstructing atrial myxoma (83)], extracardiac compression [e.g., anterior mediastinal tumors (84)], and intracardiac shunts [e.g., ventricular septal defects (VSDs) (85)]. In the event that a clear mechanism is not readily identified, performing a systematic TEE examination and keeping an open mind are important.

SPECIFIC TEE CONSIDERATIONS IN THE ICU

Septic Shock

Severe sepsis is a worldwide problem and was responsible for over 200,000 deaths in 1995 in the United States alone (86). Septic shock is the result of the complex interplay of many circulatory abnormalities that include relative and absolute volume depletion, LV systolic and diastolic dysfunction, RV dysfunction, and vasoplegia (87). In this context, establishing the correct diagnosis and initiating

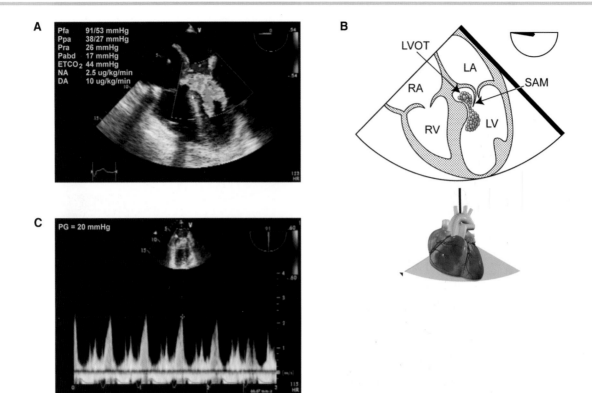

Figure 30.10 Dynamic LVOT obstruction in a 47-year-old man following cardiac arrest from RCA occlusion. (A,B) Mid-esophageal four-chamber view with flow acceleration in the LVOT with SAM. **(C)** Continuous wave Doppler showing a late-peaking systolic gradient of 20 mmHg after treatment. The LVOT obstruction was thought to be secondary to both inotropes usage and RV dilatation from the RCA occlusion. *Abbreviations*: DA, dopamine; ETCO$_2$, end-tidal carbon dioxide; LA, left atrium, LV, left ventricle; LVOT, left ventricular outflow tract obstruction; NA, noradrenaline; Pabd, abdominal pressure; Pfa, femoral arterial pressure; PG, pressure gradient; Ppa, pulmonary artery pressure; Pra, right atrial pressure; RA, right atrium; RCA, right coronary artery; RV, right ventricle; SAM, systolic anterior motion.

proper treatment can be a daunting task. Yet, this must be accomplished in a time-efficient fashion as rapid correction of the above has been shown to lead to an appreciable decrease in mortality in a randomized controlled trial (88) and meta-analysis (89).

While various monitoring devices are available to the clinician, TEE is ideally suited for this task because of its unique ability to evaluate all of the above-stated circulation abnormalities and to have an impact on the treatment (Fig. 30.11) (90). Finally, TEE can also have prognostic implications in septic shock as a hyperkinetic LV has been linked with increased mortality (91,92).

LV systolic dysfunction defined as an LVEF less than 40% to 45% was observed in 30% to 40% of septic patients (57,64,90). Interestingly, when sought, an additional 20% of septic patients developed depressed LVEF over the following 48 hours (57) (Fig. 30.12). It remains unclear if this phenomenon is due to sepsis per se or if abnormal contractility is unmasked by the increased afterload from vasopressor administration. Daily LV function reassessment should thus be considered in the first few days of septic shock in the advent of lack of response to therapy. In virtually all patients, this LV systolic dysfunction is reversible and may normalize within four to five days (57).

While the existence of sepsis-induced diastolic dysfunction has long been suspected (93), methodological issues have precluded careful analysis. With the advent of tissue Doppler imaging (TDI), LV diastolic dysfunction can be found in 20% to 40% of these patients (64,94). While most patients recover normal diastolic function, not all do and it is hypothesized that these patients had preexisting diastolic dysfunction (64). Therapeutic implications of diastolic dysfunction are unclear at present.

Often neglected, the study of RV dysfunction in septic patients has led to the reporting of a wide range of incidences (range 11–38%) (58,94). This is despite using similar methodology (RVEDA/LVEDA ratio) and probably, in part, reflects the different incidences of acute lung injury and ARDS (94) and concomitant LV systolic dysfunction in the studied populations.

Adult Respiratory Distress Syndrome

For the last 25 years, mechanical ventilation has been known to cause profound hemodynamic changes (95), including increased RV afterload. While most patients suffering from ARDS require mechanical ventilation, ARDS itself has been shown to cause increased

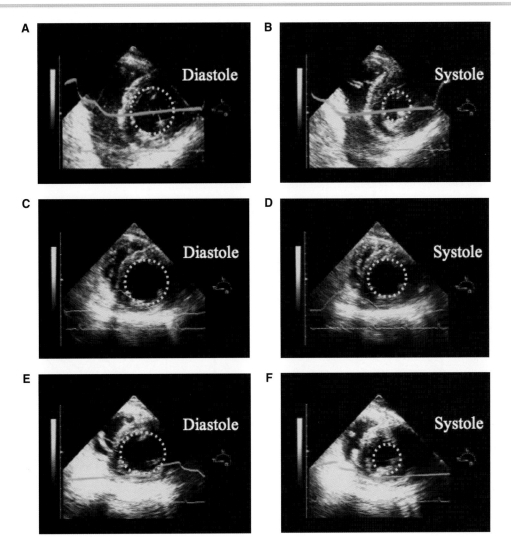

Figure 30.11 LV function in septic shock. Transgastric mid-papillary short-axis views with tracing of the LV end-diastolic and end-systolic areas for systolic function evaluation. (**A,B**) After initial resuscitation, the patient's hemodynamic status had stabilized on a norepinephrine infusion. The LV systolic function initially appears preserved. (**C,D**) The following day, hypotension and acidosis occurs without apparent reason and despite an unchanged dose of norepinephrine. Note the increased end-systolic area consistent with new diffuse LV systolic dysfunction. (**E,F**) Treatment with intravenous dobutamine led to normalization of the LV systolic function and improvement of his hemodynamic parameters. While sepsis-induced myocardial depression usually manifests during the first 24 hours, delayed occurrence over the following 48 hours is possible. *Abbreviations*: LV, left ventricular; TEE, transesophageal echocardiographic.

pulmonary vascular resistance (96). The combined afterload increasing effect of both mechanical ventilation and ARDS can lead to RV dysfunction. RV dysfunction in ARDS has been shown to cause adverse hemodynamic effects and to be a powerful factor of adverse prognosis (97).

Acute cor pulmonale is the echocardiographic manifestation of RV systolic dysfunction. Briefly, it features an increased RVEDA, an increased RVEDA/LVEDA ratio, septal flattening, and septal paradoxical motion (see Chapter 10). Improvements in mechanical ventilation have led to a decrease in its incidence from 60% to 25% (92), although up to 50% of severe ARDS cases still develop this complication (98). Doppler assessment of flow in the PA can be used to assess

the impact of mechanical ventilation on the RV (99). As a consequence of late systolic septal protrusion into the LV cavity from RV pressure overload, an abnormal LV relaxation pattern is seen in patients with acute cor pulmonale (92).

Published guidelines dealing with the ventilation of ARDS patients recommend keeping plateau pressures under 30 cmH$_2$O and tidal volumes less than 6 cc/kg (100). Despite strict adherence to these guidelines, 25% of patients still develop acute cor pulmonale and up to 50% of the most severe cases of ARDS (98). While it is likely that the majority of these cases simply reflect underlying disease severity, a contribution from mechanical ventilation cannot be excluded. Although a strategy to minimize the

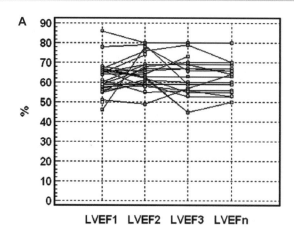

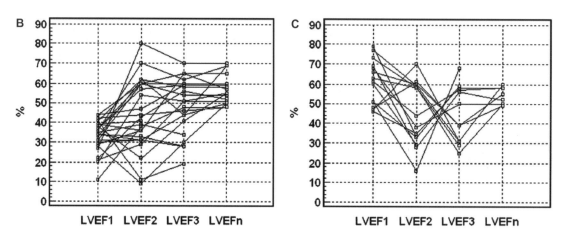

Figure 30.12 LV function in septic shock. Individual measurements of LVEF obtained on admission at day 1 (LVEF1), after 12–24 hours of vasoactive support on day 2 (LVEF2), 48 hours of vasoactive support on day 3 (LVEF3), and after weaning of vasoactive support on day n (LVEFn). (**A**) Non-hypokinetic patients (n = 27). (**B**) Primary hypokinetic patients (n = 26). (**C**) Secondary hypokinetic patients (n = 14). *Abbreviation*: LVEF, left ventricular ejection fraction. *Source*: adapted with permission from Vieillard-Baron et al., Ref. 57.

incidence of acute cor pulmonale aggressively was never tested in a randomized controlled trial, such a strategy was shown to result in identical mortality rates in patients with and without acute cor pulmonale (92).

Just like arterial blood gases are examined to adjust ventilatory parameters, echocardiographic data can play an important part in the ventilatory management of patients. When confronted with an ARDS patient having developed acute cor pulmonale, the following management strategy should be considered.

Minimizing Tidal Volume

Tidal volume insufflation has consistently been shown to impede RV ejection (101). Some have raised the possibility that limiting plateau pressure to lower than currently recommended levels may further decrease mortality (102). This mortality-lowering effect may be even more important in patients with acute cor pulmonale (103). In some cases, these patients do benefit

from further tidal volume reduction (Fig. 30.13). However, possibly stemming from its pulmonary vaso-constricting effect, hypercapnia has been associated with the occurrence of acute cor pulmonale (92). To limit the increase in PCO_2 resulting from tidal volume reduction, minimizing instrumental dead space is an interesting therapeutic avenue (104). Another option is increasing the set respiratory frequency. However, dynamic hyperinflation must be avoided as it leads to a further increase in afterload, worsening RV failure, and decreasing CO.

PEEP Titration

A controversial topic, PEEP titration, has been the recent subject of three large randomized controlled trials (105–107) with no definite answers as to the best strategy in ARDS patients. Increasing levels of PEEP have been shown to increase RV afterload and decrease CI in ARDS patients (Fig. 30.14). Increases in PEEP should thus be done very cautiously in these

TV= 400 mL Ppla = 33 cm H$_2$O

TV= 350 mL Ppla = 26 cm H$_2$O

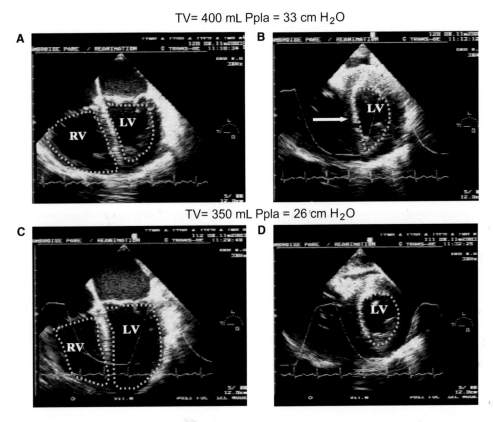

Figure 30.13 Effect of plateau pressure from mechanical ventilation on right ventricular function. Persistant hypotension (sBP 92 mmHg) in a patient with severe ARDS despite ventilation with a reduced TV of 400 mL (~6 mL/kg), associated with a Ppla of 33 cmH$_2$O. **(A)** Mid-esophageal four-chamber view and **(B)** transgastric mid-papillary view shows acute cor pulmonale with massive RV dilation, flattened ventricular septum with paradoxical motion (white arrow). **(C,D)** Further reduction in TV down to 350 mL with a Ppla to 26 cmH$_2$O immediately improved sBP up to 123 mmHg: a smaller RV and improved septal curvature were consistent with better RV systolic function. *Abbreviations*: ARDS, acute respiratory distress syndrome; LV, left ventricle; Ppla, plateau pressure; RV, right ventricle; TEE, transesophageal echocardiographic; TV, tidal volume.

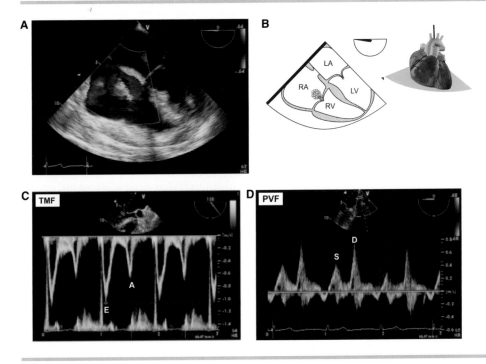

Figure 30.14 Ventricular function in a 75-year-old woman with acute hypoxic respiratory failure. (A,B) Mid-esophageal four-chamber view with RA and RV dilatation. **(C,D)** Pulsed wave Doppler of TMF and PVF are consistent with an associated moderate left ventricular diastolic dysfunction (pseudonormal pattern). However, in hypoxic respiratory failure requiring a high level of PEEP, relaxation abnormalities are more commonly reported. *Abbreviations*: A, peak late diastolic TMF velocity; D, peak diastolic PVF velocity; E, peak early diastolic TMF velocity; LA, left atrium; LV, left ventricle; PVF, pulmonary venous flow; RA, right atrium; RV, right ventricle; S, peak systolic PVF velocity; TMF, transmitral flow.

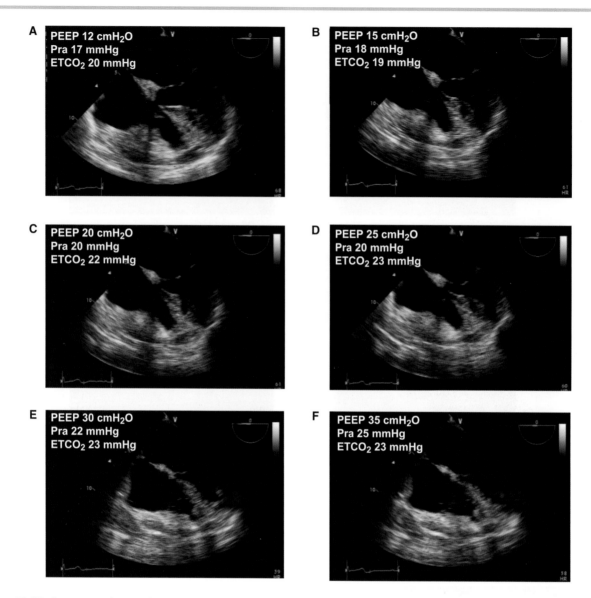

Figure 30.15 Lung recruitment in a 75-year-old woman with acute hypoxic respiratory failure. (A–F) Mid-esophageal four-chamber view. As PEEP is increased from 12 to 30 cmH_2O, a gradual increase in Pra from 17 to 25 mmHg is noted while the $ETCO_2$ increases to a maximum of 23 mmHg at 25 cmH_2O of PEEP. Reduction in the dimension of the RV and the RA were observed. *Abbreviations*: $ETCO_2$, end-tidal carbon dioxide; PEEP, positive end-expiratory pressure; Pra, right atrial pressure; RA, right atrium; RV, right ventricle.

patients and probably should not be attempted in patients with acute cor pulmonale who are at high risk of worsening RV failure. However, in cases of hypoxemic respiratory failure from massive atelectasis, lung recruitment might be beneficial. In these cases, increases in PEEP and intrathoracic pressures can be associated with reduction in right-sided cavities (Fig. 30.15) and improvement in RV function.

Prone Ventilation

Available data from randomized controlled trials (109–111) suggest a role for ventilating severe ARDS patients in the prone position. This is acknowledged by recent guidelines (100) that now suggest its use in such patients. Prone ventilation improves oxygenation, CO_2 elimination, and respiratory mechanics in the majority of ARDS patients (112). Patients with acute cor pulmonale seem to derive additional hemodynamic benefit. In a small observational study, a single session of prone ventilation was shown to decrease the severity of acute cor pulmonale and improve CO (98). Finally, high-frequency ventilation is another ventilation alternative in ARDS. We have observed improved RV function following initiation of this alternative mode of ventilation (Fig. 30.16).

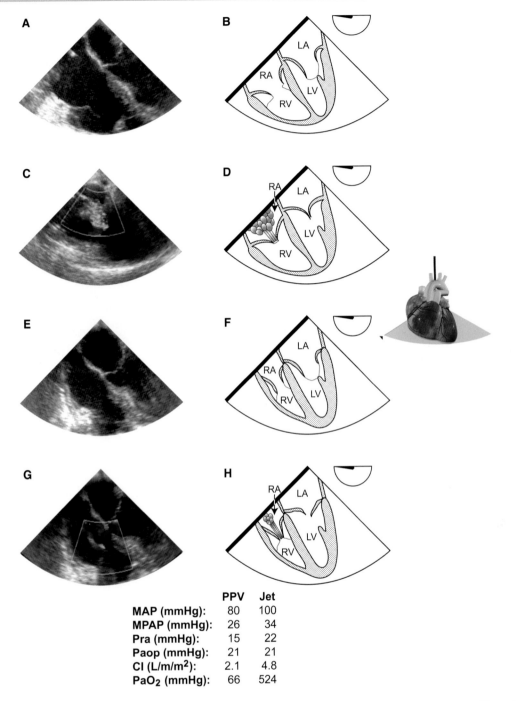

	PPV	Jet
MAP (mmHg):	80	100
MPAP (mmHg):	26	34
Pra (mmHg):	15	22
Paop (mmHg):	21	21
CI (L/m/m^2):	2.1	4.8
PaO$_2$ (mmHg):	66	524

Figure 30.16 Favorable effect of high-frequency jet ventilation on right ventricular function. Mid-esophageal four-chamber views in a 69-year-old man on PPV following cardiopulmonary bypass. (**A,B**) RV systolic dysfunction is present with RV dilatation. (**C,D**) Associated moderate tricuspid valve regurgitation. (**E,F**) With jet ventilation, right-sided cardiac chamber size decreases with better RV function. (**G,H**) Tricuspid regurgitation severity also improves, with associated increase in CI and PaO$_2$ on an inspired oxygen concentration of 100%. The reduction in pulmonary vascular resistance could be secondary to both the reduced tidal volume with jet ventilation and improved oxygenation. *Abbreviations*: CI, cardiac index; LA, left atrium; LV, left ventricle; MAP, mean arterial pressure; MPAP, mean pulmonary artery pressure; PaO$_2$, oxygen partial pressure; Paop, pulmonary artery occlusion pressure; PPV, positive-pressure ventilation; Pra, right atrial pressure; RA, right atrium; RV, right ventricle. 🖑

Stress Cardiomyopathy

Although most extensively studied in subarachnoid hemorrhage and in the apical ballooning syndrome, neurocardiac phenomena have also been described in patients suffering from other diseases such as traumatic brain injury (113,114). Emerging evidence now suggests that hyperactivity of the sympathetic limb of the autonomic nervous system is the common link between such seemingly unrelated diseases (115). While the apical ballooning syndrome and subarachnoid hemorrhage result in cardiac findings that are relatively characteristic, the prevailing view is that any acute physiological or emotional stress can, potentially, lead to variable combinations of acute systolic or diastolic LV and/or RV dysfunction.

Apical Ballooning Syndrome

Apical ballooning syndrome (also known as Tako-Tsubo cardiomyopathy) is a recently described entity that is indistinguishable from an acute coronary syndrome in its presentation (Fig. 30.17). It is estimated that 1% to 2% of all patients presenting with an acute coronary syndrome are diagnosed with apical ballooning syndrome (116,117). That number could rise

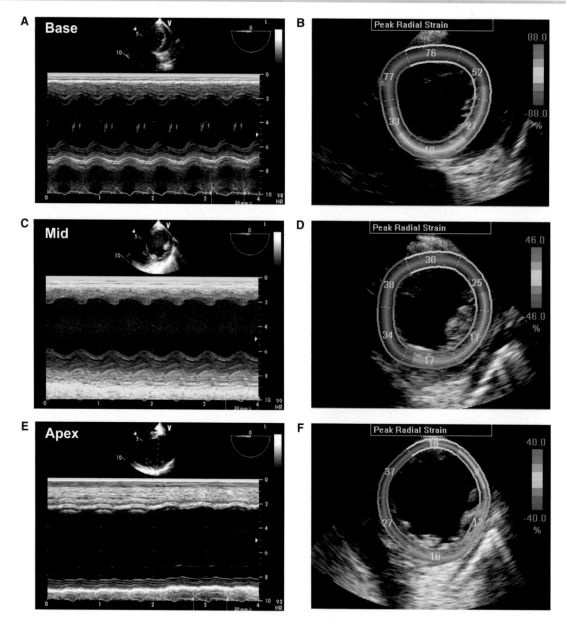

Figure 30.17 Stress cardiomyopathy (Tako-Tsubo or apical ballooning syndrome). Hemodynamically unstable 70-year-old woman after acute perforation of the duodenum. The transgastric view using M-mode and 2D speckle strain show the typically preserved basal function (**A,B**) with progressive reduction in wall motion and strain at the mid-papillary level (**C,D**) and at the apex (**E,F**). The wall motion abnormalities completely resolved the following week.

Table 30.1 Proposed Mayo Clinic Criteria for Apical Ballooning Syndrome (Tako-Tsubo or Stress Cardiomyopathy)

1. Transient hypokinesis, akinesis, or dyskinesis of the left ventricular mid segments with or without apical involvement
   - The regional wall motion abnormalities extend beyond a single epicardial vascular distribution; a stressful trigger is often but not always present[a]
2. Absence of obstructive coronary disease or angiographic evidence of acute plaque rupture[b]
3. New electrocardiographic abnormalities (either ST-segment elevation and/or T-wave inversion) or modest elevation in cardiac troponin
4. Absence of
   - Pheochromocytoma
   - Myocarditis

In all of the above circumstances, the diagnosis of ABS should be made with caution, and a clear stressful precipitating trigger must be sought.
[a]There are rare exceptions to these criteria such as those patients in whom the regional wall motion abnormality is limited to a single coronary territory.
[b]It is possible that a patient with obstructive coronary atherosclerosis may also develop ABS. However, this is very rare in our experience and in the published literature perhaps because such cases are misdiagnosed as an acute coronary syndrome.
Abbreviation: ABS, apical ballooning syndrome.
Source: From Ref. 116.

to as much as 6% in women (118) as they represent over 90% of affected patients. Other clinical features include advanced age (mean age 65–70 years), preceding emotional or physical stress (70–75%), and presenting complaint of angina-like chest pain (70–75%) or dyspnea (10–15%). The initial EKG usually features ST-elevation (60–70%) or inverted T waves. Cardiac troponins are elevated, although to a lesser extent than expected from the involved territory. Mild-to-moderate congestive heart failure is frequent (116), and frank cardiogenic shock can occur in up to 4.2% of patients (119). These patients cannot be reliably identified on the basis of the presenting symptoms or EKG (120), hemodynamic data (Fig. 30.18) and their initial management should be identical to that of an acute coronary syndrome. However, case reports of patients unnecessarily exposed to thrombolysis have been described (121), and emergent cardiac catheterization is probably a better alternative, if available, in an acutely stressed elderly woman with typical echocardiographic findings. Specific diagnostic criteria have been proposed by the Mayo Clinic (Table 30.1). Prognosis is usually good with a reported in-hospital mortality of 1% to 2%, while recurrence is thought to occur in about 10% of patients (115).

Echocardiographic findings include LV mid-segmental wall motion abnormalities with frequent apical involvement involving more than one coronary vascular territory (Fig. 30.17). As a rule, basal segments are spared. Mean initial LVEF is 35% to 40% and is expected to normalize within the first few weeks. RV involvement has been noted in 30% of cases and features a similar basal sparing pattern. Its presence is associated with a more severe form featuring a lower LVEF and an increased risk of severe congestive heart failure and prolonged hospitalization (122). Concomitant transient diastolic dysfunction has also been described (123). Significant (3+ or 4+) MR

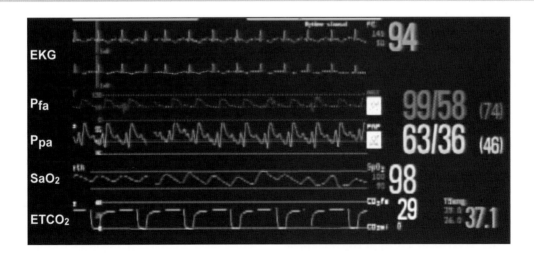

Figure 30.18 Stress cardiomyopathy (Tako-Tsubo or apical ballooning syndrome). Hemodynamically unstable 70-year-old woman after acute perforation of the duodenum. Hemodynamic waveforms show severe pulmonary hypertension. *Abbreviations*: ECG, electrocardiogram; ETCO₂, end-tidal carbon dioxide; Pfa, femoral arterial pressure; Ppa, pulmonary arterial pressure; SaO₂, oxygen saturation.

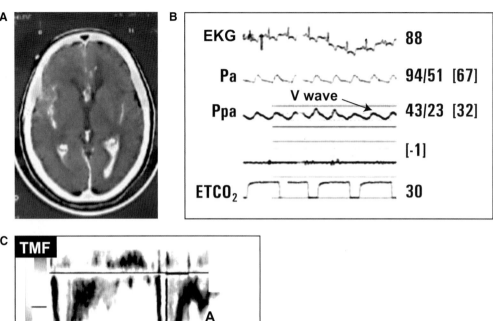

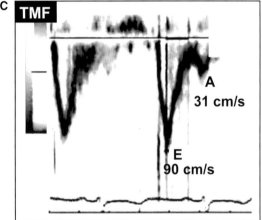

Figure 30.19 Brain-heart syndrome. Left ventricular diastolic dysfunction in a hemodynamically unstable 37-year-old woman with subarachnoid hemorrhage. (**A**) Head computed tomography scan showing intraventricular bleeding. (**B**) Hemodynamic tracing shows a heart rate of 88 beats/min systolic, and diastolic Pa of 94 and 51 mmHg, systolic, and diastolic Ppa of 43 and 23 mmHg with a prominent "V" wave on the wedged tracing. However, no significant mitral regurgitation was seen on color Doppler imaging (not shown). (**C**) Pulsed wave Doppler of TMF reveals a high E/A ratio. *Abbreviations*: A, peak late diastolic TMF velocity; E, peak early diastolic TMF velocity; EKG, electrocardiogram; $ETCO_2$, end-tidal carbon dioxide; Pa, arterial pressure; Ppa, pulmonary artery pressure; TMF, transmitral flow. *Source*: Courtesy of Dr. Nancy McLaughlin from Ref. 131.

has been observed in 20% of patients and is thought to be secondary to LV geometric changes and/or systolic anterior motion (124). Dynamic midventricular obstruction (mean peak gradient 90 mmHg) is present in 20% of patients (119). In a small clinical trial, administration of propranolol improved systolic blood pressure and LVEF (125). Other described complications include intraventricular thrombus (126), papillary muscle rupture (127), and ventricular free wall rupture (128).

Subarachnoid Hemorrhage

In the United States, 8000 people died of subarachnoid hemorrhage in 2003 (129). While most of this mortality is directly attributable to neurological deterioration, up to a quarter of patients will die of medical complications (130). Among them, cardiac-related complications, such as arrythmias, pulmonary edema, and

cardiac failure, are frequent occurrences (130) and hypothesized to be secondary to neurocardiac interactions (Fig. 30.19).

As part of such brain-heart interactions, half of patients with subarachnoid hemorrhage will present with an abnormal EKG (130). The most commonly reported abnormalities are ST-segment changes and T-wave inversions, which may mimic MI (132). Troponin levels are also elevated in 20% of these patients (133) with the proportion of troponin-positive patients increasing with more severe subarachnoid hemorrhage, although this is not a universal finding (134). Elevated troponin levels are correlated with the development of pulmonary edema and abnormal systolic function (135).

Abnormal echocardiographic findings have been described in up to 20% of patients (136) and can consist of either LV regional wall motion abnormalities (RWMA) or global LV systolic dysfunction (135). No correlation has been found between the EKG changes and evolution toward diffuse or a particular pattern of regional systolic dysfunction (132). The RWMA are not necessarily confined to a particular coronary vascular territory but will spare the apex in over 50% of cases (137). Rarely described without concomitant troponin elevation, abnormal LV systolic function was more frequent with increasingly severe subarachnoid hemorrhage (136). These changes are transient and patients improved in the following days and weeks (137). Case reports have described RV involvement (131). Diastolic dysfunction was present in 56% of patients (138) and was a good predictor of pulmonary edema development. Seemingly rare, LV thrombus has been described in case reports (139,140).

Toxicology

Acute intoxication has been the leading cause of nontraumatic deaths in the United States in individuals 13 to 40 years old between 2000 and 2005 (141). Patients who ingest more than one substance, or who attempt suicide, have a higher risk of mortality (142). In descending order of frequency, classes of substances thought to be responsible for deaths from toxic ingestion were analgesics, stimulants/street drugs, antidepressants, cardiovascular drugs, and sedatives/antipsychotics (143).

While a minority of intoxicated patients will evolve to a shock state, the AHA and the European Resuscitation Council have published guidelines for the specific care required for these patients (144,145). An important cause of shock is the direct cardiovascular toxicity of many drugs (146) and herbal medicines (147). With the exception of digoxin, which benefits from the availability of a specific antidote, care of patients who ingest substances with cardiovascular side effects is generally supportive (148).

In caring for these patients, echocardiography can greatly facilitate management issues and is a central part of some of the new proposed treatment algorithms (149). While echocardiography cannot identify an actual ingested toxin, it can sometimes suggest potential etiologies such as cocaine abuse in a young patient with RWMA. However, echocardiography is most useful in the intoxicated hemodynamically unstable patient to establish the underlying mechanism(s) of instability and assess response to treatment. Echocardiographic evaluation will allow the clinician to detect the relative hypovolemia, vasodilatation, and depressed contractility frequently responsible for drug-induced shock. Echocardiography should be repeated for any hemodynamic deterioration as possibly increasing serum levels can lead to further cardiovascular toxicity requiring a new treatment modality.

SPECIFIC TEE CONSIDERATIONS IN NONCARDIAC SURGERY

Indications

The 1996 Practice Guidelines were updated in 2010 by the American Society of Anesthesiologists (ASA) and the SCA Task Force (29). This task force on perioperative TEE included nine anesthesiologists, in both private and academic practice, from various geographic areas of the United States; two cardiologists, one representing the American College of Cardiology (ACC) and the other the American Society of Echocardiography (ASE); and two consulting methodologists from the ASA Committee on Standards and Practice Parameters (see Chapter 31). In noncardiac surgery, it was recommended that TEE be used if the nature of the surgery or the patient's known or suspected cardiovascular pathology might result in severe hemodynamic, pulmonary, or neurologic compromise. If available, TEE should also be used in cases when unexplained life-threatening circulatory instability persists despite appropriate therapy. Such cases include unexplained persistent hypotension or hypoxemia, anticipated life-threatening hypotension, lung or liver transplantation, major thoracic or abdominal trauma, and open abdominal aortic procedure. Other indications for the use of TEE in the ICU are cases when important diagnostic information altering management may not be obtained by TTE or other modalities in a timely fashion. Since then, several studies have demonstrated the implications of TEE in cardiac (see Chapter 13) and noncardiac surgeries (1,2,150–152).

Although the initial TEE data in noncardiac surgery demonstrated little incremental clinical value over other monitors (151), the European Perioperative Transesophageal Research Group showed that the use of TEE caused a significant change in overall therapeutic management, particularly in category I indications (153). Denault et al. (3) showed that for category I indications, TEE altered therapy in 60% of patients compared with 31% for category II indications and 21% for category III indications. In a study of patients presenting for noncardiac surgery, TEE had an impact on patient management in 81% of cases and resulted in the treatment of a potentially life-threatening event in 15% of cases (1). In a more recent study, TEE was described as the appropriate tool to manage hemodynamics in high-risk patients presenting for noncardiac surgery (5).

As an imaging tool, TEE is currently the most valuable hemodynamic monitor available for anesthesiologists (5). The lack of major and multicenter TEE studies in noncardiac surgery contributed to the late awakening of perioperative TEE use outside the cardiac OR. There is a need to explore TEE indications thoroughly in the noncardiac surgery population, and its advantages have to be weighed against the costs and the expertise required (154,155).

Vascular Surgery

Patients undergoing major vascular surgery are at increased risk for perioperative cardiac complications. TEE provides the anesthesiologists with a continuous real-time hemodynamic monitoring in high-risk patients. In fact, when TEE is compared with other traditional monitoring, poor correlations between the traditional monitoring and hemodynamics have been pointed out in vascular surgical patients (156–158). There is a relatively weak correlation between pulmonary capillary wedge pressure and left ventricular end-diastolic area (LVEDA) using intraoperative TEE during abdominal aortic aneurysm (AAA) repair. Furthermore, the strength of the correlation worsened during surgery, particularly after unclamping (156). This led to the conclusion that TEE is a valuable adjunct in guiding volume resuscitation of patients undergoing AAA repair (159) and thoracoabdominal aortic aneurysm (TAAA) repair (158).

As a diagnostic tool, the sensitivity of TEE, in evaluating various aortic diseases, was well recognized in many studies (160). TEE allows direct visualization and characterization of the aortic plaques, ulcerations, dissections, aneurysms, leaks, and endoleaks. Unlike angiography, TEE has the unique advantages of portability and the ability to obtain high-resolution images of the normal and abnormal anatomy of the three layers of the aortic wall and the aortic lumen (161).

It was found to be sensitive to recognition of simple aortic plaques as well more complex lesions protruding into the lumen (162) (see Chapter 23) (Fig. 30.20). TEE is also a highly sensitive and specific method of detecting injury to the thoracic aorta (163) (see Chapter 23). In addition, TEE was found to provide additional critical information during endovascular thoracic aortic aneurysm repair with impact on the early and late outcomes (see Chapter 24). Thus,

TEE is the only imaging modality that simultaneously provides the anesthesiologist with a detailed picture of both aortic pathology and cardiac function.

Thoracoabdominal Aortic Aneurysm

The hemodynamic instability associated with TAAA repair warrants the use of intraoperative TEE (150). Surgical TAAA repair can be performed by clamping the proximal aorta and suturing expeditiously. This approach relies on surgical speed to limit ischemia but is associated with a sudden increase in afterload and distal ischemia. During aortic cross clamping, significant changes in CO occur, which are associated with a reduction in left ventricular end-systolic volume (164–166). TEE was found to be a valuable supplement to pressure measurements for the evaluation of cardiac function during TAAA repair. Another approach utilizes the shunting of blood through a conduit, inserted between proximal and distal aorta, in an attempt to maintain spinal cord, renal, and lower extremity perfusion. The latter involves clamping the aorta and circulating blood to the lower body via a Gott shunt or left atrio-femoral bypass (LAFB). The use of extracorporeal circulation was found to carry less perioperative complications (167,168). In this case, TEE is essential in confirming the correct position of the LA cannula (Fig. 30.21) (158).

The LAFB flow rate determines the amount of blood diverted, and the LA pressure does not reflect the LVEDP. TEE is the only tool capable of monitoring

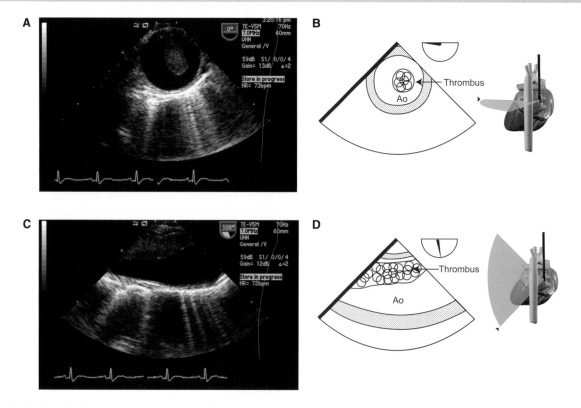

Figure 30.20 Mobile thrombus in the descending thoracic aorta. Mid-esophageal short-axis (**A,B**) and long-axis (**C,D**) views. *Abbreviation*: Ao, aorta.

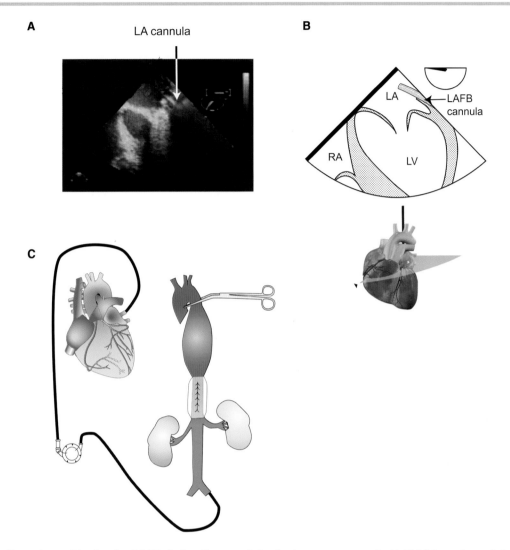

Figure 30.21 Cannula positioning for LAFB during thoracoabdominal aneurysm repair. (A,B) Mid-esophageal short-axis view at 50°: the left atrial cannula is correctly positioned in the left upper pulmonary vein. (**C**) Diagram of the LAFB circuit. *Abbreviations*: LA, left atrium; LAFB, left atrio-femoral bypass; LV, left ventricle; RA, right atrium. *Source*: Adapted with permission of Fayad et al., Ref. 158.

left ventricular end-diastolic volume in this situation. Fayad et al. (65) described the occurrence of acute intraoperative diastolic dysfunction for the first time during aortic cross clamping in patients undergoing TAAA repair. Half of the patients with intraoperative acute diastolic dysfunction developed postoperative myocardial ischemia. However, the clinical significance of intraoperative diastolic dysfunction and potential influence on perioperative management requires further investigation.

Abdominal Aortic Aneurysm

In open surgical repair of AAA, systolic and diastolic dysfunctions are common during aortic clamping and declamping (169,170). Poor correlation between the PAC and intravascular volume in patients undergoing AAA repair has been noted (150,171). In general,

patients undergoing open aortic surgery repair will benefit from TEE monitoring of cardiac function and volume status to achieve optimal hemodynamic stability.

Endovascular Repair of Aortic Aneurysm

Endovascular aortic repair is a relatively new alternative to the traditional open surgical techniques and is discussed in more detail in Chapter 24. It demonstrates a lower mortality and morbidity than the open procedures (172).

General Surgery

Patients with cardiac lesions may present for general surgical procedures with significant risk of perioperative morbidity and mortality. Patients may also

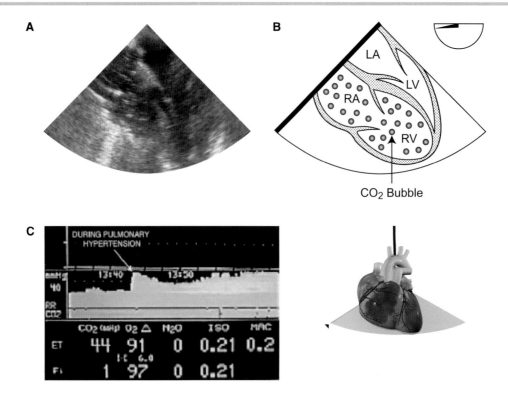

Figure 30.22 CO₂ embolism during laparoscopic intervention. A 69-year-old man undergoing laparoscopic saphenectomy suddenly became hemodynamically unstable. (**A,B**) Mid-esophageal four-chamber view showing bubbles originating from the inferior vena cava appearing in the RA and RV. This was associated with right cardiac chamber dilatation. (**C**) Hemodynamic instability coincided with an abrupt rise in end-tidal CO₂. *Abbreviations*: CO₂, carbon dioxide; LA, left atrium; LV, left ventricle; RA, right atrium; RV, right ventricle. *Source*: Adapted from Ref. 179.

present for high-risk general surgical procedures that have significant intraoperative hemodynamic instability. Both of these two categories of patients may benefit from the intraoperative use of TEE. The benefit of TEE monitoring in general surgery has been reported for the perioperative management of patients with Eisenmenger's syndrome (173), in patients with hypertrophic cardiomyopathy (174) and in obese patients undergoing general surgery procedures (175). Several studies have evaluated the hemodynamic changes during laparoscopic surgery using TEE (176–178) and its potential complications, such as CO₂ embolism and secondary RV dysfunction (Fig. 30.22). A recent clinical report demonstrated that the physiological alterations induced by laparoscopy can produce marked, if not life-threatening, hemodynamic instability in patients with hypertrophic obstructive cardiomyopathy (180).

Patients presenting for hepatic resection may also benefit from close hemodynamic monitoring with TEE, especially if portal triad clamping is required (181). In addition, the increased high risk of gas embolism during laparoscopic hepatic resection can be easily monitored and diagnosed using TEE (181). Finally, utilization of TEE in the intraoperative management

of patients undergoing pheochromocytoma resection has been described in the literature (182).

Neurosurgery

Venous air embolism (VAE) is a well-recognized complication of neurosurgical procedures requiring a sitting position (e.g., posterior fossa surgery). The incidence of Doppler-detected VAE in the sitting position is estimated to be 45% (183). However, TEE is a very sensitive detector of VAE, with reported incidence to be as high as 80% (184,185). Complications associated with VAE may vary from minimal hemodynamic changes to severe hemodynamic instability and death (Fig. 30.23). Pulmonary edema and ARDS, as a result of VAE in a patient undergoing posterior fossa craniotomy, have been reported (186).

Early detection and prompt treatment of VAE is a crucial factor in limiting morbidity and mortality. Patients with VSD or PFO are at risk of paradoxical VAE during neurosurgical procedures and development of cerebral complications. It was suggested that patients scheduled for neurosurgical procedures in the sitting position should undergo a TEE examination prior to surgery to exclude the presence of atrial

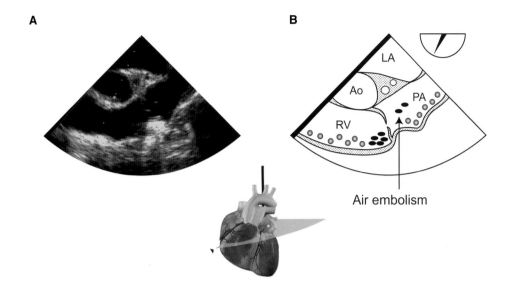

Figure 30.23 Air embolism during spinal surgery in a ventral position. A 46-year-old woman became hemodynamically unstable during the procedure. She was returned back to a supine position. (**A,B**) Mid-esophageal right ventricular outflow view disclosed the presence of residual air bubbles on the most anterior aspect of the RV, PA, and on both sides of the anterior pulmonic valve. *Abbreviations*: Ao, aorta; LA, left atrium; PA, pulmonary artery; RV, right ventricle.

or ventricular shunts. In a study of 35 patients scheduled for neurosurgical procedures in the sitting position, 3 were found to have a right-to-left shunt that led to a change in the planned surgery (187).

As discussed previously, subarachnoid hemorrhage can lead to the development of cardiac complications (Fig. 30.19). As these patients may present to the OR for the insertion of an external ventricular drain, or for surgical clipping of their aneurysm, TEE may be very valuable as a hemodynamic monitoring tool.

Ventriculoatrial (VA) shunts remain a valid option for the treatment of hydrocephalus. Correct positioning of the distal end of the catheter in the RA can be detected by TEE and results in a significant reduction in VA shunt-associated morbidity (188).

Orthopedic Surgery

Cardiopulmonary complications are well known in orthopedic surgery (Fig. 30.24). TEE detected emboli in the right heart and PA during reaming of the femoral canal and during the replacement of the femoral stem with a cemented prosthesis (189). While the clinical significance of those emboli warrants further studies with larger sample sizes, intramedullary procedures should be discontinued if paradoxical embolism is diagnosed (Fig. 30.4) (190).

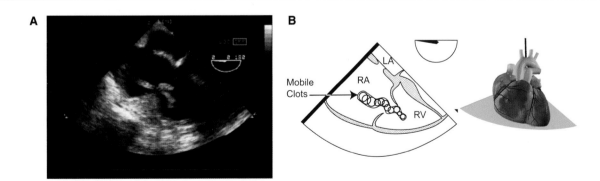

Figure 30.24 Hemodynamic instability during orthopedic surgery. An elderly woman with metastatic cancer underwent orthopedic surgery for a pathological femoral fracture. During the procedure, she became hemodynamically unstable. (**A,B**) Mid-esophageal four-chamber view reveals several mobile clots in the right-sided chambers. *Abbreviations*: LA, left atrium; RA, right atrium; RV, right ventricle. *Source*: Courtesy of Dr. Daniel Boudreault.

Total hip arthroplasty can be associated with hypotension, pulmonary hypertension, hypoxia, and severe hemodynamic instability. These intraoperative events may be related to pulmonary microembolism phenomena as a result of high intramedullary pressures generated during the insertion of the prosthesis (191). Cardiac arrest and mortality were also reported during hip surgery, leading to the suggestion that TEE should be used in high-risk patients for optimal management (192).

Another described use of TEE is to optimize volume status in patients who undergo spinal surgical procedures in the prone position. Dharmavaram et al. (193) looked at the hemodynamic changes associated with the prone position in patients undergoing spine surgery utilizing TEE. It was found that adequate fluid replacement reduced hypotension and hemodynamic instability after prone positioning with minimal effects on cardiac function. Therefore, in patients with a limited cardiac reserve, use of TEE should be considered for these procedures (193).

Urology

Renal cell carcinomas with inferior vena cava (IVC) involvement occur in 5% to 10% of patients, and in about 1% of cases the tumor thrombus extends to the level of the RA (see Fig. 25.16) (194). In these cases, the use of TEE is well documented and can provide accurate information regarding the presence of IVC thrombus, guidance for placement of a vena caval clamp, confirmation of complete removal of the IVC thrombus, and intervention using catheters for thrombectomy (195).

CONCLUSION

TEE is a safe and useful tool, to both diagnose and monitor patients, in a wide variety of clinical situations encountered during noncardiac surgery and in the ICU. The role of echocardiography for noncardiac and critical care is rapidly expanding. Although properly designed studies assessing whether the use of TEE results in an improved patient outcome are lacking, enough convincing data exist to advocate the widespread adoption of TEE, both during noncardiac surgery and in the ICU. However, widespread use should not equate to indiscriminate use and TEE should be restricted to established clinical indications or to situations in which expected benefits outweigh any risks. Training issues will also have to be resolved to ensure that enough qualified physicians are available to meet the growing demand.

ACKNOWLEDGMENTS

The author (MG) would like to dedicate this chapter to his spouse and newborn son.

REFERENCES

1. Suriani RJ, Neustein S, Shore-Lesserson L, et al. Intraoperative transesophageal echocardiography during noncardiac surgery. J Cardiothorac Vasc Anesth 1998; 12:274–280.

2. Brandt RR, Oh JK, Abel MD, et al. Role of emergency intraoperative transesophageal echocardiography. J Am Soc Echocardiogr 1998; 11:972–977.

3. Denault AY, Couture P, McKenty S, et al. Perioperative use of transesophageal echocardiography by anesthesiologists: impact in noncardiac surgery and in the intensive care unit. Can J Anaesth 2002; 49:287–293.

4. Hofer CK, Zollinger A, Rak M, et al. Therapeutic impact of intra-operative transoesophageal echocardiography during noncardiac surgery. Anaesthesia 2004; 59:3–9.

5. Brederlau J, Kredel M, Wurmb T, et al. Transesophageal echocardiography for non-cardiac surgery patients: superfluous luxury or essential diagnostic tool? Anaesthesist 2006; 55:937–940.

6. Schulmeyer MC, Santelices E, Vega R, et al. Impact of intraoperative transesophageal echocardiography during noncardiac surgery. J Cardiothorac Vasc Anesth 2006; 20: 768–771.

7. Heidenreich PA, Stainback RF, Redberg RF, et al. Transesophageal echocardiography predicts mortality in critically ill patients with unexplained hypotension. J Am Coll Cardiol 1995; 26:152–158.

8. Colreavy FB, Donovan K, Lee KY, et al. Transesophageal echocardiography in critically ill patients. Crit Care Med 2002; 30:989–996.

9. Bruch C, Comber M, Schmermund A, et al. Diagnostic usefulness and impact on management of transesophageal echocardiography in surgical intensive care units. Am J Cardiol 2003; 91:510–513.

10. Huttemann E, Schelenz C, Kara F, et al. The use and safety of transoesophageal echocardiography in the general ICU—a minireview. Acta Anaesthesiol Scand 2004; 48: 827–836.

11. Memtsoudis SG, Rosenberger P, Loffler M, et al. The usefulness of transesophageal echocardiography during intraoperative cardiac arrest in noncardiac surgery. Anesth Analg 2006; 102:1653–1657.

12. Khalil A, Helmy T, Porembka DT. Aortic pathology: aortic trauma, debris, dissection, and aneurysm. Crit Care Med 2007; 35:S392–S400.

13. Shiga T, Wajima Z, Apfel CC, et al. Diagnostic accuracy of transesophageal echocardiography, helical computed tomography, and magnetic resonance imaging for suspected thoracic aortic dissection: systematic review and meta-analysis. Arch Intern Med 2006; 166:1350–1356.

14. Delahaye F, Alla F, Beguinot I, et al. In-hospital mortality of infective endocarditis: prognostic factors and evolution over an 8-year period. Scand J Infect Dis 2007; 39:849–857.

15. Baddour LM, Wilson WR, Bayer AS, et al. Infective endocarditis: diagnosis, antimicrobial therapy, and management of complications: a statement for healthcare professionals from the Committee on Rheumatic Fever, Endocarditis, and Kawasaki Disease, Council on Cardiovascular Disease in the Young, and the Councils on Clinical Cardiology, Stroke, and Cardiovascular Surgery and Anesthesia, American Heart Association: endorsed by the Infectious Diseases Society of America. Circulation 2005; 111:e394–e434.

16. Reynolds HR, Jagen MA, Tunick PA, et al. Sensitivity of transthoracic versus transesophageal echocardiography for the detection of native valve vegetations in the modern era. J Am Soc Echocardiogr 2003; 16:67–70.

17. Lopez AD, Mathers CD, Ezzati M, et al. Global and regional burden of disease and risk factors, 2001: systematic analysis of population health data. Lancet 2006; 367:1747–1757.

18. Cardiogenic brain embolism. The second report of the Cerebral Embolism Task Force. Arch Neurol 1989; 46: 727–743.

19. Harloff A, Handke M, Reinhard M, et al. Therapeutic strategies after examination by transesophageal echocardiography in 503 patients with ischemic stroke. Stroke 2006; 37:859–864.

20. Tapson VF. Acute pulmonary embolism. N Engl J Med 2008; 358:1037–1052.

21. Guidelines on diagnosis and management of acute pulmonary embolism. Task Force on Pulmonary Embolism, European Society of Cardiology. Eur Heart J 2000; 21:1301–1336.

22. Stein PD, Fowler SE, Goodman LR, et al. Multidetector computed tomography for acute pulmonary embolism. N Engl J Med 2006; 354:2317–2327.

23. Chartier L, Bera J, Delomez M, et al. Free-floating thrombi in the right heart: diagnosis, management, and prognostic indexes in 38 consecutive patients. Circulation 1999; 99:2779–2783.

24. Torbicki A, Galie N, Covezzoli A, et al. Right heart thrombi in pulmonary embolism: results from the International Cooperative Pulmonary Embolism Registry. J Am Coll Cardiol 2003; 41:2245–2251.

25. Toosi MS, Merlino JD, Leeper KV. Prognostic value of the shock index along with transthoracic echocardiography in risk stratification of patients with acute pulmonary embolism. Am J Cardiol 2008; 101:700–705.

26. Rosenberger P, Shernan SK, Mihaljevic T, et al. Transesophageal echocardiography for detecting extrapulmonary thrombi during pulmonary embolectomy. Ann Thorac Surg 2004; 78:862–866.

27. Pierre-Justin G, Pierard LA. Management of mobile right heart thrombi: a prospective series. Int J Cardiol 2005; 99:381–388.

28. Pruszczyk P, Torbicki A, Pacho R, et al. Noninvasive diagnosis of suspected severe pulmonary embolism: transesophageal echocardiography vs spiral CT. Chest 1997; 112:722–728.

29. Practice Guidelines for Perioperative Transesophageal Echocardiography: An Updated Report by the American Society of Anesthesiologists and the Society of Cardiovascular Anesthesiologists Task Force on Transesophageal Echocardiography. Anesthesiology 2010; 112:1–13.

30. Perrier A, Tamm C, Unger PF, et al. Diagnostic accuracy of Doppler-echocardiography in unselected patients with suspected pulmonary embolism. Int J Cardiol 1998; 65:101–109.

31. Miniati M, Monti S, Pratali L, et al. Value of transthoracic echocardiography in the diagnosis of pulmonary embolism: results of a prospective study in unselected patients. Am J Med 2001; 110:528–535.

32. Kurzyna M, Torbicki A, Pruszczyk P, et al. Disturbed right ventricular ejection pattern as a new Doppler echocardiographic sign of acute pulmonary embolism. Am J Cardiol 2002; 90:507–511.

33. Nazeyrollas P, Metz D, Jolly D, et al. Use of transthoracic Doppler echocardiography combined with clinical and electrocardiographic data to predict acute pulmonary embolism. Eur Heart J 1996; 17:779–786.

34. McConnell MV, Solomon SD, Rayan ME, et al. Regional right ventricular dysfunction detected by echocardiography in acute pulmonary embolism. Am J Cardiol 1996; 78:469–473.

35. Casazza F, Bongarzoni A, Capozi A, et al. Regional right ventricular dysfunction in acute pulmonary embolism and right ventricular infarction. Eur J Echocardiogr 2005; 6:11–14.

36. Torbicki A, Kurzyna M, Ciurzynski M, et al. Proximal pulmonary emboli modify right ventricular ejection pattern. Eur Respir J 1999; 13:616–621.

37. Stevinson BG, Hernandez-Nino J, Rose G, et al. Echocardiographic and functional cardiopulmonary problems 6 months after first-time pulmonary embolism in previously healthy patients. Eur Heart J 2007; 28:2517–2524.

38. Hsiao SH, Lee CY, Chang SM, et al. Pulmonary embolism and right heart function: insights from myocardial Doppler tissue imaging. J Am Soc Echocardiogr 2006; 19:822–828.

39. Hsiao SH, Lee CY, Chang SM, et al. Usefulness of pulmonary arterial flow discordance to identify pulmonary embolism. Am J Cardiol 2007; 99:579–583.

40. Grifoni S, Olivotto I, Cecchini P, et al. Short-term clinical outcome of patients with acute pulmonary embolism, normal blood pressure, and echocardiographic right ventricular dysfunction. Circulation 2000; 101:2817–2822.

41. Mansencal N, Redheuil A, Joseph T, et al. Use of transthoracic echocardiography combined with venous ultrasonography in patients with pulmonary embolism. Int J Cardiol 2004; 96:59–63.

42. Comess KA, DeRook FA, Russell ML, et al. The incidence of pulmonary embolism in unexplained sudden cardiac arrest with pulseless electrical activity. Am J Med 2000; 109:351–356.

43. Kurkciyan I, Meron G, Sterz F, et al. Pulmonary embolism as a cause of cardiac arrest: presentation and outcome. Arch Intern Med 2000; 160:1529–1535.

44. Lin T, Chen Y, Lu C, et al. Use of transoesophageal echocardiography during cardiac arrest in patients undergoing elective non-cardiac surgery. Br J Anaesth 2006; 96:167–170.

45. Rose PS, Punjabi NM, Pearse DB. Treatment of right heart thromboemboli. Chest 2002; 121:806–814.

46. Gin KG, Fenwick JC, Pollick C, et al. The diagnostic utility of contrast echocardiography in patients with refractory hypoxemia. Am Heart J 1993; 125:1136–1141.

47. Langholz D, Louie EK, Konstadt SN, et al. Transesophageal echocardiographic demonstration of distinct mechanisms for right to left shunting across a patent foramen ovale in the absence of pulmonary hypertension. J Am Coll Cardiol 1991; 18:1112–1117.

48. Yalonetsky S, Nun AB, Shwartz Y, et al. Transcatheter closure of a patent foramen ovale prior to a pneumonectomy to prevent platypnea syndrome. Eur J Cardiothorac Surg 2006; 29:622–624.

49. Sandham JD, Hull RD, Brant RF, et al. A randomized, controlled trial of the use of pulmonary-artery catheters in high-risk surgical patients. N Engl J Med 2003; 348:5–14.

50. Costachescu T, Denault AY, Guimond JG, et al. The hemodynamically unstable patient in the intensive care unit: hemodynamic vs. transesophageal echocardiographic monitoring. Crit Care Med 2002; 30:1214–1223.

51. Benjamin E, Griffin K, Leibowitz AB, et al. Goal-directed transesophageal echocardiography performed by intensivists to assess left ventricular function: comparison with pulmonary artery catheterization. J Cardiothorac Vasc Anesth 1998; 12:10–15.

52. Grocott MP, Mythen MG, Gan TJ. Perioperative fluid management and clinical outcomes in adults. Anesth Analg 2005; 100:1093–1106.

53. Monnet X, Teboul JL. Volume responsiveness. Curr Opin Crit Care 2007; 13:549–553.

54. Maizel J, Airapetian N, Lorne E, et al. Diagnosis of central hypovolemia by using passive leg raising. Intensive Care Med 2007; 33:1133–1138.

55. Lamia B, Ochagavia A, Monnet X, et al. Echocardiographic prediction of volume responsiveness in critically ill patients with spontaneously breathing activity. Intensive Care Med 2007; 33:1125–1132.

56. Monnet X, Teboul JL. Passive leg raising. Intensive Care Med 2008; 34:659–663.
57. Vieillard-Baron A, Caille V, Charron C, et al. Actual incidence of global left ventricular hypokinesia in adult septic shock. Crit Care Med 2008; 36:1701–1706.
58. Vieillard-Baron A, Schmitt JM, Beauchet A, et al. Early preload adaptation in septic shock? A transesophageal echocardiographic study. Anesthesiology 2001; 94: 400–406.
59. Esch BT, Scott JM, Haykowsky MJ, et al. Diastolic ventricular interactions in endurance-trained athletes during orthostatic stress. Am J Physiol Heart Circ Physiol 2007; 293:H409–H415.
60. Mebazaa A, Karpati P, Renaud E, et al. Acute right ventricular failure–from pathophysiology to new treatments. Intensive Care Med 2004; 30:185–196.
61. Haddad F, Couture P, Tousignant C, et al. The right ventricle in cardiac surgery, a perioperative perspective: II. Pathophysiology, clinical importance, and management. Anesth Analg 2009; 108:422–433.
62. Abhayaratna WP, Marwick TH, Smith WT, et al. Characteristics of left ventricular diastolic dysfunction in the community: an echocardiographic survey. Heart 2006; 92:1259–1264.
63. Bhatia RS, Tu JV, Lee DS, et al. Outcome of heart failure with preserved ejection fraction in a population-based study. N Engl J Med 2006; 355:260–269.
64. Bouhemad B, Nicolas-Robin A, Arbelot C, et al. Isolated and reversible impairment of ventricular relaxation in patients with septic shock. Crit Care Med 2008; 36:766–774.
65. Fayad A, Yang H, Nathan H, et al. Acute diastolic dysfunction in thoracoabdominal aortic aneurysm surgery. Can J Anaesth 2006; 53:168–173.
66. Stugaard M, Smiseth OA, Risoe C, et al. Intraventricular early diastolic filling during acute myocardial ischemia, assessment by multigated color M-mode Doppler echocardiography. Circulation 1993; 88:2705–2713.
67. McLaughlin N, Bojanowski MW, Girard F, et al. Pulmonary edema and cardiac dysfunction following subarachnoid hemorrhage. Can J Neurol Sci 2005; 32:178–185.
68. Shi Y, Denault AY, Couture P, et al. Biventricular diastolic filling patterns after coronary artery bypass graft surgery. J Thorac Cardiovasc Surg 2006; 131:1080–1086.
69. Jardin F, Dubourg O, Bourdarias JP. Echocardiographic pattern of acute cor pulmonale. Chest 1997; 111:209–217.
70. Hsiao SH, Chang SM, Lee CY, et al. Usefulness of tissue Doppler parameters for identifying pulmonary embolism in patients with signs of pulmonary hypertension. Am J Cardiol 2006; 98:685–690.
71. Joseph G, Jose VJ. Right ventricular filling abnormalities in acute inferior wall myocardial infarction—a pulsed Doppler study. Indian Heart J 1990; 42:437–440.
72. Couture P, Denault AY, Pellerin M, et al. Milrinone enhances systolic, but not diastolic function during coronary artery bypass grafting surgery. Can J Anaesth 2007; 54:509–522.
73. Price S, Prout J, Jaggar SI, et al. "Tamponade" following cardiac surgery: terminology and echocardiography may both mislead. Eur J Cardiothorac Surg 2004; 26:1156–1160.
74. Fowler NO. Cardiac tamponade. A clinical or an echocardiographic diagnosis? Circulation 1993; 87:1738–1741.
75. Merce J, Sagrista-Sauleda J, Permanyer-Miralda G, et al. Correlation between clinical and Doppler echocardiographic findings in patients with moderate and large pericardial effusion: implications for the diagnosis of cardiac tamponade. Am Heart J 1999; 138:759–764.
76. Durand M, Lamarche Y, Denault A. Pericardial tamponade. Can J Anaesth 2009; 56:443–448.
77. Kuvin JT, Harati NA, Pandian NG, et al. Postoperative cardiac tamponade in the modern surgical era. Ann Thorac Surg 2002; 74:1148–1153.
78. Kirschner E, Berger M, Goldberg E. Hypertrophic obstructive cardiomyopathy presenting with profound hypotension. Role of two-dimensional and Doppler echocardiography in diagnosis and management. Chest 1992; 101:711–714.
79. Aurigemma G, Battista S, Orsinelli D, et al. Abnormal left ventricular intracavitary flow acceleration in patients undergoing aortic valve replacement for aortic stenosis. A marker for high postoperative morbidity and mortality. Circulation 1992; 86:926–936.
80. Bartunek J, Sys SU, Rodrigues AC, et al. Abnormal systolic intraventricular flow velocities after valve replacement for aortic stenosis. Mechanisms, predictive factors, and prognostic significance. Circulation 1996; 93:712–719.
81. Thompson CR, Buller CE, Sleeper LA, et al. Cardiogenic shock due to acute severe mitral regurgitation complicating acute myocardial infarction: a report from the SHOCK Trial Registry. SHould we use emergently revascularize Occluded Coronaries in cardiogenic shocK? J Am Coll Cardiol 2000; 36:1104–1109.
82. Jamet B, Chabert JP, Metz D, et al. Acute aortic insufficiency. Ann Cardiol Angeiol (Paris) 2000; 49:183–186.
83. Cilliers AM, van Unen H, Lala S, et al. Massive biatrial myxomas in a child. Pediatr Cardiol 1999; 20:150–151.
84. Lin CM, Hsu JC. Anterior mediastinal tumour identified by intraoperative transesophageal echocardiography. Can J Anaesth 2001; 48:78–80.
85. Menon V, Webb JG, Hillis LD, et al. Outcome and profile of ventricular septal rupture with cardiogenic shock after myocardial infarction: a report from the SHOCK Trial Registry. SHould we emergently revascularize Occluded Coronaries in cardiogenic shocK? J Am Coll Cardiol 2000; 36:1110–1116.
86. Angus DC, Linde-Zwirble WT, Lidicker J, et al. Epidemiology of severe sepsis in the United States: analysis of incidence, outcome, and associated costs of care. Crit Care Med 2001; 29:1303–1310.
87. Parrillo JE. Pathogenetic mechanisms of septic shock. N Engl J Med 1993; 328:1471–1477.
88. Rivers E, Nguyen B, Havstad S, et al. Early goal-directed therapy in the treatment of severe sepsis and septic shock. N Engl J Med 2001; 345:1368–1377.
89. Kern JW, Shoemaker WC. Meta-analysis of hemodynamic optimization in high-risk patients. Crit Care Med 2002; 30:1686–1692.
90. Vieillard-Baron A, Prin S, Chergui K, et al. Hemodynamic instability in sepsis: bedside assessment by Doppler echocardiography. Am J Respir Crit Care Med 2003; 168:1270–1276.
91. Jardin F, Fourme T, Page B, et al. Persistent preload defect in severe sepsis despite fluid loading: a longitudinal echocardiographic study in patients with septic shock. Chest 1999; 116:1354–1359.
92. Vieillard-Baron A, Schmitt JM, Augarde R, et al. Acute cor pulmonale in acute respiratory distress syndrome submitted to protective ventilation: incidence, clinical implications, and prognosis. Crit Care Med 2001; 29:1551–1555.
93. Jafri SM, Lavine S, Field BE, et al. Left ventricular diastolic function in sepsis. Crit Care Med 1990; 18:709–714.
94. Etchecopar-Chevreuil C, Francois B, Clavel M, et al. Cardiac morphological and functional changes during early septic shock: a transesophageal echocardiographic study. Intensive Care Med 2008; 34:250–256.
95. Scharf SM, Brown R, Saunders N, et al. Hemodynamic effects of positive-pressure inflation. J Appl Physiol 1980; 49:124–131.

96. Zapol WM, Snider MT. Pulmonary hypertension in severe acute respiratory failure. N Engl J Med 1977; 296:476–480.

97. Monchi M, Bellenfant F, Cariou A, et al. Early predictive factors of survival in the acute respiratory distress syndrome. A multivariate analysis. Am J Respir Crit Care Med 1998; 158:1076–1081.

98. Vieillard-Baron A, Charron C, Caille V, et al. Prone positioning unloads the right ventricle in severe ARDS. Chest 2007; 132:1440–1446.

99. Reis MD, Klompe L, Mekel J, et al. Open lung ventilation does not increase right ventricular outflow impedance: an echo-Doppler study. Crit Care Med 2006; 34:2555–2560.

100. Dellinger RP, Levy MM, Carlet JM, et al. Surviving Sepsis Campaign: international guidelines for management of severe sepsis and septic shock: 2008. Crit Care Med 2008; 36:296–327.

101. Jardin F, Delorme G, Hardy A, et al. Reevaluation of hemodynamic consequences of positive pressure ventilation: emphasis on cyclic right ventricular afterloading by mechanical lung inflation. Anesthesiology 1990; 72:966–970.

102. Hager DN, Krishnan JA, Hayden DL, et al. Tidal volume reduction in patients with acute lung injury when plateau pressures are not high. Am J Respir Crit Care Med 2005; 172:1241–1245.

103. Jardin F, Vieillard-Baron A. Is there a safe plateau pressure in ARDS? The right heart only knows. Intensive Care Med 2007; 33:444–447.

104. Prin S, Chergui K, Augarde R, et al. Ability and safety of a heated humidifier to control hypercapnic acidosis in severe ARDS. Intensive Care Med 2002; 28:1756–1760.

105. Brower RG, Lanken PN, MacIntyre N, et al. Higher versus lower positive end-expiratory pressures in patients with the acute respiratory distress syndrome. N Engl J Med 2004; 351:327–336.

106. Meade MO, Cook DJ, Guyatt GH, et al. Ventilation strategy using low tidal volumes, recruitment maneuvers, and high positive end-expiratory pressure for acute lung injury and acute respiratory distress syndrome: a randomized controlled trial. JAMA 2008; 299:637–645.

107. Mercat A, Richard JC, Vielle B, et al. Positive end-expiratory pressure setting in adults with acute lung injury and acute respiratory distress syndrome: a randomized controlled trial. JAMA 2008; 299:646–655.

108. Michard F, Teboul JL. Using heart-lung interactions to assess fluid responsiveness during mechanical ventilation. Crit Care 2000; 4:282–289.

109. Gattinoni L, Tognoni G, Pesenti A, et al. Effect of prone positioning on the survival of patients with acute respiratory failure. N Engl J Med 2001; 345:568–573.

110. Guerin C, Gaillard S, Lemasson S, et al. Effects of systematic prone positioning in hypoxemic acute respiratory failure: a randomized controlled trial. JAMA 2004; 292:2379–2387.

111. Mancebo J, Fernandez R, Blanch L, et al. A multicenter trial of prolonged prone ventilation in severe acute respiratory distress syndrome. Am J Respir Crit Care Med 2006; 173:1233–1239.

112. Vieillard-Baron A, Rabiller A, Chergui K, et al. Prone position improves mechanics and alveolar ventilation in acute respiratory distress syndrome. Intensive Care Med 2005; 31:220–226.

113. Huttemann E, Schelenz C, Chatzinikolaou K, et al. Left ventricular dysfunction in lethal severe brain injury: impact of transesophageal echocardiography on patient management. Intensive Care Med 2002; 28:1084–1088.

114. Bahloul M, Chaari AN, Kallel H, et al. Neurogenic pulmonary edema due to traumatic brain injury: evidence of cardiac dysfunction. Am J Crit Care 2006; 15:462–470.

115. Samuels MA. The brain-heart connection. Circulation 2007; 116:77–84.

116. Prasad A, Lerman A, Rihal CS. Apical ballooning syndrome (Tako-Tsubo or stress cardiomyopathy): a mimic of acute myocardial infarction. Am Heart J 2008; 155:408–417.

117. Fazio G, Barbaro G, Sutera L, et al. Clinical findings of Takotsubo cardiomyopathy: results from a multicenter international study. J Cardiovasc Med (Hagerstown) 2008; 9:239–244.

118. Elian D, Osherov A, Matetzky S, et al. Left ventricular apical ballooning: not an uncommon variant of acute myocardial infarction in women. Clin Cardiol 2006; 29:9–12.

119. Gianni M, Dentali F, Grandi AM, et al. Apical ballooning syndrome or takotsubo cardiomyopathy: a systematic review. Eur Heart J 2006; 27:1523–1529.

120. Bybee KA, Motiei A, Syed IS, et al. Electrocardiography cannot reliably differentiate transient left ventricular apical ballooning syndrome from anterior ST-segment elevation myocardial infarction. J Electrocardiol 2007; 40:38.e1–38.e6.

121. Silberbauer J, Hong P, Lloyd GW. Takotsubo cardiomyopathy (left ventricular ballooning syndrome) induced during dobutamine stress echocardiography. Eur J Echocardiogr 2008; 9:136–138.

122. Haghi D, Athanasiadis A, Papavassiliu T, et al. Right ventricular involvement in Takotsubo cardiomyopathy. Eur Heart J 2006; 27:2433–2439.

123. Cangella F, Medolla A, De Fazio G, et al. Stress induced cardiomyopathy presenting as acute coronary syndrome: Tako-Tsubo in Mercogliano, Southern Italy. Cardiovasc Ultrasound 2007; 5:36.

124. Parodi G, Del Pace S, Salvadori C, et al. Left ventricular apical ballooning syndrome as a novel cause of acute mitral regurgitation. J Am Coll Cardiol 2007; 50:647–649.

125. Yoshioka T, Hashimoto A, Tsuchihashi K, et al. Clinical implications of midventricular obstruction and intravenous propranolol use in transient left ventricular apical ballooning (Tako-tsubo cardiomyopathy). Am Heart J 2008; 155:526–527.

126. Haghi D, Papavassiliu T, Heggemann F, et al. Incidence and clinical significance of left ventricular thrombus in tako-tsubo cardiomyopathy assessed with echocardiography. QJM 2008; 101:381–386.

127. Nef HM, Mollmann H, Hilpert P, et al. Severe mitral regurgitation in Tako-Tsubo cardiomyopathy. Int J Cardiol 2009; 132:e77–e79.

128. Mafrici A, Proietti R, Fusco R, et al. Left ventricular free wall rupture in a Caucasian female with Takotsubo syndrome: a case report and a brief literature review. J Cardiovasc Med (Hagerstown) 2006; 7:880–883.

129. Shea AM, Reed SD, Curtis LH, et al. Characteristics of nontraumatic subarachnoid hemorrhage in the United States in 2003. Neurosurgery 2007; 61:1131–1137.

130. Solenski NJ, Haley EC Jr., Kassell NF, et al. Medical complications of aneurysmal subarachnoid hemorrhage: a report of the multicenter, cooperative aneurysm study. Participants of the Multicenter Cooperative Aneurysm Study. Crit Care Med 1995; 23:1007–1017.

131. McLaughlin N, Bojanowski MW, Denault AY. Early myocardial dysfunction following subarachnoid haemorrhage. Br J Neurosurg 2005; 19:141–147.

132. Macmillan CS, Grant IS, Andrews PJ. Pulmonary and cardiac sequelae of subarachnoid haemorrhage: time for active management? Intensive Care Med 2002; 28:1012–1023.

133. Tung P, Kopelnik A, Banki N, et al. Predictors of neurocardiogenic injury after subarachnoid hemorrhage. Stroke 2004; 35:548–551.

134. Horowitz MB, Willet D, Keffer J. The use of cardiac troponin-I (cTnI) to determine the incidence of myocardial ischemia and injury in patients with aneurysmal and presumed aneurysmal subarachnoid hemorrhage. Acta Neurochir (Wien) 1998; 140:87–93.

135. Parekh N, Venkatesh B, Cross D, et al. Cardiac troponin I predicts myocardial dysfunction in aneurysmal subarachnoid hemorrhage. J Am Coll Cardiol 2000; 36:1328–1335.

136. Macrea LM, Tramer MR, Walder B. Spontaneous subarachnoid hemorrhage and serious cardiopulmonary dysfunction—a systematic review. Resuscitation 2005; 65: 139–148.

137. Zaroff JG, Rordorf GA, Ogilvy CS, et al. Regional patterns of left ventricular systolic dysfunction after subarachnoid hemorrhage: evidence for neurally mediated cardiac injury. J Am Soc Echocardiogr 2000; 13:774–779.

138. Kopelnik A, Fisher L, Miss JC, et al. Prevalence and implications of diastolic dysfunction after subarachnoid hemorrhage. Neurocrit Care 2005; 3:132–138.

139. Pollick C, Cujec B, Parker S, et al. Left ventricular wall motion abnormalities in subarachnoid hemorrhage: an echocardiographic study. J Am Coll Cardiol 1988; 12:600–605.

140. Fujita K, Fukuhara T, Munemasa M, et al. Ampulla cardiomyopathy associated with aneurysmal subarachnoid hemorrhage: report of 6 patients. Surg Neurol 2007; 68:556–561.

141. Centers for Disease Control and Prevention National Center for Injury Prevention and Control (NCIPC). Electronic Citation, 2008. Available at: http://www.cdc.gov/injury/wisqars/.

142. Bronstein AC, Spyker DA, Cantilena LR Jr., et al. 2006 Annual Report of the American Association of Poison Control Centers' National Poison Data System (NPDS). Clin Toxicol (Phila) 2007; 45:815–917.

143. Lai MW, Klein-Schwartz W, Rodgers GC, et al. 2005 Annual Report of the American Association of Poison Control Centers' national poisoning and exposure database. Clin Toxicol (Phila) 2006; 44:803–932.

144. ECC Committee, Subcommittees and Task Forces of the American Heart Association. 2005 American Heart Association Guidelines for Cardiopulmonary Resuscitation and Emergency Cardiovascular Care. Part 10.2: Toxicology in ECC. Circulation 2005; 112(suppl 24):IV126–IV132.

145. Soar J, Deakin CD, Nolan JP, et al. European Resuscitation Council guidelines for resuscitation 2005. Section 7. Cardiac arrest in special circumstances. Resuscitation 2005; 67 (suppl 1):S135–S170.

146. Delk C, Holstege CP, Brady WJ. Electrocardiographic abnormalities associated with poisoning. Am J Emerg Med 2007; 25:672–687.

147. Ernst E. Cardiovascular adverse effects of herbal medicines: a systematic review of the recent literature. Can J Cardiol 2003; 19:818–827.

148. Holstege CP, Dobmeier S. Cardiovascular challenges in toxicology. Emerg Med Clin North Am 2005; 23:1195–1217.

149. Echo-in-ICU Group. Echocardiographie Doppler chez le patient en état critique: un outil de diagnostic et de monitorage. 1st ed. Issy-les-Moulineaux: Springer Masson SA, 2008.

150. Iafrati MD, Gordon G, Staples MH, et al. Transesophageal echocardiography for hemodynamic management of thoracoabdominal aneurysm repair. Am J Surg 1993; 166:179–185.

151. Eisenberg MJ, London MJ, Leung JM, et al. Monitoring for myocardial ischemia during noncardiac surgery. A technology assessment of transesophageal echocardiography and 12-lead electrocardiography. The Study of Perioperative Ischemia Research Group. JAMA 1992; 268:210–216.

152. Coletti G, Torracca L, La Canna G, et al. Diagnosis and management of cerebral malperfusion phenomena during aortic dissection repair by transesophageal Doppler echocardiographic monitoring. J Card Surg 1996; 11:355–358.

153. Kolev N, Brase R, Swanevelder J, et al. The influence of transoesophageal echocardiography on intra-operative

decision making. A European multicentre study. European Perioperative TOE Research Group. Anaesthesia 1998; 53:767–773.

154. Miller JP, Lambert AS, Shapiro WA, et al. The adequacy of basic intraoperative transesophageal echocardiography performed by experienced anesthesiologists. Anesth Analg 2001; 92:1103–1110.

155. Thys DM. Echocardiography and anesthesiology successes and challenges. Anesthesiology 2001; 95:1313–1314.

156. Gillespie DL, Connelly GP, Arkoff HM, et al. Left ventricular dysfunction during infrarenal abdominal aortic aneurysm repair. Am J Surg 1994; 168:144–147.

157. D'Angelo AJ, Kline RG, Chen MH, et al. Utility of transesophageal echocardiography and pulmonary artery catheterization during laparoscopic assisted abdominal aortic aneurysm repair. Surg Endosc 1997; 11:1099–1101.

158. Fayad A, Sawchuk C, Yang H, et al. Transesophageal echocardiography in the management of left atrio-femoral bypass during thoracoabdominal aortic aneurysm repair: a case report. Can J Anaesth 2002; 49:1081–1083.

159. Fontes ML, Bellows W, Ngo L, et al. Assessment of ventricular function in critically ill patients: limitations of pulmonary artery catheterization. Institutions of the McSPI Research Group. J Cardiothorac Vasc Anesth 1999; 13:521–527.

160. Rizzo RJ, Aranki SF, Aklog L, et al. Rapid noninvasive diagnosis and surgical repair of acute ascending aortic dissection. Improved survival with less angiography. J Thorac Cardiovasc Surg 1994; 108:567–574.

161. Willens HJ, Kessler KM. Transesophageal echocardiography in the diagnosis of diseases of the thoracic aorta: part 1. Aortic dissection, aortic intramural hematoma, and penetrating atherosclerotic ulcer of the aorta. Chest 1999; 116:1772–1779.

162. Katz ES, Tunick PA, Rusinek H, et al. Protruding aortic atheromas predict stroke in elderly patients undergoing cardiopulmonary bypass: experience with intraoperative transesophageal echocardiography. J Am Coll Cardiol 1992; 20:70–77.

163. Smith DC, Bansal RC. Transesophageal echocardiography in the diagnosis of traumatic rupture of the aorta. N Engl J Med 1995; 333:457–458.

164. Aadahl P, Saether OD, Aakhus S, et al. The importance of transesophageal echocardiography during surgery of the thoracic aorta. Eur J Vasc Endovasc Surg 1996; 12:401–406.

165. Acher CW, Wynn MM, Hoch JR, et al. Cardiac function is a risk factor for paralysis in thoracoabdominal aortic replacement. J Vasc Surg 1998; 27:821–828.

166. Eide TO, Aasland J, Romundstad P, et al. Changes in hemodynamics and acid-base balance during cross-clamping of the descending thoracic aorta. A study in patients operated on for thoracic and thoracoabdominal aortic aneurysm. Eur Surg Res 2005; 37:330–334.

167. Fehrenbacher JW, McCready RA, Hormuth DA, et al. One-stage segmental resection of extensive thoracoabdominal aneurysms with left-sided heart bypass. J Vasc Surg 1993; 18:366–370.

168. Coselli JS. Thoracoabdominal aortic aneurysms: experience with 372 patients. J Card Surg 1994; 9:638–647.

169. Dunn E, Prager RL, Fry W, et al. The effect of abdominal aortic cross-clamping on myocardial function. J Surg Res 1977; 22:463–468.

170. Gooding JM, Archie JP Jr., McDowell H. Hemodynamic response to infrarenal aortic cross-clamping in patients with and without coronary artery disease. Crit Care Med 1980; 8:382–385.

171. Roizen MF, Beaupre PN, Alpert RA, et al. Monitoring with two-dimensional transesophageal echocardiography. Comparison of myocardial function in patients

undergoing supraceliac, suprarenal-infraceliac, or infrarenal aortic occlusion. J Vasc Surg 1984; 1:300–305.

172. Dake MD, Miller DC, Semba CP, et al. Transluminal placement of endovascular stent-grafts for the treatment of descending thoracic aortic aneurysms. N Engl J Med 1994; 331:1729–1734.

173. Bouch DC, Allsager CM, Moore N. Peri-operative transoesophageal echocardiography and nitric oxide during general anaesthesia in a patient with Eisenmenger's syndrome. Anaesthesia 2006; 61:996–1000.

174. Fayad A. Left ventricular outflow obstruction in a patient with undiagnosed hypertrophic obstructive cardiomyopathy. Can J Anaesth 2007; 54:1019–1020.

175. Prior DL, Sprung J, Thomas JD, et al. Echocardiographic and hemodynamic evaluation of cardiovascular performance during laparoscopy of morbidly obese patients. Obes Surg 2003; 13:761–767.

176. Cunningham AJ, Turner J, Rosenbaum S, et al. Transoesophageal echocardiographic assessment of haemodynamic function during laparoscopic cholecystectomy. Br J Anaesth 1993; 70:621–625.

177. Derouin M, Couture P, Boudreault D, et al. Detection of gas embolism by transesophageal echocardiography during laparoscopic cholecystectomy. Anesth Analg 1996; 82: 119–124.

178. Schmandra TC, Mierdl S, Bauer H, et al. Transoesophageal echocardiography shows high risk of gas embolism during laparoscopic hepatic resection under carbon dioxide pneumoperitoneum. Br J Surg 2002; 89:870–876.

179. Martineau A, Arcand G, Couture P, et al. Transesophageal echocardiographic diagnosis of carbon dioxide embolism during minimally invasive saphenous vein harvesting and treatment with inhaled epoprostenol. Anesth Analg 2003; 96:962–964.

180. Popescu WM, Perrino AC Jr. Critical cardiac decompensation during laparoscopic surgery. J Am Soc Echocardiogr 2006; 19:1074–1076.

181. Decailliot F, Streich B, Heurtematte Y, et al. Hemodynamic effects of portal triad clamping with and without pneumoperitoneum: an echocardiographic study. Anesth Analg 2005; 100:617–622.

182. Ryan T, Timoney A, Cunningham AJ. Use of transoesophageal echocardiography to manage beta-adrenoceptor block and assess left ventricular function in a patient with phaeochromocytoma. Br J Anaesth 1993; 70:101–103.

183. Schmitt HJ, Hemmerling TM. Venous air emboli occur during release of positive end-expiratory pressure and repositioning after sitting position surgery. Anesth Analg 2002; 94:400–403.

184. Palmon SC, Moore LE, Lundberg J, et al. Venous air embolism: a review. J Clin Anesth 1997; 9:251–257.

185. Cottrell JE, Smith DS. Anesthesia and Neurosurgery. 4th ed. St. Louis: Mosby, 2001.

186. Wong AY, Irwin MG. Large venous air embolism in the sitting position despite monitoring with transoesophageal echocardiography. Anaesthesia 2005; 60:811–813.

187. Kwapisz MM, Deinsberger W, Muller M, et al. Transesophageal echocardiography as a guide for patient positioning before neurosurgical procedures in semi-sitting position. J Neurosurg Anesthesiol 2004; 16:277–281.

188. Machinis TG, Fountas KN, Hudson J, et al. Accurate placement of the distal end of a ventriculoatrial shunt with the aid of real-time transesophageal echocardiography. Technical note. J Neurosurg 2006; 105:153–156.

189. Bisignani G, Bisignani M, Pasquale GS, et al. Intraoperative embolism and hip arthroplasty: intraoperative transesophageal echocardiographic study. J Cardiovasc Med (Hagerstown) 2008; 9:277–281.

190. Bulger EM, Smith DG, Maier RV, et al. Fat embolism syndrome. A 10-year review. Arch Surg 1997; 132:435–439.

191. Pitto RP, Koessler M, Draenert K. The John Charnley Award. Prophylaxis of fat and bone marrow embolism in cemented total hip arthroplasty. Clin Orthop Relat Res 1998:23–34.

192. Li CH, Lee FJ, Shih YJ, et al. Massive pulmonary embolism during orthopedic surgery. Acta Anaesthesiol Taiwan 2007; 45:117–120.

193. Dharmavaram S, Jellish WS, Nockels RP, et al. Effect of prone positioning systems on hemodynamic and cardiac function during lumbar spine surgery: an echocardiographic study. Spine 2006; 31:1388–1393.

194. Casanova GA, Zingg EJ. Inferior vena caval tumor extension in renal cell carcinoma. Urol Int 1991; 47:216–218.

195. Oikawa T, Shimazui T, Johraku A, et al. Intraoperative transesophageal echocardiography for inferior vena caval tumor thrombus in renal cell carcinoma. Int J Urol 2004; 11:189–192.

31

Indications and Training Guidelines for Perioperative Transesophageal Echocardiography

André Martineau and Marie Arsenault
Université Laval, Quebec City, Canada

François Béïque and Annie Côté
McGill University, Montreal, Quebec, Canada

INTRODUCTION

Perioperative echocardiography is widely used in most cardiac surgery centers in North America, Europe, and around the world and has become a standard of care for many patients. Intraoperative echocardiography (IOE) is used because it provides information that significantly influences clinical management and improves clinical outcome. Several recent series have documented the usefulness of IOE in adult cardiac surgery (see Chapter 13), the intensive care unit (ICU), and noncardiac surgery (see Chapter 30). The new information obtained with IOE was examined and its impact on anesthetic or surgical management studied. In adult cardiac surgery, the incidence of new information ranged from 12.8% to 38.6%, while the impact on surgical management or medical treatment ranged from 2.2% to 14.6% (Table 31.1).

The use of IOE has also become routine in many pediatric cardiac surgery centers. Epicardial echocardiography was used before the availability of small multiplane transesophageal echocardiography (TEE) probes. Recent studies demonstrated the value of pediatric intraoperative TEE for the detection of residual defects, after cardiopulmonary bypass (CPB), which ranged from 4.4% to 12.8% (7) (Table 31.2).

These retrospective studies confirm the clinical perception that IOE provides new information on cardiac pathology in a significant number of patients and that this frequently results in changes in management. The use of TEE is not without risks as it has been associated with postoperative morbidity and complications such as swallowing dysfunction, dysphagia, esophageal ulcerations, and rupture (see Chapter 8). Therefore, the indication for performing an intraoperative TEE must be carefully evaluated and weighed against the risks. Perioperative TEE should be performed by, or in close collaboration with, a physician with advanced TEE training. The importance of physician proficiency in the use of TEE is emphasized because of the risk of adverse outcomes resulting from incorrect interpretation.

REVIEW OF PUBLISHED PRACTICE GUIDELINES

In 1996, a task force of the American Society of Anesthesiologists/Society of Cardiovascular Anesthesiologists (ASA/SCA) published their Practice Guidelines for Perioperative TEE (11). The recommendations of the task force address indications; clinical settings; and the proficiency, cognitive, and technical skills expected from the anesthesiologist who performs perioperative TEE. The guidelines were evidence-based and focused on the effectiveness of perioperative TEE in improving clinical outcomes for specific settings where it is customarily used (e.g., cardiac surgery, noncardiac surgery, critical care). The literature search conducted at that time retrieved 1844 articles, of which 588 were considered relevant to the perioperative context.

In 1997, the American Heart Association (AHA) and American College of Cardiology (ACC) published their General Guidelines for the Clinical Application of Echocardiography (12). In 2000, the AHA/ACC Task Force was reconvened to update those guidelines, and the ASE was invited to participate. A section on intraoperative echocardiography was included, based on an additional 118 articles related to the intraoperative use of echocardiography (13). The indications for IOE provided in these guidelines were based on the initial 1996 ASA/SCA guidelines as well as on the newest data available at the time. Guidelines on the appropriateness criteria for transthoracic echocardiography and TEE were published in 2007 (14) but were not limited to the role of IOE.

The 1996 practice guidelines were updated in 2010 by an ASA/SCA Task Force (15). This task force on perioperative TEE included nine anesthesiologists, in both private and academic practice, from various geographic areas of the United States, two cardiologists, one representing the ACC and the other the American Society of Echocardiography (ASE), and two consulting methodologists from the ASA Committee on Standards and Practice Parameters. The

Table 31.1 Usefulness of Intraoperative Echocardiography in Adult Cardiac Surgery

Author (Refs.)	N	New information (%)	Change in management
Eltzschig, 2008 (1)	12566		Before CPB: 7%
Click, 2000 (2)	3245	15	After CPB: 2.2[a]
			14%
Couture, 2000 (3)	851	–	14.6%
Michel-Cherqui, 2000 (4)	203	12.8	10.8%
Mishra, 1998 (5)	5016	22.9	–
Sutton, 1998 (6)	238	38.6	9.7%

[a]Apply only to change in surgical management.
Abbreviation: CPB, cardiopulmonary bypass.

Table 31.2 Usefulness of Intraoperative Echocardiography in Pediatric Cardiac Surgery

Author (Refs.)	N	Residual defects (%)
Rosenfeld, 1998 (8)	86	12.8
Sheil, 1999 (9)	200	10.5
Stevenson, 1995 (7)	667	6.6
Ungerleider, 1995 (10)	1000	4.4

literature review covered a 16-year period from 1994 through 2009. From 8000 citations initially identified, a total of 457 articles contained direct linkage-related evidence. The efficacy of TEE in detecting new abnormalities and in confirming or redefining previous diagnosis is listed in Table 31.3. Misdiagnosis or limited ability to detect pathology is also reported.

THE 2010 PERIOPERATIVE TEE GUIDELINES

Methodology

These guidelines refer to TEE performed during cardiac and noncardiac surgery, before, during and immediately after the procedure, including the critical care setting. The recommendations in the 1996 document were divided into three categories on the basis of the strength of supporting evidence, or expert opinion, that the technology improved clinical outcomes (11).

Category I are indications supported by the strongest evidence of expert opinion: TEE is frequently useful in improving clinical outcomes and is often indicated, depending on individual circumstances (e.g., patient risk and practice settings).

Category II are indications supported by weaker evidence and expert consensus: TEE may be useful in improving clinical outcomes, depending on individual circumstances, but appropriate indications are less certain.

Category III are indications in situations where the use of TEE has, so far, little current scientific or expert support: TEE is infrequently useful in improving clinical outcomes, and appropriate indications are uncertain. These recommendations refer to clinical problems rather than to individual patients who often have more than one reason for needing a perioperative TEE. Physicians must integrate these multiple variables in assessing a patient's need for TEE.

The 2010 updated practice guidelines for perioperative TEE used a different classification system that is based on both scientific (Table 31.3) and opinion evidence (15). In the scientific evidence–based evidence, four categories (A, B, C, and D) were identified with three distinct levels in each of the first three categories.

Scientific Evidence

Category A: Supportive literature. It includes randomized control trials that report statistically significant differences between clinical interventions for a specified clinical outcome.

Level 1. The literature contains multiple randomized controlled trials, and the aggregated findings are supported by meta-analysis.

Level 2. The literature contains multiple randomized controlled trials, but there is an insufficient number of studies to conduct a viable meta-analysis for the purpose of these guidelines.

Level 3. The literature contains a single randomized controlled trial.

Category B: Suggestive literature. Information from observational studies permits inference of beneficial or harmful relationships among clinical interventions and clinical outcomes.

Level 1. The literature contains observational comparisons (e.g., cohort and case-control research designs) of two or more clinical interventions or conditions and indicates statistically significant differences between clinical interventions for a specified clinical outcome.

Level 2. The literature contains noncomparative observational studies with associative (e.g., relative risks, correlation) or descriptive statistics.

Table 31.3 Sensitivity, Specificity, and Predictive Values for Perioperative TEE

Detection/diagnosis of pathology	Sensitivity (%)	Specificity (%)	PPV	NPV
Valvular disease				
Aortic, mitral, or tricuspid valvular perforation (confirmed by surgery or autopsy) (16)	95	98	a	a
Abnormal bicuspid and tricuspid aortic valve morphology (confirmed by surgery) (17)				
Biplane TEE	66	56	a	a
Multiplane TEE	87	91	a	a
Chordal rupture (confirmed by surgery) (18)	79	96	a	a
Mitral valve annular dilatation (confirmed by surgery) (18)	78	50	a	a
Mitral valve leaflet degeneration (confirmed by surgery) (18)	41	87	a	a
Mitral valve prolapse/flail (confirmed by surgery) (19)				
Bileaflet involvement or combined lesion including the commissures	20	93	a	a
Single leaflet but multiscallop involvement	57	96	a	a
Commissure involvement	11	98	a	a
Mitral valve/flail leaflet scallop (confirmed by surgery) (20)	78	92	a	a
Mitral valve regurgitation (confirmed by surgery) (21)	87	100	100%	92%
Mitral vegetation (confirmed by surgery) (21)	90	100	100%	75%
Prosthetic valve endocarditis (pathoanatomic confirmation) (22)	92	97	a	a
Prosthetic valve fistula (confirmed by surgery or necropsy) (23)	100	100	a	a
Valvular abscess (confirmed by surgery or necropsy) (23)	90	100	a	a
Coronary disease				
Myocadial infarction (confirmed by creatine kinase-MB level ≥100 ng/mL within 12 hr after operation or new Q waves on arrival in ICU or on morning of postoperative day 1) (24)	45	73	27%	86%
Pseudonaneurysm (confirmed by surgery or necropsy) (23)	100	98	a	a
Aortic disease				
Aortic dissection (confirmed by aortography, surgery, or necropsy) (25)	67	70	a	a
Aortic dissection (confirmed by double-blind readings of the images) (26)	86	67	a	a
Aortic dissection-type I or III (confirmed by CT/MRI, surgery, or autopsy) (27)	100	a	a	a
Aortic dissection-thoracic (confirmed by angiography, surgery, or autopsy) (28)	100	94	a	a
Atherosclerosis of the ascending aorta (confirmed by epiaortic scanning) (29)	100	60	34%	100%
Traumatic disruption of the aorta (confirmed by aortography, clinical findings, or both) (30)	57	91	a	a
Traumatic disruption of the aorta (confirmed by surgery) (31)	91	100	a	a
Other cardiovascular diseases				
Left ventricular outflow tract lesions (confirmed by surgery, catheter findings) (32)	94	100	a	a
Pulmonary embolus (confirmed by surgery) (33)				
Anywhere within the pulmonary arterial circulation	46	a	a	a
At one of three specific localizations	26	95	93%	32%
Confirming/refining diagnosis				
Aortic intramural hemorrhage (confirmed by surgery or follow-up changes) (34)	100	91	a	a

False positives/negatives

Preoperative TEE detected aneurysm and pericardial effusion; neither confirmed at surgery (35).
Preoperative TEE detected aortic dissection; surgery revealed Takayasu arteritis (36).
Preoperative TEE detected intramural hematoma; surgery revealed aortic dissection (37).
Preoperative TEE detected mass consistent with periannular abscess; surgery revealed coronary ostium (38).
Preoperative TEE detected type A aortic dissection; surgery revealed aortic valve commissural tear (39).
Preoperative TEE did not detect aortic outflow obstruction; surgery revealed occluded valve orifice (40).
Preoperative TEE did not detect ascending aortic dissection; revealed at surgery (41).
Preoperative TEE did not detect calcified fibrous tissue–obstructing mechanical valve inflow; detected at surgery (42).
Preoperative TEE did not detect endocarditis, aortic root abscess; revealed at surgery (43).
Preoperative TEE did not detect endocarditis; detected by intracardiac echocardiography (44).
Preoperative TEE did not detect hematoma of ascending aorta; detected by CT (45).
Preoperative TEE did not detect torn ascending aorta, detected by aortography (46).
Preoperative emergency TEE confirmed intramural hematoma; surgery revealed acute aortic intimal tear without a mobile flap (47).
Preoperative emergency TEE confirmed pericardial cyst; surgery revealed coronary arterial aneurysm (48).
Preoperative TEE confirmed ascending aorta dissection; surgery revealed chronic inflammatory aneurysm (49).
Preoperative TEE confirmed tricuspid valve mass; surgery revealed thrombus (50).
Preoperative TEE confirmed valvular tumor; surgery revealed organized thrombus when resected (51).

---

[a]No available data.
Abbreviations: CT, computed tomography; ICU, intensive care unit; MRI, magnetic resonance imaging; NPV, negative predictive value; PPV, positive predictive value; TEE, transesophageal echocardiography.
Source: From Ref. 15.

Level 3. The literature contains case reports

Category C: Equivocal literature. The literature cannot determine whether there are beneficial or harmful relationships among clinical interventions and clinical outcomes.

Level 1. Meta-analysis did not find significant differences among groups or conditions.

Level 2. There is an insufficient number of studies to conduct meta-analysis, and randomized controlled trials have not found significant differences among groups or conditions, or randomized control trials report inconsistent findings.

Level 3. Observational studies report inconsistent findings or do not permit inference of beneficial or harmful relationships.

Category D: Insufficient evidence from literature (15).

In the opinion-based evidence of the 2010 update, the data was presented in three different categories: category A represents the expert opinion; category B, a sample opinion of the ASA membership; and category C, an informal opinion from open-forum testimony, Internet-based comments, letters, and editorials. However, only findings obtained from formal surveys are reported in the 2010 updated report by the ASA/SCA Task Force (15).

These guidelines focus on the application of TEE in surgical patients in the setting of cardiac surgery, noncardiac surgery, and postoperative critical care. This chapter will review the indications for perioperative TEE according to the updated 2010 report by the ASA/SCA Task Force on perioperative TEE (15).

Practice Guidelines

Cardiac and Thoracic Aortic Procedures

There are important variations in sensitivity, specificity, or positive and negative predictive values reported in the literature for the detection of various abnormalities seen in patients undergoing cardiac and thoracic aortic procedures (Table 31.3). These variations are also reported for the TEE confirmation or refinement of diagnosis in this population (Table 31.3). There is an agreement that TEE should be used in all thoracic aortic and cardiac procedures.

Open heart surgery and thoracic aortic surgical procedures. TEE should be used in all open heart procedures and considered in coronary artery bypass surgery to

- confirm and refine the perioperative diagnosis,
- detect new or unsuspected pathologies,
- adjust the anesthetic and surgical plans accordingly, and
- assess the results of surgical intervention.

Pediatric cardiac surgery. In small children, a case-by-case analysis is required and the benefits of TEE use outweigh its potential risks.

Catheter-based intracardiac procedures. In these procedures, observational studies have confirmed the utility of TEE for

- guiding management,
- detection of unsuspected abnormalities, and
- detection of pericardial effusion.

If intracardiac ultrasound is not used, TEE is recommended in patients under general anesthesia, undergoing the following procedures:

- Septal defect closure
- Atrial appendage obliteration
- Catheter-based valve replacement and repair

Noncardiac Surgery

In noncardiac surgery, it is recommended that TEE be used if the nature of the surgery or the patient's known or suspected cardiovascular pathology might result in severe hemodynamic, pulmonary, or neurologic compromise. If available, TEE should also be used in cases when unexplained life-threatening circulatory instability persists despite appropriate therapy.

Such cases include the following:

- Unexplained persistent hypotension or hypoxemia
- Anticipated life-threatening hypotension
- Lung or liver transplantation
- Major thoracic or abdominal trauma
- Open abdominal aortic procedure

If TEE is available, it may be used in cases such as endovascular aortic procedures, neurosurgery in the sitting position, and percutaneous cardiovascular interventions, but not during orthopedic procedures.

Critical Care

In cases where persistent hypotension or hypoxemia remains unexplained, TEE should be used. Other indications for the use of TEE in the ICU are cases when important diagnostic information altering management may not be obtained by TTE or other modalities in a timely fashion.

Contraindications

In patients with previous esophagectomy or esophagogastrectomy, TEE is contraindicated (see Chapter 8). In patients with oral, esophageal, or gastric disease, TEE may be used as long as the expected benefits outweigh the risks. Necessary precautions are recommended in this population and include the following:

- Considering other imaging modalities
- Obtaining a gastroenterology consultation
- Using a smaller probe
- Limiting the examination
- Avoiding unnecessary probe manipulation
- Using the most experienced operator

Contraindications to TEE probe insertion are also discussed in the Canadian Training Guidelines in Perioperative TEE (52) and include the following:

- Patient refusal
- Esophageal or gastric pathology that would predispose to perforation
- Respiratory distress in the nonintubated patient
- Cervical spine instability
- Severe coagulopathy
  (sect. "Contraindications to TEE Probe Insertion")

TRAINING GUIDELINES FOR PERIOPERATIVE TEE

Training guidelines in echocardiography were first published by the ASE in 1987 (53). In 1992, the ASE revised these guidelines and required level 2 training in TTE to perform TEE examinations (54). Three levels of expertise were identified: level one for basic training, level two for advanced training, and level three for director of an echocardiography laboratory. These three levels of expertise in echocardiography were maintained in all subsequent training guidelines in both the United States and Canada.

Although initial guidelines focused on transthoracic echocardiography (TTE), the rapid evolution of intraoperative TEE led to the development of practice guidelines in perioperative TEE in 1996 by the ASA/SCA (11), which were updated in 2010 (15).

In 1998, the National Board of Echocardiography (NBE) established the first examination in perioperative TEE with the possibility of certification in 2000 (55). This was followed in 2002 by training guidelines in perioperative echocardiography by the ASA/SCA (56) that were later endorsed in 2003 by the ACC and AHA (13) (Table 31.4).

In the province of Quebec, in Canada, an expert consensus for training in perioperative TEE was produced in 2003 (57), but it is not until 2005 that the first Canadian guidelines for training in echocardiography were established (58). In the 2005 Canadian guidelines in echocardiography, a training pathway for TEE requires an advanced level of training in TTE, and a physician has to perform 300 TTE per year as a prerequisite to perform TEE (59). This approach was later deemed impractical for anesthesiologists and specific Canadian training guidelines were developed for perioperative TEE in 2006, using the Quebec expert consensus as a template (Table 31.5) (52,57,59). These guidelines were established by the Cardiovascular Section of the Canadian Anesthesia Society (CVCAS) and the Canadian Society of Echocardiography (CSE) (52,59). Although there are similarities with the guidelines established by the ASA/SCA on perioperative echocardiography (Tables 31.4 and 31.5), there are also other important differences as outlined in the following section (56).

Required Number of Examinations

In the CVCAS/CSE Guidelines on Perioperative TEE, the number of personally performed TEE studies is increased from 50 in the ASE/SCA basic level to 100 (52,56). At the advanced level of training, the number of examinations that are personally performed is also increased from 150 in the ASE/SCA guidelines to a total of 200. However, the total number of complete echocardiographic studies that must be reviewed by the trainee is unchanged and includes 150 for a basic level and 300 for an advanced level of training in both the CVCAS/CSE and the ASE/SCA guidelines for training in perioperative echocardiography. Considering that the focus is on perioperative TEE, the

Table 31.4 ASA/SCA Guidelines for Training in Perioperative Echocardiography (2002)

	Basic	Advanced[a]	Director[b]
Minimum no. of examinations[c]	150	300	450
Minimum no. of TEE examinations[d]	50	150	300
Duration of training	NS	NS	NS
CME hours	20	50	NS
PTE examination	NS	NS	NS
MOC: CME hours	NS	NS	NS
MOC: no. of TEE per year	50	50	50

[a]Total for basic training may be counted toward advanced training.

[b]Program director qualification includes an advanced level of training in perioperative echocardiography and an additional 150 comprehensive perioperative TEE examinations.

[c]Complete echocardiographic examinations interpreted and reported by the trainee under appropriate supervision. May include transthoracic studies recorded by qualified individuals other than the trainee.

[d]Comprehensive intraoperative TEE examinations personally performed, interpreted, and reported by the trainee under appropriate supervision.

Abbreviations: CME, continuous medical education; MOC, maintenance of competence; PTE, perioperative transesophageal echocardiography; TEE, transesophageal echocardiography.

NS: not specified.

Source: From Refs. 13, 52, 56.

Table 31.5 Canadian Guidelines for Training in Perioperative TEE (2006)

	Basic	Advanced[a]	Director[b]
Minimum no. of examinations[c]	150	300	450
Minimum no. of TEE[d]	100	200	300
Duration of training	3 mo	6 mo	9 mo
PTE examination	Yes	Yes	Yes
CME hours (accredited CME hours)[e]	50 (25)	50 (25)	100 (50)
MOC: CME hours (accredited CME hours)[f]	50 (25)	50 (25)	100 (50)
MOC: minimum no. of TEE per year	50	50	75

[a]Total for basic training may be counted toward advanced training.
[b]Program director qualification includes an advanced level of training in perioperative echocardiography and an additional 150 complete echocardiographic examination including at least 100 comprehensive perioperative TEE examinations. The trainee should also have completed a total of 100 hours of CME including 50 hours of accredited CME.
[c]Complete echocardiographic examinations interpreted by the trainee under appropriate supervision. May include transthoracic studies recorded by qualified individuals other than the trainee.
[d]Comprehensive perioperative TEE examinations personally performed, interpreted, and reported by the trainee under appropriate supervision.
[e]CME hours to achieve either a basic or an advanced level should be completed within a two-year period. The CME hours required for a director level should be completed within a four-year period.
[f]CME hours for MOC at the basic, advanced, or director level should be completed within a four-year period
Abbreviations: CME, continuous medical education; MOC, maintenance of competence; PTE, perioperative transesophageal echocardiography; TEE, transesophageal echocardiography. NS, not specified.
Source: From Refs. 52, 57.

CVCAS/CSE guidelines also include TEE studies completed in the perioperative setting outside of the operating room (OR), while only intraoperative TEE studies are considered in the ASE/SCA guidelines toward the required number of personally performed TEE studies (52,56,59).

Guidelines for performing a comprehensive intraoperative multiplane TEE examination were first established by the ASE/SCA with a total of 20 standard views (60). In the CVCAS/CSE guidelines, in addition to the views outlined in the ASE/SCA document, identification of pulmonary veins and of both atrial appendices is included in the standard views of a comprehensive TEE examination (Table 31.6). The authors would also like to recommend the addition of a mid-esophageal "five chamber view" at 0 degree in the assessment of LV and AoV function.

Role of the Physician at a Basic and Advanced Level of Expertise

In the ASE/SCA guidelines, the basic level of expertise limits the physician to patient monitoring and excludes the possibility of echocardiography-based diagnosis (13,56). The role of basic training in the CVCAS/CSE guidelines includes a limited diagnostic role that provides the physician with a new level of autonomy in the OR. The cognitive and technical skill requirement for a basic level of expertise outlined by the ASE/SCA in 2002 was, therefore, modified to reflect this new level of autonomy (Table 31.7). Although physicians with this basic level of expertise should be able to evaluate, independently, a successful valve repair or valve replacement, the presence of pathological findings that may lead to a change in the planned surgical management must be reviewed with

Table 31.6 Standard Views of a Comprehensive TEE Examination

1. Standard four- and five-chamber (0°–20°), two-chamber (80°–100°), and long axis (120°–160°) views
2. Aortic valve *five-chamber* (0°)[a], short axis (30°–60°), and long axis (120°–160°) views
3. Bicaval view of atrial septum (80°–110°)
4. Images of the mitral valve from multiple planes
   a. Four-chamber (0°–20°)
   b. Commissural (60°–70°)
   c. Two-chamber (80°–100°)
   d. Long axis (120°–160°)
5. Images of the tricuspid valve from multiple planes
   a. Four-chamber (0°–20°)
   b. Right ventricular inflow-outflow (60°–90°)
   c. Modified bicaval (110°–160°)
6. Longitudinal views of ascending aorta and pulmonary valves
7. Imaging of atrial appendices
8. Identification of pulmonary veins
9. Appropriate use of saline or other contrast agents in the setting of evaluation for interatrial shunt or abnormal venous drainage
10. Transgastric short- and long axis view for left ventricular function as well as appropriate angulated views for assessment of valves and prostheses. Specifically
    a. Basal short (0°–20°)
    b. Mid short (0°–20°)
    c. Two-chamber (80°–100°)
    d. Long axis (90°–120°)
    e. Right ventricular inflow (100°–120°)
    f. Deep transgastric (0°–20° with anteflexion)
11. Main pulmonary artery and bifurcation
12. Aorta (including ascending, arch, and descending thoracic portions)

[a]Authors' addition to the standard views outlined in both the Canadian guidelines for training in adult perioperative transesophageal echocardiography and the ASE/SCA guidelines for performing a comprehensive intraoperative multiplane TEE examination (60).
Abbreviation: TEE, transesophageal echocardiography.
Source: From Ref. 52.

Table 31.7 Recommended Training Objectives for Basic and Advanced Perioperative TEE

Basic training

Cognitive skills

1. Knowledge of the physical principles of echocardiographic image formation and blood velocity measurement
2. Knowledge of the operation of ultrasonography, including all controls that affect the quality of data displayed
3. Knowledge of the equipment handling, infection control, and electrical safety associated with the techniques of perioperative echocardiography
4. Knowledge of the indications, contraindications, and potential complications for perioperative echocardiography
5. Knowledge of the appropriate alternative diagnostic techniques
6. Knowledge of the normal tomographic anatomy as revealed by perioperative echocardiographic techniques
7. Knowledge of commonly encountered blood flow velocity profiles as measured by Doppler echocardiography
8. Knowledge of the echocardiographic manifestations of native valvular lesions and dysfunction
9. Knowledge of the echocardiographic manifestations of cardiac masses, thrombi, cardiomyopathies, pericardial effusions, and lesions of the great vessels
10. Detailed knowledge of the echocardiographic presentations of myocardial ischemia and infarction
11. Detailed knowledge of the echocardiographic presentations of normal and abnormal ventricular function
12. Detailed knowledge of the echocardiographic presentations of air embolization

Technical skills

1. Ability to operate ultrasonography including the primary controls affecting the quality of the displayed data
2. Ability to insert a TEE probe safely in the anesthetized, tracheally intubated patient
3. Ability to perform a comprehensive TEE examination and differentiate normal from markedly abnormal cardiac structures and function
4. Ability to recognize marked changes in segmental ventricular contraction indicative of myocardial ischemia or infarction.
5. Ability to recognize marked changes in global ventricular filling and ejection
6. Ability to recognize air embolization
7. *Ability to identify native and prosthetic valvular lesions or dysfunctions that would require consultation with a physician having an advanced level of training* (ability to recognize gross valvular lesions and dysfunctions)
8. *Ability to detect intracardiac masses and thrombus* (ability to recognize large intracardiac masses and thrombi)
9. *Ability to detect pericardial effusions* (ability to detect large pericardial effusions)
10. Ability to recognize common echocardiographic artifacts
11. Ability to communicate echocardiographic results effectively to healthcare professionals, the medical record, and patients
12. Ability to recognize complications of perioperative echocardiography

Advanced training

Cognitive skills

1. All the cognitive skills defined under basic training.
2. Detailed knowledge of the principles and methodologies of qualitative and quantitative echocardiography
3. Detailed knowledge of native and prosthetic valvular function, including valvular lesions and dysfunction
4. Knowledge of congenital heart disease (if congenital practice is planned, then this knowledge must be detailed)
5. Detailed knowledge of all other diseases of the heart and great vessels that is relevant in the perioperative period (if pediatric practice is planned, then this knowledge may be more general than detailed).
6. Detailed knowledge of the techniques, advantages, disadvantages, and potential complications of commonly used cardiac surgical procedures for treatment of acquired and congenital heart disease
7. Detailed knowledge of other diagnostic methods appropriate for correlation with perioperative echocardiography

Technical skills

1. All the technical skills defined under basic training
2. Ability to acquire or direct the acquisition of all necessary echocardiographic data, including epicardial and epiaortic imaging
3. Ability to recognize subtle changes in segmental ventricular contraction indicative of myocardial ischemia or infarction
4. Ability to quantify systolic and diastolic ventricular function and to estimate other relevant hemodynamic parameters
5. Ability to quantify normal and abnormal native and prosthetic valvular function.
6. Ability to assess the appropriateness of cardiac surgical plans
7. Ability to identify inadequacies in cardiac surgical interventions and the underlying reasons for the inadequacies
8. Ability to aid in clinical decision making in the operating room

Modified by the authors from the ASE/SCA Task Force Guidelines for Training in Perioperative Echocardiography 2002. The modifications are in italic and are limited to statements 7, 8, and 9 of the technical skills for basic training, with the original statement in parenthesis (56).
Abbreviation: TEE, transesophageal echocardiography.

a physician who has achieved an advanced level of expertise. The rationale for this level of autonomy at a basic training is based on the premise that the expertise required to assess a normal prosthetic valve is significantly less than the assessment and quantification of a paravalvular or valvular regurgitant jet after CPB. As most valvular repair and replacement are not associated with pathological echocardiographic findings, the level of autonomy with basic training will facilitate echocardiographic coverage of cardiac ORs. This increased level of autonomy mandates more rigorous training, and, therefore, both the number of personally performed perioperative TEE studies and number of continuous medical education (CME) hours are increased compared to the ASE/SCA guidelines (52,59).

To ensure a level of quality control, the physician must also obtain a passing score on the PTEeXAM not only for an advanced level but also for recognition of a basic level of expertise. Moreover, review of echocardiographic cases is encouraged especially at this level of expertise, and this philosophy should also apply to those with more advanced training. While the role of a physician with a basic level of expertise is different in the CVCAS/CSE and the ASE/SCA guidelines, at an advanced level of training, the role of the physician is the same in both guidelines (52,56) (Table 31.7). Since 2010, the National Board of Echocardiography is offering a new examination for basic TEE (http://www.echoboards.org/). The goal is to promote training and certification for the use of TEE in the noncardiac setting and the ICU.

Role of TTE Training

In both the CVCAS/CSE and the ASE/SCA guidelines, the complete echocardiographic examinations interpreted and reported by the trainee under appropriate supervision may include TTE studies recorded by qualified individuals other than the trainee (52,56). In the CVCAS/CSE guidelines, although training in TTE is encouraged, it is not considered essential in the learning process of perioperative TEE. The decision to exclude TTE as an absolute requirement for achieving an advanced level of expertise in perioperative TEE was based predominantly on two factors: (*i*) the problematic associated with the variability in both qualifications and access to the TTE laboratory in each training center and (*ii*) the inclusion of training requirements in TTE would also mandate maintenance of competence (MOC) criteria in TTE for expertise in perioperative TEE. At present, in the guidelines for the provision of echocardiography in Canada, MOC for an advanced level of expertise in TTE includes the performance of 300 TTE per year, which is impractical for physicians who have focused their field of interest and expertise in perioperative TEE. Although TTE training is encouraged, it is, therefore, not a prerequisite in the CVCAS/CSE training guidelines (52).

Contraindications to TEE Probe Insertion

TEE examination is associated with a 1% risk of minor complications and a 0.01% risk of major complications. Contraindications to TEE probe insertion are discussed in the 2010 practice guidelines for perioperative TEE and are based on the results of opinion surveys of ASA members and SCA consultant (15). Contraindications to TEE probe insertion are also identified in the CVCAS/CSE training guidelines for perioperative TEE section "Critical Care" (52).

CME Hours, MOC, Duration of Training, and Grandfathering

In the 2006 CVCAS/CSE Guidelines in Perioperative TEE, the importance of accredited CME hours is introduced for echocardiography (52). Duration of training in perioperative TEE for each level of expertise is only addressed in the CVCAS/CSE guidelines with the acknowledgement that this may vary depending on the training pathway and the structure of the training program (Table 31.4). Provisions for training in parallel with clinical activity is acknowledged by the NBE as a valid training pathway but this issue is only addressed in the 2006 CVCAS/CSE Training Guidelines in Perioperative TEE and is not included in the 2002 ASE/SCA training guidelines (52,56). At present, restricted grandfathering of existing practitioners for perioperative TEE has only been supported in the 2006 CVCAS/CSE training guidelines (52).

TESTAMUR STATUS AND CERTIFICATION IN PERIOPERATIVE TEE

Testamur of the NBE

A testamur is someone who has passed an examination of special competence administered by the NBE. A physician who obtains a passing score on the PTE examination becomes a testamur of the NBE. In 2009, the PTEeXAM examination is offered for the first time as a computer-based format multiple-choice examination through Prometric Testing Centers. Prometric features more than 300 professional testing centers throughout the United States, U.S. territories, and Canada (61).

Diplomate of the NBE

A testamur of the NBE who completes the certification process becomes a diplomate of the NBE. Completion of the certification process requires documented training in cardiovascular disease, extended training in echocardiography, and maintenance of these skills for a minimum of two years before applying for certification. Applicants who wish to apply for certification must also hold a valid, unrestricted license to practice medicine at the time of application and must be board certified by a board that holds membership in the American Board of Medical Specialties, the Advisory Board for Osteopathic Specialties, the American Association of Physician Specialists, or the Royal College of Physicians and Surgeons of Canada (61).

The supervised training pathway and the practice experience pathway are both recognized by the NBE for the purpose of certification. Physicians who complete their core residency training before July 1, 2009 will always be able to follow the practice experience pathway for certification in Perioperative TEE. However, the practice experience pathway will not be available to those finishing their core residency training after June 30, 2009 (61).

Fellowship Pathway

In the Fellowship Pathway, the applicants must have a minimum of 12 months of clinical fellowship training dedicated to the perioperative care of surgical patients with cardiovascular disease. The specific training or clinical experience in perioperative TEE must include 300 complete perioperative TEE examinations under appropriate supervision over a maximum period of two years. Note that the maximum duration of training is not specified in the ASE/SCA Task Force guidelines for training in perioperative echocardiography. These examinations must include a wide spectrum of cardiac diagnoses. Of the 300 examinations, at least 150 comprehensive intraoperative TEE examinations must be personally performed, interpreted, and reported by the trainee. For these 150 examinations, the supervising physician must be present for all critical aspects of the procedure, and immediately available throughout the procedure.

Those examinations that are not personally performed by the applicant must be acquired and reviewed at an institution where the applicant has performed TEEs under supervision. The required number of TEE examinations for the certification process follows the ASE/SCA Task Force guidelines for advanced training in perioperative echocardiography (Table 31.9). Documentation of compliance with the requirements of this pathway must be obtained from the institution where the examinations are performed and must be in a form acceptable to the NBE. Training obtained during the core residency (anesthesiology, internal medicine, or general surgery) may not be counted toward this requirement. For applicants finishing their core residency after June 30 2009, fellowship training in cardiothoracic or cardiovascular anesthesiology must be obtained in an Accreditation Council for Graduate of Medical Education (ACGME) accredited fellowship program (61).

Practice Experience Pathway

In the Practice Experience Pathway, applicants must have a minimum of 24 months of clinical experience dedicated to the perioperative care of surgical patients with cardiovascular disease. The experience must include perioperative care personally delivered by the applicant to at least 150 patients with cardiovas-

cular disease per year in each of the two years immediately preceding the application. Training obtained during core residency may not be counted toward this requirement. Specific training in echocardiography must include at least 300 perioperative transesophageal echocardiograms personally performed and interpreted by the applicant within four consecutive years immediately preceding the application with no less than 50 in any year in which any of the 300 echocardiograms were performed. At least 150 of the 300 transesophageal echocardiograms must be intraoperative. Physicians seeking certification by this pathway must have at least 50 hours of American Medical Association (AMA) category 1 continuing medical education devoted to echocardiography obtained during the time the physician is acquiring the requisite clinical experience in TEE (61).

Recertification Examination

The testamur status of special competence in perioperative TEE is valid for a period of 10 years. A recertification examination of special competence in perioperative TEE is currently available and to qualify for this examination, the applicant must have performed at least 50 perioperative TEE per year in two of the three years immediately preceding the application. The applicant must also have at least 15 hours of AMA category 1 CME devoted to echocardiography obtained during the three years preceding the application (61).

THE ECHOCARDIOGRAPHY REPORT

Recommendations for a standardized echocardiography report are proposed both in the CVCAS/CSE Training Guidelines in Perioperative Echocardiography (52) (Table 31.8) and by the SCA/ASE Task Force report for a standardized perioperative echocardiography (62) (Table 31.9). The report of the SCA/ASE Task Force includes a sample form (Table 31.9) that contains the following six sections: (i) demographic and other identifying information, (ii) echocardiographic and Doppler measurements, (iii) postintervention follow-up study, (iv) comments, (v) summary, and (vi) complications. It is also recognized by the SCA/ASE Task Force that this form can and should be customized to fit the specific needs of practitioners, including a computerized version (62).

CONCLUSION

The updated 2010 practice guidelines in perioperative TEE now recommend that TEE should be used in all cardiac and thoracic aortic procedures. The scope of applications in critical care and noncardiac surgery is also increased. Training guidelines are clearly outlined by both the ASE\SCA and the CSE and CV section of the CAS. In these guidelines, several pathways can be used to achieve clinical expertise in perioperative TEE, and it is essential to ensure that responsibilities are

Table 31.8   The Intraoperative Echocardiography Report

Basic components of an intraoperative transesophageal echo report *should* include the following basic demographics

1. Patient identification
2. The indication for the study
3. Surgical procedure
4. General study information including

Study date
Referring physician identification
Interpreting physician(s) identification
Media location (e.g., disk or tape number, etc.)
Location where study was performed (e.g., OR, PACU, ER, ICU)
Study technical quality (e.g., teaching quality, good, fair, poor, incomplete)

The content of the report *should* address the indications for the study and may include some or all of the following components. Reporting the following structures as normal implies a complete examination

5. Evaluation of the structure and function of the following anatomic components of the examination: (The minimum evaluation for each, and the implied meaning of a "normal" report is detailed in the next section). In patients undergoing coronary artery bypass grafting, the focus may be on the evaluation of ventricular systolic and diastolic function. In patients who are undergoing cardiac surgery other than coronary artery bypass grafting, quantitative and Doppler measurements of the surgical pathology should be performed when appropriate. However, a qualitative assessment of the other cardiac components may be sufficient in a patient with a complete preoperative TTE assessment. A more comprehensive evaluation may be required in patients without a preoperative TTE assessment or when clinically indicated

    1. Left ventricle
    2. Right ventricle
    3. Left atrium
    4. Left atrial appendage
    5. Pulmonary veins
    6. Right atrium
    7. Inferior vena cava
    8. Superior vena cava
    9. Coronary sinus
    10. Aortic valve
    11. Mitral valve
    12. Tricuspid valve
    13. Pulmonic valve
    14. Aorta
    15. Pulmonary artery
    16. Interventricular septum
    17. Interatrial septum
    18. Pericardium

6. Specific evaluation directed at the presenting problem and detected significant pathology

The study should incorporate a final assessment of the patient based on the intraoperative findings and include the following:

7. Conclusions and summary

    1. Overall interpretation/summary of findings
    2. Assessment of presenting issue
    3. Relevant comparisons to prior studies or reports as available
    4. Study limitations
    5. Recommendations regarding alternative or additional investigations and consultation where appropriate

The above constitutes a basic examination. Specific indications or pathology require further targeted imaging and/or hemodynamic assessment. A full review of the specific data required for evaluation of all possible pathologies is beyond the scope of this review, and the reader is referred to one of the many excellent comprehensive texts available.
Abbreviations: ER, emergency room; ICU, intensive care unit; OR, operating room; PACU, postoperative anesthesia care unit; TTE, transthoracic echocardiography.
Source: From Ref. 52.

Table 31.9 Recommendations of the SCA/ASE Task Force for a Standardized Perioperative Echocardiography Report

Sample Perioperative Echo Report

1. Demographic and Other Identifying Information

Name _____ Unit # _____ DOB _____ M/F _____ Date _____ Time _____

Location: ICU/OR/ER/PACU, Phys requesting Echo _____, Examiner _____

Indication _____ CPT Codes _____

ICD-9 codes _____

Intubated: Y/N, Sedated: Y/N, Insertion: Easy/Difficult/Failed Probe Type: pediatric/biplane/multiplane/epicardial/epiaortic Modalities: 2D/CFM/PWD/CWD/Contrast/Pharm/Stress Tape/OD #

2. Echocardiographic and Doppler Measurements

Aorta	Size	Diam (cm)	Dissection	Plaque thick (mm)	Plaque mobile
Ascending Ao	NL, dilated, aneur		Y/N	0–3, >3	Y/N
Ao arch	NL, dilated, aneur		Y/N	0–3, >3	Y/N
Descending Ao	NL, dilated, aneur		Y/N	0–3, >3	Y/N

Valves	Annulus	Size	Stenosis	Diam (cm)	Area/Gradient	Regurgitation	Leaflet Morphology	Leaflet Motion
Aortic valve	NL, dilated, calc, bioprosth, mechanical		No, mild, Mod, severe			0, 1+, 2+, 3+, 4+	Nl, NL, Calc, Veg, Perf, Bicuspid Thickened	Nl, NL, Prolapse Flail, Restricted NCC/RCC/LCC
Mitral valve	NL, dilated, calc, bioprosth, mechanical		No, mild, Mod, severe			0, 1+, 2+, 3+, 4+	Nl, NL, Calc, Veg Perf, Myxom Thickened	Nl, NL, Prolapse, Flail, SAM, Restricted A_1, A_2, A_3/P_1, P_2, P_3
Tricuspid	NL, dilated, calc, bioprosth, mechanical		No, mild, Mod, severe			0, 1+, 2+, 3+, 4+	Nl, NL, Calc, Veg Perf, Myxom Thickened	Nl, Prolapse Flail, Restricted
Pulmonic	NL, dilated, calc, bioprosth, mechanical		No, mild, Mod, severe			0, 1+, 2+, 3+, 4+	Nl, NL, Calc, Veg Perf, # cusps Thickened	NL, Prolapse Flail, Restricted

Atria	Size	SEC (smoke)	Thrombus	Tumor	Device
Right atrium	NL, dilated	Y/N	Y/N	Y/N	Y/N
Left atrium	NL, dilated	Y/N	Y/N	Y/N	Y/N

Left atrial appendage:

Interatrial Septum: Morphology: Normal, Aneurysm Lipomatous Hypertrophy, PFO, ASD (Primum, Secundum, Sinus Venosus, AV Canal) Shunt: (R→L, L→R, bidirectional)

Interventricular Septum Morphology: Normal, Hypertrophy, Shift, Defect (membr, musc), Shunt: (R→L, L→R)

Ventricles	Cavity size	Cavity dimension	Hypertrophy	Thrombus	Global Fct	EF
RV	NL, dilated		Y/N	Y/N	Nl, ↓, ↓↓, ↓↓↓	
LV	NL, dilated		Y/N	Y/N	Nl, ↓, ↓↓, ↓↓↓	

Regional function: (1 = NL, 2 = hypokinetic, 3 = akinetic, 4 = dyskinetic)

Basal segments	Mid segments	Apical segments
Anterior	Anterior	Anterior
Anteroseptal	Anteroseptal	Septal
Inferoseptal	Inferoseptal	Inferior
Inferior	Inferior	Lateral
Inferolateral	Inferolateral	True apex
Anterolateral	Anterolateral	

Pericardium: Normal, Thickened, Effusion: mild, moderate, severe, Tamponade

Pleural: NL, effusion

Postintervention Follow-up Study: See additional report, No Change. Ventricular Fct: Global Fct: Improved, Decreased. Regional Fct: Improved, Decreased. Valve Fct: Native Valve: No Change, Improved, Normal Prosthetic Valve type _____ NL Fct?: Y/N, Valve repair: 0 leak, 1+,2+,3+, Valve area _____

3. **Comments:** _____

_____

_____

4. **Summary:** _____

_____

_____

5. **Complications:** _____

None, details: _____

Abbreviations. Aneur, aneurysm; Ao, aorta; ASD, atrial septal defect; ASE, American Society of Echocardiography; AV, atrioventricular; bioprosth, bioprosthesis; calc, calcification; CFM, continuous flow measure; CPT, Current Procedural Terminology; CWD, continuous wave Doppler; Diam, diameter; DOB, date of birth; ER, emergency room; F, female; Fct, function; ICD, International Classification of Diseases; ICU, intensive care unit; L, Left; LCC, left coronary cusp; LV, left ventricle; M, male; Membr, membranous; Musc, muscular; Myxom, myxomatous; N, no; NCC, noncoronary cusp; NI, not identified; NL, normal; OR, operating room; PACU, postoperative anesthesia care unit; Perf, perforated; PFO, patent foramen ovale; PWD, pulsed wave Doppler; R, right; RCC, right coronary cusp; RV, right ventricle; SAM, systolic anterior motion; SCA, Society of Cardiovascular Anesthesiologists; SEC, spontaneous echo contrast; Tape/OD, Tape/Optic Disk; Veg, vegetations; Y, yes.
Source: From Ref. 62.

Table 31.10 National Board of Echocardiography Exams and Certifications

Basic PTE examination objectives
1. Patient safety considerations
2. Echocardiographic imaging: acquisition and optimization
3. Normal cardiac anatomy and imaging plane correlation
4. Global ventricular function
5. Regional ventricular systolic function and recognition of pathology
6. Basic recognition of cardiac valve abnormalities
7. Identification of intracardiac masses in noncardiac surgery
8. Basic perioperative hemodynamic assessment
9. Related diagnostic modalities
10. Basic recognition of congenital heart disease in the adult
11. Surface ultrasound for vascular access

Advanced PTE examination objectives
1. Principles of ultrasound
2. Transducers
3. Imaging
4. Principles of Doppler ultrasound
5. Doppler flow profiles for normal and abnormal physiology
6. Quantitative echocardiography
7. Artifacts and pitfalls of imaging
8. Equipment, infection control, and safety
9. Normal anatomy and flow during the complete examination
10. Myocardial ischemia and segmental ventricular function
11. Ventricular function and hemodynamics
12. Recognizing intracavitary contents
13. Echocardiographic manifestations of congenital heart disease in adult patients
14. Hypertrophic obstructive cardiomyopathy
15. Dilated and restricted cardiomyopathies
16. Echocardiography for the pericardium and extracardiac anatomy
17. Echocardiography during cardiac surgery
18. Assessing heart valves during the perioperative period
19. Indications for transesophageal echocardiography
20. Non-TEE imaging and other diagnostic modalities

Abbreviations: PTE, perioperative transesophageal echocardiography; TEE, transesophageal echocardiography.
Source: Adapted from Ref. 61.

commensurate with the level of training. Advanced and basic certifications are available through the NBE (61). The goal of this manual was indeed to cover those objectives as summarized in Table 31.10.

REFERENCES

1. Eltzschig HK, Rosenberger P, Loffler M, et al. Impact of intraoperative transesophageal echocardiography on surgical decisions in 12,566 patients undergoing cardiac surgery. Ann Thorac Surg 2008; 85:845–852.
2. Click RL, Abel MD, Schaff HV. Intraoperative transesophageal echocardiography: 5-year prospective review of impact on surgical management. Mayo Clin Proc 2000; 75:241–247.
3. Couture P, Denault AY, McKenty S, et al. Impact of routine use of intraoperative transesophageal echocardiography during cardiac surgery. Can J Anaesth 2000; 47:20–26.
4. Michel-Cherqui M, Ceddaha A, Liu N, et al. Assessment of systematic use of intraoperative transesophageal echocardiography during cardiac surgery in adults: a prospective study of 203 patients. J Cardiothorac Vasc Anesth 2000; 14:45–50.
5. Mishra M, Chauhan R, Sharma KK, et al. Real-time intraoperative transesophageal echocardiography—how useful? Experience of 5,016 cases. J Cardiothorac Vasc Anesth 1998; 12:625–632.
6. Sutton DC, Kluger R. Intraoperative transoesophageal echocardiography: impact on adult cardiac surgery. Anaesth Intensive Care 1998; 26:287–293.
7. Stevenson JG. Role of intraoperative transesophageal echocardiography during repair of congenital cardiac defects. Acta Paediatr Suppl 1995; 410:23–33.
8. Rosenfeld HM, Gentles TL, Wernovsky G, et al. Utility of intraoperative transesophageal echocardiography in the assessment of residual cardiac defects. Pediatr Cardiol 1998; 19:346–351.
9. Sheil ML, Baines DB. Intraoperative transoesophageal echocardiography for paediatric cardiac surgery—an audit of 200 cases. Anaesth Intensive Care 1999; 27:591–595.
10. Ungerleider RM, Kisslo JA, Greeley WJ, et al. Intraoperative echocardiography during congenital heart operations: experience from 1,000 cases. Ann Thorac Surg 1995; 60:S539–S542.
11. Practice guidelines for perioperative transesophageal echocardiography. A report by the American Society of Anesthesiologists and the Society of Cardiovascular Anesthesiologists Task Force on Transesophageal Echocardiography. Anesthesiology 1996; 84:986–1006.
12. Cheitlin MD, Alpert JS, Armstrong WF, et al. ACC/AHA Guidelines for the Clinical Application of Echocardiography. A report of the American College of Cardiology/American Heart Association Task Force on Practice Guidelines (Committee on Clinical Application of Echocardiography). Developed in collaboration with the American Society of Echocardiography. Circulation 1997; 95:1686–1744.
13. Cheitlin MD, Armstrong WF, Aurigemma GP, et al. ACC/AHA/ASE 2003 guideline update for the clinical application of echocardiography: summary article: a report of the American College of Cardiology/American Heart Association Task Force on Practice Guidelines (ACC/AHA/ASE Committee to Update the 1997 Guidelines for the Clinical Application of Echocardiography). Circulation 2003; 108:1146–1162.
14. Douglas PS, Khandheria B, Stainback RF, et al. ACCF/ASE/ACEP/ASNC/SCAI/SCCT/SCMR 2007 appropriateness criteria for transthoracic and transesophageal echocardiography: a report of the American College of Cardiology Foundation Quality Strategic Directions Committee Appropriateness Criteria Working Group, American Society of Echocardiography, American College of Emergency Physicians, American Society of Nuclear Cardiology, Society for Cardiovascular Angiography and Interventions, Society of Cardiovascular Computed Tomography, and the Society for Cardiovascular Magnetic Resonance endorsed by the American College of Chest Physicians and the Society of Critical Care Medicine. J Am Coll Cardiol 2007; 50:187–204.
15. Practice Guidelines for Perioperative Transesophageal Echocardiography: An Updated Report by the American Society of Anesthesiologists and the Society of Cardiovascular Anesthesiologists Task Force on Transesophageal Echocardiography. Anesthesiology 2010; 112:1–13.
16. De Castro S, Cartoni D, d'Amati G, et al. Diagnostic accuracy of transthoracic and multiplane transesophageal echocardiography for valvular perforation in acute infective endocarditis: correlation with anatomic findings. Clin Infect Dis 2000; 30:825–826.

17. Espinal M, Fuisz AR, Nanda NC, et al. Sensitivity and specificity of transesophageal echocardiography for determination of aortic valve morphology. Am Heart J 2000; 139:1071–1076.

18. Hellemans IM, Pieper EG, Ravelli AC, et al. Comparison of transthoracic and transesophageal echocardiography with surgical findings in mitral regurgitation. The ESMIR Research Group. Am J Cardiol 1996; 77:728–733.

19. Muller S, Muller L, Laufer G, et al. Comparison of three-dimensional imaging to transesophageal echocardiography for preoperative evaluation in mitral valve prolapse. Am J Cardiol 2006; 98:243–248.

20. Grewal KS, Malkowski MJ, Kramer CM, et al. Multiplane transesophageal echocardiographic identification of the involved scallop in patients with flail mitral valve leaflet: intraoperative correlation. J Am Soc Echocardiogr 1998; 11:966–971.

21. Senni M, Merlo M, Sangiorgi G, et al. Mitral valve repair and transesophageal echocardiographic findings in a high-risk subgroup of patients with active, acute infective endocarditis. J Heart Valve Dis 2001; 10:72–77.

22. Morguet AJ, Werner GS, Andreas S, et al. Diagnostic value of transesophageal compared with transthoracic echocardiography in suspected prosthetic valve endocarditis. Herz 1995; 20:390–398.

23. San Roman JA, Vilacosta I, Sarria C, et al. Clinical course, microbiologic profile, and diagnosis of periannular complications in prosthetic valve endocarditis. Am J Cardiol 1999; 83:1075–1079.

24. Comunale ME, Body SC, Ley C, et al. The concordance of intraoperative left ventricular wall-motion abnormalities and electrocardiographic S-T segment changes: association with outcome after coronary revascularization. Multicenter Study of Perioperative Ischemia (McSPI) Research Group. Anesthesiology 1998; 88:945–954.

25. Kodolitsch Y, Krause N, Spielmann R, et al. Diagnostic potential of combined transthoracic echocardiography and x-ray computed tomography in suspected aortic dissection. Clin Cardiol 1999; 22:345–352.

26. Laissy JP, Blanc F, Soyer P, et al. Thoracic aortic dissection: diagnosis with transesophageal echocardiography versus MR imaging. Radiology 1995; 194:331–336.

27. Patel S, Alam M, Rosman H. Pitfalls in the echocardiographic diagnosis of aortic dissection. Angiology 1997; 48:939–946.

28. Sommer T, Fehske W, Holzknecht N, et al. Aortic dissection: a comparative study of diagnosis with spiral CT, multiplanar transesophageal echocardiography, and MR imaging. Radiology 1996; 199:347–352.

29. Konstadt SN, Reich DL, Kahn R, et al. Transesophageal echocardiography can be used to screen for ascending aortic atherosclerosis. Anesth Analg 1995; 81:225–228.

30. Minard G, Schurr MJ, Croce MA, et al. A prospective analysis of transesophageal echocardiography in the diagnosis of traumatic disruption of the aorta. J Trauma 1996; 40:225–230.

31. Vignon P, Gueret P, Vedrinne JM, et al. Role of transesophageal echocardiography in the diagnosis and management of traumatic aortic disruption. Circulation 1995; 92:2959–2968.

32. Singh GK, Shiota T, Cobanoglu A, et al. Diagnostic accuracy and role of intraoperative biplane transesophageal echocardiography in pediatric patients with left ventricle outflow tract lesions. J Am Soc Echocardiogr 1998; 11:47–56.

33. Rosenberger P, Shernan SK, Body SC, et al. Utility of intraoperative transesophageal echocardiography for diagnosis of pulmonary embolism. Anesth Analg 2004; 99:12–16.

34. Kang DH, Song JK, Song MG, et al. Clinical and echocardiographic outcomes of aortic intramural hemorrhage compared with acute aortic dissection. Am J Cardiol 1998; 81:202–206.

35. Attenhofer CH, Vogt PR, von Segesser LK, et al. Leaking giant aneurysm of the aortic root due to cystic medial necrosis with pericardial tamponade mimicking type-A aortic dissection. Thorac Cardiovasc Surg 1996; 44:103–104.

36. Theodore S, Vaidyanathan K, Jagannath BR, et al. Takayasu's arteritis mimicking acute aortic dissection. Ann Thorac Surg 2007; 83:1876–1878.

37. Berdat PA, Carrel T. Aortic dissection limited to the ascending aorta mimicking intramural hematoma. Eur J Cardiothorac Surg 1999; 15:108–109.

38. Vuille C, Trigo-Trindade P, Lerch R, et al. Common coronary ostium mimicking an aortic abscess in a case of bacterial endocarditis. J Am Soc Echocardiogr 1998; 11:80–82.

39. Kupersmith AC, Belkin RN, McClung JA, et al. Aortic valve commissural tear mimicking type A aortic dissection. J Am Soc Echocardiogr 2002; 15:658–660.

40. Akowuah EF, Onyeaka CV, Cooper GJ. A subtle sign of aortic outflow obstruction in an infected 29 year old Starr-Edward's valve. Heart 2001; 85:384.

41. Sherwood JT, Gill IS. Missed acute ascending aortic dissection. J Card Surg 2001; 16:86–88.

42. Kaneko Y, Furuse A, Takeshita M, et al. Fibrous tissue overgrowth and prosthetic valve endocarditis: report of a case. Thorac Cardiovasc Surg 1997; 45:150–152.

43. Park P, Khawly JA, Kearney DL, et al. Bilateral endogenous endophthalmitis secondary to endocarditis with negative transesophageal echocardiogram. Am J Ophthalmol 2004; 138:151–153.

44. Dalal A, Asirvatham SJ, Chandrasekaran K, et al. Intracardiac echocardiography in the detection of pacemaker lead endocarditis. J Am Soc Echocardiogr 2002; 15:1027–1028.

45. Flachskampf FA, Banbury M, Smedira N, et al. Transesophageal echocardiography diagnosis of intramural hematoma of the ascending aorta: a word of caution. J Am Soc Echocardiogr 1999; 12:866–870.

46. Lick SD, Zwischenberger JB, Mileski WJ, et al. Torn ascending aorta missed by transesophageal echocardiography. Ann Thorac Surg 1997; 63:1768–1770.

47. Beauchesne LM, Veinot JP, Brais MP, et al. Acute aortic intimal tear without a mobile flap mimicking an intramural hematoma. J Am Soc Echocardiogr 2003; 16:285–288.

48. Bauer M, Redzepagic S, Weng Y, et al. Successful surgical treatment of a giant aneurysm of the right coronary artery. Thorac Cardiovasc Surg 1998; 46:152–154.

49. Kunzli A, von Segesser LK, Vogt PR, et al. Inflammatory aneurysm of the ascending aorta. Ann Thorac Surg 1998; 65:1132–1133.

50. Paolillo V, Gastaldo D, Barretta A, et al. Idiopathic organized thrombus of the tricuspid valve mimicking valvular tumor. Tex Heart Inst J 2004; 31:192–193.

51. Konishi H, Fukuda M, Kato M, et al. Organized thrombus of the tricuspid valve mimicking valvular tumor. Ann Thorac Surg 2001; 71:2022–2024.

52. Beique F, Ali M, Hynes M, et al. Canadian guidelines for training in adult perioperative transesophageal echocardiography. Recommendations of the Cardiovascular Section of the Canadian Anesthesiologists' Society and the Canadian Society of Echocardiography. Can J Cardiol 2006; 22:1015–1027.

53. Pearlman AS, Gardin JM, Martin RP, et al. Guidelines for optimal physician training in echocardiography. Recommendations of the American Society of Echocardiography Committee for Physician Training in Echocardiography. Am J Cardiol 1987; 60:158–163.

54. Pearlman AS, Gardin JM, Martin RP, et al. Guidelines for physician training in transesophageal echocardiography: recommendations of the American Society of

Echocardiography Committee for Physician Training in Echocardiography. J Am Soc Echocardiogr 1992; 5:187–194.

55. Aronson S, Butler A, Subhiyah R, et al. Development and analysis of a new certifying examination in perioperative transesophageal echocardiography. Anesth Analg 2002; 95:1476–1482, table.

56. Cahalan MK, Abel M, Goldman M, et al. American Society of Echocardiography and Society of Cardiovascular Anesthesiologists task force guidelines for training in perioperative echocardiography. Anesth Analg 2002; 94:1384–1388.

57. Beique FA, Denault AY, Martineau A, et al. Expert consensus for training in perioperative echocardiography in the province of Quebec. Can J Anaesth 2003; 50:699–706.

58. Sanfilippo AJ, Bewick D, Chan KL, et al. Guidelines for the provision of echocardiography in Canada: recommendations of a joint Canadian Cardiovascular Society/Canadian Society of Echocardiography Consensus Panel. Can J Cardiol 2005; 21:763–780.

59. Finegan BA Progress through cooperation: securing a sound training pathway for perioperative transesophageal echocardiography. Can J Anaesth 2006; 53:969–972.

60. Shanewise JS, Cheung AT, Aronson S, et al. ASE/SCA guidelines for performing a comprehensive intraoperative multiplane transesophageal echocardiography examination: recommendations of the American Society of Echocardiography Council for Intraoperative Echocardiography and the Society of Cardiovascular Anesthesiologists Task Force for Certification in Perioperative Transesophageal Echocardiography. Anesth Analg 1999; 89:870–884.

61. The National Board of Echocardiography. Available at: http://www.echoboards.org/. 2009. Electronic Citation.

62. Savage R, Hillel Z, London M, et al. Recommendations for a Standardized Report for Adult Perioperative Echocardiography. Available at: http://www.scahq.org/sca3/Report_of_Task_Force.pdf, 2009. Electronic Citation.

Recommended Views in Transesophageal Echocardiography

Carl Chartrand-Lefebvre and André Y. Denault
Université de Montréal, Montreal, Quebec, Canada

Annette Vegas
University of Toronto, Toronto, Ontario, Canada

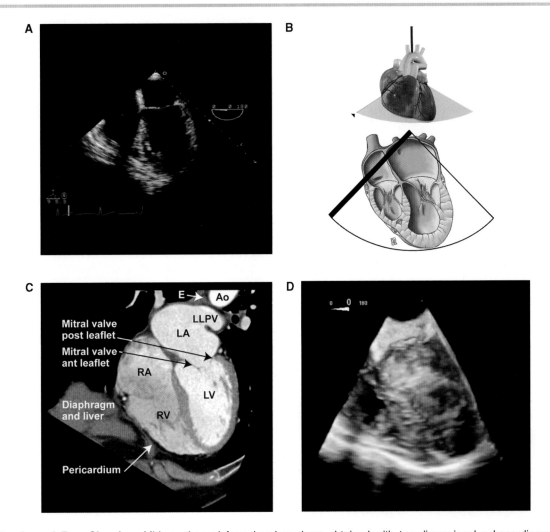

A1 Mid-Esophageal Four-Chamber. Mid-esophageal four-chamber views obtained with two-dimensional echocardiography (**A,B**), ECG-gated computed tomography (**C**), and three-dimensional echocardiography (**D**). *Abbreviations*: Ao, aorta; E, esophagus; ECG, electrocardiogram; LA, left atrium; LLPV, left lower pulmonary vein; LV, left ventricle; RA, right atrium; RV, right ventricle. *Source:* Illustration B courtesy of Gian-Marco Busato.

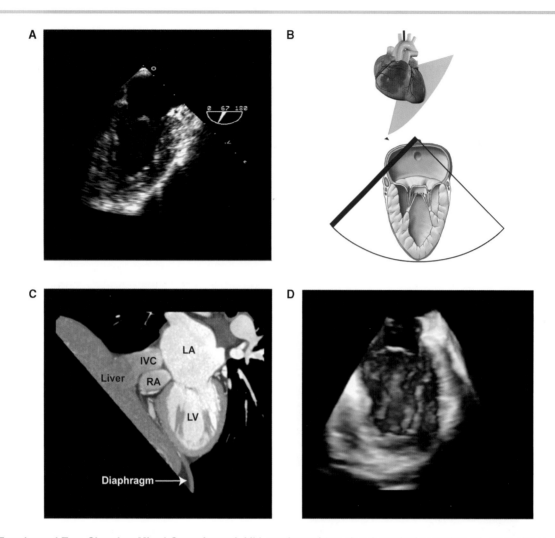

A2 Mid-Esophageal Two-Chamber Mitral Commissural. Mid-esophageal two-chamber mitral commissural views obtained with two-dimensional echocardiography (**A,B**), ECG-gated computed tomography (**C**), and three-dimensional echocardiography (**D**). *Abbreviations*: ECG, electrocardiogram; IVC, inferior vena cava; LA, left atrium; LV, left ventricle; RA, right atrium. *Source:* Illustration B courtesy of Gian-Marco Busato.

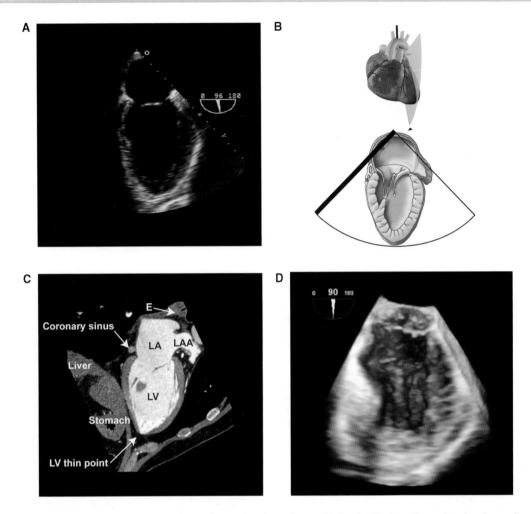

A3 Mid-Esophageal Two-Chamber. Mid-esophageal two-chamber views obtained with two-dimensional echocardiography (**A,B**), ECG-gated computed tomography (**C**), and three-dimensional echocardiography (**D**). *Abbreviations*: E, esophagus; ECG, electrocardiogram; LA, left atrium; LAA, left atrial appendage; LV, left ventricle. *Source:* Illustration B courtesy of Gian-Marco Busato.

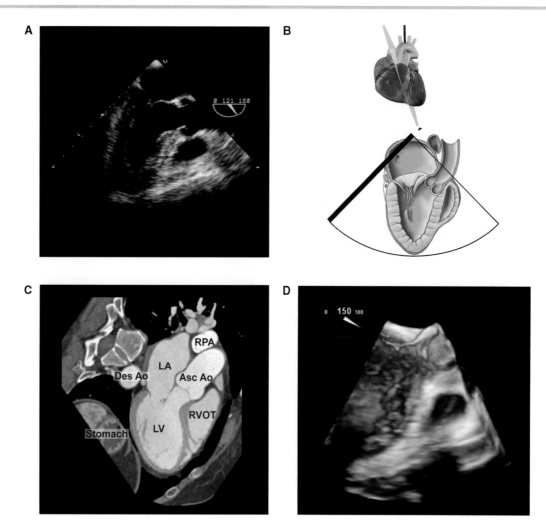

A4 Mid-Esophageal Long-Axis. Mid-esophageal long-axis views obtained with two-dimensional echocardiography (**A,B**), ECG-gated computed tomography (**C**), and three-dimensional echocardiography (**D**). *Abbreviations*: Ao, aorta; Asc, ascending; Des, descending; ECG, electrocardiogram; LA, left atrium; LV, left ventricle; RPA, right pulmonary artery; RVOT, right ventricular outflow tract. *Source*: Illustration B courtesy of Gian-Marco Busato.

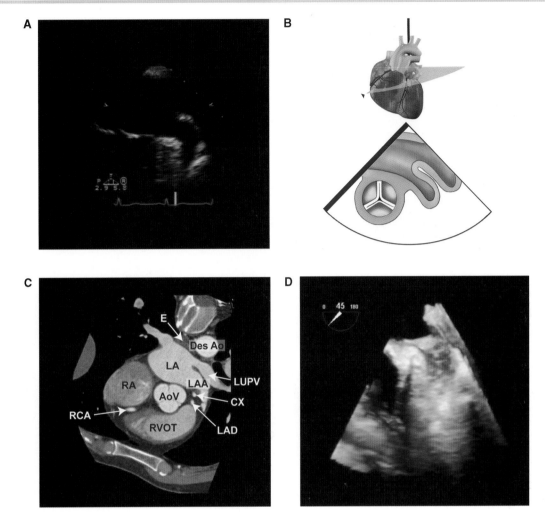

A5 Mid-Esophageal Left Atrial Appendage. Mid-esophageal left atrial appendage views obtained with two-dimensional echocardiography (**A,B**), ECG-gated computed tomography (**C**), and three-dimensional echocardiography (**D**). *Abbreviations:* Ao, aorta; AoV, aortic valve; CX, circumflex artery; Des, descending; E, esophagus; ECG, electrocardiogram; LA, left atrium; LAA, left atrial appendage; LAD, left anterior descending artery; LUPV, left upper pulmonary vein; RA, right atrium; RCA, right coronary artery; RVOT, right ventricular outflow tract. *Source:* Illustration B courtesy of Gian-Marco Busato.

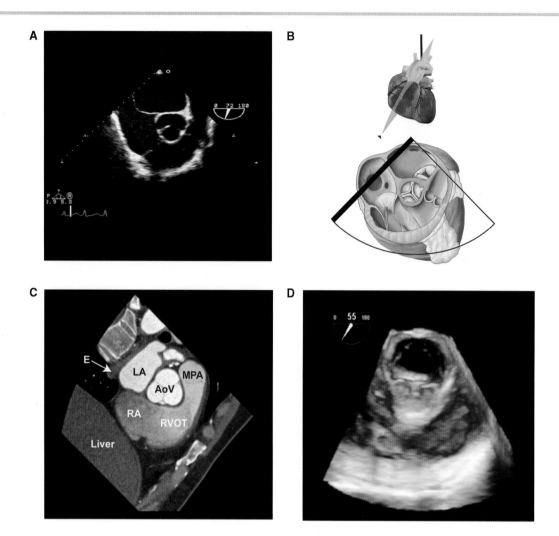

A6 Mid-Esophageal Right Ventricular Outflow Tract. Mid-esophageal right ventricular outflow tract views obtained with two-dimensional echocardiography (**A,B**), ECG-gated computed tomography (**C**), and three-dimensional echocardiography (**D**). *Abbreviations:* AoV, aortic valve; E, esophagus; ECG, electrocardiogram; LA, left atrium; MPA, main pulmonary artery; RA, right atrium; RVOT, right ventricular outflow tract. *Source*: Illustration B courtesy of Gian-Marco Busato.

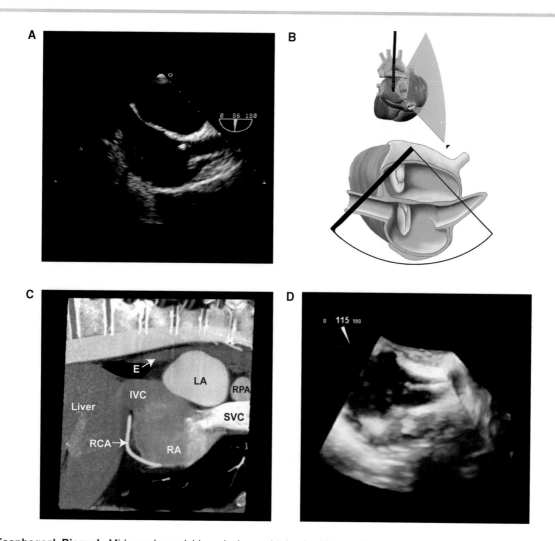

A7 Mid-Esophageal Bicaval. Mid-esophageal bicaval views obtained with two-dimensional echocardiography (**A,B**), ECG-gated computed tomography (**C**), and three-dimensional echocardiography (**D**). *Abbreviations*: E, esophagus; ECG, electrocardiogram; IVC, inferior vena cava; LA, left atrium; RA, right atrium; RCA, right coronary artery; RPA, right pulmonary artery; SVC superior vena cava. *Source*: Illustration B courtesy of Gian-Marco Busato.

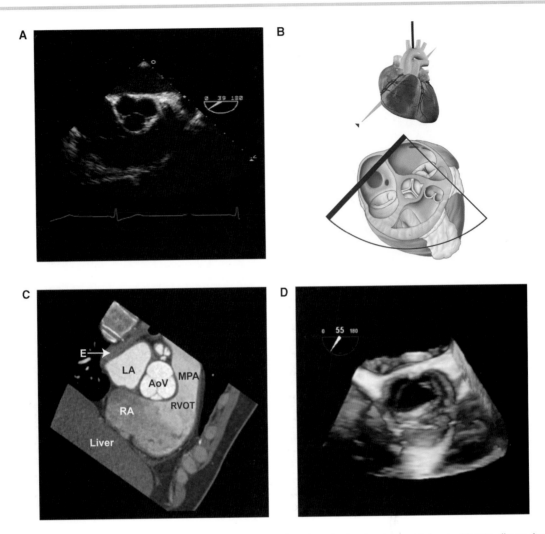

A8 Mid-Esophageal Aortic Valve Short-Axis. Mid-esophageal aortic valve short-axis views obtained with two-dimensional echocardiography (**A**,**B**), ECG-gated computed tomography (**C**), and three-dimensional echocardiography (**D**). *Abbreviations*: AoV, aortic valve; E, esophagus; ECG, electrocardiogram; LA, left atrium; MPA, main pulmonary artery; RA, right atrium; RVOT, right ventricular outflow tract. *Source*: Illustration B courtesy of Gian-Marco Busato.

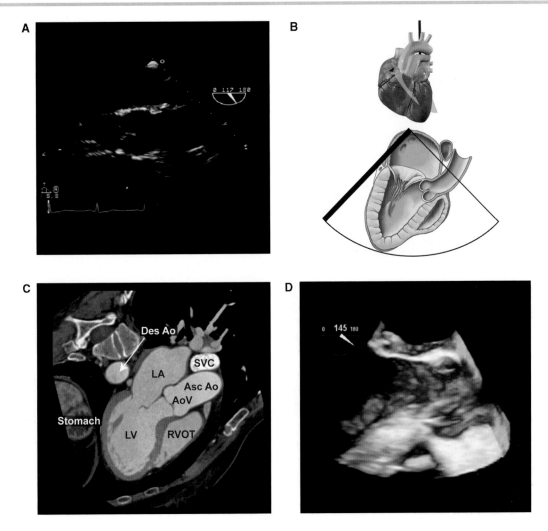

A9 Mid-Esophageal Aortic Valve Long-Axis. Mid-esophageal aortic valve long-axis views obtained with two-dimensional echocardiography (**A,B**), ECG-gated computed tomography (**C**), and three-dimensional echocardiography (**D**). *Abbreviations*: Ao, aorta; AoV, aortic valve; Asc, ascending; Des, descending; ECG, electrocardiogram; LA, left atrium; LV, left ventricle; RVOT, right ventricular outflow tract; SVC, superior vena cava. *Source*: Illustration B courtesy of Gian-Marco Busato.

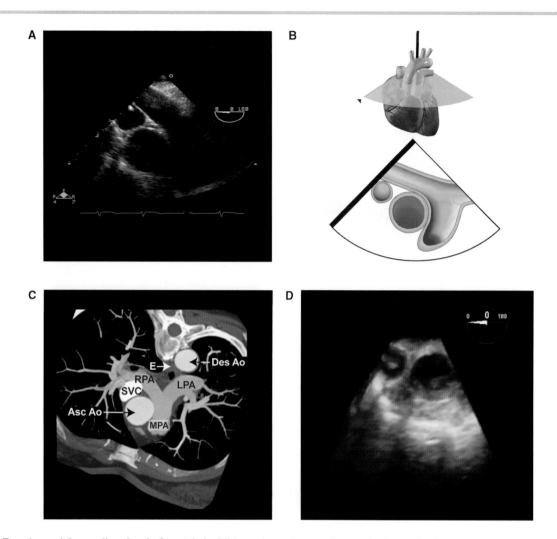

A10 Mid-Esophageal Ascending Aortic Short-Axis. Mid-esophageal ascending aortic short-axis views obtained with two-dimensional echocardiography (**A,B**), ECG-gated computed tomography (**C**), and three-dimensional echocardiography (**D**). *Abbreviations*: Ao, aorta; Asc, ascending; Des, descending; E, esophagus; ECG, electrocardiogram; LPA, left pulmonary artery; MPA, main pulmonary artery; RPA, right pulmonary artery; SVC, superior vena cava. *Source:* Illustration B courtesy of Gian-Marco Busato.

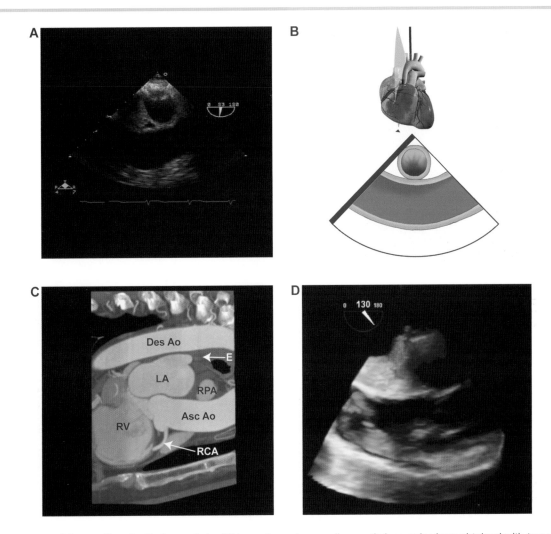

A11 Mid-Esophageal Ascending Aortic Long-Axis. Mid-esophageal ascending aortic long-axis views obtained with two-dimensional echocardiography (**A,B**), ECG-gated computed tomography (**C**), and three-dimensional echocardiography (**D**). *Abbreviations*: Ao, aorta; Asc, ascending; Des, descending; E, esophagus; ECG, electrocardiogram; LA, left atrium; RCA, right coronary artery; RPA, right pulmonary artery; RV, right ventricle. *Source:* Illustration B courtesy of Gian-Marco Busato.

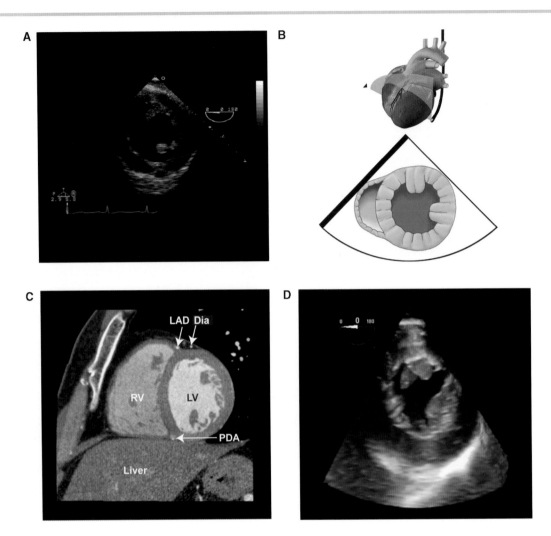

B1 Transgastric Mid-Papillary Short-Axis. Transgastric mid-papillary short-axis views obtained with two-dimensional echocardiography (**A,B**), ECG-gated computed tomography (**C**), and three-dimensional echocardiography (**D**). *Abbreviations*: Dia, diagonal artery; ECG, electrocardiogram; LAD, left anterior descending artery; LV, left ventricle; PDA, posterior descending artery; RV, right ventricle. *Source*: Illustration B courtesy of Gian-Marco Busato.

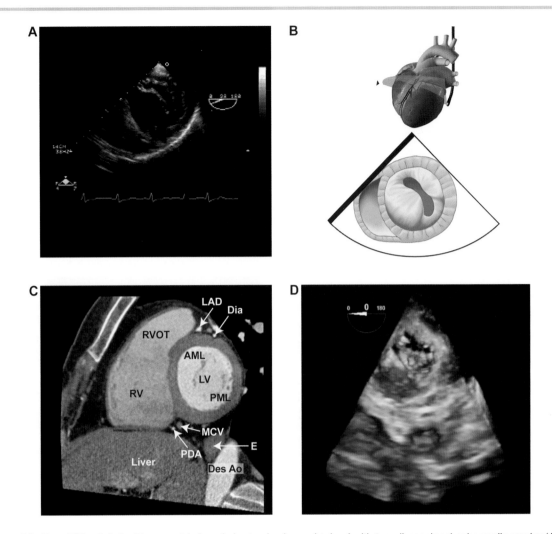

B2 Transgastric Basal Short-Axis. Transgastric basal short-axis views obtained with two-dimensional echocardiography (**A,B**), ECG-gated computed tomography (**C**), and three-dimensional echocardiography (**D**). *Abbreviations*: AML, anterior mitral leaflet; Ao, aorta; Des, descending; Dia, diagonal artery; E, esophagus; ECG, electrocardiogram; LAD, left anterior descending artery; LV, left ventricle; MCV, middle cardiac vein; PDA, posterior descending artery; PML, posterior mitral leaflet; RV, right ventricle; RVOT, right ventricular outflow tract. *Source*: Illustration B courtesy of Gian-Marco Busato.

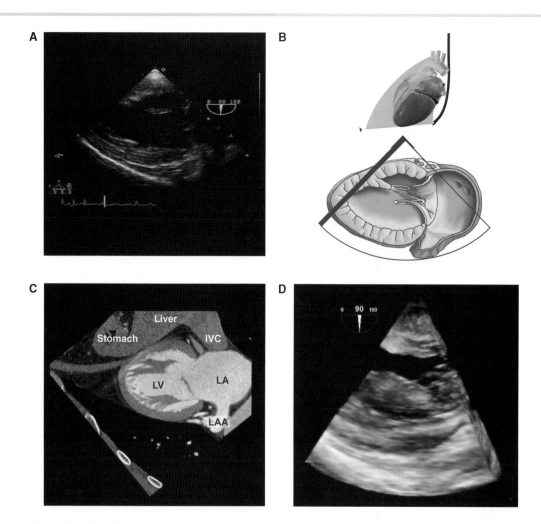

B3 Transgastric Two-Chamber. Transgastric two-chamber views obtained with two-dimensional echocardiography (**A,B**), ECG-gated computed tomography (**C**), and three-dimensional echocardiography (**D**). *Abbreviations*: ECG, electrocardiogram; IVC, inferior vena cava; LA, left atrium; LAA, left atrial appendage; LV, left ventricle. *Source*: Illustration B courtesy of Gian-Marco Busato.

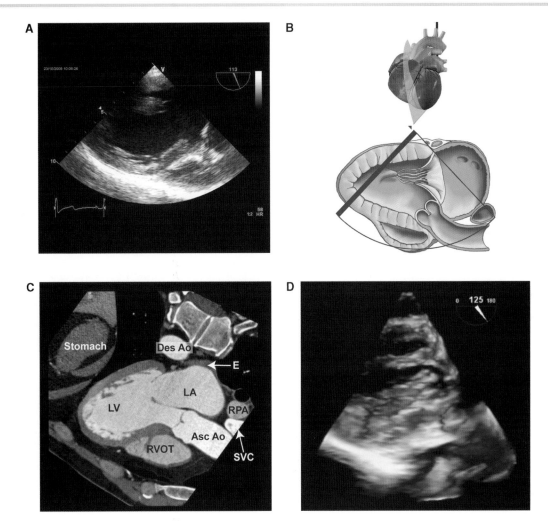

B4 Transgastric Long-Axis. Transgastric long-axis views obtained with two-dimensional echocardiography (**A,B**), ECG-gated computed tomography (**C**), and three-dimensional echocardiography (**D**). *Abbreviations*: Ao, aorta; Asc, ascending; Des, descending; E, esophagus; ECG, electrocardiogram; LA, left atrium; LV, left ventricle; RPA, right pulmonary artery; RVOT, right ventricular outflow tract; SVC, superior vena cava. *Source*: Illustration B courtesy of Gian-Marco Busato.

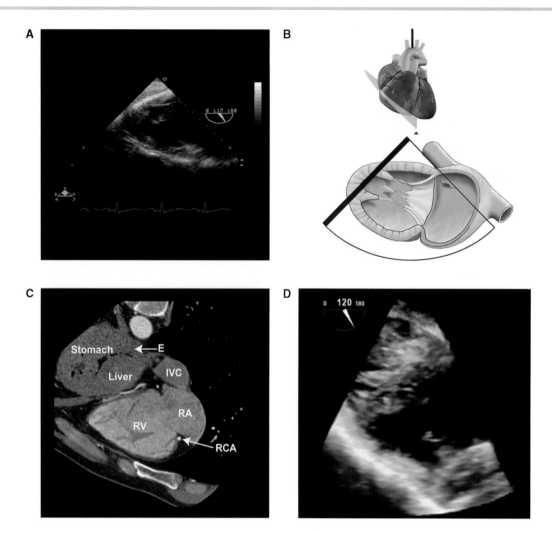

B5 Transgastric Right Ventricle. Transgastric right ventricular views obtained with two-dimensional echocardiography (**A,B**), ECG-gated computed tomography (**C**), and three-dimensional echocardiography (**D**). *Abbreviations*: E, esophagus; ECG, electrocardiogram; IVC, inferior vena cava; RA, right atrium; RCA, right coronary artery; RV, right ventricle. *Source*: Illustration B courtesy of Gian-Marco Busato.

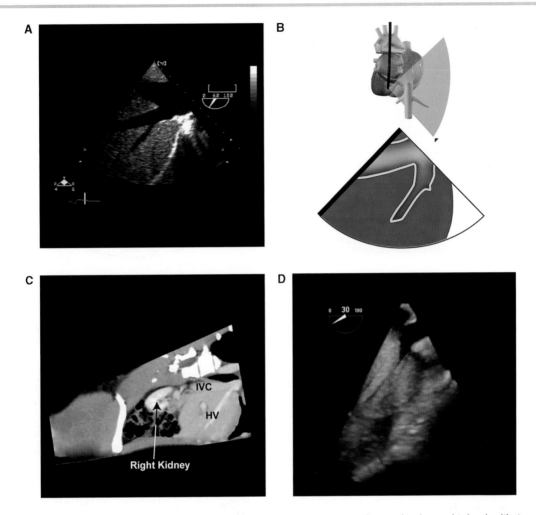

B6 Transgastric Inferior Vena Cava Long-Axis. Transgastric inferior vena cava long-axis views obtained with two-dimensional echocardiography (**A**,**B**), ECG-gated computed tomography (**C**), and three-dimensional echocardiography (**D**). *Abbreviations*: ECG, electrocardiogram; HV, hepatic vein; IVC, inferior vena cava. *Source*: Illustration B courtesy of Gian-Marco Busato.

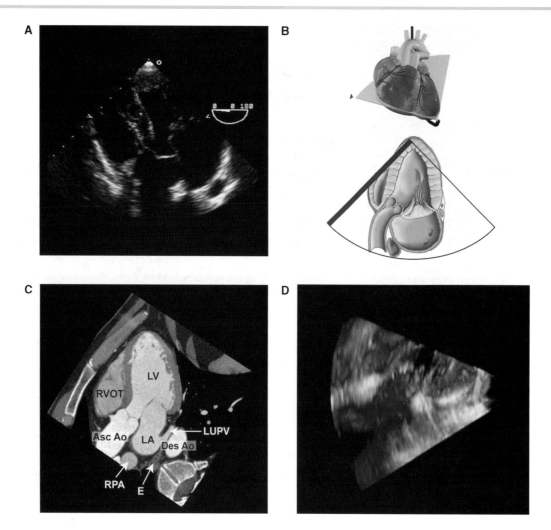

C1 Deep Transgastric. Deep transgastric views obtained with two-dimensional echocardiography (**A,B**), ECG-gated computed tomography (**C**), and three-dimensional echocardiography (**D**). *Abbreviations*: Ao, aorta; Asc, ascending; Des, descending; E, esophagus; ECG, electrocardiogram; LA, left atrium; LUPV, left upper pulmonary vein; LV, left ventricle; RPA, right pulmonary artery; RVOT, right ventricular outflow tract. *Source*: Illustration B courtesy of Gian-Marco Busato.

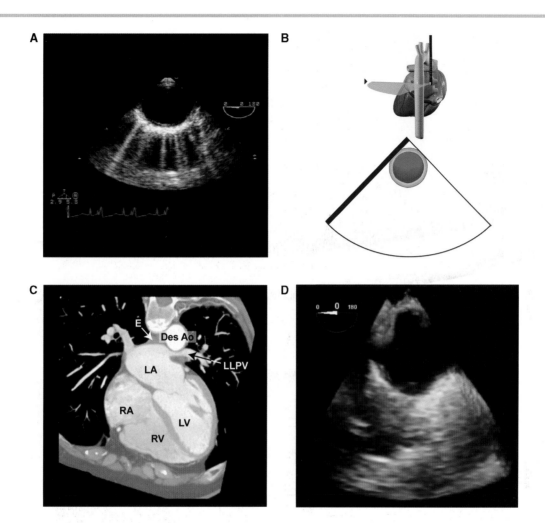

D1 Descending Aortic Short-Axis. Descending aortic short-axis views obtained with two-dimensional echocardiography (**A,B**), ECG-gated computed tomography (**C**), and three-dimensional echocardiography (**D**). *Abbreviations*: Ao, aorta; Des, descending; E, esophagus; ECG, electrocardiogram; LA, left atrium; LLPV, left lower pulmonary vein; LV, left ventricle; RA, right atrium; RV, right ventricle. *Source*: Illustration B courtesy of Gian-Marco Busato.

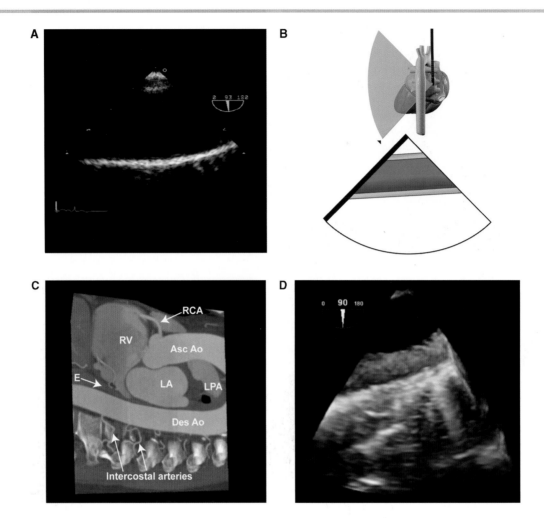

D2 Descending Aortic Long-Axis. Descending aortic long-axis views obtained with two-dimensional echocardiography (**A,B**), ECG-gated computed tomography (**C**), and three-dimensional echocardiography (**D**). *Abbreviations*: Ao, aorta; Asc, ascending; Des, descending; E, esophagus; ECG, electrocardiogram; LA, left atrium; LPA, left pulmonary artery; RCA, right coronary artery; RV, right ventricle. *Source*: Illustration B courtesy of Gian-Marco Busato.

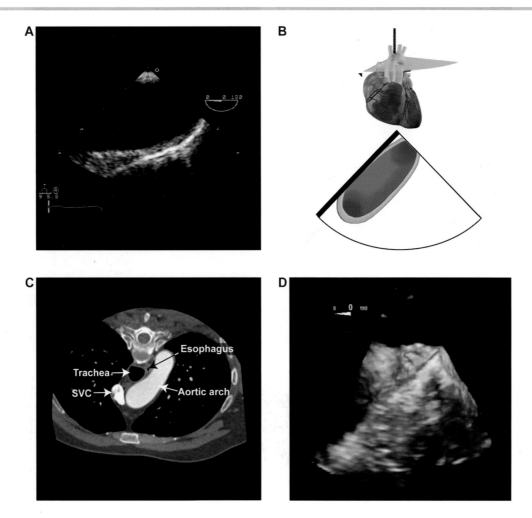

E1 Upper Esophageal Aortic Long-Axis. Upper esophageal aortic long-axis views of the aortic arch obtained with two-dimensional echocardiography (**A,B**), ECG-gated computed tomography (**C**), and three-dimensional echocardiography (**D**). *Abbreviations*: ECG, electrocardiogram; SVC, superior vena cava. *Source*: Illustration B courtesy of Gian-Marco Busato.

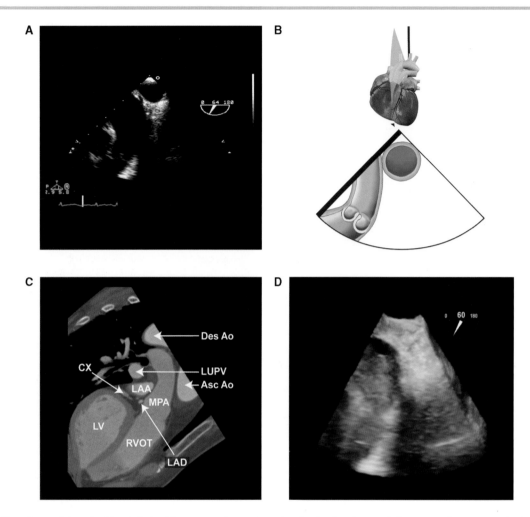

E2 Upper Esophageal Aortic Short-Axis. Upper esophageal aortic short-axis views of the ascending aorta obtained with two-dimensional echocardiography (**A,B**), ECG-gated computed tomography (**C**), and three-dimensional echocardiography (**D**). *Abbreviations*: Ao, aorta; Asc, ascending; CX, circumflex artery; Des, descending; ECG, electrocardiogram; LAA, left atrial appendage; LAD, left anterior descending artery; LUPV, left upper pulmonary vein; LV, left ventricle; MPA, main pulmonary artery; RVOT, right ventricular outflow tract. *Source*: Illustration B courtesy of Gian-Marco Busato.

Index

Note: Page numbers followed by f and t indicate figures and tables, respectively.

2D imaging. *See* Two-dimensional (2D) imaging
2D planimetry. *See* Two dimensional (2D) planimetry
3D evaluation. *See* Three-dimensional (3D) evaluation
3D imaging. *See* Three-dimensional (3D) imaging

AAA. *See* Abdominal aortic aneurysm (AAA)
Abdominal aorta, 693f
Abdominal aortic aneurysm (AAA), 761
Abscesses
  endocarditis, 402
  of pulmonic and tricuspid valves, 472
ACC. *See* American College of Cardiology (ACC)
Accelerating flow
  mitral valve orifice, 23, 25f
Accreditation Council for Graduate of Medical Education (ACGME), 778
ACGME. *See* Accreditation Council for Graduate of Medical Education (ACGME)
Acoustic impedance (Z), 4
  mismatch, 5–6, 7f
Acoustic shadowing
  imaging artifacts and, 151, 151f, 152
  reverberation and, 148f
Acquired aortic valve stenosis, 342
Acquired immunodeficiency syndrome (AIDS)
  lymphomas and, 614
ACT. *See* Activated clotting time (ACT)
Activated clotting time (ACT), 452
Acute allograft rejection
  in OHT, 557
Acute cor pulmonale, 751, 752, 753f
Acute pulmonary embolism, 681f
  diagnosis, 742, 743, 745f
  mortality, 742
  signs of, 744, 745–746
Acute respiratory distress syndrome (ARDS), 315
Acute valvular insufficiency, and hemodynamic instability, 749
Adenosine monophosphate (AMP), 320
Adult respiratory distress syndrome (ARDS)
  high-frequency ventilation in, 754, 755f
  mechanical ventilation in, 750, 751, 753f
  PEEP titration in, 752, 753f–754f, 754
  prone ventilation in, 754
  RV dysfunction in, 751
  tidal volume reduction in, 752, 753f
AF. *See* Atrial fibrillation (AF)
Afterload, 211–212
AHA. *See* American Heart Association (AHA)
AIDS. *See* Acquired immunodeficiency syndrome (AIDS)
Air detection, 327–328
Air embolism, 393f
  in lung transplantation, 669, 670f
Alferi operation, 457
Aliasing
  artifacts, 147, 148, 149f
  color Doppler, 148, 149f

[Aliasing]
  color reversal with, 22, 25f
  in computer sampling, 22, 23f
  defined, 21
  in movie image, 21–22, 22f
  prevention, 23
  PRF and, 22–23
  in spectral display, 22, 24f
  spectral Doppler, 149f
American College of Cardiology (ACC), 129, 372
American Heart Association (AHA), 129, 372
American Society of Anesthesiologists (ASA), 528, 549, 667
American Society of Anesthesiologists/Society of Cardiovascular Anesthesiologists (ASA/SCA)
  practice guidelines, 770, 771. *See also* Practice guidelines
  task force, 770
  training guidelines, 774, 774t
American Society of Echocardiography (ASE), 65, 129, 210, 398, 569
  convention for M-mode imaging, 96
American Society of Echocardiography's Guidelines and Standards Committee and Task Force on Prosthetic Valves, 380
American Society of Echocardiography/Society of Cardiovascular Anesthesiologists (ASE/SCA), 339, 774, 775, 777
AML. *See* Anterior mitral leaflet (AML)
A-mode. *See* Amplitude (A) mode
AMP. *See* Adenosine monophosphate (AMP)
Amplatzer® device, 706
  ASDs, 712f, 713f
Amplitude (A) mode, 9, 10f, 11
Anatomy
  of pulmonic valve, 460–463, 462f, 464f
  of tricuspid valve, 460–463, 461f, 464f–466f
Anesthesia
  in transcatheter aortic valve implantation, 495–496
Anesthestic drugs, 317–319
  effect of intravenous anesthetic agents on diastolic function, 318–319
  inhalation agents, 317–318
  intravenous agents on systolic function, 318
Aneurysm
  LV, 204–206, 204f, 205f, 206f
Angiosarcomas, 615, 616f, 617f
Angle dependence, 4–5, 6f
Annuloplasty, 452–454, 453f
  rings, 483, 484f
  functions of, 452–453
  tricuspid valve repair and, 483, 483f–484f, 485f
Antegrade transapical approach
  in transcatheter aortic valve implantation, 493
Anterior leaflet prolapse, 407f, 456–457
  Alferi operation and, 457
  anterior leaflet resection and, 457

[Anterior leaflet prolapse]
  chordal transfer and, 456, 456f
  papillary muscle shortening and, 456–457, 456f
  synthetic chords for, 456, 457f
Anterior leaflet resection, 457
Anterior mitral leaflet (AML), 89, 90
  perforation, 412f
  congenital, 413f
Ao. *See* Aorta (Ao)
Aorta (Ao), 86, 87–89, 633, 650. *See also* Ascending aorta
  abdominal, 693f
  anatomical considerations in, 561
  aortic aneurysms, 573–576, 574f
  aortic arch, 567–568
  aortic atherosclerosis, 568–573
  aortic dilatation, 573–576
  aortic dissection, 576–583
  ascending, 561–562, 564f
  assessment of, 139
  classification of atheromatosis of, 568f
  coarctation of, 654, 655f, 656
  descending, 562, 565f, 567
  diameter
    2D measurements of, 101, 102, 104f, 105, 105f
  echocardiographic examination of, 563f
  epiaortic scanning, 568, 569f
  evaluation of, TEE in, 498–499, 498f–499f
  ME short-axis view, 87f
  TEE, as diagnostic tool, 561
  transgastric (TG) view of, 567f
  transverse, 565f
  traumatic rupture of, 583, 584f
  upper esophageal view of, 88f
Aortic aneurysm, 573–576, 574f
  after endograft implantation, 593f
  ascending, 574f
    surgical strategy in, 583–585
  sinus of valsalva aneurysms, 573, 575f, 576, 576f
Aortic annulus
  diameter, measurement of, 379–380
Aortic arch, 567–568
  atheroma, 590f
  identification and monitoring, 595f
  upper esophageal view, 89f
Aortic atheromatosis
  intraoperative techniques for assessment of, 570, 572f, 573
Aortic atherosclerosis, 568–573
  3D view of, 572
  aortic atheromatosis, intraoperative techniques for assessment of, 570, 573
  echocardiographic findings with, 573
  outcomes after cardiac surgery, 568–570
Aortic balloon, positioning of, 520, 522, 522f, 523f, 524–525
Aortic blood flow, 597–599
Aortic cannulation, 305–306, 305f, 306f
Aortic dilatation, 573–576
Aortic dissections, 307f, 314f, 576–583, 596–597, 596f
  aortic intramural hematoma, 580, 582f
  aortic regurgitation, 740, 741f